Managing Preexisting Diabetes and Pregnancy

Technical Reviews and Consensus Recommendations for Care

John L. Kitzmiller, MD
Lois Jovanovic, MD
Florence Brown, MD
Donald Coustan, MD
Diane M. Reader, RD, CDE
EDITORS

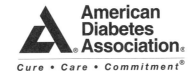

American Diabetes Association.

Cure • Care • Commitment®

Director, Book Publishing, Robert Anthony; *Managing Editor,* Abe Ogden; *Acquisitions Editor, Professional Books,* Victor Van Beuren; *Production Manager,* Melissa Sprott; Editing and *Composition,* Custom Editorial Productions, Inc.; *Cover Design,* Koncept, Inc.; *Printer,* Port City Press.

Printed in the United States of America
1 3 5 7 9 10 8 6 4 2

The suggestions and information contained in this publication are generally consistent with the Clinical Practice Recommendations and other policies of the American Diabetes Association, but they do not represent the policy or position of the Association or any of its boards or committees. Reasonable steps have been taken to ensure the accuracy of the information presented. However, the American Diabetes Association cannot ensure the safety or efficacy of any product or service described in this publication. Individuals are advised to consult a physician or other appropriate health care professional before undertaking any diet or exercise program or taking any medication referred to in this publication. Professionals must use and apply their own professional judgment, experience, and training and should not rely solely on the information contained in this publication before prescribing any diet, exercise, or medication. The American Diabetes Association—its officers, directors, employees, volunteers, and members—assumes no responsibility or liability for personal or other injury, loss, or damage that may result from the suggestions or information in this publication.

♾ The paper in this publication meets the requirements of the ANSI Standard Z39.48-1992 (permanence of paper).

ADA titles may be purchased for business or promotional use or for special sales. To purchase more than 50 copies of this book at a discount, or for custom editions of this book with your logo, contact the American Diabetes Association at the address below, at booksales@diabetes.org, or by calling 703-299-2046.

American Diabetes Association
1701 North Beauregard Street
Alexandria, Virginia 22311

Library of Congress Cataloging-in-Publication Data

Managing preexisting diabetes and pregnancy : technical reviews and consensus recommendations for care / editors, John Lee Kitzmiller ... [et al.].
    p. ; cm.
Includes bibliographical references and index.
ISBN 978-1-58040-295-8 (alk. paper)
1. Diabetes in pregnancy. I. Kitzmiller, John Lee. II. American Diabetes Association.
[DNLM: 1. Pregnancy in Diabetics—therapy—Practice Guideline. 2. Diabetes Mellitus, Type 1--therapy—Practice Guideline. 3. Diabetes Mellitus, Type 2—therapy--Practice Guideline. 4. Prenatal Care—standards--Practice Guideline. 5. Prenatal Nutrition Physiology—Practice Guideline. WQ 248 M2666 2008]

RG580.D5M38 2008
618.3--dc22
            2008009545

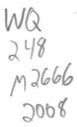

Contributors

ADA TECHNICAL REVIEWS AND CONSENSUS RECOMMENDATIONS FOR CARE

John Lee Kitzmiller, MD[1]
  (Writing Group Chair)
Jennifer M. Block, BS, RN, CDE[2]
Florence M. Brown, MD[3]
Patrick M. Catalano, MD[4]
Deborah L. Conway, MD[5]
Donald R. Coustan, MD[6]
Erica P. Gunderson, RD, PhD[7]
William H. Herman, MD, MPH[8]
Lisa D. Hoffman, MSW, LCSW[9]
Maribeth Inturrisi, RN, MS, CNS, CDE[10]
Lois Blaustein Jovanovic, MD[11]
Siri I. Kjos, MD[12]

From the [1]Division of Maternal-Fetal Medicine, Santa Clara Valley Medical Center, San Jose, California; the [2]Division of Pediatric Endocrinology, Stanford University Medical Center; the [3]Department of Internal Medicine, Joslin Diabetes Center, Boston, Massachusetts; the [4]Department of Obstetrics and Gynecology, Metrohealth Medical Center, Cleveland, Ohio; the [5]Department of Obstetrics and Gynecology, University of Texas Health Sciences Center, San Antonio, Texas; the [6]Department of Obstetrics and Gynecology, Women and Infants Hospital, Brown Medical School, Providence, Rhode Island; the [7]Epidemiology and Prevention Section, Division of Research, Kaiser Permanente Foundation, Oakland, California; the [8]Department of Medicine, University of Michigan Medical School, Ann Arbor, Michigan; the [9]Diabetes and Pregnancy Program, Obstetrix Medical Group, San Jose, California; the [10]California Diabetes and Pregnancy Program, Northcoast Region, UCSF, San Francisco, California; the [11]Sansum Diabetes Research Institute, Santa Barbara, California; the [12]Department of Obstetrics and Gynecology, Harbor/UCLA Medical Center, Torrance, California;

Robert H. Knopp, MD[13]
Martin N. Montoro, MD[14]
Edward S. Ogata, MD[15]
Pathmaja Paramsothy, MD[16]
Diane M. Reader, RD, CDE[17]
Barak M. Rosenn, MD[18]
Alyce Thomas, RD[19]
Nathaniel G. Clark, MD, MS, RD (Staff)[20]

Foreword by Steven G. Gabbe, MD[21]
Afterword by E. Albert Reece, MD, PhD, MBA[22]

---

the [13]Northwest Lipid Research Clinic, University of Washington School of Medicine, Seattle, Washington; the [14]Division of Medical Endocrinology, University of Southern California School of Medicine, Los Angeles, California; the [15]Division of Neonatology, Childrens Memorial Hospital, Northwestern University School of Medicine, Chicago, Illinois; the [16]Division of Cardiology, University of Washington School of Medicine, Seattle, Washington; the [17]International Diabetes Center, Minneapolis, Minnesota; the [18]Division of Maternal-Fetal Medicine, St Luke's Roosevelt Hospital Center, New York, New York; [19]Perinatal Nutrition Consultant, St Joseph's Regional Medical Center, Paterson, New Jersey; [20]Vice President for Clinical Affairs, American Diabetes Association, Alexandria, Virginia; [21]Dean, Vanderbilt School of Medicine and Professor of Obstetrics and Gynecology, Nashville, Tennessee; [22]Vice President, Medical Affairs, University of Maryland, Dean, School of Medicine, and Professor of Obstetrics and Gynecology, Medicine, and Biochemistry, Baltimore, Maryland.

Contents

Foreword

Over the past eight decades, management of the pregnancy complicated by diabetes mellitus has changed dramatically, as have the outcomes for these women and their babies. If women with diabetes mellitus are seen prior to pregnancy so that conception is delayed until they are in excellent glucose control and their potential vascular complications have been fully evaluated; if they receive expert care during gestation provided by a knowledgeable team including physicians, nurses, nutritionists, social workers, and pediatricians; and if they are adherent participants in their care, these women can look forward to an excellent perinatal outcome nearly identical to that of their sisters without diabetes mellitus. No longer do women with diabetes mellitus need to fear the consequences of a sudden and unexpected intrauterine fetal death, a neonatal death resulting from respiratory distress syndrome (RDS) after an elective delivery to avoid a stillbirth, or birth asphyxia or neonatal brachial plexus injury resulting from the traumatic delivery of a macrosomic infant.

What is most responsible for improved outcomes in pregnancies complicated by diabetes mellitus? Many important contributions are attributed to this success. While it has been known for some time that physiological glucose control throughout pregnancy is essential for an excellent perinatal outcome, it is only within the past 25 years that we have been able to achieve this degree of control through the availability of new techniques to assess maternal glucose levels (glucose meters, glycosylated hemoglobin measurements, continuous glucose monitoring), new insulins (rapid-acting insulin analogs), and new methods for administering insulin (continuous subcutaneous insulin infusion [CSII] or insulin pump therapy). The care of women with pregnancies complicated by diabetes mellitus has also benefited from improvements in general obstetrical and pediatric care, including techniques for antepartum fetal surveillance that have allowed confirmation of fetal well-being in the third trimester and safe prolongation of pregnancy as well as assessment of fetal pulmonary maturation through the analysis of amniotic fluid (AF) phospholipids should preterm delivery be considered. In addition, dramatic improvements in the care of the preterm infant, particularly those related to the treatment of RDS, have reduced neonatal morbidity and mortality. Finally, advances in obstetrical anesthesia have made the delivery process safer and more comfortable for our pregnant patients.

To fully appreciate how far we have come in our successful management of the pregnancy complicated by diabetes mellitus, we must go back to our roots to acknowledge two of the pioneers in this field who relied on their clinical expertise and keen insights and whose observations have served as the foundation for the success we enjoy today. Dr. Priscilla White began working at the Joslin Clinic in Boston soon after the discovery of insulin in 1921. She was charged by its director, Dr. Elliott Joslin, with the development of programs, including camps, for the care of children with diabetes mellitus and, as these young women matured, with the formation of a program for the care of the pregnant woman with diabetes mellitus. Through careful supervision of the patient's pregnancy—including hospitalizations in each trimester, most notably for the last 6–8 weeks of pregnancy to improve maternal control and reduce the risk of stillbirth—Dr. White and her colleagues prevented intrauterine fetal deaths and improved neonatal survival. Yet, when Dr. White presented her findings at other institutions, including those in Europe, she was often told that their results were just as good. She realized that, in many cases, the comparisons being made were more like comparing "apples to oranges." The Joslin Clinic patients had lived with diabetes requiring insulin treatment for many years and had often developed vasculopathy, while numerous patients from other clinics had manifested a more recent onset of diabetes. This observation led Dr. White to develop her system of maternal classification and risk assessment based on the patient's age at the onset of diabetes, the duration of the disease, and the presence of vasculopathy including hypertension, nephropathy, and retinopathy (Table A) (White 49). This risk assessment was extremely helpful in the development of improved programs of care, recognizing that patients with a more recent onset of diabetes (Classes B and C) needed greater instruction in diet and insulin use, while those women with vasculopathy (Classes D, F, R, and particularly those with nephropathy, Class F) were at the greatest risk for intrauterine growth restriction, preeclampsia, preterm delivery, and fetal death.

Several years later, Dr. Jorgen Pedersen reported his results from the Rigshospitalet in Copenhagen, Denmark (Pedersen 77). Like Dr. White, he recognized that the most effective care would be provided in a central site where the resources and expertise for management of these complicated patients could best be coordinated. He also identified four Prognostically Bad Signs in Pregnancy (PBSP) that were associated with significantly greater perinatal mortality: clinical pyelonephritis, ketoacidosis (KTA), preeclampsia, and the "neglector," those patients whose care started late in pregnancy or who were not compliant. These PBSPs significantly heightened the perinatal risk in each of the White diabetic Classes.

The findings of Drs. White and Pedersen remain as relevant today as they were nearly 60 years ago. I have found it helpful to simplify this risk assessment into two categories: the patient's blood glucose and the status of her blood vessels. Patients with excellent glucose control and no blood vessel disease will generally do well. Women with vasculopathy who have been in poor control are at significantly greater risk for poor perinatal outcomes (Landon 02).

It is my hope that this background information will enable the reader of this comprehensive text to fully appreciate and value how far we have progressed in our care of the pregnant patient with diabetes mellitus. Have all problems been solved? No, they have not. Relatively few women today receive care prior to pregnancy and thus conceive while in poor glucose control, thereby placing them at high risk for the delivery of a fetus with a major congenital malformation. Our patients continue to be challenged by social factors that impair their compliance in following the regimen of diet, insulin administration, and glucose testing that is necessary to achieve excellent control; we often see women who have

TABLE A Modified Classification of Pregnant Diabetic Women*

Class	Diabetes Onset, Age (year)		Duration (year)	Vascular Disease	Insulin Need
Gestational diabetes					
A₁	Any		Any	0	0
A₂	Any		Any	0	+
Pregestational diabetes					
B	>20		>10	0	+
C	10–19	or	10–19	0	+
Dᵛ	<10	or	<20	+	+
Fʷ	Any		Any	+	+
Rˣ	Any		Any	+	+
Tʸ	Any		Any	+	+
Hᶻ	Any		Any	+	+

The White risk classification antedated current concerns with type 1 versus type 2 diabetes, dyslipidemia, microalbuminuria, or diabetic cardiomyopathy, but included the formerly rare possibility that a woman could experience onset of diabetes under age 10 or duration of diabetes >20 years without showing signs of micro- or macrovascular disease during pregnancy.

*Based on White 49 and Landon 02.
ᵛEarly microvascular disease and chronic hypertension.
ʷNephropathy.
ˣProliferative retinopathy.
ʸRenal transplant.
ᶻCoronary heart disease.

developed vasculopathy, particularly nephropathy, who are at greater risk for the problems described earlier. Further improvement in our care of patients with pregnancies complicated by diabetes mellitus may depend upon advances that will benefit all individuals with diabetes mellitus, such as a closed-loop insulin pump system and islet cell or stem cell transplantation (Reece 04). Like our patients, I look forward to that day.

REFERENCES

Landon MB, Catalano PN, Gabbe SG: Diabetes mellitus. In: Gabbe SG, Niebyl JR, Simpson JL, eds. *Obstetrics: Normal & Problem Pregnancies.* 4th ed. Philadelphia: Churchill Livingstone; 2002:1094–1095.

Pedersen J: *The Pregnant Diabetic and Her Newborn.* 2nd ed. Baltimore: Williams & Wilkins; 1977:201–205.

Reece EA, Gabbe SG: The history of diabetes mellitus. In: Reece EA, Coustan DR, Gabbe SG, eds. *Diabetes in Women. Adolescence, Pregnancy, and Menopause.* 3rd ed. Philadelphia: Lippincott, Williams & Wilkins; 2004:1–9.

White P: Pregnancy complicating diabetes. *Am J Med* 7:609–616, 1949.

Steven G. Babbe MD

Acknowledgments

For busy clinicians, scholarly work must often be completed during "free time," and the authors are thankful for the understanding and support of their families. Regarding the long years of education and training as well as the opportunities for continued learning "on the job" that make our present work possible, we acknowledge our outstanding teachers and colleagues in conference rooms, clinics, and laboratories. We recognize the hard work and dedication of the thousands of investigators cited in this volume as they made striking advances in the art and science of diabetes care and obstetrical management. Over the years, the inspiration of our patients—who bravely cope with the burden of diabetes and the challenges of pregnancy—provided the energy for us to complete this book. We dedicate this book to them.

The senior author wishes to acknowledge the outstanding library and information services provided by Vaughn Flaming and Hella Bluhm-Stieber of Santa Clara Valley Medical Center, Nancy Firchow of Regional Medical Center in San Jose, and Janet Bruman of Natividad Medical Center in Salinas, California. The staff of the American Diabetes Association and its book department, including Victor Van Beuren, Henry H. Harrison, Sue Kirkman, and Nathaniel Clark (now with Novo Nordisk), were of great assistance in the birthing of this book. At the home office, Joan Weschler Kitzmiller provided invaluable editorial assistance. Heartfelt thanks are expressed to all who contributed to this work. For any errors or omissions, the senior author assumes sole responsibility.

DISCLOSURES

Writing group member relationships that could be construed as reflecting a possible conflict of interest.

Name	Research or Educational Grant	Speaker Honoraria	Consultant; Advisory Board	Ownership Interest
F. Brown	Harvard	Hospitals	None	None
P. Catalano	NIH	Hospitals	None	None
D. Coustan	NIH	Hospitals	RW Johnson Program	None
L. Jovanovic	Abbott, Lilly, Lifescan, Medtronic, Pfizer, Novartis	Novo Nordisk, Hemacue, Roche, Sanofe-Aventis	None	None
J. Kitzmiller	Lifescan	Lilly	None	None
S. Kjos	NIH	Hospitals	None	None
R. Knopp	Abbott, AstraZenica NIH, Takeda	Abbott, AstraZeneca	None	None
M. Montoro	None	Hospitals	None	None
E. Ogata	None	Hospitals	Bioniche Pharmaceuticals	None
P. Paramsothy	NIH, Pfizer	None	None	None
B. Rosenn	None	Hospitals	None	None

No conflicts of interest reported: J. Block, D. Conway, E. Gunderson, W. Herman, L. Hoffman, M. Inturrisi, D. Reader, A. Thomas.

NIH, National Institutes of Health.

Introduction

The purpose of this book is to provide a comprehensive resource on the evidence supporting current recommendations for the care of pregnant women with preexisting diabetes mellitus (PDM), both type 1 diabetes and type 2 diabetes. The intent is to help clinicians cope with the broad spectrum of problems that arise in the team management of diabetes and pregnancy and to note unanswered questions that stand as indicators of needed research. Whenever possible, recommendations are based on peer-reviewed publications with key references provided, recent consensus guidelines published by the American Diabetes Association (ADA) and other organizations, and expert opinion. Topics include diabetes and obstetrical management during and after pregnancy and diabetes complications, as well as cardiovascular disease (CVD), hypertension, dyslipidemias, thyroid disorders, and psychological problems—all of which can affect the outcome of diabetes and pregnancy. These Technical Reviews aim to be thorough, but they are not exhaustive reviews of the evidence from experimental and older human studies relevant to management of diabetic pregnant women. For further references, excellent multi-authored textbooks on diabetes and pregnancy have been published (Hod 03, Reece 04a, Djelmis 05, Langer 06).

In this book of Technical Reviews, the authors sought to gather dispersed prior guidelines on the many facets of diabetes and pregnancy care into one useful volume. Consensus conferees and writing group members noted the recommendations for management of PDM in pregnancy that are currently presented by the ADA in sections of the following Position Statements: Standards of Medical Care in Diabetes – 2008 (ADA 08a) and Nutrition Recommendations and Interventions for Diabetes – 2008 (ADA 08b). In addition, the ADA has published Position Statements on Preconception Care of Women with Diabetes (ADA 04a) and Gestational Diabetes (ADA 04b); they have also published Technical Reviews on preconception care of women with diabetes to prevent congenital malformations and spontaneous abortions (Kitzmiller 96) as well as evidence-based nutrition principles and recommendations for the treatment and prevention of diabetes and related complications (Franz 02). An individually edited monograph on Medical Management of Pregnancy Complicated by Diabetes is available for purchase (Jovanovic-Peterson 00). The American College of Obstetrics and Gynecology (ACOG) recently published a Practice Bulletin on Pregestational Diabetes and Pregnancy (ACOG 05) and an earlier Practice Bulletin on Gestational Diabetes (ACOG 01). The American Association of Diabetes Educators (AADE 04,06) and the American Dietetic Association (ADietA 02) have also published useful recent guidelines on management of pregnancy complicated by diabetes. We also noted the brief consensus guidelines for management of diabetes in relation to pregnancy presented by the Australasian Diabetes in Pregnancy Society (McIntyre 04, McElduff 05a) and the U.K. National Service Framework for Diabetes Standards (UKDH 01).

Additional ADA guidelines on diabetes complications include Statements on Hypertension Management in Adults with Diabetes (Arauz-Pacheco 02, ADA 04c), Nephropathy in Diabetes (ADA 04d), Retinopathy in Diabetes (Aiello 98, Fong 04), Neuropathy in Diabetes (Boulton 05), Dyslipidemia Management in Adults with Diabetes (Haffner 98, ADA 04e), Hypoglycemia in Diabetes (ADA 05), Tests of Glycemia in Diabetes (ADA 04f), and Physical Activity/Exercise and Diabetes (Wasserman 94, ADA 04g, Sigal 04,06), as well as Technical Reviews on autonomic and somatic neuropathies (Vinik 03, Boulton 04).

Pregnancy profoundly affects the management of diabetes (Kitzmiller 88, Gabbe 03, Walkinshaw 05, Jovanovic 06). Placental hormones, growth factors (GFs), and cytokines cause a progressive increase in insulin resistance, which necessitates intensive medical nutrition therapy (MNT) and frequently adjusted insulin administration to prevent dangerous hyperglycemia and worsening of diabetic vascular complications. Women with type 2 diabetes often start pregnancy with marked insulin resistance and obesity that add to the challenge of obtaining optimal glycemic control. Intensified management is also difficult because insulin-induced hypoglycemia is more common and rapid in onset during pregnancy and is a danger to the gravida, especially in patients with type 1 diabetes. The insulin resistance of pregnancy enhances the risk of KTA in response to the stress of concurrent illnesses or drugs used in the management of obstetrical complications. Severe hyperglycemia reduces fetal oxygen content and exacerbates acidosis, which can lead to fetal death. Hyperglycemia at the beginning of pregnancy increases the risk of spontaneous abortion and major congenital malformations. As pregnancy continues, intensified glycemic control is necessary to prevent fetal hyperinsulinemia, which is associated with excess fetal growth, neonatal complications such as hypoglycemia and respiratory distress, and obesity and glucose intolerance in the developing offspring. Hypertension and diabetic nephropathy (DN) are also associated with fetal hypoxia and impaired fetal growth.

These challenges led to the development of multidisciplinary patient care programs at centers of excellence that greatly reduced maternal, fetal, and neonatal complications (Hunter 93, Kitzmiller 93, Persson 93, DCCT 96, Zhu 97, Reece 98, Gunton 00, McElvy 00, Ray 01a, Langer 02, Wylie 02, Lepercq 04, Johnstone 06). However, population-based data (Table B) continue to show excess perinatal morbidity and mortality (Hanson 93, Cnattingius 94, Casson 97, Hawthorne 97, vonKries 97, Nordstrom 98, Vaarasmaki 00a, Hadden 01, Platt 02, DPGF 03, Penney 03a, Vangen 03, CDAPP 04, Evers 04, Jensen 04, CEMACH 05, Silva Idos 05, Feig 06, Yang 06, Bell 08), demonstrating that extended efforts at improved care are necessary. In the U.K., Wales, and Northern Ireland, a national survey of 2,359 pregnancies complicated by PDM in 2002 revealed four to five times higher rates of preterm delivery and perinatal mortality in the diabetic population (Casson 06, Macintosh 06). The surveys found that major congenital malformations remain two- to threefold more commonplace in infants of diabetic mothers (IDMs) and that malformations are a frequent cause of fetal or neonatal death.

TABLE B Pregnancy Outcomes in Population-Based Studies of Women with PDM Reported in 2000–2006

Author (year)	Region	Years	PDM (N)	Controls (N)	Congenital Malformations (%)	PTD (%)	Fetal Macrosomia (%)	Stillborn (%)	Infant Mortality (% of liveborn)
Vaarasmaki 2000a	N Finland	1991–95	296	NA	6.2	NA	19 LGA	2.5**	**
Hadden 2001*	N Ireland	1985–95	751	NA	6.9	NA	NA	3.5	0.8
Platt 2002	NW England	1995–99	547	Unstated	8.4 vs. 1.3			2.6	
DPGF 2003	France	2000–01	435	Unstated	4.1 vs. 2.2	38 vs. 5	17 >4kg	3.4 vs. 0.6	1.0
Penney 2003	Scotland	1998–99	219	55,433	5.9	NA	55 LGA	1.9 vs. 0.5	1.4 vs. 0.5
Vangen 2003	Norway	1988–98	2,266	570,787	2.9	21 vs. 7	6 >97.5%	2.3** vs. 1.0	**
Evers 2004	Netherlands	1999–00	324	200,679	5.5 vs. 2.6	32 vs. 7	45 LGA	2.8** vs. 0.8	**
Jensen 2004	Denmark	1993–99	1,218	70,089	5.0 vs. 2.8	42 v 6	62 LGA	2.1 vs. 0.45	1.0 vs. 0.3
CDAPP 2004***	California	2002–03	1,324	Unstated	5.6	23	22.5 LGA	2.9	NA
CEMACH 2005#	UK (Scotland)	2002–03	2,359	620,841	4.6 vs. 2.1	37#	21 >4 kg	2.7# vs. 0.6	1.0 vs. 0.4
Yang 2006	Nova Scotia	1996–02	260	62,079	10.0 vs. 3.1	28	45 LGA	1.2** vs. 0.5	**

*Includes 131 who started insulin during pregnancy but with high malformation rate.

**Total perinatal mortality.

***Includes PDM women registering at 141 affiliated diabetes and pregnancy patient education and training centers throughout the state; the number of unaffiliated patients is unknown.

#Mortality figures do not include 13 terminations of pregnancy (9 type 1 diabetes, 4 type 2 diabetes) before 20 weeks and 32 losses (22 type 1 diabetes, 9 type 1 diabetes) at 20–23 weeks: CEMACH data accessible in Casson 06 and Macintosh 06.

CDAPP, California Diabetes and Pregnancy Program; CEMACH, Confidential Enquiry into Maternal and Child Health; DPGF, Diabetes and Pregnancy Group, France; LGA, large for gestational age, >90th %; NA, not available; PDM, preexisting diabetes; PTD, preterm delivery <37 weeks.

Several European surveys reported only data on women with type 1 diabetes (Vaarasmaki 00a, Platt 02, Penney 03a, Evers 04, Jensen 04). However, the proportion of pregnancies complicated by type 2 diabetes is increasing around the globe, reflecting both the obesity epidemic and the younger age at onset of type 2 diabetes (Cheung 05, Dunne 05, Bell 08). In the U.K. survey, 28% of women with PDM were identified with type 2 diabetes (Macintosh 06) compared with 34% in France (DPGF 03), 25.1% in Italy (Botta 97), 13% in Norway (Vangen 03), 43% in Saudi Arabia (Sobande 05), 55.3% in South Africa (Huddle 05), 91.2% in Mexico (Forsbach 98), 63% in the U.S. in 1988 (Englegau 95), and 79% in California in 2001 (CDAPP 04). A growing global recognition acknowledges that outcomes in pregnant women with type 2 diabetes are equivalent to or worse than those with type 1 diabetes (Langer 88, Omori 94, Sacks 97, Brydon 00, Cundy 00, Schaefer-Graf 00, Feig 02, Dunne 03, CDAPP 04, Hieronimus 04, Clausen 05, McElduff 05b, Roland 05, Verheijen 05, Macintosh 06, Nicholson 06, Westgate 06, Cundy 07, Gonzalez 08), thereby negating the opinion that management of type 2 diabetes in pregnancy is "easier" and less fraught with risk. Problematic results with type 2 diabetes are perhaps due to later referral for intensified care, greater insulin resistance, obesity, or effects of ethnicity/social situation on access to, acceptance of, and delivery of care. Several reports refer to the relatively poor perinatal results obtained in immigrant groups with diabetes (Dunne 00, Vangen 03, Chaudhry 04, Verheijen 05). It is reassuring when investigators discover that perinatal outcome can be improved in women with type 2 diabetes when intensified medical treatment is applied before and throughout pregnancy (Hillman 06).

In the population-based survey in the Netherlands, 84% of diabetic women had planned their pregnancies; a significantly lower risk of congenital malformations was manifested in this group (Evers 04). In Denmark, 58% had received preconception guidance, but only 34% were self-measuring plasma glucose at prenatal registration (Jensen 04). Preconception care or counseling was reported in 48.5% of diabetic women in France, with significantly less perinatal mortality in this subset (DPGF 03). Northern European data appear to be better than the lower rates of adequate preparation for pregnancy in the U.K. (Casson 06) and California (CDAPP 04). In most countries, including the U.S., major public efforts are needed to enroll diabetic women in preconception care to improve pregnancy outcome. For guidelines on the prevention of major congenital malformations and early fetal loss, refer to the ADA Technical Review and Position Statement on Preconception Care of Women with Diabetes (Kitzmiller 96, ADA 04a).

Diabetes management and perinatal care are complex and require that many issues beyond glycemic control be addressed. These guidelines are intended to provide clinicians, patients, payors, and other interested people with components of care and treatment goals that can reduce morbidity and healthcare outcome costs. We also suggest areas in which further research is needed to resolve controversies and gain basic knowledge of the diabetes-related pathophysiology of pregnancy. While individual patient needs may require modification of goals, targets that are desirable for most diabetic pregnant women are provided. These guidelines are not intended to preclude more extensive evaluation and management of the pregnant patient by other specialists as needed.

This set of Technical Reviews on managing diabetes and pregnancy seeks to present an expanded point of view—not merely on the dramatic *now* of pregnancy, but also on the continuity of problems and possibilities facing diabetic women before conception, the necessary adjustments during pregnancy, and the important months and years after delivery. We think it is important to incorporate components of care designed to benefit long-term maternal health with special reference to CVD and diabetic microvascular disorders. The concept that intensified diabetes care before conception will substantially improve pregnancy outcome for both mother and baby is well supported. To obtain this result, effective contraception and pregnancy planning (reviewed in Part IV) is usually necessary. Management recommendations should encourage effective behaviors and application of pharmacotherapies through the reproductive years as well as optimal care during pregnancy. A good example is the tailoring of multifaceted treatment to fully support breast-feeding, which has profound health benefits for both mother and child. Clinicians can take advantage of the heightened motivation of pregnant diabetic women to teach them behaviors and self-management skills that are expected to control CVD risk factors. For optimal long-term outcomes, we need to find ways to foster seamless continuation of intensified management in the years after pregnancy and in preparation for the next desired conception.

The development of this book deserves comment. Members of the writing group were challenged by the ADA to develop consensus recommendations for the management of pregnant women with PDM and to present the supporting evidence in a Position Statement and a Technical Review. After months of preparation in which members focused on their assigned topics, the writing group met at the ADA Annual Scientific Meeting in June 2004 and achieved consensus on the recommendations for management. Subsequently, members prepared their sections of the document for publication and reviewed and commented on all of the sections, including modification of the recommendations based on new evidence. The editors expanded the review of the evidence and modified the language as appropriate to achieve unity in the flow of the text. The depth of the material resulted in development of four Technical Reviews including recommendations for care: Part I, Management of Preexisting Diabetes Mellitus and Pregnancy for Pregnancy; Part II, Management of Diabetic/Medical Complications in Pregnancy; Part III, Obstetrical Management of Women with Preexisting Diabetes Mellitus; and Part IV, Postpartum Management of Women with Preexisting Diabetes Mellitus. Reference citations are presented chronologically in the text as first author and year of publication so that the reader can observe the development of the evidence; full references are listed in alphabetical order at the end of each Part. An executive summary of the recommendations and evidence is simultaneously published as an ADA Statement in the journal *Diabetes Care*.

The recommendations included here are diagnostic and therapeutic actions that are known or are believed to favorably affect maternal and perinatal outcomes in pregnancies complicated by diabetes. A grading system developed by the ADA and modeled after existing methods was used to clarify and codify the evidence that forms the basis for the recommendations (ADA 08). The level of supporting evidence is listed after each recommendation by using the letters **A** (clear or supportive evidence from randomized controlled trials [RCTs]), **B** (supportive evidence from well-conducted cohort or case–control studies), **C** (supportive evidence from poorly controlled or uncontrolled studies, or conflicting evidence with the weight of the evidence supporting the recommendation), or **E** (expert consensus or clinical experience). Unfortunately there is a paucity of RCTs detailing the various aspects of the management of diabetes and pregnancy. Therefore, our recommendations are based on trials conducted in nonpregnant diabetic women and nondiabetic pregnant women, as appropriate, as well as peer-reviewed experience during pregnancy and postpartum in women with PDM.

MULTIDISCIPLINARY TEAM CARE

The complexity of issues surrounding diabetes and pregnancy and the need for excellent glycemic control require that different practitioners provide specific types of care in an integrated manner, with the patient at the center of the management team (Cousins 91, Kitzmiller 93, Miller 94, Brown 95, Brown 96, Hirsch 98a, Jovanovic-Petersen 00, Mensing 05, Thomas 06a). Comparison studies suggest that this approach will yield the best perinatal outcomes at reduced final costs (Scheffler 92, Elixhauser 93,96, Herman 99). An optimal model of care is one in which responsibility is shared and a partnership exists between the pregnant woman with diabetes, her family, and healthcare professionals (Josse 03). A diabetic pregnant woman needs to be fully aware of her risks for both maternal and infant outcomes, individualized as much as possible, and aware of the expectations for health behaviors on her part and for performance by members of the healthcare team. Numerous methods can be applied to alleviate her anxieties (Spendlove 03). Clinicians must attempt to work through the tension generated between focusing on emotional distress versus addressing the practical issues of diabetes management (Rubin 01). Emotional well-being is strongly associated with positive diabetes outcomes (ADA 08a).

In the following Technical Reviews, we use the term "clinician" broadly to include members of the diabetes self-management education (DSME) team who interact with the patient and her family. "While respecting autonomy of the pregnant woman, the health care professional's role is more than just doing what the patient wants. It includes influencing and facilitating the woman's care to achieve the outcome of a healthy baby. By agreeing with the mother that a healthy child is the desired outcome of pregnancy, the health care professional can talk through the implications of general detrimental behavior and may take 'intrusive action' such as more frequent check ups and telephone advice" (Hawthorne 03).

Ample evidence points to the benefit of DSME (Norris 01, Gary 03, Ellis 04) and the use of a coordinated team approach to patient care (Clark 01). DSME uses "a skill-based approach that focuses on helping those with diabetes make informed self-management choices." It works best when it is tailored to individual needs and preferences, addresses psychosocial issues, and includes follow-up support (ADA 08c, Funnell 08). The roles of diabetes and pregnancy team members must adapt to local needs and conditions. The patient is taught diabetes self-management skills (Thomas 06a) by a certified diabetes educator (CDE), registered nurse, or well-trained person filling this role. Skills include self-monitoring of capillary blood glucose (SMBG), insulin administration, recognition and treatment of hypoglycemia, and adjustments for illness (Mensing 05). MNT is best provided by a registered dietitian (RD) (Franz 02, Wylie-Rosett 07, ADA 08b) with experience and training in diabetes and pregnancy. MNT consists of assessment and provision of adequate nutrition for maternal and fetal health and use of an individualized food plan (Fagen 95, ADietA 02). Learning for the food plan includes carbohydrate counting, timing of meals and snacks, and prevention of hypoglycemia. Self-recording of food intake is useful to evaluate adherence to the plan and the reasons for hypo- or hyperglycemia. Regular follow-up visits are important for adjustments in the treatment plan related to stage of pregnancy, glycemic control, weight gain, and individual patient needs.

Assessment of psychosocial factors that may interfere with care is best conducted by a behavioral specialist, mental health professional, or social worker in concert with other team members. Psychosocial factors may include inadequate financial support, lack of health insurance, family strife, stress at work, denial of disease, anxiety, depression, eating disorders, and so forth. Education and counseling about the role of obstetrical testing and procedures and the influence of diabetes management on pregnancy must be provided by all team members, as appropriate. Frequent communication among team members, including physicians, about a woman's needs and any change in risk factors is essential. It is recognized that in settings with limited resources, all of these team functions may have to be provided by one or two people. In any case, careful attention to detail is required to achieve successful outcomes.

The clinician serving as obstetrician or perinatologist often has the lead role as patient advocate in securing team care and specialist referrals as well as coordinating laboratory evaluations and treatment. An integrated role for a physician focusing on diabetes management (internal medicine, endocrinology) is helpful in pregnancies complicated by PDM. Subspecialty consultations and treatment by an eye care specialist experienced in diabetic retinal disease or a nephrologist, cardiologist, podiatrist, and psychiatrist are often needed. All such physicians should be apprised of the special contingencies of pregnancy complicated by diabetes. Finally, antepartum consultations with pediatrics or neonatology can enhance the transition from fetal to neonatal life.

For optimal outcomes, the education and treatment strategies provided must be consistent with ongoing individualized patient assessments. In assessing the special needs of the woman with PDM, the diabetes and pregnancy team must take into account those cultural distinctions that may form barriers to successful care. The diabetes and pregnancy team should strive to meet the National Standards for Diabetes Self-Management and Education (AADE 00, Mensing 05). ADA-recognized DSME programs use a process of continuous quality improvement to evaluate the effectiveness of the DSME provided and identify opportunities for improvement (ADA 08c, Funnell 08).

Recommendations for organization of preconception and pregnancy care

- All women with diabetes and childbearing potential should be educated about the need for good glucose control before pregnancy and should participate in effective family planning. (E)
- Whenever possible, organize multidiscipline, patient-centered team care for women with PDM (type 1 or type 2 diabetes) in preparation for pregnancy. (B)
- Women with diabetes who are contemplating pregnancy should be evaluated and, if indicated, treated for DN, neuropathy, and retinopathy, as well as CVD, hypertension, dyslipidemia, depression, and thyroid disease. (E)
- Medications used by such women should be evaluated before conception because drugs commonly used to treat diabetes and its complications may be contraindicated or not recommended in pregnancy including statins, angiotensin-converting enzyme (ACE) inhibitors, angiotensin-receptor blockers (ARBs), and most noninsulin therapies. (E)
- Continue multidiscipline patient-centered team care throughout pregnancy and postpartum. (E)
- Regular follow-up visits are important for adjustments in the treatment plan related to stage of pregnancy, glycemic and blood pressure (BP) control, weight gain, and individual patient needs. (E)
- Educate pregnant diabetic women regarding the strong benefits of (1) long-term CVD risk factor reduction, (2) breast-feeding, and (3) effective family planning with good glycemic control prior to the next pregnancy. (E)

Managing Preexisting Diabetes Mellitus for Pregnancy

INITIAL MEDICAL EVALUATION

Depending on the extent of and proximity to preconception care, a complete medical evaluation or review should be performed to:

- classify the patient and detect the presence of diabetic or obstetrical complications
- review the history of eating patterns, physical activity/exercise, and psychosocial problems
- counsel the patient on prognosis
- set expectations for patient participation
- assist in formulating a management plan with team care members
- provide a basis for continuing care and laboratory tests

The evaluation should review the history of prior pregnancies and comorbidities such as dyslipidemias and other cardiac risk factors, hypertension, albuminuria, variant symptoms of cardiac ischemia or failure, symptoms of neuropathies (sensory, cardioautonomic, gastroparesis), hypoglycemia awareness and severe hypoglycemic episodes, bowel symptoms, celiac disease, thyroid disorders, and infectious diseases, as well as previous diabetes education, treatment, and past and present degrees of glycemic control.

In addition to appropriate obstetrical examination, physical examination should include sitting BP and orthostatic heart rate (HR) as well as BP responses, thyroid palpation, inspection for corneal arcus, auscultation for carotid and femoral bruits, palpation of dorsalis pedis and posterior tibial pulses, presence/absence of patellar and Achilles reflexes, determination of pinprick sensation, temperature/vibration perception, 10-gm monofilament pressure sensation at the distal plantar aspect of both great toes, and visual inspection of both feet. Measurement of the ankle/arm BP index (ankle/brachial index [ABI]) using normal values from women can be considered as a sign of peripheral arteriosclerotic disease (see Part II).

Laboratory tests appropriate to the evaluation of each patient's general maternal condition should be performed (Table I.1). Although some complications cannot be

TABLE I.1 Laboratory and Special Exam Components of Initial and Subsequent Evaluation of Pregnant Women with Type 1 and Type 2 Diabetes*

Initial Evaluation	Subsequent Testing	Supporting Evidence (book part, pages)
Hemoglobin A1C	Every 1–3 months	I:2–15
Fasting lipid profile,** including triglycerides and total, HDL-C, and LDL-C	As indicated	II:314–322
TSH, free T4 and thyroid peroxidase antibodies in all type 1 diabetes and selected type 2 diabetes patients**	To monitor treatment	II:285–288
ALT/AST; possible liver ultrasound	As indicated	I:83–86
Consider anti-tTG or anti-EMA plus IgA level in type 1 diabetes**	Repeat to confirm abnormal result or monitor effect of gluten-free diet.	I:76–83
Hemoglobin, serum ferritin; vitamin B12 in type 1 diabetes	To monitor treatment	I:47–49; 61–65
Random urine for albumin/creatinine ratio *or* 24-h urine collection for microalbuminuria and creatinine clearance** (measure 24-h total protein excretion if urine is dipstick positive for albumin or protein)	Every 1–3 months if abnormal (24-h urine total protein is also used for diagnosis of preeclampsia, plus CBC with platelet count, transaminase, serum uric acid)	II:379–384
Dilated retinal exam**	Every 1–6 months	II:384–292
Assess cardiac risk factors. Electrocardiogram** if diabetes mellitus ≥10 years or age ≥35 years. Consider stress electrocardiogram or stress echocardiogram with positive risk factors of hypertension, dyslipidemia, albuminuria, smoking, or family history of premature cardiovascular disease. Consider Doppler echocardiogram with indication of diabetic cardiomyopathy or diastolic heart failure.	As indicated	II:314–320

*In addition to usual prenatal laboratory tests.

**May be delayed or omitted if performed before pregnancy.

ALT, alanine aminotransferase; AST, aspartate aminotransferase; EMA, endomysial autoantibody; TSH, thyroid-stimulating hormone; tTG, tissue transglutaminase.

treated with optimal drugs during pregnancy, their identification allows for intensified management postpartum. All preconception or pregnant patients should be tested for HbA_{1C} (A1c), lipids, iron status, thyroid status, and steatosis and should be screened for albuminuria, diabetic retinopathy (DR), and diabetic neuropathy. Selected patients will need electrocardiogram (ECG) or echocardiography due to the risk of coronary heart disease associated with age and duration of diabetes or symptomatology (see Table I.1). Patients with random urine albumin/creatinine ratio (ACR) at the upper end of normal for women may benefit from a 24-h urine collection for microalbuminuria. Patients with proteinuria on dipstick should have a 24-h total urinary protein excretion and creatinine clearance (CrCl) quantified. Estimated glomerular filtration rate (GFR) based on serum creatinine, age, gender, and race (Modification of Diet in Renal Disease [MDRD] formula) is not accurate during pregnancy (Smith 08).

Patients with type 1 diabetes without recent testing should be screened for vitamin B12 status as well as thyroid disease and celiac disease because of the association with disease-producing autoimmunity. Due to possible fetal problems with subclinical hypothroidism early in pregnancy, also perform thyroid testing in women with type 2 diabetes. Given the high prevalence of celiac disease in women with type 1 diabetes, frequent absence of symptoms, difficulty arriving at the diagnosis, and potential for malabsorption of nutrients and adverse fetal outcomes, preconception screening for serological markers of celiac disease with tissue transglutaminase (tTG) or endomysial autoantibody (EMA) IgA and a quantitative serum IgA level is recommended. In the presence of antibodies, a referral should be made to a gastroenterologist for confirmation of the diagnosis and initiation of treatment.

A focus on components of the comprehensive diabetes evaluation (Table 7 in Standards of Medical Care in Diabetes—2008) (ADA 08a) will assist the healthcare team in providing optimal management of the pregnant woman with PDM.

GLYCEMIC CONTROL AND PERINATAL OUTCOME

—— Original contribution by John L. Kitzmiller MD
and Jennifer M. Block, BS RN, CDE

Excess spontaneous abortions and major congenital malformations are strongly associated with maternal hyperglycemia during the first few weeks of pregnancy (earlier studies reviewed in Kitzmiller 96; Gunton 00, Schaefer-Graf 00, Vaarasmaki 00b, Sheffield 02, Temple 02, DFSG 03, Evers 04, Jovanovic 05, Nazer 05, Nielsen 05, Verheijen 05). Apparent thresholds for the increased risk include A1C values ≥3 SDs above the normal mean (≥6.3), with risk progressively rising as glucose levels worsen (Kitzmiller 96, Nielsen 97, Schaefer 97, Suhonen 00, Langer 02, Temple 02, Wender-Ozegowska 05, Guerin 07). It is recognized that the relationship of maternal glucose to early pregnancy outcome is a continuum and that ideal results are achieved when maternal glucose concentrations are within normal limits, including limits that are not too low (Jovanovic 05). Studies of the mechanisms of experimental diabetic embryopathy generally reveal biomolecular processes similar to those thought to cause the microvascular and neurological complications of diabetes (Moley 01, Chang 03, Chugh 03, De Hertogh 03, Wentzel 03, Reece 04b).

Twelve prospective studies of intensified glycemic control both before and at the beginning of pregnancy show reduction of malformation rates to near normal (<3%), with increased rates (5–12%) in diabetic women not using intensified therapy until after organogenesis (first eight reviewed in Kitzmiller 96 and Ray 01b; DCCT 96, McElvey 00, Guerrero 04, Temple 06a). In these studies, good results were found with average premeal fingerstick glucose values <110 mg/dL, postprandial <140 mg/dL, and mean daily glucose <120 mg/dL in early pregnancy. Most of these studies were not randomized trials due to concern regarding the assignment of pregnant women to standard poor control. Large population surveys continue to show increased malformation rates in infants of mothers with diabetes of both types (Casson 97, Hawthorne 97, Nordstrom 98, Farrell 02, Platt 02, DPGF 03, Evers 04, Jensen 04, Clausen 05,

McElduff 05b, Sharpe 05), reflecting the frequency of unplanned pregnancy and lack of participation in intensified preconception care (Botta 97, Hieronimus 04, Kim 05, Roland 05, Hillman 06). These issues are analyzed in detail in the ADA's Technical Review (Kitzmiller 96) and Position Statement on Preconception Care of Diabetes in Women (ADA 04a). New clinical research studies are needed concerning suitable methods to achieve widespread good glycemic control in diabetic women at risk of becoming pregnant as well as novel therapies based on the emerging understanding of the biochemical and genetic mechanisms of diabetic embryopathy.

Fetal Macrosomia

Studies of the relationship of maternal–fetal hyperglycemia to fetal hyperinsulinemia, accelerated growth, and excess adiposity in animal models and diabetic women (Pedersen 61, Weiss 78, Sosenko 79, Lin 81, Sosenko 82, Susa 85, Salvesen 93a, Schwartz 94, Kainer 97, Weiss 98, Fallucca 00, Lindsay 03, Westgate 06) led clinical investigators to examine the influence of glycemic control throughout pregnancy on fetal macrosomia and infant birth weight (BW) (Mimouni 88a, Fraser 95, Banerjee 03, Sacks 06a, Shefali 06). Newborn macrosomia is variously defined as BW >4000–4500 gm (Langer 02). Large for gestational age (LGA) is usually defined as BW above the reference population 90th percentile for gender and gestational age. An analysis of outcomes in 8,264,308 term U.S. births with BW ≥3,000 gm indicated that BW >4,000 gm was a threshold indicator for increased risk of delivery complications, BW >4,500 was a good risk indicator for neonatal morbidity, and BW >5,000 gm was a useful indicator for newborn mortality risks. In this study, 2.5% of births were coded as maternal diabetes, and the crude odds ratio (OR) for BW >4,500 gm in the diabetic subgroup was 2.76 vs. the nondiabetic population (Boulet 03). Recent population surveys of pregnancies complicated by PDM show rates of macrosomia in IDMs to be in great excess compared with nondiabetic controls (Johnstone 06). For example, LGA rates were 26.9%, 27.6%, 55%, 45%, 62.5%, and 56% in six surveys vs. 10% in controls, respectively (DFSG 91, vonKries 97, Penney 03a, Evers 04, Jensen 04, Clausen 05), and 35% of IDMs were above the reference 95th percentile in another survey (Hawthorne 97). These European figures are similar to those found in large national U.S. surveys of >100,000 infants with "maternal diabetes" coded on the birth certificates (Kieffer 98, Mondestin 02, Boulet 03).

Macrosomia in IDMs is associated with increased rates of operative delivery and birth trauma (Nesbitt 98, Stotland 04a), fetal death (Seeds 00, Mondestin 02), and neonatal complications including hypoglycemia, hypertrophic cardiomyopathy, polycythemia, and hyperbilirubinemia (Small 87, Berk 89, Tyrala 96, Weiss 98, Johnstone 00). Subsequent childhood obesity and glucose intolerance is also more commonplace when macrosomia is due to fetal hyperinsulinemia (Vohr 80, Silverman 93,98, Forsen 00, Gray 02), which exemplies the prolonged offspring effect of intrauterine exposure to diabetes (Pettitt 83, Plagemann 97, Rodrigues 98, Dabalea 00, Hunter 04, Touger 05, Fetita 06).

Prospective observational studies at >12 weeks gestation using maternal glucose profiles as the measure of suboptimal glycemic control found a significant association with fetal macrosomia (Table I.2) (Roversi 79, Coustan 80, Schneider 80, Tevaarwerk 81, Willman 86, Landon 87, Langer 88, Jovanovic 91, Combs 92, Parfitt 92, Persson 96, Mello 97, Sacks 97, Mello 00, Raychaudhuri 00, Sturrock 01). This relationship has been more difficult to establish using only A1C measurements in some (Berk 89, Combs 92, DCCT 96, Persson 96, Koukkou 97, Nordstrom 98, Sturrock 01, Taylor 02, Wong 02, Evers 02a, Penney 03b, Kernaghan 07, Nielsen 07), but not all,

TABLE I.2 Prospective Observational Studies of Maternal Glucose Profiles in Pregnant Women with Type 2 Diabetes and/or Type 1 Diabetes Related to Perinatal Outcome

Author	Year	N	Glucose Measure	Outcome Measure	Glucose Threshold	Best Outcome
Harley	1965	113	ven BG, 3-h PP	PNM	3-h PPBG <150	PNM 7.6%
Karlsson	1972	167	ven BG, premeal	PNM	MBG <100	PNM 3.8%
Roversi	1978	213	ven BG, premeal	Birth weight	Premeal <100	LGA 8.5%
Coustan	1980	73	ven PG, pre & PP	Birth weight	MPG <110	89% <9 lb
Schneider	1980	108	ven PG, 2-h PP	PNM, birth weight	Mean PP 165	PNM 2.7% LGA 40%
Tevaarwerk	1981	110	ven PG, premeal	Birth weight, NN complic	Mean pre 117	LGA 24.6%
Hanson	1984	100	ven PG cap BG	NN complic	MBG 108	PNM 0 RDS 4%
Landon	1987	75	cap PG, premeal	Birth weight	FPG <100, premeal <120	LGA 9.3%
Langer	1988	103	cap BG, pre & PP	Birth weight	Mean pre 89, mean 2-h 109	LGA 9.7%
Jovanovic	1991	323	ven PG, cap BG, F & PP	Birth weight	1-h PG <120	LGA <20%
Combs	1992	111	cap BG, F & PP	Birth weight	1-h BG <130	LGA 13.8%
Parfitt	1992	14	cap BG, pre & PP	Birth weight	MBG 127	LGA 29%
Page	1996	29	cap BG, pre & PP	Birth weight	Mean pre 108, mean PP 144	LGA 41%
Persson	1996	113	cap BG, pre & PP	Birth weight	FBG <108, PPBG <126	AGA
Mello	1997	31	cap BG, pre & PP	NN complic	Mean pre 96, mean PP 107	No complic
Mello	2000	98	cap BG, pre & PP	Birth weight	MBG ≥95	LGA 5.4%
Raychaudhuri	2000	76	cap BG, premeal	Birth weight	Premeal <113	AGA
Sturrock	2001	45	cap BG, pre & PP	Birth weight, NN complic	Mean pre 121, 2-h PP 147	93% <4,500 g 52% NICU

Glucose = mg/dL.
AGA, appropriate for gestational age; BG, blood glucose; cap, capillary; complic, complications; FPG, fasting plasma glucose; LGA, large for gestational age; MBG, mean whole blood glucose; NICU, neonatal intensive care unit; NN, neonatal; PG, plasma glucose; PNM, perinatal mortality; PP, postprandial; PPBG, postprandial blood glucose; RDS, respiratory distress syndrome; ven, venous.

studies (Small 87, Jovanovic 91, Parfitt 92, Wyse 94, Djelmis 97, Johnstone 00, Raychaudhuri 00, Hummel 07, Kerssen 07), possibly because A1C levels are determined by low as well as high glucose values. Intensive glucose monitoring reveals a substantial proportion of postprandial glucose recordings above targets in pregnant diabetic women with near normal A1C (Kyne-Grzebalski 99, Kerssen 03). Maternal glucose thresholds for the excess risk of fetal macrosomia and associated neonatal complications in IDMs appear to be those that are slightly above levels measured in nondiabetic pregnant women (Table I.2; refer to Table I.3 in the section titled "Normoglycemia During Pregnancy") (Coustan 80, Hanson 84, Jovanovic 91, Combs 92, Persson 96, Mello 00, Raychaudhuri 00, Langer 02). Postprandial glucose values were the best predictors of excess BW in the few studies in which both pre- and postmeal glucose were measured (Jovanovic 91, Combs 92, Parfitt 92). Upward excursions of maternal hyperglycemia with pulses of fetal glucose may be the most relevant to fetal insulin secretion (Artal 83, Carver 96).

Glucose control that is too tight can result in an increase of small-for-gestational-age (SGA) babies (BW <10th percentile in the reference population), but in these series, many SGA infants were delivered by hypertensive mothers (Roversi 78, Coustan 80, Combs 92, Rosenn 00). Increased (or decreased) BW is also associated with relatively higher (or lower) maternal glucose levels in large surveys of nondiabetic pregnant women, independent of maternal weight and weight gain (Sermer 95, Scholl 01, Mello 03). Fetal growth restriction may also be a factor in subsequent obesity and glucose intolerance (Forsen 00, Gray 02).

Several investigators found the best prediction of fetal macrosomia with elevated maternal glucose in the first half of pregnancy (Peck 90, Page 96, Gold 98, Rey 99, Vaarasmaki 00b) or the middle trimester (Landon 87, Combs 92, Parfitt 92, Persson 96, Raychaud 00, Sturrock 01). There is evidence that uncontrolled diabetes in early pregnancy can enhance the expression and activity of human placental glucose transporters (Demers 72, Challier 86, Hauguel 86, Schmon 91, Hauguel-de Mouzon 94, Kniss 94, Gordon 95, Sciullo 97, Xing 98, Gaither 99, Jansson 99, Hahn 00, Illsley 00, Baumann 02, Gude 03, Li 04, Ericsson 05a,b, Jansson 06a, Mitchell 06). Because expression of human placental glucose transporters is evolving throughout pregnancy (Jansson 06b), even modest changes in maternal glucose concentrations later in gestation might still be associated with increased glucose transfer into the fetus (Desoye 02).

In any case, several programs of intensified glycemic control throughout pregnancy have achieved near-normal rates of large-for-gestational age (LGA) infants and low perinatal morbidity (Roversi 78, Coustan 80, Jovanovic 80,81, Weiss 84, Nachum 99, Howorka 01). Randomized trials are mostly lacking (Farrag 87, Walkinshaw 96) due to the previously mentioned ethical and legal risks of withholding intensified treatment from pregnant diabetic women (Kitzmiller 93, Langer 02). The bulk of observational studies suggest that the optimal glycemic targets for achieving near-normal infant body composition are fasting, premeal, and nighttime glucose values of 60–99 mg/dL, peak postprandial values of 100–129 mg/dL, mean daily glucose <100 mg/dL, and A1C <6.0 (Table I.2) (Jovanovic 91, Combs 92, Persson 96, Mello 97, Mello 00, Raychaudhuri 00, Vaarasmaki 00b, Langer 02).

One pilot study of an RCT assigned pregnant women with type 1 diabetes to target premeal capillary plasma glucose levels at 60–90 mg/dL and 1-h postprandial glucose at 120–140 mg/dL vs. less "rigid" control of premeal glucose levels at 95–115 mg/dL and 1-h postprandial glucose at 155–175 mg/dL (Sacks 06b). The study was abandoned after 3 years due to difficulty in recruiting subjects. Thirteen subjects were available for analysis in the good control group and only nine in the less-rigid control group; four women dropped out of the latter group. Baseline A1C level was not reported for the two groups, but 85% of subjects in the good control group reported preconception care vs. 44% in the less-rigid control group. In spite of the small numbers, women in the good control group had lower first-trimester A1C (6.3 ± 0.7 vs.

7.5 ± 1.5, p < 0.04), lower second-trimester mean plasma glucose (127 ± 12 mg/dL vs. 145 ± 15 mg/dL, p < 0.01), and a greater percentage of days with one or more subjective hypoglycemic episodes (64 ± 14 vs. 42 ± 12, p < 0.003). A trend was apparent for smaller BW in infants of non-overweight mothers in the good control group (3,579 vs. 3,886 gm), but the number of subjects in the trial was insufficient to evaluate perinatal outcome. No fetal or neonatal deaths occurred in either small group (Sacks 06b).

Influences on fetal growth and neonatal adiposity/metabolic homeostasis are complex (Catalano 95a,b,03), and factors such as maternal BMI and weight gain (Ehrenberg 04), vascular disease, placental size/endocrine function (Catalano 06a), and smoking also play a role in pregnancies complicated by diabetes (Willman 86, Madsen 91, Persson 96, Johnstone 00). Possible interactions between maternal glucose control, placental growth hormone, and the fetal IGF system and their effects on fetal macrosomia are difficult to unravel due to conflicting data (Milner 84, Hill 89, Davies 91, Patel 95, Culler 96, Roth 96, Yan-Jun 96, Gibson 99a, McIntyre 00, Fuglsang 03, Geary 03, Wu 03, Fuglsang 05, Loukovaara 05). Current studies of the role of maternal–fetal hyperglycemia and hyperinsulinemia on placental gene expression should increase our understanding of diabetic fetopathy (Cauzac 03, Radaelli 03, Hiden 06, Radaelli 06). Maternal diabetes seems to induce a variety of cytokine network and inflammatory signals in the placenta (Hauguel-de Mouzon 06a). One possible pathway to placental–fetal macrosomia is via interleukin (IL)-6 and IL-1 and tumor necrosis factor-α (TNF-α)–stimulated leptin production. In addition, insulin stimulation of mitogen-activated protein kinase (MAPK) phosphorylation and DNA synthesis in placental cells can result in many leptin–pleiotropic effects (Jansson 03, Varastehpour 06) leading to placental hypertrophy and fetal adiposity (Lepercq 99, Hauguel-de Mouzon 06b). Alternatively, leptin or adiponectin may activate proinflammatory cytokine release and phospholipid metabolism in the human placenta (Lappas 05a). Placental leptin mRNA and protein concentrations are increased with maternal diabetes, especially with fetal macrosomia, and most placental leptin seems to be released into maternal blood (Lepercq 98, Lea 00, Hauguel-de Mouzon 06). It is well established that elevated leptin concentrations found in the cord blood of IDMs reflects their increased adiposity (Gross 98, Maffei 98, Shekhawat 98, Persson 99, Ng 00, Tapanainen 01, Manderson 03a). Whether maternal diabetes affects placental adiponectin and its receptors is undergoing current investigation (Caminos 05, Lappas 05b, Chen 06).

Other metabolic fuels also play a role in fetal growth and development. Maternal amino acids transported across the placenta against a concentration gradient may contribute to fetal macrosomia (Johnson 88, Kalkhoff 88, McGivan 94, Moe 95, Jansson 03). Branched-chain amino acids, especially leucine, can stimulate fetal insulin production (Jozwik 01), but these amino acids are maintained at normal levels by intensified insulin therapy in pregnancy (Reece 91). Fasting total amino acids were higher than controls in three studies of women with type 1 diabetes (Kalkhoff 88, Kalhan 94, Whittaker 00), but whole-body protein breakdown to leucine and nonoxidized leucine disposal for protein synthesis did not differ in diabetic and control groups (Whittaker 00). In vitro studies in the perfused normal-term placenta showed no effect of hyperglycemic load (28 mM) on leucine transport, but "hyperglycemia" reduced transport of A-type amino acids, such as α-aminoisobutyric acid (Nandakumaran 02, Nandakumaran 05). Studies of system-A amino acid transporters in microvillous membrane vesicles from placentas of diabetic women produced conflicting results: they were not different (Dicke 88), decreased (Kuruvilla 94), or increased in activity compared with controls (Jansson 02).

Maternal as well as placental lipids may influence fetal adiposity (Szabo 74, Knopp 85,92, Kitajima 01). Diabetic women demonstrate resistance to insulin suppression of lipolysis. Triglycerides (TGs) and nonesterified fatty acids (NEFAs; aka, free fatty acids [FFAs]) are increased in the basal state and postprandially with inadequate metabolic control of diabetic pregnant women (Gillmer 77, Hollingsworth 82, Montelongo 92). TGs are not transferred across the placenta, but they deliver maternal NEFA to placental cells (Herrera 04). NEFAs, including essential polyunsaturated fatty acids (PUFAs), are taken up by the human placenta and transferred into the fetal circulation (Hendricks 85, Knopp 86, Campbell 96a, Kilby 98, Haggarty 02, Hotmire 06, Varastehpour 06). The complex multistep processes involved in placental transfer of fatty acids are discussed later in this book in the section titled "Dietary Fats: Total Fats and Fatty Acids." Additional data are needed on NEFAs, fatty acid types, and triacylglycerols in pregnancies of women with type 1 and type 2 diabetes related to glycemic control and fetal–neonatal complications. One study of intensified treatment of type 1 diabetes revealed that normalization of glucose also produced normal pregnancy levels of serum TGs, but NEFAs remained somewhat elevated compared with controls (Reece 91).

Other Effects of Glycemic Control on Pregnancy Outcome

Many other effects of maternal glycemic control are evident on the fetus, infant, and child. Studies in animals (Phillipps 82,84, Hay 89) and humans (Robillard 78, Mimouni 88b, Bradley 91, Salveson 95) demonstrate that acute or chronic fetal hyperglycemia causes fetal hypoxia and acidosis that are probably related to excess stillbirth rates still observed in poorly controlled diabetic women (Hanson 93, Casson 97, Hawthorne 97, Cundy 00, Platt 02, Temple 02, Lauenberg 03, Wood 03, McElduff 05b). Since the 1970s, it has been known that good glycemic control reduces perinatal mortality (Pedersen 56, Harley 65, Delaney 70, Karlsson 72, Gugliucci 76, Gabbe 77, Kitzmiller 78, Jervell 79, Kitzmiller 93, Wylie 02). Unsatisfactory maternal glucose levels in the third trimester are also related to neonatal hypoglycemia (Kalhan 77, Mimouni 88b, Johnstone 00, Taylor 02), hypocalcemia (Demarini 94), decreased bone mineral content (Mimouni 88c), and polycythemia (Widness 90, Green 92, Salvesen 92,93), plus abnormal fetal surfactant production and neonatal respiratory distress in most (Ylinen 87, Piper 93,98, Heimberger 99), but not all, studies (Delgado 00, Moore 02). Such morbidity in the infant markedly increases the costs of neonatal care (Elixhauser 93, Elixhauser 96, Herman 97). Attainment of optimal glucose targets throughout pregnancy to prevent excess macrosomia can also minimize these neonatal complications (Hanson 84, Mello 97, Vaarasmaki 00b, Langer 02). Finally, long-term follow-up studies (5–15 years) of IDMs suggest that aberrant maternal energy metabolism related to poor glycemic control has a negative influence on intellectual performance and psychomotor development (Rizzo 91,94, Sells 94, Rizzo 95, Ornoy 98, Silverman 98, Ratzon 00, Ornoy 01).

Tight glycemic control also may benefit the mother. Elevated glucose during pregnancy is related to progression of retinopathy and nephropathy and the frequency of superimposed preeclampsia (Jovanovic 84, Klein 90, Rosenn 92,93, Chew 95, Miodovnik 96, Lovestam 97, Hsu 98, Reece 98, Ekbom 00, Hillesma 00, Lauszus 01a, Manderson 03b, Temple 06b) and premature labor (Mimouni 88a, Rosenn 93, Kovilam 02, Lauszus 06). Of course, one cost of tight glycemic control in pregnancy is maternal hypoglycemia, with an average of two to three symptomatic reactions per week in women with type 1 diabetes (Rayburn 86, Kitzmiller 91, Kimmerle 92, Rosenn 95a,b, Hellmuth 00a, Evers 02b). Therefore, intensive patient training is necessary to minimize this problem in the interest of maternal safety. Higher glucose targets should be used in patients with hypoglycemia unawareness. In view of studies of maternal glycemic control and perinatal outcome, it seems prudent for most pregnant diabetic women and their healthcare providers to strive for premeal and postprandial glucose levels as close to normal as possible before and throughout pregnancy and delivery (refer to Table I.3 in the section titled "Normoglycemia During Pregnancy") without causing debilitating hypoglycemia.

Recommendations

- To prevent excess spontaneous abortions and major congenital malformations before pregnancy, target A1C as close to normal as possible without significant hypoglycemia. (B)
- Ensure effective contraception until stable and acceptable glycemia is achieved. (E)
- Utilize resources with referral as necessary to enhance intensified preconception diabetes care and to minimize significant hypoglycemia. (B)
- Excellent glycemic control in the first trimester continued throughout pregnancy is associated with the lowest frequency of maternal, fetal, and neonatal complications. Develop or adjust the management plan to achieve near-normal glycemia while minimizing significant hypoglycemia. (B)
- To minimize perinatal morbidity throughout pregnancy, optimal fingerstick glucose goals are premeal, bedtime, and overnight glucose levels at 60–99 mg/dL, peak postprandial glucose levels at 100–129 mg/dL, mean daily glucose <110 mg/dL, and near-normal A1C <6.0. (B)
- Higher glucose targets may be used in patients with hypoglycemia unawareness or the inability to cope with intensified management. (E)

ASSESSMENT OF GLYCEMIC CONTROL

—— *Original contribution by Lois B. Jovanovic MD and Maribeth Inturissi RN, MNS, CDE*

Normoglycemia During Pregnancy

Recent studies of intermittent capillary blood glucose and continuous interstitial glucose monitoring in normal women in their usual settings reveal a rather narrow range of glucose concentrations. Fasting plasma glucose (FPG) concentrations decline in early normal pregnancy (Mills 98). A slight, gradual rise appears in mean and postprandial glucose values throughout the second and third trimesters of normal pregnancy. In nondiabetic pregnant women, the best third-trimester reference ranges for capillary fasting, overnight, and premeal glucose calibrated to plasma levels are 50–99 mg/dL, with postmeal peak values 60–70 min after eating at 81–129 mg/dL (Table I.3) (Parretti 01, Yogev 04a). Another study of capillary gluose levels in 36 "normal" pregnant women noted slightly higher ranges, but subjects were included with plasma glucose

TABLE I.3 Normal Glucose Concentrations and A1C Levels During Third-Trimester Pregnancy, Capillary Glucose and A1C Goals for Women with PDM Before and During Early Pregnancy, and Optimal Goals During the Second and Third Trimesters

Group	Daily Mean Glucose (mg/dL)	Fasting, Premeal, Nightime Glucose	1-h Postprandial Glucose	A1C (%)
Normal pregnancy, mean ± SD				5.0 ± 0.4*
Capillary glucose by meter** (Parretti 00)	82.9 ± 5.8	69.3 ± 5.7	108.4 ± 6.0	
Continuous interstitial glucose (Yogev 04a)	83.7 ± 18	76.6 ± 11.5	105.3 ± 12	
PDM goals before and during early pregnancy	<125	60–119	100–149	<6.3
PDM goals during second and third trimesters	<110	60–99	100–129	<6.0

*O'Kane 01 and Nielsen 04.

**Adjusted to be equivalent to plasma glucose values.

PDM, preexisting diabetes mellitus.

values >140 mg/dL (<7.8 mM) 1 h after challenge with a 50-gm sugar solution who had negative glucose tolerance tests (GTTs) (by the older National Diabetes Data Group criteria) (Montaner 02).

Self-Monitoring of Capillary Blood Glucose

SMBG is an integral part of the intensified treatment of diabetes that dramatically improved pregnancy outcome over the past 25 years (Hanson 84, Kitzmiller 93, Langer 02), and this process is necessary for individuals to achieve optimal glucose goals (Goldstein 04, Silverstein 05, Kerssen 06a). Capillary blood glucose refers to the usual sample obtained by the patient. Because it is recognized that most glucose meters now calibrate capillary blood measurements to read as plasma glucose for comparability with reference laboratory measurements, use of the term SMBG in this document also implies that fact. The amount of glucose per unit of water mass is the same in whole blood and plasma. "Although erythrocytes are essentially freely permeable to glucose (glucose is taken up by facilitated transport), the concentration of water in plasma (kg/l) is ~11% higher than that of whole blood. Therefore, glucose concentrations in plasma are ~11% higher than whole blood if the hematocrit is normal" (Sacks 02a). Because this is true for glucose values measured in venous or capillary blood (Chmielewski 95, IFCC 01, Kuwa 01, Torjman 01, Buhling 03), "it is crucial that people with diabetes know whether their monitor and strips provide whole blood or plasma results" (ADA 04a). However, the recent National Academy of Clinical Biochemistry's guideline for management of diabetes adopted by the ADA (Sacks 02b) suggests that the total error when using a meter (user plus analytical) is often as much as the difference between the whole blood and plasma glucose measurement, as noted by others (Parkes 00, Boehme 03). Variance between capillary glucose measurements and a reference plasma method seems to be greatest when the glucose value is higher (Boehme 03). In studies detailing the accuracy of SMBG in the normo- to hyperglycemic range in diabetic pregnant women, usage of most home devices had a total error of <15% (Moses 97, Henry 01). In the hypoglycemic range, there may be a reduction in the accuracy of SMBG (Moberg 93, Zenobi 95, Trajanoski 96, Henry 01), perhaps due to alterations in subcutaneous blood flow during hypoglycemia (Hilsted 85, Fernqvist-Forbes 88, Aman 92).

SMBG allows the patient to evaluate her individual response to therapy and assess whether glycemic targets are being achieved. Frequent sampling is optimal in pregnancy (Kerssen 06a) due to the increased potential for rapid-onset hypoglycemia in the absence of food or presence of exercise and the exacerbated hyperglycemic responses to food ingestion, psychological stress, and intercurrent illness related to gestational insulin resistance. Use of glucose meters with memory capacity is important for verification of the reliability of patient self-testing and recording (Langer 86, Kendrick 05). The accuracy of SMBG is instrument and user dependent (Sacks 02a), and it is important for healthcare providers to evaluate each patient's monitoring technique, both initially and at regular intervals thereafter. The patient should "use calibrators and controls on a regular basis to assure accuracy of results" (Goldstein 04). Optimal use of SMBG requires proper interpretation of the data, and many patients can be taught how to use the data to adjust food intake, exercise, or insulin therapy to achieve specific glycemic goals. Health professionals regularly should evaluate the patient's ability to use data to guide therapy.

Site of Glucose Sampling

To provide less painful glucose self-testing, manufacturers developed products designed for use at alternate sites, usually the forearm or thigh (Goldstein 04). However, when glucose concentrations are rapidly rising or falling (e.g., postprandially, immediately after exercise, or with insulin-induced hypoglycemia), a lag time exists between the fingerstick capillary glucose concentration and alternative site testing of the forearm and thigh (Ellison 02, Jungheim 02). Therefore, use of alternative site testing systems in the dynamic state of pregnancy will produce different results than fingerstick testing (Goldstein 04) and is not wise. Palm and fingertip capillary glucose values are similar at different timepoints (Bina 03, Meguro 05), but these testing sites have not been compared in pregnancy.

Timing of SMBG

A randomized trial studying premeal versus postprandial glucose testing as the guide for insulin therapy in pregnant women with rather severe gestational diabetes mellitus (GDM) and fasting hyperglycemia reported lower frequencies of perinatal complications with the treatment strategy based on postmeal testing (de Veciana 95). A similar result was found in a randomized trial of premeal versus postprandial testing starting at 16 weeks' gestation in type 1 diabetes (Manderson 03b). These trials support previous observational studies in type 1 and type 2 diabetes that revealed postprandial glucose levels as the best predictor of fetal macrosomia (Jovanovic 91, Combs 92, Parfitt 92). Because most pregnant patients with type 1 and type 2 diabetes will use short-acting insulin injections before meals to prevent postprandial hyperglycemia, premeal glucose testing is useful to allow temporary adjustments of the insulin dose if the glucose level is low or elevated (Skyler 81, Miller 94, Hirsch 98b, Jovanovic-Peterson 07). Bedtime and overnight blood glucose testing is used as needed to detect hyper- or hypoglycemia at those timepoints to allow subsequent adjustment of snacks or insulin doses.

Protocols for the timing and frequency of self-monitored glucose concentrations should be designed to reflect the peak and nadir of maternal glycemia. When animal Regular insulin was prescribed previously—and even with the advent of recombinant DNA technology that made human Regular insulin available—concern that the peak action of Regular insulin might cause hypoglycemic reactions 1.5–2.5 h after the injection led to use of the 2-h postprandial timepoint. Because the available rapid-acting insulin analogs have their peak effect 45–70 min after injection and because the concern is to prevent hyperglycemia-induced fetal complications, evidence is mounting that 1-h postprandial testing may be a better choice in most pregnancies complicated by diabetes. The time to peak rise in plasma glucose after finishing a test meal was 60–80 min throughout gestation in a longitudinal study with frequent intravenous sampling postmeal in primigravid women with uncomplicated pregnancies (Stanley 95). Studies of continuous interstitial glucose monitoring in diabetic pregnant women showed mean peak postprandial glucose to average 60–90 min after beginning the meal, with considerable variation from patient to patient (Ben-Haroush 04) and high day-to-day variability (Kerssen 04a, Buhling 05). Instructing patients to test 1 h after finishing the meal should approximate these peaks.

Some pregnant patients may have delayed postprandial peak glucose excursions related to delayed gastric emptying (Samsom 03). It is also recognized that meals containing a high fat content in pregnancy may prolong the postprandial glucose excursion (Fran 02, Gentilcore 06). A study in which 68 women with GDM used SMBG at both 1- and 2-h postprandial for 1 week after diagnosis revealed a greater proportion of abnormal values at 1 h after breakfast, equivalence after lunch, but a greater proportion of abnormal values at 2 h after dinner (Sivan 01). It is optimal for individual patients to determine their own postprandial peak times after specific meals to be used in their SMBG regimen.

Continuous Monitoring of Blood Glucose

At least six continuous glucose monitoring systems have been investigated or marketed (Klonoff 05a,b). The Continuous Glucose Monitoring System (CGMS) measures subcutaneous interstitial tissue glucose by an electrochemical method. Because interstitial fluid glucose levels are 20–50% lower than blood glucose levels (Rebrin 99), calibration of CGMS with four capillary glucose levels per day corrects for this difference (Kerssen 04b). CGMS glucose concentrations are "calculated in retrospect using a regression analysis of the [capillary] blood glucose values with corresponding sensor readings for each calendar day." Therefore, CGMS readings are not used in real time by the patient, but are expected to help clinicians identify patterns and trends in glycemic control (Kerssen 04b).

Feasibility studies of CGMS in pregnancies of women with type 1 diabetes treated with multiple daily insulin injections revealed periods of both hyper- and hypoglycemia that were not detected by fingerstick testing or patient symptoms (Kerssen 03, Yogev 03a,b, Ben-Haroush 04, Buhling 04, Kerssen 04a,b, Kerssen 06a). However, interstitial glucose values failed to reflect symptomatic hypoglycemia confirmed by capillary glucose testing in 6.2% of all paired samples in a careful study of CGMS in 15 pregnant women with type 1 diabetes (Kerssen 04b). Reproducibility of glucose measurements in subjects wearing two sensors at the same time was not optimal in early studies (Metzger 02, Guerci 03, Larsen 04). When this approach was used in five pregnant women with type 1 diabetes, 95% of the data pairs had a difference <31.5 mg/dL (<1.75 mM); in 81% of nonconcordant pairs, one glucose value was hypoglycemic and one was normoglycemic (Kerssen 05). The methodology is expected to improve (Cheyne 02, DirNet 05a, Wentholt 05,06), and prospective controlled trials are needed to determine whether intermittent application of this expensive method to fine-tune glycemic control will improve perinatal outcome and maternal safety. Ancillary questions posed are which patients might benefit the most from this system and at which stages of pregnancy.

The Gluco Watch Biographer is based on reverse iontophoresis in which a low-level electric current moves glucose across the skin by electro-osmosis, and the glucose concentration is then measured by a glucose oxidase electrode detector (Sacks 02a).

This system is designed to measure glucose approximately three times per hour up to 12 h, and calibration is necessary with intermittent capillary glucose measurements (Tierney 00). Glucose readings correlate with plasma glucose values taken 10–20 min earlier. Use of the device is associated with local skin irritation (DirNet 05b), and sweating can cause falsely low glucose readings (Goldstein 04). Systematic studies of this and other systems in pregnant diabetic women are lacking.

Other Measures of Metabolic Control

Glycated Hemoglobin

GHb is the general term used to describe a series of stable minor hemoglobin components formed slowly and nonenzymatically in direct proportion to the ambient glucose concentration (ADA 04f). GHb values expressed as a percentage of total hemoglobin provide the best assessment of the degree of chronic glycemic control, reflecting the average blood glucose concentration during the preceding 6–12 weeks because the lifespan of erythrocytes is shortened to <90 days in pregnancy (Lurie 92). However, GHb can be misleading if patients balance frequent low and high plasma glucose levels because this indicator of average glucose would not reflect postprandial elevations that represent pulses of high glucose in the fetus (Kyne-Grzebalski 99, Derr 03, Kerssen 03,06a,b). Preanalytic variables important during pregnancy include decreased mean erythrocyte age (which falsely lowers the A1C result) as well as iron-deficiency anemia and hypertriglyceridemia (which falsely increases results) (Sacks 02b, Goldstein 04).

Many GHb assays are available, but hemoglobin A1C (HbA_{1C} or A1C test) has become the preferred standard for assessing glycemic control (ADA 04f). The current goal is to achieve standardization of laboratory A1C measurements (Marshall 00, Sacks 02, Goldstein 04) because a variety of reference limits have been obtained with different high performance liquid chromatography (HPLC) equipment (Parentoni 98). Manufacturers of A1C test methods can earn a certificate of traceability to the Diabetes Control and Complications Trial (DCCT) reference method (Rohlfing 02) by passing rigorous testing criteria for precision and accuracy (ADA 04f). An international consensus was reached in 2007 (1) that a new International Federation of Clinical Chemistry and Laboratory Medicine (IFCC) reference system specifically measuring the concentration of only one molecular species of glycated A1C should be used as the anchor to implement standardization of measurement, (2) that A1C results are to be reported worldwide in IFCC units (mmol/mol) and derived National Glycohemoglobin Standardization Program (NGSP) units (%), and (3) that an A1C-derived average glucose value will also be reported (ADA 07).

When maternal glycemia is elevated and rapidly brought toward normal in pregnancy, A1C has been reported to show a significant decrease within two weeks compared with the baseline elevation; thus, measurement of A1C every 2–6 weeks confirms SMBG measurements. A1C reference levels are lower during pregnancy. A sensitive, precise, and accurate HPLC A1C measurement method yielded a reference range (2.5 and 97.5 percentiles) of 3.2–5.3 for 63 healthy pregnant women compared with 3.4–5.9 in other adult women (Parentoni 98). A network of similar HPLC DCCT-linked systems at five diabetes care centers in Italy observed reproducible A1C measurements in pregnancy (coefficient of variation [CV] = 2.0%) and reported pooled reference intervals of 4.0–5.5 in 445 normal pregnant women compared with 4.8–6.2 for 384 nonpregnant controls (Mosca 06). Evaluation of DCCT-aligned ion exchange liquid chromatography assays in two studies revealed lower reference ranges for A1C in 493 and 100 healthy pregnant women of 4.1–5.9 and 4.5–5.7, respectively, compared with 4.7–6.3 in age-matched nonpregnant control women (O'Kane 01, Nielsen 04). Results were not affected by differences in body mass between groups in these two studies. In preliminary data from the global Hyperglycemia and Adverse Perinatal Outcome study, the 97.5th percentile for DCCT-aligned A1C in 19,023 gravidas was 5.7. A yet-unknown percentage of these women had mild glucose intolerance (Lappin 06). All investigators agree that pregnant women have lower A1C values and urge the use of pregnancy-specific reference levels by DCCT-linked laboratories. Trimester- and ethnic group-related differences in A1C in various stages of normal pregnancy are not of clinical significance (Parentoni 98, Hartland 99, O'Kane 01).

Glycated Serum Protein Assays

These assays correlate well with the A1C test (ADA 04f), but debate continues as to whether these measurements need to be corrected for serum albumin concentration (Goldstein 04). Although the measurement of fructosamine—an indirect measurement of glycosylated serum proteins (mostly albumin)—should theoretically reflect average blood glucose over the past week because of the rapid turnover rate of albumin (14–20 days in pregnancy), fructosamine has not proven to be useful in pregnancies complicated by diabetes. Because fructosamine assays are an indirect measurement of total glycosylated serum proteins, there is interference by reducing agents in the blood. If a pregnant woman has recently taken her prenatal vitamins, results of the fructosamine assay will then vary based on her blood concentrations of vitamin C. Vitamin C concentrations in the blood alter the fructosamine assay more than do small changes in glycemia. In addition, there is diurnal variation in serum protein concentrations in the blood. Thus, fructosamine tests must be taken at the same time for each determination or the variation in total serum proteins may be greater than the change in this measurement of average glucose concentrations.

Plasma Anhydro-D-Glucitol

This is an inverse correlate of hyperglycemic excursions that responds more rapidly than A1C and is under study as an adjunct measure of glycemic status (Kishimoto 95, McGill 04, Dungan 06). To date, this measure has undergone only preliminary experience in diabetic pregnant women (Tetsuo 90, Dworacka 06).

Ketonuria and Ketonemia

Ketone testing is important because the presence of ketones can indicate impending KTA, which may develop quickly in pregnancy with type 1 diabetes. Urine ketones should be measured periodically when the pregnant diabetic woman is ill or when any blood glucose value is >250 mg/dL. Outside of pregnancy, a value of 300 mg/dL is used, but a lower threshold is used in pregnancy because KTA can develop at lower levels of hyperglycemia in pregnant women with type 1 and type 2 diabetes (Whiteman 96). KTA is associated with a high mortality rate in the fetus (Chauhan 95). In addition, fasting ketonemia in poorly controlled pregnant diabetic women has been associated with decreased intelligence and fine motor skills in offspring (Rizzo 91,95). In early pregnancy, ketonuria sometimes occurs in women who limit their caloric intake due to nutritional recommendations or nausea and vomiting; however, it is unclear whether starvation ketosis is associated with decreased intelligence in the offspring. Women with moderate to large ketonuria associated with hyperglycemia should alert their physician immediately for determination of ketonemia. Urine ketone tests are not reliable for the firm diagnosis of KTA, which is better assessed with blood ketone testing that quantifies β-hydroxybutyric acid (ADA 04f). Home tests for β-hydroxybutyric acid are available for use on sick days (Laffel 06), but have not been evaluated systematically in pregnancy.

Recommendations

- SMBG is a key component of diabetes therapy during pregnancy in both type 1 and type 2 diabetes and should be included in the management plan. Daily SMBG with checking both before and after meals, at bedtime, and occasionally at 2–4 a.m. will provide optimal results in pregnancy. (E)
- Fingerstick SMBG is best in pregnancy because alternate site testing may not identify rapid changes in blood glucose concentrations characteristic of pregnant women with PDM. (E)
- Instruct the patient in SMBG by using meters calibrated to plasma glucose and with memory capacity. Instruct the patient to record data in a logbook. Routinely evaluate the patient's technique and ability to use data to adjust therapy. Ideally, provide the pregnant patient with the opportunity for daily telephone or electronic contact with the healthcare staff to discuss problems in management. (E)
- Postprandial capillary glucose measured 1 h after beginning the meal best approximates postmeal peak glucose measured continuously. (C)
- Due to individual differences in the time to peak postprandial glucose level related to content and time of meals, rate of gastric emptying, and possibly other factors, it may be useful for each patient to determine her own peak postprandial testing time after beginning her meals. (E)
- Check fingerstick glucose appropriately to prevent, identify, and treat hypoglycemia. (E)
- Continuous glucose monitoring may be a supplemental tool to SMBG for selected patients with type 1 diabetes, especially those with hypoglycemia unawareness. (E)
- Teach the pregnant patient to perform urine ketone measurements at times of illness or when blood glucose reaches 200 mg/dL. Positive values should be reported promptly to the healthcare professional. (E)
- Perform the A1C test, using a DCCT-aligned assay, at the initial visit during pregnancy and then monthly until target levels <6.0 are achieved. Conduct tests every 2–3 months thereafter. (E)

MEDICAL NUTRITION THERAPY

—— Original contribution by Diane M. Reader RD, CDE, Alyce M. Thomas RD, and Erica P. Gunderson RD, PhD

Medical Nutrition Therapy Goals for Pregnancy Complicated by PDM

The clinical goals of MNT are threefold: (a) to provide adequate energy and nutrients needed for normal fetal and placental development and to minimize pregnancy complications, (b) to achieve optimal glycemic control to maximize perinatal outcomes, and (c) to educate and train women with diabetes to adopt nutrition and activity behaviors that will benefit their lifelong health by reducing CVD (Howard 02, Giugliano 06). An additional goal is to maintain the pleasure of eating by making food choices based on scientific evidence and clinical outcome measures, such as plasma glucose responses and weight gain (ADA 08b). Patients with poor eating habits can often be educated to enjoy a healthy diet during the motivated time of pregnancy, and achieving these goals requires a coordinated team effort that includes the pregnant woman with diabetes. Because of the complexity of nutrition issues, it is strongly recommended that an RD—who has knowledge of the dynamic changes in nutritional needs and fuel metabolism during pregnancy and who is skilled in implementing nutrition therapy as part of diabetes education and management—should be the team member who provides MNT whenever possible. However, it is essential that all clinical team members become informed about goals and basic principles of nutrition therapy for pregnancy and support the woman with diabetes when making lifestyle changes. Optimally, these changes should be made in anticipation of pregnancy to facilitate good glycemic control during implantation and embryogenesis.

In addition to the ADA (ADA 08b), other agencies have issued recommendations on MNT for managing diabetes during pregnancy (ACOG 99,01 UKDH 01, ADietA 02, AADE 04, ACOG 05) that are aligned with the 2005 Dietary Guidelines for Americans (DGA 05, DGAr 05). Nutrition requirements for women with PDM are based on those identified by the Food and Nutrition Board of the Institute of Medicine (IOM) for women with normal and complicated pregnancies in reports on pregnancy (IOM 90,92) and on the Dietary Reference Intakes (DRIs) for all individuals (IOM 97,98,00a,01,02,04). Pages from these reports can be downloaded in pdf format.

Consistency in the timing and intake of macronutrients at meals and snacks is helpful for regulation of glycemia within the optimal target range during pregnancy. MNT for diabetes in pregnancy should incorporate an individualized food plan as discussed in more detail in a later section titled "Individualized Nutrition Therapy." Specific nutrition and food recommendations are determined and modified based on individual assessment and plasma glucose monitoring data, daily food records, the requirements of insulin therapy, and weight gain. Nutrition counseling and patient teaching will be most effective when sensitive to the personal needs and cultural preferences of the pregnant woman with diabetes (ADietA 02, ADA 08b).

Pregnancy Effects on Metabolism

The combined effects of pregnancy on maternal metabolism include accelerated starvation and facilitated anabolism (Freinkel 80, Knopp 97). These states can be considered in terms of time of day (postprandial or postabsorptive), stage of pregnancy, or with reference to carbohydrate, protein, and lipid metabolism (Butte 00, Herrera 00) and the increasing insulin resistance of pregnancy (Kirwan 02,04, Catalano 06b, McLachlan 06). These states affect changes in body composition in pregnancy and energy use both before and during exercise. Accelerated starvation characterizes the more rapid use of fuels that results in reduced fasting glucose levels and a tendency to greater lipolysis and ketosis after 12–14 h without food intake compared with the nonpregnant state (Metzger 82, Buchanan 90a). Facilitated anabolism occurs after food ingestion and results in (a) conservation of nitrogen, (b) variable deposition of maternal fat stores, and (c) higher elevations in postprandial glucose compared with the nonpregnant state (Catalano 98a, Butte 00, King 00a, Butte 04). During the first trimester, the effects of accelerated starvation and possible irregular food intake secondary to nausea and vomiting may lead to increased occurrences of hypoglycemia. During the second and third trimesters, postprandial facilitated anabolism may be more pronounced. The later pregnancy shift in lipid metabolism from anabolic adipogenesis to catabolic lipolysis (Catalano 02, Herrera 02a) allows use of ingested and stored lipids as a maternal energy source "while preserving glucose and amino acids for the fetus" (Butte 00), but excessive lipolysis and ketogenesis must be controlled in diabetic women. Fatty acids derived from the diet, circulating triacylglycerols, or adipose tissue also cross the placenta and may contribute to fetal macrosomia (Knopp 85, Butte 00, Herrera 02a, Catalano 06c). Lipolysis-increased glycerol can serve as a substrate for maternal hepatic ketogenesis, which may have harmful effects on the fetal brain (Rizzo 91,95). MNT must be modified to accommodate these changes in maternal fuel metabolism as well as the increased energy and nutrient needs during the second half of gestation.

The fetal demand for nutrients is greatest in the second half of pregnancy (King 00a). Net substrate use (percentage of total energy expenditure [TEE] by macronutrient oxidation) for gravida plus conceptus is 55% carbohydrate, 15% protein, and 30% fat (Butte 99). Energy expenditure increases during pregnancy because of the metabolic contribution of the uterus and fetus and the increased work of the heart and lungs (Butte 99). The reader is referred to several recent studies of the variables affecting energy expenditure and body composition in pregnant women (Sohlstrom 95, Prentice 96, Butte 99, Kopp-Hoolihan 99, Butte 04, Lof 05,06). The cumulative net increase in basal metabolism relates to BMI (kg/m^2), prepregnancy percentage of total body fat, and gestational weight gain (Butte 04, Lof 05). The increase in total energy costs in pregnancy (basal plus thermic effects of exercise and food) (Catalano 92a) is 14% in women with low BMI (<19.8 kg/m^2), 22% with normal BMI, and 17% with high BMI (≥26 kg/m^2) (Butte 04). Expressed as kcal/day, the change in total energy cost from baseline with normal BMI is 32, 356, and 496 kcal/day per trimester, respectively. High intersubject variability for these measures can be observed (Prentice 96, Butte 04), which is affected by rates of lipid synthesis/storage, physical activity, and ethnic group; therefore, recommendations on energy intake must be individualized (King 00a, Butte 04). Studies of energy balance in diabetic pregnant women have been limited to GDM (Hsu 97, Catalano 98a).

Individualized Nutrition Therapy

An individualized food plan is a key part of therapy for all types of diabetes (Franz 02, DUK 03) and is especially important in managing diabetes in pregnancy (Ney 81, Jovanovic-Petersen 90, Ferris 94, Gunderson 04, Reader 05, Thomas 06a,b). Most, if not all, observational studies and RCTs of MNT in hyperglycemic pregnant women have been conducted in GDM (early studies reviewed in Fagen 95, Dornhorst 02, Gunderson 04; plus Rae 00, Lauszus 01b, Romon 01). However, MNT has been an integral part of prospective observational studies of intensified glycemic control for PDM (Diamond 83, Kitzmiller 91, DCCT 96, Nachum 99, DCCT 00). Therefore, recommendations for MNT in pregnancies with PDM are based on all of those studies as well as on trials in nonpregnant diabetic women (DCCT 93a,b, Delahanty 93, Franz 95a,b, Kulkarni 98, Pastors 02) and extensive clinical experience. We recognize that RCTs of aspects of MNT are lacking in the field of PDM and pregnancy, including studies relating to the optimal food plan for obese woman with PDM. Such trials are necessary to help answer many open questions regarding effects on pregnancy and long-term outcome.

A food plan should be customized for each woman's daily eating schedule, nutrient needs, food preferences, and financial resources. The food plan, activity routine, and insulin regimen work in concert to achieve glucose targets. The food plan:

- determines the caloric needs to achieve the designated weight gain
- describes the eating pattern: times of meals and snacks
- identifies the usual amount of carbohydrate in grams or servings at specific meals and snacks
- assures that adequate protein, amino acids, specific fatty acids, minerals, and vitamins are incorporated
- contributes to selection of the insulin regimen to achieve glucose control
- is designed to prevent hypoglycemia, which is most common in early pregnancy but can be a danger to the gravida or a cause of "rebound" hyperglycemia at any stage of gestation

Historically, nutrition requirements for pregnant women have focused on the adequacy of individual nutrients, but patients plan meals and consume foods. The best nutritional intake is based on eating a "balanced diet" composed of foods from all food groups. The individualized food plan incorporates the minimal daily servings from the Food Guide Pyramid during pregnancy (ADietA 02). These include nine servings daily of the whole-grain bread, cereal, rice, and pasta group; four servings of vegetables; three servings of fruit; three servings of the milk, yogurt, and cheese group; and two servings daily of the meat, poultry, fish, dry beans, eggs, and nuts group (Shaw 00, DGA 05). For cardiovascular health and to provide sufficient fiber, the chosen foods should include whole grains, leafy green and yellow vegetables, and fruit (DGAr 05). Paying attention to food portion size and energy density (Ello-Martin 05) should help maintain glycemic control and prevent excess weight gain.

The RD and other members of the diabetes and pregnancy management team will benefit from reviewing daily food records in conjunction with records of daily SMBG. Most women can be trained to adjust food choices and insulin doses to achieve good glucose control by using the records of food intake and glucose tests both before and after eating. Consistent timing of meals and snacks is recommended throughout pregnancy and especially late in the first trimester, when hypoglycemia is most likely due to increased insulin sensitivity (Weiss 84, Haworka 01, Jovanovic 91). Three meals and two to four timely snacks are needed by most women with intensively treated PDM to prevent premeal hypoglycemia. A bedtime snack may help prevent nocturnal hypoglycemia. The role of bedtime and nocturnal snacking in preventing fasting ketonemia is inadequately studied.

Gestational Weight Gain

Due to evidence that gestational weight gain below 20 lb was associated with higher rates of low-birth-weight babies (Kramer 87), the IOM liberalized weight-gain recommendations for all pregnant women to reduce the risk of fetal growth restriction (IOM 90, Parker 92). Target gestational weight-gain ranges were based on pregravid BMI as a marker for obesity in women (Wolfe 91, Lindsay 97, Cnattingius 98). Lower gains were recommended for overweight or obese women, and higher gains were recommended for women underweight before conception (Table I.4) (IOM 92, Lederman 97). Clinicians are urged to use grids of weight gain by gestational age so that the slope of increase in an individual woman can be compared with the reference slope for her BMI

TABLE I.4 U.S. Institute of Medicine: Recommended Total Weight Gain in Pregnancy by Prepregnancy BMI*

Weight for Height (kg/m²)	(IOM BMI)	(WHO BMI)	Recommended Gain in kg (lb)	Fat Gain** (kg)	Energy Deposition** (kcal)
Underweight	(<19.8)	(<18.5)	12.5–18 (28–40)	6.0	60,726
Normal	(19.8–26.0)	(18.5–24.9)	11.5–16 (25–35)	3.8	40,376
Overweight	(26.1–29.0)	(25.0–29.9)	7–11.5 (15–25)	2.8	31,126
Obese	(>29.0)	(≥30.0)	6.8*** (15)	–0.6	–324

*In kg/m².

**Fat gains measured in 200 women with appropriate weight gain using a four-component body composition model and calculated total energy deposition (Lederman 97).

***The recommended target weight gain for obese women is at least 6.8 kg (15 lb) (IOM 90). See text for comment.

(IOM 90, Parker 92, WHO 97, NIH 98).

BMI, body mass index; IOM, Institute of Medicine; WHO, World Health Organization.

group to recognize when adjustments in nutrient intake or physical activity are indicated. Although an upper limit was not placed on weight gain for obese women, it was recognized that many obese women will not gain to the target weight and still have excellent perinatal outcomes and that fetal macrosomia and the risk of maternal weight retention may increase with weight gains in the upper ranges (IOM 90). The World Health Organization (WHO) (WHO 91,97) and the U.S. National Institutes of Health (NIH) use slightly different BMI groupings (Table I.4), and obesity is subclassified into groups of severity (Class I, 30.0–34.9; Class II, 35.0–39.9; Class III, ≥40 kg/m²) (NIH 98). It is recognized that BMI categories specific to pregnant women of Asian origin (Far East, South East, India) are needed (Deurenberg 98). The WHO recommends cutoff levels of 23.0–24.9 kg/m² for overweight in Asian and Asian-Indian adults and ≥25 kg/m² as obesity for general clinical and research use (WHO 97), but these groupings have not been validated for effects on gestational weight gain and pregnancy outcome.

Studies continue to show that maternal pregravid body size and gestational weight gain impact perinatal outcomes (Abrams 00, Cedergren 06). Inadequate weight gain in the second and third trimesters in nondiabetic women of low or normal body size may be associated with premature birth or SGA babies (Carmichael 97, Strauss 99, Abrams 00). In nondiabetic overweight/obese women, gestational weight gain above 11.4–18 kg (>25–40 lb) is associated with increased fetal macrosomia, potential birth trauma, cesarean sections (CSs) (Cogswell 95, Thorsdottir 02, Rhodes 03, Kabiru 04, Stotland 04b,05, Nielsen 06), other adverse neonatal outcomes (Hedderson 06, Stotland 06), and postpregnancy fat and weight retention (Gunderson 00, Gunderson 01, Rooney 02, Butte 03, Olson 03, Butte 04, Kac 04, Rooney 05). Studies of PDM in pregnancy have considered the influence of maternal pregravid body size and gestational weight gain (Small 87, Jovanovic 91, Madsen 91, Cundy 93, Yanigasawa 99, Ray 01a, Lepercq 02) on infant BW and other perinatal outcomes, but few accounted for caloric intake, glycemic control, insulin resistance, and comorbidities (Catalano 98a). Excess weight gain in diabetic women may contribute to overgrown infants with excess fat deposition (Berk 89, Madsen 91, Cundy 93, Bianco 98, Johnstone 00, Nielsen 07) and an increase in cesarean deliveries (Ray 01). In the large prospective Diabetes and Early Pregnancy Study of type 1 diabetes, weight gain ≥20 kg by 32 weeks gestation was independently associated with fetal macrosomia (Jovanovic 91). In general, large maternal size and gestational weight gain are both independently and interactively associated with large IDMs. Additional prospective studies are needed regarding the relationship of pregravid BMI and gestational weight gain to perinatal outcome and weight retention in diabetic women, especially in type 2 diabetes. Pending results of such studies, clinicians should target the low-range weight gain for each BMI group in diabetic pregnant women.

Weight should be monitored at each prenatal visit. In the first trimester, weight gain is often minimal (2.3 ± 2.1 kg) (Brown 02), but weight change in the first half of pregnancy is an important determinant of fetal linear growth in nondiabetic women (Li 98, Neufeld 99, Neufeld 04). Weight lost in the first trimester may be associated with smaller infant size in spite of increased feeding later in pregnancy (Stein 95, Brown 02, Dodds 06); we lack such data for diabetes and pregnancy. In the second and third trimester of nondiabetic pregnancies, recommended weight gain is ~0.45 kg (1 lb) per week for women with normal BMI. Weight loss is contraindicated; however, a minimum gain may not be necessary for obese diabetic women who are consuming adequate calories and nutrients according to ongoing review of self-recorded food records (IOM 90).

Macronutrient Intake

Intake of macronutrients (carbohydrate, fiber, protein, fat) provides energy for maternal physiological adjustments as well as fetal–placental growth and development and has strong effects on glycemic control and successful pregnancy in diabetic women. From 1997 to 2004, the Food and Nutrition Board of the IOM promulgated use of DRIs for the first time. The term DRI "refers to a set of four nutrient-based reference values that can be used for assessing and planning diets and for many other purposes … Where adequate information is available, each nutrient has a set of DRIs" (IOM 00b,03). DRIs are illustrated in Figure I.1, and the terms estimated average requirement (EAR), recommended dietary allowance (RDA), adequate intake (AI), and tolerable upper intake level (UL) are defined in the caption. Values for individual nutrients for pregnant women are listed in the table found in the following section titled "Sources of Information on Nutrient Intake." Space does not allow detailed discussion of the basis for setting reference values for pregnancy, and the reader is referred to the IOM books at *www.nap.edu*. Future research may demonstrate that DRIs should be modified for diabetic pregnant women.

For all adults, the IOM also promulgated acceptable macronutrient distribution ranges (AMDRs) for consumption of carbohydrate, protein, fat, and *n*-6 and *n*-3 PUFAs as percentage of total energy intake. AMDRs are "based on evidence from interventional trials, with support of epidemiological evidence, to suggest a role in the prevention or increased risk of chronic diseases" and to ensure sufficient intakes of essential nutrients as well as adequate energy intake and physical activity to maintain energy balance and appropriate weight (IOM 02). AMDRs function as guiding principles in the 2005 Dietary Guidelines for Americans (a parallel DGA 05 emphasis pertains to daily selection of foods from all food groups) (DGAr 05). Because the macronutrients of carbohydrate, protein, and fat are somewhat interchangeable as sources of body fuel, their ranges of proportional intake of energy consumed are broad.

The AMDR is estimated to be 45–65% of energy for carbohydrate, 10–35% for protein, and 20–35% for fat (IOM 02). The proportions selected should add up to 100%. Carbohydrate and fat proportions are based on evidence indicating a risk for

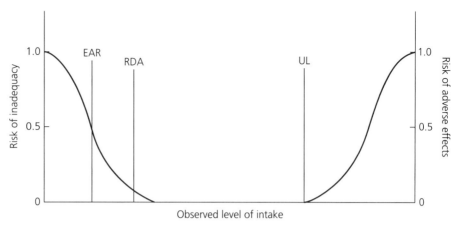

FIGURE I.1 Dietary Reference Intakes. This figure demonstrates that the estimated average requirement (EAR) is the intake of a nutrient at which the risk of inadequacy is 0.5 (50%) to a pregnant woman. The recommended dietary allowance (RDA) is the intake at which the risk of inadequacy is very small–only 0.02–0.03 (2–3%). The adequate intake (AI) does not bear a consistent relationship to the EAR or RDA because it is set when data do not allow estimation of the average requirement. It is assumed that the AI is at or above the RDA if one could be calculated. At intakes between the RDA and the tolerable upper intake level (UL), the risks of inadequacy and of excess are both close to 0. At intakes above the UL, the risk of adverse effects may increase. From the Food and Nutrition Board, IOM 03; used with permission. Copyright 2003, National Academy of Sciences.

coronary heart disease (CHD) at high intakes of carbohydrate to achieve low intakes of fat, risk of obesity and its complications with high intakes of fat, and risk of nutrient inadequacy in pregnancy with intakes below the designated ranges. The range of proportions for protein intake are based on prevention of negative nitrogen balance, but recent evidence suggests that the higher range of protein intake with reduced carbohydrate intake will lower glucose and triacylglycerol levels in type 2 diabetes (Gannon 03). No compelling evidence exists that AMDRs are not appropriate for diabetic pregnant women, although some clinicians prefer a lower proportion of carbohydrate for the short term of gestation, such as 40% of energy (ADietA 02).

Dietary assessment "compares usual nutrient intakes with estimated nutrient requirements and examines the probability of inadequate or excessive intake" (IOM 03). Errors associated with brief assessments of variable dietary intake (IOM 03) may be minimized in diabetic pregnant patients by using food records that are regularly reviewed with an RD. Dietary planning "aims for the consumption of diets that have acceptably low probabilities of inadequate or excessive nutrient intakes" (IOM 03) based on DRIs and experience in pregnancy with factors such as glycemic control and weight gain. Other considerations when setting intake goals include food preferences of the individual and the cost and availability of foods (IOM 03). It is hoped that computer programs will be developed and made accessible to clinicians to aid in the assessment and planning of nutrient intakes for individual patients. Preliminary data demonstrate the efficacy of electronic food lists for cell phones in patient assessment of carbohydrate unit amount and optimal dosage of bolus insulin (Pithova 06). Table I.5 presents the list of DRIs for pregnancy (IOM 97,98,00,01,02,04), slightly different

TABLE I.5 Dietary Reference Intake Values

Nutrient (unit)	RDA for Nonpregnant Women (19–50 years)	RDA for Pregnancy	Tolerable Upper Limit in Pregnancy	Food Label Daily Value[a]	Prenatal Supplement Range[b]	Average Diet Intake by Diabetic Pregnant Women[c,d,e,f]
EER, kcal/day	See text	+340–452	NA	2,000	NA	1774–1914
Carbohydrate, gm/day	130	175	NA	300	NA	184–214
Total fiber, gm/day	25*	28*	NA	25	NA	14–16
Linoleic acid, gm/day	12*	13*	NA	NA	NA	NA
α-Linolenic acid, gm/day	1.1*	1.4*	NA	NA	NA	NA
Protein, gm/day#	46	71	NA	50	NA	81–99
Fluids, L/day (cups/day)	2.2 (~9)	2.3 (~10)	None	NA	NA	NA
Calcium, mg/day	1,000*	1,000*	2,500	1,000	0–455	1,078
Chromium, µg/day	25*	30*	NA	NA	NA	NA
Copper, µg/day	900	1,000	10,000	2,000	0 or 2 mg	1,040
Fluoride, mg/day	3*	3*	10	NA	NA	NA
Iodine, µg/day	150	220	1,100	150	None	370**
Iron, mg/day	18	27	45	18	18–40	11.7
Magnesium, mg/day	320	350	350 suppl	400	0–150	210–375**
Manganese, mg/day	1.8*	2.0*	11	NA	NA	NA
Molybdenum, µg/day	45	50	2000	NA	NA	NA
Phosphorus, mg/day	700	700	3,500	1,000	none	1,137–1,196**
Potassium, gm/day	4.7*	4.7*	None[g]	3.5	NA	3.1**
Selenium, µg/day	55	60	400	NA	0–75	NA
Sodium, gm/day	1.5*	1.5*	2.3	2.4	NA	4.2**
Zinc, mg/day	8	11	40	15	15–25	8.5–11.0
Vitamin A, µg/day retinol activity equiv.	700	770	3,000	5,000 IU, 1,500 µg	0–4,000 IU	691**
Vitamin C, mg/day	75	85	2,000 suppl	60	50–240 mg	85

Vitamin D, µg/day cholecalciferol	5*	5*	50	10	6–10 (1 µg = 40 IU)	NA
Vitamin E, mg/day	**15**	**15**	1,000 suppl	30 IU = 20 mg[h]	0, 3.5 IU, 30 IU (1 IU = 0.45 mg)[i]	5.2
Vitamin K, µg/day	90*	50*	None	NA	None	NA
Thiamin, mg/day	1.1	**1.4**	None	1.5	1.7–4.0	1.5–1.8**
Riboflavin, mg/day	1.1	**1.4**	None	1.7	1.7–4.0	1.8–2.2**
Niacin, mg/day	14	**18**	35	20	10, 18, 20	19–24**
Vitamin B6, mg/day	1.3	**1.9**	100	2.0	2.6–50.0	1.6–1.9**
Folate, µg/day	400	**600**	1,000	400	800–1,000	NA***
Vitamin B12, µg/day	2.4	**2.6**	None	6	2, 4, 8, 12	4.9
Choline, mg/day	425*	450*	3.5 gm/day		0–25	NA

Dietary Reference Intake values for individual macro- and micronutrients in pregnancy compared with prepregnancy, food label values, range of ingredients in prenatal vitamin and mineral supplements, and range of average dietary intakes in studies of diabetic pregnant women with moderate glycemic control.

RDA values in bold.

[a]*Based on 2,000-calorie diet.*

[b]*Range of ingredients in 10 common brands of prenatal supplements.*

[c]*Diabetic data from Combs 1992.*

[d]*Diabetic data from Bates 1997.*

[e]*Diabetic data from Kaplan 1999.*

[f]*Diabetic data from Kalkwarf 2001.*

[g]*<4.7 mg/day if urinary potassium excretion is impaired.*

[h]*Natural vitamin E = d-α-tocopherol = RRR-α-tocopherol.*

[i]*Form of supplement as dl-α-tocopherol = all rac-α-tocopherol.*

**Adequate intake (AI).*

***Data from nondiabetic pregnant women.*

****After food fortification.*

[#]*Protein intake based on 0.8 gm/kg body weight for reference body weight in nonpregnaqnt woman and 1.1 gm/kg in pregnancy. (IOM 97,98,00,01,02,04, USDA 04).*

EER, estimated energy requirements; adjustments for second and third trimesters and first 6 months' lactation; NA, not applicable or not available; RDA, recommended dietary allowance.

daily values on current food labels (now under revision) (USDA 04, Fulgoni 06), prenatal supplements for nutrients relevant to diabetic pregnant women, and average dietary intakes assessed in prospective studies of diabetic pregnant women with moderate glycemic control (Combs 92, Bates 97, Kaplan 99, Kalkwarf 01).

Sources of Information on Nutrient Intake

Tables of U.S. food sources for macro- and micronutrients in 1994–1996 have been published (Cotton 04), as well as an analysis of secular trends in dietary intake and supplement use in the U.S. population in four National Health and Nutrition Examination Surveys (NHANES I, II, III, IV) conducted in 1971–1974, 1976–1980, 1988–1994, and 1999–2000 (Briefel 04). Regarding nutrient intake in pregnancy, the IOM appendixes reported (a) the NHANES III mean and selected percentiles of intakes of macro- and micronutrients in 346 apparently healthy pregnant women and (b) selected dietary intake data of 81 pregnant women in the Continuing Survey of Food Intakes by Individuals (CSFII) 1994–1996, 1998 (IOM 97,98,00a,b,02,04). Recent regional surveys of nutritional intakes in nondiabetic pregnant women in the U.S. and U.K. used food diaries and structured interviews in 63 and 693 women, respectively (Mathews 99, Turner 03) and food frequency questionnaires validated by food diaries in 95, 583, and 2,247 women, respectively (Godfrey 96, Swensen 01, Siega-Riz 02). In addition, data on average daily intakes of macronutrients, minerals, trace elements, and vitamins (dietary plus usual prenatal supplement) on 1 day at 13–21 weeks gestation in 3,125 nondiabetic North American women who remained normotensive throughout pregnancy are also used in this text (Morris 01).

Regarding the limited data available on PDM and pregnancy, macronutrient intake (Table I-5) was assessed in women with moderate glycemic control by analysis of daily food diaries throughout pregnancy in 111 women with type 1 and type 2 diabetes (Combs 92) and by 3-day food diaries in each trimester in 69 women with type 1 diabetes (Kalkwarf 01). Macro- and micronutrient intake was estimated by a 7-day dietary history interview using food photographs to estimate portion sizes compared with previously validated food frequency questionnaires in 38 women with type 1 diabetes and an equal number of matched controls in early pregnancy (Bates 97). Because food frequency questionnaires may underreport nutrient intake (IOM 03), these investigators used repeated interviews by experienced RDs to optimize the accuracy of the food diaries.

Calories for Appropriate Weight Gain and Fetal Growth

In 2002, the IOM provided a table of estimated energy requirements (EERs) to maintain balance in nonpregnant women according to age, height, BMI, and levels of physical activity (Table I.6) (IOM 02, pp. 5–58). The EER is the dietary energy intake predicted to maintain balance with TEE consistent with good health. Energy intakes above the EER before pregnancy are expected to result in weight gain.

The EER for pregnancy is derived from the sum of the TEE of the woman in the nonpregnant state plus the median change in TEE for pregnancy of 8 kcal/week (from the doubly labeled water method) plus the energy deposition during pregnancy of 180 kcal/day. This calculates to +340 kcal/day for the second trimester and +450 kcal/day for the third trimester (IOM 02). However, successful pregnancy outcomes have been reported with lower energy intakes (Durnin 87). Based on studies restricting energy intake to 1700–1800 kcal/day among women with GDM (Algert 85, Gilmer 86,

TABLE I.6 Estimated Energy Requirements for Nonpregnant Women 30 Years of Age*

Height (inches, m)	Physical Activity Level	Weight (lb [kg]) for BMI 18.5	Weight (lb [kg]) for BMI 25	EER (kcal/day) BMI 18.5	EER (kcal/day) BMI 25
59 (1.50)	Sedentary	92 (41.6)	124 (56.2)	1,625	1,762
	Low active			1,803	1,956
	Active			2,025	2,196
	Very active			2,291	2,489
65 (1.65)	Sedentary	111 (50.4)	150 (68.0)	1,816	1,982
	Low active			2,016	2,202
	Active			2,267	2,477
	Very active			2,567	2,807
71 (1.80)	Sedentary	132 (59.9)	178 (81.0)	2,015	2,211
	Low active			2,239	2,459
	Active			2,519	2,769
	Very active			2,855	3,141

For pregnancy, add 340 kcal/day for the second trimester and 450 kcal/day for the third trimester. Adapted from IOM 02 (National Academies of Science) and Trumbo 02.
For each year below 30, add 7 kcal/day; for each year above 30, subtract 7 kcal/day; BMI as kg/m².
BMI, body mass index; EER, estimated energy requirement.

Dornhorst 91, Rae 00), the woman with type 2 diabetes who is obese and insulin resistant may benefit from a similar energy intake (Gunderson 04). However, greater restriction to 1200–1600 kcal/day usually will not maintain weight and may lead to maternal oxidation of fat and hepatic generation of β-hydroxybutyrate (Magee 90, Knopp 91), with possible fetal effects resulting in childhood neurobehavioral deficits (Rizzo 91,95).

Energy intake in diabetic pregnancy should be sufficient to promote appropriate weight gain and fetal–placental growth. The high intersubject variability of energy needs in prospective studies of healthy nondiabetic pregnant women with good outcomes (Knopp 99, King 00a, Butte 04) suggests that an individual approach be used for energy intake recommendations for diabetic pregnant women based on patient preferences, physical activity, and monitored weight gain (Pitkin 99). Well-nourished women use a variety of strategies to meet the energy demands of pregnancy including a decrease in activity, an increase in energy intake, or use of deposited fat mass (Durnin 91, King 00a). During pregnancy with PDM, recommendations for energy intake should be increased for insufficient weight gain and decreased for excessive weight gain. Consideration should be given to portion sizes and the energy density of a food (kcal/100 gm), which depends on its content of carbohydrate, protein, fat, and water (DGAr 05). The goal is "to promote consumption of a wholesome, balanced diet consistent with ethnic, cultural, and financial considerations" (IOM 90) and to maintain the pleasure of eating by making food choices according to scientific evidence, weight gain, and postprandial glucose responses.

Carbohydrate Intake and Optimal Glucose Control for Pregnancy

The definitions of types of carbohydrates (sugars, starches, fibers) in fruits, vegetables, whole grains, legumes, and low-fat milk products are based on the number of sugar units (DGAr 05). Carbohydrates are classified as monosaccharides (glucose, galactose, fructose, sugar alcohols), disaccharides (sucrose, lactose, maltose, trehalose), oligosaccharides of 3–10 units (legumes and corn syrup), and polysaccharides of >10 units, such as starch (hundreds or thousands of linked units) in plants and glycogen in animals (IOM 02, Sigman-Grant 03). The di-, oligo- and polysaccharides are broken down into monosaccharides in the intestine by brush-border enzymes. Recent experimental evidence supports the role of an apical GLUT2 transporter in intestinal sugar absorption (Kellett 05). Monosaccharides pass through intestinal enterocytes and enter the portal circulation as glucose, galactose, and fructose. The latter two sugars are more efficiently taken up into hepatocytes and converted to glucose-1-phosphate or fructose-1-phosphate; more glucose remains in circulation for distribution to brain cells, erythrocytes, muscle cells, adipocytes, kidneys, placenta, and fetus to be used for energy (Sigman-Grant 03). A distinction exists between "natural" sugars (such as intrinsic sugars in the cell walls of plants, lactose in milk, and fructose in fruits) and extrinsic sugars added to foods or added at the table. U.S. food labels provide the amount of total sugars per serving without distinguishing between natural and added sugars, making it difficult for the patient to know how much has been added.

The RDA for carbohydrate is 130 grams per day for women in childbearing years based on the average minimum amount of glucose utilized by the brain. During pregnancy, the RDA is increased to 175 grams per day to provide ~33 gm/day for the fetal brain (IOM 02, Trumbo 02). With respect to the AMDR for carbohydrate for pregnancy (45–65% of energy or 40–60% for diabetic pregnancy) (Franz 02, DGAr 05), it is important to note that very low carbohydrate diets are not compatible with the goals of a healthy plan for pregnancy. At the low end of the range, it is difficult to meet the recommendations for fiber intake, vitamins, and minerals; at the high end, overconsumption of carbohydrates may raise glucose and TG levels and contribute to excess weight gain (DGAr 05). Distribution and type of carbohydrate in the food plan has been an aspect of investigations of intensive MNT for GDM (Peterson 91, Gunderson 04), but has been evaluated in few studies in PDM. Given appropriate motivation, patients with PDM can be trained (Gregory 94, Gillespie 98) to "count" food serving sizes approximating 15 gm of carbohydrate. Typical food plans for carbohydrate in three meals and three snacks would be: 15–45 gm, 15–30 gm, 30–75 gm, 15–30 gm, 30–75 gm, and 15–45 gm (main meals underlined). Adjustments can be made based on patient preferences, weight gain, insulin doses, and premeal, postprandial, and nighttime glucose values. Refer to the section titled "Insulin Therapy Used in Pregnancy" later in Part I for discussion on the use of insulin–carbohydrate ratios, which change as gestation advances. Therefore, the emphasis in pregnancy is on consistency of carbohydrate intake to achieve excellent glucose control.

Glycemic response to carbohydrates. The glycemic response to food ingestion is affected by carbohydrate type as well as amount, along with many other variables (Franz 02, Sheard 04). Ingestion of certain carbohydrate foods causes a greater rise in postprandial glucose in humans (Forst 00, Kelley 03). In experimental animals, ingestion of simple dietary sugars primes apical GLUT2 and rapidly increases carbohydrate absorption (Kellett 05). On the other hand, consumption of slowly digestible starches can improve glycemic control and lower postprandial NEFA concentrations (Ellis 05). In the high-insulin resistance state of diabetic pregnancy in which optimal glucose levels are required for normal fetal growth and well-being, high total carbohydrate intake or inclusion of excess mono- and disaccharides with the starch needed for nutrient intake in main meals often provokes postprandial hyperglycemia. Milk products and fruits are important for maternal and fetal nutrition, and they are often best consumed three times daily at the between-meal and bedtime snacks. Products with high amounts of added sugars are best avoided in the interests of good glycemic control because they do not provide essential vitamins, minerals, and fiber. If foods with added sugars are desired, portion control and postmeal testing are important to determine their impact on glucose levels. Use of nonnutritive sweeteners is discussed in the section titled "Intake of Other Substances" later in Part I.

Dietary fiber sources contain digestible carbohydrates (soluble fiber). Increasing dietary fiber content improves glycemic control and lowers cholesterol and TG levels in nonpregnant diabetic patients by delaying gastric emptying and monosaccharide absorption, increasing insulin sensitivity, increasing magnesium absorption, increasing bile acid excretion, increasing adiponectin, and decreasing cholesterol absorption (Fraser 88, Clapp 91, Chandalia 00, Coudray 03, Kelley 03, Anderson 04, Weickert 05, Qi 06a). Functional fiber "consists of isolated or extracted nondigestible carbohydrates that have beneficial physiological effects in humans" such as cellulose added to foods, guar gum, pectins added to low-calorie gelled products, psyllium, and retrograded or chemically modified resistant starches (IOM 02). Total fiber intake is the sum of both types of fiber. The reason for distinguishing between them is because it may be difficult to detect the beneficial effects of dietary fiber per se due to the presence of other beneficial nutrients, and isolated functional fiber can be more easily studied (IOM 02). The AI for total fiber in foods is based on the intake level observed to protect against CHD (IOM 02). Because "there is no evidence to suggest the beneficial effect of fiber in reducing the risk of CHD for pregnant adolescent girls or women is different," the AI for diabetic pregnant women of any age is 28 gm/day (IOM 02) or 14 g/1000 kcal/day (DGAr 05).

Four groups of investigators analyzed the association of dietary fiber intake (water soluble and insoluble) with insulin requirements and glycemic control in pregnant women with type 1 diabetes (Ney 82, Reece 95, Bates 97, Kalkwarf 01). Average fiber intake was estimated as only 15.9–18.6 gm/day in different trimesters, and most patients consumed less than the recently recommended AI (Trumbo 02). One study found no association between the amount of dietary fiber intake and premeal glucose or A1C values in any trimester (Kalkwarf 01). However, in the second and third trimesters, daily insulin dose was negatively correlated with fiber intake. This result supported previous interventional studies in type 1 diabetes and GDM that showed lower insulin dosage (Ney 82) or fewer hypoglycemic episodes (Reece 95) with high supplemented fiber intakes of 60–70 gm/day, but otherwise showed no significant effects on glycemic control.

Note that fiber content is listed on the food label. If the amount of fiber is >5 gm per food serving, it can be subtracted from the total carbohydrate amount to determine the amount of carbohydrate that is absorbed and that will affect the postmeal glucose level. In summary, pregnant women with diabetes do not need more fiber than those without diabetes, but they do need to increase intake to an AI of 28 gm/day. Generally speaking, people with diabetes are encouraged to eat a diet with fiber-containing foods such as legumes, fiber-rich cereals, fruits, vegetables, and whole-grain products.

Certain foods produce a higher glycemic response (Crapo 81, Jenkins 81, Wolever 94,96,02a,b, Ludwig 02) and may contribute to postprandial hyperglycemia in insulin-resistant pregnancies (Lock 88, Scholl 04, Moses 06). The glycemic index is a "ranking of carbohydrate exchanges according to their effect on postprandial glycemia" (Sheard 04). As measured in the laboratory, the glycemic index is defined as the increase in glucose measured over 2 h following ingestion of 50 gm of available carbohydrate (without soluble fiber) from a test food compared with a reference food, such as 50 gm glucose or white bread with equivalent grams of carbohydrate (Jenkins 02). The glycemic index is calculated as the incremental area under the glucose curve of the test food divided by the incremental area under the glucose curve of the reference test, multiplied by 100 (Wolever 85, Wolever 03, Wolever 04, Granfeldt 06). There is evidence that capillary blood sampling is optimal for determination of glycemic indexes (Hatonen 06).

Tables of the glycemic indexes of a wide variety of foods have been published (Foster-Powell 02, Henry 05). The glycemic index of a food may be the result of its effect on insulin response and action as well as carbohydrate absorption from the gut and is affected by ripeness, cooking, physical form of the food, and possibly added fat (Collier 82, d'Emden 87, Schenk 03, Galgani 06). Early and continuing studies demonstrate that use of the glycemic index concept is applicable to women with both types of diabetes (Jenkins 84, Wolever 87, Buyken 00, Mohammed 04, Panlasigui 06) in different ethnic groups and regions (Chan 01, Noriega 01, Sugiyama 03, Chan 04a, Abdelgadir 05, Diaz 05, Bove 06). Daily incorporation of low-glycemic-index carbohydrates is effective in the office setting as well as in research studies (Burani 06). Use of a personal digital assistant to help patients make low-glycemic-index food choices is under evaluation (Ma 06a). An illustration of the comparison between the glycemic index of selected foods to glucose ingestion in glucose-intolerant pregnant women is provided in Figure I.2. A weak positive correlation is shown between the individual glycemic indexes and the means of the fasting glucose levels used in their calculation. No correlation exists between the glycemic index and individual gestational age or body weight. Investigators concluded that glycemic indexes were uniform after ingestion of the test foods in spite of the known changes in gastrointestinal function in pregnancy (Lock 88).

A meta-analysis of randomized crossover or parallel-design trials comparing low-glycemic-index with high-glycemic-index standard diabetic (isocaloric) diets included six studies of type 1 diabetes subjects and nine studies in subjects with type 2 diabetes, using A1C or fructosamine values as the end point. The crossover trials used a small number of subjects (6–21), and the three parallel-design trials used 51–104 subjects in each group. The duration of time on each diet varied from 2 to 52 weeks, with 11 of the RCTs lasting <10 weeks. A total of 10 of 14 trials documented differences in the postprandial glucose profile between the two types of diet. All trials of low-glycemic-index diet reduced A1C or fructosamine, with seven studies showing a clear level of significance (Brand-Miller 03a). A subsequent parallel-design RCT compared 8 weeks on a low-glycemic-index diet of 43 glycemic index units versus a high-glycemic-index diet of 75 glycemic index units (both 1440 kcal/day, 60% carbohydrate) in overweight subjects with type 2 diabetes in Australia. In this setting of energy restriction, weight loss and improved glycemic indexes were similar in both diet groups (Heilbronn 02). A subsequent crossover RCT in Mexican subjects with type 2 diabetes found significantly reduced A1C values after a 6-week treatment period with a low-glycemic-index meal plan (Jimenez-Cruz 03).

A limitation of the glycemic index is that, by definition, it compares equal quantities of carbohydrate and measures the effect of quality but not quantity. The concept of glycemic load (GL) was developed to quantify the overall glycemic effect of a usual portion of food (Salmeron 97, Ludwig 03). The higher the GL, the greater the expected rise

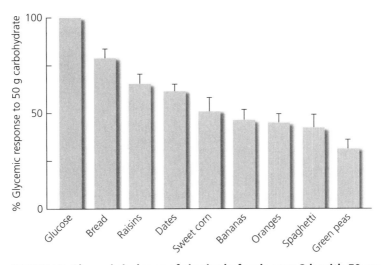

FIGURE I.2 Glycemic indexes of six single foods over 2 h with 50 gm carbohydrate compared with ingestion of 50 gm glucose in seven to nine fasting pregnant subjects with impaired glucose tolerance. Corn and peas contained 25 gm carbohydrate and were compared with 25 gm glucose in eight subjects. Plasma glucose was sampled at 30, 60, 90, and 120 min; mean + SEM. Peak glucose response was at 60 min for 50 gm glucose (Δ 110 mg/dL), 25 gm glucose (Δ 72 mg/dL), and white bread (Δ 82 mg/dL) and at 30 min for spaghetti (Δ 41 mg/dL), sweet corn (Δ 44 mg/dL), green peas (Δ 28 mg/dL), bananas (Δ 77 mg/dL), dates (Δ 78 mg/dL), oranges (Δ 83 mg/dL), and raisins (Δ 79 mg/dL). The deltas of the glucose rise above fasting are approximate and taken from Figure 1 in the reference. Adapted from Lock 88 and used with permission.

in plasma glucose and insulin secretion in response to food (Foster-Powell 02). GL is the product of the glycemic index of a food and its total amount of available carbohydrate in a serving (carbohydrate in grams × glycemic index / 100 = GL) (Brand-Miller 03b, Galgani 06, Venn 06). A low-index/high-carbohydrate food or a high-index/low-carbohydrate food can have the same GL (Barclay 05). In Table I.7, the GL of one carbohydrate serving (~15 gm carbohydrate) has been calculated using the glycemic index of each food. A food with a GL <10 is considered low, a GL of 10–19 is medium, and a GL ≥20 is high. The overall GL of a meal or the entire diet is calculated by summing the GL contributed by individual foods (Sheard 04). Foods composed mainly of protein and fat, such as chicken, fish, oil, or butter, do not contain carbohydrate, do not raise the glucose level in the immediate postprandial state, and are not considered when determining the GL. Nonstarchy vegetables, such as greens, broccoli, cabbage, and nopales, are so low in total carbohydrate (usually <5 grams of carbohydrate per 1 cup raw serving) that they do not impact the GL. For example, a meal consisting of a meat and cheese sandwich (GL of 10 for each slice of white or wheat bread), an orange (GL of 8), and a cup of skim milk (GL of 4) would have a GL of 32.

In clinical practice, postprandial glucose level has been used as a measure of the GL (the amount and type of carbohydrate) of a particular meal. Requesting the woman with diabetes to record her food intake and pre/postmeal glucose values for at least 3–5 days before each office visit will provide clinicians with valuable data to suggest food changes. Table I.7 provides a way to compare the possible postprandial

TABLE I.7 Glycemic Index and Glycemic Load for Foods Used During Pregnancy in North America

A. Starchy Foods

Cereals	Glycemic Index	One-Carb Serving Size	Glycemic Load for One-Carb Serving
Shredded Wheat	75 ± 8	1/2 cup	17.5
Cornflakes	81 ± 3	3/4 cup	15
Grape Nuts	71 ± 4	1/4 cup	15
Cheerios	74 ± 0	3/4 cup	12
Raisin Bran	61 ± 5	1/2 cup	12
All Bran	38	1/2 cup	9
Oatmeal, long cooking	58 ± 4	1/2 cup	6.1
Breads			
Baguette	95 ± 15	1-oz slice	15
Middle Eastern flat bread	97 ± 29	1-oz piece	15
Chapati, wheat	66 ± 9	1 chapati	12.5
Soda crackers	74 ± 0	8 crackers	12
Taco shell, cornmeal, hard	68 ± 0	2 shells	11
English muffin bread	77 ± 7	1 slice	11
White wheat bread	70 ± 0	1 slice	10
Pita bread	57 ± 0	1/2 piece	10
Wonder Bread	73 ± 2	1 slice	10
Whole wheat flour bread	71 ± 2	1 slice	9
Hamburger bun	61 ± 0	1/2 bun	9
Croissant	67	1-oz croissant	9
Sourdough	54	1-oz slice	8
Tortilla, corn	38	1 oz or 1 medium	5
Rye bread	50 ± 4	1 slice	4
Tortilla, wheat	30	1/3 of 10" tortilla	4
Grains and Starchy Vegetables			
Potato, mashed	74 ± 5	1/3 cup	15
Potato, instant mashed	85 ± 3	1/3 cup	17
Jasmine rice	109 ± 10	1/3 cup	15.8
Rice, Asian glutinous	92 ± 6	1/3 cup	14.7
Potato, baked russet	85 ± 12	3 oz	13.6
French Fries, frozen/reheated	75 ± 0	1 cup	12
Sweet potato, cooked	61 ± 7	1/2 cup	9.8
Udon noodles, cooked	62 ± 8	1/3 cup	8
Rice, white long grain	56 ± 2	1/3 cup	8
Sweet corn, canned	53 ± 4	1/2 cup	8
Rice noodles, dried, boiled	61 ± 6	1/3 cup	7.6
Rice, brown	55 ± 5	1/3 cup	7.5
Kidney beans, canned	52 ± 0	1/2 cup	7.5

(Continued)

TABLE I.7 (Continued)

Grains and Starchy Vegetables	Glycemic Index	One-Carb Serving Size	Glycemic Load for One-Carb Serving
Couscous, prepared	65 ± 4	1/3 cup	7.4
Macaroni, boiled	47 ± 2	1/3 cup	6
Yam, cooked	37 ± 8	1/2 cup	5.9
Spaghetti, cooked firm	44 ± 3	1/3 cup	5.4
Lentils	29 ± 1	1/2 cup	3.5
Green peas, boiled	48 ± 5	1/2 cup	3
Carrots, raw	16 ± 0	1 cup	2

B. Milk and Dairy Substitutes

Milk, Dairy, and Substitutes	Glycemic Index	One-Carb Choice	Glycemic Load for One-Carb Choice
Soy milk, full fat and reduced fat	44 ± 5	250 mL	8
Milk, skim	32 ± 5	1 cup (250 mL)	4
Milk, full fat	27 ± 4	1 cup (250 mL)	3
Yogurt, nonfat, artificially sweetened	24 ± 1	7 oz	3

C. Fruits and Juices

Fruits and Fruit Juices	Glycemic Index	One-Carb Serving Size	Glycemic Load for One-Carb Serving
Raisins	64 ± 11	2 Tbsp	9
Watermelon	72 ± 13	1 1/2 cup (190 gm)	8.6
Mango	51 ± 5	1/2 small	8
Orange	42 ± 3	1 small	8
Cranberry juice	68 ± 3	1/2 cup	8
Grapes	46 ± 3	20 small grapes	8
Banana	52 ± 4	1/2 banana	7.9
Pineapple, raw	59 ± 8	3/4 cup	7
Orange juice	57 ± 3	1/2 cup	6
Apple	38 ± 2	1 small	6
Apple juice	40 ± 1	1/2 cup	5.8
Grapefruit juice	48	1/2 cup	5.2
Prunes	29 ± 4	3 prunes	5
Grapefruit	25	1/2 grapefruit	3

D. Dessert and Sweets

Desserts/Sweets	Glycemic Index	One-Carb Serving Size	Glycemic Load for One-Carb Serving
Vanilla wafers	77	6 wafers (25 gm)	14
Snickers bar	68	1/2 of 2-oz bar	11.5
Waffle	76	1 four inch (33 gm)	10

(Continued)

TABLE I.7 (*Continued*)

Desserts/Sweets	Glycemic Index	One-Carb Serving Size	Glycemic Load for One-Carb Serving
Honey	55 ± 5	1 Tbsp (25 gm)	10
Shortbread cookies	64 ± 8	25 gm	10
Ice cream	61 ± 7	1/2 cup (50 gm)	8
Sugar	68 ± 5	1 Tbsp (10 gm)	8
Muffin, blueberry	59	1 oz (28 gm)	8
Instant pudding	44 ± 4	1/3 cup (100 gm)	7

The glycemic index ranks carbohydrate foods according to the rise in blood glucose over 2 h in healthy nonpregnant volunteers after ingestion of 50 gm of the single carbohydrate compared with ingestion of 50 gm glucose (reference level 100). The GL may be a more useful way of assessing the impact of a food's available carbohydrate on the glucose level because it takes into account the amount of carbohydrate eaten. The GL equals the glycemic index divided by 100 times the amount of carbohydrate minus fiber, in grams. A food may have a higher glycemic index, but because the amount commonly eaten is low in total carbohydrate, the GL is lower (e.g., compare All Bran with oatmeal). One carbohydrate serving = ~15 gm. A food with a low GL is <10, and a moderate GL is 11–19. The GL does not account for the interacting effect of eating mixed foods on carbohydrate absorption and stimulation of insulin secretion, nor does it account for the effect of high-sugar foods on women with glucose intolerance or absent insulin secretion. Based on Foster-Powell 02, Pennington 98, and Wheeler 03.

GL, glycemic load.

glucose response of similar foods. Note the portion size of each food because the amount consumed is often three or more servings at a meal. It is important to mention that the glycemic index of many foods has a large range of interpatient variability, so each woman needs to confirm her response to a carbohydrate source.

Epidemiological studies suggest that consumption of low-glycemic-index foods is associated with improved markers of inflammation (Qi 06b) and plasma oxidative stress (Hu 06) and lower risks of CHD in overweight women, independent of other risk factors (Liu 00). Emphasizing low-glycemic-index and low-GL diets has been shown to improve total HDL-C, LDL-C, and TG status (Luscombe 99, Liese 06, Ma 06b). These studies support national guidelines to minimize intake of refined carbohydrates and increase intakes of whole grains and less-starchy vegetables (DGA 05). Three (Pereira 04, Ebbeling 05, McMillan-Price 06) of four (Raatz 05) recent randomized trials demonstrated the benefit of low-GL diets in reducing heart disease risk factors in overweight young women. Unfortunately, few studies tested the glycemic index or GL concept in normal pregnancy (Clapp 98, Scholl 04, Moses 06), and only one study tested 28 women with GDM (Lock 88). However, these concepts are important to study because "a low-GL diet can create a more favorable glucose and insulin profile than can a high-GL diet. For those who need to use the carbohydrate exchange concept for glycemic control, there is need for a 'glycemic load exchange list' of foods that better reflects the total glucose raising potential of dietary carbohydrates" (Liu 06). Table I.7 may be helpful in that regard.

Research on the glycemic response to mixed meals is limited but important (Bantle 83, Jenkins 83, Nuttall 83, Coulston 84, Wolever 85, Colagiuri 86, Schrezenmeir 89). Some critics contend that the concept of glycemic index or GL may not persist when carbohydrate foods are incorporated into a mixed meal and that any index of metabolic response to eating should include glucose, insulin (and incretins), and be studied in individuals for whom dietary recommendations are proposed (including diabetic pregnant women) (Bantle 83, Coulston 84, Laine 87). Early studies suggested that the addition of fat and protein to a meal reduces the glycemic impact of challenges with single carbohydrate foods (Estrich 67, Collier 83, Collier 84). The presence of fat in the small intestine inhibits gastric emptying, and a recent experiment showed that consumption of fat (30 mL olive oil) 30 min before a potato meal slowed gastric emptying and delayed the rise in postprandial glucose in men with type 2 diabetes (Gentilcore 06). However, inclusion of 30% fat and 20% protein in test meals (including 94 gm of carbohydrate as apple juice) did not obviate striking differences in the incremental glycemic response over 180 min to instant potato, white bread, rice, spaghetti, and a combination of barley and lentils in insulin-treated patients with type 2 diabetes. The authors concluded that the relative glycemic effects of mixed meals can be predicted from the additive glycemic indexes of their carbohydrate components (Collier 86).

An independent study of subjects with type 2 diabetes in France confirmed the hierarchy of glycemic indexes with different carbohydrate foods in spite of 20 gm fat and 24 gm protein in the meals. The mixed meals did heighten insulinogenic responses to the different carbohydrates compared with ingestion of only carbohydrates (Bornet 87). What was not tested in these studies was variation in the amount and type of fat and protein in the mixed meals. A recent study did vary the fat (0–18 gm) and protein (0–18 gm) in a composite breakfast meal, which did not affect glucose responses in nondiabetic subjects. The authors concluded that carbohydrate content and glycemic index explained 88% of the variation in glycemic response (Wolever 06). Another study confirmed the differences between patients with type 2 diabetes in glycemic responses to the same mixed meals, although intrapatient reproducibility was good and did vary according to carbohydrate type (Brillon 06). Thus, the use of individual food records and postprandial glucose logs is important.

A recent ADA Consensus Statement on dietary carbohydrate for diabetes concluded that "a recent analysis of the randomized controlled trials that have examined the efficacy of the glycemic index on overall blood glucose control indicates that the use of this technique can provide an additional benefit over that observed when total carbohydrate is considered alone" (Sheard 04). Foods containing fiber (whole grains, leafy green and yellow vegetables) and starches rather than sugars are encouraged for the main meals in pregnancy (Jovanovic-Peterson 90, Ferris 94, Reece 95, ADietA 02, Reader 05, Thomas 06a,b). Common changes to the food plan of a pregnant woman with diabetes are to eliminate highly processed low-fiber breakfast cereals and breads at breakfast time or other meals and snacks, as well as to eliminate other processed snack foods such as cookies, pretzels, and bagels. Patients are trained to pay attention to the postprandial glycemic response to different types of carbohydrates (e.g., rice versus potato versus pasta versus types of bread versus beans/lentils versus flour or corn tortilla). We need to learn more about the effects of GL variance on postprandial glucose and lipid levels in pregnancies complicated by type 1 and type 2 diabetes.

Intake of Protein and Amino Acids

Nitrogen balance studies are used to estimate the protein intake requirement to maintain adequate concentrations of free amino acids and tissue protein in the face of constant protein turnover by degradation and synthesis. The EAR of nitrogen for healthy nonpregnant women aged 19–50 years is 0.66 gm/kg/day of protein "based on the lowest continuing intake of dietary protein that is sufficient to achieve body nitrogen equilibrium" (IOM 02). The RDA for nonpregnant women of the same age is set at

0.80 gm/kg/day. There is little evidence that intake should differ in diabetes (Franz 02, Eckel 03).

Whole body protein turnover is increased in the second half of pregnancy (Kalhan 00, Dugglesby 02). Pregnant subjects with type 1 diabetes studied in the fasting state had higher rates of protein breakdown and oxidation but similar protein synthesis rates compared with pregnant controls, which should provide increased plasma amino acids for placental–fetal use (Kalhan 94). Basal total plasma amino acids (Kalkhoff 88, Kalhan 94) and alanine, glutamine, histidine, methionine + cysteine, serine, and threonine were increased in diabetic women compared with normal pregnant controls, but leucine and isoleucine were slightly reduced (Whittaker 00). After an overnight fast, alanine turnover was similar in pregnant women with type 1 diabetes and controls (Kalhan 91), but leucine oxidation was higher with diabetes (Kalhan 94). When well-controlled pregnant type 1 diabetes subjects were studied under the anabolic conditions of a hyperinsulinemic–euglycemic clamp and amino acid infusion, protein synthesis and breakdown were increased as expected for normal pregnancy and the insulin sensitivity of amino acid turnover was not altered (Whittaker 00).

Additional protein is required during pregnancy (~21 gm/day averaged over the second and third trimesters) for maternal physiological adjustments and the support of fetal (~440 gm N) and placental (~100 gm N) growth (IOM 02). No evidence can be found that pregnant women store protein early in gestation for later fetal demands (Kin 00). Efficiency of the use of dietary protein is assumed to be 43% in pregnancy. The RDA for protein intake is set at 1.1 g/kg/day during pregnancy beginning in the second trimester, which is an average of +25 gm/day of additional protein; the value is doubled for twin gestation (IOM 02, Trumbo 02). Minimal protein requirements in pregnant women with PDM are the same as for pregnant women without diabetes. Severe malnutrition in pregnancy can stunt fetal growth, but a meta-analysis of RCTs in underprivileged populations showed no consistent benefit to maternal or fetal health from protein supplementation (Kramer 93).

Protein intake on 1 day (94–96 gm/day) at 13–21 weeks gestation did not differ in a large group of nondiabetic pregnant women in North America who remained normotensive or developed gestational hypertension or preeclampsia (Morris 01). High protein intake increases cortisol levels (Slag 81, Gibson 99b). Epidemiological evidence shows that high protein intakes in late pregnancy are associated with long-term elevated BP in adult offspring (Campbell 96b, Roseboom 01, Shiell 01, Herrick 03). Based on animal studies, the hypothesis is that high maternal cortisol levels may reset the fetal hypothalamic–pituitary–adrenal axis, resulting in elevated cortisol and hypertension in the adult.

For pregnant women with PDM, average protein intake was 81–100 gm/day in three reports (Combs 92, Bates 97, Kalkwarf 01). In the first of these studies (Combs 92), no differences in protein intake were found among diabetic mothers delivering appropriate-age, SGA, or LGA infants. The recommended protein requirement is not decreased for pregnant women with clinical nephropathy, but excessive protein intake should be avoided. No prospective studies have been conducted detailing the possible effects of high-range protein intake on glycemic control or renal function in diabetic pregnancy.

No reliable data exist on changes in individual amino acid consumption related to the outcome of normal pregnancy. Therefore, the indispensable amino acid EARs for adult nonpregnant women are multiplied by 1.33 and rounded for pregnancy,

TABLE I.8 Recommended Dietary Allowances for Indispensable Amino Acids

RDAs for Pregnancy*		Example for 80-kg (175-lb) Woman	Estimated Intake (gm/day)**	
Amino acid	mg/kg/day		Mean	(10th–90th percentile)
Histidine	18	1.4 gm	2.32	(1.75–2.94)
Isoleucine	25	2.0 gm	3.78	(2.95–4.78)
Leucine	56	4.4 gm	6.50	(4.96–8.28)
Lysine	51	4.1 gm	5.57	(4.11–7.15)
Methionine + cysteine	25	2.0 gm	2.95	(2.22–3.74)
Phenylalanine + tyrosine 44	44	3.5 gm	6.60	(5.10–8.30)
Threonine	26	2.1 gm	3.22	(2.48–4.01)
Tryptophan	7	0.56 gm	1.05	(0.80–1.30)
Valine	31	2.4 gm	4.25	(3.24–5.45)

*For pregnant women of all ages (IOM 02).

**Dietary intake by 341 pregnant women participating in the Third National Health and Nutrition Examination Survey, 1988–1994 (NHANES III) (IOM 02).

and then the RDAs are set by increasing the EARs by 24% (IOM 02). The estimated RDAs for these amino acids in pregnancy are listed in Table I.8, which also lists mean and 10th–90th–percentile amino acid intakes by 341 pregnant women in the NHANES III national survey (IOM 02). Inspection of the table shows that ~10% of the pregnant women had average intakes of histidine, leucine, lysine, methionine + cysteine, and threonine that were less than the RDA for a 100-kg woman. We lack similar data on the intake of individual amino acids in diabetic pregnant women.

Dietary protein quality is determined by digestability as well as the content and metabolic availability of the individual indispensable amino acids, which are actively transported to the fetus against individual concentration gradients (Moe 95, IOM 02). The protein quality of foods is rated by the content of a single indispensable amino acid in the diet that limits the utilization of other amino acids (e.g., lysine in wheat protein or methionine + cysteine in soy protein) (IOM 02). Studies comparing amino acid scores of common protein sources show that animal protein (beef, milk, egg) and well-processed soy protein reference sources demonstrate the highest quality compared with wheat, rice, and lupin protein sources (IOM 02). However, even in a diet composed of cereal proteins, "inclusion of relatively modest amounts of animal or other vegetable proteins, such as those from legumes and oilseeds," will remove the risk of essential amino acid inadequacy (IOM 02). Although poorly studied, it is presumed that food sources of amino acids are important to gravida and fetus in pregnancies complicated by diabetes. The "complete proteins" from animal sources (meat, poultry, fish, eggs, milk, cheese, yogurt) provide all nine indispensable amino acids. The "incomplete proteins" from plants, grains, nuts, seeds, and vegetables tend to be deficient in one or more of the indispensable amino acids (IOM 02). Thus, construction of a food plan for a vegetarian diabetic pregnant woman is an important challenge.

Dietary Fats: Total Fat and Fatty Acids

Dietary fat. Dietary fat provides energy and essential fatty acids and aids in the absorption of fat-soluble vitamins. All fat and oil sources are mixtures of fatty acids, which are almost completely absorbed (IOM 02). Dietary fat consists of 98% triacylglycerols (TGs), which consist of one glycerol molecule esterified with three fatty acid molecules. Fatty acids vary by carbon chain length (8–24 carbon atoms) and in their degree of unsaturation (number of double bonds in the carbon chain) (IOM 02). The *n*-3 to *n*-9 designation refers to the location of the first double bond from the methyl end of the fatty acid carbon chain. Saturated fatty acids (SFAs) have no double bonds. They are a source of fuel energy in pregnancy and are required for the normal function of various proteins. The *n*-9 *cis*-monounsaturated fatty acids (MUFAs), oleic acid and nervonic acid, are particularly important as membrane structural lipids in nervous tissue myelin, which are critical for fetal development. Both SFAs and MUFAs are synthesized in the body to provide for their physiological and structural functions, and therefore AIs or RDAs are not set for them (IOM 02). However, their dietary intake is an important consideration in relation to CVD. The PUFA *n*-6 *cis*-linoleic acid cannot be synthesized by humans and is essential in the diet. Linoleic acid is the precursor to arachidonic acid, which is important in maternal and fetal cell signaling pathways and is the substrate for eicosanoid production in tissues. The essential nonmarine *n*-3 α-linolenic acid is the precursor for synthesis of eicosapentaenoic acid (EPA) and docosahexaenoic acid (DHA) in animal tissues but not plant cells (IOM 02). EPA is the precursor of *n*-3 eicosanoids, which are beneficial in preventing CVD. *n*-3 PUFAs are particularly important in developing nerve tissue and the retina (IOM 02). The *trans* fatty acids are detrimental to health, and therefore no AI or RDA has been set and intake should be as low as possible (IOM 02, DGAr 05, ADietA 07).

Total fat intake. It is unclear whether dietary fat intake is related to pregnancy outcome, but the quality of dietary fat is certainly related to CHD in nondiabetic and diabetic women (DGAr 05). Discussion of evidence and recommendations for MNT of dyslipidemias in diabetic pregnant women is presented in the section on lipid disorders in Part II. Total fat intake refers to the intake of all forms of triacylglycerol as a percentage of total energy. As noted earlier, the AMDR for total fat is set at 20–35% of energy. The lower limit is set at 20% of calories to achieve recommended intakes of several nutrients and "because serum triacylglycerol concentrations increase and serum HDL cholesterol concentrations decrease when fat intake is low and carbohydrate intake is high," which may also increase the risk of CHD. Intakes of total fat above 35% of calories "result in an unacceptably high content of saturated fatty acids" (DGAr 05). No AI level or RDA is set for dietary total fat intake in nonpregnant or pregnant women of any age because "there are insufficient data to determine a defined level of fat intake at which risk of inadequacy or prevention of chronic disease occurs," and no UL is set for total fat intake because "there is no defined intake level of fat at which an adverse effect occurs" (IOM 02).

Median pregnancy total fat intake estimated by a 7-day food diary was 84.7 gm/day (upper quartile 99.2 gm/day) in 693 healthy nulliparous English women in early gestation, representing 37.8% of energy (upper quartile 40.9%) (Mathews 99). In this study, early pregnancy total fat intake was not related to infant BW or placental weight. Total fat intake on 1 day at 13–21 weeks gestation (99–108 gm/day, representing

37% of energy) was not different in 4,157 nondiabetic pregnant women in North America with or without hypertensive disorders (Morris 01). Excess fat intake is probably associated with higher caloric intake and may relate to excess maternal weight gain. In many studies, excessive maternal weight gain is associated with high-fat diets; controlling weight gain is important to prevent excessive postpartum weight retention.

Total fat intake did not differ among insulin-treated women with PDM delivering normal-weight or macrosomic infants (75.6 ± 18.8 gm/day) (Combs 92). In three other studies of pregnant women with type 1 diabetes, daily fat intake was 85 ± 23 gm/day (Kalkwarf 01) and 76.9 gm/day (Bates 97), or 37 ± 3% of energy (Lakin 98). These studies suggest that MNT in diabetic pregnant women may be successful in limiting fat intake. Studies of intentional variation of dietary fat content or its components are few in pregnancy and limited to nondiabetic women or women with GDM (Hachey 94, Ilic 99, Butte 00, Lauszus 01b, Glillen 04).

Cholesterol. Humans can synthesize sufficient cholesterol as a component of cell membranes and as a precursor of steroid hormones and bile acids; therefore, there is no evidence for its dietary requirement (IOM 02). Cholesterol absorption may be increased in type 1 diabetes, but its synthesis is decreased (Gylling 04, Miettinen 04); in type 2 diabetes, cholesterol absorption is low, but synthesis is increased (Simonen 02). Because dietary cholesterol increases serum total cholesterol (total-C) and LDL-C concentrations (Clarke 97), thus raising the risk of CHD, "cholesterol intake should be kept as low as possible, within a nutritionally adequate diet" (<300 mg/day if LDL-C is <130 mg/dL; <200 mg/day if LDL-C is >130 mg/dL) (NCEP 01, AHA 04, DGAr 05). There is no evidence that the recommendation should be different in pregnancies with or without diabetes. Mean intake of total-C was 280 mg/day in 81 presumably healthy pregnant women in the national CSFII survey (IOM 02) compared with 384 mg/day in 24-h dietary recall by 3,125 normotensive nondiabetic women at 13–21 weeks gestation (Morris 01). Cholesterol intake was not an independent predictor for risk of preeclampsia in multivariate analysis in the latter study (Morris 01). Mean cholesterol intake was 272.8 mg/day in the single available study of 38 pregnant women with type 1 diabetes compared with 241.4 mg/day in matched controls (NS, not significant) (Bates 97). Research is needed to determine whether there is any effect from cholesterol intake in diabetic pregnancy.

Fatty acids. Primary sources of SFAs are cheese, beef, whole milk, cooking oils and shortening, regular ice cream, butter, fried chicken, and fried fish (De Vriese 01, De Vriese 02, Cotton 04). Any incremental increase in SFA intake increases CHD risk (IOM 02, Sacks 02c), presumably by increasing plasma LDL-C concentrations (Howard 02). SFA intake should be as low as possible (<10% of energy intake if LDL-C <130 mg/dL; <7% of energy intake if LDL-C >129 mg/dL) while consuming a diet that provides 20–35% of calories from fat and meets recommendations for *n*-6 linoleic acid, *n*-3 α-linolenic acid, and vitamin E (DGAr 05). No evidence suggests that advice should be different for diabetic pregnant women. The mean intake of total SFA was 38 gm/day in 3,125 nondiabetic women remaining normotensive throughout gestation, representing 13% of energy intake, and did not differ in women developing gestational hypertension or preeclampsia (Morris 01). In a study of four pregnant women with type 1 diabetes, the average intake of total SFA was 47 gm/day, and the concentration of selected SFA was elevated in maternal erythrocytes and placenta compared with controls (Lakin 98). Although we lack sufficient studies of the dietary intake of cholesterol and SFA in pregnant women with PDM, their usual motivation during gestation offers an opportunity to educate and train them in cooking and eating behaviors that, if continued, may provide long-term health benefits. Recommendations for dietary cholesterol and SFA intake support the need to determine LDL-C concentrations before or at the beginning of pregnancy.

Plant sources rich in MUFAs include nuts and canola (rapeseed), olive, safflower, and sunflower oils; ~92% of dietary intake is oleic acid (IOM 02). MUFA intake can range up to 20% of calories (NCEP 02), and the ADA position is that carbohydrate and MUFAs together should provide 60–70% of energy intake to restrict saturated fat intake to <10% of calories (ADA 04b). Incorporation of almonds into a food plan lowered glycemic responses to mixed meals and may have provided antioxidants (increased serum thiol, less oxidative protein damage) (Jenkins 06a). Few studies exist of MUFA intake in pregnant women with or without diabetes. The CSFII survey (1994–1996) reported that mean intake of MUFAs was 24.3 gm/day in 2,498 adult women and 27.2 gm/day in 81 pregnant women (IOM 02); MUFAs were slightly higher at 28.6 gm/day in Belgium (De Vriese 01,02). Median intake of MUFAs was 28.5 gm/day according to a food frequency questionnaire in the midtrimester of 60 women in Vancouver, Canada, representing 10.4% of total energy, compared with 27.6 gm/day for saturated fat, representing 9.8% of total energy (Elias 02). In 38 women with type 1 diabetes in Northern Ireland, MUFA intake was 25.7 gm/day in the first trimester compared with 32.3 gm/day total saturated fat; these measurement did not differ from those in matched controls (Bates 97). In a careful study of a small sample of pregnant women with type 1 diabetes in Scotland, MUFA intake was 35 gm/day in late pregnancy (Lakin 98). All of these limited studies indicate that continuing efforts should be made to increase MUFA intake and decrease intake of SFAs in diabetic pregnant women.

An AMDR of 5–10% of energy is estimated for *n*-6 PUFAs in pregnant women because the lower boundary will meet the AI for linoleic acid; benefits or risks are unclear for intakes >10% of energy intake. Primary sources of the essential *n*-6 linoleic acid are liquid vegetable oils including soybean, corn, and safflower oils. Linoleic acid makes up 85–90% of total PUFA consumption, and arachidonic acid is ~2% (DGAr 05). The AI for intake of linoleic acid in pregnant women of any age is set at 13 gm/day, and the AMDR is 5–10% of energy (IOM 02). During pregnancy, the demand for *n*-6 fatty acids for incorporation into placental tissue and the developing fetus must be met by *n*-6 fatty acids from maternal tissues or from dietary intake (Herrera 02b, Heird 05, Innis 05). The IOM review found no evidence "that maternal dietary intervention with *n*-6 fatty acids has any effect on fetal or infant growth and development in women meeting the requirements for *n*-6 fatty acids" (IOM 02). Controversy surrounds whether higher-range intake of linoleic acid in pregnancy will reduce neonatal *n*-3 fatty acid status (Al 96, De Vriese 02). Mean intake of linoleic acid was 13.9 gm/day in 81 pregnant women in the CSFII survey, and at least 25% consumed less than the AI (IOM 02); a similar level of intake was seen in Belgium (De Vriese 02). Mean total PUFA intake was only 11.3 gm/day in pregnant women with type 1 diabetes in the 1990s in Northern Ireland (Bates 97) and was similar in Scotland (Lakin 98). Linoleic acid is significantly lower in umbilical cord plasma than in maternal plasma (Lakin 98, Herrera 04), suggesting limited placental transfer or high fetal use (Koletzko 90). Data are needed on intake of *n*-6 PUFAs in pregnant diabetic women.

An AMDR for the essential *n*-3 α-linolenic acid is estimated to be 0.6–1.2% of energy. The lower boundary meets the AI level; the upper boundary corresponds to the highest α-linolenic intakes from foods consumed by individuals in the U.S. and Canada, which may afford some protection against CVD (IOM 02). Plant sources of α-linolenic acid include canola oil, soybean oil, walnuts, and flaxseed (DGAr 05). Incorporation of walnuts into a diabetic food plan supplies *n*-3 PUFAs and improves lipid profiles (Tapsell 04, Gillen 05). The demand for *n*-3 PUFAs for incorporation into placental tissue and the developing fetus must be met by *n*-3 fatty acids from maternal tissues or by dietary intake. Due to the lack of evidence for determining a unique requirement for *n*-3 fatty acids during pregnancy, the AI for α-linolenic acid for pregnant women of any age is set at 1.4 gm/day, and the AMDR is estimated to be 0.6–1.2% of energy intake (IOM 02). Mean intake of α-linolenic acid was 1.42 gm/day in 81 pregnant women in the CSFII survey (IOM 02) and the same in four pregnant women with type 1 diabetes in Scotland (Lakin 98). We have insufficient data on the intake or effects of α-linolenic acid in pregnancies complicated by diabetes. α-linolenic acid is transferred across the placenta to fetal blood, but concentrations are lower than maternal concentrations.

Most studies of maternal–placental–fetal fatty acid disposition have focused on GDM (Wijendran 99, Loosemore 04, Dijck-Brouwer 05, Bitsanis 06, Thomas 06c). A single study investigated the fatty acid composition in midtrimester maternal and cord plasma triacylglycerols and choline phosphoglycerides in 39 controls, 32 women with type 1 diabetes, and 17 women with type 2 diabetes (Min 05). A1C values were slightly elevated in the diabetic groups, mean FPG was 121 mg/dL (6.6 ± 0.8 mM), and only one macrosomic infant was delivered. No group differences were apparent in maternal Σ SFAs (palmitic 27.5%, stearic 3.6%), Σ monoene fatty acids (oleic 35.8%, palmitoleic 3.9%), Σ *n*-6 fatty acids (linoleic 16.6%, arachidonic 1.0), and Σ *n*-3 fatty acids (α-linolenic 1.0%, EPA 0.2%, DHA 0.6%). The percentages given are the percentages of total fatty acids in plasma triacylglycerols in the women with type 1 diabetes. Fatty acid composition in cord plasma triacylglyceols did not differ except for lower perecentages for the *n*-3 series in the type 1 diabetes group versus controls (Min 05).

The active long-chain polyunsaturated fatty acid (LC-PUFA) derivatives of *n*-6 linoleic acid are *n*-6 arachidonic acid and dihomo-γ linolenic acid; LC-PUFA derivatives of *n*-3 α-linolenic acid are *n*-3 DHA and EPA. They are important structural elements of cell membranes and are "of pivotal importance for the formation of new tissue in the fetus" (Herrera 04). Arachidonic acid is an important precursor for eicosanoids (prostaglandins, prostacyclins, leukotrienes, thromboxanes) involved in vascular function and coagulation. Human placental tissue lacks both the Δ^6- and Δ^5-desaturase activities for production of *n*-6 and *n*-3 LC-PUFAs from their precursors linoleic acid and α-linolenic acid. Therefore, fetal LC-PUFAs are primarily derived from maternal plasma (Dutta-Roy 00). DHA is essential for development of the brain and retina (Haggarty 04). LC-PUFAs circulate in maternal plasma associated with low-density lipoprotein TGs and in chylomicrons and they also circulate in the form of NEFAs bound to albumin (Herrera 06a). The central nervous system (CNS) content of LC-PUFAs increases progressively during brain organogenesis (Herrera 04), and the provision of essential fatty acids and their derivatives to the fetal and neonatal brain affects development (Koletzko 90, Yavin 01, Champoux 02). Arachidonic acid and DHA show significantly higher percentage values in cord plasma total lipids compared with maternal concentrations at delivery (Herrera 04), suggesting preferential maternal–fetal transfer over their parent fatty acids or fetal synthesis in the liver (Dutta-Roy 00, Haggarty 04, Herrera 06a). The fetus/neonate has the capacity for metabolic elongation and desaturation of linoleic acid and AHA to form arachidonic acid and DHA, respectively (Herrera 04). The synthesis of *n*-3 EPA from its precursor α-linolenic acid or by retroconversion of DHA also takes place in the fetus (Greiner 96).

Placental transfer of NEFAs across placental cells occurs (1) by bidirectional diffusion; (2) by means of trophoblast lipoprotein receptors, hydrolysis by membrane lipoprotein lipases, intracellular phospholipase A-2 and intracellular lipase activities in placental cells (Bonet 92, Waterman 98, Herrera 06a); and (3) via selective uptake of NEFA by the syncytiotrophoblast, intracellular metabolic channeling, and selective export to fetal circulation (Haggarty 04). The latter complex, multistep process is under current investigation and probably involves placental plasma membrane fatty acid–binding protein (p-FABP$_{pm}$) with preference for LC-PUFAs (Dutta-Roy 00), fatty acid translocase, fatty acid transport protein-4 (FATP-4) (Larque 06), lipid droplet-associated adipophilin (Bildirici 03), and cytoplasmic H- and L-type FABPs that "may be responsible for transcytoplasmic movement of FFAs to their sites of esterification, β-oxidation, or to the fetal circulation via placental basal membranes" (Dutta-Roy 00). Trophoblast TG hydrolases show a marked preference in uptake of fatty acids from TGs compared with albumin-bound fatty acids (Bonet 92). Ligand-activated peroxisome proliferator-activated receptor (PPAR)γ and its nuclear receptor partner retinoid X receptor enhanced the expression of FATP-4 and adipophilin, and stimulated fatty acid uptake and accumulation in trophoblasts (Schaiff 05, Schild 06). A combination of insulin and oleic plus linoleic acids enhanced the expression of adipophilin and increased the accumulation of fat droplets in trophoblasts, but had no effect on FATP-4 (Elchalal 05). H-type FABP mostly binds LC-PUFAs, and L-FABP binds heterogenous ligands, including bile salts and eicosanoids (Dutta-Roy 97). Sixty percent of DHA taken up into trophoblast cells is esterified into triacylglycerol fractions (phosphatidylcholine), and 60% of the uptake of arachidonic acid is incorporated into phospholipid fractions (phosphatidylethanolamine) (Dutta-Roy 00). There are also mechanisms within the placental cells for selective incorporation of arachidonic acid into phosphoglycerides and their export to the fetal circulation to become structural membrane components (Kuhn 86).

Further studies on the regulation of fatty acid transport and metabolism in placenta may provide insight into the possible effects of diabetes on these systems. In vitro perfusion of isolated placental lobules obtained at delivery from women with type 1 diabetes revealed transport kinetics for palmitic acid that did not differ from controls (Nandakumaran 99). Both TGs and phospholipids accumulate in placental cells in diabetic pregnancies (Diamont 82), suggesting enhanced uptake of fatty acids if not decreased breakdown of intracellular TGs and fat droplets. In fact, there is increased expression of the main placental phospholipases and accumulation of *n*-3 PUFAs in diabetes and fetal obesity, perhaps stimulated by the placental cytokines leptin and TNF-α (Varastehpour 06). Microvillous membranes from pregnancies of women with type 1 diabetes show increased lipoprotein lipase (LPL) activity but no increase in placenta-specific TG hydrolase activity, plus increased L-FABP expression in placental homogenates. The authors concluded that these alterations could contribute to the enhanced lipid deposition and metabolism seen in diabetic pregnancies (Magnusson 04).

Dietary sources of long-chain PUFA derivatives. DHAs are found in all fish and shellfish, particularly fatty fish such as mackerel, salmon, trout, and tuna (1 oz = 407 mg EPA + DHA) (DGAr 05). The cardioprotective effects of fish consumption in women (Hu 02, He 04a) are apparently related to EPA and DHA (Wijendran 04), and the weekly consumption of at least two servings (~8 oz) of fish rich in EPA and DHA is suggested. Adverse effects are not seen until EPA and l EPA + DHA intake exceeds 3 gm/day (7.4 oz fish) (DGAr 05). In an observational study of 488 low-risk Icelandic pregnant women, consumption of high doses of *n*-3 LC-PUFAs in liquid cod liver oil in early pregnancy seemed to increase the risk of developing hypertensive disorders of pregnancy (Olafsdottir 06). The ADA position is that two to three servings of fish per week are recommended for diabetic women (ADA 08b), but attention must be paid to the degree of contamination of fish sources with organic mercury and polychlorinated biphenyls (PCBs) (Wilson 04) and to the dwindling fish supply (Brunner 06). Fish is also low in saturated fat and a good source of protein, B-vitamins, and minerals such as potassium, phosphorus, and selenium (DGAr 05). The potential neurotoxic effects of mercury consumption via fish and shellfish in pregnancy are considered later in Part I in the section titled "Intake of Other Substances." The hope exists that foods enriched with EPA and DHA will become a suitable alternative to achieve recommended intakes (Gebauer 06).

In the 1990s, 50% of American women consumed <0.07 gm/day of EPA + DHA, and mean intake was also 0.07 gm/day in 81 pregnant women (IOM 02). A 2005 consensus panel urged women to consume 100–300 mg/day of DHA (Akabas 06). Supplementation with fish oil during pregnancy increases DHA and EPA in both mother and infant, but decreases arachadonic acid and other *n*-6 LC-PUFAs (Dunstan 04). The IOM review concluded that there is no evidence "to show that increasing intakes of DHA in pregnant women consuming diets that meet requirements for *n*-6 and *n*-3 fatty acids have any physiologically significant benefit to the infant" (IOM 02). A recent meta-analysis of six RCTs of *n*-3 LC-PUFA supplementation of women with low-risk pregnancies demonstrated a small effect on longer pregnancy duration and increased fetal head size, with the implications for later growth and development to be determined (Szajewska 06). Small amounts of EPA and DHA can help reverse an *n*-3 fatty acid deficiency in pregnancy and can "contribute towards the AI for α-linolenic acid" (IOM 02).

In view of possible developmental problems in IDMs, research is needed on the dietary intake of PUFA, maternal metabolism, placental transfer, and fetal–neonatal metabolism/synthesis of LC-PUFA in pregnancies complicated by diabetes. In the limited studies available, *n*-6 and *n*-3 LC-PUFAs (except EPA) were reduced in maternal erythrocytes of diabetic pregnant women and in cord plasma and erythrocytes compared with controls (Lakin 98, Min 05).

***Trans* fats.** Partial hydrogenation of vegetable oils results in the formation of *trans* unsaturated fatty acids (Stender 06) that increase both LDL-C and harmful small, dense LDL particles, decrease protective HDL cholesterol, and contribute to the risk of CHD in women (Mauger 03, Mozzafarian 04, Mozaffarian 06a). The 2005 Dietary Guidelines for Americans advise all people to keep *trans* fatty acid intake as low as possible, which is ~1% of energy (DGAr 05). Elaidic acid is the predominant *trans* fatty acid found in processed fats. In 1989–1991, mean consumption of total *trans* fatty acids by American women aged 20–49 was 4.6 gm/day, or 2.6% of total energy, with the 10th–90th percentiles at 1.6–8.0 gm/day (Allison 99). They compete with LC-PUFAs for binding sites in human placental membranes (Dutta-Roy 00). *Trans* fatty acids are known to cross the placenta, with umbilical cord plasma levels similar to maternal (Koletzko 90). It is uncertain whether these levels can significantly inhibit essential fatty acid desaturation and impair synthesis of the LC-PUFAs important in fetal growth and neural development (Carlson 97, Innis 06).

An analysis of dietary sources of *trans* fatty acids among pregnant women by a food intake questionnaire in Vancouver, Canada, showed multiple sources in products consumed by diabetic women (breads 11%, pastas/grains/cereals 9%, snack foods 11%, fast foods 11%) (Elias 02). The major source of *trans* fatty acids (34%) was found in baked goods (cakes, cookies, muffins, croissants) that were less likely to be part of a diabetes and pregnancy food plan. Mean total *trans* fatty acid intake was 3.8 0.3 gm/day in mid-pregnancy of nondiabetic women (Elias 02). French fries also have a high *trans* fatty acid content (Litin 93). In a single limited study of diabetic pregnant women and controls, average intake of total *trans* fatty acids was 3.5–3.7 gm/day, but total *trans* fatty acid composition of maternal erythrocytes and placental tissue was significantly elevated in diabetic subjects, although cord blood concentrations did not differ (Lakin 98). Data are lacking on *trans* fatty acid consumption and metabolism in diabetic pregnant women.

Micronutrient Intake

Concern continues to surround the adequacy of micronutrient intake (minerals, trace elements, vitamins) (Bartley 05, Kennedy 05), its effects on pregnancy (Goldenberg 03, Merialdi 03, Villar 03), and whether dietary supplements (Picciano 03) are indicated for diabetic pregnant women. We and other authors (Keen 03, Ramakrishnan 04, Allen 05) emphasize five key issues in this overview of multiple micronutrients and long-term pregnancy outcome. First, to quote a leader in the field, "Maternal micronutrient status in the periconceptional period, and throughout pregnancy and lactation, should be viewed as a continuum; too often these 3 stages are treated and discussed separately from both a scientific and a public health perspective." (Allen 05). Second, micronutrient effects do not occur in isolation, and we must account for the strong biological interactions between them. Third, multiple micronutrient deficiencies occur together when diets are poor. Fourth, because requirements for most micronutrients are higher during gestation, the possibility of inadequate intake increases (Allen 05). Fifth, poorly controlled diabetes may cause specific deficiencies in micronutrient status (Mooradian 87, 94).

Regarding micronutrient supplementation in diabetes, the ADA position is that "there is no clear evidence of benefit from vitamin or mineral supplementation in [non-pregnant] people with diabetes (compared with the general population) who do not have underlying deficiencies. Routine supplementation with antioxidants, such as vitamins E and C and carotene, is not advised because of lack of evidence of efficacy and concern related to long-term safety" (ADA 08b). A 2006 NIH State-of-the-Science panel concluded that there is insufficient evidence to recommend either for or against the use of multivitamin/mineral supplements by the general public to prevent chronic disease, but the needs of pregnant women were not considered (NIH 06). Diabetic patients should be educated about the importance of acquiring daily vitamin and mineral requirements from natural food sources (Franz 02). To achieve an adequate intake of micronutrients, the focus should be on food groups and not single nutrients, and successive nutrient-dense foods (vegetables, fruits) must be added to major staple foods in meals and snacks (rice, refined wheat, potato, maize/bean) (Bartley 05).

According to the IOM (IOM 90) and the position of the American Dietetic Association (ADietA 02), mineral and multivitamin supplements are recommended only for pregnant women with special needs: multifetal gestations, tobacco smokers, alcohol or drug abusers, iron-deficiency anemia, and poor-quality food intake, including those who rarely consume animal products. Diabetic pregnant women were not included in the group with special needs.

Studies of micronutrient intake in women with PDM are limited. In evaluating trace element status related to intake, more information can be gained by investigating concentrations in blood cells instead of evaluating only plasma levels, which may be misleading (Kruse-Jarres 00). Existing data on dietary intake of specific micronutrients in pregnancies with or without diabetes are listed in Table I.5, with appropriate citations in this section of the book. Space does not allow a detailed discussion of the many micronutrients, and the reader is referred to the IOM books on DRIs for supporting background information. We do present summary information on the basis for the RDAs or AIs of the major micronutrients for pregnancy. Chromium deficiency has been suspected in association with glucose intolerance (Ravina 95, Jovanovic-Peterson 96), but RCTs have not shown an influence of chromium intake on glycemic control (Gunton 01, Althuis 02, Gunton 05, Kleefstra 06). Micronutrients recommended for consideration as supplements during pregnancy by the IOM (1990) include calcium, iron, zinc, folate, and vitamins B6, C, and D (ACOG 93, Trombo 02, Gunderson 03). In addition, evidence states that substantial proportions of pregnant women in the U.S. continue to have low dietary intakes of copper, magnesium, potassium, selenium, niacin, riboflavin, thiamine, choline, vitamin A, and vitamin E (Gunderson 03), and an excessive intake of sodium (de Wardener 04). Our analysis finds that dietary intake of calcium, magnesium, copper, selenium, zinc, vitamin C, vitamin D, and vitamin E may be deficient in many diabetic pregnant women. It is often practical to provide most of these micronutrients in a prenatal supplement capsule, although the clinician should be aware of the variation in content of these supplements displayed in Table I.5. It is unfortunate that information is lacking on the optimal formulation of micronutrient supplements for pregnant women (Allen 05), especially those with diabetes.

Water and Electrolytes

Water intake has not been well studied in diabetic pregnant women, but there is no evidence that the IOM recommendation for AI (~2.3 L/day = 78 fl oz; ~10 cups as total beverages, including drinking water) should differ in PDM (IOM 04). The AI is set to prevent the deleterious effects of dehydration in moderately active women in a temperate climate and to allow normal expansion of maternal intra- and extracellular spaces and the products of conception.

Sodium. Disagreement persists concerning the relationship of sodium intake to the large increases in plasma volume and interstitial space in pregnancy because the usual total sodium accretion of 2.1–2.3 gm represents an intake of a few milligrams of sodium per day (IOM 04). According to the IOM, there is lack of evidence that sodium requirements during pregnancy differ from that of nonpregnant women (IOM 04). The AI for sodium (1.5 gm/day) is set to cover possible daily losses, provide adequate intakes of other nutrients, and maintain normal function. The UL for sodium (2.3 gm/day) is set because of the risks of increased BP and perhaps should be lower for diabetic women (IOM 04). Excess sodium intake is related to BP level in nonpregnant patients (deWarderner 04), and reducing sodium intake to 2.4 gm/day sodium or 6.0 gm/day salt lowers systolic and diastolic BP (Midgley 96, Sacks 01, Franz 02, He 03, Bray 04). This information is important in diabetes because hypertension is so common and salt sensitivity (reduction in BP in response to lowered salt intake or rise in BP in response to sodium loading) is more prevalent (IOM 04). The UL is well below the mean 1-day intake of sodium of 4.2 gm/day recorded in 3,125 nondiabetic women who remained normotensive during pregnancy, 4.2 gm/day in 721 women who developed gestational hypertension, and 4.3 gm/day in 311 women who developed preeclampsia (Morris 01). Mean sodium intake was 3.5 gm/day in 346 pregnant women in NHANES III, and 90% consumed above the UL (IOM 04). Sodium intake was not measured in the few studies on nutrient intake of pregnant diabetic women, and studies of salt sensitivity in this group are lacking.

Sodium is added to canned and packaged foods. To decrease sodium in the diet, the patient should be directed to eat fresh, unprocessed foods such as fresh meat, fruits, and vegetables. A food considered low in sodium is defined as having <140 mg per serving. Foods considered to be very high in sodium (>400 mg per serving) include soups, pickles, cured meats, and many convenience and fast foods.

Potassium. Increasing potassium intake may protect against hypertension, CVD, and renal disease (Young 99, He 01, IOM 04, DGAr 05, ADA 08b). Moderate potassium restriction may add to insulin resistance (Yang 03), and increasing potassium intake may improve insulin sensitivity (Ard 04). Extensive processing of foods in Western societies can lead to insufficient potassium intake and relative potassium depletion (Demigne 04). There are no interventional trials of potassium intake on BP in pregnancy. The AI for normal or diabetic pregnancy is set at 4.7 gm/day, and a UL is not established unless there is impaired urinary excretion (IOM 04). Based on studies in nonpregnant women, intake of potassium at 4.7 gm/day "should lower BP, blunt the adverse effects of sodium chloride on BP, reduce the risk of kidney stones, and possibly reduce bone loss" (IOM 04). Beneficial effects stem from the forms of potassium found naturally in low-fat dairy products, whole grains, fruits, and vegetables (Lin 03). However, epidemiological surveys in the U.S. suggest that median potassium intake for nonpregnant women is only 2.1–2.3 gm/day (IOM 04) and 3.1 gm/day for normotensive or hypertensive pregnant women (Morris 01). We lack data on the adequacy of potassium intake in diabetic pregnant women.

Minerals and Trace Elements

Calcium. Calcium requirements do not change during pregnancy (AI 1,000 mg/day; 1,300 mg/day if aged <19) due to the increased efficiency of calcium absorption in gestation, which should take care of fetal needs (IOM 90,97, ADietA 02, Vargas-Zapata 04). The UL of 2.5 gm/day is based on risk of nephrolithiasis (IOM 97). Good sources of calcium in pregnancy include 1 cup milk (300 mg) or 1 cup yogurt (300 mg). Median calcium intake was 1,243 mg/day in a multiracial survey of 385 pregnant U.S. women, but total intake was <800 mg/day in 24% (Harville 04). In cross-sectional studies of preconception (Smith 88) among pregnant diabetic (Bates 97) and control (Morris 01) women, mean dietary calcium intake was similar, and serum and urinary calcium levels did not differ. Calcium intake did not relate to development of hypertension in pregnancy in the latter large cross-sectional study. Prospective longitudinal studies of serum total and ionized calcium in diabetic pregnant women yielded mixed results: they did not differ in any stage of pregnancy in two small studies of pregnant women with type 1 diabetes compared with controls (Cruikshank 80, Donatelli 84), but were lower in the third trimester only in larger studies of 68 and 199 type 1 diabetic women, respectively (Kuoppala 88, Mimouni 89).

Studies of calcium-regulating hormones also yield mixed results in diabetic pregnancy. Decreased calcium levels should stimulate parathyroid hormone (PTH) secretion unless there is a magnesium deficiency (Silver 02), and PTH concentrations have been reported to be normal (Donatelli 84, Mimouni 89) or reduced in diabetic pregnant women (Cruikshank 80,83, Martinez 94). Calcitonin, produced by thyroid parafollicular cells in response to hypercalcemia (DeLuca 04), has a transient, weak effect by enhancing deposition of calcium in the exchangeable bone calcium salts, which may be more pronounced in young animals due to the rapid interchange of absorbed and deposited calcium (Guyton 05). Calcitonin levels double in normal pregnancy, but did not differ in the few available small studies of diabetic pregnant women (Cruikshank 83, Donatelli 84, Ardawi 97). Vitamin D_3 is discussed later in the subsection titled "Vitamin D." Osteocalcin is a noncollagenous protein produced by osteoblasts that may be a marker for bone formation or turnover. Serum osteocalcin concentrations seem to increase in early or later normal pregnancy (Ardawi 97, Wisser 05, Ainy 06); concentrations were lower than in nonpregnant controls in a single study of diabetic pregnant women (Martinez 94).

Recent reviews of clinical trials suggested that increases in calcium intake during pregnancy and lactation improve maternal bone health (O'Brien 06, Thomas 06d); however, an RCT studying the ingestion of 1,500-mg/day calcium supplements from 20 weeks gestation conducted in a country with low calcium intake reported no significant benefit for BW, breast milk calcium concentrations, or infant growth or bone–mineral status in the first year of life (Jarjou 06). Several small RCTs in nondiabetic pregnant women (some conducted in places with low amounts of calcium in the usual diet) suggested that calcium supplementation reduces the incidence of gestational hypertension or preeclampsia (Bucher 96, Herrera 06b), but a large multicenter trial in North America showed no benefit of supplementation when calcium intake was 982 mg/day from food and usual prenatal supplements in the placebo group. The lack of benefit extended to the subgroup with the lowest dietary calcium intake (422 mg/day) (Levine 97). In a global placebo-controlled RCT, calcium supplementation of 1,500 mg/day in 4,157 women with low dietary calcium intake (<600 mg/day) did not prevent preeclampsia (4.1% vs. 4.5%) or spontaneous preterm delivery (6.9% vs. 7.2%), but did reduce preeclampsia severity and frequency of severe gestational hypertension (1.04% vs. 1.42%) (Villar 06). To our knowledge, RCTs have not been conducted in pregnant women with diabetes. The recommended calcium supplementation is 600 mg/day in diabetic pregnant women who cannot consume dairy products (IOM 90).

Phosphorus. Dietary phosphorus supports tissue growth during pregnancy and replaces excretory/dermal losses to maintain a normal level of P_i in the extracellular fluid (ECF) (IOM 97). The added efficiency in intestinal absorption of calcium due to increased concentrations of $1,25(OH)_2D$ also will lead to an ~10% increase in phosphorus absorption, which covers fetal needs (IOM 97). Daily phosphorus intake was deemed sufficient in studies of normal pregnant women (Cross 95, IOM 97, Morris 01), but it is not known whether there is an increased phosphorus requirement for multifetal or diabetic pregnancies. Serum phosphorus did not differ from pregnant controls in four studies of women with type 1 diabetes (Cruikshank 80,83, Donatelli 84, Kuoppala 88).

Magnesium. There is no evidence for conservation or increased absorption of magnesium in pregnancy. The RDA in pregnancy (350 mg/day) is an increase of 15% for the growth in lean body mass; it is set at 360 mg/day for ages >30 and at 400 mg/day for ages <19 years (IOM 97). The UL of 350 mg/day in added supplements is set to avoid diarrhea (IOM 97). Magnesium is ubiquitous in animal and plant foods, but paradoxically high levels of protein intake or of fiber in fruits, vegetables, and grains decrease magnesium absorption or retention (IOM 97). Results of cross-sectional studies of altered magnesium status in pregnant women with preterm labor, hypertension, or GDM are inconsistent (IOM 97, Durlach 04). Clinical trials of magnesium supplementation also yielded inconsistent outcomes (Villar 03), but these studies have not been conducted in diabetic women. Average dietary intake of magnesium was only 210–375 mg/day in control pregnant women (IOM 97, Swenson 01, Turner 03), with similar values in diabetic (Bates 97) or hypertensive (Morris 01) pregnant women.

Magnesium depletion is identified in inadequately controlled diabetes (Sjogren 86, Tosiello 96). Urinary magnesium excretion increased by a factor of 2.4 in type 1 diabetes patients exposed to hyperglycemia for several hours without hyperinsulinemia, and plasma magnesium decreased by 3% (Djurhuus 00, Djurhuus 01). Factors maintaining ECF concentrations of magnesium include its exchangeable bone reservoir, glomerular filtration and tubular reabsorption, and the normal intestinal absorption rate of 51–60%. An observational study of moderately controlled women with type 1 diabetes in the preconception period found urinary excretion of magnesium to be significantly higher than in matched controls, and serum magnesium was lower despite similar daily dietary intake (Smith 88). In the diabetic women, serum magnesium was negatively correlated with urinary glucose ($r = -0.758$, $p < 0.001$) and glycohemoglobin ($r = -0.603$, $p < 0.01$). In two prospective longitudinal studies during pregnancy, serum magnesium was significantly lower in insulin-dependent diabetic women compared with controls, apparently resulting from increased urinary loss and associated with lower PTH levels (Cruikshank 80, Mimouni 89). However, another study found no difference in serum magnesium in diabetic pregnant women (Kuoppala 88), and serum magnesium was only slightly lower in 12 pregnant women with type 1 diabetes intensively treated with insulin compared with normal pregnant controls by the third trimester (Wibell 85). Serum magnesium concentrations do not appear to be adequate indicators of magnesium status in pregnancy due to hemodilution (IOM 97), and tissue levels (Resnick 04) are not well studied in diabetic pregnant women. Only one report associated low serum magnesium levels in the first trimester with early fetal loss or congenital malformations, possibly confounded by elevated glycohemoglobin levels (Mimouni 87). Increased risks of hypocalcemia and hypomagnesemia in infants of inadequately controlled diabetic mothers have been partly ascribed to magnesium deficiency in the mother (Mimouni 86).

Vitamin D. Vitamin D (calciferol) is found naturally in fatty fish and egg yolks and is fortified in dairy products, cereals, and orange juice in the U.S. Dietary calciferol is incorporated into chylomicrons and absorbed into the lymphatic system, then bound to vitamin D–binding protein (DBP) or lipoproteins in circulating blood (DeLuca 04, Specker 04). Alternatively, during exposure to sunlight, ultraviolet B radiation is absorbed by 7-dehydrocholesterol in dermal cells, forming previtamin D_3, which is converted to vitamin D_3 by a temperature-dependent process that then enters the dermal capillary circulation bound to DBP (Holick 06). Vitamin D_3 is really more of a biologically inert prohormone than a typical vitamin (DeLuca 04). Above latitude 35, very little vitamin D_3 is produced in the skin from November to March (Holick 06). Circulating vitamin D_3 is dihydroxylated, first in the liver [$25(OH)D_3$] and then in the kidney to $1,25(OH)_2D_3$. This biologically active form of vitamin D, by binding to nuclear vitamin D receptors in various tissues, indirectly functions to maintain serum calcium and phosphorus via: (1) induction of the genes for proteins responsible for active intestinal calcium and phosphate absorption; (2) stimulation of osteoblasts to produce a ligand that stimulates osteoclasts, bone resorption, and calcium release in the presence of PTH; and (3) stimulation of renal tubular reabsorption of the last 1% of the filtered load of calcium, also in the presence of PTH (DeLuca 04). In the absence of dietary calcium, the other $1,25(OH)_2D_3$-PTH–dependent processes serve to maintain plasma calcium concentrations.

However, $25(OH)D_3$ is the major circulating form of vitamin D that is measured to determine vitamin D status (<15 ng/mL = rickets = childhood skeletal abnormalities; <20 ng/mL = subclinical deficiency) (DeLuca 04) because the low calcium of vitamin D deficiency leads to secondary hyperparathyroidism in the presence of magnesium, and PTH stimulates renal production of $1,25(OH)_2D_3$, thereby giving false reassurance from its blood level (Holick 06).

Vitamin D hormone also seems to have a role in the pancreatic islets and serves as an antiproliferative and prodifferentiation hormone that may be important in suppressing malignant cells and autoimmune diseases (Grant 02, Eyles 03, Cantorna 04, DeLuca 04, Holick 06). Hypovitaminosis D is associated with glucose intolerance, insulin resistance, impaired β-cell function, obesity, type 2 diabetes, and evidence of atherosclerosis (Scragg 95, Wortsman 00, Arunabh 03, Chiu 04, Hypponen 06, Targher 06).

A progressive rise in serum $1,25(OH)_2D_3$ is found during pregnancy beyond the increase in DBP. However, a significant proportion of pregnant women in many populations are found to have inadequate D_3 status (Veith 01, Datta 02, Sachan 05, Ainy 06, vanderMeer 06). Low maternal $25(OH)D_3$ in late pregnancy is associated with reduced intrauterine long bone growth and slightly shorter gestation (Morley 06). The placenta changes $25(OH)D_3$ to the active metabolite and thereby contributes to maternal and fetal $1,25(OH)_2D_3$ (Pitkin 85, IOM 97, Bezerra 02). There is some evidence that diabetes per se affects vitamin D status in pregnancy: three (Koskinen 86, Kuoppala 88, Martinez 91) of four (Donatelli 84) studies found low $25(OH)D$ levels in maternal blood or AF from diabetic pregnant women.

The AI of cholecalciferol is set to be 5 μcg/day (1 μcg = 40 IU vitamin D) before and during pregnancy to maintain normal serum $25(OH)D$ levels (IOM 97). However, higher intakes of 1,000–2,000 IU/day may be necessary to correct D_3 deficiency (Hollis 04, Holick 06). Controversy surrounds the UL for cholecalciferol (DeLuca 04). It is of interest that modern health behaviors may actually contribute to vitamin D deficiency via decreased intake of fortified milk and cereals as well as decreased exposure to sunlight for fear of the risk of skin cancer (Raiten 04). Studies of healthy pregnant women usually show dietary vitamin D intakes to be adequate (Hollis 04, Specker 04) except for women living above latitude 35 in winter, women with darker pigment or who cover their skin or use sun protection, or in South Asian women who migrate to northern countries (vanderMeer 06). In the U.K., vitamin D supplements of 400 IU/day are recommended but underused for pregnant women of ethnic minorities (Datta 02). Observational studies and intervention trials with supplements in high-risk women show that improved maternal vitamin D status is associated with better neonatal calcium balance (IOM 97) and childhood bone mass at 9 years (Javaid 06) and perhaps less islet autoimmunity in offspring (Fronczak 03). Results are inconclusive regarding effects on maternal weight gain and fetal growth (Merialdi 03, Specker 04). Vitamin D intervention trials have not been performed in pregnant women with PDM.

Copper. Copper functions as a component of many metalloenzymes that act to reduce molecular oxygen (IOM 00b). Ceruloplasmin glycoprotein is a circulating multicopper oxidase that contains >95% of the copper in plasma (Daimon 98). Copper is widespread in foods, especially organ meats, seafood, nuts, whole grains, and wheat bran cereals. The efficiency of intestinal copper absorption varies from 20 to 50%, and it may increase slightly in pregnancy (Turnland 98); iron and zinc supplementation can reduce its absorption (Keen 03). The EAR for adult women is based on a combination of indicators including plasma copper and ceruloplasmin concentrations, erythrocyte superoxide dismutase activity, and platelet copper concentration (IOM 00). The RDA for copper for pregnant women of any age (1,000 mcg/day) represents an increase of 100 μcg/d from prepregnancy to account for fetal–placental needs (Trumbo 01). The UL of 10 mg/day for copper intake is set for protection from liver damage (IOM 00). The human copper transporter hCTR1 has been identified toward the basal plasma membranes of placental syncytiotrophoblast and within the fetoplacental vascular endothelial cells; insulin can alter the intracellular localization of the transporter (Hardman 06).

Diabetes may perturb copper metabolism (Walter 91) and trigger subclinical deficiency; copper deficits can result in embryonic defects (Keen 03). Urinary copper excretion is increased in diabetic subjects in moderate to poor glycemic control (Smith 88, Cooper 05). Copper excess could also be a problem (Mooradian 87) because ceruloplasmin, an acute-phase reactant (Keen 03), may be elevated in type 2 diabetes patients with high A1C levels (Daimon 98) and free copper ions are highly redox active (Monnier 01). However, ceruloplasmin levels plateau when copper intake is adequate and are not useful for chacterizing copper excess states (Hambidge 03, Cooper 05). Increased blood cell copper levels were found in a study of adult and child subjects with type 1 diabetes (Kruse-Jarres 00). Copper intake is poorly studied in healthy and diabetic pregnant women. In the preconception period or pregnancy, 40% of adult women in the U.S. may have intakes below the RDA (Smith 88, IOM 00). In pregnant diabetic women, daily copper intake was similar to controls (104,0 20 vs. 99,9 40 μcg/d) in a single study of 38 pregnant women with type 1 diabetes in Northern Ireland; ~40% were again below the RDA (Bates 97). In two small studies, erythrocyte or maternal venous blood copper, respectively, was higher in the third trimester in diabetic compared with control women (Twardowska-Saucha 94, Al-Saleh 05). To our knowledge, no observational or interventional studies of copper intake or levels related to pregnancy outcome in women with PDM have been conducted.

Iodine. Iodine is an essential component of the thyroid hormones (T3, T4) that regulate key biochemical reactions involved in protein synthesis and enzymatic activity, especially in the developing brain, heart, muscle, kidney, and pituitary (IOM 00, Nader 04). Iodine itself is critical for myelination of the CNS, and T4 affects brain somatogenesis, neuronal differentiation, and formation of neural processes (Dunn 01). Iodine in milk or dairy products, marine fish and seaweed, and foods grown in iodine-rich soils, plus iodate added to table salt, are reduced in the gut to iodide and almost completely absorbed. Iodized salt is mandatory in Canada and used optionally by approximately one-half of the U.S. population (IOM 00). Iodide is concentrated 20- to 50-fold in the thyroid gland compared with plasma via a sodium–iodide transporter in amounts adequate for thyroid hormone production, and the remainder is excreted by the kidneys (IOM 00).

Iodine deficiency results in hypothyroidism, preferential T3 secretion, increased thyrotropin (TSH) after the first trimester, thyroid enlargement (goiter) accompanied by supranormal thyroglobulin, and, most importantly, a continuum from mild mental retardation in the child to gross neurological impairment and various growth abnormalities, including microcephaly (cretinism) (IOM 00, Dunn 01, Nader 04). To prevent cretinism, severe iodine deficiency must be corrected by the second trimester and optimally before conception (Cao 94). Mild iodine deficiency in women becoming pregnant is possible in the U.S. (IOM 00). In one study, 7% of pregnant women had urinary iodine excretion <50 mg/L, indicating relative iodine deficiency (Nader 04). The EAR for adult women is based on adequate thyroid iodine accumulation and turnover and is increased in pregnancy to account for estimated fetal uptake of 75 μcg/day. Renal clearance of iodine increases during pregnancy (Nader 04). The RDA for pregnant women of any age is 220 μcg/day, which prevents goiter and neonatal defects in women living in areas of iodine deficiency (IOM 00). Prenatal exposure to excess iodine can result in neonatal iodine goiter and hypothyroidism. Iodine-deficient individuals with autoimmune thyroid disease can respond adversely to increased iodine uptake (IOM 00). Data on iodine intake and levels in diabetic pregnant women are lacking. Given the frequency of thyroid disorders associated with diabetes, it is prudent to recommend use of iodized salt during pregnancy.

Iron balance. Oxidized iron (ferrous^{2+}, ferric^{3+}, ferryl^{4+}) is a component of many enzymes, electron-carrier cytochrome proteins, oxygen-transporting hemoglobin and oxygen-attracting myoglobin, and transport and storage proteins (serum transferrin [Tf], lactoferrin, mostly intracellular ferritin, hemosiderin). Adequate protein binding is critical because free iron acts as a pro-oxidant. Iron participates in electron transfer via interconversion of the iron oxidation states, which is also the mechanism by which iron reversibly binds ligands such as oxygen, nitrogen, and sulfur atoms (IOM 00).

Iron absorption occurs by two pathways in the upper small intestine: (a) endocytic uptake of proteolyzed heme (ferrous protoporphyrin IX) from hemoglobin and myoglobin in meat, poultry, and fish and (b) absorption of nonheme dietary iron extracted from plant and dairy foods (Fe^2 salts, Fe^2 or Fe^3 complexed with organic acids, such as citrate, or peptides, such as albumin and ferritin) (Mackenzie 05). Process (b) contributes ~88% of absorbed dietary iron in most humans and is enhanced by gastric acid and substances such as ascorbic acid in food (IOM 00, Atanasova 05). Certain foods inhibit iron absorption, which "tends to be poor from meals in which whole-grain cereals and legumes predominate. Phytates in whole-grain cereals, calcium and phosphorus in milk, tannin in tea, and polyphenols in many vegetables all inhibit iron absorption by decreasing the intestinal solubility of nonheme iron from the entire meal. The addition of even relatively small amounts of meat and ascorbic acid-containing foods substantially increases the absorption of iron from the entire meal by keeping nonheme iron more soluble" (IOM 90). Although the amount of heme iron is less in most diets, its absorption is greater and is not influenced as much by other foods.

Dietary iron is taken up by matured duodenal enterocytes (1.6–2.8 mg/day with 13–25% absorption efficiency) via the apical-to-endosomal divalent metal transporter (DMT)1 with the assistance of duodenal cytochrome b (Dcytb), which reduces ferric iron (Ponka 03, Frazer 05, Mackenzie 05). Fe^{2+} is transported across the basolateral surface by the export protein ferroportin and loaded onto transferrin receptor 1 (TfR-1) + bound Tf located on the basolateral membrane, with a ceruloplasmin-like copper oxidase (hephaestin) as cofactor (Pietrangelo 04, Wessling-Resnicke 06). Plasma iron is bound to Tf, which then docks to the ubiquitous cell-surface TfR-1 for cellular uptake of iron via receptor-mediated endocytosis, facilitated by the protein HFE (Ponka 99, Pietrangelo 04). With cellular iron deficiency, iron regulatory-binding proteins (IRP-1 and -2) bind to iron-responsive elements located at the ends of mRNA for TfR and ferritin (Hentze 04). The effect is enhanced cellular uptake of iron.

Absorption and distribution of iron are regulated by several newly discovered processes (Hentze 04, Pietrangelo 04). The protein hepcidin is synthesized by hepatocytes in response to iron excess or the inflammation cytokine IL-6. Hepcidin downregulates iron release from enterocytes, macrophages, and placental cells (Ganz 03, Leong 04, Frazer 05, Ganz 06). Hepcidin binds to ferroportin and induces its internalization and lysosomal degradation (Nemeth 04, Wessling-Resnicke 06). Hepatic transferrin receptor 2 (TfR-2) somehow senses increased diferric Tf and stimulates hepcidin production and release in the presence of HFE and hemojuvelin (Ganz 04, Johnson 04, Robb 04, Frazer 05, Ganz 06). The hepcidin–ferroportin interaction also explains how macrophage recycling of iron is regulated: more hepcidin, less ferroportin, and decreased iron export. When iron stores are low or with low oxygen levels, the gene encoding hepcidin production is suppressed and iron import increases (Nicolas 02, Ganz 06). The roles of all regulatory proteins in the possibly disordered iron homeostasis of diabetes and pregnancy are yet to be studied.

If the body need for iron is low before pregnancy, it is stored in ferritin in the enterocytes. The bulk of the remaining body iron is stored in hepatocytes (~1,000 mg) or as myoglobin in muscle cytoplasm (~300 mg), but values are lower in women with heavier menstruation. Conservation of iron is dependent on tissue macrophage recycling of about 20 mg/day from hemoglobin of senescent red cells via plasma Fe–Tf to the bone marrow for new red cells. Smaller amounts of iron from myoglobin and redox enzymes are also recycled (Ganz 06). Intestinal iron absorption increases two- to fourfold in pregnancy, perhaps due to increased duodenal expression of the iron transport molecules DMT1, Dcytb, and iron-regulated mRNA, with reduction in hepcidin, HFE protein, and TfR-2 in the liver (Millard 04). Women with depleted iron stores have greater absorption than those with ample stores (Milman 06a). How much enterocyte storage occurs in pregnancy is unknown, but the increased use of iron means that other iron stores diminish in pregnancy in the absence of supplementation (IOM 00b). Iron loss occurs by sloughing of enterocytes after 48 h (0.8 mg/day ferritin–iron) or loss of hemoglobin–iron, Tf–iron, serum ferritin–iron in blood at parturition (~250 mg iron; almost twice that for cesarean delivery), or with trauma (IOM 90,93).

The RDA for elemental iron intake in pregnancy (27 mg/day) was set by modeling the components of iron requirements (basal losses [0.9 mg/day] + iron deposited in fetus and related tissues [2.1 mg/day] + iron used [2.8 mg/day] in expansion of hemoglobin mass), estimating the requirement for absorbed iron at the 97.5th percentile, using an upper limit of 25% iron absorption, and rounding (IOM 00a, Trumbo 01). The UL for absorbed iron was specified at 45 mg/day for pregnancy to avoid gastrointestinal side effects (IOM 00). Recent estimates of average dietary iron intake in various populations of pregnant women have been 12.4–14.0 mg/day (Mathews 99, Swenson 01, Turner 03) and 11.7 mg/day in pregnant women with type 1 diabetes (Bates 97). Because dietary intake of iron is inadequate for many pregnant women, low-dose supplementation of 30 mg/day of elemental iron taken between meals or at bedtime has been recommended during the second and third trimesters to reduce loss of iron stores (ACOG 93, CDC 98a, ADietA 02). However, routine iron supplementation remains controversial (PSTF 93, Milman 99, Beard 00, Rasmussen 01, Cogswell 03a, Mahomed 04). In 1993, the IOM recommended prospective evaluation of a complex schema of selective daily supplementation with 0, 30 mg, or 60–120 mg iron depending on maternal hemoglobin and serum ferritin concentrations specific to each trimester (IOM 93). Since then, RCTs have demonstrated that 40 mg/day of ferrous iron is adequate to prevent iron deficiency in pregnant women (Milman 05). With evidence of deficient iron stores and microcytic anemia, oral elemental iron doses of 60–120 mg/day are prescribed for treatment, which necessitates additional copper (2 mg) and zinc (15 mg) intake (ACOG 93, ADietA 02).

Iron deficiency. Three stages of iron deficiency are described by the Centers for Disease Control and Prevention (CDC) and the IOM: (a) depleted iron stores reflected by serum ferritin <12 μcg/L, (b) iron-deficient erythropoiesis with Tf saturation <16%, and (c) microcytic anemia (hemoglobin <11.0 gm/dL in first trimester, <10.5 gm/dL in second trimester, <11.0 gm/dL in third trimester) (CDC 89, IOM 90,93,00b). Use of serum ferritin as a measure of iron stores in pregnancy is complicated by the fact that serum ferritin declines in gestation in spite of iron supplementation (Kaneshigi 81, Goldenberg 96) and rises as an acute-phase protein with infection/inflammation (Scholl 98) or increasing plasma glucose (IOM 00). The IOM considers low iron stores in late pregnancy to be physiological and reserves the term *iron deficiency* for stages (b) and (c) (IOM 90,93).

Anemia is more common in nonpregnant diabetic women than in controls at any level of albuminuria or GFR (Astor 02, Craig 05), and the strongest predictor of iron status in the group of diabetic women with normal renal function was Tf saturation (Thomas 03a). The soluble truncated form of cell-surface transferrin receptor (sTfR) found in serum reflects the receptor density on cells (Skikne 90, Feelders 99), and "sTfR correlates inversely with the amount of iron available for tissues, and directly with the rate of erythropoiesis" (Akkeson 02). Current research focuses on increased sTfR levels as a marker for iron deficiency in diabetes (De Block 00a, Hernandez 05) and in pregnancy (Akkeson 98, Rusia 99, Choi 00, Akkeson 02) or focuses on decreased sTfR levels as a marker of iron excess (Khumalo 98). sTfR levels are not affected by inflammation or chronic disease, and there is less day-to-day variation than seen with ferritin (Ferguson 92, Cooper 96, Punnonen 97). sTfR is not yet studied in diabetic pregnant women.

Iron deficiency in pregnancy is associated with poor weight gain, and microcytic anemia is associated with increased risk for low BW due to preterm delivery (Lieberman 88, Scholl 92,94,97, IOM 00b, Scanlon 00). However, the putative effects of iron-deficiency anemia may be confounded by many demographic or biological factors (Klebanoff 89, Allen 01). Other epidemiological data suggest that optimal pregnancy outcomes occur with a diluted midpregnancy hemoglobin concentration of 9–11 gm/dL up to 12–13 gm/dL (Murphy 86, Steer 95, Stephansson 00, Little 05) or a hematocrit of 30–38% (Knottnerus 90, Lu 91), viewed as an effect of increased plasma volume (Koller 79, Huisman 86). The incidence of hypertension increases in pregnancy as baseline hemoglobin rises above 12 gm/dL (Murphy 86). The less that hemoglobin declines (or the more it rises) per week in early pregnancy, the greater the risk of fetal growth restriction and stillbirth, even excluding cases of preeclampsia or fetal malformation (Stephansson 00). Indexes of low-iron status obtained before or in early pregnancy and before the effects of hemodilution are more reliable predictors of poor pregnancy outcome (Scholl 05). Diet-induced severe iron-deficiency anemia in pregnant rhesus monkeys had no effect on fetal growth or neurological function after birth (Golub 06). Effects of anemia in diabetic pregnancies without proteinuria are not well studied.

Recent placebo-controlled RCTs of iron supplementation in nonanemic, nondiabetic pregnant women showed significantly reduced frequencies of preterm delivery and low BW at term (Christian 03, Cogswell 03b), although a Cochrane meta-analysis of

20 RCTs of iron supplementation showed no benefit (Mahomed 04). Some think the recent studies support prenatal iron supplementation regardless of baseline iron status to improve pregnancy outcome (Rasmussen 01,03), but similar trials have not been conducted in pregnant diabetic women in whom iron excess may be more of a risk.

Iron excess. Most clinicians worry about iron deficiency, but iron excess is possible as well. Free iron can damage tissues by participating in the formation of toxic free radicals, such as hydroxide and the superoxide anion (Andrews 99, Sulieman 04). At least three mechanisms link free iron to oxidative stress and early atherosclerosis (Ramakrishna 03, Ferrera 05). First, Fe^{2+} oxidizes H_2O_2 and leads to its autooxidation and the generation of hydroxyl radical, which in turn initiate lipid peroxidation (Grinshtein 03). Second, heme can initiate the oxidation of LDL (Camejo 98). Third, iron is essential for synthesis of enzymes that play a role in atherosclerosis, such as 5-lipooxygenase and myelo peroxidase (Brennan 02, Mehrabian 02). Iron depletion may even contribute to vascular protection (Ferrera 05, Sullivan 05, Zheng 05).

Possible diabetes-related mechanisms contributing to cellular iron excess include (a) insulin resistance and hyperinsulinemia, causing increased plasma Tf (Fernadez-Real 02); (b) insulin stimulation of adipocyte iron uptake by redistributing Tf receptors to the cell membrane (Davis 86); and (c) glycation of Tf that decreases its ability to bind ferrous iron and increases the pool of free iron (Reif 92, Fujimoto 95). Nontransferrin-bound iron in plasma (Gosriwatana 99, Breuer 00, Jacobs 05) was detected in the great majority of patients with type 2 diabetes in a Korean study, even when Tf was not fully saturated (Lee 06a). Iron excess outside of pregnancy is suggested by a Tf saturation >45% and persistently elevated serum ferritin >100 mcg/L, but controversy remains as to whether serum ferritin is an appropriate marker (Lee 04a, Pietrangelo 04). Recent data suggest that relative iron excess may exist in blood and tissues of diabetic women (Lao 01, Fernandez-Real 02, Jiang 04), which could contribute to oxidative stress in the placenta (Hubel 98, Casanueva 03, Milczarek 06). Some investigators propose that excessive oral iron supplementation during pregnancy could temporarily result in iron overload and increase oxidative stress (Scholl 98, Lao 00, Lachili 01, Devrim 06). They also speculate that twice-weekly dosing would be just as effective in preventing anemia (Ridwan 96, Ekstrom 02, Pena-Rosas 04) and would avoid daily exposure of the intestinal mucosa to high luminal iron contents, which may contribute to oxidative stress at that tissue site (Casanueva 03). Clinical trials are needed in diabetic women to test these hypotheses.

Placental–fetal iron balance. Maternal Tf iron is taken up by placental TfR-1 on the brush border of syncytiotrophoblast, with rapid iron transfer to the fetus via endosome to cytoplasm (perhaps involving DMT1) (Georgieff 00, Chong 05, Gunshin 05), unknown cytoplasm transport mechanisms, and export via ferroportin (McKie 05) and copper oxidase (Danzeisen 02) to fetal Tf (Gambling 01, O'Brien 03, Bradley 04, Morris 04, Gruper 05, Bastin 06). Hepcidin action on placenta is thought to involve transcriptional downregulation of the iron uptake machinery (Martin 04). Iron is stored as ferritin in trophoblast cells (Petry 94, Georgieff 99), and there is a ferritin receptor in placental microvilli (Liao 01). Iron regulatory protein-1 (IRP-1) is a cytoplasmic apoprotein that binds to iron-responsive elements in the untranslated regions of the mRNAs for TfR-1 and ferritin, stabilizing the mRNAs by preventing binding of RNases (Eisenstein 00). In the human third-trimester placenta, IRP-1 correlated inversely with ferritin protein expression, but not with placental TfR-1 and ferroportin expression (Bradley 04). A ferritin subunit in syncytiotrophoblast appears to have immunomodulatory activity (Moroz 02, Nahum 04). Regarding maternal iron deficiency, there is upregulation of placental TfR-1, DMT1, and copper oxidase (Gambling 01), and IRP-1 mRNA is more highly expressed in iron-deficient placentae (Georgieff 99, Bradley 04). Recent evidence also demonstrates the regulation of iron transfer to the fetus at the level of the maternal intestine, which "suggests that the iron needs of the fetus take priority over maternal requirements" (O'Brien 03, Millard 06). Additional research is needed to determine whether abnormal iron balance in diabetic pregnancy or maternal–fetal hyperglycemia/hyperinsulinemia contributes to glycosylation and reduced binding affinity of placental TfR-1 (Petry 94, Georgieff 97,99) and low iron stores in infants of diabetic women (Georgieff 90, Petry 92).

Selenium. This trace element functions through an association with enzymic proteins (14 selenoproteins are known in animals) in (a) defense against oxidative stress via glutathione peroxidases and selenoprotein P, (b) regulation of thyroid hormone metabolism via iodothyronine deiodinases, and (c) regeneration of ascorbic acid from its oxidized metabolites via thioredoxin reductases (IOM 00a). Selenomethionine and selenocysteine are found in plants where selenium is present in the soil and in animal proteins and fish, and both are efficiently absorbed. Selenomethionine can substitute for methionine in humans, but the biologically active form of selenium per se is selenocysteine (IOM 00a). The body selenomethionine pool contributes to available selenocysteine via turnover of the methionine pool, and the other reserve pool is liver glutathione peroxidase that, in a state of deficiency, can provide selenium to be available for synthesis of other selenoenzymes (IOM 00a). Selenocysteine and ingested selenite and selenate are metabolized to selenide, which is (a) further metabolized to selenophosphate, the precursor of selenocysteine in selenoproteins and of selenium in transfer RNA; or (b) selenide is converted to excretory metabolites. Apparently, excretion is responsible for maintaining selenium homeostasis (IOM 00a).

The inorganic forms of selenium, selenate and selenite, are commonly used to fortify foods and as supplements (IOM 00a). The EAR for selenium is based on the criterion of maximizing plasma glutathione peroxidase activity. The major form of selenium in blood is selenoprotein P, but there is lack of an assay. The RDA for women aged 19–50 before pregnancy is 55 μg (0.7 μmol)/day, and it is increased to 60 μg (0.76 μmol)/day for pregnancy in women aged 14–50 to provide 4 μg/day for fetal deposition. The tolerable UL is based on hair and nail brittleness and loss and is 400 μg (5.1 μmol)/day for pregnancy (IOM 00a). Distribution of food from high- to low-selenium areas usually prevents dietary insufficiency in the U.S. and Canada. The 10th–90th perecentiles of dietary selenium intake were 107–174 μg/day in 211 pregnant participants in the NHANES III 1988–1994 U.S. nutritional survey based on dietary recall and food tables (IOM 00a). Serum selenium levels in nonpregnant women in this survey were well above the threshold (7–9 μg/dL; 0.8–1.1 μmol/L) for maximization of plasma selenoproteins (IOM 00). Data on selenium status during pregnancy are inconsistent (Butler 82, Swanson 83, Cenac 92, Zachara 93, Ferrer 99, Mihailovic 00, Fett 02, Chen 03, Orhan 03, Al-Saleh 04, Lorenzo 05). Late pregnancy brings good absorption of selenium and conservation by decreased urinary excretion (King 01). Evidence suggests an impaired selenium status in pregnancies complicated by diabetes (Tan 01, Hawkes 04, Al-Saleh 05). A single study of dietary intake showed decreased selenium intake (and lower serum selenium levels) in pregnant women with impaired glucose tolerance (IGT) compared with controls (Bo 05).

Examples of illness due to inadequate selenium intake coupled with another stress (IOM 00a) include lipid peroxidation, hepatic necrosis, myocarditis, Keshan's pediatric cardiomyopathy, and perhaps intrahepatic cholestasis of pregnancy (Kauppila 87, Reyes 00). Because selenoproteins act as antioxidants and peroxynitrite scavengers, investigation is ongoing into the role of selenium status in CVD (Flores-Mateo 06) and complications of diabetes (Faure 03). Studies of experimental diabetes show that selenium deficiency produces insulin resistance, cardiac contractile dysfunction, and hepatic ultrastructural pathology; selenium replacement has protective effects (Can 05, Ayaz 06, Mueller 06). Selenium plasma concentrations were lower than those of controls in patients with type 1 and type 2 diabetes, being just below or at the low range of the 7–9-µg/dL threshold (Ruiz 98, Navarro-Alarcon 99, Kljai 01). Selenium levels had an inverse relationship with A1C (Kljai 01); urinary concentration of selenium did not differ in diabetic subjects versus controls (Navarro-Alarcon 99). Selenium measurements in erythrocytes and toenails have been lower in diabetic subjects than in controls, which is associated with impaired erythrocyte glutathione peroxidase activity (Osterode 96, Kruse-Jarres 00, Kljai 01, Raipathak 05). Selenium supplementation versus placebo in subjects with type 2 diabetes raised plasma selenium and erythrocyte glutathione peroxidase activity; it also reduced the diabetes-related excess of nuclear factor-kappa B in blood mononuclear cells (a marker for oxidative stress associated with CVD) (Faure 04).

Low selenium as well as folate status after pregnancy was associated with delivery of an infant with a neural tube defect (NTD) in Spain, coupled with a marker for increased homocysteine (Hcy) transsulfuration (Martin 04). There are two reports of low selenium status in women with preeclampsia, and an RCT of low-dose selenium supplements in pregnancy is underway (Rayman 03, Atamer 05). In a small longitudinal study, erythrocyte selenium decreased during pregnancy to a greater degree in diabetic than in control women, coupled with decreased activity of glutathione peroxidase (Twardowska 94). Maternal blood selenium at delivery did not differ between diabetic women and normal pregnant controls in another study (Al-Saleh 05). Research is needed on selenium intake, metabolism, function, and excretion in diabetic pregnant women.

Zinc. Zinc is a component of catalytic enzymes involved in the maintenance of structural proteins and regulation of gene expression (IOM 00a). Zinc deficiency due to malabsorption or increased urinary zinc loss is associated with diverse clinical outcomes including impaired growth, immune dysfunction, diarrhea, dermatitis, defects in carbohydrate usage, poor wound healing in diabetes, teratogenesis, intrauterine growth restriction, and premature birth (Sandstead 97, IOM 00a, King 00b, Franz 02, Keen 03). Many investigators report increased urinary excretion of zinc with inadequately controlled diabetes (McNair 81, Heise 88, Cunningham 94, Cooper 05). However, blood cell levels of zinc were elevated in adults and children with type 1 diabetes compared with controls, and they correlated with elevated A1C (Kruse-Jarres 00). Plasma zinc level, usually tightly regulated at 65.0–97.5 µg/dL (10–15 µmol/L) in spite of decreased or increased intake, is an insensitive indicator of zinc status (King 90, King 94, IOM 00a). Lower cutoffs (2.5th percentile) have been proposed for use in pregnancy (50 µg/dL) based on reanalysis of data from NHANES II (Hotz 03). Stress, infection, and trauma can lower plasma zinc levels via the actions of cortisol and IL (IOM 00a). Other bioassays are also used to determine zinc deficiency (Sandstead 97, IOM 00a). Most total body zinc is found in skeletal muscle and bone, and circulating zinc in plasma is highly bound to albumin and α_2-macroglobulin (IOM 00a). Bioavailability of zinc is greatest from flesh foods (meat, poultry, fish) because phytate and fiber in cereals and legumes may impair absorption (Fung 97). Foods from cow milk provide ~20% of dietary zinc (Sandstead 96). Alcohol, tobacco, and iron supplementation may interfere with zinc absorption.

The pregnancy RDA for zinc (11 mg/day) is based on the minimal quantity necessary to match total daily excretion, the average rate of zinc accumulation by the maternal and fetal tissues by late pregnancy (0.73 mg/day), and a fractional absorption of 27% (IOM 00a). The UL (40 mg/day) is based on impairment of copper absorption and reduction in erythrocyte copper–zinc superoxide dismutase activity (IOM 00a). National surveys pertaining to the intake of zinc from food show that ~40% of women of reproductive age consume less than the RDA (IOM 00a), with similar findings in smaller studies of nondiabetic pregnant women (Mathews 99, Morris 01, Swenson 01, Turner 03). Mean dietary intake of zinc for pregnant women with type 1 diabetes was estimated to be 10.5 mg/day, which is significantly higher than the value of 8.7 mg/day in matched controls in a small observational study (Bates 97). Zinc supplementation has reduced low BW and prematurity and increased fetal femur length in some (Scholl 93, Goldenberg 95, Merialdi 04), but not all, interventional studies (Keen 03, Merialdi 03, Villar 03). No large-scale observational or interventional studies relating zinc status to outcome in pregnant diabetic women have been conducted.

Antioxidants and Vitamins

Vitamin C. Vitamin C (ascorbate) is an electron donor cofactor for many enzymes and provides reducing equivalents to quench a variety of reactive oxygen and nitrogen species in aqueous environments (IOM 00a). Ascorbic acid deficiency has been associated with increased infections, premature rupture of membranes, and preterm birth (IOM 00a, Casanueva 05). In pregnancy, plasma vitamin C decreases secondary to hemodilution and active transfer of the reduced form to the fetus. Further decreases are associated with tobacco smoking and preeclampsia in nonsmoking women (Mikhail 94, Chappell 02). The intestinal absorption rate of vitamin C is 70–90% before and during pregnancy up to doses of 1,000 mg; bioavailability is similar from foods and supplements. Primary food sources include citrus fruits, tomatoes, potatoes, and green and yellow vegetables. The EAR is based on adding the average requirement to obtain the near-maximal neutrophil ascorbate concentration for antioxidant protection of the nonpregnant woman to the amount necessary to transfer adequate vitamin C to the fetus (IOM 00a). No evidence states that the RDA for pregnancy (85 mg/day) should differ in diabetic women; subgroups of pregnant women using cigarettes, alcohol, aspirin, or street drugs may have a higher requirement. The UL in pregnancy (2,000 mg/day) is based on avoiding gastrointestinal disturbances (IOM 00a). Median dietary intake of vitamin C in pregnancy varied from 110 to 133 mg/day in several studies, with 8–25% of women consuming less than two-thirds of the RDA (Mathews 99, IOM 00a, Swensen 01, Turner 03). Mean intake from food *and* prenatal vitamins was 251 mg on 1 day in normotensive nondiabetic pregnant women and slightly higher in women developing gestational hypertension or preeclampsia (Morris 01). Mean dietary intake of vitamin C was estimated at 85 mg/day in 38 pregnant women with type 1 diabetes in Northern Ireland and 83 mg/day in controls (Bates 97). Intervention trials are discussed later in this section.

Vitamin E. Vitamin E (α-tocopherol) is a nonspecific chain-breaking antioxidant that reduces lipid peroxidation (IOM 00a). Intestinal absorption of vitamin E in humans is of low efficiency and is dependent on fat intake, micelle formation, and secretion of chylomicrons. Uptake of chylomicron remnants by the liver leads to secretion of α-tocopherol in VLDLs, and this process controls plasma α-tocopherol concentrations (IOM 00a). Most dietary vitamin E is present in fat, edible vegetable oils, and fortified cereals (Leonard 04). The EAR is based on maintaining a plasma α-tocopherol concentration that limits hydrogen peroxide–induced hemolysis to <13% (IOM 00a). The plasma concentration rises in pregnancy in parallel with an increase in total lipids, exhibiting relatively constant but limited placental transport (Debier 05). The RDA for pregnant and nonpregnant women of any age is set at 15 mg/day, and the UL for both groups is 1,000 mg/day of any form of supplementary α-tocopherol because there is no evidence of adverse effects from consumption of vitamin E in foods (IOM 00a). U.S. nutrition surveys revealed intakes lower than the RDA in 90% of pregnant subjects (IOM 00a). Average dietary intake of vitamin E was estimated to be only 5.8 mg/day in 683 pregnant women in southern England (Mathews 99); it was 5.2 mg/day in well-controlled Irish women with type 1 diabetes in early pregnancy and 4.9 mg/day in matched controls (Bates 97). Mean intake of vitamin E from food *and* prenatal vitamins was only 11.0 mg on 1 day in 3,125 women remaining normotensive in pregnancy in North America, with similar intakes noted in the 721 women developing gestational hypertension or 311 women diagnosed with preeclampsia (Morris 01), confirming a prior case–control study (Schiff 96). Whether "deficient" intake of vitamin E or low plasma levels of α-tocopherol are associated with poor placental growth or risk of preeclampsia remains controversial because smaller studies presented conflicting results (Wang 91, Mikhail 94, Jain 95, Schiff 96, Gratecos 98, Chappell 02). Recently, plasma α-tocopherol concentration at entry and 28 weeks gestation was positively related to fetal growth and a decreased risk of SGA births (Scholl 06). As noted, data on diabetic pregnant women are insufficient to draw conclusions.

Oxidative and nitrosative stress is increased in diabetes (Ceriello 98, Marra 02, Endemann 04, Manuel-Kenoy 05, Sies 05) and its complications (Brownlee 01, Sheetz 02, Hodgkinson 03, He 04b, Lassegue 04); in pregnancy, this stress is associated with diabetic embryopathy (Reece 04b, Hobbs 05a) and preeclampsia (Walsh 98, Roberts 99, Redman 03, Poston 04, Charles 06). Plasma antioxidants are reduced in adult female subjects with type 1 (Marra 02) and type 2 diabetes (Ceriello 98), including pregnant diabetic patients (Carrone 93, Twardowska 94, Orhan 03, Djordjevic 04, Peuchant 04, Toescu 04, Rajdl 05). Although oxidative stress contributes to atherogenesis and vascular dysfunction (Touyz 04), it is important to note that low-level reactive oxygen species (ROS) are essential to normal functioning of the cellular components of the vessel wall (Griendling 00). Intracellular and extracellular ROS levels are dependent on the balance between at least six pro-oxidant enzymes that mediate ROS production and seven enzymes involved in the removal of ROS, all of which vary in activity in different vascular cells (Griendling 05). The different sources and actions of various ROS (superoxide O_2^-, hydroxyl radical HO, NO, ROO^- [unpaired electrons in their outer orbital], oxidants H_2O_2, peroxynitrite) have been recently reviewed (Leopold 05, Mueller 05). The complexity of ROS-generating systems and cellular antioxidant defenses (Griendling 05) suggests that simplistic provision of antioxidant vitamins may not be successful, and approaches that target cellular enzymes may be helpful in reducing atherogenesis (Ceriello 06).

The question arises whether to prescribe pharmacological doses of antioxidant vitamins to pregnant women with PDM (Franz 02). Although large observational studies of nonpregnant subjects (Stanner 04) show correlations between dietary or supplemental consumption of antioxidant vitamins and various clinical outcomes (Franz 02, Costacou 06), placebo-controlled trials of vitamins C and E have generally not shown benefit in reducing CVD (Yusuf 00, PPP 01, Knekt 04, Bleys 06); whether they may cause harm is controversial (Hathcock 05, Miller 05). Vitamins C and E may not affect intracellular/organelle-generated ROS, may themselves have pro-oxidant effects by enhancing conversion of $\cdot O_2^-$ to H_2O_2 (Mueller 05), and do not scavenge H_2O_2 and HOCl (Touyz 04). Vitamin C also may interact with redox active iron in patients with diabetes (Lee 06a). Eating a well-balanced diet and emphasizing natural antioxidants in food may be more effective than use of supplements in reducing CVD (John 02, Trichopoulos 04, Blomhoff 05). Consumption of fruits, vegetables, and olive oil increases the antioxidant capacity measured in serum (Pitsavos 05), and tables of redox-active foods with ranked antioxidant contents have been published. Ginger, cinnamon, walnuts, pecans, chocolate (unsweetened), black pepper, artichokes, berries, and bran or whole-grain cereals lead the list (Halvorsen 06).

Preliminary studies showed reduction of preeclampsia with supplementation of vitamins C (1,000 mg/day) and E (180 mg/day) starting at 16–22 weeks gestation (Chappell 99). A similar trial is apparently being conducted in pregnant women with PDM (Holmes 04). Another RCT in high-risk subjects, including pregnant women with PDM, was unfortunately terminated prematurely due to lack of funding; the results suggested that 500–950 subjects would be necessary in each arm to fairly test the hypothesis of a significant reduction in preeclampsia (Beazley 05). However, large multicenter randomized trials of antioxidant vitamin therapy in nondiabetic women failed to prevent preeclampsia (Poston 06, Rumbold 06, Spinnato 07).

Two large trials of vitamin C 1,000 mg/d and vitamin E 400 IU/day starting at 21–22 weeks gestation produced negative results; the first included 1,877 nulliparous women with adequate dietary vitamin intake (Rumbold 06), and the second included 2,404 women with clinical risk factors for preeclampsia (Poston 06). In the latter RCT, preeclampsia developed in 19% of 97 diabetic women and 23% of 435 women with chronic hypertension randomized to treatment with antioxidant vitamins compared with 16% of 102 diabetic subjects and 22% of 422 chronically hypertensive subjects randomized to placebo. In the third RCT, preeclampsia developed in 13.8% of 355 women with chronic hypertension or prior preeclampsia treated daily with vitamin C (1,000 mg) and vitamin E (400 IU) starting at 20 weeks gestation, compared to a rate of 15.6% in 352 similar subjects treated with placebo (Spinnato 07). Because systemic antioxidant vitamins are ineffective, it is suggested that specific targeting of intracellular oxidative processes might be necessary to prevent cardiovascular or diabetic complications (Packer 01, Ceriello 03, Wassman 04, Ceriello 06, Yi 06, Ziegler 06); whether this approach would be helpful or harmful in gestational pathophysiology is unknown. As a further caution, a model has been proposed through which the non-antioxidant regulatory roles of vitamin E are detrimental to human pregnancy via PKC-θ activation and cytokine signaling in trophoblast and maternal immune effector cells (Banerjee 06).

Interventions with antioxidants to prevent diabetic embryopathy have been limited to studies in experimental animals (Chiang 03, Wentzel 03, Reece 04b). It is uncertain whether multivitamin supplements had any role in the beneficial effects of intensified preconception care of diabetes in reducing major malformations (Czeizel 93, Shaw 94,95, Botto 96, Kitzmiller 96, Correa 03, Botto 04, Goh 06). At this time, there is no evidence to support a recommendation for antioxidant vitamin therapy for pregnant women with PDM beyond the current suggested RDAs.

Vitamin A. Vitamin A is a fat-soluble vitamin with several dietary forms. Absorbed vitamin A is packed in chylomicrons and taken up by hepatocytes, where retinyl esters are hydrolyzed into retinol and secreted bound to retinol-binding protein (RBP) when there is a tissue need for vitamin A (Azais-Braesco 00). Circulating RBP-bound retinol is taken up by membranous receptors specific for RBP (as in retinal pigment epithelium and trophoblast) and is transformed within target cells to active retinoic acid, which controls gene transcription through nuclear receptor-mediated events. In addition to its importance for vision, vitamin A influences cell proliferation and differentiation in embryonic development (IOM 00b). Placental transfer of vitamin A is limited but constant, even at the expense of maternal stores; whether the mechanism of transfer involves RBP or lipoproteins is uncertain (Debier 04). Vitamin A deficiency leads to multiple malformations in animal models, but whether malformations are increased in regions of endemic vitamin A deficiency is controversial (Azais 00). On the other hand, it is accepted by most investigators that high doses of vitamin A are teratogenic (Martinez-Frias 90, Werler 90, Dudas 92, Rothman 95, Mills 96).

The EAR for dietary vitamin A is calculated to maintain a given body-pool size in well-nourished subjects during times of stress and low vitamin A intake. During pregnancy, the EAR is increased by 10% to allow adequate accumulation of vitamin A in the liver of the fetus (IOM 00b). The RDA for pregnant women aged 19–50 is set at 770 μcg/day retinol activity equivalents (RAE) (1,000 IU = 300 μcg RAE). The UL of preformed vitamin A intake is 3,000 μcg/day in women of reproductive age, including pregnancy, using teratogenicity as the critical adverse event (IOM 00b). The 25th percentile of intake from food in nonpregnant adult women aged 19–30 years was only 388 μcg RAE/day (428 μcg RAE/day for ages 31–50) in the NHANES III (1988–1994) nutrition survey. Thus, many of these women at potential risk of pregnancy consumed <56% of the RDA. Median intake of vitamin A from food in 346 pregnant women was only 691 μcg RAE/day in the same survey (IOM 00b). Regarding possible exposure to excess vitamin A, the 90th percentile of intake during pregnancy was 1,118 μcg RAE/day from food plus 1,120 μcg RAE/day in 118 women using supplements. These figures are similar to a median *total* intake of 1,734 μcg RAE/day in a cohort of 95 pregnant Women, Infants, and Children (WIC) public health program recipients (Swenson 01) and a mean *total* intake of 1,230 mcg RAE on 1 day at 13–21 weeks gestation in 3,125 healthy women at five centers in the U.S. (Morris 01). In a sample of 38 pregnant women with type 1 diabetes, dietary intake of both vitamin A and β-carotene was slightly above the reference nutrient intake set by the Department of Health for the U.K. in 1991 (Bates 97). Intake and status of vitamin A is poorly studied in diabetic pregnancy.

Vitamin K. Vitamin K is a coenzyme for the synthesis of proteins involved in blood coagulation and bone metabolism (osteocalcin). Phylloquinone, the plant form of the vitamin, is absorbed in the small intestine and secreted into lymph as a component of chylomicrons. It circulates in blood in VLDL and chylomicron remnants, which are taken up in the liver where phylloquinone is stored (IOM 00b). Phylloquinone is found in highest concentration in green vegetables, plant oils, and margarine. The AI for adult women is based on representative median dietary intake data from healthy individuals (90 μcg/day). Vitamin K does not cross the placenta, and there are no data on fetal content on which to estimate additional needs during pregnancy; therefore, the AI level is unchanged for pregnancy. No data suggest adverse effects from a high intake of phylloquinone; therefore, no UL is provided (IOM 00b). Intake of vitamin K and its influence on maternal health has not been assessed in diabetic pregnant women.

B-complex vitamins. The water-soluble B-complex vitamins are considered in two categories of action: (a) reactions of intermediary metabolism related to energy production and redox status and (b) transfer of single-carbon (methyl) units (IOM 98). Thiamin, riboflavin, niacin, vitamin B6, and pantothenic acid are required for various reactions in category (a), and they are also important for synthesis of amino acids, fatty acids, cholesterol, steroids, and glucose. Folate is involved in the supply of single-carbon units for DNA synthesis. Folate, vitamin B12, choline, betaine, and riboflavin are required for methyl group ($-CH_3$) transfer reactions (Mason 03) involved in the generation of Hcy. The water-soluble B-vitamins are actively transported across the placenta against a concentration gradient, and maternal B-vitamin status predicts biochemical indexes of the B-vitamins in cord sera (Obeid 05). If usable experimental data were lacking to set specific EARs and RDAs or AIs for these vitamins in pregnancy, the IOM based the recommended values on obligatory fetal transfer and maternal needs related to increases in energy or protein metabolism (IOM 98). U.S. nutrition surveys from 1988 to 1996 revealed that 15–25% of 379 pregnant subjects consumed less than the RDA values from food sources for thiamine, riboflavin, niacin, and vitamin B6, and >95% consumed inadequate folate (IOM 98 appendixes).

Thiamin. Thiamin (B1) is absorbed at low efficiency, mainly in the jejunum, and is carried in the blood in erythrocytes and plasma. The major U.S. food sources for thiamin are fortified or whole-grain bread products and ready-to-eat cereals (IOM 98). The basis for estimating the adult EAR combines erythrocyte transketolase activity, urinary thiamin excretion, and other findings. Clinical signs of deficiency (beriberi, anorexia and weight loss, enlarged heart, mental changes) occur at thiamin intakes <0.3 mg/1,000 kcal/day. The RDA for pregnant women of any age is 1.4 mg/day of thiamin, an increase of 30% from preconception based on increased growth in maternal and fetal compartments and a small increase in energy usage (IOM 98). Data concerning adverse effects of high doses of thiamin were not sufficient to set a UL. Thiamine and its derivatives are increasingly studied for beneficial effects on diabetes complications by decreasing metabolic cycling through a variety of pathways of glucose-related damage (Brownlee 01, Hammes 03, Bloomgarden 05). The only study of dietary intake of thiamin in diabetic pregnant women (Bates 97) showed that a small percentage of subjects consumed less than the RDA. Mean thiamin intake from food *and* prenatal vitamins was estimated to be 5.5 mg on 1 day in a large survey of normotensive nondiabetic pregnant women (Morris 01). No thiamine intervention studies in diabetic pregnant women have been conducted.

Riboflavin. Most dietary riboflavin (B2) is consumed in a complex with food protein. Gastric acidification releases riboflavin coenzymes that are hydrolyzed to riboflavin, which is absorbed in the proximal small intestine by a saturable rapid transport system (IOM 98). In the U.S., the greatest contribution to riboflavin intake comes from milk beverages, bread products, and fortified cereals. The adult EAR is based on a combination of erythrocyte glutathione reductase activity and urinary riboflavin excretion. Clinical signs of deficiency (stomatitis, dermatitis, anemia) appear at intakes <0.6 mg/day. The RDA for riboflavin for pregnant women of any age is 1.4 mg/day, which is an increase of ~27% from preconception based on increased maternal and fetal compartments and a small increase in energy usage. Data concerning adverse effects from high doses of riboflavin were not sufficient for setting a UL. Only a small percentage of healthy pregnant women (Turner 03) and diabetic women (Bates 97) consumed less than the RDA in studies of dietary intake, and mean intake of riboflavin from food, drink, and prenatal vitamins was estimated to be 3.9 mg/day in 3,125 normotensive nondiabetic pregnant women (Morris 01). No riboflavin intervention studies in diabetic pregnant women have been conducted.

Niacin. The term niacin (B3) refers to nicotinamide, nicotinic acid, and derivatives that have the biological activities of nicotinamide (IOM 98). Niacin is rapidly absorbed from the stomach and intestine. In the U.S., the major food sources of niacin are mixed dishes high in meat, fish, or poultry; enriched and whole-grain bread products; and fortified ready-to-eat cereals. The primary criterion used to estimate the EAR for adult females is urinary excretion of niacin metabolites (IOM 98). Clinical signs of deficiency (pellagra: localized pigmented rash, gastroenteritis, and neurologic deficits, including cognitive decline) may appear with an intake <10 mg/2,500 kcal/day. It is estimated that the need for niacin increases by 27% in pregnancy to cover increased energy use and maternal–fetal growth. The RDA for pregnant women of any age is 18 mg/day of niacin equivalents. The UL for niacin doses in pregnant women is 35 mg/day based on flushing as the critical adverse event.

Intake of niacin from food in healthy pregnant women was 19 and 24 mg/day for the 25th and 75th percentiles in a sample of women using WIC services (Turner 03), and mean intake from food plus supplements was 47 mg on 1 day in a large survey of normotensive, nondiabetic women (Morris 01). Mean dietary intake of niacin was estimated to be 17.8 mg/day in a sample of pregnant women with type 1 diabetes in Northern Ireland, which was significantly higher than 14.7 mg/day in matched controls (Bates 97). Observational studies of the relationship between niacin intake and the outcome of pregnancy are inadequate in both healthy and diabetic pregnant women. The only interventional studies of niacin in pregnancy are sporadic reports of treatment of hypertriglyceridemia.

Vitamin B6. Vitamin B6 comprises a group of six compounds, but the major form in humans is pyridoxal 5′ phosphate (PLP). Large doses are well absorbed in the gut by passive diffusion. PLP is protein bound in plasma, erythrocytes, and tissues, which protects it from the action of phosphatases (IOM 98). Main food sources of vitamin B6 in the U.S. are fortified cereals; mixed foods with meat, fish, or poultry as the main ingredient; starchy vegetables; and noncitrus fruits (IOM 98). The criterion used to estimate the EAR for adult women (1.1 mg/day of vitamin B6 in food) is the intake needed to maintain the plasma PLP level at ≥20 nmol/L (IOM 98). Clinical signs of B6 deficiency (seborrheic dermatitis, microcytic anemia, convulsions, depression, confusion) may appear with intakes <0.5 mg/day. The RDA for pregnancy (1.9 mg/day) is set 33% higher than preconception to cover the increased metabolic needs and weight of the gravida and fetal–placental requirements. The UL for pyridoxine supplementation for pregnant women ≥19 years is 100 mg/day based on the risk of sensory neuropathy (IOM 98).

Blood indicators of B6 status progressively decrease to a greater extent than explained by hemodilution during pregnancy, and the fetus sequesters PLP at concentrations much higher than maternal (IOM 98). However, the IOM found little evidence of clinical problems related to B6 status in pregnancy except for reports of even lower PLP levels in patients with preeclampsia, perhaps due to the reduced action of placental enzymes involved in PLP synthesis (IOM 98). Two small surveys of dietary intake of vitamin B6 in healthy pregnant women reported median levels of 1.9 mg/day (Turner 03) and 2.0 mg/day (Swensen 01), while the mean intake from food plus prenatal vitamins was 8.7 mg on 1 day at 13–21 weeks in 3,125 normotensive, nondiabetic women (Morris 01). Mean intakes were almost identical in women developing gestational hypertension or preeclampsia. Vitamin B6 intakes are not reported in pregnant women with PDM, and there are no intervention trials of pyridoxine except for sporadic reports of treatment for hyperemesis gravidarum.

Folate. Folate is a generic term for the water-soluble vitamin that exists in many chemical forms (IOM 98). Food folates (polyglutamate derivatives) are most commonly found in green vegetables, grains, and citrus fruits. Folic acid itself is uncommon in food, but it is the stable form used in vitamin supplements and fortified food products. Since 1998, all enriched cereal grains (bread, pasta, flour, breakfast cereal, rice) in the U.S. are required to be fortified with folic acid, so those foods have become the largest source of folate for women of reproductive age. Folate deficiency first leads to a decrease in serum folate concentration; it then leads to decreased erythrocyte folate, a rise in Hcy concentration, and megaloblastic changes "in the bone marrow and other tissues with rapidly dividing cells," followed by macrocytic anemia (IOM 98). The EAR for adults is based on quantities of consumed folate that will maintain normal blood concentrations of erythrocyte folate, plasma or serum folate, and plasma Hcy.

The effect of folate on human reproduction has been well reviewed (Bailey 05, Tamura 06). Randomized trials indicate that periconception supplementation with folic acid in addition to dietary folate intake will reduce the frequency of midline embryonic neurulation defects (IOM 98, Bailey 03), including those in IDMs (Correa 06). Due to the risk of NTDs (CDC 92,98), "it is recommended that women capable of becoming pregnant consume 400 μcg of folic acid daily from supplements, fortified foods, or both, in addition to consuming food folate from a varied diet" (IOM 98). Hypotheses stating that impaired absorption of polyglutamate folates (Boddie 00, Molloy 00), maternal obesity (Ray 05), or autoantibodies against folate receptors (Rothenberg 04) may be factors in NTDs have not been tested in diabetic women. Folic acid supplementation may mask symptoms of vitamin B12 deficiency by maintaining a normal mean cell volume. It is optimal to obtain baseline B12 levels in diabetic women with folic acid intake higher than the RDA.

During pregnancy, folate requirements increase substantially due to expansion of maternal erythrocyte number, uterine enlargement, placental development, and fetal growth (IOM 98). Folate is actively transferred to the fetus. The RDA for folate for pregnant women of any age (600 μcg/day of dietary folate equivalents) is based on maintenance of maternal erythrocyte folate and serum folate adjusted for hemodilution in pregnancy (Bailey 00). This intake should be adequate to maintain normal folate status in 97.5% of pregnant women with diabetes (Kaplan 99). The UL of 1,000 μcg/day of folate from fortified foods or supplements is set to avoid the risk of permanent neurological damage in vitamin B12–deficient individuals (IOM 98), as with type 1 diabetes (complete vegetarians, lack of gastric intrinsic factor, intestinal problems with absorption of B12). Comprehensive studies suggest that folate deficiency during gestation is associated with impaired cellular growth and replication resulting in megaloblastic anemia, spontaneous abortions, fetal malformations, placental abruption, and preterm delivery and low BW independent of birth defects (Giles 71, IOM 90, Scholl 96, Shaw 97, Ray 99, Frenkel 00, George 02, Siega-Riz 04, Bailey 05). Folic acid fortification may have decreased the NTD rate by ~50% (Mills 04). On the other hand, folic acid supplementation may increase the rate of dizygotic twinning (Kallen 04, Signore 05).

Prior to fortification of enriched grains, mean or median dietary intake of folate was only 217–294 mcg/day in nondiabetic (Mathews 99, Swenson 01) and diabetic pregnant women (Bates 97, Kaplan 99). Mean estimated intake of folate from food plus prenatal vitamins was 584 μcg on 1 day at 13–21 weeks gestation prior to food fortification in a large sample of normotensive, nondiabetic pregnant women in a U.S. multicenter study (Morris 01). In diabetic women using prenatal supplements, erythrocyte and serum folate levels were significantly higher than in supplemented pregnant controls (Kaplan 99). This is the only observational study to evaluate whether maternal folate status is affected by diabetes, and few dietary intake data in pregnant diabetic women have been reported since food fortification. In view of the increased frequency of pregnancy loss and preterm labor in diabetic women, observational and interventional studies are needed in this high-risk population. Food fortification of grains in North America has raised the average folic acid intake by 76–240 mcg/day (Choumenkovitch 02, Quinlavan 03, Dietrich 05). Still, one-third of pregnant women in Canada (Sherwood 06) and >50% of American women (especially in ethnic minorities) (Bentley 06, Yang 07) may not have adequate folate intake. In a study of urban pregnant women using prenatal vitamins after fortification of the food supply, dietary folate equivalents rarely exceeded 1,000 mcg/day (Stark 05). However, prenatal vitamins with a 1,000 mcg folic acid/dose would result in a total folate intake in excess of the UL in U.S. women eating fortified foods.

U.S. (ACOG 03) and Canadian obstetrical societies (Allen 07) have recommended high-dose folic acid supplementation (4–5 mg/day) in diabetic women before and during pregnancy based on the increased risk of congenital malformations in their babies. The reader should note that prospective preconception care programs generally did not use such high-dose supplementation of folic acid when they achieved low rates of congenital malformations in IDMs (Ray 01b). Other authors caution that high doses of folic acid may aggravate B12 vitamin deficiency and promote neoplasia in diabetic women (Capel 07).

Vitamin B12. Vitamin B12 (cobalamin) is essential for normal formation of erythrocytes and optimal neurological function and has a role in Hcy metabolism. Adult women obtain vitamin B12 from meat, fish, or poultry; eggs; milk beverages; and fortified ready-to-eat cereals (IOM 98). Small amounts of B12 are absorbed via an active process that requires an intact stomach, parietal cell intrinsic factor, pancreatic sufficiency, and a normally functioning terminal ileum (IOM 98). In the small intestine, B12 binds with intrinsic factor, and the complex moves into the enterocyte. Vitamin B12 enters the circulation bound to specific plasma proteins known as transcobalamins and is taken up by cells via transcobalamin receptors (IOM 98).

The EAR for B12 in adult women (2 μg/day) is based on the amount needed to prevent or correct anemia and to maintain normal plasma or serum B12 values >120–180 pM (>170–275 pg/mL), depending on the laboratory method. Gastrointestinal absorption is estimated at 50%. The RDA (2.4 μg/day) is 120% of the EAR to cover the needs of 97.5% of individuals in a group. Serum methylmalonic acid (MMA) concentrations rise >260–500 nM when the supply of B12 is low, but the MMA assay is laborious and used for research (IOM 98, Refsum 01, Monsen 03). Total serum or plasma Hcy levels are another indicator of B12 status. In pregnancy, absorption of vitamin B12 may increase, but serum levels of total B12 usually decline throughout pregnancy in excess of hemodilution effects (Fernandes-Costa 82). The placenta concentrates the newly absorbed B12 that is then actively transferred to the fetus, with fetal serum B12 levels higher than maternal (Frery 92, IOM 98). The RDA is increased in pregnancy by

10% to 2.6 μg/day to account for fetal deposition throughout gestation and prevent subsequent B12 deficiency in infants (IOM 98). No adverse effects are associated with excess B12 intake from food or supplements in healthy individuals; therefore, there is no UL. Estimated dietary intake of vitamin B12 was 4.2 and 4.9 μcg/day in healthy and diabetic pregnant women, respectively (Bates 97, Turner 03), and was 8.7 μcg/day from food plus prenatal vitamins in a large sample of normotensive, nondiabetic pregnant women (Morris 01). We lack data on B12 intake in vegetarian diabetic women, in whom B12 supplementation should be used. B12 administration also should be considered in pregnant diabetic women who have the possibility of malabsorption.

In a recent study of 406 healthy pregnant women in Denmark, the median value of plasma cobalamin was 161 pM (median MMA 130 nM), and levels of cobalamin at 39 weeks were <150 pM in 43% of subjects (Milman 06b). Maternal B12 concentrations <185 pM were associated with a 3.5-fold risk of spina bifida in a case–control study in the Netherlands, in spite of no differences in folate status between the two groups (Groenen 04). These recent studies indicate that marginal to inadequate B12 status is not uncommon and is not found only in undeveloped countries (Baker 06). As a further example, vitamin B12 deficiency of presumed nutritional origin is described in pregnant women from Brazil (Giugliani 84), China (Ma 04), Malaysia (Sindhu 74), Nepal (Bondevik 01), Turkey (Ackurt 95), and in 55% of pregnant immigrants from India to the U.K. (Roberts 73). Vitamin B12 deficiency was independently associated with preterm birth in China (Ronnenberg 02) and fetal growth restriction in urban India (Muthayya 06). A single study of cobalamin status is available in diabetic pregnant women. The investigators reported normal serum vitamin B12 levels (493 ± 275 pg/mL) in early pregnancy in 15 unsupplemented diabetic women; even in this small group, serum B12 concentration had a significant direct relationship to maternal A1C ($r < 0.6$, $p < 0.05$) (Kaplan 04). We must conclude that vitamin B12 status (as well as folate status) is insufficiently studied in pregnant diabetic women.

Vitamin B12 deficiency classically presents as a megaloblastic, macrocytic anemia indistinguishable from that of folate deficiency, plus various gastrointestinal complaints and neurological complications in 75–90% of affected individuals (IOM 98, Toh 04). Latent forms of B12 deficiency are various, insidious, and not rare (2.6–4.0%) in type 1 diabetes (Ungar 68, Irvine 70, Riley 82, Davis 92, De Block 99, Liu 02). Vitamin B12 deficiency can result from insufficient B12 intake (as witnessed in complete vegetarians), autoimmune atrophic oxyntic gastritis and lack of gastric intrinsic factor (IF) (as in diabetes) (Kokkonen 80), and problems in the small intestine (IOM 98). Billions of oxyntic glands or pits are found within the gastric mucosa in the fundus and body of the stomach. Near the entry to the pits are the mucous neck cells; the parietal cells secreting hydrochloride and IF are deeper in the glands. The peptic (chief) or zymogenic cells secreting pepsinogen are at the base of the glands. Many cases of B12 deficiency are identified as pernicious anemia (PA) due to parietal cell or anti-IF autoantibodies that (a) reduce gastric acid secretion, cause loss of gastric parietal cells, and prevent production of IF; and (b) also "bind to the B12 binding site on intrinsic factor and prevent the formation of the B12-intrinsic factor complex" (IOM 98). Most studies of PA have focused on women of European origin, but a significant prevalence of B12 deficiency is described in China (Chiu 01), Bangladesh (Gamble 05), and India (Refsum 01), with PA noted in Africa (Lothe 69, Mwanda 99), Israel (Zimran 83), India (Britt 71), Japan (Haruma 95), and China (Wun 06). Younger black and Latino women may be more likely to have anti-IF than anti-parietal cell antibodies (PCAbs) (Carmel 92). PA is more common in women than men, usually appearing at >50 years of age, but can be found in younger pregnant women, especially black, Hispanic, and Asian Indian females in the U.S. (Hibbard 70,

Carmel 78, Houston 85, Carmel 87,99,02). Iron-deficiency anemia can be an early marker for autoimmune oxyntic gastritis in 30- to 50-year-old women (Hersshko 06). Recent meta-analyses of limited clinical trials conclude that high-dose oral vitamin B12 is as effective as intramuscular injections in treating B12 deficiency (Vidal-Alaball 05, Butler 06a).

Evidence suggests that the autoantigen in autoimmune oxyntic gastritis and PA is the gastric parietal cell H^+/K^+ ATPase (proton pump) recognized by CD4+ T-cells, which produce TNF-α, help B-cell immunoglobulin production, express cytotoxicity against antigen-presenting cells, and induce apoptosis in target cells (Karlsson 88, Toh 00, D'Elios 01, Bergman 03, D'Elios 05). PCAbs are targeted against the gastric proton pump (Burman 89); thus, there is diminished gastric acid secretion, which decreases iron absorption (Shearman 96). Besides antibodies to H^+/K^+ ATPase and parietal cells, other markers for autoimmune gastritis of the oxyntic gland mucosa include low serum pepsinogen I (reflecting the secretory activity of the glands) (Carmel 87, Lindgren 98a) and elevated gastrin from the G-cells in the antral (pyloric) glands (Lindgren 98b, Rembiasz 05). In type 1 diabetes, hypo- or hyperglycemia can also lead to elevated serum gastrin levels (De Block 99). Although high serum MMA is an indicator of cobalamin deficiency, it is not specific because it can be elevated from impaired renal function in diabetes (Lindgren 02, Herrmann 05a). The role of *Helicobacter pylori* infection as a trigger for the autoimmune process that results in severe atrophic gastritis and PA is uncertain (Fong 91, Ma 94, Annibale 97, Barrio 97, De Block 02a, Hersshko 06).

In type 1 diabetes, observational studies revealed PCAbs in 7–26% of women of European origin <40 years of age (Goldstein 70, Irvine 70, Kokkonen 80, Riley 82, Landin-Olsson 92). In one of the largest series of 245 unselected female outpatients with type 1 diabetes in Belgium, PCAbs were identified in 8 of 46 (17.4%) women aged 20–29, 15 of 72 (20.8%) women aged 30–39, and 15 of 61 (24.6%) women aged 40–49; of 14 PCAb+ patients with gastric symptoms who had gastroscopy, 93% had atrophic gastritis. Of the total PCAb+ group, 34% were positive for antithyroid peroxidase, 27% had hypergastrinemia, 15% had hypochromic microcytic anemia, and 10.5% had PA (De Block 99). Further gastric biopsy studies in this population showed that autoimmune gastritis was present in 57% of 47 PCA+ patients (23% PA) compared with 10% of 41 PCA− patients (2% PA). *H. pylori* infection was present in 53% of the total group, but it did not influence corpus histology or gastrinemia. Concentrations of gastrin correlated strongly with H^+/K^+ ATPase antibody levels and inversely with the percentage of parietal cells per gland. Premalignant lesions were identified in 26% of diabetic PCA+ subjects: enterochromaffin-like cell (ECL) hyperplasia (most had high gastrin levels) or corpus intestinal metaplasia (De Block 03). Gastric emptying was not significantly prolonged in the PCA+ group of type 1 diabetes patients (De Block 02b). In an unselelected group of 91 Spanish women with type 1 diabetes at age 32 ± 10 years, 25% were PCA+. Only 1.6% of the diabetic cohort had cobalamin concentrations <250 pg/mL. Pepsinogen <30 µg/L was noted in 15% and elevated gastrin >100 ng/L in 11%. The authors used low pepsinogen as the indicator for latent PA, but only one-half were PCA+. Nine patients of both sexes had both low pepsinogen and high gastrin; all had PCAs of high titer (>1:640) and focal mucosal atrophy in the gastric body (five with metaplastic intestinal glands and negative *H. pylori* infection status) (Alonso 05).

These and other results support a policy of screening type 1 diabetes patients of European origin for autoimmune gastritis. Data on its prevalence are lacking for women with type 1 diabetes in other ethnic groups. Immunogenetic links between autoimmune diabetes and PA are uncertain (De Block 00b,01). PA found in type 1 diabetes is often associated with autoimmune thyroid disease in both white and black patients (Irvine 70, Davis 92, De Block 99, Perros 00). In the era prior to fetal monitoring, women with type 1 diabetes who later developed PA were noted to have excessive early and late fetal mortality (Beral 84). We are not aware of modern perinatal outcome data in diabetic women with autoimmune gastritis or PA. Gastric autoantibodies cross the placenta, and anti-IF antibody has been associated with vitamin B12 deficiency in the infant (Bar-Shany 67, Fisher 67).

Choline. Choline is an essential dietary component that is a (1) substrate for acetylation to acetylcholine in the terminals of cholinergic neurons, placenta, and elsewhere (neurotransmitter involved in memory storage, muscle function, and much else), (2) precursor for the universal membrane components phosphatidylcholine and sphingomyelin, (3) precursor for platelet-activating factor (potent messenger molecule), and (4) methyl donor upon choline oxidation to betaine (trimethylglycine) (IOM 98, Zeisel 00, Niculescu 02, Zeisel 06a). Thus, choline is essential for cholinergic neurotransmission, the structural integrity of membranes and transmembrane signaling, the role of phosphatidylcholine in the export of excess TG from hepatic cells, the role of betaine in endothelial and renal cell adaption to osmotic stress, and betaine remethylation of Hcy that produces methionine and demethylglycine for single-carbon recycling (IOM 98, Zeisel 00,06a). The interaction of choline, methionine, and folate metabolism occurs at the point of Hcy conversion to methionine (by two parallel pathways: using methyl groups from methyltetrahydrofolate [methyl-THF] or using methyl groups from betaine that are derived from choline) (Zeisel 06a). Transmethylation metabolic pathways closely interconnect choline, methionine, methyl-THF, and vitamins B6 and B12 (Figure I.3). "Perturbing the metabolism of one of these pathways results in compensatory changes in the others. ..... When animals and humans are deprived of choline, they use more methyl-THF to remethylate homocysteine in the liver and increase dietary folate requirements. Conversely, when they are deprived of folate, they use more methyl groups from choline, increasing the dietary requirement form choline" (Niculescu 02).

Choline is found in many foods as free choline and also in esterified forms (especially the phosphatidylcholine-rich fraction lecithin, a food additive). Eggs, milk, liver, and peanuts are rich sources of choline (IOM 98, Zeisel 03,04). Dietary intake of choline is estimated at 0.3–1.0 gm/day and that of betaine at 0.5–2.0 gm/day, so there is at least a twofold variation among subjects (Zeisel 06a). Higher-range intakes of choline and betaine are related to modestly lower total homocysteine (tHcy) concentrations, especially in the setting of low folate intake (Holm 05, Cho 06). Foods that are rich in betaine include wheat, spinach, shellfish, and sugar beets (Zeisel 03, Ueland 05). Excess betaine intake or supplementation will raise serum lipids, perhaps by enhanced synthesis of phosphatidylcholine, which enhances transport of VLDL from hepatocytes (Ueland 05). Considering the human dietary intake of methyl groups, the major sources of methyl groups in foods are from choline or its metabolite betaine (~30 mmol/day), methionine (~10 mmol/day), and from one-carbon metabolism via methylfolate (~5–10 mmol/day) (IOM 98, Niculescu 02).

Pancreatic enzymes digest the esterified forms and liberate free choline, which is absorbed from the lumen of the small intestine via transporter proteins in the enterocytes and enters the portal circulation (IOM 98). Phosphatidylcholine also enters the circulation via lymph in chylomicrons. Choline enters tissues by diffusion and specific carrier mechanisms, including use by trophoblast and active transport across the placenta (Sweiry 85,86, Garner 93) and by high-capacity uptake into fetal brain

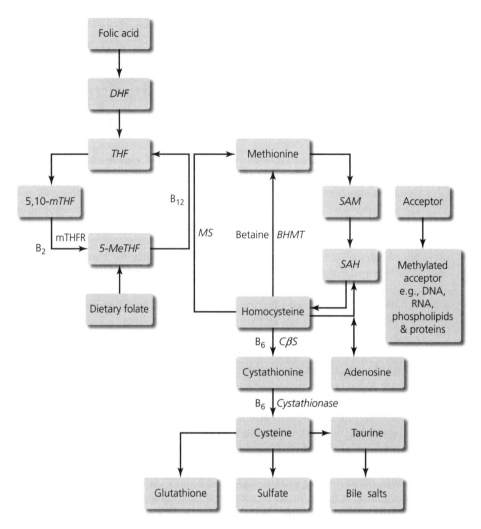

FIGURE I.3 Metabolism of folate, methionine, betaine, and homocysteine showing points of action of cofactors vitamins B2 (riboflavin), B6, and B12. The transmethylation pathway on the right converts methionine to homocysteine. The transsulfuration pathway shown at the bottom involves the breakdown of homocysteine and production of cysteine. On the left, the remethylation (recycling) pathway involves the folic acid cycle, which provides the methyl donor and carboxyl group to convert homocysteine back into methionine. The *BHMT* reaction shown in the center for remethylation of methionine is independent of folate/B12. *Enzymes* in italics: 5-MeTHF, 5-methyltetrahydrofolate; *BHMT, betaine-homocysteine methyltransferase; CβS, cystathionine β-synthase*; DHF, dihydrofolate; *MS, methionine synthase; mTHF, methylenetetrahydrofolate; mTHFR, methylenetetrahydrofolate reductase;* SAH, S-adenosylhomocysteine; SAM, S-adenosylmethionine; THF, tetrahydrofolate. Modified from Moat 2004a; used with permission.

(Zeisel 06b). A significant proportion of choline is oxidized in liver and kidney mitochondria to form betaine, an important source of methyl groups for S-adenosylmethionine (SAM)–dependent methylation reactions in the cytosol. These reactions are crucial for regulation of DNA expression, protein functions, and intermediary metabolism (Figure I.3) (IOM 98). With increased need for choline, as in pregnancy, hepatic de novo synthesis of phosphatidylcholine via *phosphatidylethanolamine-N-methyltransferase* (*PEMT*) and THF-dependent SAM is an important endogenous source of choline (IOM 98, Ueland 05, Zeisel 06b). Indeed, choline and folate metabolism are codependent (and affected by the B-vitamins), and individual deficiencies increase the requirement for the other nutrient (IOM 98, Niculescu 02, Holm 05, Melse-Boonstra 05, Verhoef 05).

With choline deprivation, animals, men, and some women develop fatty liver (hepatosteatosis), liver cell apoptosis, muscle damage from fragile membranes or cellular apoptosis, and DNA damage and apoptosis in lymphocytes (daCosta 05). A decreased capacity to methylate Hcy ensues, and subjects develop an elevated Hcy concentration after a methionine load (Zeisel 06a,b). Women of reproductive age may have partial protection from choline deficiency because estrogen seems to augment the *PEMT* pathway of endogenous generation of phosphatidylcholine (Zeisel 06a,b). Choline is critical for embryonic and fetal development; has an influence on the risk for NTDs (Fisher 01a, Shaw 04) and orofacial clefts (Shaw 06), stem cell proliferation and apoptosis, and life-long memory; and alters the brain and spinal cord structure and function (Zeisel 06a,b).

Presumably due to the fetal–placental need for choline, hepatic stores of choline diminish in pregnancy (Zeisel 04). Serum-free choline and phospolipid-bound choline rise during pregnancy (Ozarda 02), but plasma betaine and tHcy paradoxically decrease, showing an inverse relationship with choline with advancing gestation in a longitudinal study. The authors speculated that increasing estrogen and cortisol levels in gestation enhance *betaine-homocysteine methyltransferase* (*BHMT*)–catalyzed Hcy remethylation (Figure I.3), contributing to pregnancy-associated decreases in tHcy (Velzing-Aarts 05). In contrast, a cross-sectional study of uncomplicated pregnancies at delivery observed a positive relationship between choline and betaine as well as DMG and total plasma Hcy in maternal blood. In a multiple-regression model, choline was a positive predictor of maternal total plasma Hcy, whereas betaine and vitamin B12 were negative predictors. The authors speculated that upregulated activity of the *PEMT* pathway generating both *S*-adenosylhomocysteine (SAH) and phosphatidylcholine could explain the association between choline and Hcy (Molloy 05). Further research on these transmethylation systems should improve our understanding of their roles during pregnancy and whether they contribute to gestational complications (Vollset 00, Zeisel 05).

Data are inadequate to establish an EAR and RDA for choline. The IOM used the criterion of prevention of liver damage as assessed by measuring serum alanine aminotransferase (ALT) levels to establish the AI for choline at 425 mg/day for women of any age. The AI is increased to 450 mg/day for pregnant women of any age based on placental and fetal accumulation of choline. The UL for choline is set at 3.5 gm/day for pregnant and nonpregnant women on the basis of prevention of hypotension, cholinergic effects, and fishy body odor (IOM 98). National dietary surveys do not provide data on choline intake (IOM 98). A small study used food frequency questionnaires to estimate choline intake at 10–15 weeks gestation in 16 pregnant women in Jamaica (Gossell-Williams 05). Most subjects reported consumption of diets providing less than the AI for pregnancy; mean intake was 279 mg/day, and mean plasma choline concentration was 8.4 μmol/L, which is similar to levels of 5–12 μmol/L reported at 8–16 weeks gestation on the island of Curacao (Velzing-Aarts 05). In a population-based case–control study of NTDs in California, the lower and upper quartiles of maternal periconceptional choline intake assessed by food frequency questionnaires were <290 mg/day and >499 mg/day, respectively. The group in the lowest quartile had a significantly greater risk of infants with NTDs, even adjusting for supplemental folic acid and periconceptional vitamin intake, dietary folate, dietary methionine, and maternal weight and education level. NTD risk estimates were lowest when maternal diets were rich in choline, betaine, and methionine (Shaw 04). Additional studies of choline, betaine, and methionine status in normal and complicated pregnancies are needed, including pregnant women with diabetes.

Betaine. Betaine is also important in the diet (Sakamoto 02, Craig 04, Slow 05, Verhoef 05). Betaine is an organic osmolyte that accumulates in renal medullary cells and endothelial cells to balance extracellular hypertonicity (Alfieri 02, Kempson 04, Ueland 05). In healthy subjects, plasma betaine is not related to urinary excretion of betaine, which is <5% of creatinine excretion (Lever 94a, Ueland 05). Plasma betaine increases minimally in renal disease in contrast to large increases in plasma choline and dimethylglycine (DMG) (McGregor 01, Holm 04). Plasma betaine is normal in diabetes, but its urinary excretion is increased markedly in patients with proximal tubular dysfunction or high A1C (Lever 94b, Dellow 99a). However, glucose infusion does not increase betaine excretion (Dellow 99b).

B-Complex Vitamins, Methyl Group Transfer, and Homocysteine

Complex interactions among folate, riboflavin, vitamin B6, vitamin B12, choline, and betaine affect plasma Hcy levels (Figure I.3) (IOM 98, Kluijtmans 03, Holm 04,05). The possible role of Hcy in vascular and pregnancy complications is controversial. Hcy is formed in two steps (enzymes in italics): first, ATP and a *transferase* activate methionine to form S-adenosylmethionine (SAM; AdoMet), the primary methyl donor for essential *methyltransferase* reactions to acceptor proteins and histones; second, after methyl transfer, SAM is converted to S-adenosylhomocysteine (SAH; AdoHcy) by *glycine N-methyltransferase (GNMT)*, and SAH undergoes hydrolysis to Hcy with the production of adenosine. An efficient reverse reaction also occurs from Hcy to the synthesis of SAH, which accumulates with elevated Hcy concentrations.

Hcy concentrations can increase due to decreased catabolism. The kidney is thought to be a major site for the clearance, tubular reabsorption, and subsequent metabolism of circulating Hcy, whose concentration is influenced by the GFR (Cusworth 68, Bostom 95, Bostom 99); however, one study reported no net renal extraction of Hcy in fasting humans (vanGuldener 98). Renal uptake of Hcy during postprandial elevations of tHcy is possible (Guttormsen 94). Excess cellular Hcy is catabolized via the vitamin B6–dependent transsulfuration pathway to cysteine by *cystathione β-synthase (CβS)* and *cystathione lyase (CL)* (Nieman 04). Two parallel pathways also remethylate and convert Hcy back to methionine by (1) using methyl groups from methyl-THF and the ubiqitous *methionine synthase* or (2) in liver and kidney, by transfer of a methyl group from betaine (partly produced from choline in the mitochondria) to Hcy, converting them to DMG and methionine, respectively, in a reaction catalyzed by cytosolic *BHMT* (Figure I.2) (Niculescu 02). DMG contributes two methyl groups to the folate pool through the formation of 5,10-methylenetetrahydrofolate in the mitochondria (Ueland 05). Hcy concentrations "reflect the collective balance between production from AdoMet-dependent transmethylation reactions, remethylation to methionine, and catabolism via the transsulfuration pathway" (Nieman 04).

Remethylation is a more important pathway than transsulfuration in adult vascular cells (Chen 99).

In addition to the need for folate and B-vitamins, optimal metabolism of methyl groups and Hcy is dependent on an adequate dietary source of methyl groups, such as methionine and choline (Nieman 04, Verhoef 05). Deficiencies of any of three enzyme activities (*CβS, methionine synthase, methylenetetrahydrofolate reductase [mTHFR]*) can lead to excess Hcy (Moat 04a), which can be reduced by supplementation with folic acid and B-vitamins (HLTC 98, Rimm 98, Riddell 00, Doshi 02). Gene polymorphisms for the enzymes are found in human populations and affect these interrelated metabolic pathways (Loktionov 03). Impaired regeneration of methionine can lead to deficiencies in vasculoprotective adenosine. A high-protein load transiently increases methionine and Hcy levels (Verhoef 05). Methionine excess decreases the activity of the folate-dependent *methionine synthase,* but increases hepatic *BHMT,* which would remove excess choline, betaine, or Hcy (Ueland 05).

Basal or methionine-induced homocysteinemia in human subjects is associated with oxidized LDL-C and increased expression of inflammatory cytokines, which can be prevented by antioxidants (Antoniades 06, Ferriti 06, Solini 06, Taniguchi 06). Homocysteinylation of LDL-C induces alteration of functional properties and nitric oxide (NO) metabolism in human endothelial cells, plus increased peroxynitrite production (Vignini 04). Methionine loading produces increased asymmetrical dimethyl-arginine (ADMA), which inhibits endothelial NO synthase (eNOS) and impairs endothelial function (Antoniades 06). Experimental dietary methionine excess causes endothelial dysfunction and atherogenesis (Lentz 96, Troen 00). SAH, increasingly synthesized when Hcy is elevated and not removed, is a product inhibitor of cellular *methyltransferases* with resulting hypomethylation of DNA (Yi 00) and altered gene expression, cell differentiation, and apoptosis during embryogenesis–organogenesis (Ehrlich 03, Hobbs 05b).

Hyperhomocysteinemia is currently investigated for its relationship to atherosclerosis (Taylor 99, Clarke 02, Wald 02, Hankey 04, Moat 04b, Splaver 04, Kullo 06a); vascular complications of diabetes (Stehouwer 99, Hoogeveen 00, Davies 01, Okumura 03, Soinio 04, Soedamah-Muthu 05, Godsland 06, Ndrepepa 06); pregnancy complications, including early fetal loss and preeclampsia (Rajkovic 97, Ray 99, Sorensen 99, Nelen 00, Vollset 00, Cotter 01, Ray 02, Ronnenberg 02, Cotter 03, El-Khairy 03, Kamudhamas 04, Patrick 04, Raijmakers 04b, Herrmann 05b, Lindblad 05, Refsum 06, Vadachkoria 06); and congenital malformations (Mills 95, Kapusta 99, vanRooij 03, Hobbs 05b, Zhao 06a). Alternatively, hyperhomocysteinemia may simply be a reflection of poor nutrition, inflammation, vascular repair, oxidative degradation of folates, or associated with another atherogenic product of methionine metabolism (Christen 00, Moat 04a,b, Kullo 06b).

Two trials of folic acid, vitamin B6, and vitamin B12 supplementation to lower plasma tHcy reduced the rate of coronary restenosis after percutaneous coronary angioplasty (Schnyder 01) and decreased mortality within 1 year after angioplasty (Schnyder 02); subgroup analyses were not completed. A similar trial showed an increase of in-stent restenosis after 6 months in nondiabetic patients in the vitamin group versus placebo, but showed no change in mortality or myocardial infarction (MI) in the target vessel by 250 days. In-stent restenosis tended to be less likely with vitamin therapy in women, diabetic patients, and subjects with markedly elevated tHcy levels ≥ 15 μmol/L (Lange 04). Other much larger RCTs of secondary prevention failed to show reduction in cardiac events or deaths from modest Hcy lowering by supplementation of folic acid and vitamins B6 and B12 in high-risk patients with vascular disease, and the Hcy hypothesis was declared dead (Toole 04, Bonaa 06, HOPE 06). Subgroup analysis showed no treatment effect in the diabetic subjects or in women. Discussants raised the possibility of harmful vascular effects from high doses of interacting B-vitamins that could offset the effects of lowering Hcy (Loscalzo 06, Wang 06). Although other trials are ongoing and when considered with the previously noted results with antioxidant vitamins, recent results suggest that a simplistic approach to vitamin therapy (Kullo 06b, Maron 06) will not solve the complex atherogenesis problem. Cell- and enzyme-targeted antioxidant therapies will be evaluated. As a mark of the complexity, Hcy stimulates the proliferation of smooth-muscle cells (Tsai 94), but a folate-rich diet in the absence of hyperhomocysteinemia is associated with intimal hyperplasia (Lange 04, Loscalzo 06). In the meantime, a well-balanced diet, physical activity, and lowering of excess glucose, BP, and lipids are of proven benefit in reducing CVD.

Insulin may be a regulator of methionine and Hcy metabolism in humans because insulin deficiency in type 1 diabetes decreases remethylation but increases transsulfuration (Abu-Lebdeh 06). In experimental diabetes, there is increased activity of the enzymes *BHMT* and *CβS* (Jacobs 98, Nieman 04, Wijekoon 05, Ratnam 06), which may explain the decreased fasting plasma tHcy concentrations reported in these animals and in diabetic patients without nephropathy (Robillon 94, Cronin 98, Pavia 00, Wiltshire 01). Plasma SAH and tHcy are inversely related to changes in GFR (Wollesen 99, Davies 01, Diakoumopoulou 05, Veldman 05, Jabs 06, Schafer 06). The 5th to 95th percentiles for tHcy concentration in 358 vitamin-replete nonpregnant women aged 20–39 years in the U.S. NHANES III (1991–1994) were 3.7–10.4 μM. Sixty-nine percent of the women in the top 5th percentile for tHcy had low folate and vitamin B12 levels (Selhub 99). Although it is claimed that tHcy concentrations declined in the U.S. population (NHANES 1999–2002) due to fortification of food with folic acid (Ganji 06), direct comparison between the two surveys is problematic due to methodologic changes (Pfeiffer 00).

Plasma tHcy decreases during pregnancy—at least in regions with folate enrichment—with a rise in late gestation (Andersson 92, Cikot 01, Molloy 02, Holmes 05, Velzing-Aarts 05). Investigators suggest upper-limit reference ranges for fasting tHcy levels in plasma or serum of 8 μM in folate-supplemented diabetic pregnant women and 10 μM in unsupplemented women (Hankey 04, Moat 04a, Refsum 04). In a longitudinal study of 404 unsupplemented pregnant Danish women, folate status declined throughout gestation, and mean tHcy increased slightly from 6.4 to 7.7 μM compared with 10.8 μM 8 weeks postpartum. The prevalence of hyperhomocysteinemia (>13 μM) rose during pregnancy and reached 17% pospartum (Milman 06c). Caffeine consumption is associated with higher tHcy levels in pregnant smokers (Carlsen 05). Plasma tHcy may be an inconsistent marker for B-vitamin deficiency in pregnancy due to the multiple interrelationships of betaine–methionine metabolism as well as the effects of hemodilution (Bonnette 98, IOM 98, Walker 99) and those of renal hyperfiltration. Mothers with tHcy >14 μM after pregnancy in the Netherlands had a 2.9-fold increased risk of having delivered a child with congenital heart disease in spite of adequate folate status in the case children (Verkleij-Hagoort 06), confirming U.S. reports (Hobbs 06). As noted earlier, several observational studies report elevated tHcy in women with preeclampsia (11–13 vs. 6–8 μM) (Raijmakers 00, Makedos 06, Roes 06), and tHcy has been inversely related to insulin sensitivity in preeclamptic women (Laivuori 99). Although tHcy is cleared by renal excretion, increased levels of tHcy in preeclampsia in one study (4.4 μM vs. 3.2 μM) were not associated with decreased renal clearance of Hcy (Powers 04).

Hcy has not been well investigated in diabetic pregnant women. Serum tHcy levels were 6.9 ± 5.9 μM at 10.6 ± 7.2 weeks gestation in a single observational study of 31 pregnant women with type 1 diabetes, one-half of whom were using multivitamins. In 15 unsupplemented diabetic subjects, mean tHcy was 8.0 ± 8.1 μM vs. 6.5 ± 1.9 μM in 34 nondiabetic, unsupplemented pregnant controls. No analysis of the proportion of diabetic women with elevated tHcy and pregnancy outcome was conducted in this small study (Kaplan 99). Prospective studies are needed regarding the possible relationship of methyl-donor metabolism, nutrient intake, and Hcy to pregnancy complications in diabetic women (Picciano 00).

Intake of Other Substances

Sugar Substitutes (nonnutritive sweeteners)

The U.S. Food and Drug Administration (FDA) has approved four nonnutritive sweeteners (Table I.9) for general-purpose use in addition to saccharin, including moderate use in diabetic pregnant women, and regulates them as food additives (ADietA 02, Franz 02, ADietA 04). Approvals are based on studies of chronic dietary toxicity, mutagenicity, carcinogenicity, teratogenicity, multigenerational reproductive toxicity in laboratory animals, and studies of toxicity, metabolism, and pharmacokinetics in humans (ADietA 04). Human studies on the effects of nonnutritive sweeteners on pregnancy outcome and child development are mostly lacking.

Saccharin. Saccharin is derived from naphthalene and has been used as an artificial sweetener since the 1880s. Saccharin is excreted unchanged by the kidney. In the 1970s, the FDA proposed labeling on products stating that saccharin caused cancer in laboratory animals (ADietA 04), specifically bladder tumors in male rat offspring exposed in utero (Jensen 82). In 1985, the Council on Scientific Affairs of the American Medical

TABLE I.9 Nonnutritive Sweeteners Approved for General-Purpose Use in the U.S., Including Moderate Use During Pregnancy

Nonnutritive Sweetener	FDA Approval (year)	Brand Name	Sweetness Potency Compared with Sucrose	Acceptable Daily Intake (mg/kg/day)
Saccharin	2002 for beverages; table-top additive; processed foods	Sweet and Low, Necta Sweet, Sucaryl, Sugar Twin	200–700 ×	12 mg/fl oz; package = 20 mg sugar; 30 mg/serving processed foods
Aspartame	1983, 1996	Equal, Nutrasweet	160–220 ×; reduced with heating	50; ~225 mg in typical diet soda
Acesulfame-K	1988	Sunett, Sweet & Safe, Sweet One	200 ×	15
Sucralose	1999	Splenda	600 ×	5
Neotame	2002		8,000 ×	18

Modified from the American Dietetic Association 04.

Association recommended (a) continuation of saccharin availability because there was no evidence of increased risk of bladder cancer in humans, (b) careful consideration of saccharin use by pregnant women, and (c) continued monitoring of adverse health effects (AMA 85). In 2001, saccharin was removed from the list of potential carcinogens (ADietA 04). Saccharin crosses the placenta and may remain in fetal tissue due to slow fetal clearance (Pitkin 71).

Aspartame. Aspartame is hydrolyzed by intestinal esterases to absorbable aspartic acid, phenylalanine, and methanol, which are metabolized. After ingestion of aspartame, plasma aspartic acid levels do not increase, but plasma phenylalanine can rise to symptomatic levels in individuals with the inborn error of metabolism known as phenylketonuria (ADietA 04). Controversy has surrounded aspartame and the possible risks of free methanol and its metabolite, formic acid; tissue accumulation of formaldehyde adducts (Trocho 98); headaches (Schiffman 87) and neurobehavioral effects (Shaywitz 94, Smith 01); brain tumors in adults (Olney 96); or fetal optic nerve damage associated with aspartame use (Steinman 90). However, Health Canada, the Scientific Committee on Food of the European Commission, the United Kingdom Food Standards Agency, and the French Food Safety Agency reported their extensive reviews in 2002–2003 and stated that there was no evidence that aspartame use in conjunction with a healthy diet would pose a health hazard to consumers (CCC 04). Minimal placental transfer of aspartate occurs in pregnant monkeys with oral doses of aspartame at twice the human accepted daily intake (Stegink 79). Phenylalanine plasma levels after aspartame ingestion are far below those associated with adverse effects on the fetus–neonate (Levy 83). It is possible that methanol is concentrated on the fetal side of the placenta, but due to the small quantity of methanol available from the usual dose of aspartame, "this metabolite appears safe for pregnant women" (London 88). Aspartame use in laboratory animals showed no risk to the fetus when ingested in amounts at least three times the accepted daily intake (Sturtevant 85).

Acesulfame potassium. Acesulfame potassium (acesulfame-K) is excreted unchanged in the urine and does not provide energy or potassium (ADietA 04). It is often blended with other sweeteners. Acesulfame-K also crosses the placenta, but is considered safe during pregnancy based on studies in laboratory animals and the absence of evidence to the contrary in humans. Sucralose is a disaccharide that is poorly absorbed (11–27%), not metabolized, and excreted unchanged in the feces (ADietA 04). The FDA reviewed a large number of studies in humans and animals and concluded that this high-intensity sweetener does not pose carcinogenic, reproductive, or neurological risk to human beings (Grice 00). An RCT showed no effect over 3 months on glucose balance in type 2 diabetes (Grotz 03). Neotame is a derivative of the dipeptide that is composed of aspartic acid and phenylalanine, but the peptidase that breaks their peptide bond is blocked by the 3,3-dimethylbutyl moiety, which reduces the bioavailability of phenylalanine (ADietA 04). Rapid metabolism in humans by hydrolysis of the methyl ester by esterases yields neotame and methanol, and the latter is considered to be in exceedingly small amounts compared with methanol derived from fruits and vegetables and their juices. Use of neotame in type 2 diabetes showed no effect on fasting glucose or insulin levels (ADietA 04). Specific studies of newer nonnutritive sweeteners are lacking in diabetic pregnant women.

Ethanol
Ethanol use in pregnancy is one of the leading causes of infant morbidity and mortality (AAP 00, Hanigan 00). Fetal growth restriction, mental retardation, and fetal alcohol

syndrome malformations are associated with heavy alcohol use, and moderate drinking may have behavioral or neurocognitive consequences in the offspring. Moderate drinking is defined as ≤1 drink/day for women (12 oz beer, 5 oz wine, 1.5 oz. distilled spirits) and heavy drinking as >1 drink/day (DGAe 05). Women have increased alcohol bioavailability after drinking compared with men based on decreased gastric first-pass metabolism and decreased gastric alcohol dehydrogenase activity (Frezza 90). The U.S. Surgeon General advises pregnant women to abstain from all forms of alcohol because no safe level has been established. The recommendation that alcohol should be avoided applies to diabetic women who might become pregnant (because early pregnancy may be unrecognized) (DGAe 05). All pregnant and lactating women need to be informed of the harmful effects of alcohol to the fetus and breast-feeding infant (PSTF 04). Use of alcohol must be managed carefully by diabetic women who are not at risk of pregnancy because intake without food can be associated with hypoglycemia (Kerr 90, Franz 02). Consumption with meals will slow alcohol absorption. Some evidence indicates that alcohol can impair hormonal counterregulatory responses to low plasma glucose (Kerr 93) as well as reduce cognitive performance and recognition of the onset of hypoglycemia (Cheyne 04, Richardson 05). Alcohol use on the previous night is associated with increased frequency of hypoglycemia the next day (Turner 01, Richardson 05).

Caffeine

Caffeine is known to cross the placenta and to stimulate fetal breathing and HR, but human studies have not found caffeine consumption to be teratogenic. Caffeine intakes >300 mg/day in the first trimester had been inconsistently linked to an increase in spontaneous abortions (Cnattingius 00, Signorello 04). However, in the most recent prospective cohort study, 1,063 consenting women were interviewed by 15 weeks gestation. The adjusted hazard ratio for miscarriage at >8 weeks was 1.72 (1.01–2.92) for <200 mg/day caffeine consumption (all sources) and 2.79 (1.46–5.34) for >200 mg/day compared with 1.0 for zero consumption (Weng 08). An increased risk of stillbirth was found in pregnant women who drank >8 cups of coffee per day during pregnancy compared with women who did not drink coffee (adjusted OR 2.2 [1.0–4.7]) (Wisborg 03). A limit of <300 mg/day is now advised during pregnancy by the March of Dimes (MOD 08), but many clinicians now advise a nearly zero consumption of caffeine in preparation for pregnancy. Table I.10 delineates the quantity of caffeine in beverages consumed by diabetic pregnant women (Barrone 96).

Caffeine or chlorogenic acid polyphenols in coffee may acutely reduce insulin sensitivity and raise both glucose and insulin levels in normal and diabetic subjects (Pizziol 98, Graham 01, Greer 01, Keijzers 02, Johnston 03, Lane 04, vanDam 04, Lane 08). Chronic, regular caffeine use may not affect glycemic control because humans develop tolerance to caffeine (Colton 68, Robertson 81). Indeed, chronic heavy consumption of filtered coffee, perhaps via antioxidant effects, seems to have beneficial effects on women's health (Lopez-Garcia 06), including reducing the risk of developing type 2 diabetes (Salazar-Martinez 04, Tuomilehto 04, Greenberg 06, Smith 06, vanDam 06). Caffeine intake (250-mg dose or 200 mg twice daily) may also enhance recognition of hypoglycemia by increasing the intensity of warning symptoms (Debrah 96, Watson 00). Conversely, chronic coffee use is associated with increased BP (Noordzij 05) and serum LDL. Trials using filtered coffee demonstrated little increase in serum cholesterol (Jee 01).

Consumption of Chinese oolong tea with a high concentration of polymerized polyphenols and 352 mg/day caffeine for 30 days reduced fasting glucose and

TABLE I.10 Caffeine Quantity in Common Beverages Used by Diabetic Women

Beverage	Serving Size	Caffeine (mg/serving)
Brewed coffee	8 oz	135
Instant coffee	8 oz	95
Espresso	1 oz	35
Coffee Tall, Starbucks	12 oz	375
Coffee Short, Starbucks	8 oz	250
Tea, black	8 oz	50
Tea, iced	16 oz	18–40
Tea, green	8 oz	30
Diet cola	12 oz	35
Hot chocolate	8 oz	5
Chocolate milk	1 oz	5

Sources: Nutrition Action Healthletter, Barone 96.

fructosamine levels in women with type 2 diabetes (Hosoda 03). We are not aware of studies on the metabolic effects of caffeine, coffee, or tea in diabetic pregnant women.

Methylmercury

A strong association exists between dietary total mercury intake and blood organic mercury (methylmercury [MeHg]), with a risk for neurological changes (Mahaffey 98). Elemental mercury is emitted as a combustion byproduct of fossil fuels (NRC 00). Mercury accumulates in streams and oceans from rainfall and turns into MeHg in water. Large fish that have lived a long time generally absorb the highest quantities of MeHg as they feed. Exposure to inorganic mercury (I-Hg) mainly occurs through release of mercury vapor from dental amalgam fillings. Both forms of mercury are neurotoxic, especially to the developing brain (NRC 00), and both readily cross the placenta (Cernichiari 95, Ramirez 00, Ask 02, Bjornberg 05). Approximately 95% of mercury measured in blood is the methylated form compared with 80% in hair, which represents exposure over weeks or months (McDowell 04); the hair-to-blood mercury ratio is >200 in women of reproductive age (McDowell 04). The concentration of mercury is nearly twofold higher in cord blood than maternal blood (Vahter 00, Mahaffey 04a, Sakamoto 04, Bjornberg 05). The amount of fish consumed relates to mercury levels in maternal blood or hair and umbilical cord blood or tissue in several studies conducted in all parts of the globe (Stern 01, Bjornberg 03, Morrissette 04, Sato 06). Low levels of I-Hg in umbilical cord blood (0.03–0.53 μg/L) correlate with an increasing number of maternal dental amalgam fillings (Bjornberg 03).

MeHg is associated with neurological effects in the fetus and developmental changes in the child in many, but not all, cross-sectional studies (Crump 98, NRC 00, Ramirez 03, Jedrychowski 06, Spurgeon 06). Long-term child development studies show a persistent effect of prenatal MeHg exposure on neurobehavioral function in infancy (Steuerwald 00), at 7 years (Grandjean 97), and at 14 years of age in the Faroe Islands in the North Atlantic (Debes 06), but not in children born in the Seychelles in the Indian Ocean (Davidson 98, Myers 03, Davidson 06). The mercury content of ocean fish near the Seychelles is similar to that in other oceans (Myers 03), but marine food includes pilot whale in the Faroes (Steuerwald 00). The 95% CI for mercury concentrations in umbilical cord blood was 4–128 μg/L in the Faroes (Grandjean 05). The Seychelles studies measured mercury levels in maternal hair and determined that maternal levels of 17–22 ppm (μcg/gm) were safe (vanWijngaarden 06). The WHO limit on total hair mercury is <10 μcg/gm (ICPS 90). In Arctic Canada, 56% of Inuit cord blood mercury levels were >5.8 μg/L compared with only 5% in Dene/Metis women, who also had lower maternal blood mercury concentrations than the Inuit (Butler 06b). Considering the Pacific Ocean, consumption of fish or seafood more than once per week in Honolulu was associated with elevated cord blood mercury levels of 6–14 μg/L (Sato 06). In Japan, fish consumption also correlates with mercury levels in maternal blood or hair and in umbilical cord blood or tissue (Murata 04, Kim 06, Sakamoto 07). We are not aware of studies on the effects of maternal diabetes on mercury toxicity.

The U.S. Environmental Protection Agency recommendation is to keep blood MeHg levels <5.8 μg/L (Rice 03,04, Stern 05). Blood mercury levels were <5 μg/L in 90% of women of reproductive age consuming fish no more than once/week compared with 28% of women whose levels were ≥5 μg/L when eating fish ≥2 times/week (Mahaffey 04a). In a recent survey of 286 pregnant women, the 90th-percentile geometric mean total blood mercury concentration was 4.8 mcg/L (Schober 03). Assuming 1:1 conversion of total hair mercury as ppm to μg/gm, the 95th percentile for total hair mercury in 295 pregnant women sampled across the U.S. was 1.84 μg/gm. In the total population of 1,726 women aged 16–49, the frequency of fish and shellfish consumption was indeed related to low-level mercury accumulation in the hair (McDowell 04). All pregnant and lactating women are advised to avoid the consumption of certain marine fish (shark, swordfish, Gulf of Mexico tilefish and mackerel) that have been found to contain high MeHg levels (≥0.7 ppm) and to limit albacore (white) tuna to 6 oz (1 average meal) per week (FDA 04a,b). Fish from American lakes and rivers is also of concern for organic mercury and other toxins (Knobeloch 05).

Higher maternal fish consumption was associated with better infant cognition in a Massachusetts cohort of 135 mother–infant pairs (presumably related to *n*-3 fatty acids) as long as maternal mercury levels were low (Oken 05). In a much larger British population, umbilical tissue mercury was low, and the amount of maternal fish intake during pregnancy correlated positively with child development scores at 15–18 months of age (Daniels 04). The message is to eat fish uncontaminated with mercury. Fortunately, there is minimal association between *n*-3 fatty acids and mercury concentrations in marine fish species; Atlantic mackerel, sardines, herring, and salmon are high in the former and low in mercury (Kris-Etherton 02, Mahaffey 04b, Mozaffarian 06b). Information about the safety of locally caught fish and shellfish is available at the U.S. Environmental Protection Agency's Fish Advisory Website (*www.epa.gov/waterscience/fish*) and the FDA's Food Safety Website (*www.cfsan.fda.gov/seafood1.html*).

Organochlorines: Polychlorinated Biphenyls and Dioxins

PCBs and pesticides are environmentally persistent contaminants that concentrate in the food chain as well as in human adipose tissue (Larsen 06) and readily cross the placenta (Sagiv 07). PCBs contaminate fish in the Great Lakes and elsewhere (Stewart 99, Weisskopf 05, Turyk 06) and are associated with childhood intellectual impairment (Jacobson 96a, Winneke 98, Darvill 00, Grandjean 01, Arisawa 05) and possibly with fetal and postnatal growth restriction (Karmaus 04, Lamb 06). In Japan, the background level of polychlorinated dioxins (rather than PCBs) was associated with impaired motor development of 6-month-old infants (Nakajima 06). Using stored sera, PCB levels during U.S. pregnancies in 1959–1965 did not correlate with infant behavioral scores overall, but a negative relationship was found at some centers in the Collaborative Perinatal Project (CPP) (Daniels 03). In these data, in utero exposure to background levels of PCBs was not associated with lower IQ at age 7 years (Gray 05). It is of interest that maternal serum levels of PCBs were ~30% higher in 44 pregnant diabetic women than in 2,201 control subjects in the CPP. The authors speculated that the pharmacokinetics of PCBs could be altered among patients with diabetes (Longnecker 01) and that PCBs could induce changes in thyroid metabolism (Koopman-Esseboom 94, Brouwer 99, Osius 99). Increased blood levels of PCBs and dioxins have been reported in nonpregnant women with diabetes (Remillard 02, Fierens 03, Hokanson 04), especially in younger participants, Mexican-Americans, and the obese (Lee 06b). Increased PCB exposure during pregnancy in the Faroes was associated with desaturase inhibition in maternal and cord sera and decreased arachidonic acid concentrations. Because arachidonic acid is of key importance for growth and development, the authors speculated that such interference with fetal LC-PUFA utilization could attenuate the beneficial effects of the essential lipids contained in seafood (Grandjean 03).

Listeriosis
Listeriosis is a serious bacterial infection caused by eating contaminated foods. Pregnant women are 20 times more likely to be infected than nonpregnant women. Being infected with listeriosis increases the risk for miscarriage, stillbirth, preterm delivery, and an infected infant (Smith 03, Pofsay-Barbe 04, Huang 06). Case reports of listeria septicemia causing influenza-like disease (Solomon 78) and bacterial endocarditis (Holshauser 78) in diabetic pregnant women have been published.

To prevent becoming infected with listeriosis (MacDonald 05, Ogunmodede 05), pregnant women are advised not to consume:

- deli meats, hot dogs, or luncheon meats unless reheated until steaming hot
- soft cheeses such as feta, Brie, Camembert, blue-veined, *queso blanco*, and *queso fresco* (hard cheeses and pasteurized cheeses are recommended)
- refrigerated paté or meat spreads (canned or shelf-stable paté and meat spreads can be consumed)
- refrigerated smoked seafood unless cooked
- raw or unpasteurized milk

Herbal Medicines and Dietary Supplements
Herbal medicines and dietary supplements may be substituted for prescription medications, and their use has proliferated in recent years (Yeh 03). Diabetic pregnant women of certain cultures might not inform their healthcare providers of their use of supplements, including herbal teas, and may be unaware of potential adverse effects to the fetus (Stevens 02). Few RCTs have evaluated the effect of alternative therapies during pregnancy. The American Dietetic Association's Position Paper on pregnancy lists many herbal and botanical supplements that may not be safe for use during pregnancy (ADietA 02).

Special Nutritional Circumstances

Vegetarian Diets

Vegetarian diets can meet guidelines for the treatment of diabetes (Franz 02) and reduction of CVD (Sabate 03), but the vegetarian diabetic pregnant woman needs special attention to provide appropriate intake of essential amino acids, fatty acids, and micronutrients. Lacto-ovo-vegetarian and complete vegan diets can meet the energy needs of pregnant women, and infant BWs are generally similar to controls (ADietA 03). In the 1994–1998 CSFII, 120 vegetarians who ate no meat, poultry, or fish reported intakes of carbohydrate as 60% of energy, protein as 12%, and total fat as 25% (Haddad 03). Intake of linoleic acid may be greater in vegetarian women, which could inhibit Δ6 desaturation and decrease the proportion of DHA in the fetal brain (Sanders 99). It is prudent to ensure that vegetarian diets do not contain excessive amounts of linoleic acid and that the ratio of n-6 linoleic acid to n-3 α-linolenic acid is kept around 4:1 (Lakin 98, Sanders 99, Davis 03). Vegetable oils, such as corn and sunflower oils, have high proportions of linoleic acid to α-linolenic acid, and the partial hydrogenation of canola and soybean oils reduces the quantity of α-linolenic acid (Sanders 99). Nuts, seeds, and avocado are good sources of n-3 fats for vegetarians (Messina 03). Regarding micronutrients, mean daily intake was less than the RDA for calcium, magnesium, nonheme iron, zinc, niacin, folate, and vitamin B12 for vegans in the CSFII (Haddad 03). Supplementation of these nutrients plus vitamin D and vitamin B12 (5 mcg/day or 2,000 mcg/week) will often be needed (ADietA 03, Hunt 03). The American Dietetic Association recently published a useful new food guide for North American vegetarians (Messina 03). For pregnant vegans, the minimal number of daily servings in specific food groups is as follows: four servings of B12-rich foods, seven servings of beans/nuts/seeds, and eight servings of calcium-rich foods, which can be included among nine servings of whole grains and four servings of vegetables (ADietA 02, Messina 03).

Celiac Disease

Celiac disease (gluten-sensitive enteropathy, celiac sprue) is a cellular and humoral autoimmune response in the proximal small intestine to the consumption of wheat gluten (gliadin protein fraction, glutenin peptides) and similar proteins found in rye (secalin) and barley (hordein) in susceptible individuals (Collin 02, Alaedini 05, Branski 06). We use the term *gluten* generically to mean any of these grain proteins–peptides that are rich in glutamine and proline (Vader 02). Eating oats (avenin) does not typically cause sensitivity (Janatiunem 95, Picarelli 01a, Hogberg 04, Haboubi 06, Hollen 06, Holm 06). Recent evidence states that at least one 33-amino-acid (33-mer) peptide survives the gut proteolytic enzymes to reach the small intestine carrying three epitopes that are immunogenic in celiac disease (Shan 02). Homologs of this peptide are found in food grain proteins that are toxic to patients with celiac disease but not in corn, oats, or rice (Piper 02). In sensitized individuals, the consumption of gluten induces inflammation of the small intestine and blunting of the small intestinal villi, causing increased fluid loss (loose stools to chronic diarrhea) and impaired absorption of both micro- and macronutrients (Hill 02, Troncone 04, Dewar 05, Chand 06). The extent of injury is variable, ranging from 1% to nearly 100% of the small intestine (Murray 03), and may also involve the terminal ileum (Hopper 06). Subtle clinical features of celiac disease in young people and adults include mild abdominal pain and bloating or extraintestinal features such as short stature, delayed puberty, anemia, or increased soluble Tf receptor/ferritin index (de Caterina 05), thyroid disorders (Ventura 00), dermatitis herpetiformis, cardiomyopathies, diminished bone mineralization, neuropathy, and ataxia (Murray 99, Collin 02, Pengiran 02, Chin 03, Fasano 03, Cerutti 04, Alaedini 05, Barker 06). However, many cases are relatively asymptomatic or "silent."

The definitive diagnosis of celiac disease is made when an intestinal biopsy shows small bowel mucosal villous atrophy, increased density of intraepithelial and lamina densa lymphocytes, and crypt hyperplasia, all of which revert to normal on a gluten-free diet (GFD) (Hill 02, Cerutti 04, Dewar 05). Formerly thought to be a rare disease, the estimated prevalence of celiac disease now approaches 1% based on population screening (Hill 00, Fasano 03, Maki 03, Bingley 04, Tommasini 04) and is even more common in both children (Acerini 98, Fraser-Reynolds 98, Carlsson 99, Gillett 01, Kaspers 04) and adults (Collin 89, Cronin 97a,b, Seissler 99, Kordonouri 00) with type 1 diabetes, reaching a prevalence of 4–12% (Not 01, Valerio 02, Mahmud 05, Barker 06, Hansen 06). Prevalence of celiac disease is not increased in patients with type 2 diabetes (Cerutti 04).

Although most reports of celiac disease concern European populations, it is diagnosed globally in many other ethnic groups (Dawood 81, Ashabani 03, Freeman 03, Green 03a, Baptista 05, Brar 05, Butterworth 05, Kaur 06). The risk of celiac disease is higher among first-degree relatives (1:10–22) than second-degree relatives (1:40) (Fasano 03, Chand 06), and there is 75% concordance in monozygotic twins (Greco 02). There exists a close genetic linkage of celiac disease to the human leukocyte antigen (HLA) genotypes DR3-DQ2 and DR4-DQ8 (Louka 03), which are shared predictors for type 1 diabetes (Bao 99, Chand 06). About 95% of patients with celiac disease have the DQ2 marker, and the DQ8 marker is found in most of the remainder (Howell 86, Sollid 89). The DQ2 and DQ8 molecules confer susceptibility to celiac disease by presenting specific gluten peptides to gluten-specific CD4+ T-cells in the intestinal lamina propria and other T-cells in the epithelium (Alaedini 05, Kagnoff 05). However, celiac disease develops in a minority of HLA-DQ2 and HLA-DQ8 individuals. If there is normal induction and maintenance of immune tolerance to dietary components and commensal gut flora, it is unknown why tolerance is not established or broken in patients with celiac disease (Stepniak 06). Proinflammatory triggers may include gastrointestinal infections or early exposure to gluten during weaning (Kagnoff 05).

The pathogenesis of celiac disease is under study and is currently viewed as a series of three phases (Figure I.4) (Kagnoff 05). The *first phase* relates to uptake and processing of gluten peptides (Dewar 04). The luminal and early mucosal events may reflect the innate immune response to gluten (within hours) and consist of interactive changes in surface epithelial cells with activation of intraepithelial lymphocytes, upregulation of IL-15, and changes in permeability (Maiuri 00,01, Cerf-Bensussan 03, Maiuri 03, Matysiak-Budnik 03). Gluten peptides reach the intestinal lamina propria when intestinal permeability increases (Fasano 00, Clemente 03), as after gastrointestinal infection (El-Asmar 02, Green 03a). The *second phase* is an adaptive immune response to the gluten peptides (Cerf-Bensussan 03). The intruding peptides gain increased immunostimulatory potential by deamidation of particular glutamine residues (Vader 02) by tTG (transglutaminase 2, which is expressed on the subepithelial layer and released by gut fibroblasts in the setting of inflammation) and then by complexing with tTG (Schuppan 00, Alaedini 05). The peptide–tTG complexes encounter APCs expressing DQ2 or DQ8 and together induce human DQ2- or DQ8-restricted CD4+ T-cells (Kagnoff 05). Thus, tTG is considered

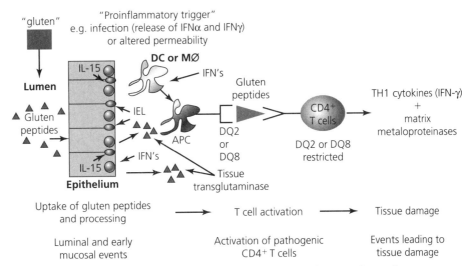

FIGURE I.4 Pathogenesis of celiac disease described as three major series of events. During the luminal and early mucosal events, key features include the ingestion of "gluten" (proteins and peptides in wheat, rye, and barley) by a genetically susceptible individual. Gluten is not fully digested because of its high proline content, and this gives rise to a number of large undigested gluten peptides. The peptides gain access across the epithelial barrier to the lamina propria, where they encounter tTG and APCs (macrophages, dendritic cells, B-cells) that express DQ2 or DQ8 that are ideally suited to bind the deamidated (by tTG) proline-rich peptides. In a further series of events, the APCs present some of these peptides to DQ2- or DQ8-restricted populations of CD4+ T-cells, which become activated and release mediators that ultimately lead to tissue damage. Many unknowns still exits, including the mechanism by which gluten peptides cross the epithelial barrier, the role of IL-15 and type-1 interferons (IFNs) in disease pathogenesis, and the underlying basis for the release of tTG that leads to deamidation of gluten peptides. IEL, intraepithelial lymphocytes. Adapted from Kagnoff 05 and used with permission.

the major autoantigen of celiac disease (Dieterich 97, Molberg 98, Arentz-Hansen 00, Korpony-Szabo 00, Molberg 00, Marzari 01, McManus 03, Molberg 03, Maiuri 05). The 33-mer peptide reacts with tTG with great selectivity and induces gut-derived T-cells of patients with celiac disease but not controls (Shan 02, Kagnoff 05). The *third phase* concerns the molecular–cellular events leading to tissue damage (Kagnoff 05). Recognition of the HLA-bound gluten peptides by T-cells leads to their activation and release of cytokines that drive the clonal expansion of B-cells that (1) produce antibodies (anti-tTG, anti-endomysial, anti-reticulin, anti-gliadin); (2) promote inflammatory mechanisms, including secretion of damaging matrix metalloproteinases by fibroblasts and inflammatory cells; and (3) lead to intraepithelial lymphocyte-mediated destruction of epithelial cells and mucosal damage (Alaedini 05).

Many cases of celiac disease in type 1 diabetes are clinically unrecognized without autoantibody screening due to lack of dramatic gastrointestinal symptoms. For that reason, most identified cases have been diagnosed within 10 years after diagnosis of type 1 diabetes (Saukkonen 96, Chand 06). Multicenter screening programs of new-onset type 1 diabetes reveal that 60–80% of patients with celiac disease already have autoimmunity at diagnosis, and the remainder test positive on subsequent annual testing (Jaeger 01, Barera 02, Peretti 04). Celiac disease is more common with younger onset of type 1 diabetes, in females, and in those with thyroid autoimmunity (Cerutti 04, Sumnik 06). Type 1 diabetic children with silent celiac disease identified by autoantibody screening and confirmed by biopsy showed no obvious effects on metabolic control, but did have lower weight gain and body mass than diabetic controls (Rami 05). However, other studies linked celiac disease to problems with glycemic control in young diabetic patients, especially unexplained hypoglycemia (Iafusco 98, Mohn 01). Several small observational studies (total: 50 diabetic patients) suggested benefit from a GFD on symptoms and growth characteristics (Amin 02, Saadah 04, Sanchez-Albisua 05). A cohort of 33 diabetic children aged 2–16 years was identified by universal autoantibody screening in southern Denmark (prevalence of celiac disease: 12.3%). Only five of the children had a diagnosis of celiac disease prior to screening, even though 48% of the cohort reported abdominal pain, 27% bloating, 24% tiredness, 21% loose and/or frequent stools, 21% arthralgias, and 9% constipation at baseline. All of these symptoms were much more common than in diabetic patients without celiac disease. Anemia was present at baseline in 12% of the children and low serum ferritin in 27%. Treatment with a GFD for 2 years lowered autoantibodies and improved symptoms, growth, hemoglobin, serum calcium, ferritin, and folate, suggesting the benefit of screening for celiac disease (Hansen 06).

Celiac disease has long been associated with failure to thrive in children (Hoffenberg 04), but new research demonstrates an increased prevalence of undiagnosed celiac disease with intestinal villous atrophy in adults in the general population (Green 05). The demographics and presentation of celiac disease in adults differ from that in children. Relatively asymptomatic patients may be detected by screening protocols (Lee 06c, Rampertab 06). In adults, a higher prevalence of celiac disease is detected in females by a ratio of 3 to 1; approximately one-third of patients are underweight (Green 01, Murray 04). Women are younger at presentation and have a longer duration of symptoms than males (Lo 03). Peak age at diagnosis is between 40 and 60 years of age; patients with symptoms report that their onset preceded diagnosis by an average of 11 years (Green 01). Many patients experience alternating diarrhea and constipation, often associated with nausea, abdominal pain, and bloating, that usually resolve with a strict GFD over a period of 4 months (Murray 04). Celiac disease may well be detected in adults during evaluation for irritable bowel syndrome (Sanders 01). Adults may present with a single symptom, such as unexplained iron-deficiency anemia (Ransford 02) with low cholesterol (Ciacci 99), chronic diarrhea, or unexplained weight loss (Green 05). Additional symptoms and associated pathologies include history of delayed puberty, dermatitis herpetiformis (itchy, blistery skin rash most frequently found on major joints), arthritis, thyroid disorders, dental enamel hypoplasia, liver disease, osteopathy, neuropathy, ataxia, and gastrointestinal malignancies (Murray 99, Collin 02,03, Green 03b, Peters 03, Adaelini 05, Dewar 05, Lee 06c). Celiac disease is also associated with depression, anxiety, migraines, epilepsy, and vitamin and protein deficiencies (Hill 02). In longitudinal observational studies, a GFD is associated with recovery from subclinical hypothyroidism (Sategna-Guidetti 01) and deficiencies of iron (Annabale 01) and vitamin B12 (Dahele 01) in adults. Some evidence exists for a protective role of a GFD in reducing the risk of gastrointestinal cancer, but perhaps not that of non-Hodgkins lymphoma (Holmes 89, Green 03b).

In adults with type 1 diabetes, diabetes is usually recognized before diagnosis of celiac disease. A landmark early description noted that unstable glycemic control and troublesome hypoglycemia often improved with adherance to a GFD (Walsh 78). Recent screening studies of groups of "asymptomatic" adults with type 1 diabetes revealed a prevalence of biopsy-proven celiac disease of 2.6–12% (Sategna-Guidetti 94, Rensch 96, Cronin 97a, Talal 97, Sjoberg 98, Not 01, Schuppan 01, Li 02, Mahmud 05). Possibly due to insufficient recognition of the problems of celiac disease in the adult population in the U.S., there are no RCTs of the value of diagnosis or treatment with a GFD in adults with diabetes.

Screening for celiac disease is recommended by the ADA for patients with type 1 diabetes soon after diagnosis of diabetes (Silverstein 05, ADA 08a) by testing for circulating IgA autoantibodies to human tTG (Dieterich 99, Baldas 00, Kordonouri 00, Fabiani 01, Hill 04, Barker 05, Liu 05), with subsequent testing with limited growth, failure to gain weight, weight loss, or gastroenterological symptoms (Holmes 02, Freemark 03). As noted earlier, mucosal surface tTG is considered the autoantigen of celiac disease, with production of autoantibodies in the gut mucosa stimulated by gliadin-specific T-cells (Dieterich 99, Marzari 01, Maiuri 05). Some authorities rescreen young type 1 diabetes patients with negative antibody levels every 1–2 years over a course of 6–8 years (Barker 06, Hansen 06). Patients with elevated levels of anti-tTG (Barker 05, Liu 05) should be referred for consideration of intestinal biopsy and therapy with a GFD by a dietitian experienced in the management of both diabetes and celiac disease (Silverstein 05, ADA 08a).

For screening in adults, sensitivity of the human tTG assay is >95% with a specificity of 98% in meta-analyses of studies in nondiabetic patients (Alaedini 05, Rostom 05). If the tTG assay is not available, the more cumbersome assay for endomysial autoantibody ([EMA], which also targets tTG) against human umbilical vein antigen may be used (sensitivity >90%; 99% specificity) (Volta 95, Picarelli 01b). The less-sensitive and less-specific anti-gliadin antibody test is no longer recommended for screening. A quantitative serum IgA level should be obtained at the time of testing because IgA deficiency is present in 1–3% of patients with celiac disease, causing falsely low levels of the IgA tTG or EMA assay (Green 01). If IgA deficiency is found, measurement of IgG-class anti-tTG or anti-EMA is recommended (Korponay-Szabo 03).

The NIH Consensus Development Conference in June 2004 recommended screening in adults with type 1 diabetes when subtle symptoms consistent with celiac disease are present (Collin 05), such as unexplained hypoglycemia (NIH 05). Consideration should be given to screening women with type 1 diabetes who are planning or entering pregnancy who have not been tested for celiac disease (Silverstein 05, ADA 08a). Given the presumed high prevalence in this population (~5%) and frequent absence of symptoms, screening and diagnosis may be warranted to allow treatment to improve the nutritional state, begin the process of recovery for the small intestine, and perhaps improve fetal outcomes. No prospective studies of celiac disease associated with diabetic pregnancy are available to evaluate this hypothesis. Because the definitive diagnosis of celiac disease requires a duodenal biopsy examination obtained during routine upper gastrointestinal endoscopy (Dewar 05), its screening and diagnosis is best performed before conception. Failing that, patients with high-titer anti-tTG or anti-EMA may be treated with a GFD as a test of response during pregnancy, with endoscopy delayed until after gestation.

In the first-trimester and term placenta, tTG is identified in the syncytial microvillous membrane, fibroblasts, and extracellular matrix, suggesting the possibility of autoimmune responses in this important tissue (Hager 97, Robinson 06). Several studies are available regarding pregnancies of nondiabetic women with celiac disease. Small case–control studies of consecutive pregnant women with celiac disease suggested that there were more spontaneous abortions, growth-restricted fetuses, and stillbirths associated with untreated celiac disease (Molteni 90, Sher 94, Kotze 04). Problems with the onset or worsening of diarrhea and weight loss during pregnancy were noted (Smecuol 96). Pregnant women with celiac disease on a GFD had fewer spontaneous abortions and heavier babies than did untreated patients in early observational analyses (Ogburn 75, Ferguson 82) and subsequent nonrandomized studies (Sher 94, Smecuol 96, Kotze 04, Ciacci 05).

A historical cohort study using a birth registry in Denmark showed that the rate of fetal growth restriction at term was greater in 132 women giving birth well before their first hospitalization for celiac disease compared with babies delivered to 43 mothers after treatment for celiac disease (8.3% vs. 0% vs. 2.4% in healthy controls; OR 3.4; 95% CI 1.6–7.2) (Norgard 99). In a screening study of 845 consecutive obstetrical admissions in Italy, 12 women were positive (1.4%) on EMA and later intestinal biopsy; of these women, five delivered SGA babies at term and three delivered preterm at 24, 26, and 36 weeks (Martinelli 00). A case–control study compared 31 GFD-treated women with 94 untreated patients and found a ninefold higher relative abortion risk and sixfold higher risk of low BW in the untreated group (Ciacci 96). Crude fertility rates were similar in a larger population-based cohort study of 1,521 women with celiac disease compared with 7,732 age- and practice-matched women without celiac disease in the U.K., but the miscarriage rate was moderately higher with celiac disease (relative risk [RR] 1.31; 95% CI 1.06–1.61). No differences were found in stillbirths (Tata 05).

A national register-based cohort study in Sweden compared outcomes of 1,018 women diagnosed with celiac disease prior to pregnancy with 370 women diagnosed after the infant birth. After adjusting for smoking, maternal age, parity, nationality, infant sex, and calendar period, undiagnosed celiac disease increased the risk of low BW (<2,500 g) and very low BW (<1,500 g), as well as preterm birth and CS when compared with women who were diagnosed prior to pregnancy (Table I.11). The group diagnosed after pregnancy (and therefore not treated during gestation) had an increased risk of fetal growth restriction (OR = 1.62; 95% CI 1.22–2.15), preterm birth (OR = 1.71; 95%

TABLE I.11 Fetal Outcomes in Women with Celiac Disease

Parameter	No CD	CD Diagnosed Prior to Pregnancy	CD Diagnosed After Pregnancy
Number	1,785,448	1,018	370
FGR (<2 SDs)	2.6%	3.5%	3.8%
Low BW (<2,500 gm)	3.2%	3.9%	7.8%*
Very low BW (<1,500 gm)	0.5%	0.5%	1.6%**
Preterm birth	5.0%	6.2%	10.2%*

Adjusted for maternal age, parity, weight, smoking, national origin, calendar period, and newborn gender.

$*p < 0.001$.

$**p < 0.01$.

BW, birth weight; CD, celiac disease; FGR, fetal growth restriction.

Table adapted from Ludvigsson 05.

CI 1.35–2.17), and very low BW (OR = 2.45; 95% CI 1.35–4.43) (Ludvigsson 05). Another retrospective comparison of pregnancy outcomes in 48 deliveries of patients with known celiac disease and 143,663 pregnancies of patients without known celiac disease in Israel showed a higher prevalence of fetal growth restriction with celiac disease (6.3% vs. 2.1%; p = 0.04), but no significant difference in perinatal mortality. Investigators assumed that the pregnant women with celiac disease were treated with a GFD (Sheiner 06). Possible bias might have affected all of these retrospectively controlled studies, but there is enough pathology to suggest the need for prospective evaluation of the benefit of screening for celiac disease in undiagnosed pregnant women with type 1 diabetes and treating them with a GFD.

Management of celiac disease in pregnancy. Six key elements for management of celiac disease have been identified (NIH 05) that can best be remembered by the mnemonic CELIAC:

C: Consultation with a skilled dietitian
E: Education about celiac disease
L: Lifelong adherence to a GFD
I: Identification and treatment of nutrition deficiencies
A: Access to a support group
C: Continuous long-term follow-up

Excellent, practical, and detailed references on the nutritional management of celiac disease are available (Kupper 05, See 06). "The goal of the gluten-free diet is to achieve healing and maintain health through the adoption of a well-balanced, varied diet that avoids gluten" (Murray 04). The grain proteins stimulating celiac disease can originate from wheat, barley, rye, spelt, kamut, triticale, and perhaps oats contaminated with other grains in the production process. Therefore, it may be more useful to inquire whether a food has an ingredient that is in any way derived from or processed with these grains than to ask, "Is this food gluten free?" (Murray 99). Hidden sources of "gluten" are frequently present in hydrolyzed vegetable protein, modified food starch, malt, vegetable gum, mono- and diacylglycerols, and natural flavorings (See 06). It is also important that patients with celiac disease be educated about nonfood sources of gluten such as vitamins, supplements, medications, toothpaste, mouthwash, lipstick, and postage stamps. Gluten in nonfood sources can be hard to identify and often necessitates contacting the manufacturer to determine whether or not "gluten" is present (See 06). It is possible to obtain flour substitutes from reliable sources that cater to patients with celiac disease. Secondary lactose intolerance usually resolves on the GFD once damage to the gut has healed (Murray 99).

Because the GFD is hard to maintain, patients who are active members of a local or national support group will have better results (Murray 99, Pietzak 05). Self-taught patients may overly restrict their diets, resulting in nutritional deficiencies that can be a special problem in pregnancy. It is well documented that untreated celiac disease is associated with nutrient malabsorption. As an example, iron and vitamin B12 status should be known before folic acid replacement is started (Dickey 02). Not so well known is that unfortified gluten-free products are often low in B-vitamins, calcium, vitamin D, iron, zinc, magnesium, and fiber. "Because of the nutritional risks associated with celiac disease, a registered dietitian must be part of the health care team that monitors the patient's nutritional status and compliance on a regular basis" (Kupper 05). A dietitian skilled in the management of celiac disease may be located through use of the American Dietetic Association's National Center for Nutrition and Dietetics Consumer Nutrition Hotline at 1-800-366-1655 or accessed on the Web at *www.eatright.org*.

Maintenance of a GFD in a patient with diabetes presents further challenges because glucose levels may fluctuate as the ability of the intestine to absorb foods changes and because many gluten-free foods are higher in carbohydrate and lower in fiber (See 06). Conflicting data attest to the impact of a diagnosis of celiac disease and initiation of a GFD on glycemic control in adults (Acerini 98, Kaukinen 99, Holmes 01, Mohn 01, Amin 02, Hill 02, Chand 06). Untreated celiac disease can be associated with increased frequency of hypoglycemia and progressive reduction in insulin requirements. Introduction of a GFD can increase absorption of nutrients and improve weight gain, with increased insulin requirements. Episodic poor adherence to the GFD can reverse these trends and result in hypoglycemia. The difficulties of treatment of celiac disease can be magnified in diabetic pregnancy due to the increased frequency of hypoglycemia, nausea and vomiting, delayed gastric emptying, and constipation.

The good news is that many gluten-free foods are whole and not processed, which tends to facilitate the intake of fresh fruits and vegetables, meats, and dairy products. The bad news is that the limited choice of grains in the diet and the presence of "intolerance" to other foods mean that patients on a GFD may be at higher risk for low intake of protein, healthy fats, fiber, calcium, iron, folate, and vitamins, and supplements are therefore usually needed.

In the future, innovative treatments may obviate the need for a strict GFD. Approaches for investigation include blocking IL-15 (Mention 03, Di Sabatino 06), introducing recombinant IL-10 to suppress gliadin-dependent T-cell activation (Salvati 05), boosting immunoregulatory Tr-1 T-cells (Gianfrani 06), and exploring gene therapy (Londei 01). Whether these hypothetical approaches would provide cost-effective advantages to a GFD will need to be determined in clinical trials, and concern for the fetal safety of therapies used during pregnancy is always a factor.

Nonalcoholic Fatty Liver Disease in Diabetic Women

The spectrum of nonalcoholic fatty liver disease extends from simple steatosis (macrovesicular triacylglycerol accumulation in hepatocytes) to the features of liver cell injury (hepatocyte ballooning and necrosis, mixed inflammatory-cell and microvesicular-pattern fatty infiltration, fibrosis) called nonalcoholic steatohepatitis (NASH), sometimes then progressing to cryptic cirrhosis, liver failure, and even hepatocellular carcinoma (Paradis 01, Angulo 02, Angelico 03, Caldwell 04, El-Serag 04, Trombetta 05, Farrell 06). Symptoms of steatosis and NASH are vague, and the physical examination for hepatomegaly may be difficult in pregnancy. Steatosis is visualized as bright echogenicity on ultrasound (US) of the liver (Saverymutta 86, Mishra 07), but US, computed tomography (CT), or magnetic resonance imaging (MRI) techniques are not good at detecting progression (Mathiesen 02, Saadeh 02). NASH is diagnosed by liver biopsy (Joy 03, Brunt 04, Sorrentino 04).

Common risk factors for steatosis and NASH include increased adipocyte mass (obesity), insulin resistance and hyperinsulinemia, hypertriglyceridemia, dietary excess of saturated fat, and type 2 diabetes (Neuschwander-Tetri 03, Browning 04, Tolman 04, Hamiguchi 05, Neuschwander-Tetri 05, Powell 05, Roden 06, Utzschneider 06). Liver fat content is a predictor of myocardial insulin resistance in women with type 2 diabetes and CHD (Lautamaki 06). Insulin resistance in type 1 diabetes is not associated with hepatic fat deposition (Perseghin 05). The prevalence of steatosis in overweight women of reproductive age with type 2 diabetes is probably >80%, with steatohepatitis found in at least one-half (Tolman 04).

Increased plasma ALT above aspartate aminotransferase (AST) levels are useful but imperfect markers of fatty liver disease (Kaplan 02, Prati 02, Ionnou 06), and an AST/ALT ratio >1 may indicate progression to fibrosis or cirrhosis; a ratio >2 is strongly suggestive of alcoholic liver disease (Sorbi 99, Angulo 02, de Ledinghen 04, Amarapurka 06). Type 2 diabetes in children is frequently associated (29%) with unexplained ALT elevations that are more than twice the normal range (Nadeau 05). Indeed, NASH is increasingly diagnosed in nondiabetic children (Fishbein 03, Chan 04b, Patton 06, Roberts 06) as part of the global rising tide of obesity. Increased transaminase levels are also found in 15% of women with polycystic ovary syndrome (PCOS) (Setji 06). Unfortunately, we lack prevalence data on steatosis and NASH in diabetic pregnant women, but there is no reason to believe that these conditions would be less common based on the expected gestational increases in lipolysis, NEFA (FFA), and TGs.

The pathogenesis of steatosis originates in poor glycemic control in spite of hyperinsulinemia (increased hepatic glucose production, decreased peripheral glucose disposal), insulin resistance in adipocytes causing increased hormone-sensitive lipase (HSL) activity, unrestrained TG lipolysis, and elevated FFA levels (Tolman 04). Increased hepatic uptake of FFA overloads the mitochondrial β-oxidation system, and preferential esterification to triacylglycerol (TGs) occurs for storage or incorporation into VLDL particles. A current model of the metabolic alterations resulting in hepatic TG accumulation is illustrated in Figure I.5 (Browning 04, Tamura 05). Hyperinsulinemia and hyperglycemia also induce hepatic transcription factors that activate lipogenic genes and increase conversion of excess glucose into FFA. The contribution of hepatic lipogenesis to TG secretion is increased in hyperinsulinemic patients with steatosis compared with controls (Diraison 03a). A multiple stable-isotope study of patients with NASH tracked the pathways of lipid flux through the liver; 59% of hepatic triacylglycerol arose from serum NEFA, 26% from de novo lipogenesis, and 15% from dietary fat. The pattern of labeling in VLDL was similar to that in the liver (Donnelly 05).

Knowledge of the mechanisms by which hepatic steatosis progresses to NASH is largely based on animal models that incompletely model the human disease (Browning 04). Accumulation of fatty acids in the cytosol increases fatty acid oxidation in the peroxisomes and endoplasmic reticulum with excess generation of reactive oxygen species (Robertson 01), and impaired mitochondrial respiratory chain activity directly leads to production of superoxide anions and hydrogen peroxide (Perez-Carreras 03). Oxidative stress and lipid peroxidation are thought to (1) generate inflammatory cytokines (TNF-α and IL-8) and neutrophil chemotaxis, (2) lead to fibrosis and hepatic stellate cell activation, and (3) cause cellular DNA and protein damage and apoptosis (Browning 04).

Nutritional management of fatty liver disease is based on evidence that high carbohydrate intake (including high fructose) stimulates hepatic fatty acid synthesis (Schwarz 95, Hudgins 96, Diraison 03b, Schwarz 03). Dietary intake of high-glycemic-index carbohydrates is associated with high-grade liver steatosis in insulin-resistant subjects (Valtuena 06). Low-glycemic-index meals result in lower serum NEFA levels in the late postprandial period (Ludwig 02, Jenkins 06b). Caloric restriction reduced hepatic lipogenesis in obese subjects (Diraison 02), and a moderate weight loss over 2–3 months

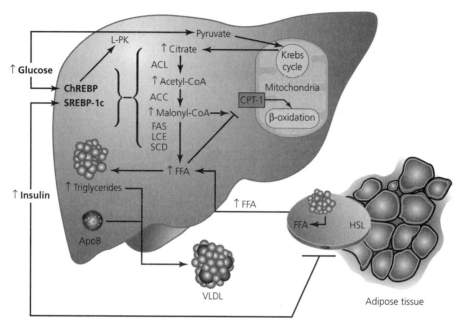

FIGURE I.5 Metabolic alterations resulting in hepatic triglyceride accumulation in insulin-resistant states. Increased hormone-sensitive lipase (HSL) activity results in elevated rates of triglyceride (TG) lipolysis and enhanced free fatty acid (FFA) flux to the liver. Hyperinsulinemia induces hepatic sterol regulatory element-binding protein 1-c (SREBP-1c) expression, leading to transcriptional activation of lipogenic genes. Hyperglycemia activates carbohydrate response element-binding protein (ChREBP), which transcriptionally activates liver-type pyruvate kinase (L-PK), which then stimulates both glycolysis and lipogenesis and facilitates the conversion of glucose to fatty acids under conditions of energy excess. Adapted from Browning 04 and used with permission.

produced a striking reduction of intrahepatic lipid and improved hepatic insulin resistance in obese subjects (Hickman 04) and middle-aged patients with type 2 diabetes (Petersen 05). A 12-month pilot study of MNT (40–45% carbohydrate, 35–40% fat, 15–20% protein) emphasizing complex carbohydrates with fiber and mono- and polyunsaturated fats showed reduction of the histologic changes of NASH in 9 of 15 patients (Huang 05). In addition to MNT, RCTs of metformin (Bugianesi 05) and pioglitazone (Belfort 06) have decreased liver fat and improved histology in patients with NASH. Clinical trials of ursodiol (± vitamin E) have shown reductions in transaminase levels without necessarily improving liver fat or histology (Laurin 96, Santos 03, Lindor 04, Mendez-Sanchez 04, Dufour 06).

As noted earlier, we are not aware of studies regarding the course of steatosis or the short- or long-term impact of NASH or its treatment in pregnancies complicated by diabetes; this appears to be a fruitful area for research. In the meantime, if the diagnosis of steatosis is suspected based on transaminase levels and liver US, the dietary principles of controlled intake of carbohydrate and fats as well as the prevention of excess weight gain can be applied. Intensified glycemic control achieved with multiple-dose insulin regimens might also reduce hepatic lipogenesis. The apparently separate, fortunately uncommon problem of the devastating late-pregnancy acute fatty liver (Usta 94, Bacq 98, Castro 99, Fesenmeier 05) does not appear to be particularly associated with maternal diabetes.

Pregnancy After Bariatric Surgery for the Treatment of Obesity

The link between the obesity epidemic and type 2 diabetes in women means that patients coming to pregnancy may have had bariatric surgery (Wittgrove 98, Martin 00, Clegg 03, Stocker 03). The most common procedures are the open or laparoscopic Roux-en-Y gastric bypass, the laparoscopic adjustable gastric band, and the complex biliopancreatic diversion that is occasionally still performed. Gastric bypass creates a very small gastric pouch that is attached directly to the jejunum with a narrow anastomosis. Vomiting of solid food is very common in the first few months after surgery, and stomal stenosis may need to be treated with baloon dilation (Huang 03). If fluids are mixed with food, symptoms of the dumping syndrome (fatigue, light-headedness, sweating, occasional diarrhea) are more pronounced. This syndrome is due to osmotic overload from foods with increased sugar content reaching the small intestine, with increased luminal fluid causing a vagal reaction (Fujioka 05). Dehydration also occurs frequently. Fluids should be taken separately from food with frequent sipping throughout the day, and digestable food should be taken in six to nine small feedings daily (Fujioka 05), thereby attempting to meet the nutritional guidelines for diabetes and pregnancy. Longer-term nutritional problems in these patients include iron-deficiency anemia (Avinoah 92) requiring intravenous iron therapy, vitamin B12 deficiency treated with 25,000 units sublingual B12 twice a week (Provenzale 92, Fujioka 05), and secondary hyperparathyroidism and bone demineralization (Goode 04) requiring higher-dose calcium and vitamin D supplementation (Fujioka 05).

Ulcers at the margin of the gastrojejunostomy anastomois can cause blood loss and/or abdominal pain (Huang 03). Nonsteroidal anti-inflammatory drugs and cyclooxygenase-2 inhibitors must not be used by gastric bypass patients (Fujioka 05). Formation of gallstones is common during surgery-induced weight loss; therefore, gallstones are removed at the time of surgery, and patients are placed on a gallstone solubilizing agent (Wudel 02). An important surgical complication during the first year after surgery is small bowel obstruction secondary to intra-abdominal adhesions or internal hernias into abnormal spaces created by gastrointestinal surgery (Higa 00,03, Liu 03). These complications, including gastrointestinal hemorrhage, can occur during pregnancy (Ramirez 95, Kakarla 05). Several studies have examined pregnancy outcome after bariatric surgery, although not in diabetic women. Fetal growth restriction; anemia due to iron, folate, and vitamin B12 deficiencies; and cesarean deliveries are significantly more common after bariatric surgery, with no difference between open and laparoscopic procedures (Rand 89, Granstrom 90, Martin 00, Dixon 01, Sheiner 04). It is claimed that adjustability of gastric bands during pregnancy results in improved outcomes (Dixon 05, Bar-Zohar 06), but RCTs have not been performed.

Recommendations

- Assess pregravid BMI and target individual gestational weight gain at the lower range of the IOM recommendations according to BMI group. (E)
- Base energy intake on BMI group physical activity level, fetal growth pattern, and desire to prevent excess maternal weight gain and postpartum weight retention. (E)
- Recognize that many obese diabetic women will not gain much weight in spite of adequate food intake and if problems with fetal well-being are not detected. Optimal gestational weight gain is not established for obese diabetic women with regard to perinatal outcome and long-term maternal health. (E)

- Develop the food plan (daily meal and snack pattern) based on individual preferences. Include (1) appropriate calorie level; (2) adequate consumption of protein (1.1 gm/kg/day), fats, and micronutrients; (3) consumption of 175 gm/d digestible carbohydrate; and (4) distribution of carbohydrate intake that will promote optimal glycemic control and avoidance of hypoglycemia and ketonemia. (E)
- Instruct the woman with diabetes to estimate the quantity of carbohydrate per serving and per meal/snack and to select the type of carbohydrates that will contribute to postprandial glucose control; encourage fiber intake (28 gm/day) by use of whole grains, fruits, and vegetables. (E)
- Use of the glycemic index and glycemic load may provide a modest additional benefit for glycemic control over that observed when total carbohydrate is considered alone. (B)
- Select a well-balanced nutrient intake, choosing foods high in fiber and including foods from all food groups. (A)
- Emphasize consistent timing of meals and snacks on a daily basis to minimize hypoglycemia, and in proper relation to insulin doses to prevent hyperglycemia. (E)
- Encourage patients to record all food and beverage intake continuously or for at least 1 week prior to each visit for assessment of adequacy of nutrient intake and comparison of carbohydrate intake with SMBG records. (E)
- Teach patients to control fat intake in the interest of long-term maternal health; encourage consumption of unsaturated fatty acids including, the *n*-6 and *n*-3 fatty acids; limit saturated fat to <10% of energy intake and *trans* fats to the minimal amount possible. (A)
- Reduce risk for CVD in diabetic women with consumption of two oily fish meals per week (of low-risk for excess mercury; fish oil 1 gm/day may be substituted, but effects on the offspring are uncertain). (A)
- Monitor weight gain, nutrient intake, and SMBG levels throughout gestation, and modify the food plan to accommodate changes in metabolic status and increased energy and nutrient needs that occur as gestation progresses. Use a grid of weight gain per time in gestation, showing normative curves for pregravid BMI groups, to facilitate assessment of appropriate weight gain. (E)
- Encourage 2.3 L/day (10 cups) fluid intake and consumption of potassium from all sources; limit sodium intake to 1.5–2.3 gm/day. (E)
- Consume folate at 600 μg/day in the periconception and prenatal periods through supplementation or fortified food sources. (A)
- Supplement mineral, trace element, and vitamin intake to achieve AI or RDA levels recommended by the IOM during all trimesters of pregnancy. (E)
- Pregnant women with diabetes should receive individualized MNT as needed to achieve treatment goals, preferably by an RD familiar with the components of diabetes and pregnancy MNT, in concert with the other clinical team members, who should also understand and support the individualized food plan. (B)
- The FDA has determined that nonnutritive sweeteners approved for general-purpose use are safe during pregnancy in moderate amounts. (A)
- Avoid all alcoholic beverages during pregnancy. (A)
- It is difficult to establish a safe level of caffeine intake during pregnancy, but the upper limit probably should be <200 mg/day. (E)

- Patients with evidence suggesting celiac disease should be referred when possible to a multidisciplinary team, including a gastroenterologist and RD specializing in celiac disease, to ensure adequate education, adherence to a GFD, and assessment of nutritional deficits. (E)
- Educate patients with evidence of hepatic steatosis about long-term risks, the benefits of controlling their intake of carbohydrates and fats, and the possibility of pharmacological therapy after pregnancy. (E)
- Promote consumption of a wholesome, balanced diet consistent with ethnic, cultural, and financial considerations. Maintain the pleasure of eating by selecting food choices according to scientific evidence, weight gain, and postprandial glucose responses. (E)

INSULIN THERAPY

—— *Original contribution by Florence M. Brown MD and Lois B. Jovanovic MD*

Insulin Regimens

Exogenous insulin administration is the mainstay of intensified therapy for PDM in pregnancy (type 1 and type 2 diabetes) (Gottlieb 02, Gonzalez 05, Lapolla 05, Homko 06, Jovanovic 08a). Multiple daily injections (MDIs) of insulin with either three or four injections per day (Coustan 80, Jovanovic 80,81, Weiss 84, Homko 96, Nachum 99, Haworka 01, Kitzmiller 03, Homko 06, Jovanovic 08a) or CSIIs with an external pump (Potter 81, Rudolf 81, Kitzmiller 85, Caruso 87, Leveno 88, Gabbe 00, Simmons 02) are necessary in most women with type 1 diabetes to achieve optimal glucose control (Table I.3) for pregnancy. Although some women with type 2 diabetes can achieve treatment goals by using conventional mixed/split dose regimens (Table I.12), women who eat their largest meal at midday may not be able to maintain optimal postprandial glucose levels without an injection of short-acting insulin before lunch. In patients with type 1 diabetes, an initial period of increased insulin sensitivity at 10–14 weeks gestation may be seen in well-controlled patients (Weiss 84, Haworka 01, Jovanovic 01). After that time, insulin requirements are expected to rise sequentially as much as 60–200% throughout pregnancy in type 1 diabetes, with rather wide individual variation (Rayburn 85, Langer 88, Haworka 01, Fuglsang 03). The insulin requirement often levels off or declines after 35 weeks (Weiss 84, McManus 92, Steel 94). In women with type 2 diabetes, insulin requirements may double or triple during the course of pregnancy (Rigg 80, Langer 88).

In studies of insulin kinetics, the disappearance rate of single intravenous injections of insulin is not accelerated or delayed in normal pregnancy (Burt 74, Bellmann 75, Lind 77), suggesting that placental degradation of insulin is not a factor in the progressive insulin resistance of pregnancy (Rigg 80, Cowett 83, Gray 84, Ryan 85, Schmitz 85, Buchanan 90b, Catalano 91,92,93, Sivan 97, Catalano 99). Insulin sensitivity decreases at least 40% as estimated by peripheral glucose uptake in the second and third trimesters in nondiabetic pregnant women (Sivan 97, Catalano 99). Conflicting results emerge regarding whether changed insulin clearance occurs during pregnancy when using insulin infusion/glycemic clamp techniques (Gray 84, Catalano 98b). Investigators using a hypoglycemic clamp (to 40 mg/dL) in women with type 1 diabetes found a 24% lower metabolic clearance rate of insulin in the third trimester compared with the same patients

TABLE I.12 Regimens of Insulin Treatment for Preexisting Diabetes During Pregnancy

Parameter	Conventional Mixed/Split Dose	Intensive Multiple Daily Injections	Continuous Subcutaneous Insulin Infusion
Insulin administration technique	Injections before breakfast and dinner	3–4 injections before meals, bedtime	External programmable insulin pump
Type of insulin	Mixed intermediate, short-acting	Mixed in a.m., short-acting before meals, NPH at bedtime	Short-acting only
Typical dosing ratios*	2/3 a.m.: short:NPH 1:2 1/3 p.m.: short:NPH 1:1-3	50% NPH: a.m.:p.m. 1–2:1 50% short: 3:2:2	50% basal rate units/h 50% boluses before meals and snacks: 3:1:2:1:2:1
Glucose monitoring	Fasting, after meals	Fasting, after meals, before dinner or bedtime	Before and after meals, bedtime, 3 a.m. prn
Grade of control	Average to poor	Good unless "brittle" type 1 diabetes	Good, especially for daytime or nocturnal hypoglycemia; dawn phenomenon; variable carbohydrate intake
Problematic application	—	Insufficient motivation; inappropriate personality	Insufficient motivation; inappropriate personality; inability to master mechanics of monitoring and dose adjustments

*Fixed ratio insulin preparations (intermediate/short-acting) typically do not provide sufficient dose-adjustment flexibility for use in intensified treatment in pregnancy.

CSII, continuous subcutaneous insulin infusion; MDI, multiple daily injection.
Modified from Homko 96 and Kitzmiller 03.

tested 5–13 months after delivery (Bjorklund 98). The authors reasoned that this result could be due to altered blood-flow distribution and decreased hepatic insulin extraction, as well as a relative increase in body fat during pregnancy, and that the lowered insulin clearance rate would contribute to the risk for serious hypoglycemic events in type 1 diabetes patients during gestation.

Both MDI and CSII use the concept of basal and bolus insulin replacement to approximate physiological delivery of insulin during fasting and eating (DeWitt 93a,b). Basal insulin is used to cover the fasting and postabsorptive insulin requirements, and bolus doses are used to control postprandial glucose excursions. Patients are taught which glucose targets are affected by individual doses of insulin. Tailoring of insulin doses by "daily pattern management" rather than "after-the-fact catch-up doses" is recommended because this approach yields smoother glycemic control (Homko 96). Detailed algorithms are available for teaching self-adjustment of insulin doses during pregnancy based on premeal glucose levels, anticipated food choices, and intercurrent illness (Skyler 81, Miller 94, Hirsch 98b, Jovanovic-Peterson 07, Haworka 01, Jovanovic 08b). A relationship exists between the premeal insulin dose and the postprandial response to the amount and type of carbohydrate in the meal (Franz 02, ADA 08a,b).

Insulin-to-carbohydrate ratios allow the woman with diabetes to adjust the premeal dose of insulin for the anticipated number of carbohydrate grams, exchanges, or servings eaten per meal; as the pregnancy progresses, the insulin requirements change and so will the insulin-to-carbohydrate ratio. Because the ratio changes repeatedly during pregnancy, many clinicians ignore it and simply increase insulin doses as needed, comparing food records with pre- and postprandial glucose readings. Although the insulin-to-carbohydrate ratio allows for flexibility in food intake, eating consistent amounts of carbohydrate in the dynamic state of pregnancy is beneficial to many women in achieving optimal glucose control and preventing hypoglycemia.

Insulin should be started as soon as possible in patients with type 2 diabetes who have been taking oral medications prior to pregnancy. Oral medications should be stopped. When converting patients with type 2 diabetes to insulin therapy in early pregnancy, an initial total daily dose of 0.7 units/kg present body weight is often effective, adjusted according to subsequent glucose levels (Homko 96, Kitzmiller 03, Jovanovic 08a). The insulin dosage may initially be divided ~50/50 between basal and bolus needs. One method of initiating insulin is to use bedtime NPH insulin 0.2 units/kg and premeal rapid- or short-acting insulin 0.25 units/kg divided over three meals. Basal and bolus insulin doses are adjusted empirically according to pre- and postmeal blood glucose levels (Jovanovic 08b). Morning or lunchtime NPH (basal insulin) may be added if prelunch, predinner, or bedtime glucose levels are above target. Titration of insulin doses should proceed rapidly, with patients reporting glucose values and insulin doses every 2–3 days so that adjustments can be made.

Types of Insulin Used in Pregnancy

NPH Insulin

In MDI therapy, intermediate-acting NPH insulin is used two to four times/day to provide basal coverage. It is assumed that the time-actions of injected human-like insulins (Hirsch 98b, DeWitt 03b, Mooradian 06) are unchanged during pregnancy (Miller 94, Jovanovic 07). NPH has an onset of action at 1–4 h, peaks at 4–10 h, and has an end of action at 11–17 h (Lepore 00, DeWitt 03b), with some day-to-day and intersubject variability of subcutaneous absorption (Bolli 89). The larger the insulin dose, the more prolonged the absorption (Binder 84). Ultra-lente (U-L) is a long-acting insulin with an onset of action at 1–4 h, peak action at 8–14 h, and end of action at 18–30 h after injection (Hirsch 98b, Lepore 00). However, because U-L has such an unpredictable absorption pattern, its use is rarely beneficial in pregnancy. Historically, NPH was preferred over Lente (a mixture of semi-Lente and ultra-Lente) because NPH produced less intra- and intersubject variability of insulin concentrations after injection (Lindstrom 00). The relatively short peak-action profile of NPH may contribute to the risk of nocturnal hypoglycemia in pregnancy (Kimmerle 92), even when taken at bedtime; a bedtime snack is used to reduce this risk. Middle-of-the-night glucose levels should be spot-checked one or more times per week to rule out hypoglycemia and certainly checked when fasting glucose is above or below the target range. Another consideration to avoid fasting hyperglycemia is to awaken within 8–10 h after the bedtime dose, test FPG levels and administer the a.m. insulin doses as the nighttime insulin concentration is waning. Dosing of NPH in the early evening should be avoided except in patients with documented stable nocturnal and fasting glucose levels. A lunchtime injection of intermediate insulin may be needed to prevent presupper or bedtime hyperglycemia in some patients.

Insulin Glargine

The long-acting analog-variant insulin glargine is less soluble at neutral pH due to a shift in its isoelectric point and has delayed dissociation into monomers; this results in a slow but sustained release of subcutaneous insulin into the circulation (Lepore 00, Rosenstock 00). Glargine provides steadier serum levels than NPH or U-L over 24 h in patients who are not pregnant, with an onset of action at 1.2–1.8 h after injection and an end of action at 18–26 h (Heinemann 00, Lepore 00). Glargine can be injected once daily at breakfast, dinner, or bedtime with equivalent results (Hamann 03), and there is no effect on absorption from exercise (Peter 05). A possible advantage is that glargine induces less hypoglycemia than NPH (Ratner 00, Rosenstock 05).

Information regarding the use of insulin glargine in pregnancy is limited to case reports (Devlin 02a, Holstein 03, Dolci 05, Al-Shaikh 06) and short observational series (Di Cianni 05, Wooderink 05, Poyhoenen-Alho 07, Price 07, Torlone 07, Gallen 08), including <300 patients with no untoward results reported. Due to the need for frequent adjustment of basal insulin doses in pregnancy and diurnal variation in basal insulin needs that is potentiated in pregnancy, the effect of insulin glargine may be too flat. Thus, insulin glargine may be less useful than NPH because of glargine's long half-life and the amount of time necessary to reach steady-state equilibrium. Bedtime NPH may produce better fasting glucose levels. Lack of controlled data on safety in pregnancy (Hofmann 02) suggests that insulin glargine should not be used in pregnancy except in clinical trials. Glargine demonstrates six- to tenfold increased binding to the IGF-1 receptor and mitogenic potency compared with native insulin (Kurtzhals 00, Ciaraldi 01, Zib 06, Jovanovic 07). IGF-1 receptors are more abundant than insulin receptors in human macro- and microvascular cells (Chisalita 04). The role of possible enhanced activation of IGF-1 receptors in retinal angiogenesis or placental function in pregnancies complicated by diabetes is unknown. It is also unknown whether insulin glargine crosses the placenta.

Insulin Detemir

Insulin detemir is another insulin analog variant with a prolonged pharmacodynamic profile due to lack of precipitation after injection and its ability to self-associate into hexamers and bind reversibly to albumin (Morales 07). Detemir's duration of action (6–23 h) is dependent on dose (Plank 05a), and it has much higher serum concentrations at 6–12 h compared with NPH insulin (Danne 03). Insulin detemir has less affinity to insulin receptors and IGF-1 receptors and less mitogenic potency than human insulin (Kurtzhals 00, Jovanovic 07). We lack data on detemir's efficacy and safety in pregnancy and whether it crosses the placenta; therefore, its use in pregnancy should be limited to clinical trials.

Regular Insulin U-500

Human Regular insulin given by bolus injection 20–40 min before meals (Dimitriadis 83, Lean 85) has been the standard type of insulin used for postprandial glucose control during pregnancy. Onset of action for Regular is 30–60 min, peak of action is 2–3 h, and effective duration of action is 5–8 h (Hirsch 98b, DeWitt 03b). Subcutaneous injection into fat rolls of the abdomen or hip provides the most rapid and consistent absorption of short-acting insulin and avoids the variation in insulin absorption caused by proximity to exercising muscle in the arm or leg (Witt 83, Bantle 93). Bolus insulin treatment is coupled to ingestion of meals or snacks (Jovanovic 08b). Short- or rapid-acting insulin is given before carbohydrate is ingested, either with a set food plan that involves consistent carbohydrate at meals and snacks or based on a predetermined insulin–carbohydrate ratio that allows for more flexible carbohydrate intake. A one-time correction dose based on an empiric adjustment scale or calculated sensitivity factor may be given to account for elevated or low premeal glucose values (Miller 94, Hirsch 98b). Continuing adjustments of bolus doses are based on trends of postprandial glucose values. This approach to bolus insulin treatment is used with both MDI and CSII.

Regular insulin U-500 (500 units/mL) may be used to reduce the volume of insulin required at a single bolus injection in patients with severe insulin resistance (Cochrane 05, Neal 05, Ballani 06, Wafa 06). This insulin may be preferable for women taking >100 units at one time because it reduces the number of required injections; patients are often taught to divide large-volume insulin injections into two or three sites to improve insulin absorption. Regular insulin U-500 may also be used in CSII when very large volumes of insulin are required in patients with type 2 diabetes (Knee 03, Hatipoglu 06). The pharmacokinetics of Regular U-500 are similar to repository insulins, but individual responses may vary. Slower absorption and longer duration appear to be related to the preparation's higher concentration (Cochrane 05). Clinicians and patients should be very clear about dosing, such as 50 units of Regular U-500 in a U-100 insulin syringe equals 250 units of insulin.

Rapid-Acting, Genetically Modified Human Insulin Analog Variants

Insulin lispro (H), insulin aspart (NL), and insulin glulisine do not self-aggregate in solution as does human Regular insulin, thus leading to much more rapid absorption (DiMarchi 94, DeWitt 03b, Jovanovic 07). Onset of action is 5–15 min after injection, peak action is 30–90 min, and effective duration is 4–5 h (DeWitt 03b, Guerci 05, Hirsch 05); it is assumed that these pharmacodynamic measures do not differ in pregnancy. Subcutaneous abdominal injection of insulin lispro in healthy subjects results in faster absorption and shortened duration of action compared with deltoid or femoral injections as well as higher serum insulin concentrations (98 μU/ml, 589 pM) compared with Regular insulin (47 μU/ml, 281 pM) (terBraak 96). Subcutaneous abdominal injection of insulin aspart in nondiabetic subjects also results in higher peak serum insulin levels compared with human Regular insulin injected at the same site (75 vs. 31.5 μU/ml; 450 vs. 190 pM) (Mudaliar 99). Insulin glulisine has similar pharmacokinetics to other analogs (Danne 05, Rave 06) and is comparable to human insulin in binding to the IGF-1 receptor and stimulation of thymidine uptake in human skeletal muscle cells (Ciaraldi 05).

Insulins lispro or aspart injected 5 min before or during meals (Anderson 97, Brunelle 98, Strachan 98, Chatterjee 99) may improve patient compliance, decrease postmeal glucose excursions, and lower the risk of premeal and nocturnal hypoglycemia during pregnancy (Garg 03, Mecacci 03, Carr 04). For consistent long-term improvement in overall glycemic control using these shorter-acting insulin analog variants, doses of basal insulin need to be increased (Ebeling 97, Del Sindaco 98, Colombel 99). A meta-analysis of 42 RCTs that assessed the effect of rapid-acting insulin analogs compared with Regular insulin revealed a minor benefit in A1C values in adults with type 1 diabetes, but no benefit in type 2 diabetes (Plank 05b).

Although large RCTs of insulin lispro in pregnant women with PDM are not available (Carr 06), several retrospective and small prospective clinical trials support the effectiveness and safety of insulins lispro and aspart in pregnancy (Jovanovic 99a, Bhattacharyya 01, Persson 02, Scherbaum 02, Masson 03, Garg 03, Mecacci 03, Carr 04, Cypryk 04, Lapolla 08). One RCT of insulin aspart in 322 pregnant women with type 1 diabetes has been reported. There was no increase in maternal (Mathiesen 07) or fetal complications (Hod 08a) compared with human insulin. Use of insulin aspart produced improved postprandial glucose control at the end of the first and third trimesters (Mathiesen 07), and there was a trend toward fewer preterm deliveries in this study with limited power to discriminate differences in outcome (Hod 08a). Insulin aspart did not cross the placenta into fetal blood in preliminary studies (Jovanovic 07).

Insulin lispro does not appear to cross the human placenta (Jovanovic 99a) unless serum concentrations are >200 μU/ml (1,200 pM) (Boskovic 03), but high concentrations of insulin lispro did accumulate in human placental tissue in an in vitro study (Holcberg 04). Insulin lispro does not appear to cause an increased incidence of congenital malformations when used at the beginning of pregnancy (Diamond 97, Bhattacharyya 01, Scherbaum 02, Masson 03, Wyatt 05, Lapolla 08), although RCTs are lacking. We are not aware of experience with insulin glulisine during pregnancy.

Insulin lispro has 156% binding affinity and insulin aspart has 81% binding affinity to the solubilized human IGF-1 receptor compared with human insulin (Kurtzhals 00). IGF-1 receptors are five to sevenfold more abundant than insulin receptors in human micro- and macroendothelial cells (Chisalita 04). Due to the much larger binding affinity of free IGF-1 than any insulin for the IGF-1 receptor, the IGF-1 receptor probably does not play a role in mediating the effects of insulin at normal physiological levels of insulin. Yet at supraphysiological insulin concentrations as attained in treatment of insulin-resistant patients, insulin might exert mitogenic effects via the IGF-1 receptor (King 85, Kurtzhals 00, Chisalita 04). Insulin and IGF-1 may contribute to retinal neovascularization (Merimee 97, Reiter 03) "in part, by modulating the expression of various vascular mediators" (Bronson 03). Several recent studies continue to suggest a role for IGF-1 in the pathogenesis of proliferative diabetic retinopathy (PDR) (Boulton 97, Chantelau 98, Burgos 00, Spranger 00, Simo 02, Lauszus 03, Guidry 04) and in experimental models of retinal neovascularization (Smith 99, Poulaki 02, Kondo 03, Poulaki 04, Ruberte 04), perhaps by enhancement of the effects of vascular endothelial growth factor (VEGF) (Punglia 97, Miele 00). Although insulin lispro and insulin glargine have increased binding to the IGF-I receptor, premarketing trials did not suggest that their use was associated with increased rates or worsening of PDR.

Hybrid insulin/IGF-1 receptors exist when a αβ segment of the insulin receptor is crosslinked to a αβ segment of the homologous IGF-1 receptor (Reiter 03). Hybrid receptors are widely distributed in human tissues and could be more responsive to insulins with IGF-1 activity (Soos 93, Seely 95, Bailyes 97, Federici 97a, Pandini 02, Sakai 03). Insulin/IGF-1 hybrid receptor expression and content increases with hyperglycemia or hyperinsulinemia (Federici 96,97b,99). The role of hybrid insulin/IGF-1 receptors in retinal neovascularization (Reiter 03) and in placental responses (Bailyes 97, Valensise 96) to insulin treatment during pregnancy is unknown.

One anecdotal report involves the development of retinal neovascularization by late pregnancy in three of ten poorly controlled diabetic women switched from Regular insulin to insulin lispro at the end of the first trimester (Kitzmiller 99). This is a rare finding because the patients had no clinical retinopathy in early pregnancy. Hyperglycemic patients may have subclinical retinal ischemia/hypoxia at the initiation of intensified treatment, so the development of neovascularization in these women has been ascribed to rapid improvement of glycemic control (Chantelau 97, Jovanovic 99b). However, intensified treatment with Regular insulin has been necessary in early pregnancy in countless diabetic women that did not develop de novo PDR. Intensification of insulin treatment increases free IGF-1 (Attia 99) and exacerbates diabetic blood–retinal barrier breakdown (Poulaki 02). Data on so-called "early worsening" of DR with intensified glycemic control in pregnancy are included in Part II in the section titled "Diabetic Retinopathy and Pregnancy."

Regarding insulin lispro, subsequent retrospective (Bhattacharyya 99, Buchbinder 00, Masson 03) and prospective (Persson 02, Loukovaara 03) studies in 110 patients using insulin lispro before conception did not confirm an association with development of PDR either during or after pregnancy. Studies after the initial report found that only 12 women were changed to insulin lispro in early pregnancy due to poor glycemic control; of these, none developed PDR de novo or from nonproliferative diabetic retinopathy (NPDR). Only one of these studies was a randomized trial, with approximately eight subjects with poor glycemic control in each treatment group (Persson 02). Data are insufficient to conclude whether conversion to insulin lispro therapy in diabetic pregnant women with poor glycemic control is associated with development of serious retinopathy by the end of pregnancy—at a frequency no different than that found with use of human Regular insulin—in the absence of a large randomized trial.

Insulin Delivery Systems

Syringes with short ultrafine needles are most commonly used in pregnancy due to low cost. Use of the lowest-dose syringe possible (0.3 cc − 30 units; 0.5 cc − 50 units; 1.0 cc − 100 units) may increase the accuracy of administration (DeWitt 03b). Insulin pens (Jovanovic 08a) are easiest to use, but often at increased cost (Homko 96, DeWitt 03b). Nasal and aerosolized inhaled insulins (Schatz 04, Freemantle 05, Rave 05, Skyler 05, Barnett 06, Ceglia 06) remain experimental in pregnancy.

CSII delivered by an external insulin pump delivers a predetermined small amount of rapid- or short-acting insulin per hour for basal levels of insulin (e.g., 0.1–2.0 units/h). Progammed adjustment of the hourly basal insulin dose is based on clinician and patient analysis of premeal, bedtime, and overnight glucose values because serial fasting is not conducted during pregnancy to determine insulin requirements. During pregnancy, basal doses may need adjustment ranging from every few days to 1–2 weeks. Bolus doses determined by the patient and given before meals are adjusted based on (a) the previous pattern of postprandial glucose values, (b) the immediate premeal glucose value, and (c) expected carbohydrate intake (Jovanovic 08b). Clinical trials of MDI and CSII in pregnancy generally showed equivalent glycemic control and perinatal outcome (Carta 86, Coustan 86, Burkart 88, Lapolla 03, Hieronimus 05, Chen 07, Farrar 07, Gimenez 07), but the multiple programmable basal rates offered by CSII can be especially useful for patients with daytime or nocturnal hypoglycemia or a prominent dawn phenomenon (increased insulin requirement between 4 and 8 a.m.) (Bolli 93, Simmons 02). Disadvantages of CSII (DeWitt 03a, Gabbe 04) are cost and the potential for marked hyperglycemia and risk of diabetic KTA as a consequence of insulin delivery failure. Although this is an unusual occurrence, it can happen when technical problems arise with the pump or, more frequently, when there is kinking of the catheter, an air bubble in the tubing that displaces insulin, or failure to change the insertion site every 3 days. Frequent glucose testing is necessary to identify these problems.

Recommendations

- For optimal glycemic control in pregnancy in women with type 1 or type 2 diabetes, provision of basal and prandial insulin needs with intensified insulin regimens usually provides the best results (multiple dose regimens of subcutaneous long- and short-acting insulins, or continuous subcutaneous insulin infusion - CSII). (E)

- Basal insulin is best provided by injections of NPH two to four times daily or by adjustable hourly basal insulin infusion of rapid-acting insulin with CSII. (E)

- Patients who are taking a daily dose of insulin detemir or insulin glargine should be transitioned to a twice- or three-times-daily dosing of NPH, preferably prior to pregnancy or at the first prenatal visit, pending clinical trials proving efficacy and safety. (E)

- Consider matching prandial insulin doses to carbohydrate intake, premeal blood glucose, and anticipated activity. (E)

- Rapid-acting insulin analogs, such as lispro or aspart, may produce better postprandial control with less hypoglycemia compared with use of premeal Regular insulin in some pregnant women with PDM. (E)

- Injections should be given in the abdomen or hips for consistency of absorption. (E)

- Consider teaching patients to correct high postmeal or nighttime blood glucose levels (>250 mg/dL) with an injection of rapid-acting insulin according to an individualized scale. (E)

- Patients using CSII should be trained in careful operation and checking of the insulin delivery system and should check fingerstick glucose frequently. Those with postmeal or nighttime glucose ≥250 mg/dL in the absence of urine or blood ketones should administer a supplemental bolus dose of rapid-acting insulin by syringe and recheck within 2 h to ensure that glucose levels are improving. Capillary glucose ≥200 mg/dL in the presence of urine ketones should be treated immediately with a subcutaneous injection of short-acting insulin via syringe. Capillary glucose and urine ketones should be checked hourly. The infusion setup should be changed and glucose levels carefully reevaluated. (E)

ORAL MEDICATIONS FOR TYPE 2 DIABETES IN PREGNANCY

—— Original contribution by Deborah L. Conway MD and
William H. Herman MD, MPH

Insulin therapy remains the standard method of PDM treatment in pregnancy. Oral antihyperglycemic agents (Merlob 02) are not generally used to treat pregnant women with type 2 diabetes for two primary reasons. First, fears over fetal harm due to transplacental passage of drug, both during organogenesis and later fetal development, have led to most of these medications being avoided during pregnancy. The second reason is related to increased insulin resistance during pregnancy. Added to the existing insulin resistance of type 2 diabetes, these gestation-related changes make it unlikely that optimal glycemic targets can be met by using oral agents during pregnancy (Ekpebegh 07).

Sulfonylureas

These agents bind to specific receptors (SURs) on pancreatic β-cells, hepatocytes, skeletal muscle, and cardiac and vascular cells. Endogenous ligands of the SURs "are presumed to be gastrointestinal peptides released following ingestion of meals" (Melander 04). Drug binding to SURs is linked to closure of ATP-dependent K$^+$ ion channels (K$_{ATP}$) in the cell membrane, depolarization, increased calcium ion influx, and exocytosis of insulin from β-cells (Kamp 03, Melander 04, Ling 06). The primary clinical effect of sulfonylureas is attributable to promotion of insulin secretion, although they also increase glucose uptake (Groop 91). The extrapancreatic effects of sulfonylureas are of uncertain clinical significance (Belfiore 00). Striking differences exist among sulfonylureas in pharmacokinetics, affinity, potency and effective plasma levels, rates of absorption and onset of action, elimination and duration of action, and risk of long-lasting hypoglycemia (Melander 04). Few of these characteristics have been studied systematically in pregnant patients (Anderson 05, Hebert 07).

First-generation sulfonylureas (acetohexamide, chlorpropamide, tolazamide, tolbutamide) cross the placenta and are highly bound to fetal plasma albumin, causing a long plasma half-life (Miller 62, Elliott 94, Christesen 98, Garcia-Bournissen 03). They stimulate neonatal insulin secretion and were associated with prolonged neonatal hypoglycemia in early studies (Zucker 68, Kemball 70). Effectiveness was not established with use of these agents in type 2 diabetes and GDM in pregnancy (Notelovitz 71, Sutherland 74, Coetzee 80, Tran 04).

Second-generation sulfonylureas (glibenclamide/glyburide, glipizide, glimepiride) have increased affinity to SURs (a 1,000-fold increase compared with first generation, but a 100-fold increase in hypoglycemic activity), resulting in lower effective doses in the range of 1–10 mg and lower effective plasma levels of 50–100 nM (peak level: ~105 ng/mL for glyburide) (Melander 04). Of these agents, glyburide has the slowest absorption, which is further delayed during hyperglycemia (Groop 89, Hoffman 94). Glyburide is eliminated by hepatic metabolism, with a half-life of 15–24 h (including active metabolites) (Jonsson 94). Prolonged exposure to higher-range plasma levels of these sulfonylureas downregulates SUR sensitivity so that, at some point, increasing the dosage for persisting hyperglycemia can be counterproductive (Stenman 93, Jonsson 01). Apparently, sulfonylureas operate within a fairly narrow range of plasma concentrations, with little evidence of further increases in plasma insulin levels or glucose uptake above glyburide or glipizide doses of 10 mg/day in the nonpregnant patient (Groop 91, Stenman 93, Melander 04).

SUR sensitivity is unstudied during pregnancy, but biotransformation of glyburide by the hepatic cytochrome P450 oxidase system (CYP2C9 isoform) (Kirkheiner 02, Niemi 02, Wilkinson 02) is likely to be progressively enhanced (25–47%) throughout gestation (Anderson 05, Tracy 05). Therefore, glyburide concentrations are likely to be lower in pregnancy than postpartum, and dosage may need to be greater (Hebert 07). Genetic polymorphisms of CYP2C9 are fairly common and can influence the clinical pharmacokinetics of glyburide (Kirkheiner 02, Niemi 02, Wilkinson 05) and its drug–drug interactions (Rettie 05). CYP2C9 is widely expressed in nonhepatic tissues, including endothelium (Rettie 05), but not placenta (Hakkola 96a,b,98). Human and baboon placental microsomes metabolize glyburide in vitro, but with much less activity and different specificity than the corresponding hepatic CYP isozymes (Ravindran 06, Zharikova 07).

It is noteworthy that SUR1 belongs to the ATP-binding cassette (ABC) protein superfamily that includes the efflux pump P-glycoprotein that is important in extrusion of drugs from many cell types (Payen 01, Lee 04b). P-glycoprotein is localized to the maternal surface brush border of human trophoblasts (Nakamura 97, Ushigome 00). Glyburide is a substrate for or will inhibit P-glycoprotein activity (Golstein 99, Payen 00), and pharmacological blockade of placental P-glycoprotein by glyburide might increase fetal exposure to other drugs in early pregnancy (Smit 99, Molso 05).

Radiolabeled glyburide crossed the placenta well at midpregnancy in rats, resulting in a fetal tissue–maternal blood ratio of radioactivity similar to that for freely diffused diazepam (Sivan 95). The role of SUR/K_{ATP} channels in placental effects of glyburide is unknown. Glyburide does block K_{ATP} channels in human fetoplacental arteries, resulting in increased vascular tone and perfusion pressure (Bisseling 05). However, in an ex vivo system using isolated human-term placenta cotyledons, perfusion of the maternal side with glyburide and glipizide in an albumin-containing solution produced limited cumulative placental transport over 2 h of 2.4% and 5.6%, respectively, compared with 11.0% for chlorpropamide and 22.8% for tolbutamide (Elliott 94). Pharmacokinetic considerations suggest that differences in placental transfer of these drugs are not related to pKa, molecular weight, or lipid solubility (Koren 01). The "insignificant transfer" of glyburide (Elliott 91) was presumably due to the short in vivo elimination half-life of 4–6 h and to its very high binding to maternal protein (99.8% for glyburide vs. 96.0% for tolbutamide), leaving 0.2% glyburide free to cross the placenta compared with 4.0% for tolbutamide (a 20-fold difference). In a subsequent preliminary report of a clinical study of glyburide dosing in pregnancies complicated by GDM, the umbilical vein/maternal plasma ratio of glyburide at birth was 0.58 ± 0.24 (Hebert 07), casting doubt on the relevance of the ex vivo studies.

After an initial randomized trial (Langer 00), glyburide has been used safely in the treatment of GDM (Chmait 04, Conway 04, Kremer 04, Langer 05) but without proof that it is better or equal to insulin therapy in reducing neonatal complications of maternal diabetes (Jacobson 05, Cheng 06, Rochon 06). In fact, the most recent small observational studies suggest that neonatal outcome may be worsened with glyburide rather than with insulin treatment (Holt 07, Ramos 07). Glyburide was not associated with excess neonatal hypoglycemia compared with maternal insulin therapy in the only RCT (Langer 00). Additional RCTs are needed in hyperglycemic women with GDM to answer uncertainties about neonatal outcome, with careful monitoring of glycemic control, weight gain, and other variables that can affect perinatal results. However, it is unlikely that glyburide would be effective in the presence of the impaired insulin secretion and stronger insulin resistance of type 2 diabetes in pregnancy (Langer 05, Kahn 06). There is anecdotal evidence of glyburide use in addition to insulin therapy in type 2 diabetes patients with extreme degrees of insulin resistance in pregnancy, but we need properly controlled trials to determine whether glyburide or similar agents will play a role in the care of pregnant women with type 2 diabetes. Glyburide induces multiple defects in glucagon and growth hormone responses to insulin-induced hypoglycemia (Landstedt-Hallin 99, terBraak 02), which may contribute to the problem of clinical hypoglycemia associated with its use (Ferner 88, Stahl 99, Yogev 04b).

Concerns over harm from sulfonylureas to the early fetus originate primarily from studies dating back several decades. The quality of these studies precludes drawing meaningful conclusions from them regarding the association between drug exposure and congenital anomalies (Gutzin 03). Many are case reports or uncontrolled series (Comess 69, Sutherland 74, Soler 76, Coetzee 84, Ramos-Arroyo 92, Hellmuth 94,00b,

Tran 04), and the degree of hyperglycemia in early pregnancy (teratogenic in itself) (Kitzmiller 96) was either high or unable to be discerned from the information provided. Tolbutamide given in vivo to several species of pregnant laboratory animals produced embryonic malformations independent of maternal hypo- or hyperglycemia (Smithberg 63, McColl 67), but glibenclamide in large doses produced no excess malformations (Hebold 69). Mouse embryos exposed to chlorpropamide or tolbutamide concentrations of therapeutic range in whole embryo culture demonstrated NTDs and cardiac defects (Smoak 92,93). It is uncertain whether glyburide or glipizide would achieve significant exposure to human embryos in vivo.

In women, a retrospective cohort study of 16 type 2 diabetes patients exposed to sulfonylureas during early pregnancy revealed an increased rate of anomalies (4 major; 6 minor [4 were ear defects]) compared with five major anomalies in 40 matched women with type 2 diabetes who used insulin therapy at the beginning of pregnancy (Piaquadio 91). However, the exposed babies also had higher rates of polycythemia and hyperbilirubinemia at birth (many months after medication had been stopped), suggesting overall worse glycemic control in these women compared with the patients on insulin. A larger retrospective cohort study of 147 women who took chlorpropamide, glyburide, or glipizide at any time in the first 8 weeks of pregnancy used a prospectively collected database initiated at 13.4 ± 1.5 weeks (Towner 95). Investigators found no significant difference in the rate of major anomalies between infants of type 2 diabetic women using sulfonylurea treatment, insulin, or diet therapy in early pregnancy (9.5%, 11.7%, 14.4%, respectively). First-trimester A1C level was the only independent predictor of the risk of anomalies by stepwise regression analysis. The authors concluded that risk of major malformations was associated with poor glycemic control in early pregnancy and not with use of sulfonylureas (Towner 95). However, data are inadequate to conclude that sulfonylurea use is safe during human organogenesis. On the other hand, stopping sulfonylurea treatment at diagnosis of pregnancy without immediate conversion to adequate insulin therapy may be more dangerous due to the expected worsening of glycemic control during embryogenesis/organogenesis (weeks 3–10 from last menstrual period).

Biguanides

Phenformin and metformin are biguanide drugs with similar antihyperglycemic actions but different degrees of lactic acidosis–provoking toxicity based on their kinetics-effect relationships (Melander 04). Phenformin is hydrophobic, weakly basic, and nonpolar and is inactivated by a hepatic cytochromal enzyme. This enzyme has low activity in some women and is competitively bound by other common medications, resulting in dangerous accumulation of the biguanide drug. Metformin is hydrophilic, strongly basic, polar, unbound to plasma proteins, and is mainly excreted by renal filtration and tubular secretion, the latter probably via organic cation transporter 2 (OCT2) (Wang 02). OCT1 seems to be responsible for hepatic and intestinal uptake of metformin, at least in the rat (Wang 02). Judicious use of metformin can avoid drug-induced lactic acidosis (Melander 04). Effective doses are 0.5–1.5 gm/day, with plasma levels at 0.05–0.1 mg/dL (Belfiore 00). Renal OCT2 may be inhibited by progesterone in pregnancy, whereas renal filtration is increased in pregnancy. The net effect may be lowered metformin concentrations during pregnancy (Hughes 06a). One limited study suggested that the pharmacokinetics of metformin in late pregnancy were similar to those in nonpregnant patients, with mean maternal clearance at 28 L/h/70 kg and mean volume of distribution at 190 L/70 kg (Charles 06).

Recent research identifies OCT1 and OCT3 in amnion epithelial cells (Hayer-Zillgen 02); OCT2 was found to be weakly expressed in placenta (Zhang 98) and OCT3 to be abundantly expressed (Kekuda 98). OCT2 is also detected at a low level in the intima of fetoplacental veins (Bottalico 04). The role of these OCTs in transport or elimination of metformin into or out of the fetoplacental unit is unknown. However, metformin readily crosses the human placenta in late pregnancy in in vivo (Hague 03) and ex vivo experiments as rapidly as antipyrine (Nanovskaya 06), with fetal concentrations approaching those of the gravida (Vanky 05, Charles 06).

The antihyperglycemic effect of metformin is mainly due to enhanced hepatic insulin sensitivity, reduced hepatic glucose output, and increased fasting glucose clearance (Kirpichnikov 02, Natali 06). Whether metformin facilitates insulin-stimulated glucose uptake in skeletal muscle and whole body glucose disposal is controversial (Galuska 94, Kumar 02, Karlsson 05, Natali 06). Metformin suppresses hepatic gluconeogenesis from many substrates, presumably by increasing mitochondrial levels of calcium and interfering with respiratory oxidation in mitochondria (Owen 00). Metformin enhances AMP-activated protein kinase signaling in hepatocytes and skeletal muscle (Musi 02), which can ameliorate lipid-induced insulin resistance in the liver (Cleasby 04). FFA levels and their oxidation by tissue are reduced by metformin (Perriello 94). This effect can improve insulin sensitivity and help correct FFA-impaired insulin secretion by β-cells (Kirpichnikov 02). Metformin decreases apoptosis of β-cells and improves the redox state of pancreatic islets isolated from patients with type 2 diabetes (Marchetti 04).

Metformin decreases intestinal absorption of glucose, but increases intestinal consumption of glucose and production of lactate. Absorption of vitamin B12 and folate is also reduced by metformin, leading to a 5% increase in serum homocysteine (Wulffele 03); however, this malabsorptive effect can be reversed by an increased calcium intake of 1 gm/day (Baumann 00). Other effects of metformin include facilitation of weight loss, improved lipoprotein profiles, and decreased levels of plasminogen activator inhibitor-1. Finally, metformin decreases vasoconstriction and improves cardiac diastolic relaxation by enhancing sodium pump activity and nitric acid production, causing a decrease in intracellular calcium levels (Kirpichnikov 02). These direct and indirect effects may explain cardiovascular protection by metformin therapy.

Because metformin crosses the human placenta, concern arises about possible protean effects of the drug (Lenhard 97) on the function of fetal cells and systems. Metformin had no effect on human placental glucose uptake or transport in experiments using the isolated, perfused, single-cotyledon model (Elliott 97). However, in mouse blastocysts, metformin increased glucose uptake and decreased apoptosis (Eng 04). Mouse embryos exposed to phenformin in tissue culture exhibited open neural tubes, craniofacial hypoplasia, and embryolethality, but metformin at concentrations of 0.5–1.8 mg/mL in culture media only temporarily slowed closure of the neuropores and produced no major malformations or alterations in embryonic growth (Denno 94). Reported exposures of fetuses of diabetic mothers to biguanides in uncontrolled studies in early pregnancy are quite limited. Of 16 fetuses exposed to phenformin, two major malformations were found and no perinatal mortality (Coetzee 84, Piaquadio 91). Of 28 fetuses exposed to metformin in early pregnancy, there were no major malformations (Coetzee 84, Piaquadio 91, Hellmuth 94).

Clinical experience regarding the use of metformin later in diabetic pregnancies is quite limited (Hague 02). In South Africa, 33 women with type 2 diabetes or GDM were started on metformin in the second or third trimester. There were no stillbirths, two neonatal deaths, three cases of neonatal hypoglycemia, and jaundice requiring phototherapy in ten babies (Coetzee 79). In Copenhagen, 50 similar patients (31 GDM, 19 type 2 diabetes) were treated with metformin, with most starting in the third trimester. Four stillborn infants and 16 cases of preeclampsia occurred, and both complications seemed more common than in a retrospective insulin-treated cohort (Hellmuth 00a). It is difficult to evaluate the potential roles of glycemic control, advanced maternal age, and obesity in this uncontrolled study. Another retrospecive analysis found high rates of perinatal complications in 32 women with type 2 diabetes taking metformin through-out pregnancy, as well as in 61 women who stopped metformin during pregnancy, and 121 women with type 2 diabetes who never used metformin in pregnancy. Thus, it was impossible to determine an effect of the drug (Hughes 06b). Hopefully, ongoing RCTs of metformin in GDM will contribute to this evaluation (Moore 07, Rowan 07).

In recent years, metformin has been used to treat nondiabetic insulin-resistant women with PCOS (LaMarca 05) and has been continued throughout pregnancy in relatively small, poorly controlled studies. Investigators report a decrease in early pregnancy loss that is often associated with this syndrome (Glueck 02a, Heard 02, Jakubowicz 02, Thatcher 06) and note the expected frequencies of preeclampsia, congenital malformations, and other neonatal morbidities that would be seen in an untreated PCOS population (de Vries 98, Glueck 02b, Glueck 04). In one small RCT of metformin for PCOS, GDM and preeclampsia developed in similar numbers of subjects who were treated with placebo compared with metformin (Vanky 04). With this limited experience in mind, an Australasian Diabetes in Pregnancy Society Ad Hoc Working Party recommended against routine use of metformin in pregnancies complicated by diabetes, but "when the potential harm from metformin therapy is likely to be outweighed by the benefits of metformin use, metformin therapy should be considered after discussion. Such situations include a requirement for large doses of insulin, and refusal of the patient to use insulin" (Simmons 04). Other writers argue for or against the use of metformin in pregnant women with diabetes (Hague 02, Brown 06, Hawthorne 06, Lilja 06) without benefit of clinical trial data. We believe that metformin should only be used in the setting of properly controlled trials during pregnancy in type 2 diabetes until there is ample evidence of efficacy and safety. Such trials should include a focus on infant long-term development and metabolic function.

Thiazolidinediones and "Glitazones"

These potent insulin-sensitizing agents (pioglitazone, rosiglitazone) activate a nuclear hormone receptor (the transcription factor PPARγ) that regulates gene expression in response to specific ligands in adipose tissue, cardiac and skeletal muscle, liver, and placenta (Bhatia 06). Other ligands for PPARγ include fatty acids, prostaglandins, and nonsteroidal anti-inflammatory drugs, such as indomethacin and ibuprofen (Bocos 95, Kliewer 97, Lehmann 97, Olefsky 00). Thiazolidinediones (TZDs, or gli-tazones) have beneficial effects on metabolic balance by increasing peripheral glucose utilization in skeletal muscle and adipose tissue, reducing hepatic glucose production, increasing fatty acid uptake, and reducing lipolysis in fat cells (Miyazaki 01, O'Moore-Sullivan 02, Wallace 04). The eventual result (3–4 months) in patients with insulin resistance, IGT, and type 2 diabetes is reduction in fasting and postprandial glucose, insulin, and circulating FFA levels (Boden 06). One adverse effect of TZD treatment is fluid retention and weight gain, and they should not be used if there is elevation of hepatic transaminase enzymes (O'Moore-Sullivan 02, Boden 06). TZDs have been shown to reduce TG accumulation, inflammation, and fibrosis in human nonalcoholic fatty liver disease (Buckingham 05), even though liver PPARγ activation contributes to steatosis in animal models (Chao 00, Boelsterli 02, Gavrilova 03).

The effects of glitazones on fat cells and lipids are striking (Wilson-Fritch 04, Goldberg 05). TZDs stimulate adipocyte differentiation that results in increased and smaller fat cells (Boden 06), stimulate adipogenesis in subcutaneous fat depots (Adams 97, Spiegelman 98), increase adiponectin production, and increase circulating lipoproteins, although the increase in LDL-C is mostly in the larger, more buoyant, and less atherogenic particles (O'Moore-Sullivan 02). Pioglitazone reduces serum TG levels (O'Moore-Sullivan 02, Boden 06). TZDs also reduce inflammatory cytokine production by adipocytes (Hammerstedt 05) and improve vascular dysfunction (Parulkar 01, Marx 04a, Vinik 06a.b). However, recent epidemiologic evidence suggests that TZD use in older patients with diabetes may increase congestive heart failure (Masoudi 05, Aguilar 07, Lago 07) and myocardial infarction (Lipscombe 07).

According to manufacturer's product reports, TZDs cross the placenta in animal studies, and treatment of the midpregnancy rat results in increased fetal loss, retarded fetal development, and suppression of postnatal growth (O'Moore-Sullivan 02). A glitazone administered to rats in late pregnancy decreased maternal TG levels by 47% without effect on maternal glucose and was associated with fetal hyperinsulinemia without a change in fetal plasma glucose, TG, NEFA, or ketone bodies. Maternal treatment with the glitazone raised neonatal glucose and insulin and enhanced lipolysis and ketogenesis in the pups; it also impaired the growth of the neonates due to insulin resistance and reduced IGF-1 in spite of adequate amounts of neonatal fuels (Sevillano 05). These studies demonstrate the complexity of possible metabolic effects of glitazones in the murine maternal–placental–fetal unit. It should be noted that experimental models of diabetes in pregnant rats do not mimic the full metabolic changes found in the human condition (Herrera 85, Martin 91, Caluwaerts 03, Lopez-Soldado 03).

The presence of PPARγ affects development of the murine placenta (Asami-Miyagishi 04, Shalom-Barak 04). PPARγ modulates human trophoblast differentiation in a ligand-specific manner (Schaiff 00, Waite 00, Handschuh 06, Schild 06, Fournier 07). The presumed endogenous PPARγ ligand is 15ΔProstaglandinJ2 (Forman 95), which diminished human trophoblast differentiation and promoted apoptosis, while a glitazone enhanced biochemical and morphological trophoblast differentiation (Schaiff 00). PPARγ expression was similar in term placental tissue from women with PDM compared with controls, but 15ΔPGJ2 levels were reduced. Nevertheless, 15ΔPGJ2 was active in placental explants from diabetic women in reducing NO overproduction (nitrate and nitrite concentrations) (Jawerbaum 04). Extreme hyperglycemia in vitro and experimental diabetes enhanced PPARγ expression in human and mouse placenta, respectively. However, these effects were attenuated by PPARγ ligands that also increased VGEF expression (Suwaki 07).

PPARγs have an important role in regulating the expression of fatty acid–metabolizing enzymes in the mammalian placenta (Xu 07). PPARγ stimulation is involved in fatty acid uptake by human trophoblast cells (Bildirici 03, Duttaroy 04, Schaiff 05). Oxidized lipids enhance the activity of PPARγ in primary human trophoblasts (Schild 02). Could use of PPARγ activators increase placental uptake, accumulation, and transfer of lipids in diabetic pregnancies? Alternatively, PPARγ activators could have protective effects on the placenta. Glitazones have been shown to reduce the release of cytokines from human amnion, choriodecidual, and placental tissue (Lappas 02,04,06) and to attenuate hypoxia-induced injury in cultured term human trophoblasts (Elchalal 04).

Minimal human placental transfer and fetal accumulation of rosiglitazone (dissolved in a solution containing 30 gm/L albumin) was seen in an ex vivo perfusion study using term placentas from uncomplicated pregnancies (Holmes 06). Maternal rosiglitazone concentrations were 216–692 ng/mL, as expected after an 8-mg oral dose, with a median half-life of 1.5 h. Fetal accumulation reached 16.4 ng/mL in one experiment and was nil in four others. Rosiglitazone is highly bound to serum albumin and may be metabolized by *N*-demethylation and hydroxylation by the placenta (Holmes 06). A few case reports detailed inadvertent use of glitazones during the first weeks of pregnancy with normal pregnancy outcome (Yaris 04, Kalyoncu 05). Registry data should be collected on unplanned pregnancies in women with type 2 diabetes using glitazones during embryogenesis/organogenesis prior to onset of prenatal care. Such patients should be converted to insulin with effective glycemic control prior to conception. Experimental studies in primates should be performed and evaluated prior to RCTs of glitazones in diabetic pregnant women. However, the need for TZDs in pregnancies complicated by type 2 diabetes is arguable because intensified insulin therapy produces excellent clinical results.

Meglitinide Analogs: "Glinides"

These quickly absorbed insulinotropic agents (nateglinide, repaglinide) bind to SURs slightly differently than sulfonylureas and rapidly increase early-phase insulin secretion in response to glucose (Dornhorst 01). Their relatively short-acting effects may help in postprandial glucose control, with reduced risk of delayed post-prandial hypoglycemia. They are used primarily in combination therapy in type 2 diabetes. It is unknown to what degree they cross the human placenta and whether they cause fetal or maternal harm or benefit. Studies in pregnant rats showed a no-toxic-effect (NTE) level of 0.5 mg/kg in teratogenicity studies and 5 mg/kg in perinatal–postnatal studies, with the major effect being reduction of long bone growth after organogenesis. Small fibrotic foci were formed in the area of dislocation of the epiphyseal plate (Viertel 00). Only two cases of repaglinide use (1.5–2.5 mg/day) at the beginning of unplanned but well-controlled pregnancies have been reported, with resultant normal outcomes (Napoli 06). No evidence supports the use of glinides during pregnancy.

α-Glucosidase Inhibitors

These agents (acarbose, miglitol) inhibit α-glucosidase at the brush border of the small intestine, interfering with conversion of disaccharides to monosaccharides. Thus, they slow absorption of carbohydrates from the intestine and may help with postprandial glucose control (Fujisawa 05, van de Laar 05, Shimabukuro 06). Acarbose has limited absorption into circulating blood (1–2% in humans), although there is slow absorption of microbial degradation products from the intestine, which are distributed into the tissues of experimental animals (Ahr 89a,b). Miglitol is absorbed after oral dosing, and [14C]miglitol crossed the placenta slowly and to a limited extent in pregnant rats (Ahr 97). Acarbose might be safe to use in pregnancy due to its limited absorption, but gastrointestinal side effects limit their acceptance (Zarate 00). A single report referred to 19 women with GDM who were assigned to treatment with acarbose compared with 27 using insulin and 24 using glyburide, and glucose control was "not achieved" in 42% of patients using acarbose (Bertini 05).

Incretins

Glucagon-like peptide (GLP-1) is secreted by the gut in response to ingestion of food, stimulates insulin secretion, inhibits glucagon secretion (Edwards 05), and moderates postprandial glucose homeostasis (Edwards 99). Continuous infusion of GLP-1 lowers plasma glucose in type 2 diabetes, inhibits gastric emptying, and reduces appetite (Vella 00, Zander 02). Thus, the GLP-1 system is a possible therapeutic target in diabetes (Edwards 05, Joy 05). Studies of GLP-1 in pregnancy are very limited. Secretion of GLP-1 was normal in women with GDM (Cypryk 07) and was reduced compared with controls in only one of two studies after pregnancies with GDM (Forbes 05, Meier 05).

The GLP-1 receptor agonist exenatide is injected at 5–10 µg twice daily to resist gut proteolysis. Exenatide also slows gastric emptying, suppresses glucagon, potentiates nutrient-stimulated insulin secretion, promotes satiety, and is sometimes associated with nausea (Riddle 06). Negligible passage of exenatide was seen across the ex vivo term perfused placenta (fetal-to-maternal ratio 0.017 at equilibrium) (Hiles 03). We are not aware of studies of treatment with exenatide during pregnancies complicated by diabetes.

Islet amyloid peptide, or amylin, is co-secreted with insulin by β-cells (the predominant source of circulating amylin) in response to nutrient stimuli, glucagon, GLP-1, and cholinergic agonists and is also secreted by the somatostatin-producing δ-cells. Amylin immunoreactivity and mRNA are also present throughout the gut as well as in the lung and CNS. Amylin inhibits gastric emptying and gastric acid secretion and reduces short-term food intake; its analog, pramlintide, lowers meal-related glucose excursions (Riddle 06). Increased amylin secretion is experienced in pregnancy, especially in glucose-intolerant women (Kautsky-Willer 97, Wareham 98, Kinalski 04). Amylin co-localizes with insulin and glucagon in fetal pancreatic cells (Portela-Gomez 99), and amylin levels were strikingly elevated in umbilical cord sera of 31 IDMs (Kairamkonda 05).

Pramlintide is approved for injection at doses of 15–60 µg 15 min before meals in patients with type 1 diabetes and 60–120 µg in type 2 diabetes. Slow titration of doses over 4–6 weeks can minimize the side effects of nausea, vomiting, and insulin-induced hypoglycemia (Riddle 06). Negligible passage of pramlintide was seen across the ex vivo perfused human term placenta, with a fetal-to-maternal ratio of 0.006 at equilibrium (Hiles03). We are not aware of studies of treatment with pramlintide in pregnancies complicated by diabetes.

Recommendations

- Oral medications for treatment of type 2 diabetes should be stopped, and insulin should be initiated and titrated to achieve acceptable glucose control prior to conception. (E)

- An expedited appointment should be made for women who become pregnant while taking oral medications to start insulin as soon as possible. It may be inferred from limited first-trimester data that metformin and glyburide can be continued until insulin is started to avoid severe hyperglycemia, which is a known teratogen. (E)

- Controlled trials are needed to determine whether glyburide treatment of women with type 2 diabetes (alone or in combination with insulin) is safe in early pregnancy or effective later in gestation. (E)

- Metformin should currently be used only in the setting of properly controlled trials during pregnancy in type 2 diabetes until there is ample evidence of efficacy and safety. Such trials should include a focus on long-term development and metabolic function of the infants. (E)
- There is insufficient evidence to support a recommendation for or against use of alpha-glucosidase inhibitors in pregnancy. (E)
- Thiazolidinediones, meglitinide inhibitors, and incretins should be used during pregnancy only in the setting of approved clinical trials. (E)

PHYSICAL ACTIVITY/EXERCISE AND MANAGEMENT OF PREGNANT WOMEN WITH PREEXISTING DIABETES MELLITUS

—— Original contribution by Patrick M. Catalano MD and
Jennifer M. Block BS, RN, CDE

To reduce the risk of chronic disease, the 2005 Dietary Guidelines for Americans recommends accumulated physical activity of moderate intensity at least 30 min/day for all adults capable of participating. To prevent unhealthy body weight gain, the guideline is "approximately 60 minutes of moderate- to vigorous-intensity activity most days of the week while not exceeding caloric intake requirements" (DGA 05). The recommendation for pregnant women without medical or obstetrical complications is to "incorporate 30 minutes or more of moderate-intensity physical activity on most, if not all, days of the week," while avoiding activities with a high risk of falling or abdominal trauma (DGA 05). This recommendation is also promulgated by the ACOG (ACOG 02) and can be adopted by most pregnant women with PDM in the absence of specific complications. The amount of exercise may be modified if there is poor weight gain or evidence of fetal growth restriction. Daily activity can be completed in segments, as with pregnant women with diabetes who walk after meals.

The 2005 Dietary Guidelines for Americans Advisory Committee classified physical activity into three groups of intensity (DGAr 05):

- *Sedentary*—light physical activity of day-to-day life
- *Moderately active*—addition of activity equivalent to walking ~1.5–3 miles/day at 3–4 miles/h, which would meet the lower end of the recommendation for adults (minimum of 30 min of at least moderate-intensity physical activity)
- *Active*—addition of activity equivalent to walking >3 miles/day at 3–4 miles/h, which meets the full recommendation for a minimum of 60 min of at least moderate-intensity physical activity

Following the 1996 U.S. Surgeon General report on *Physical Activity and Health* (DHHS 96), the ADA defined physical activity "as bodily movement produced by the contraction of skeletal muscle that requires energy expenditure in excess of resting energy expenditure. Exercise is a subset of physical activity: planned, structured, and repetitive bodily movement performed to improve or maintain one or more component of physical fitness. Aerobic exercise consists of rhythmic, repeated, and continuous movements of the same large muscle groups for at least 10 min at a time. Examples include walking, bicycling, jogging, swimming, water aerobics, and many sports. Resistance exercise consists of activities that use muscular strength to move a weight or work against a resistive load. Examples include weight lifting and exercises using weight machines" (ADA 08a). The ADA further classified physical activity intensity up to 60 min as "moderate" if maximal heart rate (HR_{max}) is 55–70% (VO_{2max} 40–59%) and as "hard" (or "vigorous" [Sigal 04]) if HR_{max} is >70% (VO_{2max} >60%) (ADA 04g). If not determined by a maximal graded exercise test, HR_{max} is approximated in nonpregnant women by subtracting the age from 220.

To improve glycemic control, assist with weight maintenance, and reduce risk of CVD, the ADA recommends at least 150 min/week of moderate-intensity aerobic physical activity and/or at least 90 min/week of vigorous aerobic exercise. Physical activity should be distributed over at least 3 days per week with no more than two consecutive days without physical activity (ADA 08a). The effects of a single bout of aerobic exercise on insulin sensitivity lasts 24–72 h in patients with type 2 diabetes depending on the duration and intensity of the activity (Wallberg-Henriksson 98, Sigal 06). In adults with glucose intolerance or type 2 diabetes, resistance exercise improves insulin sensitivity to about the same extent as aerobic exercise (Ivy 97, Sigal 06). The benefits of exercise on long-term glycemic control and cardiorespiratory fitness are best documented in patients with type 2 diabetes (Boule 01,03, Thomas 06). Studies of exercise in young patients with type 1 diabetes have produced inconsistent results in reducing A1C, and large randomized trials are lacking (Wasserman 94, Mosher 98, Roberts 02, Lisle 06, Ramalho 06).

Hyperglycemia (glucose >180 mg/dL; >10 mM) prior to aerobic exercise did not affect exercise capacity in subjects with type 1 diabetes (Stettler 06), nor did it influence exercise-induced increments in growth hormone, IGF-1, glucagon, epinephrine, or cortisol (Galassetti 06). In the setting of insufficient insulin with ketosis in patients with type 1 diabetes, exercise can worsen severe hyperglycemia and ketonemia (Berger 77). Studies are needed regarding the influence of antecedent glucose level on metabolic responses to exercise in pregnant women with diabetes.

In individuals using insulin or insulin secretogogues, physical activity can cause hypoglycemia if medication dose or carbohydrate consumption is not altered (ADA 08a). In young people with type 1 diabetes, aerobic daytime exercise lowers glucose at least 25% from baseline (in spite of a rise in counterregulatory hormones, which may be greater with intermittent exercise) (Guelfi 05a,b) and increases the risk of hypoglycemia during the night (Tsalikian 05, McMahon 06). In a multicenter study, the chance of young patients with type 1 diabetes needing treatment for hypoglycemia during and after exercise varied with the baseline glucose level: 86% if <120 mg/dL (<6.7 mM), 13% if 120–180 mg/dL (6.7–10 mM), and 6% if >180 mg/dL (>10 mM) (DirNet 06a). Studies on the risk of exercise-induced hypoglycemia experienced 1–3 h after breakfast and injection of insulins NPH and lispro in subjects with type 1 diabetes suggest that the same precautions are needed at either 1 or 3 h (Dube 06) and that an estimated 40 gm of a liquid glucose supplement ingested 15 min prior to exercise should maintain safe glucose levels (Dube 05). Due to the complexity of variables, experts agree that the management of glucose and insulin before, during, and after exercise depends on the trial-and-error method (Ertl 04, DirNet 06a). However, patients with type 1 diabetes using insulin pumps may have less trouble with hypoglycemia if they suspend the basal insulin infusion during exercise (Admon 05, DirNet 06b). The ADA recommends adding extra carbohydrate before exercise if plasma glucose is <100 mg/dL (<5.6 mM) (ADA 08a); for young patients with type 1 diabetes, a safer threshold might be 120 mg/dL (6.7mM).

Exercise causes blunted autonomic and metabolic responses to subsequent hypoglycemia in patients with type 1 diabetes (Sandoval 04,06), but the effects of prior exercise are greater in men than in women (Galassetti 01). With experimental hypoglycemia (50 mg/dL [2.8 mM] for 2 h) 1 day prior to exercise, the secretion of counterregulatory hormones, endogenous glucose production, and lipolytic responses to exercise were reduced by 40–80% in subjects with type 1 diabetes (Galassetti 03,06). Thus, hypoglycemic episodes can exacerbate subsequent hypoglycemic responses to exercise in type 1 diabetes. However, gender differences may play a role in neuroendocrine and metabolic responses to exercise after prior hypoglycemia in normal and diabetic individuals (Cryer 00, Davis 00a,b). Prior prolonged experimental hypoglycemia (two 2-h bouts, morning and afternoon, at ~50 mg/dL, 2.9 mM) reduced glucagon, epinephrine, norepinephrine, growth hormone, and glucose kinetic responses to next-day exercise more significantly in men than in women with type 1 diabetes (Galassetti 04). The authors speculated that these gender differences on counterregulatory responses to exercise after antecedent hypoglycemia could explain the DCCT finding that women with type 1 diabetes had a lowered risk of severe hypoglycemia during intensified insulin treatment compared with men (DCCT 91,97). If prior hypoglycemia exists, there is an ~40% increase in the amount of exogenous glucose required to maintain euglycemia during exercise in women with type 1 diabetes (Galassetti 04). We do not know how pregnancy would modify these metabolic responses to interchanging the timing of exercise and hypoglycemia in diabetic women.

Medical evaluation is important for patients with diabetes prior to starting an exercise program. A graded exercise test with ECG monitoring should be seriously considered before undertaking aerobic physical activity with an intensity exceeding the demands of everyday living (more intense than brisk walking) in previously sedentary diabetic individuals aged ≥35 years whose 10-year risk of a coronary event is likely to be >10% (ADA 04g). Patients with diabetes should be assessed for conditions that might contraindicate certain types of exercise or predispose them to injury such as uncontrolled hypertension, severe autonomic neuropathy, severe peripheral neuropathy, severe NPDR, PDR, or macular edema (ADA 08a). Non–weight-bearing activities may be best in the presence of peripheral neuropathy with decreased pain sensation in the extremities. Due to the many risks of exercise-induced injury in diabetic patients with autonomic neuropathy, they should undergo cardiac evaluation before beginning physical activity more intense than that to which they are accustomed (ADA 08a). Albuminuria will increase with physical activity, but there is no evidence that exercise increases the progression of DN (ADA 08a). Vigorous aerobic or resistance exercise may be contraindicated in the presence of PDR or severe NPDR due to the risk of triggering vitreous hemorrhage or retinal detachment (Aiello 98,01, Fong 04). Pregnancy-related relative contraindications to exercise are discussed later in this section.

The presence of autonomic neuropathy "may limit an individual's physical activity capacity and increase risk of an adverse cardiovascular event during physical activity" (ADA 04g). Cardiac autonomic neuropathy may be indicated by a resting HR >110 bpm (in the absence of anemia or hyperthyroidism) or a fall in systolic BP >20 mmHg upon standing. Additional information regarding appropriate tests of cardiovascular function can be found in Part II in the section titled "Cardiovascular Autonomic Neuropathy." The ADA Position Statement on physical activity/exercise (ADA 04g) notes the following additional criteria that indicates an increased risk for underlying CVD in diabetic women of reproductive age:

- Age >35 years
- Age >25 years and duration of type 1 diabetes >15 years or duration of type 2 diabetes >10 years
- Presence of any additional risk factor for coronary artery disease
- Presence of retinopathy or nephropathy, including microalbuminuria
- Signs or symptoms of peripheral arterial disease

During pregnancy, physiological adaptations of gestation must be taken into consideration (Lotgering 91, Revelli 92, Artal 95, Jaque-Fortunato 96, Khodiguian 96, Soultanakis 96, Spinnewijn 96, Lotgering 98, Carpenter 03, Wolfe 03a). Systolic BP and HR rise during moderate exercise in pregnant women (Artal 81). Because resting HR increases during gestation and HR_{max} is attenuated during exercise testing (suggesting reduction in HR_{max} reserve), the HR method of prescribing exercise intensity is less precise during pregnancy (Lotgering 92, Pivarnik 02, Wolfe 03b). Although VO_{2max} is well preserved in pregnancy, there is a decrease in aerobic work capacity in late gestation (Soultanakis 96). A rating of perceived exertion (RPE) of 12–14 ("somewhat hard") from a possible 20 corresponds to moderate-intensity physical activity (Borg 82, DHHS 96, Davies 03, ADA 04g) and is recommended for use in pregnancy (Wolfe 03b). The "talk test" can also be used "as a final test to avoid over-exertion—the exercising pregnant woman should be able to carry on a verbal conversation; if she cannot, the exercise intensity is too high" (Wolfe 03b).

The hormonal–metabolic changes of exercise are important considerations in the pregnancy complicated by diabetes. In pregnant women with type 2 diabetes (Artal 85) as well as in controls (Artal 81, Rauramo 82, Bonen 92, Revelli 92, McMurray 98, Bessinger 02), concentrations of catecholamines and glucagon increase in circulating blood during exercise, but cortisol does not. During the third trimester, both the sympathoadrenal and glucagon response is somewhat blunted (Bonen 92, Bessinger 02). As oxygen consumption increases, energy for the working skeletal muscle is initially supplied by "its own stores of glycogen and triglycerides, as well as free fatty acids (FFAs) derived from the breakdown of adipose tissue triglycerides and glucose released from the liver" (ADA 04g). With prolonged and more intense activity, an increase in energy is derived from carbohydrate use and a decrease in energy from lipid oxidation (Brooks 94, Bessinger 03, Sigal 04). Exercise increases muscle glucose uptake by (a) increasing blood flow and capillary recruitment, (b) increasing muscle membrane glucose transport with translocation of GLUT4 to the muscle cell surface, and by (c) enhanced intracellular glucose phosphorylation by hexokinase (Sigal 04). Some studies show that carbohydrate use during exercise does not differ in pregnancy, but glucose levels decline to a greater extent (Soultanakis 96, Clapp 98, Bessinger 02). As noted, we lack data on endocrine/metabolic responses to exercise in pregnant women with type 1 diabetes.

A decrease in plasma insulin and the presence of glucagon are needed to increase hepatic glucose production during physical activity. Increases in plasma glucagon and catecholamines are important for sustained glucose production (ADA 04g) in the shift from hepatic glycogenolysis to gluconeogenesis (Sigal 04). Because these hormonal adaptations may be lacking in some patients with type 1 diabetes, unregulated exercise can disturb glycemic balance. The problem of exercise-induced hypoglycemia may be exacerbated in pregnant women with diabetes due to the increase in non–insulin-mediated glucose disposal from mother to fetus with advancing gestation. On the other hand, in the presence of inadequate insulin levels, "an excessive release of counterinsulin hormones may increase already high levels of glucose and ketone bodies and can even precipitate ketoacodosis" (ADA 04g). Pregnancy further complicates these issues as insulin sensitivity increases in early gestation and then decreases in late pregnancy, accompanied by increased insulin clearance.

For most pregnant women with type 1 and type 2 diabetes, daily physical activity may help metabolic balance; however, care must be taken to ensure that glycemic control is achieved peri-exercise. An important precaution is to check the fingerstick glucose before and after exercise and even during exercise if symptoms of hypoglycemia are noted. Adjustments in glucose control through pre- and postexercise glucose monitoring as well as adequate carbohydrate provision are essential to avoid serious hypoglycemia (Wasserman 94, Devlin 02b, Sigal 04). The recommendation is to consume added carbohydrate before, during, and after physical activity only as needed to avoid hypoglycemia, especially if glucose levels are <100 mg/dL. Active exercise should be avoided during peak insulin action or if glucose levels are ≥250 mg/dL (ADA 04g). Prior to engaging in moderate-intensity exercise, pregnant diabetic women should include a proper warm-up of low-intensity aerobic activity for 5–10 min to prepare the skeletal muscles, heart, and lungs for a progressive increase in exercise intensity. Additionally, before or after gentle stretching of the used muscle groups, a cool-down period of 5–10 min that is structured similarly to the warm-up is recommended (ADA 04g). Other precautions include prevention of trauma to the feet and adequate hydration before, during, and after physical activity.

The potential substantial benefits of exercise for pregnant women include a sense of well-being, controlled weight gain, improved glucose levels, decreased BW/adiposity of their babies, and an improved tolerance of labor (Artal 99, ACOG 02, Polley 02, Carpenter 03, Davies 03, Kramer 06, Haaksted 07). In individuals with diabetes, moderate exercise helps decrease glucose concentrations via non–insulin-mediated glucose disposal. In type 2 diabetes, increased physical activity may help prevent the progression of obesity and increased insulin resistance as well as the associated problems of insulin resistance syndrome, such as hypertension and hyperlipidemia (Sigal 04). In pregnancy, it is unknown whether regular exercise may reduce manifestations of the metabolic syndrome such as increased weight gain (Roessner 99), hyperlipidemia, oxidative stress, and development of preeclampsia. Randomized clinical trials are needed to further study these issues. A Cochrane review of exercise for diabetic pregnant women focused on four trials involving 114 subjects with GDM, but none with PDM. The reviewers concluded that there was insufficient evidence to recommend or advise against exercise as therapy for women with diabetes (Ceysens 06).

The risks of exercise in pregnancy include the possibility of decreased placental transfer of oxygen and substrates to the fetus and a transient increase in uterine contractions. The potential for competition between contracting maternal skeletal muscle and the fetus for oxygenated blood flow and glucose is probably highest in late gestation; therefore, "the second trimester is the best time to progressively increase the amount of physical activity" (Wolfe 03b). Submaximal steady-state cycling for 5 min had a transient deleterious effect on umbilical artery Doppler flow in a subset of women with uteroplacental vascular insufficiency (Chadda 05). Results of epidemiological studies of a possible association between maternal physical activity and spontaneous abortion (Madsen 07, Blohm 08) or preterm birth and low BW are conflicting (ACOG 02,

Morris 05, Dwarkanath 07, Juhl 08). Prospective controlled trials with large numbers of subjects and precise measurements of exercise and outcomes will be necessary to resolve these questions (Chasan-Taber 07).

Because maternal hyperthermia >39.2°C from fever or immersion may be damaging to the fetus, concern arose that, during exercise, pregnant women could drive their core temperature up to dangerous levels, especially in hot weather (Clapp 91). Subsequent studies of low-impact aerobics have not confirmed this risk (Soultanakis 96, Lindqvist 03, Larsson 05, Morris 05). Pregnant women should avoid the supine position during exercise after the first trimester to avoid relative obstruction of venous return and resultant decreased cardiac output (CO) and orthostatic hypotension (ACOG 02). Motionless standing may also be associated with a significant decrease in CO (Clark 91). Additionally, alterations in a woman's shape occur with advancing gestation that require compensatory adjustments in factors such as balance and strain on vertebral muscle and ligaments (Artal 99).

The ACOG (ACOG 02) and the Society of Obstetricians and Gynecologists of Canada (Davies 03) have presented similar lists of contraindications to aerobic exercise during pregnancy (Table I.13).

Both organizations also list additional warning signs for pregnant women to stop exercising and seek medical attention:

- Dyspnea prior to exertion or excessive shortness of breath
- Chest pain
- Dizziness or headache
- Calf pain or swelling (rule out thrombophlebitis)
- Vaginal bleeding or leakage of amniotic fluid
- Painful uterine contractions

TABLE I.13 Contraindications to Aerobic Exercise During Pregnancy

- Hemodynamically significant heart disease
- Restrictive lung disease
- Incompetent cervix
- Multiple gestation at risk for preterm labor; higher-order multiple gestation
- Persistent second- or third-trimester bleeding
- Placenta previa after 26 weeks gestation
- Premature labor or ruptured membranes during the current pregnancy
- Preeclampsia or uncontrolled hypertension
- Poorly controlled seizure disorder or hyperthyroidism (R)
- Hemoglobin <10 gm/dL (R)
- Extreme morbid obesity (R)
- Heavy smoker (R)
- Previous spontaneous abortions or preterm births (R)

Relative contraindications are marked (R).
Modified from statements of the American College of Obstetricians and Gynecologists (ACOG 02) and the Society of Obstetricians and Gynecologists of Canada (Davies 02).

Recommendations

- Educate women with type 1 and type 2 diabetes as to the benefits of appropriate daily physical activity. (A)
- Evaluate specific types of physical activity practiced prior to conception. Evaluate all pregnant women with PDM for medical complications such as CVD, retinopathy, nephropathy, and neuropathy. If present, modifications in physical activity may need to be made. (E)
- Encourage pregnant women with type 1 or type 2 diabetes without contraindications to use physical activity as part of their overall diabetes management for at least 30 minutes per day. (E)
- Advise patients that no compelling evidence has been found that adverse pregnancy outcomes are increased for healthy exercising women, although controlled trials have not been conducted in diabetic women. (B)
- Women should be taught to monitor the intensity of physical activity. (E)
- Monitor capillary glucose closely around times of exercise, consider adjustments in carbohydrate and insulin requirements, and maintain good hydration before, during, and after exercise. (E)
- Women should choose activities that will avoid the supine position and minimize the risk of loss of balance and fetal trauma. (E)
- Note the published specific contraindications for physical activity in pregnancy, and teach patients the warning signs to determine when to terminate exercise and seek medical attention. (E)

BEHAVIORAL THERAPY

—— Original contribution by Lisa D. Hoffman MSW, LCSW and
John L. Kitzmiller MD

Women with PDM who become pregnant will face many months of hard work and likely will need to make significant lifestyle changes to have a successful outcome. Due to the need for intensified diabetes management during gestation, it is crucial to make a thorough assessment of psychosocial issues that may influence a patient's ability to respond to treatment (Lorenz 96, Peyrot 05, Carbone 07, Delahanty 07, Nouwen 07, Funnell 08) and collaborate with the diabetes and pregnancy care team (ADietA 02, AADE 04, Kendrick 04, AADE 06, ACOG 06a). Healthy coping is identified as a behavior change strategy that needs additional emphasis during DSME (Zgibor 07).

Psychosocial screening should include but is not limited to (a) attitudes about diabetes and the pregnancy, (b) expectations for management and outcomes, (c) affect/mood, (d) quality of life and resources (financial, social, emotional), and (e) psychiatric/eating behavior history (ADA 08a). A short psychosocial screening tool promulgated by the ACOG and modified for diabetes and pregnancy is presented in Table I.14 (ACOG 06a). Efficient assessment allows effective interaction with members of the care team and timely referral for further evaluation by a mental health specialist familiar with diabetes and pregnancy management (ADA 08a), preferably a member of the team. Even with thorough education about nutrition and medication, women may find the demands of intensified treatment overwhelming. Behavioral assessment of self-management skills is strongly recommended (ADA 08a). Concurrent with the medical

TABLE I.14 Psychosocial Screening Tool

Yes	No	Do you have any problems (e.g., job, transportation) that prevent you from keeping your health care appointments?
Yes	No	Do you feel unsafe where you live?
Yes	No	In the past 2 months, have you used any form of tobacco?
Yes	No	In the past 2 months, have you used drugs or alcohol (including beer, wine, or mixed drinks)?
Yes	No	In the past year, have you been threatened, hit, slapped, or kicked by anyone you know?
Yes	No	Has anyone forced you to perform any sexual act that you did not want to do?
Yes	No	Does having diabetes still make you angry?
Yes	No	Do you feel overwhelmed by the need to test your blood glucose and inject insulin?
Yes	No	Do you have any problem eating food?

On a 1-to-5 scale, how do you rate your current stress level?

1   2   3   4   5

Low   High

How many times have you moved in the past 12 months? _____

If you could change the timing of this pregnancy, would you want it

earlier   later   not at all   no change

Modified and reprinted with permission from the American College of Obstetricians and Gyenecologists and Florida's Healthy Start Prenatal Risk Screening Instrument. ACOG 2006a; Florida Department of Health, Tallahassee, FL, 1997, DH 3134.

regimen, it is also important to explore the psychosocial challenges that women bring with them (Welch 97, Snoek 00, Polonsky 05, Hermanns 06, Knight 06, Weinger 06). "Emotional wellbeing is a part of diabetes management ... It is preferable to incorporate psychological treatment into routine care rather than waiting for identification of a specific problem or deterioration in psychological status ... Screening tools can facilitate this goal" (ADA 08a).

Psychosocial therapies are of proven benefit in the co-management of type 1 and type 2 diabetes (Glasgow 99a, Steed 03, van Dam 05, Peyrot 06,07). Successful approaches include behavioral modification, intensive interactive psychotherapy, other types of cognitive behavior therapy, and psychiatric medication. Cognitive behavior therapy covers "a wide range of psychological techniques designed to bring about change in thinking patterns and behaviors," including relaxation training (Ismail 04). The most effective interventions incorporate "individually tailored strategies to change behavior," such as increasing the patient's sense of empowerment and self-management skills (Anderson 95, Clement 95, Delamater 01). Psychological disorders that affect glycemic control are detectable in up to one-third of patients (Blanz 93, Jacobson 96b, Lustman 00a, Weinger 01, Anderson 02, Bryden 03, Thomas 03b, Hassan 06, Nakahara 06), which includes diabetic women who may find themselves pregnant. Although preconception care is the goal, most pregnancies of patients with PDM are unplanned. The patient and treatment team will often be met with the challenge of rapidly optimizing glycemic control. Obstacles to care may be concrete including financial hardship, inadequate transportation, and lack of childcare or language/cultural barriers. Emotional issues, such as depression, guilt, anger, or perceived lack of control, can also affect a patient's ability to successfully engage in care. Of the myriad of issues that can block successful management, depression, stress or anxiety, and disordered eating may frequently be encountered.

Depression

Depression in Diabetes

Depression is a commonly encountered comorbidity with type 1 or type 2 diabetes (Eaton 02, Engum 05, Ali 06, Egede 06, Hood 06), especially in women of reproductive age (Katon 04, Zhao 06b). In type 2 diabetes, depression often precedes the diagnosis of diabetes (Knol 06). Meta-analyses of studies in adults with diabetes reported an 11–12% prevalence of major depression based on psychiatric interviews compared with 3.2% in control subjects as well as depression symptoms in 31% based on use of depression-related scales (Anderson 01, Barnard 06). Subsequent population studies yielded prevalence figures of 11.2%, 23.1%, and 23.9% for clinical depression in diabetic women, respectively (Egede 03, Nichols 03, Goldney 04). Depression is a common but often unrecognized and untreated comorbidity with diabetes in minority groups (Egede 02a,b, Cherrington 06, de Groot 06, Wagner 07). Rates of major depressive disorder in the adult female reference population in North America have ranged from 7% to 13 % (Bennett 04).

Depression is viewed as either a response to the psychosocial stress caused by diabetes and other life stresses (Fisher 01b) or as a response to the biochemical changes related to diabetes and its treatment (Lustman 92). Whatever the probable bidirectional relationship (Jacobson 93, Talbot 00), depression in diabetic women is strongly associated with poor self care (Lin 04, Morse 06) and glycemic control (Gary 00, Lustman 05), micro- and macrovascular complications (de Groot 01), neuropathy (Vileikyte 05), panic attacks (Ludman 06), and increased healthcare expenditures (Ciechanowski 00, Egede 02a). Structured psychotherapy can be a useful first-line therapy for mild depression, but pharmacotherapy is added for severe depression (Mann 05). RCTs demonstrated the benefit of both cognitive behavior therapy (Lustman 98) and the antidepressor drugs nortriptyline (Lustman 97) and fluoxetine (Lustman 00b) in decreasing the severity of depression and improving glycemic control in women with diabetes (Lustman 02).

Depression in Pregnancy

Although there are few published data on rates of depression in pregnant women with PDM, a systematic review of 21 observational studies of nondiabetic pregnant women through 2002 yielded prevalence rates of 10.7–14.8 (95% CI) for the second trimester and 7.4–16.7 for the third trimester (Bennett 04). In these studies, the Edinburgh Postnatal Depression scale (Murray 90) was as efficient in assessment as structured clinical interviews and better than the Beck Depression Inventory (Holcomb 96) (refer to the Edinburgh Postnatal Depression scale in Part IV in the section titled "Postpartum Mood Disturbances"). Great heterogeneity was found among the studies (Bennett 04), but we can conclude that approximately 7–15% of nondiabetic pregnant women struggle with depression (Dietz 07); however, only 2.0–7.6% of all pregnant women were using antidepressant drugs in recent surveys (Ververs 06, Andrade 08). The prevalence of depression might be higher in women with poorly controlled chronic diabetes. In another survey of 3,472 obstetrics patients, 20% obtained a high score on the Center for Epidemiologic Studies Depression Scale; however, 86% of the pregnant women with depressive symptoms did not receive any treatment, and >50% had stopped antidepressant medication when pregnancy was diagnosed (Marcus 03).

It is clear that pregnancy does not protect against depression as was originally believed. On the contrary, hormonal changes and other stresses of pregnancy are thought to increase vulnerability for the onset or return of depression (Wisner 99, Burt 02, O'Keane 07). Symptoms of depression that can directly impact a patient's ability to appropriately care for herself include appetite disturbance, lethargy, feelings of hopelessness, sleep disruption, and in severe cases, suicidal ideation. Women with a current or preexisting history of depression are at increased risk for postpartum depression and should be counseled about signs, symptoms, and available support services. Referral to a licensed mental health provider for further assessment and treatment of depression is an important component of team care. A Cochrane review of psychosocial and psychological interventions for the treatment of antenatal depression was inconclusive as to its benefit due to an inadequate number of studies (Dennis 07).

A systematic review of 37 studies of depression during pregnancy through April 2003 concluded that untreated depression was associated with variable perinatal risks, but that most investigators focused on the potential risks of psychotropic medication and not on the possibility of biological dysregulation caused by gestational depression (Bonari 04). Another set of reviewers concluded that the risk of fetal exposure to untreated major depressive disorder is a greater cause for concern than fetal antidepressant exposure (Henry 04). Depression and its pharmacotherapy prior to and during 972 pregnancies compared with 3,878 unexposed controls in a population survey in Saskatchewan was associated with increased rates of stillbirth (adjusted OR 2.2), delivery <37 weeks (adjusted OR 1.6), BW <2,500 gm (adjusted OR 1.6), and neonatal seizures (adjusted OR 3.9) (Wen 06). These results are similar to those found in other observational studies (Chambers 96, Hendrick 03, Lattimore 05, Davis 07, Suri 07). On the other hand, a recent case–control (Pearson 07) and prospective controlled cohort investigation (Maschi 08) found no evidence of major increases in adverse obstetrical or neonatal outcomes following prenatal exposure to antidepressants. It is difficult to determine whether antidepressant drug therapy in general hazards perinatal outcomes beyond the effects of clinical depression itself.

Discontinuing antidepressant treatment was associated with relapse of major depression during pregnancy in 68% of patients compared with a 26% relapse rate in those who maintained their medication, in a prospective investigation of a multicenter cohort of women considered stable on medication prior to pregnancy (Cohen 06). Regarding bipolar disorder, discontinuation of a mood stabilizer during pregnancy carried a high risk for new morbidity, especially for early depressive and dysphoric states (Viguera 07).

Specific Antidepressant Drugs in Pregnancy

Tricyclic antidepressants are effective in the treatment of depression in pregnancy (Goldberg 94). No evidence suggests that these drugs are teratogenic, but they do cross the placenta (Heikkinen 01, Davis 07). Transient withdrawal or anticholinergic symptoms can be seen in infants of mothers treated in the third trimester (Altshuler 96, Gentile 05), but follow-up studies are limited. *Monoamine oxidase inhibitors* should be avoided in pregnant women due to the risk of hypertensive crisis (Hendrick 02).

Use of *selective serotonin-reuptake inhibitors* (SSRIs) in early pregnancy is generally not associated with increased spontaneous abortions or congenital malformations in most studies (Kulin 98, Hendrick 02, Gentile 05, Wen 06, Berard 07, Davis 07, Louik 07). In a 3-year population survey of British Columbia (119,547 live births), the risk for atrial septal defect was significantly higher following SSRI monotherapy compared with no exposure, after adjustment for maternal covariates. Use of SSRIs combined with benzodiazepines was associated with a higher risk for congenital heart disease in general (Oberlander 08). In the same population survey, SSRI use was associated with low BW and increased neonatal respiratory distress compared with offspring of mothers with depression who were not on antidepressants. The concern that outcomes might reflect worsened depression in treated gravidas was addressed by use of a severity of maternal illness scale (Oberlander 06). One study found a significant association between use of sertraline and omphalocele and cardiac septal defects, but the absolute risks were small (Louik 07). Inconsistent evidence exists for increased rates of omphalocele or cardiac defects in infants exposed to paroxetine in early pregnancy (Mills 06, Davis 07, Louik 07), but first-trimester exposure to a dose >25 mg/day was associated with a threefold risk of major cardiac malformations in a 6.5-year survey of all births in the province of Quebec (Berard 07). High doses of fluoxetine (40–80 mg/day) were associated with low BW at term in one recent cohort study (Hendrick 03). In a case-control analysis of 377 infants with primary pulmonary hypertension of the newborn (PPHN), use of SSRIs after 20 weeks gestation was associated with PPHN in the offspring (adjusted OR 6.1). The authors estimated a low absolute risk of PPHN of 6–12 per 1,000 SSRI users (Chambers 06). A separate review of cohort studies found that only 1 of 313 full-term infants exposed to SSRIs in utero required intubation in the neonatal intensive care unit (NICU) (Moses-Kolko 05).

Poor neonatal adaptation or "SSRI withrawal syndrome" was only occasionally noted in some, but not all, of the first studies of infants exposed to SSRIs in the third trimester (six studies [1996–2004] describing negative effects of SSRIs in infants reviewed by Ruchkin 05). However, 93 suspected cases of SSRI-induced neonatal withdrawal syndrome (convulsions, irritability, abnormal crying, tremor) were reported to the WHO database of adverse drug reactions from nine countries from 1995 through 2003; the large denominator of exposed fetuses is unknown (Sanz 05). A prospective cohort study in Vancouver described transient neonatal signs of a "discontinuation syndrome" (mild respiratory symptoms or hypotonia) in 30% of infants exposed to fluoxetine, paroxetine, or sertraline in the second and third trimesters (Oberlander 04). A subsequent cohort study of 60 neonates exposed to SSRIs in utero also reported a 30% frequency of "neonatal abstinence syndrome," with 8 of 18 infants showing severe symptoms (Levinson-Castiel 06). Another systematic study of neurobehavior in 17 healthy full-term SSRI-exposed infants compared with controls showed increased tremulousness, greater numbers of startles or sudden arousals, less flexible and dampened-state regulation, and greater autonomic dysregulation. The authors question whether the behaviors are due to a "withdrawal syndrome" or to serotonin toxicity. One limitation of the investigation is that no infants of untreated depressed mothers were studied (Zeskind 04). The few follow-up studies of SSRI-exposed infants suggest subtle effects on motor development, but no effects on language development or behavior (Casper 03). Considerably more research is needed on this important question because maternal depression itself both during and after pregnancy can affect child development (Henry 04).

Bupropion is an aminoketone that is chemically unrelated to other antidepressants and is a relatively weak inhibitor of the neuronal uptake of norepinephrine, serotonin, and dopamine (Ascher 95). This amphetamine is also used for smoking cessation. In the manufacturer's registry of pregnancies exposed to bupropion in the first trimester, there was a higher-than-expected frequency of neonatal cardiac malformations (BupReg 05). A separate study of bupropion use in the first trimester in 136 women demonstrated no increase in malformations, as well as no increase in prematurity or perinatal mortality in 45 women who continued to use the drug throughout pregnancy, compared with 89 women using other antidepressants (Chun-Fai-Chan 05). Neonatal behavior was not assessed. Analysis of 1,213 infants (from a large U.S. healthcare plan) exposed to bupropion in the first trimester revealed a prevalence of 10.7/1,000 for major cardiac malformations, which was not a significant increase compared with that in 4,743 infants exposed to other antidepressants or in 1,049 infants exposed to bupropion outside the first trimester (Cole 07).

We conclude that psychopharmacological treatment should be continued only in diabetic pregnant women "with histories of rapid and severe relapse of major depressive episodes after medication discontinuation" (Hendrick 02) and otherwise should be initiated in pregnant patients with severe depression for whom psychotherapy has proven unsuccessful after careful risk–benefit analysis and informed consent (Hendrick 03, ACOG 06b).

Stress and Anxiety Disorders

Stress and anxiety disorders have been shown to negatively impact self-care in women with diabetes (Anderson 02, Wiesli 05, Shaban 06), and stress management training improves long-term glycemic control in type 2 diabetes (Surwit 02). During gestation, the need for increased glycemic and fetal monitoring, strict meal planning, and medication changes can significantly add to the usual stressors of pregnancy. Family conflict surrounding the tasks of diabetes care may interfere with treatment outcomes (Anderson 90, Gerstle 01, ADA 08a). Whether acute or chronic, stress can adversely affect eating and sleeping patterns as well as motivation levels. Having patients record times of stress on the glucose log can assist in evaluating how stress affects individual glycemic control. Helping patients identify previous times of stress and their coping mechanisms provides another opportunity to look at successful and problematic strategies that have been used. Instruction in stress management techniques, such as visualization, muscle relaxation, and relaxation breathing, provides patients with tools to manage stressors.

Anxiety is even more common than depression in community samples of pregnant women (Ross 06, Lee 07). Antenatal anxiety predicts the increased risk of postnatal depression, even when controlling for antenatal depression, in studies conducted in different parts of the world (Heron 04, Austin 07, Lee 07). It is not known whether specific treatment of anxiety disorders in pregnancy will improve perinatal outcome or reduce postpartum morbidity. Three studies reported increased anxiety in pregnancies complicated by PDM (Barglow 85, York 96, Langer 98), but no controlled trials of interventions in this population have been conducted. Tricyclic antidepressants are recommended for panic disorders in pregnancy rather than benzodiazepines, which can result in "floppy baby syndrome" or neonatal withdrawal symptoms (Goldberg 94, Altshuler 96).

Eating Disorders

For women who have never come to terms with their diabetes, the diagnosis of pregnancy can bring special challenges. For some patients, pregnancy will be the first time that they make a concerted effort to achieve glycemic control, which may necessitate considerable changes in their relationship to food. Numerous studies find a relationship between type 1 and type 2 diabetes and eating disorders (Bryden 99, Goebel-Fabbri 02, Colton 04, Grylli 05, Mannucci 05, Pollock-BarZiv 05, Battaglia 06, Allison 07, Colton 07). Prevalence rates of disordered eating behaviors vary from 5.4% to 29% in young diabetic women (Rydall 97, Herpertz 98,01, Rodin 02, Peveler 05). Predictors of disturbed eating behaviors in preteen girls with type 1 diabetes included lower self esteem, higher BMI, and more disturbed attachment to one's mother (Colton 07). Comorbid eating disorders are associated with anxiety disorders (Kaye 04) as well as greater risks of poor glycemic control and diabetic complications (Steel 87, Rydall 97, Peveler 05). Young women with diabetes are especially likely to have unhealthy weight control practices and misuse insulin to help control their weight (Engstrom 99, Neumark-Sztainer 02, Peveler 05). Additional information is needed concerning eating disorders in women of reproductive age and with type 2 diabetes.

In pregnancy, nondiabetic women with active eating disorders are also more likely to have an increased incidence of hyperemesis, preterm delivery, low BW at term, microcephaly, and postpartum depression (Conti 98, Bulik 99, Morgan 99, Franko 01, Sollid 04, Kouba 05, Morgan 06, Milcali 07). A Swedish study of 1,000 women who had previously been hospitalized for anorexia nervosa showed no influence on subsequent birth outcomes compared with the general population (Ekeus 06). Although no studies were found examining the prevalence or perinatal effects of eating disorders in pregnant women with PDM, the confluence of these factors can present unique challenges for the patient and treatment team.

Questioning diabetic pregnant women regarding a history of anorexia nervosa, bulimia, or binge eating is an important assessment, but it is recognized that women with eating disorders are reluctant to disclose symptoms to healthcare providers (Franko 00). Additional warning signs during pregnancy are hyperemesis gravidarum and lack of weight gain in the second trimester (Franko 00). The American Dietetic Association Position Statement on nutrition intervention in the treatment of eating disorders is an excellent resource on diagnostic criteria as well as nutritional considerations (ADietA 06). In addition, a reliable and well-validated interview is available (Eating Disorder Examination; Fairburn 93a) that differentiates normative discontent, previous dieting, and eating concerns from more dysfunctional behaviors and attitudes (Franko 00). Detection instruments that have been validated in young women with type 1 diabetes include the Eating Discovery Inventory (Engstrom 99) and the Diabetes Eating Problems Survey (Neumark 02). Specific questions regarding previous or current omission of insulin for weight reduction, binging, and/or use of laxatives will aid in detection of eating disorders. Questions such as "Are you satisfied with your eating patterns?" and "Do you eat in secret?" differentiated women with bulimia nervosa from healthy controls in a primary care setting (Freund 93). Desire for a healthy baby may provide women with the incentive to address this problem and/or create added stress and struggle. While some women will have a diagnosable eating disorder, others will fall into the category of disordered eating. Helping women to examine the role that food plays in their lives—whether as a means of comfort, stress reduction, and/or emotional avoidance—can increase their ability to successfully manage the nutritional component of any diabetes and pregnancy program. For those women with an active eating disorder, referral to a mental health clinician specializing in its treatment is important (Peveler 92).

The intensification of diabetes management that is required for pregnancy involving strict adherence to a food plan "may exacerbate weight and shape concerns, and trigger a full blown eating disorder. When the introduction of intensive diabetes management produces a paradoxical deterioration in metabolic control, the health care providers should question whether an eating disturbance may be at the root of the deterioration" (Daneman 98). For diabetic pregnant patients with "full-blown bulimia nervosa or anorexia nervosa, a specific eating disorder treatment program is required," and aggressive interventions, such as total parenteral nutrition (TPN), may be needed for pregnancy to be successful. Various treatment approaches are described, but "the success rate is likely to be lower than that in nondiabetic females with an eating disorder. In milder cases, a clinic-based approach to changing eating attitudes and behavior may be successful" (Daneman 98). Important principles of management include (a) addressing factors that may have triggered the expression of disordered eating, namely, dietary restraint and excessive weight gain, (b) family involvement, (c) instruction in the use of regular meal and snack times and responding to hunger and satiety cues at mealtimes, and (d) nondeprivational approaches to eating (Daneman 98). Recent evidence-based U.K. guidelines on interventions for eating disorders emphasize psychological approaches of proven benefit (Mussell 00) for women with anorexia nervosa as well as specifically adapted cognitive behavior therapy (Fairburn 93b) for women with bulimia nervosa or binge-eating disorder, which may be supplemented with antidepressants and SSRIs (Wilson 05).

Other Issues

Pregnancy presents a unique opportunity to help women address a variety of concerns that may impact their diabetes management (Jovanovic 07). A woman entering a diabetes and pregnancy program will have a history of self-management that may not meet the expectations of the care provider. Most women experience a normal level of anxiety while pregnant. For women with PDM, feelings of anxiety, guilt, and responsibility are heightened. Acknowledging steps to make positive changes while encouraging more intensive self-management is vital to establishing a strong patient–clinician relationship (Glasgow 99b). These relationships are invaluable if behavior modification is needed for the cessation of smoking (ACOG 00, Lumley 04, Melvin 04) or use of alcohol or other drugs (Whitlock 04) during pregnancy. Inclusion of a licensed clinical social worker or other licensed mental health clinician as part of the interdisciplinary team allows for an established means of addressing psychological issues that arise. The DCCT team provided an analysis of practical lessons on changing behavior as a crucial part of achieving intensified glycemic control (Lorenz 96). Recognizing psychosocial challenges as well as medical issues creates an environment where the patient feels that all of her needs are being addressed. Establishing a relationship based on trust and mutual goals will assist the patient in openly discussing concerns and may empower her to better handle the challenges of diabetes management.

Recommendations

- Incorporate psychological assessment and treatment into routine care rather than waiting for identification of a specific problem or deterioration in psychological status. (E)
- Strive to include a mental health professional in the diabetes and pregnancy team to facilitate access to care and interprofessional communication. (E)
- Psychosocial screening and follow-up should include, but not be limited to, attitudes about diabetes, expectations for medical management and outcomes,

affect/mood, general and diabetes-related quality of life, resources (financial, social, emotional), and psychiatric history. (E)

- Screen diabetic pregnant women for depression, anxiety/stress, and disordered eating habits and adjust the team management plan as appropriate. (E)
- Use structured psychotherapy for first-line treatment of mild depression. (A)
- Continue or initiate psychopharmacological treatment for major depressive disorder during pregnancy only after appropriate consultation, risk–benefit analysis, and informed consent. (E)
- Instruct patients in stress management techniques. (E)
- Consider intensified interventions for diabetic pregnant women with current anorexia nervosa to ensure adequate prenatal nutrition and fetal development. (E)
- Offer specifically adapted cognitive behavior therapy to women with bulimia nervosa or binge-eating disorder. (A)

Part 1 Reference

AADE—American Association of Diabetes Educators: The scope of practice for diabetes educators and the standards of practice for diabetes educators. *Diabetes Educ* 26:25–31, 2000.

AADE—American Asssociation of Diabetes Educators. Slocum J, Barcio L, Darany J, Friedley K, Homko C, Mills JJ, Roberts D, Seifert H; Pregnancy/Reproductive Health Specialty Practice Group Education Task Force: Preconception to postpartum: management of pregnancy complicated by diabetes. *Diabetes Educ* 30:740–753, 2004.

AADE—American Association of Diabetic Educators. Mensing C, Cypress M, Halstensen C, McLaughlin S, Walker EA, eds: *The Art and Science of Diabetes Self-Management Education. A Desk Reference for Healthcare Professionals.* Chicago: American Association of Diabetes Educators; 2006.

AAP—American Academy of Pediatrics: Fetal alcohol syndrome and alcohol-related neurodevelopmental disorders. *Pediatrics* 106:358–360, 2000.

Abdelgadir M, Abbas M, Jarvi A, Elbagir M, Eltom M, Berne C: Glycaemic and insulin responses of six traditional Sudanese carbohydrate-rich meals in subjects with type 2 diabetes mellitus. *Diabet Med* 22:213–217, 2005.

Abrams, B, Altman, SL, Pickett, KE. Pregnancy weight gain: still controversial. *Am J Clin Nutr* 71 (Suppl):1233S-1241S, 2000.

Abu-Lebdeh HS, Barazzoni R, Meek SE, Bigelow ML, Persson X-MT, Nair KS: Effects of insulin deprivation and treatment on homocysteine metabolism in people with type 1 diabetes. *J Clin Endocrinol Metab* 91:3344–3348, 2006.

Acerini CL, Ahmed ML, Ross KM, Sullivan PB, Bird G, Dunger DB: Celiac disease in children and adolescents with IDDM: clinical characteristics and response to gluten-free diet. *Diabet Med* 15:38–44, 1998.

Ackurt F, Wetherilt H, Loker M, Hacibekiroglu M: Biochemical assessment of nutritional status in pre- and post-natal Turkish women and outcome of pregnancy. *Eur J Clin Nutr* 49:613–622, 1995.

ACOG—American College of Obstetricians and Gynecologists: Nutrition during pregnancy. Technical bulletin # 179. *Int J Gynecol Obstet* 43:67–74, 1999.

ACOG—American College of Obstetricians and Gynecologists: Smoking cessation during pregnancy. Educational bulletin # 260. *Obstet Gynecol* 96:1–4, 2000.

ACOG—American College of Obstetricians and Gynecologists: Gestational diabetes. ACOG practice bulletin # 30. *Obstet Gynecol* 98:525–537, 2001.

ACOG—American College of Obstetricians and Gynecologists: Exercise during pregnancy and the post partum period. Committee opinion # 267. *Obstet Gynecol* 99:171–173, 2002.

ACOG—American College of Obstetricians and Gynecologists, Committee on Practice Bulletins: Neural tube defects. Clinical management guidelines for obstetrician-gynecologists. ACOG practice bulletin # 44. *Obstet Gynecol* 102:203–213, 2003.

ACOG—American College of Obstetricians and Gynecologists: Pregestational diabetes mellitus. ACOG practice bulletin # 60. *Obstet Gynecol* 105:675–685, 2005.

ACOG—American College of Obstetricians and Gynecologists, Committee on Health Care for Underserved Women: Psychosocial risk factors: perinatal screening and intervention. ACOG Committee opinion # 343. *Obstet Gynecol* 198:469–477, 2006a.

ACOG—American College of Obstetricians and Gynecologists, Committee on Obstetric Practice: Treatment with selective serotonin reuptake inhibitors during pregnancy. Committee opinion # 354. *Obstet Gynecol* 108:1601–1603, 2006b.

ADA—American Diabetes Association: Preconception care of women with diabetes. Position statement. *Diabetes Care* 27 (Suppl 1):S76–S78, 2004a.

ADA—American Diabetes Association: Gestational diabetes mellitus. Position statement. *Diabetes Care* 27 (Suppl.1):S88–S90, 2004b.

ADA—American Diabetes Association: Hypertension management in adults with diabetes. Position statement. *Diabetes Care* 27 (Suppl.1):S65–S67, 2004c.

ADA—American Diabetes Association: Nephropathy in diabetes. Position statement. *Diabetes Care* 27 (Suppl.1):S79–S83, 2004d.

ADA—American Diabetes Association: Dyslipidemia management in adults with diabetes. Position statement. *Diabetes Care* 27 (Suppl.1):S68–S71, 2004e.

ADA—American Diabetes Association: Tests of glycemia in diabetes. Position statement. *Diabetes Care* 27 (Suppl 1):S91–S93, 2004f.

ADA—American Diabetes Association: Physical activity/exercise and diabetes. Position statement. *Diabetes Care* 27 (Suppl.1):S58–S62, 2004g.

ADA—American Diabetes Association Workgroup on Hypoglycemia: Defining and reporting hypoglycemia in diabetes. *Diabetes Care* 28:1245–1249, 2005.

ADA—American Diabetes Association, European Association for the Study of Diabetes, International Federation of Clinical Chemistry and Laboratory Medicine, and the International Diabetes Federation: Consensus statement on the worldwide standardization of the HbA1C measurement. *Diabetologia* 50:2042–2043, 2007; *Diabetes Care* 30:2399–2400, 2007.

ADA—American Diabetes Association: Standards of medical care in diabetes—2008. Position statement. *Diabetes Care* 31 (Suppl.1):S12–S54, 2008a.

ADA—American Diabetes Association: Nutrition recommendations and interventions for diabetes. Position statement. *Diabetes Care* 31 (Suppl 1):S61–S78, 2008b.

Adams M, Montague CT, Prins JB, Holder JC, Smith SA, Sanders L, Digby JE, Sewter CP, Lazar MA, Chatterjee VK, O'Rahilly S: Activators of peroxisome proliferator-activated receptor gamma have depot-specific effects on human preadipocyte differentiation. *J Clin Invest* 100:3149–53, 1997.

ADietA—American Dietetic Association: Nutrition and lifestyle for a healthy pregnancy outcome. Position statement. *J Am Diet Assoc* 102:1479–1490, 2002.

ADietA—American Dietetic Association and Dietitians of Canada: Vegetarian diets. Position statement. *J Am Diet Assoc* 103:748–765, 2003.

ADietA—American Dietetic Association: Use of nutritive and nonnutritive sweeteners. Position statement. *J Am Diet Assoc* 104:255–275, 2004.

ADietA—American Dietetic Association: Nutrition intervention in the treatment of anorexia nervosa, bulimia nervosa, and other eating disorders. Position statement. *J Am Diet Assoc* 106:2073–2082, 2006.

ADietA—American Dietetic Association and Dietitians of Canada: Dietary fatty acids. Position statement. *J Am Diet Assoc* 107:1599–1611, 2007.

Admon G, Weinstein Y, Falk B, Weintrob N, Benzaquen H, Ofan R, Fayman G, Zigel L, Constantini N, Phillip M: Exercise with and without an insulin pump among children and adolescents with type 1 diabetes mellitus. *Pediatrics* 116: e348–e355, 2005.

Aguilar D, Bozkurt B, Pritchett A, Petersen NJ, Deswal A: The impact of thiazolidinedione use on outcomes in ambulatory patients with diabetes mellitus and heart failure. *J Am Coll Cardiol* 50:32–36, 2007.

AHA—American Heart Association Expert Panel/Writing Group, Mosca L (chair): Evidence-based guidelines for cardiovascular disease prevention in women. *Circulation* 109:672–693, 2004.

Ahr HJ, Boberg M, Brendel E, Krause HP, Steinke W: Pharmacokinetics of miglitol. Absorption, distribution, metabolism, and excretion following administration to rats, dogs, and man. *Arzneimittelforschung* 47:734–745, 1997.

Ahr HJ, Boberg M, Krause HP, Maul W, Muller FO, Ploschke HJ, Weber H, Wunsche C: Pharmacokinetics of acarbose. Part I: Absorption, concentration in plasma, metabolism and excretion after single administration of [14C] acarbose to rats, dogs and man. *Arzneimittelforschung* 39:1254–1260, 1989a.

Ahr HJ, Krause HP, Siefert HM, Steinke W, Weber H: Pharmacokinetics of acarbose. Part II: Distribution to and elimination from tissues and organs following single or repeated administration of [14C] acarbose to rats and dogs. *Arzneimittelforschung* 39:1261–1267, 1989b.

Aiello LP, Gardner TW, King GL, Blankenship G, Cavallerano JD, Ferris FL III, Klein R: Diabetic retinopathy. ADA technical review. *Diabetes Care* 21:143–156, 1998.

Aiello LP, Cahill MT, Wong JS: Systemic considerations in the management of diabetic retinopathy. *Am J Ophthalmol* 132:760–776, 2001.

Ainy E, Ghazi AA, Arizi F: Changes in calcium, 25(OH) vitamin D_3 and other biochemical factors during pregnancy. *J Endocrinol Invest* 29:303–307, 2006.

Akabas SR, Deckelbaum RJ: Summary of a workshop on n-3 fatty acids: current status of recommendations and future directions. *Am J Clin Nutr* 83 (Suppl): 1536S–1538S, 2006.

Akkeson A, Bjellerup P, Berglund M, Bremme K, Vahter M: Serum transferrin receptor: a specific marker of iron deficiency in pregnancy. *Am J Clin Nutr* 68:1241–1246, 1998.

Akkeson A, Bjellerup P, Berglund M, Bremme K, Vahter M: Soluble transferrin receptor: longitudinal assessment from pregnancy to postlactation. *Obstet Gynecol* 99:260–266, 2002.

Al MD, Badart-Smook A, von Houwelingen AC, Hasaart TH, Hornstra G: Fat intake of women during normal pregnancy: relationship with maternal and neonatal essential fatty acid status. *J Am Coll Nutr* 15:49–55, 1996.

Alaedini A, Green PHR: Narrative review: celiac disease: understanding a complex autoimmune disorder. *Ann Intern Med* 142:289–298, 2005.

Alfieri RR, Cavazzoni A, Petronini PG, Bonelli MA, Caccamo AE, Borghetti AF, Wheeler KP: Compatible osmolytes modulate the response of porcine endothelial cells to hypertonicity and protect them from apoptosis. *J Physiol* 540:499–508, 2002.

Algert S, Shragg P, Hollingsworth DR: Moderate caloric restriction in obese women with gestational diabetes. *Obstet Gynecol* 65:487–491, 1985.

Ali S, Stone MA, Peters JL, Davies MJ, Khunti K: The prevalence of co-morbid depression in adults with type 2 diabetes: a systematic review and meta-analysis. *Diabet Med* 23:1165–1173, 2006.

Allen LH: Biological mechanisms that might underly iron's effects on fetal growth and preterm birth. *J Nutr* 131:581S–589S, 2001.

Allen LH: Multiple micronutrients in pregnancy and lactation: an overview. *Am J Clin Nutr* 81 (Suppl):1206S–1212S, 2005.

Allen VM, Armson BA, Wilson RD, Blight C, Gagnon A, Johnson JA, Langlois S, Summers A, Wyatt P, Farine D, Crane J, Delisle MF, Keenan-Lindsay L, Morin V, Schneider CE, Van Aerde J; Society of Obstetricians and Gynecologists of Canada: Teratogenicity associated with preexisting and gestational diabetes. *J Obstet Gynecol Can* 29:927–944, 2007.

Allison DB, Egan SK, Barraj LM, Caughman C, Infante M, Heimbach JT: Estimated intakes of *trans* fatty and other fatty acids in the U.S. population. *J Am Diet Assoc* 99:166–174, 1999.

Allison KC, Crow SJ, Reeves RR, West DS, Foreyt JP, Dilillo VG, Wadden TA, Jeffery RW, Van Dorsten B, Stunkard AJ: Binge eating disorder and night eating syndrome in adults with type 2 diabetes. *Obesity* 15:1287–1293, 2007.

Alonso N, Granada L, Salinas I, Lucas AM, Reverter JL, Junca J, Oriol A, Sanmarti A: Serum pepsinogen I: an early marker of pernicious anemia in patients with type 1 diabetes. *J Clin Endocrinol Metab* 90:5254–5258, 2005.

Al-Saleh E, Nandakumaran M, Al-Shammari M, Al-Fatah F, Al-Harouny A: Assessment of maternal-fetal status of some essential trace elements in pregnant women in late gestation: relationship with birth weight and placental weight. *J Matern Fetal Neonatal Med* 16:9–14, 2004.

Al-Saleh E, Nandakumaran M, Al-Shammari M, Makhseed M, Sadan T, Harouny A: Maternal-fetal status of copper, iron, molybdenum, selenium and zinc in insulin-dependent diabetic pregnancies. *Arch Gynecol Obstet* 271:212–217, 2005.

Al-Shaikh AA: Pregnant women with type 1 diabetes mellitus treated by glargine insulin. *Saudi Med J* 27:563–565, 2006.

Althuis MD, Jordan NE, Ludington EA, Wittes JT: Glucose and insulin responses to dietary chromium supplements: a meta-analysis. *Am J Clin Nutr* 76:148–155, 2002.

Altshuler LL, Cohen L, Szuba MP, Burt VK, Gitlin M, Mintz J: Pharmacologic management of psychiatric illness during pregnancy: dilemmas and guidelines. *Am J Psychiatry* 153:592–606, 1996.

AMA—American Medical Association, Council on Scientific Affairs: Saccharin. Review of safety issues. *JAMA* 254:2622–2624, 1985.

Aman J, Berne C, Ewald U, Tuvemo T: Cutaneous blood flow during a hypoglycemic clamp in insulin-dependent diabetic patients and healthy subjects. *Clin Sci* 82:615–618, 1992.

Amarapurka DN, Amarapurkar AD, Patel ND, Agal S, Baigal R, Gupte P, Pramanik S: Nonalcoholic steatohepatitis (NASH) with diabetes: predictors of liver fibrosis. *Ann Hepatol* 5:30–33, 2006.

Amin R, Murphy N, Edge J, Ahmed M, Acerini C, Dunger D: A longitudinal study of the effects of a gluten-free diet on glycemic control and weight gain in subjects with type 1 diabetes and celiac disease. *Diabetes Care* 25:1117–1122, 2002.

Anderson BJ, Auslander WF, Jung KC, Miller JP, Santiago JV: Assessing family sharing of diabetes responsibilities. *J Pediatr Psychol* 15:477–492, 1990.

Anderson RM, Funnell M, Butler P, Arnold M, Fitzgerald J, Feste C: Patient empowerment: results of a randomized controlled trial. *Diabetes Care* 18: 943–949, 1995.

Anderson JH Jr, Brunelle RL, Koivisto VA, Pfutzner A, Trautmann ME, Vignati L, DiMarchi R; Insulin Lispro Study Group: Reduction of postprandial hyperglycemia and frequency of hypoglycemia in IDDM patients on insulin-analog treatment. *Diabetes* 46:265–270, 1997.

Anderson RJ, Freedeland KE, Clouse RE, Lustman PJ: The prevalence of comorbid depression in adults with diabetes. *Diabetes Care* 24:1069–1078, 2001.

Anderson RJ, Grigsby AB, Freedland KE, de Groot M, McGill JB, Clouse RE, Lustman PJ: Anxiety and poor glycemic control: a meta-analytic review of the literature. *Int J Psychiatry Med* 32:235–247, 2002.

Anderson JW, Randles KM, Kendall CWC, Jenkins DJA: Carbohydrate and fiber recommendations for individuals with diabetes: a quantitative assessment and meta-analysis of the evidence. *J Am Coll Nutr* 23:5–17, 2004.

Anderson GD: Pregnancy-induced changes in pharmacokinetics: a mechanistic-based approach. *Clin Pharmacokinet* 44:989–1008, 2005.

Andersson A, Hultberg B, Brattstrom I, Isaksson A: Decreased serum homocysteine in pregnancy. *Eur J Clin Chem Clin Biochem* 30:377–379, 1992.

Andrade SE, Raebel MA, Brown J, Lane K, Livingston J, Boudreau D, Rolnick SJ, Roblin D, Smith DH, Willy ME, Staffa JA, Platt R: Use of antidepressant medications during pregnancy: a multisite study. *Am J Obstet Gynecol* 198:194e1–e5, 2008.

Andrews NC: Disorders of iron metabolism. *N Engl J Med* 341:1986–1995, 1999.

Angelico F, Del Ben M, Conti R, Francioso S, Feole K, Maccioni D, Antonini TM, Alessandri C: Non-alcoholic fatty liver syndrome: a hepatic consequence of common metabolic diseases. *J Gastroenterol Hepatol* 18:588–594, 2003.

Angulo P: Nonalcoholic fatty liver disease. *N Engl J Med* 346:1221–1231, 2002.

Annibale B, Marignani M, Azzoni C, D'Ambra G, Caruana P, D'Adda T, Delle Fave G, Bordi C: Atrophic body gastritis: distinct features associated with *Helicobacter pylori* infection. *Helicobacter* 2:57–64, 1997.

Annibale B, Severi C, Chistolini A, Antonelli G, Lajner E. Marcheggiano A, Iannoni C, Monarca B, Delle Fave G: A longitudinal study of the effects of a gluten-free diet alone on recovery from iron deficiency in adult celiac patients. *Am J Gastroenterol* 96:132–137, 2001.

Antoniades C, Tousoulis D, Marinou K, Vasiliadou C, Tentolouris C, Bouras G, Pitsavos C, Stefanadis C: Asymmetrical dimethylarginine regulates endothelial function in methionine-induced but not in chronic homocystinemia in humans: effect of oxidative stress and proinflammatory cytokines. *Am J Clin Nutr* 84:781–788, 2006.

Arauz-Pacheco C, Parrott MA, Raskin P: The treatment of hypertension in adult patients with diabetes. ADA technical review. *Diabetes Care* 25:134–147, 2002.

Ard JD, Brambow SC, Liu D, Slentz CA, Kraux WE, Svetkey LP: The effect of the PREMIER intervention on insulin sensitivity. *Diabetes Care* 27:340–347, 2004.

Ardawi MS, Nasrat HA, BA'Aqueel HS: Calcium-regulating hormones and parathyroid hormone-related peptide in normal human pregnancy and postpartum: a longitudinal study. *Eur J Endocrinol* 137:402–409, 1997.

Arentz-Hansen H, Korner R, Molberg O, Quarsten H, Vader W, Kooy YMC, Lundin KEA, Koning F, Roepstorff P, Sollid LM, McAdam SN: The intestinal T cell response to α-gliadin in adult celiac disease is focused on a single deamidated glutamine targeted by tissue transglutaminase. *J Exp Med* 191:603–612, 2000.

Arisawa K, Takeda H, Mikasa H: Background exposure to PCDDs/PCDFs/PCBs and its potential health effects: a review of epidemiologic studies. *J Med Invest* 52: 10–21, 2005.

Artal R, Platt LD, Sperling M, Kammula RK, Jilek J, Nakamura R: I. Maternal cardiovascular and metabolic responses in normal pregnancy. *Am J Obstet Gynecol* 140:123–127, 1981.

Artal R, Golde SH, Dorey F, McCllan SN, Gratacos JA, Lierette T, Montoro M, Wu PYK, Anderson B, Mestman J: The effect of plasma glucose variation on neonatal outcome in the pregnant diabetic. *Am J Obstet Gynecol* 147:537–541, 1983.

Artal R, Wiswell R, Romem Y: Hormonal responses to exercise in diabetic and nondiabetic pregnant patients. *Diabetes* 34 (Suppl 2):78–80, 1985.

Artal R, Fortunato V, Welton A, Constantino N, Khodiguian N, Villalobos L, Wiswell R: A comparison of cardiopulmonary adaptations to exercise in pregnancy at sea level and altitude. *Am J Obstet Gynecol* 172:1170–1180, 1995.

Artal R, Sherman C: Exercise during pregnancy: safe and beneficial for most. *Phys Sports Med* 27:51–52, 54, 57–58, 1999.

Arunabh S, Pollack S, Yeh J, Aloia JF: Body fat content and 25-hydroxyvitamin D levels in healthy women. *J Clin Endocrinol Metab* 88:157–161, 2003.

Asami-Miyagishi R, Iseki S, Usui M, Uchida K, Kubo H, Morita I: Expression and function of PPAR-γ in rat placental development. *Biochem Biophys Res Commun* 315:497–501, 2004.

Ascher JA, Cole JO, Colin JN, Feighner JP, Ferris RM, Fibiger HC, Golden RN, Martin P, Potter WZ, Richelson E, Sulser F: Bupropion: a review of its mechanism of antidepressant activity. *J Clin Psychiatry* 56:395–401, 1995.

Ashabani A, Abushofa U, Abusrewill S, Abdelazez M, Tuckova L, Tlaskalova-Hogenova H: The prevalence of celiac disease in Libyan children with type 1 diabetes mellitus. *Diabetes Metab Res Rev* 19:69–75, 2003.

Ask K, Akesson A, Berglund M, Vahter M: Inorganic mercury and methylmercury in placentas of Swedish women. *Environ Health Perspect* 110:523–526, 2002.

Astor BC, Muntner P, Levin A, Eustace JA, Coresh J: Association of kidney function with anemia: the Third National Health and Nutrition Examination Survey (1988–1994). *Arch Intern Med* 162:1401–1408, 2002.

Atamer Y, Kocyigit Y, Yokus B, Atamer A, Erden AC: Lipid peroxidation, antioxidant defense, status of trace metals and leptin levels in preeclampsia. *Eur J Obstet Gynecol Reprod Biol* 119:60–66, 2005.

Atanasova BD, Li ACY, Bjarnason I, Tzatchev KN, Simpson RJ: Duodenal ascorbate and ferric reductase in human iron deficiency. *Am J Clin Nutr* 81:130–133, 2005.

Attia N, Caprio S, Jones TW, Heptulla R, Holcombe J, Silver D, Sherwin RS, Tamborlane WV: Changes in free insulin-like growth factor-1 and leptin concentrations during acute metabolic decompensation in insulin withdrawn patients with type 1 diabetes. *J Clin Endocrinol Metab* 84:2324–2328, 1999.

Austin MP, Tully L, Parker G: Examing the relationship between antenatal anxiety and postnatal depression. *J Affect Disord* 101:169–174, 2007.

Avinoah E, Ovnat A, Charuzi I: Nutritional status seven years after Roux-en-Y gastric bypass surgery. *Surgery* 111:137–142, 1992.

Ayaz M, Turan B: Selenium prevents diabetes-induced alterations in [Zn2+]I and metallothionein level of rat heart via restoration of cell redox cycle. *Am J Physiol* 290:H1070–H1080, 2006.

Azais-Braesco V, Pascal G: Vitamin A in pregnancy: requirements and safety limits. *Am J Clin Nutr* 71 (Suppl):1325S–1333S, 2000.

Bacq Y: Acute fatty liver of pregnancy. *Semin Perinatol* 22:134–140, 1998.

Bailey LB: New standard for dietary folate intake in pregnant women. *Am J Clin Nutr* 71 (Suppl):1304S–1307S, 2000.

Bailey LB, Rampersaud GC, Kauwell GPA: Folic acid supplements and fortification affects the risk for neural tube defects, vascular disease and cancer: evolving science *J Nutr* 133:1961S–1968S, 2003.

Bailey LB, Berry RJ: Folic acid supplementation and the occurrence of congenital heart defects, orofacial clefts, multiple births, and miscarriage. *Am J Clin Nutr* 81:1213S–1217S, 2005.

Bailyes EM, Nave BT, Soos MA, Orr SR, Hayward AC, Siddle K: Insulin receptor/ IGF-I receptor hybrids are widely distributed in mammalian tissues:

quantification of individual receptor species by selective immunoprecipitation and immunoblotting. *Biochem J* 327:209–215, 1997.

Baker H, DeAngelis B, Holland B, Gittens-Williams L, Barrett T Jr: Vitamin profile of 563 gravidas during trimesters of pregnancy. *J Am Coll Nutr* 21:33–37, 2006.

Baldas V, Tommasini A, Trevisiol C, Berti I, Fasano A, Sblattero D, Bradbury A, Marzari R, Barillari G, Ventura A, Not T: Development of a novel rapid non-invasive screening test for celiac disease. *Gut* 47:628–631, 2000.

Ballani P, Tran MT, Navar MD, Davidson MB: Clinical experience with U-500 regular insulin in obese, markedly insulin-resistant type 2 diabetic patients. *Diabetes Care* 29:2504–2505, 2006.

Banerjee S, Ghosh US, Banerjee D: Fetomaternal complications in pregnancies with diabetes mellitus: association with the amount of insulin requirement, mean terminal blood glucose and HbA1C levels. *J Indian Med Assoc* 101:728, 730–732, 740, 2003.

Banerjee S, Chambers AE, Campbell S: Is vitamin E a safe prophylaxis for preeclampsia? *Am J Obstet Gynecol* 194:1228–1233, 2006.

Bantle JP, Laine DC, Castle GW, Thomas JW, Hoogwerf BJ, Goetz FC: Postprandial glucose and insulin responses to meals containing differenct carbohydrates in normal and diabetic subjects. *N Engl J Med* 309:7–12, 1983.

Bantle JP, Lonzette N, Frankamp LM: Effects of anatomical region used for insulin injections on glycemia in in type 1 diabetes subjects. *Diabetes Care* 16: 1592–1597, 1993.

Bao F, Yu L, Babu S, Wang T, Hoffenberg EJ, Rewers M, Eisenbarth GS: One third of HL DG2 homozygous patients with type 1 diabetes express celiac disease-associated transglutaminase autoantibodies. *J Autoimmun* 13:143–148, 1999.

Baptista ML, Koda YK, Mitsunori R, Nisihara, Ioshii SO: Prevalence of celiac disease in Brazilian children and adolescents with type 1 diabetes mellitus. *J Pediatr Gastroenterol Nutr* 41:621–624, 2005.

Barclay AW, Brand-Miller JC, Wolever TMS: Glycemic index, glycemic load, and glycemic response are not the same. *Diabetes Care* 28:1839–1840, 2005.

Barera G, Bonfanti R, Viscardi M, Bazzigalupi E, Calori G, Meschi F, Bianchi C, Chiumello G: Occurrence of celiac disease after onset of type 1 diabetes: a 6-year prospective longitudinal study. *Pediatrics* 109:833–838, 2002.

Barglow P, Hatcher R, Berndt DS, Phelps R: Psychosocial child bearing stress and metabolic control in pregnant diabetics. *J Nerv Ment Dis* 173:615–620, 1985.

Barker CC, Mitton C, Jevon G, Mock T: Can tissue transglutaminase antibody titers replace small-bowel biopsy to diagnose celiac disease in select pediatric populations? *Pediatrics* 115:1341–1346, 2005.

Barker JM: Type 1 diabetes-associated autoimmunity: natural history, genetic associations, and screening. *J Clin Endocrinol Metab* 91:1210–1217, 2006.

Barnard KD, Skinner TC, Peveler R: The prevalence of co-morbid depression in adults with type 1 diabetes: a systematic review. *Diabet Med* 23:445–448, 2006.

Barnett AH, Dreyer M, Lange P, Serdarvic-Pehar M; on behalf of the Exubera Phase III Study Group: An open, randomized, parallel-group study to compare the efficacy and safety profile of inhaled human insulin (Exubera) with glibenclamide as adjunctive therapy in patients with type 2 diabetes poorly controlled on metformin. *Diabetes Care* 29:1818–1825, 2006.

Barone JJ, Roberts HR: Caffeine consumption. *Food Chem Toxicol* 34:119–129, 1996.

Barrio R, Roldan MB, Alonso M, Canton R, Camarero C: *Heliobacter pylori* infection with parietal cell antibodies in children and adolescents with insulin dependent diabetes mellitus. *J Pediatr Endocrinol Metab* 10:511–516, 1997.

Bar-Shany S, Herbert V: Transplacentally acquired antibody to intrinsic factor with vitamin B12 deficiency. *Blood* 30:777–784, 1967.

Bartley KA, Underwood BA, Deckelbaum RJ: A life cycle micronutrient perspective for women's health. *Am J Clin Nutr* 81 (Suppl):1188S–1193S, 2005.

Bar-Zohar D, Azem F, Klausner J, Abu-Abeid S: Pregnancy after laparoscopic adjustable gastric banding: perinatal outcome is favorable also for women with relatively high gestational weight gain. *Surg Endosc* 20:1580–1583, 2006.

Bastin J, Drakesmith H, Rees M, Sargent I, Townsend A: Localisation of proteins of iron metabolism in the human placenta and liver. *Br J Hematol* 134:532–543, 2006.

Bates JH, Young IS, Galway L, Traub AI, Hadden DR: Antioxidant status and lipid peroxidation in diabetic pregnancy. *Br J Nutr* 78:523–532, 1997.

Battaglia MR, Alemzadeh R, Katte H, Hall PL, Perlmuter LC: Brief report: disordered eating and psychosocial factors in adolescent females with type 1 diabetes mellitus. *J Pediatr Psychol* 31:552–556, 2006.

Bauman WA, Shaw SS, Javatilleke E, Spungen AM, Herbert V: Increased intake of calcium reverses vitamin B12 malabsorption induced by metformin. *Diabetes Care* 23:1227–1231, 2000.

Baumann MU, Deborde S, Illsley NP: Placental glucose transfer and fetal growth. *Endocrine* 19:13–22, 2002.

Beard JL: Effectiveness and strategies of iron supplementation during pregnancy. *Am J Clin Nutr* 71 (Suppl):1288S–1294S, 2000.

Beazley D, Ahokas R, Livingston J, Griggs M, Sibai BM: Vitamin C and E supplementation in women at high risk for preeclampsia: a double-blind, placebo-controlled trial. *Am J Obstet Gynecol* 192:520–521, 2005.

Belfiore F, Iannello S: Insulin secretion and its pharmacological stimulation. In: Belfiore F, Mogensen CE, eds. *New Concepts in Diabetes and Its Treatment.* Basel, Switzerland: Karger; 2000:20–37.

Belfort R, Harrison SA, Brown K, Darland C, Finch J, Hardies J, Balas B, Gastaldelli A, Tio F, Pulcini J, Berria R, Ma JZ, Dwivedi S, Havranek R, Fincke C, DeFronzo R, Bannayan GA, Schenker S, Cusi K: A placebo-controlled trial of pioglitazone in subjects with nonalcoholic steatohepatitis. *N Engl J Med* 355:2297–2307, 2006.

Bell R, Bailey K, Cresswell T, Hawthorne G, Critchley J, Lewis-Barned: the Northern Diabetic Pregnancy Survey Steering Group: Trends in prevalence and outcomes of pregnancy in women with preexisting type I and type II diabetes. *BJOG* 115:445–452, 2008.

Bellmann O, Hartman M: Influence of pregnancy on the kinetics of insulin. *Am J Obst Gynecol* 122:829–832, 1975.

Ben-Haroush A, Yogev Y, Chen R, Rosenn B, Hod M, Langer O: The postprandial glucose profile in the diabetic pregnancy. *Am J Obstet Gynecol* 191:576–581, 2004.

Bennett HA, Einarson A, Taddio A, Koren G, Einarson TR: Prevalence of depression during pregnancy: systematic review. *Obstet Gynecol* 103:698–709, 2004.

Bentley TG, Willett WC, Weinstein MC, Kuntz KM: Population-level changes in folic acid intake by age, gender, and race/ethnicity after folic acid fortification. *Am J Public Health* 96:2040–2047, 2006.

Beral V, Roman E, Colwell L: Poor reproductive outcome in insulin-dependent diabetic women associated with later development of other endocrine disorders in the mothers. *Lancet* 1:4–7, 1984.

Berard A, Ramos E, Rey E, Blais L, St-Andre M, Oraichi D: First trimester exposure to paroxetine and risk of cardiac malformations in infants: the importance of dosage. *Birth Defects Res B Dev Reprod Toxicol* 80:18–27, 2007.

Berger M, Berchtold P, Cuppers HJ, Drost H, Klev HK, Muller WA, Wiegelmann W, Zimmerman-Telschow H, Gries FA, Kruskemper HL, Zimmermann H: Metabolic and hormonal effects of muscular exercise in juvenile type diabetics. *Diabetologia* 13:355–365, 1977.

Bergman MP, Amedei A, D'Elios MM, Azzurri A, Benagiano M, Tamburini C, van der Zee R, Vandenbroucke-Grauls CM, Appelmelk BJ, Del Prete G: Characterization of H+, K+-ATPase T cell epitopes in human autoimmune gastritis. *Eur J Immunol* 33:539–545, 2003.

Berk MA, Mimouni F, Miodovnik M, Hertzberg V, Valuck J: Macrosomia in infants of insulin-dependent diabetic mothers. *Pediatrics* 86:1029–1034, 1989.

Bertini AM, Silva JC, Taborda W, Becker F, Lemos Bebber FR, Zucco Viesi JM, Aquim G, Engel Ribeiro T: Perinatal outcomes and the use of oral hypoglycemic agents. *J Perinat Med* 33:519–523, 2005.

Bessinger RC, McMurray RG, Hackney AC: Substrate utilization and hormonal responses to moderate intensity exercise during pregnancy and after delivery. *Am J Obstet Gynecol* 186:757–764, 2002.

Bessinger RC, McMurray RG: Substrate utilization and hormonal responses to exercise in pregnancy. *Clin Obstet Gynecology* 46:467–478, 2003.

Bezerra FF, Laboissiere FP, King JC, Donangelo CM: Pregnancy and lactation affect markers of calcium and bone metabolism differently in adolescent and adult women with low calcium intake. *J Nutr* 132:2183–2187, 2002.

Bhatia V, Viswanathan P: Insulin resistance and PPAR insulin sensitizers. *Curr Opin Investig Drugs* 7:891–897, 2006.

Bhattacharyya A, Vice PA: Insulin lispro, pregnancy and retinopathy. *Diabetes Care* 22:2101–2102, 1999.

Bhattacharyya A, Brown S, Hughes S, Vice PA. Insulin lispro and regular insulin in pregnancy. *Q JM* 94:255–260, 2001.

Bildirici I, Roh C-R, Schaiff WT, Lewkowski BM, Nelson DM, Sadovsky Y: The lipid droplet-associated protein adophilin is expressed in human trophoblasts and is regulated by peroxisomal proliferator-activated receptor-γ/retinoid X receptor. *J Clin Endocrinol Metab* 88:6056–6062, 2003.

Bina DM, Anderson RL, Johnson ML, Bergenstal RM, Kendall DM: Clinical impact of prandial state, exercise, and site preparation on the equivalence of alternative-site blood glucose testing. *Diabetes Care* 26:981–985, 2003.

Binder C, Lauritzen T, Faber O, Pramming S: Insulin pharamacokinetics. *Diabetes Care* 7:188–199, 1984.

Bingley PJ, Williams AJK, Norcross AJ, Unsworth DJ, Lock RJ, Ness AR, Jones RW; on behalf of the Avon Longitudinal Study of Parents and Children Study Team: Undiagnosed celiac disease at age seven: population bases prospective birth cohort study. *BMJ* 328:322–323, 2004.

Bisseling TM, Versteegen MG, van der Wal S, Copius Peereboom-Stegeman JJH, Borggreven JMPM, Steegers EAP, van der Laak JAWM, Russel FGM, Smits P: Impaired KATP channel function in the fetoplacental circulation of patients with type 1 diabetes mellitus. *Am J Obstet Gynecol* 192:973–979, 2005.

Bitsanis D, Ghebremeskel K, Moodley T, Crawford MA, Djahanbakhch O: Gestational diabetes mellitus enhances arachidonic and docosahexaenoic acids in placental phospholipids. *Lipids* 41:341–346, 2006.

Bjorklund AO, Adamson UKC, Lins P-E, Westgren LMR: Diminished insulin clearance during late pregnancy in patients with type 1 diabetes mellitus. *Clin Sci* 95:317–323, 1998.

Bjornberg KA, Vahter M, Petersson-Grawe K, Glynn A, Cnattingius S, Darnerud PO, Atuma S, Becker W, Berglund M: Methyl mercury and inorganic mercury in Swedish pregnant women and in cord blood: influence of fish consumption. *Environ Health Perspect* 111:637–641, 2003.

Bjornberg KA, Vahter M, Berglund B, Niklasson B, Blennow M, Sandborgh-Englund G: Transport of methylmercury and inorganic mercury to the fetus and breast-fed infant. *Environ Health Perspect* 113:1381–1385, 2005.

Blanz BJ, Rensch-Riemann BS, Fritz-Sifmund DI, Schmidt MH: IDDM is a risk factor for adolescent psychiatric disorders. *Diabetes Care* 16:1579–1587, 1993.

Bleys J, Miler ER III, Pastor-Barriuso R, Appel LJ, Guallar E: Vitamin-mineral supplementation and the progression of atherosclerosis: a meta-analysis of randomized controlled trials. *Am J Clin Nutr* 84:880–887, 2006.

Blohm F, Friden B, Milsom I: A prospective longitudinal population-based study of clinical miscarriage in an urban Sedish population. *BJOG* 115:176–183, 2008.

Blomhoff R: Dietary antioxidants and cardiovascular disease. *Curr Opin Lipidol* 16:47–54, 2005.

Bloomgarden ZT: EASD thiamine symposium. The European Association for the Study of Diabetes. Perspectives on the news. *Diabetes Care* 28:1253–1257, 2005.

Bo S, Lezo A, Menato G, Gallo ML, Bardelli C, Signorite A, Berutti C, Massobrio M, Pagano GF: Gestational hyperglycemia, zinc, selenium, and antioxidant vitamins. *Nutrition* 21:186–191, 2005.

Bocos C, Gottlicher M, Gearing K, Banner C, Enmark E, Teboul M, Crickmore A, Gustafsson JA: Fatty acid activation of peroxisome proliferator-activated receptor (PPAR). *J Steroid Biochem Mol Biol* 53:467–473, 1995.

Boddie AM, Dedlow ER, Nackashi JA, Opalko FJ, Kauwell GPA, Gregory JF III, Bailey LB: Folate absorption in women with a history of neural tube defect-affected pregnancy. *Am J Clin Nutr* 72:154–158, 2000.

Boden G, Zhang M: Recent findings concerning thiazolidinediones in the treatment of diabetes. *Expert Opin Investig Drugs* 15:243–250, 2006.

Boehme P, Floriot M, Sirveaux M-A, Durain D, Ziegler O, Drouin P, Guerci B: Evolution of analytical performance in portable glucose meters in the last decade. *Diabetes Care* 26:1170–1175, 2003.

Boelsterli UA, Bedoucha M: Toxicological consequences of altered peroxisome proliferator-activated receptor gamma (PPARgamma) expression in the liver: insights from models of obesity and type 2 diabetes. *Biochem Pharmacol* 63:1–10, 2002.

Bolli GB: The pharmacokinetic basis of insulin therapy in diabetes mellitus. *Diabetes Res Clin Pract* 6:S3–S16, 1989.

Bolli GB, Perriello G, Fanelli CG, De Feo P: Nocturnal blood glucose control in type 1 diabetes mellitus. *Diabetes Care* 16 (Suppl 3):71–89, 1993.

Bonaa KH, Njolstad I, Ueland PM, Schirmer H, Tverdal A, Steigen T, Wang H, Nordrehaug JE, Arnesen E, Rasmussen K; NORVIT Trial Investigators: Homocysteine lowering and cardiovascular events after acute myocardial infarction. *N Engl J Med* 354:1578–1588, 2006.

Bonari L, Pinto N, Ahn E, Einarson A, Steiner M, Koren G: Perinatal risks of untreated depression during pregnancy. *Can J Psychiatry* 49:726–735, 2004.

Bondevik GT, Schneede J, Refsum H, Lie RT, Ulstein M, Kvale G: Homocysteine and methylmalonic acid levels in pregnant Nepali women. Should cobalamin supplementation be considered? *Eur J Clin Nutr* 55:856–864, 2001.

Bonen A, Campagna P, Gilchrist L, Young DC, Beresford P: Substrate and endocrine responses during exercise at selected stages of pregnancy. *J Appl Physiol* 73:134–142, 1992.

Bonet B, Brunzell JD, Gown AM, Knopp RH: Metabolism of very low density lipoprotein triglyceride by human placental cells: the role of lipoprotein lipase. *Metabolism* 41:596–603, 1992.

Bonnette RE, Caudill MA, Boddie AM, Hutson AD, Kauwell GP, Bailey LB: Plasma homocysteine concentrations in pregnant and nonpregnant women with controlled folate intake. *Obstet Gynecol* 92:167–170, 1998.

Borg GAV: Psychophysical bases of perceived exertion. *Med Sci Sports Exerc* 14:377–381, 1982.

Bornet FR, Costagliola D, Rizkalla SW, Blayo A, Fontvieille AM, Haardt MJ, Letanoux M, Tchobroutsky G, Slama G: Insulinemic and glycemic indexes of six starch-rich foods taken alone and in a mixed meal by type 2 diabetic subjects. *Am J Clin Nutr* 45:588–595, 1987.

Boskovic R, Feig DS, Derewlany L, Knie B, Portnoi G, Koren G: Transfer of insulin lispro across the human placenta: in vitro perfusion. *Diabetes Care* 26:1390–1394, 2003.

Bostom A, Brosnan JT, Hall B, Nadeau MR, Selhub J: Net uptake of plasma homocysteine by the rat kidney in vivo. *Atherosclerosis* 116:59–62, 1995.

Part 1 Reference **133**

Bostom AG, Bausserman L, Jacques PF, Liaugaudas G, Selhub J, Rosenberg IH: Cystatin C as a determinant of fasting plasma total homocysteine levels in coronary artery disease patients with normal serum creatinine. *Arterioscler Thromb Vasc Biol* 19:2241–2244, 1999.

Botallico B, Larsson I, Brodszki J, Hernandez-Andrade E, Casslen B, Marsal K, Hansson SR: Norepinephrine transporter (NET), serotonin transporter (SERT), vesicular monoamine transporter (VMAT2) and organic cation transporters (OCT1, 2 and EMT) in human placenta from preeclamptic and normotensive pregnancies. *Placenta* 25:518–529, 2004.

Botta RM: Congenital malformation in infants of 517 pregestational diabetic mothers. *Ann Ist Super Sanita* 33:307–311, 1997.

Botto LD, Khoury MJ, Mulinare J, Erickson JD: Periconceptional multivitamin use and the occurrence of conotruncal heart defects: results from a population-based, case-control study. *Pediatrics* 98:911–917, 1996.

Botto LD, Olney RS, Erickson JD: Vitamin supplements and the risk for congenital anomalies other than neural tube defects. *Am J Med Genet C Semin Med Genet* 125:12–21, 2004.

Boule NG, Haddad E, Kenny GP, Wells GA, Sigal RJ: Effects of exercise on glycemic control and body mass in type 2 diabetes mellitus: a meta-analysis of controlled clinical trials. *JAMA* 186:1218–1227, 2001.

Boule NG, Kenny GP, Haddad E, Wells GA, Sigal RJ: Meta-analysis of the effect of structured exercise training on cardiorespiratory fitness in type 2 diabetes mellitus. *Diabetologia* 46:1071–1081, 2003.

Boulet SL, Alexander GR, Salihu HM, Pass M-A: Macrosomic birth in the United States: determinants, outcomes, and proposed grades of risk. *Am J Obstet Gynecol* 188:1372–1378, 2003.

Boulton M, Gregor Z, McLeod D, Charteris D, Jarvis-Evans J, Moriarty P, Khaliq A, Foreman D, Allamby D, Bardsley B: Intravitreal growth factors in proliferative diabetic retinopathy: correlation with neovascular activity and glycemic management. *Br J Ophthalmol* 81:228–233, 1997.

Boulton AJ, Malik RA, Arrezo JC, Sosenko JM: Diabetic somatic neuropathies. ADA technical review. *Diabetes Care* 27:1458–1486, 2004.

Boulton AJM, Vinik AI, Arezzo JC, Bril V, Feldman EL, Freeman R, Malik RA, Maser RE, Sosenko JM, Ziegler D: Diabetic neuropathies. A statement by the American Diabetes Association. *Diabetes Care* 28:956–962, 2005.

Bove A, Hebreo J, Wylie-Rosett, Isasi CR: Burger King and Subway: key nutrients, glycemic index, and glycemic load of nutritionally promoted items. *Diabetes Educ* 32:675–690, 2006.

Bradley RJ, Brudenell JM, Nicolaides KH: Fetal acidosis and hyperlacticemia diagnosed by cordocentesis in pregnancies complicated by diabetes mellitus. *Diabet Med* 8:464–468, 1991.

Bradley J, Leibold EA, Harris ZL, Wobken JD, Clarke S, Zumbrennen KB, Eisenstein RS, Georgieff MK: Influence of gestational age and fetal iron status on IRP activity and iron transporter protein expression in third-trimester human placenta. *Am J Physiol* 287:R894–R901, 2004.

Brand-Miller J, Hayne S, Petocz P, Colagiuri S: Low-glycemic index diets in the management of diabetes. A meta-analysis of randomized controlled trials. *Diabetes Care* 26:2261–2267, 2003a.

Brand-Miller JC, Thomas M, Swan V, Ahmad ZI, Petocz P, Colagiuri S: Physiological validation of the concept of glycemic load in lean young adults. *J Nutr* 133:2728–2732, 2003b.

Branski D, Fasano A, Troncone R: Latest developments in the pathogenesis and treatment of celiac disease. *J Pediatr* 149:295–300, 2006.

Brar P, Lee AR, Lewis SK, Bjagat G, Green PH: Celiac disease in African-Americans. *Dig Dis Sci* 51:1012–1015, 2005.

Bray GA, Vollmer WM, Sacks FM, Obarzanek E, Svetkey LP, Appel LJ; DASH Collaborative Research Group: A further subgroup analysis of the effects of the DASH diet and three dietary sodium levels on blood pressure: results of the DASH-Sodium trial. *Am J Cardiol* 94:222–227, 2004.

Brennan ML, Wu W, Fu X, Shen Z, Song W, Frost H, Vadseth C, Narine V, Lenkiewicz E, Borchers MT, Lusis AJ, Lee JJ, Lee NA, Abu-Sond HM, Ischiropoulos H, Hazen SL: A tale of two controversies: i) Defining the role of peroxidases in nitrotyrosine formation in vivo using eosinophil peroxidase and myeloperoxidase deficient mice; and ii) defining the nature of peroxidase-generated reactive nitrogen species. *J Biol Chem* 277:17415–17427, 2002.

Breuer W, Herschko C, Cabantchik ZI: The importance of non-transferrin-bound iron in disorders of iron metabolism. *Transfus Sci* 23:185–192, 2000.

Briefel RR, Johnson CL: Secular trends in dietary intake in the United States. *Annu Rev Nutr* 24:401–431, 2004.

Brillon DJ, Sison CP, Salbe AD, Poretsky L: Reproducibility of a glycemic response to mixed meals in type 2 diabetes mellitus. *Horm Metab Res* 38:536–542, 2006.

Britt RP, Harper C, Spray GH: Megaloblastic amaemia among Indians in Britain. *Q J Med* 40:499–520, 1971.

Bronson SK, Reiter CEN, Gardner TW: An eye on insulin. Commentary. *J Clin Invest* 111:1817–1819, 2003.

Brooks GA, Mercier J: Balance of carbohydrate and lipid utilization during exercise: the "crossover" concept. *J Appl Physiol* 76:2253–2261, 1994.

Brouwer A, Longnecker MP, Birnbaum LS, Cogliano J, Kostvniak P, Moore J, Schantz S, Winneke G: Characterization of potential endocrine-related health effects at low-dose levels of exposure to PCBs. *Environ Health Perspect* 107 (Suppl 4):639–649, 1999.

Brown FM, Hare JW: *Diabetes Complicating Pregnancy: The Joslin Clinic Method.* 2nd ed. Wilmington, DE: Wiley-Liss; 1995.

Brown CJ, Dawson A, Dodds R, Gamsu H, Gillmer M, Hall M, Hounsome B, Knopfler A, Ostler J, Peacock I, Rothman D, Steel J: Report of the pregnancy and neonatal care group. British Diabetic Association. *Diabet Med* 13:S43–S53, 1996.

Brown JE, Murtaugh MA, Jacobs DR Jr, Margellos HC: Variation in newborn size according to pregnancy weight change by trimester. *Am J Clin Nutr* 76:205–209, 2002.

Brown FM, Wyckoff J, Rowan JA, Jovanovic L, Sacks DA, Briggs GG: Metformin in pregnancy. Its time has not yet come. *Diabetes Care* 29:485–486, 2006.

Browning JD, Horton JD: Molecular mediators of hepatic steatosis and liver injury. *J Clin Invest* 114:147–152, 2004.

Brownlee M: Biochemistry and molecular cell biology of diabetic complications. *Nature* 414:813–820, 2001.

Brunelle BL, Llewelyn J, Anderson JH Jr, Gale EAM, Koivisto VA: Meta-analysis of the effect of insulin lispro on severe hypoglycemia in patients with type 1 diabetes. *Diabetes Care* 21:1726–1731, 1998.

Brunner E: Oily fish and omega 3 fat supplements. Health recommendations conflict with concerns about dwindling supply. *BMJ* 332:739–740, 2006.

Brunt EM: Nonalcoholic steatohepatitis. *Semin Liver Dis* 24:3–20, 2004.

Bryden KS, Neil A, Mayou RA, Peveler RC, Fairburn CG, Dunger DB: Eating habits, body weight, and insulin misuse. A longitudinal study of teenagers and young adults with type 1 diabetes. *Diabetes Care* 22:1956–1960, 1999.

Bryden KS, Dunger DB, Mayou RA, Peveler RC, Neil HAW: Poor prognosis of young adults with type 1 diabetes. A longitudinal study. *Diabetes Care* 26: 1052–1057, 2003.

Brydon P, Smith T, Proffitt M, Gee H, Holder R, Dunne F: Pregnancy outcome in women with type 2 diabetes mellitus needs to be addressed. *Int J Clin Pract* 54:418–419, 2000.

Buchanan TA, Metzger BE, Freinkel N: Accelerated starvation in late pregnancy: a comparison between obese women with and without gestational diabetes. *Am J Obstet Gynecol* 162:1015–1020, 1990a.

Buchanan TZ, Metzger BE, Freinkel N, Bergman RN: Insulin sensitivity and β-cell responsiveness to glucose during late pregnancy in lean and moderately obese women with normal glucose tolerance or mild gestational diabetes. *Am J Obstet Gynecol* 162:1008–1014, 1990b.

Buchbinder A, Miodovnik M, McElvy S, Rosenn B, Kranias G, Khoury J, Siddiqi TA. Is insulin lispro associated with the development or progression of diabetic retinopathy during pregnancy? *Am J Obstet Gynecol* 183:162–165, 2000.

Bucher HC, Guyatt GH, Cook RJ, Hatala R, Cook DJ, Lang JD, Hunt D: Effect of calcium supplementation on pregnancy-induced hypertension and preeclampsia: a meta-analysis of randomized controlled trials. *JAMA* 275: 1113–1117, 1996.

Buckingham RE: Thiazolidinediones: pleiotropic drugs with potent anti-inflammatory properties for tissue protection. *Hepatol Res* 33:167–170, 2005.

Bugianesi E, Gentilcore E, Manini R, Natale S, Vanni E, Villanova N, David E, Rizzetto M, Marchesini G: A randomized controlled trial of metformin versus vitamin E or prescriptive diet in nonalcoholic fatty liver disease. *Am J Gastroenterol* 100:1082–1090, 2005.

Buhling KJ, Henrich W, Kjos SL, Siebert G, Starr E, Dreweck C, Stein U, Dudenhausen JW: Comparison of point-of-care-testing glucose meters with standard laboratory measurement of the 50 g-glucose-challenge test (GCT) during pregnancy. *Clin Biochem* 36:333–337, 2003.

Buhling KJ, Kurzidim B, Wolf C, Wohlfarth K, Mahmoudi M, Wascher C, Siebert G, Dudenhausen JW: Introductory experience with the Continuous Glucose Monitoring System (CGMS; Medtronic Minimed) in detecting hyperglycemia by comparing the self-monitoring of blood glucose (SMBG) in non-pregnant women and in pregnant women with impaired glucose tolerance and gestational diabetes. *Exp Clin Endocrinol Diabetes* 112:556–560, 2004.

Buhling KJ, Winkel T, Wolf C, Kurzidim B, Mahmoudi M, Wohlfarth K, Wascher C, Schink T, Dudenhausen JW: Optimal timing for postprandial glucose measurement in pregnant women with diabetes and a non-diabetic pregnant population evaluated by the Continuous Glucose Monitoring System (CGMS). *J Perinat Med* 33:125–131, 2005.

Bulik CM, Sullivan PF, Fear JL, Pickering A, Dawn A, McCullin M: Fertility and reproduction in women with anorexia nervosa: a controlled study. *J Clin Psychiatry* 60:130–135, 1999.

BupReg—Buproprion Registry: Buproprion (amfebutamone): caution during pregnancy. *Prescrire Int* 14:225, 2005.

Burani J, Longo PJ: Low-glycemic index carbohydrates: an effective behavioral change for glycemic control and weight management in patients with type 1 and 2 diabetes. *Diabetes Educ* 32:78–88, 2006.

Burgos R, Mateo C, Canton A, Hernandez C, Mesa J, Simo R: Vitreous levels of IGF-I, IGF binding protein 1, and IGF binding protein 3 in proliferative diabetic retinopathy. A case-control study. *Diabetes Care* 23:80–83, 2000.

Burkart W, Hanker JP, Schneider HP: Complications and fetal outcome in diabetic pregnancy: intensified conventional versus insulin pump therapy. *Gynecol Obstet Invest* 26:104–112, 1988.

Burman P, Mardh S, Norberg L, Karlsson FA: Parietal cell antibodies in pernicious anemia inhibit H+/K+ adenosine triphosphatase, the proton pump of the stomach. *Gastroenterology* 96:1434–1438, 1989.

Burt RL, Davidson IWF: Insulin half-life and utilization in normal pregnancy. *Obstet Gynecol* 43:161–170, 1974.

Burt VK, Stein K: Epidemiology of depression throughout the female life cycle. *J Clin Psychiatry* 63:9–15, 2002.

Butler JA, Whanger PD, Tripp MJ: Blood selenium and glutathione peroxidase activity in pregnant women. Comparative assays in primates and other animals. *Am J Clin Nutr* 36:15–23, 1982.

Butler CC, Vidal-Alaball J, Cannings-John R, McCaddon A, Hood K, Papaioannou A, McDowell I, Goringe A: Oral vitamin B_{12} versus intramuscular vitamin B_{12} for vitamin B_{12} deficiency: a systematic review of randomized controlled trials. *Fam Pract* 23:279–285, 2006a.

Butler WJ, Houseman J, Seddon L, McMullen E, Tofflemire K, Mills C, Corriveau A, Weber JP, LeBlanc A, Walker M, Donaldson SG, Van Oostdam J: Maternal and umbilical cord blood levels of mercury, lead, cadmium, and essential trace elements in Arctic Canada. *Environ Res* 100:295–318, 2006b.

Butte NF, Hopkinson JM, Mehta N, Moon JK, Smith EO: Adjustments in energy expenditure and substrate utilization during late pregnancy and lactation. *Am J Clin Nutr* 69:299–307, 1999.

Butte NF: Carbohydrate and lipid metabolism in pregnancy: normal compared with gestational diabetes mellitus. *Am J Clin Nutr* 71 (Suppl):1256S–1261S, 2000.

Butte NF, Ellis KJ, Wong WW, Hopkinson JM, O'Brian Smith E: Composition of gestational weight gain impacts maternal fat retention and infant birth weight. *Am J Obstet Gynecol* 189:1423–1432, 2003.

Butte NF, Wong WW, Treuth MS, Ellis KJ, O'Brian Smith E: Energy requirements during pregnancy based on total energy expenditure and energy deposition. *Am J Clin Nutr* 79:1078–1087, 2004.

Butterworth JR, Iqbal TH, Cooper BT: Celiac disease in South Asians resident in Britain: comparison with white Caucasian celiac patients. *Eur J Gastroenterol Hepatol* 17:541–545, 2005.

Buyken AE, Toeller M, Heitkamp G, Irsigler K, Holler C, Santeusanio F, Stehle P, Fuller JH; EURODIAB Complications Study Group: Carbohydrate sources and glycemic control in type 1 diabetes mellitus. *Diabet Med* 17:351–359, 2000.

Caldwell SH, Crespo DM: The spectrum expanded: cryptogenic cirrhosis and the natural history of non-alcoholic fatty liver disease. *J Hepatol* 40:578–584, 2004.

Caluwaerts S, Holemans K, van Bree R, Verhaeghe J, van Assche FA: Is low-dose streptozotocin in rats an adequate model for gestational diabetes mellitus? *J Soc Gynecol Investig* 10:216–221, 2003.

Camejo G. Halberg C, Manschik-Lundin A, Hurt-Camejo E, Rosengren B, Olsson H, Hansson GI, Forsberg GB, Yilhen B: Hemin binding and oxidation of lipoproteins in serum: mechanisms and effect on the interaction of LDL with human macrophages. *J Lipid Res Apr* 39:755–766, 1998.

Caminos JE, Nogueiras R, Gallego R, Bravo S, Tovar S, Garcia-Caballero T, Casnueva FF, Dieguez C: Expression and regulation of adiponectin and receptor in human and rat placenta. *J Clin Endocrinol Metab* 90:4276–4286, 2005.

Campbell FM, Gordon MJ, Dutta-Roy AK: Preferential uptake of long chain polyunsaturated fatty acids by isolated human placental membranes. *Moll Cell Biochem* 155:77–83, 1996a.

Campbell DM, Hall MH, Barker DJ, Cross J, Shiell AW, Godfrey KM: Diet in pregnancy and the offspring's blood pressure 40 years later. *Br J Obstet Gynecol* 103:273–280, 1996b.

Can B, Ulusu NN, Kiline K, Levia Acan N, Saran Y, Turan B: Selenium treatment protects diabetes-induced biochemical and ultrastructural alterations in liver tissue. *Biol Trace Elem Res* 105:135–150, 2005.

Cantorna MT, Zhu Y, Froicu M, Wittke A: Vitamin D status, 1,25-dihydroxyvitamin D_3, and the immune system. *Am J Clin Nutr* 80 (Suppl):1717S–1720S, 2004.

Cao X-Y, Jiang X-M, Dou Z-H, Rakeman MA, Zhang M-L, O'Donnell K, Tai M, Amette K, DeLong N, DeLong R: Time of vulnerability of the brain to iodine deficiency in endemic cretinism. *N Engl J Med* 331:1739–1744, 1994.

Capel I, Corcoy R: What dose of folic acid should be used for pregnant diabetic women? *Diabetes Care* 30:e63, 2007.

Carbone ET, Rosal MC, Torres MI, Goins KV, Bermudez OI: Diabetes self-management: perspectives of Latino patients and their health care providers. *Patient Educ Couns* 66:202–210, 2007.

Carlsen SM, Jacobsen G, Vatten L, Romundstad P: In pregnant women who smoke, caffeine consumption is associated with an increased level of homocysteine. *Acta Obstet Gynecol Scand* 84:1049–1054, 2005.

Carlson SE, Clandinin MT, Cook HW, Emken EA, Filer LJ Jr: *trans* Fatty acids: infant and fetal development. Report of the Expert Panel. *Am J Clin Nutr* 66:17S–36S, 1997.

Carlsson AK, Axelsson IE, Borulf SK, Bredberg AC, Lindberg BA, Sjoberg KG, Ivarsson SA: Prevalence of IgA-antiendomysium and IgA-antigliadin autoantibodies at diagnosis of insulin-dependent diabetes mellitus in Swedish children and adolescents. *Pediatrics* 103:1248–1252, 1999.

Carmel R, Johnson CS: Racial patterns in pernicious anemia: early age at onset and increased frequency of intrinsic-factor antibody in black women. *N Engl J Med* 298:647–650, 1978.

Carmel R, Johnson CS, Weiner JM: Pernicious anemia in Latin America is not a disease of the elderly. *Arch Intern Med* 147:1995–1996, 1987.

Carmel R: Reassessment of the relative prevalences of antibodies to gastric parietal cell and to intrinsic factor in patients with pernicious anemia: influence of patient age and race. *Clin Exp Immunol* 89:74–77, 1992.

Carmel R: Ethnic and racial factors in cobalamin metabolism and its disorders. *Semin Hematol* 36:88–100, 1999.

Carmel R, Mallidi PV, Vinarskiy S, Brar S, Frouhar Z: Hyperhomocysteinemia and cobalamin deficiency in young Asian Indians in the United States. *Am J Hematol* 70:107–114, 2002.

Carmichael SL, Abrams B: A critical review of the relationship between gestational weight gain and preterm delivery. *Obstet Gynecol* 89:865–873, 1997.

Carpenter MW: Exercise in normal and diabetic pregnancies. In: Reece EA, Coustan DR, Gabbe SG, eds *Diabetes in Women. Adolescence, Pregnancy, and Menopause.* Philadelphia: Lippincott Williams & Wilkins; 2003:283–298.

Carr KJE, Idama TO, Masson EA, Ellis K, Lindow SW: A randomized controlled trial of insulin lispro given before or after meals in pregnant women with type 1 diabetes—the effect on glycemic excursion. *J Obstet Gynecol* 24:382–386, 2004.

Carr KJ, Lindow SW, Masson EA: The potential for the use of insulin lispro in pregnancy complicated by diabetes. *J Matern Fetal Neonatal Med* 19:323–329, 2006.

Carroll MF, Izard A, Riboni K, Burge MR, Schade DS: Control of postprandial hyperglycemia: optimal use of short-acting insulin secretagogues. *Diabetes Care* 25:2147–2152, 2002.

Carrone D, Loverro G, Greco P, Capuano F, Selvaggi L: Lipid peroxidation products and antioxidant enzymes during normal and diabetic pregnancy. *Eur J Obstet Gynecol Reprod Biol* 51:103–109, 1993.

Carta Q, Meriggi E, Trossarelli GF, Catella G, Dal Molin V, Menato G, Gagliardi L, Massobrio M, Vitelli A: Continuous subcutaneous insulin infusion versus intensive conventional insulin therapy in type 1 and type 2 diabetic pregnancy. *Diabetes Metab* 12:121–129, 1986.

Caruso A, Lanzone V, Biancji M, Massidda M, Castelli MP, Fulghesu AM, Mancuso S: Continuous subcutaneous insulin infusion (CSII) in pregnant diabetic patients. *Prenat Diagn* 7:41–50, 1987.

Carver TD, Anderson SM, Aldoretto PW, Hay WW: Effect of low-level basal plus marked 'pulsatile' hyperglycemia on insulin secretion in fetal sheep. *Am J Physiol* 271:E865–E871, 1996.

Casanueva E, Viteri FE: Iron and oxidative stress in pregnancy. *J Nutr* 133: 1700S–1708S, 2003.

Casanueva E, Ripoll C, Tolentino M, Morales RM, Pfeffer F, Vilchis P, Vadillo-Ortega F: Vitamin C supplementation to prevent premature rupture of the chorioamniotic membranes: a randomized trial. *Am J Clin Nutr* 81:859–863, 2005.

Casper RC, Fleisher BE, Lee-Ancajas JC, Gilles A, Gaylor E, DeBattista A, Hoyme HE: Follow-up of children of depressed mothers exposed or nor exposed to antidepressant drugs during pregnancy. *J Pediatr* 142:402–408, 2003.

Casson IF, Clarke CA, Howard CV, McKendrick O, Pennycook S, Pharoah POD, Platt MJ, Stanisstreet M, van Velszen D, Walkinshaw S: Outcomes of pregnancy in insulin dependent diabetic women: results of a five year population cohort study. *BMJ* 315:275–278, 1997.

Casson IF: Pregnancy in women with diabetes—after the CEMACH report, what now? *Diabet Med* 23:481–484, 2006.

Castro MA, Fassett MJ, Reynolds TB, Shaw KJ, Goodwin TM: Reversible peripartum liver failure: a new perspective on the diagnosis, treatment, and cause of acute fatty liver of pregnancy, based on 28 consecutive cases. *Am J Obstet Gynecol* 181:389–395, 1999.

Catalano PM, Tyzibir ED, Roman NM, Amini SB, Sims EAH: Longitudinal changes in insulin resistance in non-obese pregnant women. *Am J Obstet Gynecol* 165:1667–1672, 1991.

Catalano PM, Hollenbeck C: Energy requirements in pregnancy: a review. *Obstet Gynecol Surv* 47:368–372, 1992a.

Catalano PM, Tyzbir ED, Wolfe RR, Roman NM, Amini SB, Sims EAH: Longitudinal changes in basal hepatic glucose production and suppression during insulin infusion in normal pregnant women. *Am J Obstet Gynecol* 167:913–919, 1992b.

Catalano PM, Tyzbir ED, Wolfe RR, Calles J, Roman NM, Amini SB, Sims EAH: Carbohydrate metabolism during pregnancy in control subjects and women with gestational diabetes. *Am J Physiol* 264:E60–E67, 1993.

Catalano PM, Drago NM, Amini SB: Factors affecting fetal growth and body composition. *Am J Obstet Gynecol* 172:1459–1463, 1995a.

Catalano PM, Drago NM, Amini SB: Maternal carbohydrate metabolism and its relationship to fetal growth and body composition. *Am J Obstet Gynecol* 172:1464–1470, 1995b.

Catalano PM, Roman-Drago NM, Amini SB, Sims EAH: Longitudinal changes in body composition and energy balance in lean women with normal and abnormal glucose tolerance during pregnancy. *Am J Obstet Gynecol* 179:156–165, 1998a.

Catalano PM, Drago NM, Amini SB: Longitudinal changes in pancreatic β-cell function and metabolic clearance rate of insulin in pregnant women with normal and abnormal glucose tolerance. *Diabetes Care* 21:403–408, 1998b.

Catalano PM, Huston L, Amini SB, Kalhan SC: Longitudinal changes in glucose metabolism during pregnancy in obese women with normal glucose tolerance and gestational diabetes. *Am J Obstet Gynecol* 180:903–916, 1999.

Catalano PM, Nizielski SE, Shao J, Preston L, Qiao L, Friedman JE: Downregulated IRS-1 and PPARγ in obese women with gestational diabetes: relationship to FFA during pregnancy. *Am J Physiol* 282:E522–E533, 2002.

Catalano PM, Thomas A, Huston-Presley L, Amin SB: Increased fetal adiposity: a very sensitive marker of abnormal in utero development. *Am J Obstet Gynecol* 189:1698–1704, 2003.

Catalano PM, Huston-Presley L, Haugel-DeMouzon S: Placental size at term: a function of early pregnancy insulin response? *Diabetes* 55:A40, 2006a.

Catalano PM, Hoegh M, Minium J, Huston-Presley L, Bernard S, Kalhan S, Haugel-De Mouzon S: Adiponectin in human pregnancy: implications for regulation of glucose and lipid metabolism. *Diabetologia* 49:1677–1685, 2006b.

Catalano PM, Huston-Presley L, Kalhan S: Decreases in maternal lipid sensitivity in late pregnancy are related to fetal adiposity. *Diabetes* 55 (Suppl 1):A40, 2006c.

Cauzac M, Czuba D, Girard J, Haugel-de Mouzon S: Transduction of leptin growth signals in placental cells is independent of JAK-STAT activation. *Placenta* 24:378–384, 2003.

CCC—Calorie Control Council: Aspartame archives. 2004. Available at: www .aspartame.org/aspartame_archive.html. Accessed Mar 13, 2008.

CDAPP—California Diabetes and Pregnancy Program, Department of Health: Data report for deliveries between January 1, 2002, and December 31, 2002, and between January 1, 2003, and Dec 31, 2003. Sacramento, State of California; 2004.

CDC—Centers for Disease Control and Prevention: CDC. Criteria for anemia in children and childbearing-aged women. *MMWR Morb Mortal Wkly Rep* 38: 400–404, 1989.

CDC—Centers for Disease Control and Prevention, U.S. Department of Public Health: Recommendations for the use of folic acid to reduce the number of cases of spina bifida and other neural tube defects. *MMWR Morb Mortal Wkly Rep* 41:1–7, 1992.

CDC—Centers for Disease Control: Recommendations to prevent and control iron deficiency in the United States. *MMWR Morb Mortal Wkly Rep* 47:1–36, 1998a.

CDC—Centers for Disease Control and Prevention, U.S. Department of Public Health: Use of folic acid-containing supplements among women of childbearing age—United States, 1997. *MMWR Morb Mortal Wkly Rep* 47:131–134, 1998b.

Cedergren M: Effects of gestational weight gain and body mass index on obstetric outcome in Sweden. *Int J Gynecol Obstet* 93:269–274, 2006.

Ceglia L, Lau J, Pittas AG: Meta-analysis: efficacy and safety of inhaled insulin therapy in adults with diabetes mellitus. *Ann Intern Med* 145:665–675, 2006.

CEMACH—Confidential Enquiry into Maternal and Child Health: *Pregnancy in Women with Type 1 and Type 2 Diabetes in 2002–2003, England, Wales and Northern Ireland.* London: CEMACH; 2005.

Cenac A, Simonoff M, Moretto P, Djibo A: A low plasma selenium is a risk factor for peripartum cardiomyopathy. A comparative study in Sahelian Africa. *Int J Cardiol* 36:57–59, 1992.

Cerf-Bensussan N, Cellier C, Heyman M, Brousse N, Schmitz J: Celiac disease: an update on facts and questions based on the 10th International Symposium on Celiac Disease. *J Pediatr Gastroenterol Nutr* 37:412–421, 2003.

Ceriello A, Bortolotti N, Motz E, Crescentini A, Lizzio S, Russo A, Tonutti L, Taboga C: Meal-generated oxidative stress in type 2 diabetic patients. *Diabetes Care* 21:1529–1533, 1998.

Ceriello A: New insights on oxidative stress and diabetic complications may lead to a 'causal' antioxidant therapy. *Diabetes Care* 26:1589–1596, 2003.

Ceriello A: Controlling oxidative stress as a novel molecular approach to protecting the vascular wall in diabetes. *Curr Opin Lipidol* 17:510–518, 2006.

Cernichiari E, Brewer R, Myers GJ, Marsh DO, Lapham LW, Cox C, Shamlave CF, Berlin M, Davidson PW, Clarkson TW: Monitoring methylmercury during pregnancy: maternal hair predicts fetal brain exposure. *Neurotoxicology* 16: 705–710, 1995.

Cerutti F, Bruno G, Chiarelli F, Lorini R, Meschi F, Sacchetti C; Diabetes Study Group of the Italian Society of Pediatric Endocrinology and Diabetology: Younger age at onset and sex predict celiac disease in children and adolescents with type 1 diabetes. An Italian multicenter study. *Diabetes Care* 27:1294–1298, 2004.

Ceysens G, Rouiller D, Boulvain M: Exercise for diabetic pregnant women. *Cochrane Database Syst Rev* 2006;(3):CD004225.

Chadda V, Simchen MJ, Hornberger LK, Allen VM, Fallah S, Coates AL, Roberts A, Wilkes DL, Schneiderman-Walker J, Jaeggi E, Kingdom JCP: Fetal response to maternal exercise in pregnancies with uteroplacental insufficiency. *Am J Obstet Gynecol* 193:995–999, 2005.

Challier JC, Haugel S, Desmaizieres V: Effects of insulin on glucose uptake and metabolism in the human placenta. *J Clin Endocrinol Metab* 62:803–807, 1986.

Chambers CD, Johnson KA, Dick LN, Felix RJ, Jones KL: Birth outcomes in pregnant women taking fluoxetine. *N Engl J Med* 335:1010–1015, 1996.

Chambers CD, Hernandez-Diaz S, Van Marter LJ, Werler MM, Louik C, Jones KL, Mitchell AA: Selective serotonin-reuptake inhibitors and risk of persistent pulmonary hypertension of the newborn. *N Engl J Med* 354:579–587, 2006.

Champoux M, Hibbeln JR, Shannon C, Majchrzak S, Suomi S, Salem N Jr, Higley JD: Fatty acid formula supplementation and neuromotor development in Rhesus monkey neonates. *Pediatr Res* 51:273–281, 2002.

Chan HM, Brand-Miller JC, Holt SH, Wilson D, Rozman M, Petocz P: The glycaemic index values of Vietnamese foods. *Eur J Clin Nutr* 55:1076–1083, 2001.

Chan EM, Cheng WM, Tiu SC, Wong LL: Postprandial glucose response to Chinese foods in patients with type 2 diabetes. *J Am Diet Assoc* 104:1854–1858, 2004a.

Chan DF, Li AM, Chu WC, Chan MH, Wong EM, Liu EK, Chan IH, Yin J, Lam CW, Fok TF, Nelson EA: Hepatic steatosis in obese Chinese children. *Int J Obes Relat Metab Disord* 28:1257–1263, 2004b.

Chand N, Mihas AA: Celiac disease: current concepts in diagnosis and treatment. *J Clin Gastroenterol* 40:3–14, 2006.

Chandalia M, Garg A, Lutjohann D, von Bergmann K, Grundy SM, Brinkley LJ: Beneficial effects of high dietary fiber intake in patients with type 2 diabetes. *N Engl J Med* 342:1392 1398, 2000.

Chang TI, Horal M, Jain SK, Wang F, Patel R, Loeken MR: Oxidant regulation of gene expression and neural tube development: insights gained from diabetic pregnancy on molecular causes of neural tube defects. *Diabetologia* 46:538–545, 2003.

Chantelau E, Kohner EM: Why some cases of retinopathy worsen when diabetic control improves. *BMJ* 315:1105–1106, 1997.

Chantelau E: Evidence that upregulation of serum IGF-1 concentration can trigger acceleration of diabetic retinopathy. *Br J Opthalmol* 82:719–721, 1998.

Chao L, Marcus-Samuels B, Mason MM, Moitra J, Vinson C, Arioglu E, Gavrilova O, Reitman ML: Adipose tissue is required for the antidiabetic, but not for the hypolipidemic, effect of thiazolidinediones. *J Clin Invest* 106:1221–1228, 2000.

Chappell LC, Seed PY, Briley AL, Kelly FJ, Lee R, Hunt BJ, Parmar K, Bewley SJ, Shennan AH, Steer PJ, Poston L: Effect of antioxidants on the occurrence of pre-eclampsia in women at increased risk: a randomized trial. *Lancet* 354:810–816, 1999.

Chappell LC, Seed PT, Kelly FJ, Briley A, Hunt BJ, Charnock-Jones DS, Mallet A, Poston L: Vitamin C and E supplementation in women at risk of preeclampsia is associated with changes in indices of oxidative stress and placental function. *Am J Obstet Gynecol* 187:777–784, 2002.

Charles B, Norris R, Xiao X, Hague W: Population pharmacokinetics of metformin in late pregnancy. *Ther Drug Monit* 28:67–72, 2006.

Chasan-Taber L, Evenson KR, Sternfeld B, Kengeri S: Assessment of recreational physical activity during pregnancy in epidemiologic studies of birthweight and length of gestation: methodologic aspects. *Womens' Health* 45:85–107, 2007.

Chatterjee S, Gallen JW, Sandler L: Two-year prospective audit of the effect of the introduction of insulin lispro in patients with specific clinical indications. *Diabetes Care* 22:1226–1227, 1999.

Chaudhry T, Ghani AM, Mehrali TH, Taylor RS, Brudon PA, Gee H, Barnett AH, Dunne FP: A comparison of fetal and labor outcomes in Caucasian and Afro-Caribbean women with diabetes in pregnancy. *Int J Clin Pract* 58:932–936, 2004.

Chauhan SP, Perry KG Jr: Management of diabetic ketoacidosis in the obstetric patient. *Obstet Gynecol Clin North Am* 22:143–155, 1995.

Chen P, Poddar R, Tipa EV, Dibello PM, Moravec CD, Robinson K, Green R, Kruger WD, Garrow TA, Jacobsen DW: Homocysteine metabolism in cardiovascular cells and tissues: implications for hyperhomocysteinemia and cardiovascular disease. *Adv Enzyme Regul* 39:93–109, 1999.

Chen X, Scholl TO, Leskiw MJ, Donaldson MR, Stein TP: Association of glutathione peroxidase activity with insulin resistance and dietary fat intake during normal pregnancy. *J Clin Endocrinol Metab* 88:5963–5968, 2003.

Chen J, Tan B, Karteris E, Zervou S, Digby J, Hillhouse EW, Vatish M, Randeva HS: Secretion of adiponectin by human placenta: a differential modulation of adiponectin and its receptors by cytokines. *Diabetologia* 49:1292–1302, 2006.

Chen R, Ben-Haroush A, Weissman-Brenner A, Melamed N, Hod M, Yogev Y: Level of glycemic control and pregnancy outcome in type 1 diabetes: a comparison between multiple daily insulin injections and continuous subcutaneous insulin infusions. *Am J Obstet Gynecol* 197:404.e.1–404.e.5, 2007.

Cheng Y, Chung J, Block-Kurbisch I, Inturrisi M, Caughey A: Treatment of gestational diabetes mellitus: oral hypoglycemic agents compared to subcutaneous insulin therapy. *Am J Obstet Gynecol* 195 (Suppl):S36, 2006.

Cherrington A, Ayala GX, Sleath B, Corbie-Smith G: Examining knowledge, attitudes, and beliefs about depression among Latino adults with type 2 diabetes. *Diabetes Educ* 32:603–613, 2006.

Cheung NW, McElduff A, Ross GP: Type 2 diabetes in pregnancy: a wolf in sheep's clothing. *Aust N Z J Obstet Gynecol* 45:479–483, 2005.

Chew EY, Mills JL, Metzger BE, Remaley NA, Jovanovic-Peterson L, Knopp RH, Conley M, Rand L, Simpson JL, Holmes LB, Aarons JH; NICHHD: Metabolic control and progression of retinopathy. The Diabetes in Early Pregnancy Study. *Diabetes Care* 18:631–637, 1995.

Cheyne EH, Cavan DA, Kerr D: Performance of a Continuous Glucose Monitoring System during controlled hypoglycemia in healthy volunteers. *Diabetes Technol Therapeut* 4:607–613, 2002.

Cheyne EH, Sherwin RS, Lunt MJ, Cavan DA, Thomas PW, Kerr D: Influence of alcohol on cognitive performance during mild hypoglycemia: implications for type 1 diabetes. *Diabet Med* 21:230–237, 2004.

Chiang TI, Horal M, Jain SK, Wang F, Patel R, Loeken MR: Oxidant regulation of gene expression and neural tube development: insights gained from diabetic pregnancy on molecular causes of neural tube defects. *Diabetologia* 46:538–545, 2003.

Chin RL, Sander HW, Brannagan TH, Green PH, Hays AP, Alaedini A, Latov N: Celiac neuropathy. *Neurology* 60:1581–1585, 2003.

Chisalita SI, Arnqvist HJ: Insulin-like growth factor I receptors are more abundant than insulin receptors in human micro- and macrovascular endothelial cells. *Am J Physiol* 286:E896–E901, 2004.

Chiu CH, Lau FY, Wong R, Soo OY, Lam CK, Lee PW, Leung HK, So CK, Tsoi WC, Tang N, Lam WK, Cheng G: Vitamin B$_{12}$ deficiency—need for a new guideline. *Nutrition* 17:917–920, 2001.

Chiu KC, Chu A, Go VLW, Saad MF: Hypovitaminosis D is associated with insulin resistance and β cell dysfunction. *Am J Clin Nutr* 79:820–825, 2004.

Chmait R, Dinise T, Moore T: Prospective observational study to establish predictors of glyburide success in women with gestational diabetes mellitus. *J Perinatol* 24:617–622, 2004.

Chmielewski SA: Advances and strategies for glucose monitoring. *Am J Clin Pathol* 104 (Suppl 1):S59–S71, 1995.

Cho E, Zeisel SH, Jacques P, Selhub J, Dougherty L, Colditz GA, Willett WC: Dietary choline and betaine assessed by food-frequency questionnaire in relation to plasma total homocysteine concentration in the Framingham Offspring Study. *Am J Clin Nutr* 83:905–911, 2006.

Choi JW, Im MW, Pai SH: Serum transferrin receptor concentrations during normal pregnancy. *Clin Chem* 46:725–727, 2000.

Chong WS, Kwan PC, Chan LY, Chiu PY, Cheung TK, Lau TK: Expression of divalent metal transporter 1 (DMT1) isoforms in first trimester human placenta and embryonic tissues. *Hum Reprod* 20:3532–3538, 2005.

Choumenkovitch SF, Selhub J, Wilson PW, Rader JI, Rosenberg IH, Jacques PF: Folic acid intake from fortification in United States exceeds predictions. *J Nutr* 132:2792–2798, 2002.

Christen WG, Ajani UA, Glynn RJ, Hennekens CH: Blood levels of homocysteine and increased risks of cardiovascular disease. Causal or casual? *Arch Intern Med* 160:422–434, 2000.

Christesen HB, Melander A: Prolonged elimination of tolbutamide in a premature newborn with hyperinsulinemic hypoglycemia. *Eur J Endocrinol* 138:698–701, 1998.

Christian P, Khatry SK, Katz J, Pradhan EK, LeClerq SC, Shrestha SR, Adhikari RK, Sommer A, West PW Jr: Effects of alternative maternal micronutrient supplements on low birth weight in rural Nepal: double blind randomized community trial. *BMJ* 326:571–574, 2003.

Chugh SS, Wallner EI, Kanwar YS: Renal development in high-glucose ambience and diabetic embryopathy. *Semin Nephrol* 23:583–592, 2003.

Chun-Fai-Chan B, Koren G, Fayez I, Kalra S, Voyer-Lavigne S, Boshier A, Shakir S, Einarson A: Pregnancy outcome of women exposed to bupropion during pregnancy: a prospective comparative study. *Am J Obstet Gynecol* 192:932–936, 2005.

Ciacci C, Cirillo M, Auriemma G, Di Dato G, Sabbatini F, Mazzacca G: Celiac disease and pregnancy outcome. *Am J Gastroenterol* 91:718–722, 1996.

Ciacci C, Cirillo M, Giorgetti G, Alfinito F, Franchi A, Mazzetti di Pietralata M, Mazzacca G: Low plasma cholesterol: a correlate of nondiagnosed celiac disease in adults with hypochromic anemia. *Am J Gastroenterol* 94:1888–1891, 1999.

Ciacci C, Iovino P, Amoruso D, Siniscalchi M, Tortora R, Di Gilio A, Fusco M, Mazzacca G: Grown-up celiac children: the effects of only a few years on a gluten-free diet in childhood. *Aliment Pharmacol Ther* 15:421–429, 2005.

Ciaraldi TP, CarterL, Seipke G, Mudaliar S, Henry RR. Effects of the long-acting insulin glargine on cultured human skeletal muscle cells: comparisons to insulin and IGF-1. *J Clin Endocrinol Metab* 86:5838, 2001.

Ciaraldi TP, Phillips SA, Carter L, Aroda V, Mudaliar S, Henry RR: Effects of the rapid-acting insulin analog glulisine on cultured human skeletal muscle cells: comparisons with insulin and insulin-like growth factor I. *J Clin Endocrinol Metab* 90:5551–5558, 2005.

Ciechanowski PS, Katon WJ, Russo JE: Depression and diabetes: impact of depressive symptoms on adherence, function, and costs. *Arch Intern Med* 160:3278–3285, 2000.

Cikot RJ, Steegers-Theunissen RP, Thomas CM, de Boo TM, Merkus HM, Steegers EA: Longitudinal vitamin and homocysteine levels in normal pregnancy. *Br J Nutr* 85:49–58, 2001.

Clapp JFD: The changing thermal response to endurance exercise during pregnancy. *Am J Obstet Gynecol* 165:1684–1689, 1991.

Clapp JF III: Effect of dietary carbohydrate on the glucose and insulin response to mixed caloric intake and exercise in both nonpregnant and pregnant women. *Diabetes Care* 21:B107–B112, 1998.

Clark SL, Cotton DB, Pivarnik JM, Lee W, Hankins GD, Benedetti TJ, Phelan JP: Position change and central hemodynamic profile during normal third-trimester pregnancy and postpartum. *Am J Obstet Gynecol* 164:883–887, 1991 [erratum 165:241].

Clark CM Jr, Fradkin JE, Hiss RG, Lorenz RA, Vinicor F, Warren-Boulton E: The National Diabetes Education Program, changing the way diabetes is treated. Comprehensive diabetes care. *Diabetes Care* 24:617–618, 2001.

Clarke R, Frost C, Collins R, Appleby P, Peto R: Dietary lipids and blood cholesterol: quantitative meta-analysis of metabolic ward studies. *BMJ* 314:112–117, 1997.

Clarke R, Collins R, Lewington S, Donals A, Alfthan G, Tuomilehto J: Homocysteine and the risk of ischemic heart disease and stroke: a meta-analysis. *JAMA* 288:2015–2022, 2002.

Clausen TD, Mathiesen E, Ekbom P, Hellmuth E, Mandrup-Poulsen T, Damm P: Poor pregnancy outcome in women with type 2 diabetes. *Diabetes Care* 28: 323–328, 2005.

Cleasby ME, Dzamko N, Hegarty BD, Cooney GJ, Kraegen EW, Ye J-M: Metformin prevents the development of acute lipid-induced insulin resistance in the rat through altered hepatic signaling mechanisms. *Diabetes* 53:3258–3266, 2004.

Clegg A, Colquitt J, Sidhu M, Royle P, Walker A: Clinical and cost effectiveness of surgery for morbid obesity: a systematic review and economic evaluation. *Int J Obes Relat Metab Disord* 27:1167–1177, 2003.

Clement S: Diabetes self-management education. *Diabetes Care* 18:1204–1214, 1995.

Clemente MG, De Virgiliis S, Kang JS, Macatagney R, Musu MP, Di Pierro MR, Drago S, Congia M, Fasano A: Early effects of gliadin on enterocyte intracellular signaling involved in intestinal barrier function. *Gut* 52:218–223, 2003.

Cnattingius S, Berne C, Nordstrom M-L: Pregnancy outcome and infant mortality in diabetic patients in Sweden. *Diabet Med* 11:696–700, 1994.

Cnattingius S, Bergstrom R, Lipworth L, Kramer MS: Prepregnancy weight and the risk of adverse pregnancy outcomes. *N Engl J Med* 338:147–152, 1998.

Cnattingius S, Signorelo LB, Anneren G, Clausson B, Ekbom A, Ljunger E, Blot W, McLaughlun JK, Petersson G, Rane A, Granath F. Caffeine intake and the risk of first trimester spontaneous abortion. *N Engl J Med* 3343:1839–1845, 2000.

Cochrane E, Musso C, Gorden P: The use of U-500 in patients with extreme insulin resistance. *Diabetes Care* 28:1240–1241, 2005.

Coetzee EJ, Jackson WPU: Metformin in management of pregnant insulin-independent diabetics. *Diabetologia* 16:241–245, 1979.

Coetzee EJ, Jackson WP: Pregnancy in established non-insulin-dependent diabetics. *S Afr Med J* 58:795–802, 1980.

Coetzee EJ, Jackson WPU: Oral hypoglycemics in the first trimester and fetal outcome. *S Afr Med J* 66:635–637, 1984.

Cogswell ME, Serdula MK, Hungerford DW, Yip R: Gestational weight gain among average-weight and overweight women. What is excessive? *Am J Obstet Gynecol* 172:705–712, 1995.

Cogswell ME, Kettel-Khan L, Ramakrishnan U: Iron supplement use among women in the United States: science, policy and practice. *J Nutr* 133:1974S–1977S, 2003a.

Cogswell ME, Parvanta I, Ickes L, Yip R, Brittenham GM: Iron supplementation during pregnancy, anemia, and birth weight: a randomized controlled trial. *Am J Clin Nutr* 78:773–781, 2003b.

Cohen LS, Altshuler LL, Harlow BL, Nonacs R, Newport DJ, Viguera AC, Suri R, Burt VK, Hendrick V, Reminick AM, Loughead A, Vitonis AF, Stowe ZN: Relapse of major depression during pregnancy in women who maintain or discontinue antidepressant treatment. *JAMA* 295:499–507, 2006.

Colagiuri S, Miller JJ, Holliday JL, Phelan E: Comparison of plasma glucose, serum insulin, and C-peptide responses to three isocaloric breakfasts in non-insulin-dependent diabetic subjects. *Diabetes Care* 9:250–254, 1986.

Cole JA, Modell JG, Haight BR, Cosmatos IS, Stoler JM, Walker AM: Buproprion in pregnancy and the prevalence of congenital malformations. *Pharmacoepidemiol Drug Saf* 16:474–484, 2007.

Collier G, O'Dea K: Effect of physical form of carbohydrate on the postprandial glucose, insulin, and gastric inhibitory polypeptide responses in type 2 diabetes. *Am J Clin Nutr* 36:10–14, 1982.

Collier G, O'Dea K: The effect of coingestion of fat on the glucose, insulin, and gastric inhibitory polypeptide responses to carbohydrate and protein. *Am J Clin Nutr* 37:941–944, 1983.

Collier G, McLean A, O'Dea K: Effect of co-ingestion of fat on the metabolic responses to slowly and rapidly absorbed carbohydrates. *Diabetologia* 26:50–54, 1984.

Collier GR, Wolever TM, Wong GS, Josse RG: Prediction of glycemic response to mixed meals in noninsulin-dependent diabetic subjects. *Am J Clin Nutr* 44:349–352, 1986.

Collin P, Salmi J, Halstrom O, Oksa H, Oksala H, Maki M: High frequency of celiac disease in adult patients with type 1 diabetes. *Scand J Gastroenterol* 24:81–84, 1989.

Collin P, Kaukinen K, Valimaki M, Salmi J: Endocrinological disorders and celiac disease. *Endocr Rev* 23:464–483, 2002.

Collin P, Reunala T: Recognition and management of the cutaneous manifestations of celiac disease: a guide for dermatologists. *Am J Clin Dermatol* 4:13–20, 2003.

Collin P: Should adults be screened for celiac disease? What are the benefits and harms of screening? *Gastroenterology* 128:S104–S108, 2005.

Colombel A, Murat A, Krempf M, Kuchly-Anton B, Charbonnel B: Improvement of blood glucose control in type 1 diabetic patients treated with lispro and multiple NPH injections. *Diabet Med* 16:319–24, 1999.

Colton T, Gosselin RE, Smith RP: The tolerance of coffee drinkers to caffeine. *Clin Pharmacol Ther* 9:31–39, 1968.

Colton P, Olmsted M, Daneman D, Rydall A, Rodin G: Disturbed eating behavior and eating disorders in preteen and early teenage girls with type 1 diabetes. A case-controlled study. *Diabetes Care* 27:1654–1659, 2004.

Colton PA, Olmstead MP, Daneman D, Rydall AC, Rodin GM: Natural history and predictors of disturbed eating behavior in girls with type 1 diabetes. *Diabet Med* 24:424–429, 2007.

Combs CA, Gavin LA, Gunderson E, Main EK, Kitzmiller JL: Relationship of fetal macrosomia to maternal postprandial glucose control during pregnancy. *Diabetes Care* 15:1251–1257, 1992.

Comess LJ, Bennett PH, Man MB, Burch TA, Miller M: Congenital anomalies in the Pima Indians of Arizona. *Diabetes* 18:471–477, 1969.

Conti J, Abraham S, Taylor A: Eating behavior and pregnancy outcome. *J Psychosom Res* 44:465–477, 1998.

Conway DL, Gonzales O, Skiver D: Use of glyburide for the treatment of gestational diabetes: the San Antonio experience. *J Matern Fetal Neonatal Med* 15:51–55, 2004.

Cooper MJ, Zlotkin SH: Day-to-day variation of transferrin receptor and ferritin in healthy men and women. *Am J Clin Nutr* 64:738–742, 1996.

Cooper GJS, Chan Y-K, Dissanayake AM, Leahy FE, Keogh GF, Frampton CM, Gamble GD, Brunton DH, Baker JR, Poppitt SD: Demonstration of a hyperglycemia-driven pathogenic abnormality of copper homeostasis in diabetes and its reversibility by selective chelation. Quantitative comparisons between the biology of copper and eight other nutritionally essential elements in normal and diabetic individuals. *Diabetes* 54:1468–1476, 2005.

Correa A, Botto L, Liu Y, Mulinare J, Erickson JD: Do multivitamin supplements attenuate the risk for diabetes-associated birth defects? *Pediatrics* 111:1146–1151, 2003.

Cotter AM, Molloy AM, Scott JM, Daly SF: Elevated plasma homocysteine in early pregnancy: a risk factor for the development of severe preeclampsia. *Am J Obstet Gynecol* 185:781–785, 2001.

Cotter AM, Molloy AM, Scott JM, Daly SF: Elevated plasma homocysteine in early pregnancy: a risk factor for the development of nonsevere preeclampsia. *Am J Obstet Gynecol* 189:391–394, discussion 396, 2003.

Cotton PA, Subar AF, Friday JE, Cook A: Dietary sources of nutrients among U.S. adults, 1994 to 1996. *J Am Diet Assoc* 104:921–930, 2004.

Coudray C, Demigne C, Rayssiguier Y: Effects of dietary fibers on magnesium absorption in animals and humans. *J Nutr* 133:1–4, 2003.

Coulston AM, Hollenbeck CB, Liu GC, Williams RA, Starich GH, Mazzaferri EL, Reaven GM: Effect of source of dietary carbohydrate on plasms glucose, insulin, and gastric inhibitory polypeptide responses to test meals in subjects with noninsulin-dependent diabetes mellitus. *Am J Clin Nutr* 40:965–70, 1984.

Cousins L: The California Diabetes and Pregnancy Program: a statewide collaborative program for the preconception and prenatal care of diabetic women. *Bailliere's Clin Obstet Gynecol* 5:443–459, 1991.

Coustacou T, Zgibor JC, Evans RW, Tyurina YY, Kagan VE, Orchard TJ: Antioxidants and coronary artery disease among individuals with type 1 diabetes: findings from the Pittsburgh Epidemiology of Diabetes Complications Study. *J Diabetes Complications* 20:387–394, 2006.

Coustan DR, Berkowitz RL, Hobbins JC: Tight metabolic control of overt diabetes in pregnancy. *Am J Med* 68:845–852,1980.

Coustan DR, Reece EA, Sherwin RS, Rudolf MC, Bates SE, Sockin SM, Holford T, Tamborlane WV: A randomized clinical trial of the insulin pump versus intensive conventional therapy in diabetic pregnancies. *JAMA* 255:631–636, 1986.

Cowett RA, Susa JB, Kahn CB, Giletti B, Oh W, Schwartz R: Glucose kinetics in nondiabetic and diabetic women during the third trimester of pregnancy. *Am J Obstet Gynecol* 146:773–780, 1983.

Craig SA: Betaine in human nutrition. *Am J Clin Nutr* 80:539–549, 2004.

Craig KJ, Williams JD, Riley SG, Smith H, Owens DR, Worthing D, Cavill I, Phillips AO: Anemia and diabetes in the absence of nephropathy. *Diabetes Care* 28:1118–1123, 2005.

Crapo PA, Insel J, Sperling M, Kolterman OG: Comparison of serum glucose, insulin, and glucagons responses to different types of complex carbohydrates in noninsulin-dependendent diabetic patients. *Am J Clin Nutr* 34:184–190, 1981.

Cronin CC, Feighery A, Ferriss JB, Liddy C, Shanahan F, Feighery C: High prevalence of celiac disease among patients with insulin-dependent (type 1) diabetes mellitus. *Am J Gastroenterol* 92:2210–2212, CC 1997a.

Cronin CC, Shanaha F: Insulin-dependent diabetes mellitus and celiac disease. *Lancet* 349:1096–1097, 1997b.

Cronin CC, McPartlin JM, Barry DG, Ferriss JB, Scott JM, Weir DG: Plasma homocysteine concentrations in patients with type 1 diabetes. *Diabetes Care* 21:1843–1847, 1998.

Cross NA, Hillman LS, Allen SH, Krause GF: Calcium homeostasis and bone metabolism during pregnancy, lactation, and postweaning: a longitudinal study. *Am J Clin Nutr* 61:514–523, 1995.

Cruikshank DP, Pitkin RM, Reynolds WA, Williams GA, Hargis GK: Altered maternal calcium homeostasis in diabetic pregnancy. *J Clin Endocrinol Metab* 50:264–267, 1980.

Cruikshank DP, Pitkin RM, Varner MW, Williams GA, Hargis GK: Calcium metabolism in diabetic mother, fetus, and newborn infant. *Am J Obstet Gynecol* 145:1010–1016, 1983.

Crump KS, Kjellstrom T, Shipp AM, Silvers A, Stewart A: Influence of prenatal mercury exposure upon scholastic and psychological test performance: benchmark analysis of a New Zealand cohort. *Risk Anal* 18:701–713, 1998.

Cryer PE: Are gender differences in the responses to hypoglycemia relevant to iatrogenic hypoglycemia in type 1 diabetes? Editorial. *J Clin Endocrinol Metab* 85:2145–2147, 2000.

Culler FL, Yung RF, Jansons RA, Mosier HD: Growth-promoting peptides in diabetic and non-diabetic pregnancy: interactions with trophoblastic receptors and serum carrier proteins. *J Pediatr Endocrinol Metab* 9:21–29, 1996.

Cundy T, Gamble G, Manuel A, Townend K, Roberts A: Determinants of birth-weight in women with established and gestational diabetes. *Aust N Z J Obstet Gynecol* 33:249–254, 1993.

Cundy T, Gamble G, Townend K, Henley PG, MacPherson P, Roberts AB: Perinatal mortality in type 2 diabetes. Diabet Med 17:33–39, 2000.

Cundy T, Gamble G, Neale L, Elder R, McPherson P, Henley P, Rowan J: Differing causes of pregnancy loss in type 1 and type 2 diabetes. *Diabetes Care* 30: 2603–2607, 2007.

Cunningham JJ, Fu A, Mearkle PL, Brown RG: Hyperzincuria in individuals with insulin-dependent diabetes mellitus: concurrent zinc status and the effect of high-dose zinc supplementation. *Metabolism* 43:1558–1562, 1994.

Cusworth DC, Gattereau A: Inhibition of renal tubular absorption of homocysteine by lysine and arginine. *Lancet* 2:916–917, 1968.

Cypryk K, Sobczak M, Pertynska-Marczewska M, Zawodniak-Szalapaka M, Szymczak W, Wilczynski J, Lewinski A: Pregnancy complications and perinatal outcome in diabetic women treated with humalog (insulin lispro) or regular human insulin during pregnancy. *Med Sci Monit* 10:129–132, 2004.

Cypryk K, Vilsbell T, Nadel I, Smyczynska J, Holst JJ, Lewinski A: Normal secretion of the incretin hormones glucose-dependent insulinotropic polypeptide and glucagons-like peptide-1 during gestational diabetes. *Gynecol Endocrinol* 23: 58–62, 2007.

Czeizel AE: Prevention of congenital abnormalities by periconceptional multivitamin supplementation. *BMJ* 306:1645–1648, 1993.

D'Elios MM, Bergman MP, Azzurri A, Amedei A, Benagiano M, DePont JJ, Cianchi F, Vandenbroucke-Grauls CM, Romagnani S, Appelmelk BJ, Del Prete G: H(+), K(+)-atpase (proton pump) is the target autoantigen of Th1-type cytotoxic T cells in autoimmune gastritis. *Gastroenterology* 120:377–86, 2001.

D'Elios MM, Amedei A, Azzurri A, Benagiano M, Del Prete G, Bergman MP, Vandenbroucke-Grauls CM, Appelmelk BJ: Molecular specificity and functional properties of autoreactive T-cell response in human gastric autoimmunity. *Int Rev Immunol* 24:111–22, 2005.

d'Emden MC, Marwick TH, Dreghorn J, Howlett VL, Cameron DP: Postprandial glucose and insulin responses to different types of spaghetti and bread. *Diabetes Res Clin Pract* 3:221–226, 1987.

Dabalea D, Hanson RL, Lindsay RS, Pettitt DJ, Imperatore G, Gabir MM, Roumain J, Bennett PH, Knowler WC: Intrauterine exposure to diabetes conveys risks for type 2 diabetes and obesity: a study of discordant sibships. *Diabetes* 49: 2208–2211, 2000.

daCosta KA, Gaffney CE, Fischer LM, Zeisel SH: Choline deficiency in mice and humans is associated with increased plasma homocysteine concentration after a methionine load. *Am J Clin Nutr* 81:440–444, 2005.

Dahele A, Ghosh S: Vitamin B$_{12}$ deficiency in untreated celiac disease. *Am J Gastroenterol* 96:745–750, 2001.

Daimon M, Susa S, Yamatani K, Manaka H, Hama K, Kimura M, Ohnuma H, Kata T: Hyperglycemia is a factor for an increase in serum ceruloplasmin in type 2 diabetes. *Diabetes Care* 21:1525–1528, 1998.

Daneman D, Olmsted M, Rydall A, Maharaj S, Rodin G: Eating disorders in young women with type 1 diabetes. Prevalence, problems and prevention. *Horm Res* 50 (Suppl 1):79–86, 1998.

Daniels JL, Longnecker MP, Klebanoff MA, Gray KA, Brock JW, Zhou H, Chen Z, Needham LL: Prenatal exposure to low-level polychlorinated biphenyls in relation to mental and motor development at 8 months. *Am J Epidemiol* 157:485–492, 2003.

Daniels JL, Longnecker MP, Rowland AS, Golding J; ALSPAC Study Team: University of Bristol Institute of Child Health: Fish intake during pregnancy and early cognitive development of offspring. *Epidemiology* 15:394–402, 2004.

Danne T, Lupke K, Walte K, von Schuetz W, Gall M-A: Insulin detemir is characterized by a consistent pharmacokinetic profile across age-groups in children, adolescents, and adults with type 1 diabetes. *Diabetes Care* 26: 3087–3092, 2003.

Danne T, Becker RH, Heise T, Bittner C, Frick AD, Rave K: Pharmacokinetics and safety of insulin glulisine in children and adolescents with tyoe 1 diabetes. *Diabetes Care* 28:2100–2105, 2005.

Danzeisen R, Fosset C, Chariana Z, Page K, David S, McArdle HJ: Placental ceruloplasmin homolog is regulated by iron and copper and is implicated in iron metabolism. *Am J Physiol* 282:C472–C478, 2002.

Darvill T, lonky E, Reihman J, Stewart P, Pagano J: Prenatal exposure to PCBs and infant performance on the Fagan test of infant intelligence. *Neurotoxicity* 21:1029–1038, 2000.

Datta S, Alfaham M, Davies D, Dunstan F, Woodhead S, Evans J, Richards B: Vitamin D deficiency in pregnant women from a non-European ethnic minority population—an interventional study. *BJOG* 109:905–908, 2002.

Davidson PW, Myers GJ, Cox C, Axtell C, Shamlaye C, Sloane-Reeves J, Cernichiari E, Needham L, Choi A, Wang Y, berlin M, Clarkson TW: Effects of prenatal and postnatal methylmercury exposure from fish consumption on neurodevelopment: outcomes at 66 months of age in the Seychelles Child Development Study. *JAMA* 280:701–707, 1998.

Davidson PW, Myers GJ, Cox C, Wilding GE, Shamlaye CF, Huang LS, Cernichiari E, Sloane-Reeves J, Palumbo D, Clarkson TW: Methylmercury and neurodevelopment: longitudinal analysis of the Seychelles child development cohort. *Neurotoxicol Teratol* 28:529–535, 2006.

Davies SC, Holly JM, Coulson VJ, Cotterill AM, Abdulla AF, Whittaker PG, Chard T, Wass JA: The presence of cation-dependent proteases for insulin-like growth factor binding proteins does not alter the size distribution of insulin-like growth factors in pregnancy. *Clin Endocrinol (Oxf)* 34:501–506, 1991.

Davies L, Wilmshurst EG, McElduff A, Gunton J, Clifton-Bligh P, Fulcher GR: The relationship among homocysteine, creatinine clearance, and albuminuria in patients with type 2 diabetes. *Diabetes Care* 24:1805–1809, 2001.

Davies GAL, Wolfe LA, Mottola MF, MacKinnon C; SOGC Clinical Practice Obstetrics Committee; Canadian Society for Exercise Physiology Board of Directors: Exercise in pregnancy and the postpartum period. *J Obstet Gynecol Can* 25:516–529, 2003.

Davis RJ, Corvera S, Czech MP: Insulin stimulates cellular iron uptake and causes the redistribution of intracellular transferrin receptors to the plasma membrane. *J Biol Chem* 261:8708–8711, 1986.

Davis RE, McCann VJ, Stanton KG: Type 1 diabetes and latent pernicious anemia. *Med J Aust* 156:160–162, 1992.

Davis SN, Galassetti P, Wasserman DH, Tate D: Effects of antecedent hypoglycemia on subsequent counterregulatory resonses to exercise. *Diabetes* 49:73–81, 2000a.

Davis SN, Galassetti P, Wasserman DH, Tate D: Effects of gender on neuroendocrine and metabolic counterregulatory responses to exercise in normal man. *J Clin Endocrinol Metab* 85:224–230, 2000b.

Davis BC, Kris-Etherton PM: Achieving optimal essential fatty acid status in vegetarians: current knowledge and practical implications. *Am J Clin Nutr* 78 (Suppl):640S–646S, 2003.

Davis RL, Rubanowice D, McPhillips H, Raebel MA, Andrade SE, Smith D, Yood MU, Platt R; HMO Research Network Center for Education, Research in Therapeutics: Risks of congenital malformations and perinatal events among infants exposed to antidepressant medications during pregnancy. *Pharmacoepidemiol Drug Saf* 16:1086–1094, 2007.

Dawood FH, Jabbar AA, Al-Mudaris AF, Al-Hasani MH: Association of HLA antigens with celiac disease among Iraqi children. *Tissue Antigens* 18:35–39, 1981.

DCCT—Diabetes Control and Complications Trial Research Group: Epidemiology of severe hypoglycemia in the Diabetes Control and Complications Trial. *Am J Med* 90:450–459, 1991.

DCCT—Diabetes Control and Complications Trial Research Group: Expanded role of the dietitian in the Diabetes Control and Complications Trial: implications for practice. *J Am Diet Assoc* 93:758–757, 1993a.

DCCT—Diabetes Control and Complications Trial Research Group: Nutrition interventions for intensive therapy in the Diabetes Control and Complications Trial. *J Am Diet Assoc* 93:768–772, 1993b.

DCCT—Diabetes Control and Complications Trial Research Group: Pregnancy outcomes in the Diabetes Control and Complications Trial. *Am J Obst Gynecol* 174:1343–1353, 1996.

DCCT—Diabetes Control and Complications Trial Research Group: Hypoglycemia in the Diabetes Control and Complications Trial. *Diabetes* 46:271–286, 1997.

DCCT—Diabetes Control and Complications Trial Research Group: Effect of pregnancy on microvascular complications in the Diabetes Control and Complications Trial. *Diabetes Care* 23:1084–1091, 2000.

De Block CEM, De Leeuw IH, Van Gaal LF; Belgian Diabetes Registry: High prevalence of manifestations of gastric autoimmunity in parietal cell antibody-positive type 1 (insulin-dependent) diabetic patients. *J Clin Endocrinol Metab* 84:4062–4067, 1999.

De Block CEM, Van Campenhout CMV, De Leeuw IH, Keenoy BM, Martin M, Van Hoof V, Van Gaal LF: Soluble transferrin receptor level. A new marker of iron deficiency anemia, a common manifestation of gastric autoimmunity in type 1 diabetes. *Diabetes Care* 23:1384–1388, 2000a.

De Block CE, De Leeuw IH, Rooman RP, Winnock F, Du Caju MV, Van Gaal LF: Gastric parietal cell antibodies are associated with glutamic acid decarboxylase-65 antibodies and the HLA DQA1*0501-DQB1*0301 haplotype in type 1 diabetes mellitus. Belgian Diabetes Registry. *Diabet Med* 17:618–22, 2000b.

De Block CE, De Leeuw IH, Vertommen JJ, Rooman RP, Du Caju MV, Van Campenhout CM, Weyler JJ, Winnock F, Van Autreve J, Gorus FK; Belgian Diabetes Registry: Beta-cell, thyroid, gastric, adrenal and celiac autoimmunity and HLA-DQ types in type 1 diabetes. *Clin Exp Immunol* 126:184–186, 2001.

De Block CEM, De Leeuw IH, Bogers JJ, Pelckmans PA, Ieven MM, Van Marck EA, Van Hoof V, Maday E, Van Acker KL, Van Gaal LF: *Heliobacter pylori*, parietal cell antibodies and autoimmune gastropathy in type 1 diabetes mellitus. *Aliment Pharmacol Ther* 16:281–289, 2002a.

De Block CEM, De Leeuw IH, Pelckmans PA, Callens D, Emoke M, Van Gaal LF: Delayed gastric emptying and gastric autoimmunity in type 1 diabetes. *Diabetes Care* 25:912–917, 2002b.

De Block CEM, De Leeuw IH, Bogers JJPM, Pelckmans PA, Ieven MM, Van Marck EAE, Van Acker KL, Van Gaal LF: Autoimmune gastropathy in type 1 diabetic patients with parietal cell antibodies. *Diabetes Care* 26:82–88, 2003.

de Caterina M, Grimaldi E, Di Pascale G, Salerno G, Rosiello A, Passaretti M, Scopacasa F: The soluble transferrin receptor (sTfR)-ferritin index is a potential predictor of celiac disease in children with refractory iron deficiency anemia. *Clin Chem Lab Med* 43:38–42, 2005.

de Groot M, Anderson R, Freedland KE, Clouse RE, Lustman PJ: Association of depression and diabetes complications: a meta-analysis. *Psychosom Med* 63: 619–630, 2001.

de Groot M, Pinkerman B, Wagner J, Hockman E: Depression treatment and satisfaction in a multicultural sample of type 1 and type 2 diabetic patients. *Diabetes Care* 29:549–553, 2006.

De Hertogh R, Casi AL, Hinck L: Pre-implantation embryopathy and maternal diabetes. In: Hod M, Jovanovic L, Di Renzo GC, de Leiva A, Langer O, eds. *Textbook of Diabetes and Pregnancy.* London: Martin Dunitz; 2003:241–252.

de Ledinghen V, Combes M, Trouette H, Winnock M, Amouretti M, de Mascarel A, Couzigou P: Should a liver biopsy be done in patients with subclinical chronically elevated transaminases? *Eur J Gastroenterol Hepatol* 16:879–883, 2004.

de Veciana M, Major CA, Morgan MA, Asrat T, Toohey JS, Lien JM, Evans AT: Postprandial versus preprandial blood glucose monitoring in women with gestational diabetes mellitus requiring insulin therapy. *N Engl J Med* 333: 1237–1241, 1995.

de Vries MJ, Dekker GA, Schoemaker J: Higher risk of preeclampsia in the polycystic ovary syndrome. A case control study. *Eur J Obstet Gynecol Reprod Biol* 76:91–95, 1998.

De Vriese SR, De Henauw S, De Backer G, Dhont M, Christophe AB: Estimation of dietary fat intake of Belgian pregnant women. Comparison of two methods. *Ann Nutr Metab* 45:273–278, 2001.

De Vriese SR, Matthys C, De Henauw S, De Backer G, Dhont M, Christophe AB: Maternal and umbilical fatty acid status in relation to maternal diet. *Prostaglandins Leukot Essent Fatty Acids* 67:389–396, 2002.

de Wardener HE, He FJ, MacGregor GA: Plasma sodium and hypertension. *Kidney Int* 66:2454–2466, 2004.

Debes F, Budtz-Jorgensen E, Weihe P, White RF, Grandjean P: Impact of prenatal methylmercury exposure on neurobehavioral function at age 14 years. *Neurotoxicol* 28:363–375, 2006.

Debier C, Larondelle Y: Vitamins A and E: metabolism, roles and transfer to offspring. *Br J Nutr* 93:153–174, 2005.

Debrah K, Sehrwin RS, Murphy J, Kerr D: Effect of caffeine on recognition of and physiological responses to hypoglycemia in insulin-dependent diabetes. *Lancet* 347:19–24, 1996.

Del Sindaco P, Ciofetta M, Lalli C, Perriello G, Pampanelli S, Torlone E, Brunetti P, Bolli GB: Use of the short-acting insulin analogue lispro in intensive treatment of type 1 diabetes mellitus: importance of appropriate replacement of basal insulin and time-interval injection-meal. *Diabet Med* 15:592–600, 1998.

Delahanty LM, Halford BN: The role of diet behaviors in achieving glycemic control in intensively treated patients in the Diabetes Control and Complications Trial. Diabetes Care 16:1453–1458, 1993.

Delahanty LM, Grant RW, Wittenberg E, Bosch JL, Wexler DJ, Cagliero E, Meigs JB: Association of diabetes-related emotional distress with diabetes treatment in primary care patients with type 2 diabetes. *Diabet Med* 24:48–54, 2007.

Delamater AM, Jacobson AM, Anderson B, Cox, D, Fisher L, Lustman P, Rubin R, Wysocki T: Psychosocial therapies in diabetes. Report of the Psychosocial Therapies Working Group. *Diabetes Care* 24:1286–1292, 2001.

Delaney JJ, Ptacek J: Three decades of experience with diabetic pregnancies. *Am J Obstet Gynecol* 106:550–556, 1970.

Delgado JC, Greene MF, Winkelman JW, Tanasijevic MJ: Comparison of disaturated phosphatidylcholine and fetal lung maturity surfactant/albumin ratio in diabetic and nondiabetic pregnancies. *Am J Clin Pathol* 113:233–239, 2000.

Dellow WJ, Chambers ST, Lever M, George PM, Robson RA, Chambers ST: Elevated glycine betaine excretion in diabetes mellitus patients is associated with proximal tubular dysfunction and hyperglycemia. *Diabetes Res Clin Pract* 43: 91–99, 1999a.

Dellow WJ, Chambers ST, Barrell GK, Lever M, Robson RA: Glycine betaine excretion is not directly linked to plasma glucose concentrations in hyperglycemia. *Diabetes Res Clin Pract* 43:91–99, 1999b.

DeLuca HF: Overview of general physiologic features and functions of vitamin D. *Am J Clin Nutr* 80 (Suppl):1689S–1696S, 2004.

Demarini S, Mimouni F, Tsang RC, Khoury J, Hertzberg V: Impact of metabolic control of diabetes during pregnancy on neonatal hypocalcemia: a randomized study. *Obstet Gynecol* 83:918–922, 1994.

Demers LM, Gabbe SG, Villee CA, Greep RO: The effects of insulin on human placental glycogenesis. *Endocrinology* 91:270–275, 1972.

Demigne C, Sabboh H, Remesy C, Meneton P: Protective effects of high dietary potassium: nutritional and metabolic aspects. *J Nutr* 134:2903–2906, 2004.

Dennis CL, Ross LE, Grigoriadis S: Psychosocial and psychological interventions for treating antenatal depression. *Cochrane Database Syst Rev* Jul 18 2007;(3): CD006309.

Denno KM, Sadler TW: Effects of the biguanide class of oral hypoglycemic agents on mouse embryogenesis. *Teratology* 49:260–266, 1994.

Derr R, Garrett E, Stacy GA, Suadek CD: Is HbA1c affected by glycemic instability? *Diabetes Care* 26:2728–2733, 2003.

Desoye G, Korgun ET, Ghaffari-Tabrizi N, Hahn T: Is fetal macrosomia in inadequately controlled diabetic women the result of a placental defect? A hypothesis. *J Matern Fetal Neonatal Med* 11:258–261, 2002.

Deurenberg P, Yap N, Van Staveren WA: Body mass index and percent body fat: a meta-analysis among different ethnic groups. *Int J Obes Relat Metab Disord* 22:1164–1171, 1998.

Devlin JT, Hothersall L, Wilkis JL: Use of insulin glargine during pregnancy in a type 1 diabetic woman. *Diabetes Care* 25:1095–1096, 2002a.

Devlin JT, Ruderman N: Diabetes and exercise: the risk-benefit profile revisited. In: Ruderman N, Devlin JT, Schneider SH, Krisra A, eds. *Handbook of Exercise in Diabetes.* Alexandria VA: American Diabetes Association; 2002b.

Devrim E, Tarhan I, Erguder IB, Durak I: Oxidant/antioxidant status of placenta, blood, and cord blood samples from pregnant women supplemented with iron. *J Soc Gynecol Investig* 13:502–505, 2006.

Dewar D, Pereira SP, Ciclitira PJ: The pathogenesis of celiac disease. *Int J Biochem Cell Biol* 36:17–24, 2004.

Dewar DH, Ciclitira PJ: Clinical features and diagnosis of celiac disease. *Gastroenterology* 128:S19–S24, 2005.

DeWitt DE, Dugdale DC: Using new insulin strategies in the outpatient treatment of diabetes. Clinical applications. *JAMA* 289:2265–2269, 2003a.

DeWitt DE, Hirsch IB: Outpatient insulin therapy in type 1 and type 2 diabetes. Scientific review. *JAMA* 289:2254–2264, 2003b.

DGA—U.S. Department of Agriculture, U.S. Department of Health and Human Services: Dietary guidelines for Americans, 2005. 6th ed. Washington, DC: U.S.

Government Printing Office; 2005. Available at: www.healthierus.gov/dietaryguidelines. Accessed Mar 13, 2008.

DGAe—U.S. Department of Agriculture, U.S. Department of Health and Human Services: 2005 Dietary Guidelines Advisory Committee report, Part D: science base, section 8: ethanol. Washington, DC: 2005; 1–14. Available at: www.health.gov/dietaryguidelines/dga2005/report. Accessed Mar 13, 2008.

DGAr—U.S. Department of Agriculture, U.S. Department of Health and Human Services: 2005 Dietary Guidelines Advisory Committee report. Washington, DC: 2005. Available at: www.health.gov/dietaryguidelines. Accessed Mar 13, 2008.

DHHS—U.S. Department of Health and Human Services: Physical activity and health: a report of the Surgeon General. Washington, DC: U.S. Government Printing Office; 1996.

Di Cianni G, Volpe L, Lencioni C, Chatzianagnostou K, Cuccuru I, Ghio A, Benzi L, Del Prato S: Use of insulin glargine during the first weeks of pregnancy in five type 1 diabetic women. *Diabetes Care* 28:982–983, 2005.

Di Sabatino A, Ciccocioppo R, Cupelli F, Cinque B, Millimaggi D, Clarkson MM, Paulli M, Cifone MG, Corazza GR: Epithelium derived interleukin 15 regulates intraepithelial lymphocyte Th1 cytokine production, cytotoxicity, and survival in celiac disease. *Gut* 55:469–477, 2006.

Diakoumopoulou E, Tentolouris N, Kirlaki E, Perrea D, Kitsou E, Psallas M, Doulgerakis D, Katsilambros N: Plasma homocysteine levels in patients with type 2 diabetes in a Mediterannean population: relation with nutritional and other factors. *Nutr Metab Cardiovasc Dis* 15:109–117, 2005.

Diamond MP, Vaughn WK, Salyer SL, Cotton RB, Fields LM, Boehm FH: Efficacy of outpatient management of insulin-dependent diabetic pregnancies. *Am J Perinatol* 5:2–8, 1983.

Diamond TD, Kormas N: Possible fetal effect of insulin lispro. *N Engl J Med* 337:1009–1010, 1997.

Diamont YZ, Metzger BE, Freinkel N, Shafrir E: Placental lipid and glycogen content in human and experimental diabetes mellitus. *Am J Obstet Gynecol* 144:5–11, 1982.

Diaz VA, Mainous AG 3rd, Koopman RJ, Geesey ME: Are ethnic differences in insulin sensitivity explained by variation in carbohydrate intake? *Diabetologia* 48:1264–1268, 2005.

Dicke JM, Henderson GI: Placental amino acid uptake in normal and complicated pregnancies. *Am J Med Sci* 295:223–227, 1988.

Dickey W: Low serum vitamin B$_{12}$ is common in celiac disease and is not due to autoimmune gastritis. *Eur J Gastroenterol Hepatol* 14:425–427, 2002.

Dieterich W, Ehnis T, Bauer M, Donner P, Volta U, Riecken EO, Schuppan D: Identification of tissue transglutaminase as the autoantigen of celiac disease. *Nat Med* 3:797–801, 1997.

Dieterich W, Ehnis T, Bauer M, Donner P, Volta U, Riecken EO, Schuppen D: Autoantibodies to human tissue transglutaminase identify silent celiac disease in type 1 diabetes. *Diabetologia* 42:1440–1441, 1999.

Dietrich M, Brown CJ, Block G: The effect of folate fortification of cereal-grain products on blood folate status, dietary folate intake, and dietary folate sources among adult nonsupplement users in the United States. *J Am Coll Nutr* 24: 266–274, 2005.

Dietz PM, Williams SB, Callaghan WM, Bachman DJ, Whitlock EP, Hornbrook MC: Clinically identified maternal depression before, during, and after pregnancies ending in live births. *Am J Psychiatry* 164:1515–1520, 2007.

Dijck-Brouwer DA, Hadders-Algra M, Bouwstra H, Decsi T, Boehm G, Martini IA, Rudy Boersma E, Muskiet FA: Impaired maternal gluose homeostasis during pregnancy is associated with low status of long-chain polyunsaturated fatty acids (LCP) and essential fatty acids (EFA) in the fetus. *Prostaglandins Leukot Essent Fatty Acids* 73:85–87, 2005.

DiMarchi RD, Chance RE, Long HB, Shields JE, Slieker LJ: Preparation of an insulin with improved pharmacokinetics relative to human insulin through consideration of structural homology with insulin-like growth factor-1. *Horm Res* 41 (Suppl 2):93–96, 1994.

Dimitriadis GD, Gerich JE: Importance of timing of preprandial subcutaneous insulin administration in the management of diabetes mellitus. *Diabetes Care* 6:374–377, 1983.

Diraison F, Dusserre E, Vidal H, Sothier M, Beylot M: Increased hepatic lipogenesis but decreased expression of lipogenic gene in adipose tissue in human obesity. *Am J Physiol Endocrinol Metab* 282:E46–E51, 2002.

Diraison F, Moulin Ph, Beylot M: Contribution of hepatic de novo lipogenesis and reesterification of plasma non esterified fatty acids to plasma triglyceride synthesis during non-alcoholic fatty liver disease. *Diabetes Metab* 29:478–485, 2003a.

Diraison F, Yankah V, Letexier D, Dusserre E, Jones P, Beylot M: Differences in the regulation of adipose tissue and liver lipogenesis by carbohydrates in humans. *J Lipid Res* 44:846–853, 2003b.

DirNet—Diabetes Research in Children Network Study Group: Accuracy of the modified Continuous Glucose Monitoring System (CGMS) sensor in an outpatient setting: results from a Diabetes Research in Children Network (DirecNet) study. *Diabetes Technol Therapeut* 7:109–114, 2005a.

DirNet—Diabetes Research in Children Network Study Group: A randomized multicenter trial comparing the GlucoWatch Biographer with standard glucose monitoring in children with type 1 diabetes. *Diabetes Care* 28:1101–1106, 2005b.

DirNet—Diabetes Research in Children Network Study Group: The effects of aerobic exercise on glucose and counterregulatory hormone concentrations in children with type 1 diabetes. *Diabetes Care* 29:20–25, 2006a.

DirNet—Diabetes Research in Children Network Study Group; Tsalikian E, Kollman C, Tamborlane WB, Beck RW, Fiallo-Scharer R, Fox L, Janz KF, Ruedy KJ, Wilson D, Xing D, Weinzimer SA: Prevention of hypoglycemia during exercise in children with type 1 diabetes by suspending basal insulin. *Diabetes Care* 29:2200–2204, 2006b.

Dixon JB, Dixon ME, O'Brien PE: Pregnancy after lap-band surgery: management of the band to achieve healthy weight outcomes. *Obes Surg* 11:59–65, 2001.

Dixon JB, Dixon ME, O'Brien PE: Birth outcomes in obese women after laparoscopic adjustable gastric banding. *Obstet Gynecol* 106:965–972, 2005.

Djelmis J, Blajic J, Bukovic D, Pfeifer D, Ivanisevic M, Kendic S, Votava-Raic A: Glycosylated hemoglobin and fetal growth in normal, gestational and insulin dependent diabetes mellitus pregnancies. *Coll Antropol* 21:621–629, 1997.

Djelmis J, Desoye G, Ivanisevic M, eds: *Diabetology of Pregnancy.* Basel, Switzerland: Karger; 2005.

Djordjevic A, Spasic S, Jovanovic-Galovic A, Djordjevic R, Grubor-Lajsic G: Oxidative stress in diabetic pregnancy: SOD,CAT and GSH-Px activity and lipid peroxidation products. *J Matern-Fetal Med* 16:367–372, 2004.

Djurhuus MS, Skott P, Vaag A, Hother-Nielsen O, Andersen P, Parving HH, Klitgaard NA: Hyperglycemia enhances renal magnesium excretion in type 1 diabetic patients. *Scand J Clin Lab Invest* 60:403–409, 2000.

Djurhuus MS: New data on the mechanisms of hypermagnesuria in type 1 diabetes mellitus. *Magnes Res* 14:217–223, 2001.

Dodds L, Fell DB, Joseph KS, Allen VM, Butler B: Outcomes of pregnancies complicated by hyperemesis gravidarum. *Obstet Gynecol* 107:285–292, 2006.

Dolci M, Mori M, Baccetti F: Use of glargine insulin before and during pregnancy in a woman with type 1 diabetes and Addison's Disease. *Diabetes Care* 28: 2084–2085, 2005.

Donatelli M, Bucalo ML, Russo V, Cerasola GA: Calcium hormones in diabetic pregnancy. *Boll Soc Ital Biol Sper* 60:1503–1508, 1984.

Donnelly KL, Coleman SI, Schwarzenberg SJ, Jessurun J, Boldt MD, Parks EJ: Sources of fatty acids stored in liver and secreted via lipoproteins in patients with nonalcoholic fatty liver disease. *J Clin Invest* 115:1343–1351, 2005.

Dornhorst A, Nicholls JSD, Probst F, Paterson CM, Hollier KL, Elkeles RS, Beard RW: Calorie restriction for the treatment of gestational diabetes. *Diabetes* 40:161–164, 1991.

Dornhorst A: Insulinotropic meglitinide analogues. *Lancet* 358:1709–1715, 2001.

Dornhorst A, Frost G: The principles of dietary management of gestational diabetes: reflection on current advice. *J Hum Nutr Diet* 15:145–156, 2002.

Doshi SN, Moat SJ, McDowell IF, Lewis MJ, Goodfellow J: Lowering plasma homocysteine with folic acid in cardiovascular disease: what will the trials tell us? *Atherosclerosis* 165:1–3, 2002.

DPGF—Diabetes and Pregnancy Group, France: French multicentric survey of outcome of pregnancy in women with pregestational diabetes. *Diabetes Care* 26:2990–2993, 2003.

Dube MC, Weisnagel SJ, Prud'homme D, Lavoie C: Exercise and newer insulins: how much glucose supplement to avoid hypoglycemia? *Med Sci Sports Exerc* 37:1276–1282, 2005.

Dube MC, Weisnagel SJ, Prud'homme D, Lavoie C: Is early and late post-meal exercise so different in type 1 diabetic lispro users? *Diabetes Res Clin Pract* 72:128–134, 2006.

Dudas I, Czeizel AE: Use of 6000 IU vitamin A during early pregnancy without teratogenic effect. *Teratology* 45:335–336, 1992.

Dufour JF, Oneta CM, Gonvers JJ, Bihl F, Cerny A, Cereda JM, Zala JF, Helbling B, Steuerwald M, Zimmerman A; Swiss Association for the Study of the Liver:

Randomized placebo-controlled trial of ursodeoxycholic acid with vitamin e in nonalcoholic steatohepatitis. *Clin Gastroenterol Hepatol* 4:1537–1543, 2006.

Dugglesby SC, Jacjson AA: Protein, amino acid and nitrogen metabolism during pregnancy: how might the mother meet the needs of her fetus? *Curr Opin Clin Nutr Metab Care* 5:503–509, 2002.

DUK—Diabetes UK Nutrition Subcommittee of the Diabetes Care Advisory Committee: The implementation of nutritional advice for people with diabetes. *Diabet Med* 20:786–807, 2003.

Dungan KM, Buse JB, Largay J, Kelly MM, Button EA, Kato S, Wittlin S: 1, 5-anhydroglucitol and postprandial hyperglycemia as measured by Continuous Glucose Monitoring System in moderately controlled patients with diabetes. *Diabetes Care* 29:1214–1219, 2006.

Dunn JT, Delange F: Damaged reproduction: the most important consequence of iodine deficiency. Commentary. *J Clin Endocrinol Metab* 86:2360–2363, 2001.

Dunne FP, Brydon PA, Proffitt M, Smith T, Gee H, Holder RL: Fetal and maternal outcomes in Indo-Asian compared to Caucasian women with diabetes in pregnancy. *QJM* 93:813–818, 2000.

Dunne F, Brydon P, Smith K, Gee H: Pregnancy in women with type 2 diabetes: 12 years outcome data 1990–2002. *Diabet Med* 20:734, 2003.

Dunne F: Type 2 diabetes and pregnancy. *Semin Fetal Neonatal Med* 10:333–339, 2005.

Dunstan JA, Mori TA, Barden A, Beilin LJ, Holt PG, Calder PC, Taylor AL, Prescott SL: Effects of *n*-3 polyunsaturated fatty acid supplementation in pregnancy on maternal and fetal erythrocyte fatty acid composition. *Eur J Clin Nutr* 58: 429–437, 2004.

Durlach J: New data on the importance of gestational Mg deficiency. *J Am Coll Nutr* 23:694S–700S, 2004.

Durnin JVGA: Energy requirements of pregnancy: an integration of the longitudinal data from the five-country study. *Lancet* 2:1131–1133, 1987.

Durnin JVGA: Energy requirements of pregnancy. *Diabetes* 40 (Suppl 2):152–156, 1991.

Dutta-Roy AK: Fatty acid transport and metabolism in the feto-placental unit and the role of fatty acid binding protein. *J Nutr Biochem* 8:548–557, 1997.

Dutta-Roy AK: Transport mechanisms for long-chain polyunsaturated fatty acids in the human placenta. *Am J Clin Nutr* 71:315S–322S, 2000.

Duttaroy AK: Fetal growth and development: roles of fatty acid transport proteins and nuclear transcription factors in human placenta. *Indian J Exp Biol* 42: 747–757, 2004.

Dwarkanath P, Muthayya S, Vaz M, Thomas T, Mhaskar A, Mhaskar R, Thomas A, Bhat S, Kurpad A: The relationship between maternal physical activity during pregnancy and birth weight. *Asia Pac J Clin Nutr* 16:704–710, 2007.

Dworacka M, Wender-Ozegowska E, Winiarska H, Borowska M, Zawiejska A, Pietryga M, Brazert J, Szczawinska K, Bobkiewicz-Kozlowska T: Plasma anhydro-D-glucitol (1.5-AG) as an indicator of hyperglycemic excursions in pregnant women with diabetes. *Diabet Med* 23:171–175, 2006.

Eaton W: Epidemiologic evidence on the comorbidity of depression and diabetes. *J Psychosom Res* 53:903–906, 2002.

Ebbeling CB, Leidig MM, Sinclair KB, Seger-Shippee LG, Feldman HA, Ludwig DS: Effects of an ad libitum low-glycemic load diet on cardiovascular disease risk factors in obese young adults. *Am J Clin Nutr* 81:976–982, 2005.

Ebeling P, Jansson PA, Smith U, Lalli C, Bolli GB, Koivisto VA: Strategies toward improved control during insulin lispro therapy in IDDM. Importance of basal insulin. *Diabetes Care* 20:1287–1289,1997.

Eckel RH: A new look at dietary protein in diabetes. Editorial. *Am J Clin Nutr* 78:671–672, 2003.

Edwards CM, Todd JF, Mahmoudi M, Wang Z, Wang RM, Ghatei MA, Bloom SR: Glucaon-like peptide 1 has a physiological role in the control of postprandial glucose in humans: studies with the antagonist exendin 9-39. *Diabetes* 48:86–93, 1999.

Edwards CM: The GLP-1 system as a therapeutic target. *Ann Med* 37:314–322, 2005.

Egede LE, Zheng D, Simpson K: Co-morbid depression is associated with increased health care use and expenditures in individuals with diabetes. *Diabetes Care* 25:464–470, 2002a.

Egede LE: Beliefs and attitudes of African Americans with type 2 diabetes toward depression. *Diabetes Educ* 28:258–268, 2002b.

Egede LE, Zheng D: Independent factors associated with major depressive disorder in a national sample of individuals with diabetes. *Diabetes Care* 26:104–111, 2003.

Egede LE: Disease-focused or integrated treatment: diabetes and depression. *Med Clin North Am* 90:627–646, 2006.

Ehrenberg HM, Mercer BM, Catalano PM: The influence of obesity and diabetes on the prevalence of macrosomia. *Am J Obstet Gynecol* 191:964–968, 2004.

Ehrlich M: Expression of various genes is controlled by DNA methylation during mammalian development. *J Cell Biochem* 88:899–910, 2003.

Eisenstein RS: Iron regulatory proteins and the molecular control of mammalian iron metabolism. *Ann Rev Nutr* 20:627–662, 2000.

Ekbom P, Damm P, Nogaard K, Clausen P, Feldt-Rasmussen U, Feldt-Rasmussen B, Nielsen LH, Molsted-Pedersen L, Mathiesen ER: Urinary albumin excretion and 24-hour blood pressure as predictors of preeclampsia in type 1 diabetes. *Diabetologia* 43:927–931, 2000.

Ekeus C, Lindberg L, Lindblad F, Hjern A: Birth outcomes and pregnancy complications in women with a history of anorexia nervosa. *BJOG* 113:925–929, 2006.

Ekpebegh CO, Coetzee EJ, van der Merwe L, Levitt NS: A 10-year retrospective analysis of pregnancy outcome in pregestational type 2 diabetes: comparison of insulin and oral glucose-lowering agents. *Diabet Med* 24:253–258, 2007.

Ekstrom EC, Hyder SM, Chowdhury AM, Chowdhury SA, Lonnerdal B, Habicht J-P, Person LA: Efficacy and trial effectiveness of weekly and daily iron supplementation among pregnant women in Bangladesh: disentangling the issues. *Am J Clin Nutr* 76:1392–1400, 2002.

El-Asmar R, Panigrahi P, Bamford P, berti I, Not T, Coppa GV, Catassi C, Fasano A: Host-dependent zonulin secretion causes the impairment of the small intestine barrier function after bacterial exposure. *Gastroenterology* 123:1607–1615, 2002.

Elchalal U, Humphrey RG, Smith SD, Hu C, Sadovsky Y, Nelson DM: Troglitazone attenuates hypoxia-induced injury in cultured term human trophoblasts. *Am J Obstet Gynecol* 191:2154–2159, 2004.

Elchalal U, Schaiff WT, Smith SD, Rimon E, Bildirici I, Nelson DM, Sadovsky Y: Insulin and fatty acids regulate the expression of fat droplet-associated protein adipophilin in primary human trophoblasts. *Am J Obstet Gynecol* 193: 1716–1723, 2005.

Elias SL, Innis SM: Bakery foods are the major dietary source of *trans*-fatty acids among pregnant women with diets providing 30 percent energy from fat. *J Am Diet Assoc* 102:46–51, 2002.

Elixhauser A, Weschler JM, Kitzmiller JL, Marks JS, Bennert HW Jr, Coustan DR, Gabbe SG, Herman WH, Kaufmann RC, Ogata ES, Sepe SJ: Cost-benefit analysis of preconception care of women with established diabetes mellitus. *Diabetes Care* 16:1146–1157, 1993.

Elixhauser A, Kitzmiller JL, Weschler JM: Short-term cost benefit of preconception care for diabetes. *Diabetes Care* 19:384, 1996.

El-Khairy L, Volset SE, Refsum H, Ueland PM: Plasma total cysteine, pregnancy complications, and adverse pregnancy outcomes: the Hordaland Homocysteine Study. *Am J Clin Nutr* 77:467–472, 2003.

Elliott BD, Langer O, Schenke S, Johnson RF: Insignificant transfer of glyburide occurs across the human placenta. *Am J Obstet Gynecol* 165:807–812, 1991.

Elliott BD, Schenker S, Langer O, Johnson R, Prihoda T: Comparative placental transport of oral hypoglycemic agents in humans: a model of human placental drug transfer. *Am J Obstet Gynecol* 171:653–660, 1994.

Elliott BD, Langer O, Schuessling F: Human placental glucose uptake and transport are not altered by the oral antihyperglycemic agent metformin. *Am J Obstet Gynecol* 176:527–530, 1997.

Ellis SE, Speroff T, Dittus RS, Brown A, Pichert JW, Elasy TA: Diabetes patient education: a meta-analysis and meta-regression. *Patient Educ Couns* 52:97–105, 2004.

Ellis LJ, Seal CJ, Kettlitz B, Bal W, Mathers JC: Postprandial glycemic, lipemic and hemostatic responses to ingestion of rapidly and slowly digested starches in healthy young women. *Br J Nutr* 94:948–955, 2005.

Ellison JM, Stegman JM, Colner SL, Michael RH, Sharma MK, Ervin KR, Horwitz DL: Rapid changes in postprandial blood glucose produce concentration differences at finger, forearm, and thigh sampling sites. *Diabetes Care* 25: 961–964, 2002.

Ello-Martin JA, Ledikwe JH, Rolls BJ: The influence of food portion size and energy density on energy intake: implications for weight management. *Am J Clin Nutr* 82 (Suppl):236S–241S, 2005.

El-Serag HB, Tran T, Everhart JE: Diabetes increases the risk of chronic liver disease and hepatocellular carcinoma. *Gastroenterology* 126:460–468, 2004.

Endemann DH, Schiffrin EL: Nitric oxide, oxidative excess, and vascular complications of diabetes melllllitus. *Curr Hypertens Rep* 6:85–89, 2004.

Eng GS, Chi MMY, Moley KH: Metformin increases glucose uptake by mouse blastocysts leading to decreased apoptosis. *Diabetes* 63 (Suppl 2): A17, 2004.

Englegau MM, Herman WH, Smith PJ, German RR, Aubert RE: The epidemiology of diabetes and pregnancy in the U.S., 1988. *Diabetes Care* 18:1029–1033, 1995.

Engstrom I, Kroon M, Arvidsson C-G, Segnestam K, Snellman K, Aman J: Eating disorders in adolescent girls with insulin-dependent diabetes mellitus: a population-based case-control study. *Acta Pediatr* 88:175–180, 1999.

Engum A, Mykletun A, Midthjell K, Holen A, Dahl AA: Depression and diabetes. A large population-based study of sociodemographic, lifestyle, and clinical factors associated with depression in type 1 and type 2 diabetes. *Diabetes Care* 28: 1904–1909, 2005.

EPA—U.S. Environmental Protection Agency: Mercury levels in commercial fish and shellfish. Updated February 2006. Available at: http://www.cfsan.fda.gov/~frf/sea-mehg.html. Accessed Mar 14, 2008.

Ericsson A, Hamark B, Jansson N, Johansson BR, Powell TL, Jansson T: Hormonal regulation of glucose and system A amino acid transport in first trimester placental villous fragments. *Am J Physiol* 288:R656–R662, 2005a.

Ericsson A, Hamark B, Powell TL, Jansson T: Glucose transporter isoform 4 is expressed in the syncytiotrophoblast of first trimester human placenta. *Hum Reprod* 20:521–530, 2005b.

Ertl AC, Davis SN: Evidence for a vicious cycle of exercise and hypoglycemia in type 1 diabetes mellitus. *Diabetes Metab Res Rev* 20:124–130, 2004.

Estrich D, Ravnik A, Schlierf G, Fukayama G, Kinsell L: Effects of co-ingestion of fat and protein upon carbohydrate-induced hyperglycemia. *Diabetes* 16:232–237, 1967.

Evers IM, de Valk HW, Mol BWJ, ter Braak EWMT, Visser GHA: Macrosomia despite good glycaemic control in type 1 diabetic pregnancy; results of a nationwide study in the Netherlands. *Diabetologia* 45:1484–1489, 2002a.

Evers IM, ter Braak E W, de Valk H W, van der Schoot B, Janssen N, Visser G H: Risk indicators predictive for severe hypoglycemia during the first trimester of type 1 diabetic pregnancy. *Diabetes Care* 25: 554–559, 2002b.

Evers IM, de Valk HW, Visser GHA: Risk of complications of pregnancy in women with type 1 diabetes: nationwide prospective study in the Netherlands. *BMJ* 328:915–918, 2004.

Eyles D, Brown J, MacKay-Sim A, McGrath J, Feron F: Vitamin D3 and brain development. *Neuroscience* 118:641–653, 2003.

Fabiani E, Catassi C; International Working Group: The serum IgA class anti-tissue transglutaminase antibodies in the diagnosis and follow up of celiac disease. Results of an international multi-centre study. International Working Group on Eu-tTG. *Eur J Gastroenterol Hepatol* 13:659–665, 2001.

Fagen C, King JD, Erick M: Nutrition management in women with gestational diabetes mellitus: a review by the American Dietetic Association's Diabetes Care and Education Dietetic Practice Group. *J Am Diet Assoc* 95:460–467, 1995.

Fairburn CG, Cooper Z: The eating disorder examination. In: Fairburn CG, Wilson GT, eds. *Binge Eating: Nature, Assessment, and Treatment.* 12th ed. New York: Guilford Press; 1993a:317–356.

Fairburn CG, Marcus MD, Wilson GT: Cognitive behavioral therapy for binge eating and bulimia nervosa: a comprehensive treatment manual. In: Fairburn CG, Wilson GT, eds. *Binge Eating: Nature, Assessment, and Treatment.* 12th ed. New York: Guilford Press; 1993b:361–404.

Falluca F, Sabbatini A, Di Biase N, Borrello E, Napoli A, Sciullo E: Fetal pancreatic function in infants of diabetic and rhesus-isoimmunized women. *Obstet Gynecol* 95:195–198, 2000.

Farrag OAM: Prospective study of 3 metabolic regimens in pregnant diabetics. *Aust N Z J Obstet Gynecol* 27:6–9, 1987.

Farrar D, Tuffnell DJ, West J: Continuous subcutaneous insulin infusion versus multiple daily injections of insulin for pregnant women with diabetes. *Cochrane Database Syst Rev* July 18, 2007;(3):CD005542.

Farrell T, Neale L, Cundy T: Congenital anomalies in the offspring of women with type 1, type 2 and gestational diabetes. *Diabet Med* 19:322–326, 2002.

Farrell GC, Larter CZ: Nonalcoholic fatty liver disease: from steatosis to cirrhosis. *Hepatology* 43 (2 Suppl 1):S99–S112, 2006.

Fasano A, Not T, Wang W, uzzau S, Berti I, Tommasini A, Goldblum SE: Zonulin, a newly discovered modulator of intestinal permeability, and its expression in celiac disease. *Lancet* 355:1518–1519, 2000.

Fasano A, Berti I, Gerarduzzi T, Not T, Colletti RB, Drago S, Elitsur Y, Green PH, Guandalini S, Hill ID, Pietzak M, Ventura A, Thorpe M, Kryszak D, Fornaroli F, Wasserman SS, Murray JA, Horvath K: Prevalence of celiac disease in at-risk and not-at-risk groups in the United States: a large multicenter study. *Arch Intern Med* 163:286–292, 2003.

Faure P: Protective effects of antioxidant micronutrients (vitamin E, zinc and selenium) in type 2 diabetes mellitus. *Clin Chem Lab Med* 41:995–998, 2003.

Faure P, Ramon O, Favier A, Halimi S: Selenium supplementation decreases nuclear factor-kappa B activity in peripheral blood mononuclear cells from type 2 diabetic patients. *Eur J Clin Invest* 34:475–481, 2004.

FDA—Food and Drug Administration, Center for Food Safety and Applied Nutrition: What you need to know about mercury in fish and shellfish. March, 2004a. Available at: www.cfsan.fda.gov/~dms/admegh3.html. Accessed Mar 14, 2008.

FDA—Food and Drug Administration, Center for Food Safety and Applied Nutrition: Mercury in fish: FDA monitoring program (1990–2003). March, 2004b. Available at: http://www.cfsan.fda.gov/~frf/seamehg2.html. Accessed Mar 14, 2008.

Federici M, Zucaro L, Porzio O, Massoud R, Borboni P, Lauro D, Sesti G: Increased expression of insulin/insulin-like growth factor-I hybrid receptors in skeletal muscle of noninsulin-dependent diabetes mellitus subjects. *J Clin Invest* 98:2887–2893, 1996.

Federici M, Porzio O, Zucaro L, Fusco A, Borboni P, Lauro D, Sesti G: Distribution of insulin/insulin-like growth factor-I hybrid receptors in human tissues. *Mol Cell Endocrinol* 129:121–126, 1997a.

Federici M, Porzio O, Zucaro L, Giovannone B, Borboni P, Marini MA, Lauro D, Sesti G: Increased abundance of insulin/insulin-like growth factor-I hybrid receptors in adipose tissue from NIDDM patients. *Mol Cell Endocrinol* 135:41–47, 1997b.

Federici M, Giaccari A, Hribal ML, Giavannone B, Lauro D, Morviducci L, Pastore L, Tamburrano G, Lauro R, Sesti G: Evidence for glucose/hexosamine in vivo regulation of insulin/IGF-I hybrid receptor assembly. *Diabetes* 48:2277–2285, 1999.

Feelders RA, Kuiper-Kramer EP, van Eijk HG: Structure, function and clinical significance of transferrin receptors. *Clin Chem Lab Med* 37:1–10, 1999.

Feig DS, Palda VA: Type 2 diabetes in pregnancy: a growing concern. *Lancet* 359:1690–1692, 2002.

Feig DS, Razzaq A, Sykora K, Hux JE, Anderson GM: Trends in deliveries, prenatal care, and obstetrical complications in women with pregestational diabetes. A population-based study in Ontario, Canada, 1996–2001. *Diabetes Care* 29:232–235, 2006.

Ferguson R, Holmes GK, Cooke WT: Celiac disease, fertility, and pregnancy. *Scand J Gastroenterol* 17:65–68, 1982.

Ferguson BJ, Skikne BS, Simpson KM, Baynes RD, Cook JD: Serum transferrin receptor distinguishes the anemia of chronic disease from iron deficiency anemia. *J Lab Clin Med* 119:385–390, 1992.

Fernandes-Costa F, Metz J: Levels of transcobalamins I, II, and III during pregnancy and in cord blood. *Am J Clin Nutr* 35:87–94, 1982.

Fernandez-Real JM, Lopez-Bermejo A, Ricart W: Perspectives in diabetes. Cross-talk between iron metabolism and diabetes. *Diabetes* 51:2348–2354, 2002.

Ferner RE, Neil HA: Sulphonylureas and hypoglycemia. *BMJ* 296:949–950, 1988.

Fernqvist-Forbes E, Linde B, Gunnarsson R: Insulin absorption and subcutaneous blood flow in normal subjects during hypoglycemia in man. *J Clin Endocrinol Metab* 67:619–623, 1988.

Ferrer E, Alegria A, Barbera R, Farre R, Lagarda MJ, Monleone J: Whole blood selenium content in pregnant women. *Sci Total Environ* 227:139–143, 1999.

Ferrera DE, Taylor WR: Iron chelation and vascular function. In search of the mechanisms. Editorial. *Aterioscler Thromb Vasc Biol* 25:2235–2237, 2005.

Ferretti G, Bacchetti T, Rabini RA, Vignini A, Nanetti L, Moroni C, Mazzanti L: Homocysteinylation of low-density lipoproteins (LDL) from subjects with type 1 diabetes: effect on oxidative damage of human endothelial cells. *Diabet Med* 23:808–813, 2006.

Ferris AM, Reece EA: Nutritional consequences of chronic maternal conditions during pregnancy and lactation: lupus and diabetes. *Am J Clin Nutr* 59 (Suppl):465S–473S, 1994.

Fesenmeier MF, Coppage KH, Lambers DS, Barton JR, Sibai BM: Acute fatty liver of pregnancy in 3 tertiary care centers. *Am J Obstet Gynecol* 192:1416–1419, 2005.

Fetita LS, Sobngwi E, Serradas P, Calvo F, Gautier JF: Consequences of fetal exposure to maternal diabetes in offspring. *J Clin Endocrinol Metab* 91:3714–3724, 2006.

Fett JD, Ansari AA, Sundstrom JB, Combs GF: Peripartum cardiomyopathy: a selenium disconnection and an autoimmune connection. *Int J Cardiol* 86: 311–316, 2002.

Fierens S, Mairesse H, Heilier JF, De Burbure C, Focant JF, Eppe G, De Pauw E, Bernard A: Dioxin/polychlorinated biphenyl body burden, diabetes and endometriosis: findings in a population-based study in Belgium. *Biomarkers* 8:529–534, 2003.

Fishbein MH, Miner M, Mogren C, Chalekson J: The spectrum of fatty acid liver in obese children and the relationship of serum amionotransferases to severity of steatosis. *J Pediatr Gastroenterol Nutr* 36:54–61, 2003.

Fisher JM, Taylor KB: Placental transfer of gastric antibodies. *Lancet* 1(7492): 695–698, 1967.

Fisher MC, Zeisel SH, Mar MH, Sadler TW: Inhibitors of choline uptake and metabolism cause developmental abnormalities in neuralating mouse embryos. *Teratology* 64:114–122, 2001a.

Fisher L, Chesla CA, Mullan JT, Skaff MM, Kanter RA: Contributors to depression in Latino and European-American patients with type 2 diabetes. *Diabetes Care* 24:1751–1757, 2001b.

Flores-Mateo G, Navas-Acien A, Pastr-Barriuso R, Guallar E: Selenium and coronary heart disease: a meta-analysis. *Am J Clin Nutr* 84:762–773, 2006.

Fong TL, Dooley CP, Dehesa M, Cohen H, Carmel R, Fitzgibbons PL, Perez-Perez GI, Blaser MJ: *Heliobacter pylori* infection in pernicious anemia: a prospective controlled study. *Gastroenterology* 100:328–332, 1991.

Fong DS, Aiello L, Gardner TW, King GL, Blankenship G, Cavallerano JD, Ferris FL III, Klein R: Retinopathy in diabetes. Position statement. *Diabetes Care* 27 (Suppl.1):S84–S87, 2004.

Forbes S, Moonan M, Robinson S, Anyaoku V, Patterson M, Murphy KG, Ghatei MA, Bloom SR, Johnston DG: Impaired circulating glucagon-like peptide-1 response to oral glucose in women with previous gestational diabetes. *Clin Endocrinol (Oxf)* 62:51–55, 2005.

Forman BM, Tontonoz P, Chen J, Brun RP, Spiegelman BM, Evans RM: 15-Deoxy-delta 12, 14-prostaglandin J2 is a ligand for the adipocyte determination factor PPAR gamma. *Cell* 83:803–812, 1995.

Forsbach G, Vasquez-Lara J, Alvarez-Garcia C, Vasquez-Rosales J: Diabetes and pregnancy in Mexico. *Rev Invest Clin* 50:227–231, 1998.

Forsen T, Eriksson J, Tuomilehto J, Reunanen A, Osmond C, Barker D: The fetal and childhood growth of persons who develop type 2 diabetes. *Ann Intern Med* 133:176–182, 2000.

Forst G, Dornhorst A: The relevance of the glycemic index to our understanding of dietary carbohydrates. *Diabet Med* 17:336–345, 2000.

Foster-Powell K, Holt SH, Brand-Miller JC: International tables of glycemic index and glycemic load values: 2002. *Am J Clin Nutr* 76:5–56, 2002.

Fournier T, Tsatsaris V, Handschuh K, Evain-Brion D: PPARs and the placenta. *Placenta* 28:65–76, 2007.

Franko DL, Spurrell EB: Detection and management of eating disorders during pregnancy. *Obstet Gynecol* 95:942–946, 2000.

Franko DL, Blais MA, Becker AE, Delinsky SS, Greenwood DN, Flores AT, Ekeblad ER, Eddy KT, Herzog DB: Pregnancy complications and neonatal outcomes in women with eating disorders. *Am J Psychiatry* 158:1461–1466, 2001.

Franz MJ, Monk A, Barry B, McClain K, Weaver T, Cooper N, Upham P, Bergenstal R, Mazze RS: Effectiveness of medical nutrition therapy provided by dietitians in the management of non-insulin-dependent diabetes mellitus: a randomized controlled trial. *J Am Diet Assoc* 95:1009–1017, 1995a.

Franz MJ, Splett PL, Monk A, Barry B, McClain K, Weaver T, Upham P, Bergenstal R, Mazze RS: Cost-effectiveness of medical nutrition therapy provided by dietitians for persons with non-insulin-dependent diabetes mellitus. *J Am Diet Assoc* 95:1018–1024, 1995b.

Franz MJ, Bantle JP, Beebe CA, Brunzell JD, Chiasson J-L, Garg A, Holzmeister LE, Hoogwerf B, Mayer-Davis E, Mooradian AD, Purnell JQ, Wheeler M: Evidence-based nutrition principles and recommendations for the treatment and prevention of diabetes and related complications. ADA technical review. *Diabetes Care* 25:148–198, 2002.

Fraser RB, Ford FA, Lawrence GF: Insulin sensitivity in third trimester pregnancy. A randomized study of dietary effects. *Br J Obstet Gynecol* 95:223–229, 1988.

Fraser R: Diabetic control in pregnancy and intrauterine growth of the fetus. *Br J Obstet Gynecol* 102:275–277, 1995.

Fraser-Reynolds KA, Butzner JD, Stephure DK, Trussell RA, Scott RB: Use of immunoglobulin A-antiendomysial antibody to screen for celiac disease in North American children with type 1 diabetes. *Diabetes Care* 21:1985–1989, 1998.

Frazer DM, Anderson GJ: Iron imports. I. Intestinal iron absorption and its regulation. *Am J Physiol* 289:G631–G635, 2005.

Freeman HJ: Biopsy-defined adult celiac disease in Asian-Canadians. *Can J Gastroenterol* 17:433–436, 2003.

Freemantle N, Blonde L, Duhot D, Hompesch M, Eggertsen R, Hobbs FDR, Martinez L, Ross S, Bolinder B, Stridde E: Availability of inhaled insulin promotes greater perceived acceptance of insulin therapy in patients with type 2 diabetes. *Diabetes Care* 28:427–428, 2005.

Freemark M, Levitsky LL: Screening for celiac disease in children with type 1 diabtetes. *Diabetes Care* 26:1932–1939, 2003.

Freinkel N: The Banting lecture 1980: of pregnancy and progeny. *Diabetes* 29:1023–1035, 1980.

Frenkel EP, Yardley DA: Clinical and laboratory features and sequelae of deficiency of folic acid (folate) and vitamin B12 (cobalamin) in pregnancy and gynecology. *Hematol Oncol Clin North Am* 14:1079–1100, 2000.

Frery N, Huel G, Leroy M, Moreau T, Savard R, Blot P, Lellouch J: Vitamin B12 among parturients and their newborns and its relationship with birthweight. *Eur J Obstet Gynecol Reprod Biol* 45:155–163, 1992.

Freund KM, Graham SM, Lesky LG, Moskowitz MA: Detection of bulimia in a primary care setting. *J Gen Intern Med* 8:236–242, 1993.

Frezza M, di Padova C, Pozzato G, Terpin M, Baraona E, Lieber CS: High blood alcohol levels in women. The role of decreased gastric alcohol dehydrogenase activity and first-pass metabolism. *N Engl J Med* 322:95–99, 1990.

Fronczak CM, Baron AE, Chase HP, Ross C, Brady HL, Hoffman M, Eisenbarth GS, Rewers M, Norris JM: In utero dietary exposures and risk of autoimmunity in children. *Diabetes Care* 26:3237–3242, 2003.

Fuglsang J, Lauszus F, Flyvbjerg A, Ovesen P: Human placental growth hormone, insulin-like growth factor I and II, and insulin requirements during pregnancy in type 1 diabetes. *J Clin Endocrinol Metab* 88:4355–4361, 2003.

Fuglsang J, Lauszus FF, Fisker S, Flyvbjerg A, Ovesen P: Growth hormone binding protein and maternal body mass index in relation to placental growth hormone and insulin requirements during pregnancy in type 1 diabetic women. *Growth Horm IGF Res* 15:223–230, 2005.

Funnell MM, Brown TL, Childs BP, Haas LB, Hosey GM, Jensen B, Maryniuk M, Peyrot M, Piette JD, Reader D, Siminerio LM, Weinger K, Weiss MA: National standards for diabetes self-management education. *Diabetes Care* 31 (Suppl 1): S97–S104, 2008.

Fujimoto S, Kawakami N, Ohara A: Nonenzymatic glycation of transferrin: decrease of iron-binding capacity and increase of oxygen radical production. *Biol Pharm Bull* 18:396–400, 1995.

Fujioka K: Follow-up of nutritional and metabolic problems after bariatric surgery. *Diabetes Care* 28:481–484, 2005.

Fujisawa T, Ikegami H, Inoue K, Kawabata Y, Ogihara T: Effect of α-glucosidase inhibitors, voglibose and acarbose, on postprandial hyperglycemic correlates with subjective abdominal symptoms. *Metab Clin Exper* 54:387–390, 2005.

Fulgoni VL III, Miller GD: Dietary reference intakes for food labeling. *Am J Clin Nutr* 83 (Suppl):1215S–1216S, 2006.

Fung EB, Ritchie LD, Woodhouse LR, Roehl R, King JC: Zinc absorption in women during pregnancy and lactation: a longitudinal study. *Am J Clin Nutr* 66:80–88, 1997.

Gabbe SG, Mestman JH, Freeman RK, Goebelsmann UT, Lowensohn RI, Nochimson D, Cetrulo C, Quilligan EJ: Management and outcome of pregnancy in diabetes mellitus, classes B to R. *Am J Obstet Gynecol* 129:723–732, 1977.

Gabbe SG, Holing E, Temple P, Brown ZA: Benefits, risks, costs, and patient satisfaction associated with insulin pump therapy for the pregnancy complicated by type 1 diabetes mellitus. *Am J Obstet Gynecol* 182:1283–1291, 2000.

Gabbe SG, Graves C: Management of diabetes mellitus complicating pregnancy. *Obstet Gynecol* 102:857–868, 2003.

Gaither K, Quraishi AN, Illsley NP: Diabetes alters the expression and activity of the human placental GLUT1 glucose transporter. *J Clin Endocrinol Metab* 84: 695–701, 1999.

Galassetti P, Neill AR, Tate D, Ertl AC, Wasserman DH, Davis SN: Sexual dimorphism in counterregulatory responses to hypoglycemia after antecedent exercise. *J Clin Endocrinol Metab* 86:3516–3524, 2001.

Galassetti P, Tate D, Neill RA, Morrey S, Wasserman DH, Davis SN: Effect of antecedent hypoglycemia on counterregulatory responses to subsequent euglycemic exercise in type 1 diabetes. *Diabetes* 52:1761–1769, 2003.

Galassetti P, Tate D, Neill RA, Morrey S, Wasserman DH, Davis SN: Effect of sex on counterregulatory responses to exercise after antecedent hypoglycemia in type 1 diabetes. *Am J Physiol* 287:E16–E24, 2004.

Galassetti P, Tate D, Neill RA, Richardson A, Leu SY, Davis SN: Effect of differing antecedent hypoglycemia on counterregulatory responses to exercise in type 1 diabetes. *Am J Physiol Endocrinol Metab* 290:E1109–E1117, 2006.

Galgani J, Aguirre C, Diaz E: Acute effect of meal glycemic index and glycemic load on blood glucose and insulin responses in humans. *Nutr J* 5:22, 2006.

Gallen IW, Jaap AJ, Roland JM, Chirayath HH: Survey of glargine use in 115 pregnant women with type 1 diabetes. *Diabet Med* 25:165–169, 2008.

Galuska D, Nolte LA, Zierath JR, Wallberg-Henriksson H: Effect of metformin on insulin-stimulated glucose transport in isolated skeletal muscle obtained from patients with NIDDM. *Diabetologia* 37:826–832, 1994.

Gamble MV, Ahsan H, Liu X, Factor-Litvak P, Ilievski V, Slavkovich V, Parvez F, Graziano JH: Folate and cobalamin deficiencies and hyperhomocysteinemia in Bangladesh. *Am J Clin Nutr* 81:1372–1377, 2005.

Gambling L, Danzeisen R, Gair S, Lea RG, Charania Z, Solanky N, Joory KD, Srai SKS, McArdle HJ: Effect of iron deficiency on placental transfer of iron and expression of iron transport proteins in vivo and in vitro. *Biochem J* 356: 883–889, 2001.

Ganji V, Kafai MR: Population reference values for plasma total homocysteine concentrations in U.S. adults after the fortification of cereals with folic acid. *Am J Clin Nutr* 84:989–994, 2006.

Gannon MC, Nuttall FQ, Saeed S, Jordan K, Hoover H: An increase in dietary protein improves the blood glucose response in persons with type 2 diabetes. *Am J Clin Nutr* 78:734–741, 2003.

Ganz T: Hepcidin, a key regulator of iron metabolism and mediator of anemia of inflammation. *Blood* 102:783–788, 2003.

Ganz T: Is TfR2 the iron sensor? Commentary. *Blood* 104:3829–3830, 2004.

Ganz T, Nemeth E: Iron imports. IV. Hepcidin and regulation of body iron metabolism. *Am J Physiol* 290:G199–G203, 2006.

Garcia-Bournissen F, Feig DS, Koren G: Maternal-fetal transport of hypoglycemic drugs. *Clin Pharmacokinet* 42:303–313, 2003.

Garg SK, Frias JP, Sunitha A, Gottlieb PA, MacKenzie T, Jackson WE: Insulin lispro therapy in pregnancies complicated by type 1 diabetes: glycemic control and maternal and fetal outcomes. *Endocr Pract* 9:187–193, 2003.

Garner SC, Chou SC, Mar MH, Coleman RA, Zeisel SH: Characterization of choline metabolism and secretion by human placental trophoblasts in culture. *Biochim Biophys Acta* 1168:358–364, 1993.

Gary TL, Crum RM, Cooper-Patrick L, Ford D, Brancati FL: Depressive symptoms and metabolic control in African-Americans with type 2 diabetes. *Diabetes Care* 23:23–29, 2000.

Gary TL, Genkinger JM, Guallar E, Pevrot M, Brancati FL: Meta-analysis of randomized educational and behavioral interventions in type 2 diabetes. *Diabetes Educ* 29:488–501, 2003.

Gavrilova O, Haluzik M, Matsusue K, Cutson JJ, Johnson L, Dietz KR, Nicol CJ, Vinson C, Gonzalez FJ, Reitman ML: Liver peroxisome proliferators-activated receptor β contributes to hepatic steatosis, triglyceride clearance, and regulation of body fat mass. *J Biol Chem* 278:34268–34276, 2003.

Geary MP, Pringle PJ, Rodeck CH, Kingdom JC, Hindmarsh PC: Sexual dimorphism in the growth hormone and insulin-like growth factor axis at birth. *J Clin Endocrinol Metab* 88:3708–3714, 2003.

Gebauer SK, Psota TL, Harris WS, Kris-Etherton PM: n-3 Fatty acid dietary recommendations and food sources to achieve essentiality and cardiovascular benefits. *Am J Clin Nutr* 83 (Suppl):1526S–1535S, 2006.

Gentilcore D, Chaikomin R, Jones KL, Russo A, Feinle-Bisset C, Wishart JM, Rayner CK, Horowitz M: Effects of fat on gastric emptying of and the glycemic, insulin, and incretin responses to a carbohydrate meal in type 2 diabetes. *J Clin Endocrinol Metab* 91:2062–2067, 2006.

Gentile S: The safety of newer antidepressants in pregnancy and breastfeeding. *Drug Saf* 28:137–152, 2005.

George L, Mills JL, Johansson ALV, Olander B, Granath F, Cnattinguis S: Plasma folate levels and risk for spontaneous abortions. *JAMA* 288:1867–1873, 2002.

Georgieff MK, Landon MB, Mills MM, Hedlund BE, Faassen AE, Schmidt RL, Ophoven JJ, Widness JA: Abnormal iron distribution in infants of diabetic mothers: spectrum and maternal antecedents. *J Pediatr* 117:455–461, 1990.

Georgieff MK, Petry CD, Mills MM, McKay H, Wobken JD: Increased N-glycosylation and reduced transferrin binding capacity of transferrin receptor isolated from placentas of diabetic mothers. *Placenta* 18:563–568, 1997.

Georgieff MK, Berry SA, Wobken JD, Leibold EA: Increased placental iron regulatory protein-1 expression in diabetic pregnancies complicated by fetal iron deficiency. *Placenta* 20:87–93, 1999.

Georgieff MK, Wobken JK, Welle J, Burdo JR, Connor JR: Identification and localization of divalent metal transporter-1 (DMT-1) in term human placenta. *Placenta* 21:799–804, 2000.

Gerstle JF, Varenne H, Contento I: Post-diagnosis family adaptation influences glycemic control in women with type 2 diabetes mellitus. *J Am Diet Assoc* 101:918–922, 2001.

Gianfrani C, Levings MK, Sartirana C, Mazzarella G, Barba G, Zanzi D, Camarca A, Iaquinto G, Giardullo N, Auricchio S, Troncone R, Roncarolo MG: Gliadin-specific type 1 regulatory T cells from the intestinal mucosa of treated celiac patients inhibit pathogenic T cells. *J Immunol* 177:4178–4186, 2006.

Gibson JM, Westwood M, Lauszus FF, Klebe JG, Flyvbjerg A, White A: Phosphorylated insulin-like growth factor binding protein 1 is increased in pregnant diabetic subjects. *Diabetes* 48:321–326, 1999a.

Gibson EL, Checkley S, Papadopoulos A, Poon L, Daley S, Wardle J: Increased salivary cortisol reliably induced by a protein-rich midday meal. *Psychosom Med* 61:214–224, 1999b.

Giles PFH, Harcourt AG, Whiteside MG: The effect of prescribing folic acid during pregnancy on birth weight and duration of pregnancy: a double-blind trial. *Med J Aust* 2;17–21, 1971.

Gillen LJ, Tapsell LC, Patch CS, Owen A, Batterham M: Structured dietary advice incorporating walnuts achieves optimal fat and energy balance in patients with type 2 diabetes mellitus. *J Am Diet Assoc* 105:1087–1096, 2005.

Gillespie SJ, Kulkarni KD, Daly AE: Using carbohydrate counting in diabetes clinical practice. *J Am Diet Assoc* 98:897–905, 1998.

Gillett PM, Gillett HR, Israel DM, Metzger DL, Stewart L, Chanoine JP, Freeman HJ: High prevalence of celiac disease in patients with type 1 diabetes detected by antibodies to endomysium and tissue transglutaminase. *Can J Gastroenterol* 15:297–301, 2001.

Gillmer MD, Beard RW, Oakley NW, Brooke F, Elphick MC, Hull D: Diurnal plasma free fatty acid profiles in normal and diabetic pregnancies. *Br Med J* 2:670–673, 1977.

Gilmer MD, Maresh M, Beard RW, Elkeles RS, Alderson C, Bloxham B: Low energy diets in the treatment of gestational diabetes. *Acta Endocrinol* 277 (Suppl):44–49, 1986.

Gimenez M, Conget I, Nicolau J, Levy I: Outcome of pregnancy in women with type 1 diabetes intensively treated with continuous subcutaneous insulin infusion or conventional therapy. A case-control study. *Acta Diabetol* 44:34–37, 2007.

Giugliani ER, Jorge SM, Goncalves AL: Folate and vitamin B12 deficiency among parturients from Porto Alegre, Brazil. *Rev Invest Clin* 36:133–136, 1984.

Giugliano D, Ceriello A, Esposito K: The effects of diet on inflammation. Emphasis on the metabolic syndrome. State-of-the-art paper. *J Am Coll Cardiol* 48: 677–685, 2006.

Glasgow RE, Fisher EB, Anderson BJ, La Greca A, Marrero D, Johnson SB, Rubin RR, Coc DJ: Behavioral science in diabetes. *Diabetes Care* 22:832–843, 1999a.

Glasgow RE, Anderson RM: Moving from compliance to adherence is not enough. *Diabetes Care* 22:2090–2092, 1999b.

Glueck CJ, Wang P, Goldenberg N, Sieve-Smith L: Pregnancy outcomes among women with polycystic ovary syndrome treated with metformin. *Hum Reprod* 17:2858–2864, 2002a.

Glueck CJ, Wang P, Kobayashi S, Phillips H, Sieve-Smith L: Metformin therapy throughout pregnancy reduces the development of gestational diabetes in women with polycystic ovary syndrome. *Fertil Steril* 77:520–525, 2002b.

Glueck CJ, Bornovali S, Pranikoff J, Goldenberg N, Dharashivkar S, Wang P: Metformin, pre-eclampsia, and pregnancy outcomes in women with polycystic ovary syndrome. *Diabet Med* 21:829–836, 2004.

Godfrey K, Robinson S, Barker DJP, Osmond C, Cox V: Maternal nutrition in early and late pregnancy in relation to placental and fetal growth. *BMJ* 312:410–414, 1996.

Godsland IF, Elkeles RS, Feher MD, Nugara F, Rubens MB, Richmond W, Khan M, Donovan J, Anyaoku V, Flather MD; the Predict Study Group: Coronary calcification, homocysteine, C-reactive protein and the metabolic syndrome in type 2 diabetes: the Prospective Evaluation of Diabetic Ischemic Heart Disease by Coronary Tomography (PREDICT) Study. *Diabet Med* 23:1192–1200, 2006.

Goebel-Fabbri AE, Fikkan J, Connell A, Vangsness L, Anderson BJ: Identification and treatment of eating disorders in women with type 1 diabetes mellitus. *Treat Endocrinol* 1:155–162, 2002.

Goh YI, Bollano E, Einarson TR, Koren G: Prenatal multivitamin supplementation and rates of congenital anomalies: a meta-analysis. *J Obstet Gynecol Can* 28: 680–689, 2006.

Gold AE, Reilly R, Little J, Walker JD. The effect of glycemic control in the preconception period and early pregnancy on birth weight in women with IDDM. *Diabetes Care* 21:535–528, 1998.

Goldberg HL, Nissim R: Psychotropic drugs in pregnancy and lactation. *Int J Psychiatr Med* 24:129–149, 1994.

Goldberg RB, Kendall DM, Deeg MA, Buse JB, Zagar AJ, Pinaire JA, Tan MH, Khan MA, Perez AT, Jacober SJ; GLAI Study Investigators: A comparison of lipid and glycemic effects of pioglitazone and rosiglitazone in patients with type 2 diabetes and dyslipidemia. *Diabetes Care* 28:1547–1554, 2005.

Goldenberg RL, Tamura T, Neggers Y, Copper RI, Johnston KE, DuBard MB, Hauth JC: The effect of zinc supplementation on pregnancy outcome. *JAMA* 274: 463–468, 1995.

Goldenberg RL, Tamura T, DuBard M, Johnston KE, Copper RL, Neggers Y: Plasma ferritin and pregnancy outcome. *Am J Obstet Gynecol* 175:1356–1359, 1996.

Goldenberg RL: The plausibility of micronutrient deficiency in relationship to perinatal infection. *J Nutr* 133:1645S–1648S, 2003.

Goldney RD, Phillips PJ, Fisher LJ, Wilson DH: Diabetes, depression, and quality of life. A population study. *Diabetes Care* 27:1066–1070, 2004.

Goldstein DE, Drash A, Gibbs J, Blizzard RM: Diabetes mellitus: the incidence of circulating antibodies against thyroid, gastric, and adrenal tissue. *J Pediatr* 77:304–306, 1970.

Goldstein DE, Little RR, Lorenz RA, Malone JI, Nathan D, Peterson CM, Sacks DB: Tests of glycemia in diabetes. Technical review. *Diabetes Care* 27:1761–1773, 2004.

Golstein PE, Boom A, van Geffel J, Jacobs P, Masereel B, Beauwens R: P-glycoprotein inhibition by glibenclamide and related compounds. *Pflugers Arch* 437:652–660, 1999.

Golub MS, Hogrefe CE, Tarantal AF, Germann SL, Beard JL, Georgieff MK, Calatroni A, Lozoff B: Diet-induced iron deficiency anemia and pregnancy outcome in rhesus monkeys. *Am J Clin Nutr* 83:647–656, 2006.

Gonzalez C, Santoro S, Salzberg S, Di Girolamo G, Alvarinas J: Insulin analogue therapy in pregnancies complicated by diabetes mellitus. Expert Opin Pharmacother 6:735–742, 2005.

Gonzalez NL, Ramirez O, Mozas J, Melchor J, Armas H, Garcia-Hernandez JA, Caballero A, Hernandez M, Diaz-Gomez MN, Jimenez A, Parache J, Bartha JL: Factors influencing pregnancy outcome in women with type 2 versus type 1 diabetes mellitus. *Acta Obstet Gynecol Scand* 87:43–49, 2008.

Goode LR, Brolin RE, Hasina A: Bone and gastric bypass surgery: effects of dietary calcium and vitamin D. *Obes Res* 12:40–46, 2004.

Gordon MC, Zimmerman PD, Landon MB, Gabbe SG, Kniss DA: Insulin and glucose modulate glucose transporter messenger ribonucleic acid expression and glucose uptake in trophoblasts isolated from first-trimester chorionic villi. *Am J Obstet Gynecol* 173:1089–1097, 1995.

Gosriwatana I, Loreal O, Lu S, Brissot P, Porter J, Hider RC: Quantification of non-transferrin-bound iron in the presence of unsaturated transferrin. *Anal Biochem* 273:212–220, 1999.

Gossell-Williams M, Fletcher H, McFarlane-Anderson N, Jacob A, Patel J, Zeisel S: Dietary intake of choline and plasma choline concentrations in pregnant women in Jamaica. *West Indian Med J* 54:355–359, 2005.

Gottlieb PA, Frias JP, Peters KA, Chillara B, Garg SK: Optimizing insulin therapy in pregnant women with type 1 diabetes mellitus. *Treat Endocrinol* 1:235–240, 2002.

Graham TE, Sathasivam P, Rowland M, Marko N, Greer F, Battram D: Caffeine ingestion elevates plasma insulin response in humans during an oral glucose tolerance test. *Can J Physiol Pharmacol* 79:559–565, 2001.

Grandjean P, Weihe P, White RF, Debes F, Araki S, Yokoyama K, Murata K, Sorensen N, Dahl R, Jorgensen PJ: Cognitive deficit in 7-year-old children with prenatal exposure to methylmercury. *Neurotoxicol Teratol* 19:417–428, 1997.

Grandjean P, Weihe P, Burse VW, Needham LL, Storr-Hansen E, Heinzow B, Debes F, Murata J, Simonsen H, Ellefsen P, Budtz-Jorgensen E, Keidling N, White RF: Neurobehavioral deficits associated with PCB in 7-year-old children prenatally exposed to seafood neurotoxicants. *Neurotoxicol Teratol* 23:305–317, 2001.

Grandjean P, Weihe P: Arachidonic acid status during pregnancy is associated with polychlorinated biphenyl exposure. *Am J Clin Nutr* 77:715–719, 2003.

Grandjean P, Budtz-Jorgensen E, Jorgensen PJ, Weihe P: Umbilical cord mercury concentration as biomarker of prenatal exposure to methylmercury. *Environ Health Perspect* 113:905–908, 2005.

Granfeldt Y, Wu X, Bjorck I: Determination of glycaemic index; some methodological aspects related to the analysis of carbohydrate load and characterisitics of the previous evening meal. *Eur J Clin Nutr* 60:104–112, 2006.

Granstrom L, Granstrom L, Backman L: Fetal growth retardation after gastric banding. *Acta Obstet Gynecol Scand* 69:533–536, 1990.

Grant WB: Am estimate of premature cancer mortality in the U.S. due to inadequate doses of solar ultraviolet-B radiation. *Cancer* 94:1867–1875, 2002.

Gratecos E, Casals E, Deulofeu R, Cararach V, Alonso PL, Fortuny A: Lipid peroxide and vitamin E patterns in pregnant women with different types of hypertension in pregnancy. *Am J Obstet Gynecol* 178:1072–1076, 1998.

Gray RS, Cowan P Steel JM, Johnstone FD, Clarke BF, Duncan LJP: Insulin action and pharmacokinetics in insulin treated diabetics during the third trimester of pregnancy. *Diabet Med* 1:273–278, 1984.

Gray KA, Klebanoff MA, Brock JW, Zhou H, Darden R, Needham L, Longnecker MP: In utero exposure to background levels of polychlorinated biphenyls and cognitive functioning among school-age children. *Am J Epidemiol* 162:17–26, 2005.

Gray IP, Cooper PA, Cory BJ, Toman M, Crowther NJ: The intrauterine environment is a strong determinant of glucose tolerance during the neonatal period, even in prematurity. *J Clin Endocrinol Metab* 87:4252–4256, 2006.

Greco L, Romino R, Coto I, Di Cosmo N, percopo S, Maglio M, Paparo F, Gasperi V, Limongelli MG, Cotichini R, D'Agate C, Tinto N, Sacchetti L, Tosi R, Stazi MA: The first large population based twin study of celiac disease. *Gut* 50: 624–628, 2002.

Green DW, Khoury J, Mimouni F: Neonatal hematocrit and maternal glycemic control in insulin-dependent diabetes. *J Pediatr* 120:302–305, 1992.

Green PHR, Stavropoulos SN, Panagi SG, Goldstein SL, Mcmahon DJ, Absan H, Neugut AI: Characteristics of adult celiac disease in the USA: results of a national survey. *Am J Gastroenterol* 96:126–131, 2001.

Green PH, Jabri B: Celiac disease. *Lancet* 362:383–391, 2003a.

Green PH, Fleischauer AT, Bhagat G, Goyal R, Jabri B, Neugut AI: Risk of malignancy in patients with celiac disease. *Am J Med* 115:191–195, 2003b.

Green PHR: The many faces of celiac disease: clinical presentation of celiac disease in the adult population. *Gastroenterology* 128:S74–S78, 2005.

Greenberg JA, Boozer CN, Geliebter A: Coffee, diabetes, and weight control. *Am J Clin Nutr* 84:682–693, 2006.

Greer F, Hudson R, Ross R, Graham T: Caffeine ingestion decreases glucose disposal during a hyperinsulinemic-euglycemic clamp in sedentary humans. *Diabetes* 50:2349–2354, 2001.

Gregory RP, Davis DL: Use of carbohydrate counting for meal planning in type 1 diabetes. *Diabetes Educ* 20:406–409, 1994.

Greiner RCS, Zhang Q, Goodman KJ, Glussani DA, Nathanielsz PW, Brenna JT: Linoleate, α-linolenate, and docosahexaenoate recycling into saturated and monounsaturated fatty acids is a major pathway in pregnant or lactating adults and fetal or infant Rhesus monkeys. *J Lipid Res* 37:2675–2686, 1996.

Grice HC, Goldsmith LA: Sucralose: an overview of the toxicity data. *Food Chem Toxicol* 38 (Suppl 2):S1–S6, 2000.

Griendling KK, Sorescu D, Ushio-Fukai M: NAD(P)H oxidase: role in cardiovascular biology and disease. *Circ Res* 86:494–501, 2000.

Griendling K: ATVB in focus: redox mechanisms in blood vessels. *Arterioscler Thromb Vasc Biol* 25:272–273, 2005.

Grinshtein N, Bamm VV, Tsemakhovich VA, Shaklai N: Mechanism of low-density lipoprotein oxidation by hemoglobin-derived iron. *Biochemistry* 42:6977–6985, 2003.

Groenen PM, van Rooij IA, Peer PG, Gooskens RH, Zielhuis GA, Steegers-Theunissen RP: Marginal maternal vitamin B12 status increases the risk of offspring with spina bifida. *Am J Obstet Gynecol* 191:11–17, 2004.

Groop L, DeFronzo R, Luzi L, Melander A: Hyperglycemia and absorption of sulfonylurea drugs. *Lancet* 2:129–130, 1989.

Groop LC, Barzalai N, Ratheiser K, Luzi L, Wahlin-Boll E, Melander A, DeFronzo RA: Dose-dependent effects of glyburide on insulin secretion and glucose uptake in humans. *Diabetes Care* 14:724–727, 1991.

Gross GA, Solenberger T, Philpott T, Holcomb WL Jr, Landt M: Plasma leptin concentrations in newborns of diabetic and nondiabetic mothers. *Am J Perinatol* 15:243–247, 1998.

Grotz VL, Henry RR, McGill JB, Prince MJ, Shamoon H, Trout JR, Pi-Sunyer FX: Lack of effect of sucralose on glucose homeostasis in subjects with type 2 diabetes. *J Am Diet Assoc* 103:1607–1612, 2003.

Gruper Y, Bar J, Bacharach E, Ehrlich R: Transferrin receptor co-localizes and interacts with the hemochromatosis factor (HFE) and the divalent metal transporter-1 (DMT1) in trophoblast cells. *J Cell Physiol* 204:901–912, 2005.

Grylli V, Wagner G, Hafferi-Gattermayer A, Schober E, Karwautz A: Disturbed eating attitudes, coping styles, and subjective quality of life in adolescents with type 1 diabetes. *J Psychosom Res* 59:65–72, 2005.

Gude NM, Stevenson JL, Rogers S, Best JD, Kalionis B, Huisman MA, Erwich JJ, Timmer A, King RG: GLUT 12 expression in human placenta in first trimester and term. *Placenta* 24:566–570, 2003.

Guelfi KJ, Jones TW, Fournier PA: Intermittent high-intensity exercise does not increase the risk of early postexercise hypoglycemia in individuals with type 1 diabetes. *Diabetes Care* 28:416–418, 2005a.

Guelfi KJ, Jones TW, Fournier PA: The decline in blood glucose levels is less with intermittent high-intensity compared with moderate exercise in individuals with type 1 diabetes. *Diabetes Care* 28:1289–1294, 2005b.

Guerci B, Floriot M, Boehme P, Durain D, Benichou M, Jelliman S, Drouin P: Clinical performance of CGMS in type 1 diabetic patients treated by continuous subcutaneous glucose insulin infusion using insulin analogs. *Diabetes Care* 26:582–589, 2003.

Guerci B, Sauvanet JP: Subcutaneous insulin: pharmacokinetic variability and glycemic variability. *Diabetes Metab* 31:4S7–4S24, 2005.

Guerin A, Nisenbaum R, Ray JG: Use of maternal GHb concentration to estimate the risk of congenital anomalies in the offspring of women with prepregnancy diabetes. *Diabetes Care* 30:1920–1925, 2007.

Guerrero R, Vasquez M, Amaya M, Dios E, Quijada D, Garcia-Hernandez N, Acosta D, Astorga R: Pregnancy planning and morbidity in pregnancies complicated by pregestational diabetes mellitus. *Diabetologia* 47 (Suppl 1):A361, 2004.

Gugliucci CL, O'Sullivan MJ, Opperman W, Gordon M, Stone ML: Intensive care of the pregnant diabetic. *Am J Obstet Gynecol* 125:435–441, 1976.

Guidry C, Feist R, Morris R, Hardwick CW: Changes in IGF activities in human diabetic vitreous. *Diabetes* 53:2428–2435, 2004.

Gunderson EP, Abrams B: Epidemiology of gestational weight gain and body weight changes after pregnancy. *Epidemiol Rev* 22:261–274, 2000.

Gunderson EP, Abrams B, Selvin S: The relative importance of gestational gain and maternal characteristics associated with the risk of becoming overweight after pregnancy. *Int J Obes Relat Metab Disord* 24:1660–1668, 2001.

Gunderson EP: Nutrition during pregnancy for the physically active woman. *Clin Obstet Gynecol* 46:390–402, 2003.

Gunderson EP: Gestational diabetes and nutritional recommendations. *Curr Diab Rep* 4:377–386, 2004.

Gunshin H, Fujiwara Y, Custodio AO, DiRenzo C, Robine S, Andrews NC: SIc11a2 is required for intestinal iron absorption and erythropoiesis but dispensable in placenta and liver. *J Clin Investig* 115:1258–1266, 2005.

Gunton JE, McElduff A, Sulway M, Stiel J, Kelso I, Boyce S, Fulcher G, Robinson B, Clifton-Bligh P, Wilmshurst E: Outcome of pregnancies complicated by pre-gestational diabetes mellitus. *Aust N Z J Obstet Gynecol* 40:38–43, 2000.

Gunton JE, Hams G, Hitchman R, McElduff A: Serum chromium does not predict glucose intolerance in late pregnancy. *Am J Clin Nutr* 73:99–104, 2001.

Gunton JE, Cheung NW, Hitchman R, Hams G, O'Sullivan C, Foster-Powell K, McElduff A: Chromium supplementation does not improve glucose tolerance, insulin sensitivity, or lipid profile. A randomized, placebo-controlled, double-blind trial of supplementation in subjects with impaired glucose tolerance. *Diabetes Care* 28:712–713, 2005.

Guttormsen AB, Schneede J, Fiskerstrand T, Ueland PM, Refsum H: Plasma concentrations of homocysteine and other aminothiol compounds are related to food intake in healthy human subjects. *J Nutr* 124:1934–1941, 1994.

Gutzin SJ, Kozer E, Magee LA, Feig DS, Koren G: The safety of oral hypoglycemic agents in the first trimester of pregnancy: a meta-analysis. *Can J Clin Pharmacol* 10:179–183, 2003.

Guyton AC, Hall JE: Parathyroid hormone, calcitonin, calcium and phosphate metabolism, vitamin D, bone, and teeth. In: *Textbook of Medical Physiology.* 11th ed. Elsevier; 2005:899–915.

Gylling H, Tuominen JA, Koivisto VA, Miettinen TA: Cholesterol metabolism in type 1 diabetes. *Diabetes* 53:2217–2222, 2004.

Haakstad LA, Voldner N, Henriksen T, Bo K: Physical activity level and weight gain in a cohort of pregnant Norwegian women. *Acta Obstet Gynecol Scand* 86: 559–564, 2007.

Haboubi NY, Taylor S, Jones S: Celiac disease and oats: a systematic review. *Postgrad Med J* 82:672–678, 2006.

Hachey DL: Benefits and risks of modifying maternal fat intake in pregnancy and lactation. *Am J Clin Nutr* 59 (Suppl):454S–464S,1994.

Haddad EH, Tanzman JS: What do vegetarians in the United States eat? *Am J Clin Nutr* 78 (Suppl):626S–632S, 2003.

Hadden DR, Alexander A, McCance DR, Traub AI: Obstetric and diabetic care for pregnancy in diabetic women: 10 years outcome analysis, 1985–1995. *Diabet Med* 18:546–553, 2001.

Haffner SM: Management of dyslipidemia in adults with diabetes. ADA technical review. *Diabetes Care* 21:160–178, 1998.

Hager H, Gliemann J, Hamilton-Dutoit S, Ebbesen P, Koppelhus U, Jensen PH: Developmental regulation of tissue transglutaminase during human placentation and expression in neoplastic trophoblast. *J Pathol* 181:106–110, 1997.

Haggarty P: Placental regulation of fatty acid delivery and its effect on fetal growth—a review. *Placenta* 23:S28–S38, 2002.

Haggarty P: Effect of placental function on fatty acid requirements during pregnancy. *Eur J Clin Nutr* 58:1559–1570, 2004.

Hague WM, Davoren PM, Oliver J, Rowan J: Metformin may be useful in gestational diabetes. *BMJ* 326:762–763, 2002.

Hague WM, Davoran PM, McIntyre HD, Norris R, Xiaonian X, Charles B: Metformin crosses the placenta: a modulator for fetal insulin resistance? *BMJ* rapid response letter, Dec 3, 2003. Published online. Available at: www.bmj.bmjjournals.com/cgi/eletters/327/7420/880. Accessed Mar 14, 2008.

Hahn T, Hahn D, Blaschutz A, Korgun ET, Desoye G, Dohr G: Hyperglycemia-induced subcellular redistribution of GLUT1 glucose transporters in cultured human term placental trophoblast cells. *Diabetologia* 43:173–180, 2000.

Hakkola J, Raunio H, Purkunen R, Pelkonen O, Saarikoski S, Cresteil T, Pasanen M: Detection of cytochrome P450 gene expression in human placenta in first trimester of pregnancy. *Biochem Pharmacol* 52:379–383, 1996a.

Hakkola J, Pasanen M, Hukkanen J, Pelkonen O, Maenpaa J, Edwards RJ, Boobis AR, Raunio H: Expression of xenobiotic-metabolizing cytochrome P450 forms in human full-term placenta. *Biochem Pharmacol* 51:403–411, 1996b.

Hakkola J, Pelkonen O, Oasanen M, Raunio H: Xenobiotic-metabolizing cytochrome P450 enzymes in the human fetoplacental unit: role in intrauterine toxicity. *Crit Rev Toxicol* 28:35–72, 1998.

Halvorsen BL, Carlsen MH, Phillips KM, Bohn SK, Holte K, Jacobs DR Jr, Blomhoff R: Content of redox-active compounds (i.e., antioxidants) in foods consumed in the United States. *Am J Clin Nutr* 84:95–135, 2006.

Hamann A, Matthaei S, Rosak C, Silvestre L; for the HOE901/4007 Study Group: A randomized clinical trial comparing breakfast, dinner, or bedtime administration of insulin glargine in patients with type 1 diabetes. *Diabetes Care* 26:1738–1744, 2003.

Hambidge M: Biomarkers of trace mineral intake and status. *J Nutr* 133:948S–955S, 2003.

Hamiguchi M, Kojima T, Takeda N, Nakagawa T, Taniguchi H, Fujii K, Omatsu T, Nakajima T, Sarui H, Shimazaki M, Kato T, Okuda J, Ida K: The metabolic syndrome as a predictor of nonalcoholic fatty liver disease. *Ann Intern Med* 143:722–728, 2005.

Hammarstedt A, Andersson CX, Rotter Sopasakis V, Smith U: The effect of PPARgamma ligands on the adipose tissue in insulin resistance. *Prostaglandins Leukot Essent Fatty Acids* 73:65–75, 2005.

Hammes HP, Du X, Edelstein D, Taguchi T, Matsumura T, Ju Q, Lin J, Bierhaus A, Nawroth P, Hannak D, Neumaier M, Bergfeld R, Giardino I, Brownlee M: Benfotiamine blocks three major pathways of hyperglycemic damage and prevents experimental diabetic retinopathy. *Nat Med* 9:294–299, 2003.

Handschuh K, Guibourdenche J, Guesnon M, Laurendeau I, Evain-Brion D, Fournier T: Modulation of PAPP-A expression by PPARgamma in human first trimester trophoblast. *Placenta* 27 (Suppl A):S127–34, 2006.

Hankey GJ, Eikelboom JW, Ho WK, van Bockxmeer FM: Clinical usefulness of plasma homocysteine in vascular disease. *Med J Aust* 181:314–318, 2004.

Hannigan JH, Armant DR: Alcohol in pregnancy and neonatal outcome. *Semin Neonatal* 5:243–254, 2000.

Hansen D, Brock-Jacobsen B, Lund E, Bjorn C, Hansen LP, Nielsen C, Fenger C, Lillevang ST, Husby S: Clinical benefit of a gluten-free diet in type 1 diabetic children with screening-detected celiac disease. A population-based screening study with 2 years' follow-up. *Diabetes Care* 29:2452–2456, 2006.

Hanson U, Persson B, Enochsson E, Lennerhagen P, Lindgren F, Lundstrom V, Lunell N-O, Nilsson BA, Nilsson L, Stangenberg M, Thalme B, Tillinger K-G, Ofverholm U: Self-monitoring of blood glucose by diabetic women during the third trimester of pregnancy. *Am J Obstet Gynecol* 150:817–821, 1984.

Hanson U, Persson B: Outcome of pregnancies complicated by type 1 insulin-dependent diabetes in Sweden: acute pregnancy complications, neonatal mortality and morbidity. *Am J Perinatol* 10:330–333, 1993.

Hardmann B, Manuelpillai U, Wallace EM, Monty JF, Kramer DR, Kuo YM, Mercer JF, Ackland ML: Expression, localization and hormone regulation of the human copper transporter HCTR1 in placenta and choriocarcinoma Jeg-3 cells. *Placenta* 27:968–977, 2006.

Harley JMG, Montgomery DAD: Management of pregnancy complicated by diabetes. *Br Med J* 1:14–18, 1965.

Hartland AJ, Smith JM, Clarke PMS, Webber J, Chowdhury T, Dunne F: Establishing trimester- and ethnic group-related reference ranges for fructosamine and HBA1c in non-diabetic pregnant women. *Ann Clin Biochem* 36:235–237, 1999.

Haruma K, Komoto K, Kawaguchi H, Okamoto S, Yoshihara M, Sumii K, Kajiyama G: Pernicious anemia and *Heliobacter pylori* infection in Japan: evaluation in a country with a high prevalence of infection. *Am J Gastroenterol* 90:1107–1110, 1995.

Harville EW, Schramm M, Watt-Morse M, Chantala K, Anderson JJB, Hertz-Picciotto I: Calcium intake during pregnancy among white and African-American pregnant women in the United States. *J Am Coll Nutr* 23:43–50, 2004.

Hassan K, Loar R, Anderson BJ, Heptulla RA: The role of socioeconomic status, depression, quality of life, and glycemic control in type 1 diabetes mellitus. *J Pediatr* 149:526–531, 2006.

Hathcock JN, Azzi A, Blumberg J, Bray T, Dickinson A, Frei B, Jialal I, Johnston CS, Kelly FJ, Kraemer K, Packer L, Parthasarathy S, Sies H, Traber MG: Vitamins E and C are safe across a broad range of intakes. *Am J Clin Nutr* 81:736–745, 2005.

Hatipoglu B, Soni S, Espinosa V: Glycemic control with continuous subcutaneous insulin infusion with use of U-500 insulin in a pregnant patient. *Endocr Pract* 12:542–544, 2006.

Hatonen KA, Simila ME, Virtamo JR, Eriksson JG, Hannila M-L, Sinkko HK, Sundvall JE, Mykkanen HM, Valsta LM: Methodologic considerations in the measurement of glycemic index: glycemic response to rye bread, oatmeal porridge, and mashed potato. *Am J Clin Nutr* 84:1055–1061, 2006.

Hauguel S, Desmaizieres V, Challier JC: Glucose uptake, utilization, and transfer by the human placenta as functions of maternal glucose concentration. *Pediatr Res* 20:269–273, 1986.

Hauguel-de Mouzon S, Leturque A, Alsat E, Loizeau M, Evain-Brion D, Girard J: Developmental expression of Glut-1 glucose transporter and *c-fos* genes in human placental cells. *Placenta* 15:35–46, 1994.

Hauguel-de Mouzon S, Guerre-Millo M: The placenta cytokine network and inflammatory signals. *Placenta* 27:794–798, 2006a.

Hauguel-de Mouzon S, Lepercq J, Catalano P: The known and unknown of leptin in pregnancy. *Am J Obstet Gynecol* 194:1537–1545, 2006b.

Hawkes WC, Alkan Z, Lang K, King JC: Plasma selenium decrease during pregnancy is associated with glucose intolerance. *Biol Trace Elem Res* 100:19–29, 2004.

Haworka K, Pumprla J, Gabriel M, Feiks A, Schlusche C, Nowotny C, Schober E, Waldhoer T, Langer M: Normalization of pregnancy outcome in pregestational diabetes through functional insulin treatment and modular out-patient education adapted for pregnancy. *Diabet Med* 18:965–972, 2001.

Hawthorne G, Robson S, Ryall EA, Sen D, Roberts SH, Platt MP: Prospective population based survey of outcome of pregnancy in diabetic women: results of the Northern Diabetic Pregnancy Audit, 1994. *BMJ* 315:279–181, 1997.

Hawthorne G: Influencing care to achieve a successful outcome. Commentary to Josse J et al. *Pract Diab Int* 20:293, 2003.

Hawthorne G: Metformin use and diabetic pregnancy—has its time come? *Diabet Med* 23:223–227, 2006.

Hay WW, DiGiacomo JE, Meznarich HK, Hirst K, Zerbe G: Effects of glucose and insulin on fetal glucose oxidation and oxygen consumption. *Am J Physiol* 256: E704–E713, 1989.

Hayer-Zillgen M, Bruss M, Bonisch H: Expression and pharmacologic profile of the human organic cation transporters hOCT1, hOCT2 and hOCT3. *Br J Pharmacol* 136:829–836, 2002.

He F, McGregor GA: Beneficial effects of potassium. *BMJ* 323:497–501, 2001.

He FJ, MacGregor GA: How far should salt intake be reduced? *Hypertension* 42:1093–1099, 2003.

He K, Song Y, Daviglus ML, Liu K, Van Horn L, Dyer AR, Greenland P: Accumulated evidence on fish consumption and coronary heart disease mortality. A meta-analysis of cohort studies. *Circulation* 109:2705–2711, 2004a.

He Z, King GL: Microvascular complications of diabetes. *Endocrinol Metab Clin North Am* 33:215–238, 2004b.

Heard MJ, Pierce A, Carson SA, Buster JE: Pregnancies following use of metformin for ovulation induction in patients with polycystic ovary syndrome. *Fertil Steril* 77: 669–673, 2002.

Hebert MF, Naraharsetti SB, Ma X, Krudys KM, Umans J, Hankins GDV, Caritis S, Miodovnik M, Mattison DR, Unadkat J, Easterling TR, Vicini P: Are we guessing glyburide dosage in the treatment of gestational diabetes? The pharmacological evidence for better clinical practice. *Am J Obstet Gynecol* 197 (suppl):S25, 2007.

Hebold G, Scholz J, Schutz E, Czerwek H, Sakaguchi T, Brunk R, Nothdurft H, Kief H, Baeder C, Hartig F: Experimental investigations of the new sulfonylurea derivative glibenclamide (HB 419). *Horm Metab Res* 1(Suppl):4–10, 1969.

Hedderson MM, Weiss NS, Sacks DA, Pettitt DJ, Selby JV, Quesenberry CP, Ferrara A: Pregnancy weight gain and risk of neonatal complications: macrosomia, hypoglycemia, and hyperbilirubinemia. *Obstet Gynecol* 108:1153–1161, 2006.

Heikkinen T, Ekblad U, Laine K: Transplacental transfer of amitriptyline and nortriptyline in isolated perfused human placenta. *Psychopharmacology* 153: 450–454, 2001.

Heilbronn LK, Noakes M, Clifton PM: The effect of high- and low-glycemic index energy restricted diets on plasma lipid and glucose profiles in type 2 diabetic subjects with varying glycemic control. *J Am Coll Nutr* 21:120–127, 2002.

Heimberger CM, Ghidini A, Lewis KM, Spong CY: Glycosylated hemoglobin as a predictor of fetal pulmonic maturity in insulin dependent diabetes at term. *Am J Perinatol* 16:257–260, 1999.

Heinemann L, Linkeschova R, Rave K, Hompesch B, Sedlak M, Heise T: Time-action profile of the long-acting insulin analog insulin glargine (HOE901) in comparison with those of NPH insulin and placebo. *Diabetes Care* 23:644–649, 2000.

Heird WC, Lapillonne A: The roe of essential fatty acids in development. *Annu Rev Nutr* 25:549–571, 2005.

Heise CC, King JC, Costa FM, Kitzmiller JL: Hyperzincuria in IDDM women. Relationship to measures of glycemic control, renal function, and tissue catabolism. *Diabetes Care* 11:780–786, 1988.

Hellmuth E, Damm P, Molsted-Pedersen L: Congenital malformations in offspring of diabetic women treated with oral hypoglycemic agents during embryogenesis. *Diabetic Med* 11:471–474, 1994.

Hellmuth E, Damm P, Mølsted-Pedersen L, Bendtson I: Prevalence of nocturnal hypoglycemia in first trimester of pregnancy in patients with insulin treated diabetes mellitus. *Acta Obstet Gynecol Scand* 79:958–962, 2000a.

Hellmuth E, Damm P, Mølsted-Pedersen L: Oral hypoglycaemic agents in 118 diabetic pregnancies. *Diabet Med* 17:507–511, 2000b.

Hendrick V, Altshuler L: Management of major depression during pregnancy. *Am J Psychiatry* 159:1667–1673, 2002.

Hendrick V, Smith LM, Suri R, Hwang S, Haynes D, Altshuler L: Birth outcomes after prenatal exposure to antidepressant medication. *Am J Obstet Gynecol* 188:812–815, 2003.

Hendrickse W, Stammers JP, Hull D: The transfer of free fatty acids across the human placenta *Br J Obstet Gynecol* 92:945–952, 1985.

Henry MJ, Major CA, Reinsch S: Accuracy of self-monitoring of blood glucose: impact on diabetes management decisions during pregnancy. *Diabetes Educ* 27:521–529, 2001.

Henry AL, Beach AJ, Stowe ZN, Newport DJ: The fetus and maternal depression: implications for antenatal treatment guidelines. *Clin Obstet Gynecol* 47:535–546, 2004.

Henry CJ, Lightowler HJ, Strik CM, Renton H, Halis S: Glycaemic index and glycaemic load values of commercially available products in the UK. *Br J Nutr* 94:922–930, 2005.

Hentze MW, Muckenthaler MU, Andrews NC: Balancing acts: molecular control of mammalian iron metabolism. *Cell* 117:285–297, 2004.

Herman WH, Janz NK, Becker MP, Charron-Prochownik D: Preconception care, pregnancy outcomes, resource utilization and costs. *J Reprod Med* 44:33–38, 1999.

Hermanns N, Kulzer B, Krichbaum M, Kubiak T, Haak T: How to screen for depression and emotional problems in patients with diabetes: comparison of screening characteristics of depression questionnaires, measurement of diabetes-specific emotional problems and standard clinical assessment. *Diabetologia* 49:469–477, 2006.

Hernandez C, Lecube A, Carrera A, Simo R: Soluble transferrin receptors and ferritin in type 2 diabetic patients. *Diabet Med* 22:97–101, 2005.

Heron J, O'Connor TG, Evans J, Golding J, Glover V; ALSPAC Study Team: The course of anxiety and depression through pregnancy and the postpartum in a community sample. *J Affect Disord* 80:65–73, 2004.

Herpertz S, Wagener R, Albus C, Kocnar M, Wagner R, Best F, Schleppinghoff BS, Filz HP, Forster K, Thomas W, Mann K, Kohle K, Senf W: Diabetes mellitus and eating disorders: a multicenter study on the comorbidity of the two diseases. *J Psychosom Res* 44:503–515, 1998.

Herpertz S, Albus C, Wagener R, Kocnar M, Wagner R, Henning A, Best F, Foerster H, Schleppinghoff BS, Thomas W, Kohle K, Mann K, Senf W: Comorbidity of diabetes and eating disorders. *J Psychosom Res* 51:673–678, 2001.

Herrera E, Palacin M, Martin A. Lasuncion MA: Relationship between maternal and fetal fuels and placental glucose transfer in rats with maternal diabetes of varying severity. *Diabetes* 34 (Suppl 2):42–46, 1985.

Herrera E: Metabolic adaptations in pregnancy and their implications for the availability of substrates to the fetus. *Eur J Clin Nutr* 54 (Suppl 1):S47–S51, 2000.

Herrera E: Lipid metabolism in pregnancy and its consequences in the fetus and newborn. *Endocr Rev* 19:43–55, 2002a.

Herrera E: Implications of dietary fatty acids during pregnancy on placental, fetal and postnatal development—a review. *Placenta* 23:S9–S19, 2002b.

Herrera E, Ortega H, Alvino G, Giovanni N, Amusquivar E, Cetin I: Relationship between plasma fatty acid profile and antioxidant vitamins during normal pregnancy. *Eur J Clin Nutr* 58:1231–1238, 2004.

Herrera E, Amusquivar E, Lopez-Soldado I, Ortega H: Maternal lipid metabolism and placental lipid transfer. *Horm Res* 65 (Suppl 3):59–64, 2006a.

Herrera JA, Arevalo-Herrera M, Shahabuddin AKM, Ersheng G, Herrera S, Garcia RG, Lopez-Jaramillo P: Calcium and conjugated linoleic acid reduces pregnancy-induced hypertension and decreases intracellular calcium in lymphocytes. *Am J Hypertens* 19:381–387, 2006b.

Herrick K, Phillips DI, Haselden S, Shiell AW, Campbell-Brown M, Godfrey KM: Maternal consumption of a high-meat, low-carbohydrate diet in late pregnancy: relation to adult cortisol concentrations in the offspring. *J Clin Endocrinol Metab* 88:3554–3560, 2003.

Herrmann W, Schorr H, Obeid R, Makowski J, Fowler B, Kuhlmann MK: Disturbed homocysteine and methionine cycle intermediates S-adenosylhomocysteine and S-adenosylmethionine are related to degree of renal insufficiency in type 2 diabetes. *Clin Chem* 51:891–897, 2005a.

Herrmann W, Isber S, Obeid R, Herrmann M, Jouma M: Concentrations of homocysteine, related metabolites and asymmetric dimethylarginine in preeclamptic women with poor nutritional status. *Clin Chem Lab Med* 43: 1139–1146, 2005b.

Hersshko C, Ronson A, Souroujon M, Maschler I, Heyd J, Patz J: Variable hematologic presentation of autoimmune gastritis: age-related progression from iron deficiency to cobalamin depletion. *Blood* 107:1673–1679, 2006.

Hibbard ED, Spencer WJ: Low serum B12 levels and latent Addisonian anemia in pregnancy. *J Obstet Gynecol Br Cwlth* 77:52–57, 1970.

Hickman IJ, Jonsson JR, Prins JB, Ash S, Purdie DM, Clouston AD, Powell EE: Modest weight loss and physical activity in overweight patients with chronic liver disease results in sustained improvements in alanine aminotransferase, fasting insulin, and quality of life. *Gut* 53:413–419, 2004.

Hiden U, Maier A, Bilban M, Ghaffari-Tabrizi N, Wadsack C, Lang I, Dohr G, Desoye G: Insulin control of placental gene expression shifts from mother to fetus over the course of pregnancy. *Diabetologia* 49:123–131, 2006.

Hieronimus S, Cupelli C, Durand-Reville M, Bongain A, Fenichel P: Pregnancy and type 2 diabetes: which fetal prognosis? *Gynecol Obstet Fertil* 32:23–27, 2004.

Hieronimus S, Cupelli C, Bongain A, Durand-Reville M, Berthier F, Fenichel P: Pregnancy in type 1 diabetes: insulin pump versus intensified conventional therapy. *Gynecol Obstet Fertil* 33:389–394, 2005.

Higa KD, Boone KB, Tienchin H: Complications of the laparoscopic Roux-en-Y gastric bypass: 1040 patients—what have we learned? *Obes Surg* 10:509–513, 2000.

Higa KD, Tienchin H, Boone KB: Internal hernias after Roux-en-Y gastric bypass: incidence, treatment and prevention. *Obes Surg* 13:350–354, 2003.

Hiles RA, Bawdon RE, Petrella EM: Ex vivo human placental transfer of the peptides pramlintide and exenatide (synthetic exendin-4). *Hum Exp Toxicol* 22:623–628, 2003.

Hill WC, Peile-Day G, Kitzmiller JL, Spencer EM: Insulin-like growth factors in fetal macrosomia with and without maternal diabetes *Horm Res* 32:178–182, 1989.

Hill I, Fasano A, Schwartz R, Counts D, Glock M, Horvath K: The prevalence of celiac disease in at-risk groups of children in the United States. *J Pediatr* 140:379–380, 2000.

Hill ID, Bhatnagar S, Cameron DJ, De Rosa S, Maki M, Russell GJ, Troncone R: Celiac disease: Working Group Report of the first World Congress of Pediatric Gastroenterology, Heptatology, and Nutrition. *J Pediatr Gastroenterol Nutr* 35 (Suppl 2):S78–88, 2002.

Hill PG, Forsyth JM, Semeraro D, Holmes GK: IgA antibodies to human tissue transglutaminase: audit of routine practice confirms high diagnostic accuracy. *Scand J Gastroenterol* 39:1078–1082, 2004.

Hillesmaa V, Suhonen L, Teramo K: Glycemic control is associated with preeclampsia but not with pregnancy-induced hypertension in women with type 1 diabetes mellitus. *Diabetologia* 43:1534–1539, 2000.

Hillman N, Herranz L, Vaquero PM, Villarroel A, Fernandez A, Pallardo LF: Is pregnancy outcome worse in type 2 than in type 1 diabetic women? *Diabetes Care* 29:2557–2558, 2006.

Hilsted J, Bonde-Petersen F, Madsbad S, Parving HH, Christensen NJ, Adelhoj B, Bigler D, Sjontoft E: Changes in plasma volume, in transcapillary escape rate of albumin and in subcutaneous blood flow during hypoglycemia in man. *Clin Sci* 69:273–277, 1985.

Hirsch IB: The status of the diabetes team. *Clin Diabetes* 16:145–146, 1998a.

Hirsch IB: Intensive treatment of type 1 diabetes. *Med Clin North Am* 82:689–719, 1998b.

Hirsch IB: Insulin analogues. *N Engl J Med* 352:174–183, 2005.

HLTC—Homocysteine Lowering Trialists' Collaboration: Lowering blood homocysteine with folic acid based supplements: meta-analysis of randomized trials. *BMJ* 316:894–898, 1998.

Hobbs CA, Cleves MA, Zhao W, Melnyk S, James SJ: Congenital heart defects and maternal biomarkers of oxidative stress. *Am J Clin Nutr* 82:598–604, 2005a.

Hobbs CA, Cleves MA, Melnyk S, Zhao W, James SJ: Congenital heart defects and abnormal maternal biomarkers of methionine and homocysteine metabolism. *Am J Clin Nutr* 81:147–153, 2005b.

Hobbs CA, James SJ, Jernigan S, Melnyk S, Lu Y, Malik S, Cleves MA: Congenital heart defects, maternal homocysteine, smoking, and the 677 C > T polymorphism in the methylenetetrahydrofolate reductase gene: evaluating gene-environment interactions. *Am J Obstet Gynecol* 194:218–224, 2006.

Hod M, Jovanovic L, Di Renzo GC, de Leiva A, Langer O, eds: *Textbook of Diabetes and Pregnancy.* London: Martin and Dunitz; 2003.

Hod M, Damm P, Kaaja R, Visser GHA, Dunne F, Demidova I, Hansen A-S P, Mersebach H; the Insulin Aspart Pregnancy Study Group: Fetal and perinatal outcomes in type 1 diabetes pregnancy: a randomized study comparing insulin aspart with human insulin in 322 subjects. *Am J Obstet Gynecol* 198:186.e1–186. e7, 2008a.

Hod M, Jovanovic L, Di Renzo GC, de Leiva A, Langer O, eds: *Textbook of Diabetes and Pregnancy.* 2nd ed. London: Informa Healthcare; 2008b.

Hodgkinson AD, Bartlett T, Oates PJ, Millward BA, Demaine AG: The response of antioxidant genes to hyperglycemia is abnormal in patients with type 1 diabetes and diabetic nephropathy. *Diabetes* 52:846–851, 2003.

Hoffenberg EJ, Emery LM, Barriga KJ, Bao F, Taylor J, Eisenbarth GS, Haas JE, Sokol RJ, Taki I, Norris JM, Rewers M: Clinical features of children with screening-identified evidence of celiac disease. *Pediatrics* 113:1254–1259, 2004.

Hoffman A, Fischer Y, Gilhar D, Raz I: The effect of hyperglycemia on the absorption of glibenclamide in patients with non-insulin-dependent diabetes mellitus. *Eur J Clin Pharmacol* 47:53–55, 1994.

Hofmann T, Horstmann G, Stammberger I: Evaluation of the reproductive toxicity and embryotoxicity of insulin glargine (LANTUS) in rats and rabbits. *Int J Toxicol* 21:181–189, 2002.

Hogberg L, Laurin P, Falth-Magnusson K, Grant C, Grodzinsky E, Jansson G, Ascher H, Browaldh L, Hammersjo JA, Lindberg E, Myrdal U, Stenhammar L: Oats to children with newly diagnosed celiac disease: a randomized double blind study. *Gut* 53:649–654, 2004.

Hokanson R, Miller S, Hennessey M, Flesher M, Hanneman W, Busbee D: Disruption of estrogen-regulated gene expression by dioxin: downregulation of a gene associated with the onset of non-insulin dependent diabetes mellitus (type 2 diabetes). *Hum Exp Toxicol* 23:555–564, 2004.

Holcberg G, Tsadkin-Tamir M, Sapir O, Wiznizer A, Segal D, Polachek H, Ben Zvi Z: Transfer of insulin lispro across the human placenta. *Eur J Obstet Gynecol Reprod Biol* 115:117–118, 2004.

Holcomb WL, Stone LS, Lustman PJ, Gavard JA, Mostello DJ: Screening for depression in pregnancy: characteristics of the Beck Depression Inventory. *Obstet Gynecol* 88:1021–1025, 1996.

Holick MF: Resurrection of vitamin D deficiency and rickets. *J Clin Invest* 116:2062–2072, 2006.

Hollen E, Holmgren Peterson K, Sundqvist T, Grodzinsky E, Hogberg L, Laurin P, Stenhammar L, Faith-Magnusson K, Magnusson KE: Celiac children on a gluten-fre diet with or without oats display equal antiavenin antibody titers. *Scand J Gastroenterol* 41:42–47, 2006.

Hollingsworth DR, Grundy SM: Pregnancy-associated hypertriglyceridemia in normal and diabetic women. Differences in insulin-dependent, non-insulin-dependent, and gestational diabetes. *Diabetes* 31:1092–1097, 1982.

Hollis BW, Wagner CL: Assessment of dietary vitamin D requirements during pregnancy and lactation. *Am J Clin Nutr* 79:717–726, 2004.

Holm PI, Bleie O, Ueland PM, Lien EA, Refsum H, Nordrehaug JE, Nygard O: Betaine as a determinant of postmethionine load total plasma homocysteine before and after B-vitamin supplementation. *Arterioscler Thromb Vasc Biol* 24:301–307, 2004.

Holm PI, Ueland PM, Vollset SE, Mudttum O, Blom HJ, Keijzer MBAJ, den Heijer M: Betaine and folate status as cooperative determinants of plasma homocysteine in humans. *Arterioscler Thromb Vasc Biol* 25:379–385, 2005.

Holm K, Maki M, Vuolteenaho N, Mustalahti K, Ashorn M, Ruuka T, Kaukinen K: Oats in the treatment of childhood celiac disease: a 2-year controlled trial and a long-term clinical follow-up study. *Aliment Pharmacol Ther* 23:1463–1472, 2006.

Holmes GK, Prior P, Lane MR, Pope D, Allan RN: Malignancy in celiac disease—effect of a gluten free diet. *Gut* 30:333–338, 1989.

Holmes GKT: Screening for celiac disease in type 1 diabetes. *Arch Dis Child* 87: 495–499, 2002.

Holmes VA, Young IS, Maresh MJA, Pearson DWM, Walker JD, McCance DR; on behalf of the DAPIT Study Group: The Diabetes and Preeclampsia Intervention Trial. *Int J Obstet Gynecol* 87:66–71, 2004.

Holmes VA, Wallace JM, Alexander HD, Gilmore WS, Bradbury I, Ward M, Scott JM, McFaul P, McNulty H: Homocysteine is lower in the third trimester of pregnancy in women with enhanced folate status from continued folic acid supplementation. *Clin Chem* 51:629–634, 2005.

Holmes HJ, Casey BM, Bawdon RE: Placental transfer of rosiglitazone in the ex vivo human perfusion model. *Am J Obstet Gynecol* 195:1715–1719, 2006.

Holshauser CA, Ansbacher R, McNitt T, Steele R: Bacterial endocarditis due to Listeria monocytogenes in a pregnant diabetic. *Obstet Gynecol* 51:9s–10s, 1978.

Holstein A, Plaschke A, Egberts E-H: Use of insulin glargine during embryogenesis in a pregnant woman with type 1 diabetes. *Diabet Med* 20:777–780, 2003.

Holt RI, Clarke P, Parry EC, Coleman MA: The effectiveness of glibenclamide in women with gestational diabetes. *Diabetes Obes Metab* Dec 17, 2007 [Epub ahead of print].

Homko CJ, Khandelwal M: Glucose monitoring and insulin therapy during pregnancy. *Obstet Gynecol Clin North Am* 23:47–74, 1996.

Homko CJ, Reece EA: Insulins and oral hypoglycemic agents in pregnancy. *J Matern Fetal Neonatal Med* 19:679–686, 2006.

Hood KK, Huestis S, Maher A, Butler D, Volkening L, Laffel LMB: Depressive symptoms in children and adolescents with type 1 diabetes. Association with diabetes-specific characteristics. *Diabetes Care* 29:1389–1391, 2006.

Hoogeveen EK, Kostense PJ, Jakobs C, Dekker JM, Nijpels G, Heine RJ, Bouter LM, Stehouwer CD: Hyperhomocysteinemia increases risk of death, especially in type 2 diabetes: 5-year follow-up of the Hoorn study. *Circulation* 101: 1505–1511, 2000.

HOPE—Heart Outcomes Prevention Evaluation 2 Investigators: Homocysteine lowering with folic acid and B vitamins in vascular disease. *N Engl J Med* 354:1567–1577, 2006.

Hopper AD, Hurlstone DP, Leeds JS, McAlindon ME, Dube AK, Stephenson TJ, Sanders DS: The occurrence of terminal ileal histological abnormalities in patients with celiac disease. *Dig Liver Dis* 38:815–819, 2006.

Hosoda K, Wang M-F, Liao M-L, Chuang C-K, Iha M, Clevidence B, Yamamoto S: Antihyperglycemic effect of Oolong tea in type 2 diabetes. *Diabetes Care* 26:1714–1718, 2003.

Hotmire K, Minium J, Catalano P, Hauguel-de Mouzon S: Differential regulation of placenta fatty acid fluxes by leptin. *Diabetes* 55:A41, 2006.

Hotz C, Peerson JM, Brown KH: Suggested lower cutoffs of serum zinc concentrations for assessing zinc status: reanalysis of the second National Health and Nutrition Examination Survey data (1976–1980). *Am J Clin Nutr* 78: 756–764, 2003.

Houston GA, Files JC, Morrison FS: Race, age, and pernicious anemia. *South Med J* 78:69–70, 1985.

Howard BV: Dietary fat and diabetes: a consensus view. *Am J Med* 113(9B):38S–40S, 2002.

Howell MD, Austin RK, Kelleher D, Nepom GT, Kagnoff MF: A HLA-D region restriction fragment length polymorphism associated with celiac disease. *J Exp Med* 164:333–338, 1986.

Hsu, HW, Butte NF, Wong WW, Moon JK, Ellis KJ, Klein PD, Moise KJ: Oxidative metabolism in insulin-treated gestational diabetes. *Am J Physiol* 272:E1099–1107, 1997.

Hsu C-D, Hong S-F, Nickless NA, Copel JA: Glycosylated hemoglobin in insulin-dependent diabetes mellitus related to preeclampsia. *Am J Perinatol* 15:199–202, 1998.

Hu FB, Bronner L, Willett WC, Stampfer MJ, Rexrode KM, Albert CM, Hunter D, Manson JE: Fish and omega-3 fatty acid intake and risk of coronary heart disease in women. *JAMA* 287:1815–1821, 2002.

Hu Y, Block G, Norkus EP, Morrow JD, Dietrich M, Hudes M: Relations of glycemic index and glycemic load with plasma oxidative stress markers. *Am J Clin Nutr* 84:70–76, 2006.

Huang CS, Forse RA, Jacobsone BC, Farraye FA: Endoscopic findings and their clinical correlations in patients with symptoms after gastric bypass surgery. *Gastrointest Endosc* 58:859–866, 2003.

Huang MA, Greenson JK, Chao C, Anderson L, Peterman D, Jacobson J, Emick D, Lok AS, Conjeevaram HS: One-year intense nutritional counseling results in histological improvement in patients with nonalcoholic steatohepatitis: a pilot study. *Am J Gastroenterol* 100:1072–1081, 2005.

Huang YT, Chen SU, Wu MZ, Chen CY, Hsieh WS, Tsao BN, Horng CJ, Hsueh PR: Molecular evidence for vertical transmission of listerosis, Taiwan. *J Med Microbiol* 55:1601–1603, 2006.

Hubel CA: Dyslipidemia, iron, and oxidative stress in preeclampsia: assessment of maternal and feto-placental interactions. *Semin Reprod Endocrinol* 16:75–92, 1998.

Huddle KR: Audit of the outcome of pregnancy in diabetic women in Soweto, South Africa, 1992–2002. *S Afr Med J* 95:789–794, 2005.

Hudgins LC, Hellerstein M, Seidman C, Neese R, Diakun J, Hirsch J: Human fatty acid synthesis is stimulated by a eucaloric low fat, high carbohydrate diet. *J Clin Invest* 97:2081–2091, 1996.

Hughes RC, Rowan JA: Pregnancy in women with type 2 diabetes: who takes metformin and what is the outcome? *Diabet Med* 23:318–322, 2006a.

Hughes RC, Gardiner SJ, Begg EJ, Zhang M: Effect of pregnancy on the pharmacokinetics of metformin. *Diabet Med* 23:323–326, 2006b.

Huisman A, Aarnoudse JG: Increased 2nd trimester hemoglobin concentration later complicated by hypertension and growth retardation. Early evidence of a reduced plasma volume. *Acta Obstet Gynecol Scand* 65:605–608, 1986.

Hummel M, Marienfeld S, Huppmann M, Knopff A, Voigt M, Bonifacio E, Ziegler A-G: Fetal growth is increased by maternal type 1 diabetes and HLA DR4-related gene interactions. *Diabetologia* 50:850–858, 2007.

Hunt JR: Bioavailability of iron, zinc, and other trace minerals from vegetarian diets. *Am J Clin Nutr* 78 (Suppl): 633S–639S, 2003.

Hunter DJS, Burrows RF, Mohide PT, Whyte RK: Influence of maternal insulin-dependent diabetes mellitus on neonatal morbidity. *Can Med Assoc J* 149:47–51, 1993.

Hunter WA, Cundy T, Rabone D, Hofman PL, Harris M, Regan F, Robinson E, Cutfield WS: Insulin sensitivity in the offspring of women with type 1 and type 2 diabetes. *Diabetes Care* 27:1148–1152, 2004.

Hypponen E, Power C: Vitamin D status and glucose homeostasis in the 1958 British birth cohort. The role of obesity. *Diabetes Care* 29:2244–2246, 2006.

Iafusco D, Rea F, Prisco F: Hypoglycemia and reduction of the insulin requirement as a sign of celiac disease in children with IDDM. *Diabetes Care* 21:1379–1381, 1998.

ICPS—International Program on Chemical Safety: Methylmercury. Environmental health criteria 101. Geneva: World Health Organization; 1990. Available at: http://www.inchem.org/documents/ehc/ehc/ehc101.htm. Accessed Mar 14, 2008.

IFCC—International Federation of Clinical Chemistry and Laboratory Medicine, Scientific Division Working Group on Selective Electrodes: IFCC recommendation on reporting results for blood glucose. *Clin Chim Acta* 307:205–209, 2001.

Ilic S, Jovanovic L, Pettitt D: Comparison of the effect of saturated and monounsaturated fat on postprandial plasma glucose and insulin concentration in women with gestational diabetes mellitus. *Am J Perinatol* 16:489–495, 1999.

Illsley NP: Glucose transporters in the human placenta. *Placenta* 21:14–22, 2000.

Innis SM: Essential fatty acid transfer and fetal development. *Placenta* 26 (Suppl A, Trophoblast Res 19):S70–S75, 2005.

Innis SM: Trans fatty acid intakes during pregnancy, infancy and early childhood. *Atheroscler Suppl* 7:17–20, 2006.

IOM—Institute of Medicine, Food and Nutrition Board, National Academy of Sciences (US): *Nutrition During Pregnancy: Weight Gain and Nutrient Supplements. Report of the Committee on Nutritional Status During Pregnancy and Lactation.* Washington, DC: National Academies Press; 1990. Available at: http://www.nap.edu/catalog.php?record_id=1451, Accessed Apr 4, 2008.

IOM—Institute of Medicine, Food and Nutrition Board, National Academy of Sciences. Subcommittee for a Clinical Application Guide, Committee on Nutritional Status During Pregnancy and Lactation: *Nutrition During Pregnancy and Lactation: An Implementation Guide.* Washington, DC: National Academies Press; 1992. Available at: http://www.nap.edu/catalog.php?record_id=1984. Accessed Mar 14, 2008.

IOM—Institute of Medicine, Food and Nutrition Board: *Iron Deficiency Anemia: Recommended Guidelines for the Prevention, Detection, and Management Among U.S. Children and Women of Childbearing Age.* Washington DC: National Academies Press; 1993. Available at: http://www.nap.edu/catalog.php?record_id=2251. Accessed Mar 14, 2008.

IOM—Institute of Medicine, Food and Nutrition Board: *Dietary Reference Intakes for Calcium, Phosphorus, Magnesium, Vitamin D, and Fluoride.* Washington, DC: National Academies Press; 1997, revised 2000. Available at: http://www.nap.edu/catalog.php?record_id=5776. Accessed Mar 12, 2008.

IOM—Institute of Medicine, Food and Nutrition Board: *Dietary Reference Intakes for Thiamin, Riboflavin, Niacin, Vitamin B6, Folate, Vitamin B12, Pantothenic Acid, Biotin, and Choline.* Washington, DC: National Academies Press; 1998. Available at: http://www.nap.edu/catalog.php?record_id=6015. Accessed Mar 12, 2008.

IOM—Institute of Medicine, Food and Nutrition Board: *Dietary Reference Intakes for Vitamin C, Vitamin E, Selenium, and Carotenoids.* Washington, DC: National Academies Press; 2000a Available at: http://www.nap.edu/catalog.php?record_id=9810. Accessed Mar 12, 2008.

IOM—Institute of Medicine, Food and Nutrition Board: *Dietary Reference Intakes: Applications in Dietary Assessment.* Washington, DC: National Academies Press; 2000b. Available at: http://www.nap.edu/catalog.php?record_id=9956. Accessed Mar 14, 2008.

IOM—Institute of Medicine, Food and Nutrition Board: *Dietary Reference Intakes for Vitamin A, Vitamin K, Arsenic, Boron, Chromium, Copper, Iodine, Iron, Manganese, Molybdenum, Nickel, Silicon, Vanadium, and Zinc.* Washington, DC: National Academies Press; 2001. Available at: http://www.nap.edu/catalog.php?record_id=10026. Accessed Mar 12, 2008.

IOM—Institute of Medicine, Food and Nutrition Board: *Dietary Reference Intakes: Energy, Carbohydrates, Fiber, Fat, Fatty Acids, Cholesterol, Protein, and Amino Acids (Macronutrients).* Washington, DC: National Academies Press; 2002. Available at: http://www.nap.edu/catalog.php?record_id=10490. Accessed Mar 12, 2008.

IOM—Institute of Medicine, Food and Nutrition Board: *Dietary Reference Intakes: Applications in Dietary Planning.* Washington, DC: National Academies Press; 2003. Available at: http://www.nap.edu/catalog.php?record_id=10609. Accessed Mar 14, 2008.

IOM—Institute of Medicine, Food and Nutrition Board: *Dietary Reference Intakes for Water, Potassium, Sodium, Chloride, and Sulfate.* Washington, DC: National Academies Press; 2004. Available at: http://www.nap.edu/catalog.php?record_id=10925. Accessed Mar 12, 2008.

Ionnou GN, Boyko EJ, Lee SP: The prevalence and predictors of elevated serum aminotransferase activity in the Unoted States in 1999–2002. *Am J Gastroenterol* 101:76–82, 2006.

Irvine WJ, Scarth L, Clarke BF, Cullen DR, Duncan LJP: Thyroid and gastric autoimmunity in patients with diabetes mellitus. *Lancet* 2 (7665):163–168, 1970.

Ismail K, Winkley K, Rabe-Hesketh S: Systematic review and meta-analysis of randomized controlled trials of psychological interventions to improve glycemic control in patients with type 2 diabetes. *Lancet* 363:1589–1597, 2004.

Ivy JL: Role of exercise training in the prevention and treatment of insulin resistance and non-insulin-dependent diabetes mellitus. *Sports Med* 24:321–336, 1997.

Jabs K, Koury MJ, Dupont WD, Wagner C: Relationship between plasma S-adenosylhomocysteine concentration and glomerular filtration rate in children. *Metabolism* 55:252–257, 2006.

Jacobs RL, House JD, Brosnan ME, Brosnan JT: Effects of streptozotocin-induced diabetes and of insulin treatment on homocysteine metabolism in the rat. *Diabetes* 47:1967–1970, 1998.

Jacobs EM, Hendricks JC, van Tits BL, Evans PJ, Breuer W, Liu DY, Jansen EH, Jauhianen K, Sturm B, Porter JB, Scheiber-Mojdehkar B, von Bonsdorff L, Cabantchik ZI, Hider RC, Swinkels DW: Results of an international round robin for the quantification of serum non-transferrin-bound iron: need for defining standardization and a clinically relevant isoform. *Anal Biochem* 341:241–250, 2005.

Jacobson AM: Depression and diabetes. Commentary. *Diabetes Care* 16:1621–1623, 1993.

Jacobson JL, Jacobson SW: Intellectual impairment in children exposed to polychlorinated biphenyls in utero. *N Engl J Med* 335:783–789, 1996a.

Jacobson AM: The psychological care of patients with insulin-dependent diabetes mellitus. *N Engl J Med* 334:1249–1253, 1996b.

Jacobson GF, Ramos GA, Ching JY, Kirby RS, Ferrara A, Field DR: Comparison of glyburide and insulin for the management of gestational diabetes in a large managed care organization. *Am J Obstet Gynecol* 193:118–124, 2005.

Jaeger C, Hatziagelaki E, Petzoldt R, Bretzel RG: Comparative analysis of organ-specific autoantibodies and celiac disease-associated antibodies in type 1 diabetic patients, their first-degree relatives, and healthy control subjects. *Diabetes Care* 24:27–32, 2001.

Jain SK, Wise R: Relationship between elevated lipid peroxides, vitamin E deficiency, and hypertension in preeclampsia. *Mol Cell Biochem* 151:33–38, 1995.

Jakubowicz DJ, Iurno MJ, Jakubowicz S, Roberts KA, Nestler JE: Effects of metformin on early pregnancy loss in the polycystic ovary syndrome. *J Clin Endocrinol Metab* 87:524–529, 2002.

Janatiunem EK, Pikkarainen PH, Kemppainen TA, Kosma VM, Jarvinen RM, Uusitupa MI, Julkunen RJ: A comparison of diets with and without oats in adults with celiac disease. *N Engl J Med* 333:1033–1037, 1995.

Jansson T, Wennergren M, Powell TL: Placental glucose transport and GLUT-1 expression in insulin-dependent diabetes. *Am J Obstet Gynecol* 180:163–168, 1999.

Jansson T, Ekstrand Y, Bjorn C, Wennergren M, Powell TL: Alterations in the activity of placental amino acid transporters in pregnancies complicated by diabetes. *Diabetes* 51:2214–2219, 2002.

Jansson N, Greenwood SL, Johansson BR, Powell TL, Jansson T: Leptin stimulates the activity of the system A amino acid transporter in human placental villous fragments. *J Clin Endocrinol Metab* 88:1205–1211, 2003.

Jansson T, Powell TL: Human placental transport in altered fetal growth: does the placenta function as a nutrient sensor? A review. IFPA 2005 Award in Placentology lecture. *Placenta* 27 (Suppl A):S91–S97, 2006a.

Jansson T, Cetin I, Powell TL, Desoye G, Radaelli T, Ericsson A, Sibley CP: Placental transport and metabolism in fetal overgrowth—a workshop report. *Placenta* 27 (Suppl A):S109–S113, 2006b.

Jaque-Fortunato SV, Wiswell RA, Khodiguian N, Artal R: A comparison of the ventilatory responses to exercise in pregnant, postpartum, and non-pregnant women. *Semin Perinatol* 20:263–276, 1996.

Jarjou LMA, Prentice A, Sawo Y, Laskey MA, Bennett J, Goldberg GR, Cole TJ: Randomized, placebo-controlled, calcium supplementation study in pregnant Ganbian women: effects on breast-milk calcium concentrations and infant birth weight, growth, and bone mineral accretion in the first year of life. *Am J Clin Nutr* 83:657–666, 2006.

Javaid M, Crozier S, Harvey N, Gale CR, Dennison EM, Boucher BJ, Arden NK, Godfrey KM, Cooper C; Princess Anne Hospital Study Group: Maternal vitamin D status during pregnancy and childhood bone mass at age 9 years: a longitudinal study. *Lancet* 367:36–43, 2006.

Jawerbaum A, Capobianco E, Pustovrh C, White V, Baier M, Salzberg S, Pesaresi M, Gonzalez E: Influence of peroxisome proliferator-activated receptor gamma activation by its endogenous ligand 15-deoxy Delta12,14 prostaglandin J2 on nitric oxide production in term placental tissues from diabetic women. *Mol Hum Reprod* 10:671–676, 2004.

Jedrychowski W, Janowski J, Flak E, Skarupa A, Mroz E, Sochacka-Tatara E, Lisowska-Miszczyk I, Szpanowska-Wohn A, Rauh V, Skolicki Z, Kaim I, Perera F: Effects of prenatal exposure to mercury on cognitive and psychomotor function in one-year-old infants: epidemiologic cohort study in Poland. *Ann Epidemiol* 16:439–447, 2006.

Jee SH, He J, Appel LJ, Whelton PK, Suh I, Klag MJ: Coffee consumption and serum lipids: a meta-analysis of randomized controlled clinical trials. *Am J Epidemiol* 153:353–362, 2001.

Jenkins DJ, Wolever TM, Taylor RH, Barker H, Fielden H, Baldwin JM, Bowling AC, Newman HC, Jenkins AL, Goff DV: Glycemic index of foods: a physiological basis for carbohydrate exchange. *Am J Clin Nutr* 34:362–366, 1981.

Jenkins DJ, Wolever TM, Jenkins AL, Thorne MJ, Lee R, Kalmusky J, Reichert R, Wong GS: The glycaemic index of foods tested in diabetic patients: a new basis for carbohydrate exchange favouring the use of legumes. *Diabetologia* 24:257–264, 1983.

Jenkins DJ, Wolever TM, Wong GS, Kenshole A, Josse RG, Thompson LU, Lam KY: Glycemic responses to foods: possible differences between insulin-dependent and non-insulin-dependent diabetic patients. *Am J Clin Nutr* 40:971–981, 1984.

Jenkins DJ, Kendall CW, Augustin LS, Franceschi S, Hamidi M, Marchie A, Jenkins AL, Axelsen M: Glycemic index: overview of implications in health and disease. *Am J Clin Nutr* 76:266S-273S, 2002.

Jenkins DJ, Kendall CW, Josse AR, Salvatore S, Brighenti F, Augustin LS, Ellis PR, Vidgen E, Rao AV: Almonds decrease postprandial glycemia, insulinemia, and oxidative damage in healthy individuals. *J Nutr* 136:2987–2992, 2006a.

Jenkins DJA, Josse AR, Labelle R, Marchie A, Augustin LSA, Kendall CWC: Nonalcoholic fatty liver, nonalcoholic steatohepatitis, ectopic fat, and the glycemic index. *Am J Clin Nutr* 84:3–4, 2006b.

Jensen OM, Kamby C: Intra-uterine exposure to saccharin and risk of bladder cancer in man. *Int J Cancer* 15:507–509, 1982.

Jensen DM, Damm P, Molsted-Pedersen L, Ovesen P, Westergaard JG, Moeller M, Beck-Nielsen H: Outcomes in type 1 diabetic pregnancies. A nationwide, population-based study. *Diabetes Care* 27:2819–2823, 2004.

Jervell J, Moe N, Skaeraasen J, Blystad W, Egge K: Diabetes mellitus and pregnancy—management and results at Rikshospitalet, Oslo, 1970–1977. *Diabetologia* 16:151–155, 1979.

Jiang R, Manson JE, Meigs JB, Ma J, Rifai N, Hu FB: Body iron stores in relation to risk of type 2 diabetes in apparently healthy women. *JAMA* 291:711–717, 2004.

Jimenez-Cruz A, Bacardi-Gascon M, Turnbull WH, Rosales-Garay P, Severino-Lugo I: A flexibile, low-glycemic index Mexican-style diet in overweight and obese subjects with type 2 diabetes improves metabolic parameters during a 6-week treatment period. *Diabetes Care* 26:1967–1970, 2003.

John JH, Ziebland S, Yudkin P, Roe LS, Neil HAW: Effects of fruit and vegetable consumption on plasma antioxidant concentrations and blood pressure: a randomized controlled trial. *Lancet* 359:1969–1973, 2002.

Johnson LW, Smith CH: Neutral amino acid transport systems of microvillous membrane of human placenta. *Am J Physiol* 254:C773–C780, 1988.

Johnson M, Enns C: Diferric transferrin regulates transferrin receptor 2 protein stability. *Blood* 104:4287–4293, 2004.

Johnston KL, Clifford MN, Morgan LM: Coffee acutely modifies gastrointestinal hormone secretion and glucose tolerance in humans: glycemic effects of chlorogenic acid and caffeine. *Am J Clin Nutr* 78:728–733, 2003.

Johnstone FD, Mao J-H, Steel JM, Prescott RJ, Hume R: Factors affecting fetal weight distribution in women with type 1 diabetes. *Br J Obstet Gynecol* 107:1001–1006, 2000.

Johnstone FD, Lindsay RS, Steel J: Type 1 diabetes and pregnancy: trends in birth weight over 40 years at a single clinic. *Obstet Gynecol* 107:1297–1302, 2006.

Jonsson A, Rydberg T, Ekberg G, Hallengren B, Melander A: Slow elimination of glyburide in NIDDM subjects. *Diabetes Care* 17:142–145, 1994.

Jonsson A, Hallengren B, Rydberg T, Melander A: Effects and serum levels of glibenclamide and its active metabolites in patients with type 2 diabetes. *Diabetes Obes Metab* 3:403–409, 2001.

Josse J, James J, Roland J: Diabetes control in pregnancy: who takes responsibility for what? *Pract Diab Int* 20:290–293, 2003.

Jovanovic L, Peterson CM, Saxena BB, Dawood MY, Saudek CD: Feasibility of maintaining euglycemia in insulin-dependent diabetic women. *Am J Med* 68:105–112, 1980.

Jovanovic L, Druzin M, Peterson CM. Effect of euglycemia on the outcome of pregnancy in insulin-dependent diabetic women as compared with normal control subjects. *Am J Med* 71:921–927, 1981.

Jovanovic R, Jovanovic L: Obstetric management when normoglycemia is maintained in diabetic pregnant women with vascular compromise. *Am J Obstet Gynecol* 149:617–623, 1984.

Jovanovic L, Peterson CM, Reed GF, Metzger BE, Mills JL, Knopp Rh, Aarons JH: Maternal postprandial glucose levels and infant birth weight: the Diabetes in Early Pregnancy Study. *Am J Obstet Gynecol* 164:103–111, 1991.

Jovanovic L, Ilic S, Pettitt D, Hugo K, Gutierrez M, Bowsher RR, Bastyr EJ: Metabolic and immunologic effects of insulin lispro in gestational diabetes. *Diabetes Care* 22:1422–1427, 1999a.

Jovanovic L: Commentary. Retinopathy risk: what is responsible? Hormones, hyperglycemia, or Humalog? *Diabetes Care* 22:846–848, 1999b.

Jovanovic L, Knopp RH, Kim H, Cefalu WT, Zhu X-D, Lee YJ, Simpson JL, Mills JL; for the Diabetes in Early Pregnancy Study Group: Elevated pregnancy losses at high and low extremes of maternal glucose in early normal and diabetic pregnancy. Evidence for a protective adaptation in diabetes. *Diabetes Care* 28:1113–1117, 2005.

Jovanovic L, Nakai Y: Successful pregnancy in women with type 1 diabetes: from preconception through postpartum care. *Endocrinol Metab Clin North Am* 35:79–97, 2006.

Jovanovic L, Pettitt DJ: Treatment with insulin and its analogs in pregnancies complicated by diabetes. *Diabetes Care* 30 (Suppl 2):S220–S224, 2007.

Jovanovic L, Kitzmiller JL: Insulin therapy in pregnancy. In: Hod M, Jovanovic L, Di Renzo GC, de Leiva A, Langer O, eds. *Textbook of Diabetes and Pregnancy.* 2nd ed. London: Informa Healthcare; 2008a:205–216.

Jovanovic LG: Using meal-based self-monitoring of blood glucose as a tool to improve outcomes in pregnancy complicated by diabetes. *Endocr Pract* 14:239–247, 2008b.

Jovanovic-Peterson L, Peterson CM: Dietary manipulation as a primary treatment strategy for pregnancies complicated by diabetes. *J Am Coll Nutr* 9:320–325, 1990.

Jovanovic-Peterson L, Peterson CM: Vitamin and mineral deficiencies which may predispose to glucose intolerance of pregnancy. *J Am Coll Nutr* 15:14–20, 1996.

Jovanovic-Peterson L, ed: *Medical Management of Pregnancy Complicated by Diabetes.* Alexandria, VA: American Diabetes Association; 2007.

Joy D, Thava VR, Scott BB: Diagnosis of fatty liver disease: is biopsy necessary? *Eur J Gastroenterol Hepatol* 15:539–543, 2003.

Joy SV, Rodgers PT, Scates AC: Incretin mimetics as emerging treatments for type 2 diabetes. *Ann Pharmacother* 39:110–118, 2005.

Jozwik M, Teng C, Wilkening RB, Meschia G, Tooze J, Chung M, Battaglia FC: Effects of branched-chain amino acids on placental amino acid transfer and insulin and glucagon release in the ovine fetus. *Am J Obstet Gynecol* 185:487–495, 2001.

Juhl M, Andersen PK, Olsen J, Madsen M, Jorgensen T, Nehr EA, Andersen AM: Physical exercise during pregnancy and the risk of preterm birth: a study within the Danish National Birth Cohort. *Am J Epidemiol* Feb 25, 2008 [Epub ahead of print].

Jungheim K, Koschinsky T: Glucose monitoring in the arm. Risky delays of hypoglycemia and hyperglycemia detection. *Diabetes Care* 25:956–960, 2002.

Kabiru W, Raynor BD: Obstetric outcomes associated with increase in BMI category during pregnancy. *Am J Obstet Gynecol* 191:928–932, 2004.

Kac G, Benicio MHDA, Velasquez-Mendez G, Valente JG, Struchiner J: Gestational weight gain and prepregnancy weight influence postpartum weight retention in a cohort of Brazilian women. *J Nutr* 134:661–666, 2004.

Kagnoff MF: Overview and pathogenesis of celiac disease. *Gastroenterology* 128: S10–S18, 2005.

Kahn BF, Davies JK, Lynch AM, Reynolds RM, Barbour LA: Predictors of glyuride failure in the treatment of gestational diabetes. *Obstet Gynecol* 107:1303–1309, 2006.

Kainer F, Weiss PA, Huttner V, Haas J, Reles M: Levels of amniotic fluid insulin and profiles of maternal blood glucose in pregnant women with diabetes type-1. *Early Hum Dev* 49:97–105, 1997.

Kairamkonda V, Deorukhkar A, Coombs R, Fraser R, Mayer T: Amylin peptide levels are raised in infants of diabetic mothers. *Arch Dis Child* 90:1279–1282, 2005.

Kakarla N, Dailey C, Marino T, Shikora SA, Chelmow D: Pregnancy after gastric bypass surgery and internal hernia formation. *Obstet Gynecol* 105:1195–1198, 2005.

Kalhan SC, Savin SM, Adam PAS: Attenuated glucose production rate in newborn infants of insulin-dependent diabetic mothers. *N Engl J Med* 296:375–376, 1977.

Kalhan SC, Hertz RH, Rossi KQ, Savin SM: Glucose-alanine relationship in diabetes in human pregnancy. *Metabolism* 40:629–633, 1991.

Kalhan SC, Denne SC, Patel DM, Nuamah IF, Savin SM: Leucine kinetics during a brief fast in diabetes in pregnancy. *Metabolism* 43:378–384, 1994.

Kalhan SC: Protein metabolism in pregnancy. *Am J Clin Nutr* 71:1249S–1255S, 2000.

Kalkhoff RK, Kandaraki E, Morrow PG, Mitchell TH, Kelber S, Borkowf HI: Relationship between neonatal birth weight and maternal plasma amino acid profiles in lean and obese nondiabetic women and in type 1 diabetic pregnant women. *Metabolism* 37:234–239, 1988.

Kalkwarf HJ, Bell RC, Khoury JC, Gouge AL, Miodovnik M: Dietary fiber intakes and insulin requirements in pregnant women with type 1 diabetes. *J Am Diet Assoc* 101:305–310, 2001.

Kallen B: Use of folic acid supplementation and risk for dizygotic twinning. *Early Hum Dev* 80:143–151, 2004.

Kalyoncu NI, Yaris F, Ulku C, Kadioglu M, Kesim M, Unsal M, Dikici M, Yaris E: A case of rosiglitazone exposure in the second trimester of pregnancy. *Reprod Toxicol* 19:563–564, 2005.

Kamp F, Kizilbash N, Corkey BE, Berggren P-O, Hamilton JA: Sulfonylureas rapidly cross phospholipid bilayer membranes by a free-diffusion mechanism. *Diabetes* 52:2526–2531, 2003.

Kamudhamas A, Pang L, Smith SD, Sadovsky Y, Nelson DM: Homocysteine thiolactone induces apoptosis in cultured human trophoblasts: a mechanism for homocysteine-mediated placental dysfunction? *Am J Obstet Gynecol* 191: 563–571, 2004.

Kaneshigi E: Serum ferritin as an assessment of iron stores and other hematologic parameters during pregnancy. *Obstet Gynecol* 57:238–242, 1981.

Kaplan JS, Iqbal S, England BG, Zawacki CM, Herman WH: Is pregnancy in diabetic women associated with folate deficiency? *Diabetes Care* 22:1017–1021, 1999.

Kaplan MM: Alanine aminotransferase levels: what's normal? *Ann Intern Med* 137:49–51, 2002.

Kapusta L, Haagmans ML, Steegers EA, Cuypers MH, Blom HJ, Eskes TK: Congenital heart defects and maternal derangement of homocysteine metabolism. *J Pediatr* 135:773–774, 1999.

Karlsson K, Kjellmer I: The outcome of diabetic pregnancies in relation to the mother's blood sugar level. *Am J Obstet Gynecol* 112:213–220, 1972.

Karlsson FA, Burman P, Loof L, Mardh S: Major parietal cell antigen in autoimmune gastritis with pernicious anemia is the acid producing H+/K+ adenosine triphosphatase of the stomach. *J Clin Invest* 81:475–479, 1988.

Karlsson HKR, Hallsten K, Bjornholm M, Tsuchida H, Chibalin AV, Virtanen KA, Heinonen OJ, Lonnqvist F, Nuutila P, Zierath JR: Effects of metformin and rosiglitazone treatment on insulin signaling and glucose uptake in patients with newly diagnosed type 2 diabetes. A randomized controlled study. *Diabetes* 54:1459–1467, 2005.

Karmaus W, Zhu X: Maternal concentration of polychlorinated bephenyls and dichlorodiphenyl dichlorethylene and birth weight in Michigan fish eaters: a cohort study. *Environ Health* 3:1, 2004.

Kaspers S, Kordonouri O, Schober E, Grabert M, Hauffa BP, Holl RW; German Working Group for Pediatric Diabetology: Anthropometry, metabolic control, and thyroid autoimmunity in type 1 diabetes with celiac disease: a multicenter survey. *J Pediatr* 145:790–795, 2004.

Katon W, Von Korff M, Ciechanowski P, Russo J, Lin E, Simon G, Ludman E, Walker E, Bush T, Young B: Behavioral and clinical factors associated with depression among individuals with diabetes. *Diabetes Care* 27:914–920, 2004.

Kaukinen K, Salmi J, Lahtela J, Siljamaki-Ojansuu U, Koivisto AM, Oksa H, Collin P: No effect of gluten-free diet on the metabolic control of type 1 diabetes in patients with diabetes and celiac disease. *Diabetes Care* 22:1747–1748, 1999.

Kauppila A, Korpela H, Makila UM, Yrjanheikki E: Low selenium concentration and glutathione peroxidase activity in intrahepatic cholestasis of pregnancy. *Br Med J* 294:150–152, 1987.

Kaur G, Rapthap CC, Kumar S, Bhatnagar S, Bhan MK, Mehra NK: Polymorphism in L-selectin, E-selectin and ICAM-1 genes in Asian pediatric patients with celiac disease. *Hum Immunol* 67:634–638, 2006.

Kautsky-Willer A, Thomaseth K, Ludvik B, Nowotny P, Rabensteiner D, Waldhausl W, Pacini G, Prager R: Elevated islet amyloid pancreatic polypeptide and proinsulin in lean gestational diabetes. *Diabetes* 46:607–614, 1997.

Keen CL, Clegg MS, Hanna LA, Lanoue L, Rogers JM, Daston GP, Oteiza P, Uriu-Adams JY: The plausibility of micronutrient deficiencies being a significant contributing factor to the occurrence of pregnancy complications. *J Nutr* 133:1597S–1605S, 2003.

Keijzers GB, De Galan B, Tack CJ, Smits P: Caffeine can decrease insulin sensitivity in humans. *Diabetes Care* 25:364–369, 2002.

Kekuda R, Prasad PD, Wu X, Wang H, Fei Y-J, Leibach FH, Ganapathy V: Cloning and functional characterization of a potential-sensitive, polyspecific organic cation transporter (OCT3) most abundantly expressed in placenta. *J Biol Chem* 273:15971–15979, 1998.

Kellett GL, Brot-Laroche E: Apical GLUT2. A major pathway of intestinal sugar absorption. *Diabetes* 54:3056–3062, 2005.

Kelley DE: Sugars and starch in the nutritional management of diabetes mellitus. *Am J Clin Nutr* 78 (Suppl):858S–864S, 2003.

Kemball ML, McIver C, Milner RDG, Nourse CH, Schiff D, Tiernan JR: Neonatal hypoglycemia in infants of diabetic mothers given sulphonylurea drugs in pregnancy. *Arch Dis Child* 45:696–701, 1970.

Kempson SA, Montrose MH: Osmotic regulation of renal betaine transport: transcription and beyond. *Pflugers Arch* 449:227–234, 2004.

Kendrick JM: Periconception care of women with diabetes. *J Perinat Neonatal Nurs* 18:14–25, 2004.

Kendrick JM, Wilson C, Elder RF, Smith CS: Reliability of reporting self-monitoring of blood glucose in pregnant women. *J Obstet Gynecol Neonatal Nurs* 34: 329–334, 2005.

Kennedy E, Meyers L: Dietary reference intakes: development and uses for assessment of micronutrient status of women—a global perspective. *Am J Clin Nutr* 81 (Suppl):1194S–1197S, 2005.

Kernaghan D, Penney GC, Pearson DW; Scottish Diabetes in Pregnancy Study Group: Birth weight and maternal glycated hemoglobin in pregnancies complicated by type 1 diabetes. *Scott Med J* 52:9–12, 2007.

Kerr D, Macdonald IA, Heller SR, Tattersall RB: Alcohol causes hypoglycemic unawareness in healthy volunteers and patients with type 1 (insulin-dependent) diabetes. *Diabetologia* 33:216–221, 1990.

Kerr D: Drugs and alcohol. In: Frier BM, Fisher M, eds. *Hypoglycemia and Diabetes.* London: Hodder and Stoughton; 1993:328–336.

Kerssen A, Evers IM, de Valk HW, Visser GHA: Poor glucose control in women with type 1 diabetes mellitus and 'safe' hemoglobin A1c values in the first trimester of pregnancy. *J Matern Fetal Neonatal Med* 13:309–313, 2003.

Kerssen A, de Valk HW, Visser GHA: Day-to-day glucose variability during pregnancy in women with type 1 diabetes mellitus: glucose profiles measured with the Continuous Glucose Monitoring System. *BJOG* 111:919–924, 2004a.

Kerssen A, de valk HW, Visser GHA: The Continuous Glucose Monitoring System during pregnancy of women with type 1 diabetes mellitus: accuracy assessment. *Diabetes Technol Ther* 6:645–651, 2004b.

Kerssen A, De Valk HW, Visser GH: Validation of the Continuous Glucose Monitoring System (CGMS) by the use of two CGMS simultaneously in pregnant women with type 1 diabetes mellitus. *Diabetes Technol Ther* 7:699–706, 2005.

Kerssen A, de valk HW, Visser GH: Do HbA(1)c levels and the self-monitoring of blood glucose levels adequately reflect glycemic control during pregnancy in women with type 1 diabetes mellitus? *Diabetologia* 49:25–28, 2006a.

Kerssen A, de Valk HW, Visser GH: Forty-eight-hour first-trimester glucose profiles in women with type 1 diabetes mellitus: a report of three cases of congenital malformation. *Prenat Diagn* 26:123–127, 2006b.

Kerssen A, de Valk HW, Visser GHA: Increased second trimester maternal glucose levels are related to extremely large-for-gestational-age infants in women with type 1 diabetes. *Diabetes Care* 30:1069–1074, 2007.

Khodiguian N, Jaque-Fortunato SV, Wiswell RA, Artal R: A comparison of cross-sectional and longitudinal methods of assessing the influence of pregnancy on cardiac function during exercise. *Semin Perinatol* 20:232–241, 1996.

Khumalo H, Gomo ZAR, Moyo VM, Gordeuk VR, Saungweme T, Raoult TA, Gangaidzo IT: Serum transferrin receptors are decreased in the presence of iron overload. *Clin Chem* 44:40–44, 1998.

Kieffer EC, Alexander GR, Kogan MD, Himes JH, Herman WH, Mor JM, Hayashi R: Influence of diabetes during pregnancy on gestational age-specific newborn weight among US black and US white infants. *Am J Epidemiol* 147:1053–1061, 1998.

Kilby MD, Neary RM, Mackness MI, Durrington PN: Fetal and maternal lipoprotein metabolism in human pregnancy complicated by type I diabetes mellitus. *J Clin Endocrinol Metab* 83:1736–1741, 1998.

Kim C, Ferrara A, McEwen LN, Marrero DG, Gerzoff RB, Herman WH; the TRIAD Study Group: Preconception care in managed care: the translating research into action for diabetes study. *Am J Obstet Gynecol* 192:227–232, 2005.

Kim EH, Kim IK, Kwon JY, Kim SW, Park YW: The effect of fish consumption on blood mercury levels of pregnant women. *Yonsei Med J* 47:626–633, 2006.

Kimmerle R, Heineman L, Delecki A, Berger M: Severe hypoglycemia: incidence and predisposing factors in 85 pregnancies of type 1 diabetic women. *Diabetes Care* 15:1034–1037, 1992.

Kinalski M, Sledziewski A, Telejko B, Straczkowski M, Kretowski A, Kinalska I: Post-partum evaluation of amylin in lean patients with gestational diabetes mellitus. *Acta Diabetol* 41:1–4, 2004.

King GL, Goodman AD, Buzney S, Moses A, Kahn CR: Receptors and growth-promoting effects of insulin and insulinlike growth factors on cells from bovine retinal capillaries and aorta. *J Clin Invest* 75:1028–1036, 1985.

King JC: Assessment of zinc status. *J Nutr* 120:1474–1479, 1990.

King JC, Hambridge KM, Westcott JL, Kern DL, Marshall G: Daily variation in plasma zinc concentrations in women fed meals at six-hour intervals. *J Nutr* 124:508–516, 1994.

King JC: Physiology of pregnancy and nutrient metabolism. *Am J Clin Nutr* 71 (Suppl):1218S–1225S, 2000a.

King JC: Determinants of maternal zinc status during pregnancy. *Am J Clin Nutr* 71 (Suppl):1334S–1343S, 2000b.

King JC: Effect of reproduction on the bioavailability of calcium, zinc and selenium. *J Nutr* 131:1355S–1358S, 2001.

Kirchheiner J, Brockmoller J, Meineke I, Bauer S, Rohde W, Meisel C, Roots I: Impact of *CYP2C9* amino acid polymorphisms on glyburide kinetics and on the insulin and glucose response in healthy volunteers. *Clin Pharmacol Ther* 71:286–296, 2002.

Kirpichnikov D, McFarlane SI, Sowers JR: Metformin: an update. *Ann Intern Med* 137:25–33, 2002.

Kirwan JP, Hauguel-de Mouzon S, Lepercq J, Challier JC, Huston-Presley L, Friedman JE, Kalhan SC, Catalano PM: TNF-α is a predictor of insulin resistance in human pregnancy. *Diabetes* 51:2207–2213, 2002.

Kirwan JP, Varastehpour A, Jing M, Presley L, Shao J, Friedman JE, Catalano PM: Reversal of insulin resistance postpartum is linked to enhanced skeletal muscle signaling. *J Clin Endocrinol Metab* 89:4678–4684, 2004.

Kishimoto M, Yamasaki Y, Kubota M, Arai K, Morishima T, Kawamori R, Kamata T: 1,5-anhydro-D-glucitol evaluates daily glycemic excursions in well-controlled NIDDM. *Diabetes Care* 18:1156–1159, 1995.

Kitajima M, Oka S, Yasuhi I, Fukuda M, Rii Y, Ishimaru T. Maternal serum triglyceride at 24-32 weeks' gestation and newborn weight in nondiabetic women with positive diabetic screens. *Obstet Gynecol* 97:776–780, 2001.

Kitzmiller JL, Cloherty JP, Younger MD, Tabatabaii A, Rothchild SB, Sosenko I, Epstein MF, Singh S, Neff RK: Diabetic pregnancy and perinatal morbidity. *Am J Obstet Gynecol* 131:560–580, 1978.

Kitzmiller JL, Younger MD, Hare JW, Phillippe M, Vignati L, Farcnoli B, Grause A: Continuous subcutaneous insulin therapy during early pregnancy. *Obstet Gynecol* 66:606–611, 1985.

Kitzmiller JL, Gavin LA, Gin GD, Iverson M, Gunderson E, Farley P: Managing diabetes and pregnancy. *Curr Prob Obstet Gynecol Fertil* 11:105–167, 1988.

Kitzmiller JL, Gavin LA, Gin GD, Jovanovic Peterson L, Main EK, Zigrang WD: Preconception care of diabetes: glycemic control prevents congenital anomalies. *JAMA* 265:731–736, 1991.

Kitzmiller JL: Sweet success with diabetes: the development of insulin therapy and glycemic control for pregnancy. *Diabetes Care* 16 (Suppl 3):107–121, 1993.

Kitzmiller JL, Buchanan TA, Kjos S, Combs CA, Ratner RE: Pre-conception care of diabetes, congenital malformations, and spontaneous abortions. ADA technical review. *Diabetes Care* 19:514–541, 1996.

Kitzmiller JL, Main E, Ward B, Theiss T, Peterson DL: Insulin lispro and the development of proliferative diabetic retinopathy in pregnancy. *Diabetes Care* 22:874–876, 1999.

Kitzmiller JL, Jovanovic L: Insulin therapy in pregnancy. In: Hod H, Jovanovic L, Di Renzo GC, de Leiva A, Langer O, eds. *Textbook of Diabetes and Pregnancy.* New York: Martin Dunitz; 2003:359–378.

Klebanoff MA, Shiono PH, Berendes HW, Rhoads GG: Facts and artifacts about anemia and preterm delivery. *JAMA* 262:511–515, 1989.

Kleefstra N, Houweling ST, Jansman FGA, Groenier KH, Gans ROB, Meyboom-de Jong B, Bakker SJL, Bilo HJG: Chromium treatment has no effect in patients with poorly controlled, insulin treated type 2 diabetes in an obese western population. A randomized, double-blind, placebo-controlled trial. *Diabetes Care* 29:521–525, 2006.

Klein BEK, Moss SE, Klein R: Effect of pregnancy on progression of diabetic retinopathy. *Diabetes Care* 13:34–40, 1990.

Kliewer SA, Sundseth SS, Jones SA, Brown PJ, Wisely GB, Koble CS, Devchand P, Wahli W, Willson TM, Lenhard JM, Lehmann JM: Fatty acids and eicosanoids regulate gene expression through direct interactions with peroxisome proliferator-activated receptors α and β. *Proc Natl Acad Sci U S A* 94:4318–4323, 1997.

Kljai K, Runje R: Selenium and glycogen levels in diabetic patients. *Biol Trace Elem Res* 83:223–229, 2001.

Klonoff DC: Continuous glucose monitoring. Roadmap for 21st century diabetes therapy. *Diabetes Care* 28:1231–1239, 2005a.

Klonoff DC: A review of continuous glucose monitoring technology. *Diabetes Technol Ther* 7:770–775, 2005b.

Kluijtmans LAJ, Young IS, Boreham CA, Murray L, McMaster D, McNulty H, Strain JJ, McPartlin J, Scott JM, Whitehead AS: Genetic and nutritional factors contributing to hyperhomocysteinemia in young adults. *Blood* 101:2483–2488, 2003.

Knee TS, Seidensticker DF, Walton JL, Solberg LM, Lasseter DH: A novel use of U-500 insulin for continuous subcutaneous insulin infusion in patients with insulin resistance: a case series. *Endocr Pract* 9:181–186, 2003.

Knekt P, Ritz J, Pereira MA, O'Reilly EJ, Augustsson K, Fraser GE, Goldbourt U, Heitmann BL, Hallmans G, Liu S, Pietinen P, Spiegelman D, Stevens J, Virtamo J, Willett WC, Rimm EB, Ascherio A: Antioxidant vitamins and coronary heart disease risk: a pooled analysis of 9 cohorts. *Am J Clin Nutr* 80:1508–1520, 2004.

Knight KM, Dornan T, Bundy C: The diabetes educator: trying hard, but must concentrate more on behaviour. *Diabet Med* 23:485–501, 2006.

Kniss DA, Shubert PJ, Zimmerman PD, Landon MB, Gabbe SG: Insulin-like growth factors: their regulation of glucose and amino acid transport in placental trophoblasts isolated from first trimester chorionic villi. *J Reprod Med* 39: 249–256, 1994.

Knobeloch L, Anderson HA, Imm P, Peters D, Smith A: Fish consumption, advisory awareness, and hair mercury levels among women of childbearing age. *Environ Res* 97:220–227, 2005.

Knol MJ, Twisk JW, Beekman AT, Heine RJ, Snoek FJ, Pouwer F: Depression as a risk factor for the onset of type 2 diabetes mellitus. A meta-analysis. *Diabetologia* 49:837–845, 2006.

Knopp RH, Bergelin RO, Wahl PW, Walden CE: Relationships of infant birth size to maternal lipoproteins, apoprotein, fuels, hormones, clinical chemistries and body weight at 36 weeks gestation. *Diabetes* 34:71–77, 1985.

Knopp RH, Warth MR, Charles D, Childs M, Li JR, Mabuchi H, Van Allen MI: Lipoprotein metabolism in pregnancy, fat transport to the fetus, and the effects of diabetes. *Biol Neonate* 50:297–317, 1986.

Knopp RH, Magee MS, Raisys V, Benedetti T: Metabolic effects of hypocaloric diets in management of gestational diabetes. *Diabetes* 40:165–171, 1991.

Knopp RH, Magee MS, Walden CE, Bonet B, Benedetti TJ: Prediction of infant birth weight by GDM screening tests. Importance of plasma triglyceride. *Diabetes Care* 15:1605–1613, 1992.

Knopp RH: Hormone-mediated changes in nutrient metabolism in pregnancy: a physiological basis for normal fetal development. *Ann N Y Acad Sci* 817: 251–271, 1997.

Knottnerus JA, Delgado LR, Knipschild PG, Essed GG, Smits F: Hematologic parameters and pregnancy outcome. A prospective cohort study in the third trimester. *J Clin Epidemiol* 43:461–466, 1990.

Kokkenen J: Parietal cell antibodies and gastric secretion in children with diabetes mellitus. *Acta Paediatr Scand* 69:485–489, 1980.

Koletzko B, Muller J: *Cis-* and *trans-*isomeric fatty acids in plasma lipids of newborn infants and their mothers. *Biol Neonate* 57:172–178, 1990.

Koller O, Sagen N, Ulstein M, Vaula D: Fetal growth retardation associated with inadequate hemodilution in otherwise uncomplicated pregnancy. *Acta Obstet Gynecol Scand* 58:9–13, 1979.

Kondo T, Vicent D, Suzuma K, Yanagisawa M, King GL, Holzenberger M, Kahn CR: Knockout of insulin and IGF-1 receptors on vascular endothelial cells protects against retinal neovascularization. *J Clin Invest* 111:1835–1842, 2003.

Koopman-Esseboom C, Morse DC, Weisglas-Kuperus N, Lutkeschipholt IJ, Van der Paauw CG, Tuinstra LG, Brouwer A, Sauer PJ: Effects of dioxins and polychlorinated bphenyls on thyroid hormone status of pregnant women and their infants. *Pediatr Res* 36:468–473, 1994.

Kopp-Hoolihan L, van Loan MD, Wong WW, King JC: Longitudinal assessment of energy balance in well-nourished pregnant women. *Am J Clin Nutr* 69:697–704, 1999.

Kordonouri O, Dieterich W, Schuppan D, Webert G, Muller C, Sarioglu N, Becker M, Danne T: Autoantibodies to tissue transglutaminase are sensitive serological parameters for detecting silent celiac disease in patients with Type 1 diabetes mellitus. *Diabet Med* 17:441–444, 2000.

Koren G: Glyburide and fetal safety: transplacental pharmacokinetic considerations. *Reprod Toxicol* 15:227–229, 2001.

Korpony-Szabo IR, Sulkanen S, Halttunen T, Maurano F, Rossi M, Mazzarella G, Laurila K, Troncone R, Maki M: Tissue transglutaminase is the target in both rodent and primate tissues for celiac disease-specific autoantibodies. *J Pediatr Gastroenterol Nutr* 31:520–527, 2000.

Korponay-Szabo IR, Dahlbom I, Laurila K, Koskinen S, Woolley N, Partanen J, Kovacs JB, Maki M, Hansson T: Elevation of IgG antibodies against tissue transglutaminase as a dianostic tool for celiac disease in selective IgA deficiency. *Gut* 52:1567–1571, 2003.

Koskinen T, Kuoppala T, Tuimala R: Amniotic fluid 25-hydroxyvitamin D concentrations in normal and complicated pregnancy. *Eur J Obstet Gynecol Reprod Biol* 21:1–5, 1986.

Kotze LM: Gynecologic and obstetric findings related to nutritional status and adherence to a gluten-free diet in Brazilian patients with celiac disease. *J Clin Gastroenterol* 38:567–574, 2004.

Kouba S, Hallstrom T, Lindholm C, Hirschberg AL: Pregnancy and neonatal outcomes in women with eating disorders. *Obstet Gynecol* 105:255–260, 2005.

Koukkou E, Young P, Lowy C: The effect of maternal glycemic control on fetal growth in diabetic pregnancies. *Am J Perinatol* 14:547–552, 1997.

Kovilam O, Khoury J, Miodovnik M, Chames M, Spinnoto J, Sibai B: Spontaneous preterm delivery in the type 1 diabetic pregnancy: the role of glycemic control. *J Matern Fetal Neonatal Med* 111: 245–248, 2002.

Kraemer J, Klein J, Lubetsky A, Koren G: Perfusion studies of glyburide transfer across the human placenta: implications for fetal safety. *Am J Obstet Gynecol* 195:270–274, 2006.

Kramer MS: Determinants of low birth weight: methodological assessment and meta-analysis. *WHO Bull* 65:663–737, 1987.

Kramer MS: Effects of energy and protein intakes on pregnancy outcome: an overview of the research evidence from controlled clinical trials. *Am J Clin Nutr* 58:627–635, 1993.

Kramer MS, McDonald SW: Aerobic exercise for women during pregnancy. *Cochrane Database Syst Rev* 2006 Jul 19;(3):CD000180.

Kremer CJ, Duff P: Glyburide for the treatment of gestational diabetes. *Am J Obstet Gynecol* 190:1438–1439, 2004.

Kris-Etherton PM, Harris WS, Appel LJ: Fish consumption, fish oil, omega-3 fatty acids and cardiovascular disease. *Circulation* 106:2747–2757, 2002.

Kruse-Jarres JD, Rukgauer M: Trace elements in diabetes mellitus. Peculiarities and clinical validity of determinations in blood cells. *J Trace Elem Biol* 14:21–27, 2000.

Kuhn DC, Crawford M: Placental essential fatty acid transport and prostaglandin synthesis. *Prog Lipid Res* 25:345–353, 1986.

Kulin NA, Pastuszak A, Sage SR, Schick-Boschetto B, Spivey G, Feldkamp M, Ormond K, Matsui D, Stein-Schechman AK, Cook L, Brochu J, Rieder M, Koren G: Pregnancy outcome following maternal use of the new selective serotonin reuptake inhibitors: a prospective controlled multicenter study. *JAMA* 279:609–610, 1998.

Kulkarni K, Castle G, Gregory R, Holmes A, Leontos C, Powers M, Snetselaar L, Splett P, Wylie-Rosett J: Nutrition practice guidelines for type 1 diabetes mellitus positively affect dietitian practices and patient outcomes. *J Am Diet Assoc* 98: 62–70, 1998.

Kullo IJ, Li G, Bielak LF, Bailey KR, Sheedy PF 2nd, Peyser PA, Turner ST, Kardia SL: Association of plasma homocysteine with coronary artery calcification in different categories of coronary heart disease risk. *Mayo Clin Proc* 81:177–182, 2006a.

Kullo I: HOPE 2: can supplementation with folic acid and B vitamins reduce cardiovascular risk? *Nat Clin Pract Cardiovasc Med* 3:414–415, 2006b.

Kumar N, Dey CS: Metformin enhances insulin signaling in insulin-dependent and -independent pathways in insulin resistant muscle cells. *Br J Pharmacol* 137: 329–336, 2002.

Kuoppala T: Alterations in vitamin D metabolites and minerals in diabetic pregnancy. *Gynecol Obstet Invest* 25:99–105, 1988.

Kupper C: Dietary guidelines and implementation for celiac disease. *Gastroenterology* 128 (Suppl 1):S121–S127, 2005.

Kurtzhals P, Schaffer L, Sorensen A, Kristensen C, Jonassen I, Schmid C, Trub T: Correlations of receptor binding and metabolic and mitogenic potencies of insulin analogs designed for clinical use. *Diabetes* 49:999–1005, 2000.

Kuruvilla AG, D'Souza SW, Glazier JD, Mahendran D, Maresh J, Sibley CP: Altered activity of the system A amino acid transporter in microvillous membrane vesicles from placenta of macrosomic babies born to diabetic women. *J Clin Invest* 94:689–695, 1994.

Kuwa K, Nakayama T, Hoshino T, Tominaga M: Relationships of glucose concentrations in capillary whole blood, venous whole blood and venous plasma. *Clin Chim Acta* 307:187–192, 2001.

Kyne-Grzebalski D, Wood L, Marshall SM, Taylor R: Episodic hyperglycemia in pregnant women with well-controlled type 1 diabetes mellitus: a major potential factor underlying macrosomia. *Diabet Med* 16:702–706, 1999.

La Marca A, Artensio AC, Stabile G, Volpe A: Metformin treatment of PCOS during adolescence and the reproductive period. *Eur J Obstet Gynecol Reprod Biol* 121: 3–7, 2005.

Lachilli B, Hininger I, Faure H, Arnaud J, Richard MJ, Favier A, Roussel AM: Increased lipid peroxidation in pregnant women after iron supplementation. *Biol Trace Elem Res* 83:103–110, 2001.

Laffel LM, Wentzell K, Loughlin C, Tovar A, Moltz K, Brink S: Sick day management using blood 3-hydroxybutyrate (3-OHB) compared with urine ketone monitoring reduces hospital visits in young people with T1DM: a randomized clinical trial. *Diabet Med* 23:278–284, 2006.

Lago RM, Singh PP, Nesto RW: Congestive heart failure and cardiovascular death in patients with prediabetes and type 2 diabetes given thiazolidinediones: a meta-analysis of randomized clinical trials. *Lancet* 370:1129–1136, 2007.

Laine DC, Thomas W, Levitt MD, Bantle JP: Comparison of predictive capabilities of diabetic exchange lists and glycemic index of foods. *Diabetes Care* 10: 387–394, 1987.

Laivuori H, Kaaka R, Turpeinen U, Viinikka L, Ylikorkala O: Plasma homocysteine levels elevated and inversely related to insulin sensitivity in preeclampsia. *Obstet Gynecol* 93:489–493, 1999.

Lakin V, Haggarty P, Abramovich DR, Ashton J, Moffat CF, McNeill G, Danielian PJ, Grubb D: Dietary intake and tissue concentration of fatty acids in omnivore, vegetarian and diabetic pregnancy. *Prostaglandins, Leukot Essent Fatty Acids* 59:209–220, 1998.

Lamb MR, Taylor S, Liu X, Wolff MS, Borrell L, Matte TD, Susser ES, Factor-Litvak P: Prenatal exposure to polychlorinated bephenyls and postnatal growth: a structural analysis. *Environ Health Perspect* 114:779–785, 2006.

Landin-Olsson M, Karlsson FA, Lernmark A, Sundkvist G; the Diabetes Incidence Study in Sweden Group: Islet cell and thyrogastric antibodies in 633 consecutive

15- to 34-yr-old patients in the Diabetes Incidence Study in Sweden. *Diabetes* 41:1022–1027, 1992.

Landon MB, Gabbe SG, Piana R, Mennuti RT, Elliot K: Neonatal morbidity in pregnancy complicated by diabetes mellitus: predictive value of maternal glycemic profiles. *Am J Obstet Gynecol* 156:1086–1095, 1987.

Landstedt-Hallin L, Adamson U, Lins PE: Oral glibenclamide suppresses glucagon secretion during insulin-induced hypoglycemia in patients with type 2 diabetes. *J Clin Endocrinol Metab* 84:3140–3145, 1999.

Lane JD, Barkauskas CE, Surwit RS, Feinglos MN: Caffeine impairs glucose metabolism in type 2 diabetes. *Diabetes Care* 27:2047–2048, 2004.

Lane JD, Feinglos MN, Surwit RS: Caffeine increases ambulatory glucose and postprandial responses in coffee drinkers with type 2 diabetes. *Diabetes Care* 31:221–222, 2008.

Lange H, Suryapranata H, De Luca G, Borner C, Dille J, Kallmayer K, Pasalary MN, Scherer E, Dambrink JH: Folate therapy and in-stent restenosis after coronary stenting. *N Engl J Med* 350:2673–2681, 2004.

Langer O, Mazze RS: Diabetes in pregnancy: evaluating self-monitoring performance and glycemic control with memory-based reflectance meters. *Am J Obstet Gynecol* 155:635–637, 1986.

Langer O, Anyaegbunam A, Brustman L, Guideti D, Levy J, Mazze R: Pregestational diabetes: insulin requirements throughout pregnancy. *Am J Obstet Gynecol* 159:616–621, 1988.

Langer N, Langer O: Pre-existing diabetics: relationship between glycemic control and emotional status in pregnancy. *J Matern-Fetal Med* 7:257–263, 1998.

Langer O, Conway DL, Berkus MD, Xenakis EMJ, Gonzales O: A comparison of glyburide and insulin in women with gestational diabetes mellitus. *New Engl J Med* 343:1134–1138, 2000.

Langer O: A spectrum of glucose thresholds may effectively prevent complications in the pregnant diabetic patient. *Semin Perinatol* 26:196–205, 2002.

Langer O, Yogev Y, Xenakis EMJ, Rosenn B: Insulin and glyburide therapy: dosage, severity level of gestational diabetes, and pregnancy outcome. *Am J Obstet Gynecol* 192:134–139, 2005.

Langer O, ed: *The Diabetes in Pregnancy Dilemma: Leading Change With Proven Solutions.* Lanham, MD: University Press of America; 2006.

Lao TT, Tam KF, chan LY: Third trimester iron status and pregnancy outcome in non-anemic women: pregnancy unfavorably affected by maternal iron excess. *Hum Reprod* 15:1843–1848, 2000.

Lao TT, Chan PL, Tam KF: Gestational diabetes mellitus in the last trimester—a feature of maternal iron excess? *Diabet Med* 18:218–223, 2001.

Lapolla A, Dalfra MG, Masin M, Bruttomesso D, Piva I, Crepaldi C, Tortul C, Dalla Barba B, Fedele D: Analysis of outcome of pregnancy in type 1 diabetics treated with insulin pump or conventional insulin therapy. *Acta Diabetol* 40:143–149, 2003.

Lapolla A, Dalfra MG, Fedele D: Insulin therapy in pregnancy complicated by diabetes: are insulin analogs a new tool? *Diabetes Metab Res Rev* 21:241–252, 2005.

Lapolla A, Dalfra MG, Spezia R, Anichini R, Bonomo M, Bruttomesso D, Di Cianni G, Franzetti I, Galluzzo A, Mello G, Menato G, Napoli A, Noacco G, Parretti E, Santini C, Scaldaferri E, Songini M, Tonutti L, Torlone E, Gentilella R, Rossi A, Valle D: Outcome of pregnancy in type 1 diabetic patients treated with insulin lispro or regular insulin: an Italian experience. *Acta Diabetol* 45: 61–66, 2008.

Lappas M, Permezel M, Georgiou HM, Rice GE: Regulation of proinflammatory cytokines in human gestational tissues by peroxisome proliferator-activated receptor-γ: effect of 15-deoxy-Δ(12,14)-PGJ(2) and troglitazone. *J Clin Endocrinol Metab* 87:4667–4672, 2002.

Lappas M, Permezel M, Ho PW, Moseley JM, Wlodek ME, Rice GE: Effect of nuclear factor-kappa B inhibitors and peroxisome proliferators-activated receptor-gamma ligands on PTHrP release from human fetal membranes. *Placenta* 25:699–704, 2004.

Lappas M, Permezel M, Rice GE: Leptin and adiponectin stimulate the release of proinflammatory cytokines and prostaglandins from human placenta and maternal adipose tissue via nuclear factor-kappaB peroximal proliferators-activated receptor-gamma and exracellularly regulated kinase 1/2. *Endocrinol* 146:3334–3342, 2005a.

Lappas M, Yee K, Permezel M, Rice GE: Release and regulation of leptin, resistin and adiponectin from human placenta, fetal membranes, and maternal adipose tissue and skeletal muscle from normal and gestational diabetes mellitus-complicated pregnancies. *J Endocrinol* 186:457–465, 2005b.

Lappas M, Permezel M, Rice GE: 15-Deoxy-delta (12,14)-prostaglandin J(2) and troglitazone regulation of the release of phospholipid metabolites, inflammatory cytokines and proteases from human gestational tissues. *Placenta* 27:1060–1072, 2006.

Lappin TR, Savage GA, Metzger BE, Lowe LP, Haggan SA, Dyer AR: Normative values of hemoglobin A1C (HbA1C) in non-diabetic pregnancy: data from the Hyperglycemia and Adverse Pregnancy Outcome study. Abstract. *Diabetes* 55 (Suppl 1):A217, 2006.

Larque E, Krauss-Etschmann S, Campoy C, Hartl D, Linde J, Klingler M, Demmelmair H, Cano A, Gil A, Bondy B, Koletzko B: Docasahexaenoic acid supply in pregnancy affects placental expression of fatty acid transport protins. *Am J Clin Nutr* 84:853–861, 2006.

Larsen J, Ford T, Lyden E, Colling C, Mack-Shipman L, Lane J: What is hypoglycemia in patients with well-controlled type 1 diabetes treated by subcutaneous insulin pump with use of the Continuous Glucose Monitoring System? *Endocr Pract* 10:324–329, 2004.

Larsen JC: Risk assessments of polychlorinated dibenzo- p-dioxins, polychlorinated dibenzofurans, and dioxin-like polychlorinated biphenyls in food. *Mol Nutr Food Res* 50:885–896, 2006.

Larsson L, Lindqyist PG: Low-impact exercise during pregnancy—a study of safety. *Acta Obstet Gynecol Scand* 84:34–38, 2005.

Lassegue B, Griendling KK: Reactive oxygen species in hypertension. An update. *Am J Hypertens* 17:852–860, 2004.

Lattimore KA, Donn SM, Kaciroti N, Kemper AR, Neal CR Jr, Vasquez DM: Selective serotonin reuptake inhibitor (SSRI) use during pregnancy and effects on the fetus and newborn: a meta-analysis. *J Perinatol* 25:595–604, 2005.

Lauenberg J, Mathiesen E, Ovesen P, Westergaard JG, Ekbom P, Molsted-Pedersen L, Damm P: Audit on stillbirths in women with pregestational type 1 diabetes. *Diabetes Care* 26:1385–1389, 2003.

Laurin J, Lindor KD, Crippin JS, Gossard A, Gores GJ, Ludwig J, Rakela J, McGill DB: Ursodeoxycholic acid or clofibrate in the treatment of non-alcohol steatohepatitis: a pilot study. *Hepatology* 23:1464–1467, 1996.

Lauszus F, Rasmussen O, Henriksen J, Klebe JG, Jensen L, Lauszus KS, Hermansen K: Effect of a high monounsaturated fatty acid diet on blood pressure and glucose metabolism in women with gestational diabetes mellitus. *Eur J Clin Nutr* 55:436–443, 2001b.

Lauszus FF, Rasmussen OW, Lousen T, Klebe TM, Klebe JG: Ambulatory blood pressure as predictor of preeclampsia in diabetic pregnancies with respect to urinary albumin excretion rate and glycemic regulation. *Acta Obstet Gynecol Scand* 80:1096–1103, 2001a.

Lauszus FF, Klebe JG, Bek T, Flyvbjerg A: Increased serum IGF-I during pregnancy is associated with progression of diabetic retinopathy. *Diabetes* 52:852–856, 2003.

Lauszus FF, Fuglsang J, Flyvbjerg A, Klebe JG: Preterm delivery in normoalbuminuric, diabetic women without preeclampsia: the role of metabolic control. *Eur J Obstet Gynecol Reprod Biol* 124:144–149, 2006.

Lautamaki R, Borra R, Iozzo P, Komu M, Lehtimaki T, Salmi M, Jalkanen S, Airaksinen KE, Knuuti J, Parkkola R, Nuutila P: Liver steatosis coexists with myocardial insulin resistance and coronary dysfunction in patients with type 2 diabetes. *Am J Physiol Endocrinol Metab* 291:E282–290, 2006.

Lea RG, Howe D, Hannah LT, Bonneau O, Hunter L, Hoggard N: Placental leptin in normal, diabetic and fetal growth-retarded pregnancies. *Mol Hum Reprod* 6:763–769, 2000.

Lean MEJ, Ng LL, Tennison BR: Interval between insulin injection and eating in relation to blood glucose control in adult diabetics. *Br Med J* 290:105–108, 1985.

Lederman SA, Paxton A, Heymsfield SB, Wang J, Thornton J, Pierson RN: Body fat and water changes during pregnancy in women with different body weight and weight gain. *Obstet Gynecol* 90:483–488, 1997.

Lee DH, Jacobs DR Jr: Serum markers of stored body iron are not appropriate markers of health effects of iron: a focus on serum ferritin. *Med Hypotheses* 62:442–445, 2004a.

Lee W, Kim RB: Transporters and renal drug elimination. *Annu Rev Pharmacol Toxicol* 44:137–166, 2004b.

Lee DH, Liu DY, Jacobs DR Jr, Shin H-R, Song K, Lee I-K, Kim B, Hider RC: Common presence of non-transferrin-bound iron among patients with type 2 diabetes. *Diabetes Care* 29:1090–1095, 2006a.

Lee DH, Lee IK, Song K, Steffes M, Toscano W, Baker BA, Jacobs DR Jr: A strong dose-response relation between serum concentrations of persistent organic pollutants and diabetes: results from the National Health and Examination Survey 1999–2002. *Diabetes Care* 29:1638–1644, 2006b.

Lee SK, Green PH: Celiac sprue (the great modern-day imposter). *Curr Opin Rheumatol* 18:101–107, 2006c.

Lee AM, Lam SK, Sze Mun Lau SM, Chong CS, Chui HW, Fong DY: Prevalence, course, and risk factors for antenatal anxiety and depression. *Obstet Gynecol* 110:1102–1112, 2007.

Lehmann JM, Lenhard JM, Oliver BB, Ringold GM, Kliewer SA: Peroxisome proliferator-activated receptors alpha and gamma are activated by indomethacin and other non-steroidal anti-inflammatory drugs. *J Biol Chem* 272:3406–10, 1997.

Lenhard JM, Kliewer SA, Paulik MA, Plunket KD, Lehmann JM, Weiel JE: Effects of troglitazone and metformin on glucose and lipid metabolism: alterations of two distinct molecular pathways. *Biochem Pharmacol* 54:801–808, 1997.

Lentz SR, Sobey CG, Piegors DJ, Bhopatkar MY, Faraci FM, Malinow MR, Heistad DD: Vascular dysfunction in monkeys with diet-induced hyperhomocysteinemia. *J Clin Invest* 98:24–29, 1996.

Leonard SW, Good CK, Gugger ET, Traber MG: Vitamin E bioavailability from fortified breakfast cereal is greater than that from encapsulated supplements. *Am J Clin Nutr* 79:86–92, 2004.

Leong W-I, Lonnerdal B: Hepcidin, the recently identified peptide that appears to regulate iron absorption. *J Nutr* 134:1–4, 2004.

Leopold JA, Loscalzo J: Oxidative Enzymopathies and vascular disease. *Arterioscler Thromb Vasc Biol* 25:1332–1340, 2005.

Lepercq J, Cauzac M, Lahlou J, Timsit J, Girard J, Auwerx J, Hauguel-de Mouzon S: Overexpression of placental leptin in diabetic pregnancies: a critical role for insulin. *Diabetes* 47:847–850, 1998.

Lepercq J, Lahlou N, Timsit J, Girard J, Hauguel-de Mouzon S: Macrosomia revisited: ponderal index and leptin delineate subtypes of fetal overgrowth. *Am J Obstet Gynecol* 181:621–625, 1999.

Lepercq J, Coste J, Theau A, Dubois-Laforgue D, Timsit J: Factors associated with preterm delivery in women with type 1 diabetes. A cohort study. *Diabetes Care* 27:2824–2828, 2004.

Lepore M, Pampanelli S, Fanelli C, Porcellati F, Bartocci L, Di Vicenzo A, Cordoni C, Costa E, Brunetti P, Bolli GM: Pharmacokinetics and pharmacodynamics of subcutaneous injection of long-acting insulin analog glargine, NPH insulin and ultralente human insulin and continuous subcutaneous infusion of insulin lispro. *Diabetes* 49:42–48, 2000.

Leveno KJ, Fortunato SJ, Raskin P, Williams ML, Whalley PJ: Continuous subcutaneous insulin infusion during pregnancy. *Diabetes Res Clin Pract* 4:257–268, 1988.

Lever M, Sizeland PC, Bason LM, Hayman CM, Chambers ST: Glycine betaine and proline betaine in human blood and urine. *Biochim Biophys Acta* 1200:259–164, 1994a.

Lever M, Sizeland PC, Bason LM, Hayman CM, Robson RA, Chambers ST: Abnormal glycine betaine content of the blood and urine of diabetic and renal patients. *Clin Chim Acta* 230:69–79, 1994b.

Levine RJ, Hauth JC, Curet LB, Sibai BM, Catalano PM, Morris CD, DerSimonian R, Esterlitz JR, Raymond EG, Bild DE, Clemens JD, Cutler JA: Trial of calcium to prevent preeclampsia. *N Engl J Med* 337:69–76, 1997.

Levinson-Castiel R, Merlob P, Linder N, Sirota L, Klinger G: Neonatal abstinence syndrome after in utero exposure to selective serotonin reuptake inhibitors in term infants. *Arch Pediatr Adolesc Med* 160:173–176, 2006.

Levy HL, Waisbren SE: Effects of untreated maternal phenylketonuria and hyperphenylalaninemia on the fetus. *N Engl J Med* 309:1269–1274, 1983.

Li R, Hass JD, Habicht J-P: Timing of the influence of maternal nutritional status during pregnancy on fetal growth. *Am J Hum Biol* 10:529–539, 1998.

Li H, Gu Y, Zhang Y, Lucas MJ, Wang Y: High glucose levels down-regulate glucose transporter expression that correlates with increased oxidative stress in placental trophoblast cells in vitro. *J Soc Gynecol Investig* 11:75–81, 2004.

Li Voon Chong JS, Leong KS, Wallymahmed M, Sturgess R, MacFarlane IA: Is celiac disease more prevalent in young adults with coexisting type 1 diabetes mellitus and autoimmune thyroid disease compared with those with type 1 diabetes mellitus alone? *Diabet Med* 19:334–337, 2002.

Liao QK, Kong PA, Gao J, Li FY, Qian ZM: Expression of ferritin receptor in placental microvilli membrane in pregnant women with different iron status at mid-term gestation. *Eur J Clin Nutr* 55:651–656, 2001.

Lieberman E, Ryan KS, Minon RR, Schoenbaum SC: Association of maternal hematocrit with premature labor. *Am J Obstet Gynecol* 159:107–114, 1988.

Liese AD, Gilliard T, Schulz M, D'Agostino RB Jr, Wolever TM: Carbohydrate nutrition, glycaemic load, and plasma lipids: the Insulin Resistance Atherosclerosis Study. *Eur Heart J* 28:80–87, 2006.

Lilja AE, Mathiesen ER: Polycystic ovary syndrome and metformin in pregnancy. *Acta Obstet Gynecol Scand* 85:861–868, 2006.

Lin C-C, River P, Moawad AH, Lowensohn RI, Blix PM, Abraham M, Rubinstein AH: Prenatal assessment of fetal outcome by amniotic fluid C-peptide levels in pregnant diabetic women. *Am J Obst Gynecol* 141:671–676, 1981.

Lin EHB, Katon W, Von Korff M, Rutter C, Simon GE, Oliver M, Ciechanowski P, Ludman EJ, Bush T, Young B: Relationship of depression and diabetes self-care, medication adherence, and preventive care. *Diabetes Care* 27:254–260, 2004.

Lind T, Bell S, Gilmore E, Huisjes HJ, SchallY AV: Insulin disappearance rate in pregnant and non-pregnant women, and in non-pregnant women given GHRIH. *Eur J Clin Invest* 7:47–51, 1977.

Lindblad B, Zaman S, Malik A, Martin H, Ekstrom AM, Amu S, Holmgren A, Norman M: Folate, vitamin B12, and homocysteine levels in South Asian women with growth-retarded fetuses. *Acta Obstet Gynecol Scand* 84:1055–1061, 2005.

Lindgren A, Burman P, Kilander AF, Nilsson O, Lindstedt G: Serum antibodies to H+, K+-ATPase, serum pepsinogen A and *Heliobacter pylori* in relation to gastric mucosa morphology in patients with low or low-normal concentrations of serum cobalamins. *Eur J Gastroenterol Hepatol* 10:583–588, 1998a.

Lindgren A, Lindstedt G, Kilander AF: Advantages of serum pepsinogen A combined with gastrin or pepsinogen C as first-line analytes in the evaluation of suspected cobalamin deficiency: a study in patients previously not subjected to gastrointestinal surgery. *J Intern Med* 244:341–349, 1998b.

Lindgren A: Elevated serum methylmalonic acid. How much comes from cobalamin deficiency and how much comes from the kidneys? *Scand J Clin Lab Invest* 62:15–19, 2002.

Lindor KD, Kowdley KV, Heathcote EJ, Harrison ME, Jorgensen R, Angulo P, Lymp JF, Burgart L, Colin P: Ursodeoxycholic acid for treatment of nonalcoholic steatohepatitis: results of a randomized trial. *Hepatology* 39: 770–778, 2004.

Lindqvist PG, Marsal K, Merlo J, Pirhonen JP: Thermal response to submaximal exercise before, during and after pregnancy: a longitudinal study. *J Matern Fetal Neonatal Med* 13:152–156, 2003.

Lindsay CA, Huston L, Amini SB, Catalano PM: Longitudinal changes in the relationship between body mass index and percent body fat in pregnancy. *Obstet Gynecol* 89:377–382, 1997.

Lindsay RS, Walker JD, Halsall I, Hales CN, Calder AA, Hamilton BA: Insulin and insulin propeptides at birth in offspring of diabetic mothers. *J Clin Endocrinol Metab* 88:1664–1671, 2003.

Lindstrom T, Olsson PO, Arnqvist HJ. The use of human ultralente is limited by great intraindividual variability in overnight plasma insulin profiles. *Scand J Clin Lab Invest* 60:341–347, 2000.

Ling Z, Wang Q, Stange G, Veld PI, Pipeleers D: Glibenclamide treatment recruits β-cell subpopulation into elevated and sustained basal insulin synthetic activity. *Diabetes* 55:78–85, 2006.

Lipscombe LL, Gomes T, Levesque LE, Hux JE, Juurlink DN, Alter DA: Thiazolidinediones and cardiovascular outcomes in older patients with diabetes. *JAMA* 298:2634–2643, 2007.

Lisle DK, Trojian TH: Managing the athlete with type 1 diabetes. *Curr Sports Med Rep* 5:93–98, 2006.

Litin L, Sacks F: Trans-fatty-acid content of common foods. *N Engl J Med* 329: 1969–1970, 1993.

Little MP, Brocard P, Elliott P, Steer PJ: Hemoglobin concentration in pregnancy and perinatal mortality: a London-based cohort study. *Am J Obstet Gynecol* 193: 220–226, 2005.

Liu S, Willett WC, Stampfer MJ, Hu FB, Franz M, Sampson L, Hennekens CH, Manson J: A prospective study of dietary glycemic load, carbohydrate intake, and risk of coronary heart disease in U.S. women. *Am J Clin Nutr* 71:1455–1461, 2000.

Liu E, Eisenbarth GS: Type 1A diabetes mellitus-associated autoimmunity. *Endocr Metab Clin North Am* 31:391–410, 2002.

Liu JH, Zingmond D, Etzioni DA, O'Connell JB, Maggard MA, Livingston EH, Liu CD, Ko CY: Characterizing the performance and outcomes of obesity surgery in California. *Am Surg* 69:823–828, 2003.

Liu E, Li M, Bao F, Miao D, Rewers MJ, Eisenbarth GS, Hoffenberg EJ: Need for quantitative assessment of transglutaminase autoantibodies for celiac disease in screening-identified children. *J Pediatr* 146:494–499, 2005.

Liu S: Lowering dietary glycemic load for weight control and cardiovascular health. A matter of quality. Editorial. *Arch Intern Med* 166:1438–1439, 2006.

Lo W, Sano K, Lebwohl B, Diamond B, Green PH: Changing presentation of adult celiac disease. *Dig Dis Sci* 48:395–398, 2003.

Lock DR, Bar-Eyal A, Voet H, Madar Z: Glycemic indexes of various foods given to pregnant diabetic subjects. *Obstet Gynecol* 71:180–183, 1988.

Lof M, Olausson H, Bostrom K, Janerot-Sjoberg B, Sohlstrom A, Forsum E: Changes in basal metabolic rate during pregnancy in relation to changes in body weight and composition, cardiac output, insulin-like growth factor I, and thyroid hormones and in relation to fetal growth. *Am J Clin Nutr* 81:678–685, 2005.

Lof M, Forsum E: Activity pattern and energy expenditure due to physical activity before and during pregnancy in healthy Swedish women. *Br J Nutr* 95:296–302, 2006.

Loktionov A: Common gene polymorphisms and nutrition: emerging links with pathogenesis of multifactorial chronic diseases. Review. *J Nutr Biochem* 14: 426–451, 2003.

Londei M, Quaratino S, Maiuri L: Celiac disease: a model autoimmune disease with gene therapy applications. *Gene Ther* 10:835–843, 2003.

London R: Saccharin and aspartame. Are they safe to consume during pregnancy? *J Reprod Med* 33:17–21, 1988.

Longnecker MP, Klebanoff MA, Brock JW, Zhou H: Polychlorinated biphenyl serum levels in pregnant subjects with diabetes. *Diabetes Care* 24:1099–1101, 2001.

Loosemore ED, Judge MP, Lammi-Keefe CJ: Dietary intake of essential and long-chain polyunsaturated fatty acids in pregnancy. *Lipids* 39:421–424, 2004.

Lopez-Garcia E, van Dam RM, Qi L, Hu FB: Coffee consumption and markers of inflammation and endothelial dysfunction in healthy and diabetic women. *Am J Clin Nutr* 84:888–893, 2006.

Lopez-Soldado I, Herrera E: Different diabetogenic response to moderate doses of streptozotocin in pregnant rats, and its long-term consequences in the offspring. *Exp Diabesity Res* 4:107–118, 2003.

Lorenz RA, Bubb J, Davis D, Jacobson A, Jannasch K, Kramer J, Lipps J, Schlundt D: Changing behavior. Practical lessons from the Diabetes Control and Complications Trial. *Diabetes Care* 19:648–652, 1996.

Lorenzo Alonzo MJ, Bermejo Barrera A, Cocho de Juan JA, Fraga Bermudez JM, Bermejo Barrera P: Selenium levels in related biological samples: human placenta, maternal and umbilical cord blood, hair and nails. *J Trace Elem Med Biol* 19:49–54, 2005.

Loscalzo J: Homocysteine trials? Clear outcomes for complex reasons. Editorial. *N Engl J Med* 354:1629–1632, 2006.

Lotgering FK, Van Doorn MB, Struijk PC, Pool J, Wallenburg HC: Maximal aerobic exercise in pregnant women: heart rate, O2 consumption, CO2 production, and ventilation. *J Appl Physiol* 70:1016–1023, 1991.

Lotgering FK, Struijk PC, van Doorn MB, Wallenburg HC: Errors in predicting maximal oxygen consumption in pregnant women. *J Appl Physiol* 72:562–567, 1992.

Lotgering FK, Spinnewijn WE, Struijk PC, Boomsma F, Wallenburg HC: Respiratory and metabolic responses to endurance cycle exercise in pregnant and postpartum women. *Int J Sports Med* 19:193–198, 1998.

Lothe F, Patel KM, Tozer RA: Megaloblastic anaemia in Uganda. *Trans R Soc Trop Med Hyg* 63:393–397, 1969.

Louik C, Lin AE, Werler MM, Hernandez-Diaz S, Mitchell AA: First-trimester use of selective serotonin-reuptake inhibitors and the risk of birth defects. *N Engl J Med* 356:2675–2683, 2007.

Louka AS, Sollid LM: HLA in celiac disease: unraveling the complex genetics of a complex disorder. *Tissue Antigens* 61:105–117, 2003.

Loukovaara S, Immonen I, Teramo KA, Kaaja R: Progression of retinopathy during pregnancy in type 1 diabetic women treated with insulin lispro. *Diabetes Care* 26:1193–1198, 2003.

Loukovaara M, Leinonen P, Teramo K, Nurminen E, Anderson S, Rutanen EM: Effect of maternal diabetes on phosphorylation of insulin-like growth factor binding protein-1 in cord serum. *Diabet Med* 22:434–439, 2005.

Lovestam-Adrian M, Agardh CD, Aberg A, Agardh E: Preeclampsia is a potent risk factor for deterioration of retinopathy during pregnancy in type 1 diabetic patients. *Diabet Med* 14:1059–1065, 1997.

Lu ZM, Gondenberg RL, Cliver SP, Cutter G, Blankson M: The relationship between maternal hematocrit and pregnancy outcome. *Obstet Gynecol* 77:190–194, 1991.

Ludman E, Katon W, Russo J, Simon G, Von Korff M, Lin E, Ciechanowski P, Kinder L: Panic episodes among patients with diabetes. *Gen Hosp Psychiatry* 28:475–481, 2006.

Ludvigsson JF, Montgomery SM, Ekbom A: Celiac disease and risk of adverse fetal outcome: a population-based cohort study. *Gastroenterology* 129:454–463, 2005.

Ludwig DS: The glycemic index. Physiological mechanisms relating to obesity, diabetes, and cardiovascular disease. *JAMA* 287:2414–2423, 2002.

Ludwig DS: Glycemic load comes of age. Commentary. *J Nutr* 133:2695–2696, 2003.

Lumley J, Oliver SS, Chamberlain C, Oakley L: Interventions for promoting smoking cessation during pregnancy. *Cochrane Database Syst Rev* 2004: CD001055.

Lurie S, Danon D: Life span of erythrocytes in late pregnancy. *Obstet Gynecol* 80:123–126, 1992.

Luscombe ND, Noakes M, Clifton PM: Diets high and low in glycemic index versus high monounsaturated fat diets: effects on glucose and lipid metabolism in NIDDM. *Eur J Clin Nutr* 53:473–478, 1999.

Lustman PJ, Griffith LS, Gavard JA, Clouse RE: Depression in adults with diabetes. *Diabetes Care* 15:1631–1639, 1992.

Lustman PJ, Griffith LS, Clouse RE, Freedland KE, Eisen SA, Rubin EH, Carney RM, McGill JB: Effects of nortriptyline on depression and glucose regulation in diabetes: results of a double-blind, placebo-controlled trial. *Psychosom Med* 59:241–250, 1997.

Lustman PJ, Griffith LS, Freedland KE, Kissel SS, Clouse RE: Cognitive behavior therapy for depression in type 2 diabetes mellitus. A randomized, controlled trial. *Ann Intern Med* 129:613–621, 1998.

Lustman PJ, Anderson RJ, Freedland KE, de Groot M, Carney RM, Clouse RE: Depression and poor glycemic control: a meta-analytic review of the literature. *Diabetes Care* 23:934–942, 2000a.

Lustman PJ, Freedland KE, Griffith LS, Clouse RE: Fluoxetine for depression in diabetes. A randomized double-blind placebo-controlled trial. *Diabetes Care* 23:618–623, 2000b.

Lustman P, Clouse R: Treatment of depression in diabetes: impact on mood and medical outcome. *J Psychosom Res* 53:917–924, 2002.

Lustman PJ, Clouse RE: Depression in diabetic patients: the relationship between mood and glycemic control. *J Diabetes Complications* 19:113–122, 2005.

Ma JY, Borch K, Sjostrand E, Janzon L, Mardh S: Positive correlation between H,K-adenosine triphosphatse antibodies and *Heliobacter pylori* antibodies in patients with pernicious anemia. *Scand J Gastroenterol* 29:961–965, 1994.

Ma AG, Chen XC, Wang Y, Xu RX, Zheng MC, Li JS: The multiple vitamin status of Chinese pregnant women with anemia and nonanemia in the last trimester. *J Nutr Sci Vitaminol (Tokyo)* 50:87–92, 2004.

Ma Y, Li Y, Chiriboga DE, Olendzki BC, Hebert JR, Li W, Leung K, Hafner AR, Ockene IS: Association between carbohydrate intake and serum lipids. *J Am Coll Nutr* 25:155–163, 2006b.

Ma Y, Olendzki BC, Chiriboga D, Rosal M, Sinagra E, Crawford S, Hafner AR, Pagoto SL, Magner RP, Ockene IS: PDA-assisted low glycemic index dietary intervention for type II diabetes: a pilot study. *Eur J Clin Nutr* 60:1235–1243, 2006a.

MacDonald PD, Whitwam RE, Boggs JD, MacCormack JN, Anderson KL, Reardon JW, Saah JR, Graves LM, Hunter SB, Sobel J: Outbreak of listerosis among Mexican immigrants as a result of consumption of illicitly produced Mexican-style cheese. *Clin Infect Dis* 40:677–682, 2005.

Macintosh MCM, Fleming KM, Bailey JA, Doyle P, Modder J, Acolet D, Golightly S, Miller A: Perinatal mortality and congenital anomalies in babies of women with type 1 or type 2 diabetes in England, Wales, and Northern Ireland: population based study. *BMJ* 333:177, 2006.

Mackenzie B, Garrick MD: Iron imports. II. Iron uptake at the apical membrane in the intestine. *Am J Physiol* 289:G981–G986, 2005.

Madsen H, Ditzel J: The influence of maternal weight, smoking, vascular complications and glucose regulation on the birth weight of infants of type 1 diabetic women. *Eur J Obstet Gynecol Reprod Biol* 39:175–179, 1991.

Madsen M, Jorgensen T, Jemsen ML, Juhl M, Olsen J, Andersen PK, Nybo Andersen AM: Leisure time physical exercise during pregnancy and the risk of miscarriage: a study within the Danish National Birth Cohort. *BJOG* 114:1419–1426, 2007.

Maffei M, Volpe L, Di Cianni G, Bertacca A, Ferdeghini M, Murru S, Teti G, Casadidio I, Cecchetti P, Navalesi R, Benzi L: Plasma leptin levels in newborns from normal and diabetic mothers. *Horm Metab Res* 30:575–580, 1998.

Magee MS, Knopp RH, Benedetti TJ: Metabolic effects of a 1200 kcal diet in obese pregnant women with gestational diabetes. *Diabetes* 39:234–240, 1990.

Magnusson AL, Waterman TJ, Wennergren M, Jansson T, Powell TL: Triglyceride hydrolase activities and expression of fatty acid binding proteins in the human placenta in pregnancies complicated by intrauterine growth restriction and diabetes. *J Clin Endocrinol Metab* 89:4607–4614, 2004.

Mahaffey KR: Methylmercury exposure and neurotoxicity. *JAMA* 280:737–738, 1998.

Mahaffey KR, Clickner RP, Bodurow CC: Blood organic mercury and dietary mercury intake: National Health and Nutrition Examination Survey, 1999–2000. *Environ Health Perspect* 112:562–570, 2004a.

Mahaffey KR: Fish and shellfish as dietary sources of methylmercury and the omega-3 fatty acids, icosahexaenoic acid and docosahexaenoic acid: risks and benefits. *Environ Res* 95:414–428, 2004b.

Mahmud FH, Murray JA, Kudva YC, Zinmeister AR, Dierkhising RA, Lahr BD, Dyck PJ, Kyle RA, El-Youssef M, Burgart LJ, Van Dyke CT, Brogan DL, Melton LJ 3rd: Celiac disease in type 1 diabetes in a North American community: prevalence, serologic screening, and clinical features. *Mayo Clin Proc* 80: 1429–1434, 2005.

Mahomed K: Iron supplementation in pregnancy. *The Cochrane Review.* Oxford, UK: Update Software; 2004:CD001135.

Maiuri L, Ciacci C, Auricchio S, Brown V, Quaratino S, Londei M: Interleukin 15 mediates epithelial changes in celiac disease. G*astroenterology* 119:996–1006, 2000.

Maiuri L, Ciacci C, Vacca L, Ricciardelli I, Auricchio S, Quaratino S, Londei M: IL-15 drives the specific migration of CD94+ and TCR-gammadelta+ intraepithelial lymphocytes in organ cultures of treated celiac patients. *Am J Gastroenterol* 96:150–156, 2001.

Maiuri L, Ciacci C, Ricciardelli I, Vacca L, Raia V, Auricchio S, Picard J, Osman M, Quaratino S, Londei M: Association between innate response to gliadin and activation of pathologic T cells in celiac disease. *Lancet* 362:30–37, 2003.

Maiuri L, Ciacci C, Ricciardelli I, Vacca L, Raia V, Rispo A, Griffin M, Issekutz T, Quaratino S, Londei M: Unexpected role of surface transglutaminase type II in celiac disease. *Gastroenterology* 129:1400–1413, 2005.

Makedos G, Papanicolaou A, Hitoglou A, Kalogiannidis I, Makedos A, Vrazioti V, Goutzioulis M: Homocysteine, folic acid and B12 serum levels in pregnancy complicated with preeclampsia. *Arch Gynecol Obstet* 275:121–124, 2007.

Maki M, Mustalahti K, Kokkonen J, Kulmala P, Haapalahti M, Karttunen T, Ilonen J, Laurila K, Dahlbom I, Hansson T, Hopfl P, Knip M: Prevalence of celiac disease among children in Finland. *N Engl J Med* 348:2517–2524, 2003.

Manderson J, Patterson C, Haden D, Traub A, Leslie H, McCance D: Leptin concentration in maternal serum and cord blood in diabetic and nondiabetic pregnancy. *Am J Obstet Gynecol* 188:1326–1332, 2003a.

Manderson JG, Patterson CC, Hadden DR, Traub AI, Ennis C, McCance DR: Preprandial versus postprandial blood glucose monitoring in type 1 diabetic pregnancy: a randomized controlled clinical trial. *Am J Obst Gynecol* 189: 507–512, 2003b.

Mann JJ: The medical management of depression. *N Engl J Med* 353:1819–1834, 2005.

Mannucci E, Rotella F, Ricca V, Moretti S, Placidi GF, Rotella CM: Eating disorders in patients with type 1 diabetes: a meta-analysis. *J Endocrinol Invest* 28:417–419, 2005.

Manuel-Kenoy B, Van Campenhout A, Aerts P, Vertommen J, Abrams P, Van Gaal LF, Van Gils C, De Leeuw IH: Time course of oxidative stress status in the postprandial and postabsorptive states in type 1 diabetes mellitus: relationship to glucose and lipid changes. *J Am Coll Nutr* 24:474–485, 2005.

Marchetti P, Del Guerra S, Marselli L, Lupi R, Masini M, Pollera M, Bugliani M, Boggi U, Vistoli F, Mosca F, Del Prato S: Pancreatic islets from type 2 diabetic patients have functional defects and increased apoptosis that are ameliorated by metformin. *J Clin Endocrinol Metab* 89:5535–5541, 2004.

Marcus SM, Flynn HA, Blow FC, Barry KL: Depressive symptoms among pregnant women screened in obstetrics settings. *J Womens Health* 12:373–380, 2003.

Maron BA, Loscalzo J: Homocysteine. *Clin Lab Med* 26:591–609, 2006.

Marra G, Cotroneo P, Pitocco D, Manto A, Di Leo MAS, Ruotolo V, Caputo S, Girdina B, Ghirlanda G, Santini SA: Early increase of oxidative stress and reduced antioxidant defenses in patients with uncomplicated type 1 diabetes. A case for gender difference. *Diabetes Care* 25:370–375, 2002.

Marshall SM, Barth JH: Standardization of HbA1c measurements: a consensus statement. *Diabet Med* 17:5–6, 2000.

Martin A, Herrera E: Different responses to maternal diabetes during the first and second half of gestation in the streptozotocin-treated rat. *Isr J Med Sci* 27:442–448, 1991.

Martin LF, Finigan KM, Nolan TE: Pregnancy after adjustable gastric banding. *Obstet Gynecol* 95:927–930, 2000.

Martin ME, Nicolas G, Hetet G, Vaulont S, Grandchamp B, Beaumont C: Transferrin receptor 1 mRNA is downregulated in placenta of hepcidin transgenic embryos. *FEBS Lett* 574:187–191, 2004.

Martinelli P, Troncone R, Pararo F, Torre P, Trapanese E, Fasano C, Lamberti A, Budillon G, Nardone G, Greco L: Celiac disease and unfavorable outcome of pregnancy. *Gut* 46:332–335, 2000.

Martinez ME, Catalan P, Balaguer G, Lisbona A, Quero J, Reque A, Pallardo LF: 25(OH)D levels in diabetic pregnancies: relation with neonatal hypoglycemia. *Horm Metab Res* 23:38–41, 1991.

Martinez ME, Catalan P, Lisbona A, Sanchez-Cabezudo MJ, Pallardo F, Jans I, Bouillon R: Serum osteocalcin concentrations in diabetic pregnant women and their newborns. *Horm Metab Res* 26:338–342, 1994.

Martinez-Frias ML, Salvador J: Epidemiologic aspects of prenatal exposure to high doses of vitamin A in Spain. *Eur J Epidemiol* 6:118–123, 1990.

Marx N, Walcher D, Ivanova N, Rautzenberg K, Jung A, Friedl R, Hombach V, de Caterina R, Basta G, Wautier M-P, Wautiers J-L: Thiazolidinediones reduce endothelial expression of receptors for advanced glycation end products. *Diabetes* 53:2662–2668, 2004a.

Marx N, Duez H, Fruchart JC, Staels B: Peroxisome proliferator-activated receptors and atherogenesis: regulators of gene expression in vascular cells. *Circ Res* 94:1168–1178, 2004b.

Marzari R, Sblattero D, Florian F, Tongiorgi E, Not T, Tommasini A, Ventura A, Bradbury A: Molecular dissection of the tissue transglutaminase autoantibody response in celiac disease. *J Immunol* 166:4170–4176, 2001.

Maschi S, Clavenna A, Campi R, Schiavetti B, Bernat M, Bonati M: Neonatal outcome following pregnancy exposure to antidepressants:a prospective controlled cohort study. *BJOG* 115:283–289, 2008.

Mason JB: Biomarkers of nutrient exposure and status in one-carbon (methyl) metabolism. *J Nutr* 133:941S–947S, 2003.

Masoudi FA, Inzucchi SE, Wang Y, Havranek EP, Foody JM, Krumholz HM: Thiazolidinediones, metformin, and outcomes in older patients with diabetes and heart failure: an observational study. *Circulation* 111:583–590, 2005.

Masson EA, Patmore JE, Brash PD, BaxterM, Caldwell G, Galens, Price PA, Vice PA, Walker JD, Lindow SW. Pregnancy outcome in type 1 diabetes mellitus treated with insulin lispro (Humalog). *Diabet Med* 20:46–50, 2003.

Mathews F, Yudkin P, Neil A: Influence of maternal nutrition on outcome of pregnancy: prospective cohort study. *BMJ* 319:339–343, 1999.

Mathiesen UL, Franzen LE, Aselius H, Resjo M, Jacobsson L, Foberg U, Fryden A, Bodemar G: Increased liver echogenicity at ultrasound examination reflects degree of steatosis but not of fibrosis in asymptomatic patients with mild/moderate abnormalities of liver transaminases. *Dig Liver Dis* 34:516–522, 2002.

Mathiesen E, Kinsley B, Amiel SA, Heller S, McCance D, Duran S, Bellaire S, Raben A; Insulin Aspart Pregnancy Study Group: Maternal glycemic control and hypoglycemia in type 1 diabetic pregnancy: a randomized trial of insulin aspart versus human insulin in 322 pregnant women. *Diabetes Care* 30: 771–776, 2007.

Matysiak-Budnik T, Candalh C, Dugave C, Namane A, Cellier C, Cerf-Bensussan N, Heyman M: Alterations in the intestinal transport and processing of gliadin peptides in celiac disease. *Gastroenterology* 125:696–707, 2003.

Mauger J-F, Lichtenstein AH, Ausman LM, Jalbert SM, Jauhiainen M, Ehnholm C, Lamarche B: Effect of different forms of dietary hydrogenated fats on LDL particle size. *Am J Clin Nutr* 78:370–375, 2003.

McColl JD, Robinson S, Globus M: Effect of some therapeutic agents on the rabbit fetus. *Toxicol Appl Pharmacol* 10:244–252, 1967.

McDowell MA, Dillon CF, Osterloh J, Bolger PM, Pellizzari E, Fernando R, Montes de Oca R, Schober SE, Sinks T, Jones RL, Mahaffey KR: Hair mercury levels in U.S. children and women of childbearing age: reference data from NHANES 1999–2000. *Environ Health Perspect* 112:1165–1171, 2004.

McElduff A, Cheung NW, McIntyre HD, Lagstrom JA, Oats JJN, Ross GP, Simmons D, Walters BNJ, Wein P: The Australasian Diabetes in Pregnancy Society consensus guidelines for the management of type 1 and type 2 diabetes in relation to pregnancy. Position statement. *Med J Aust* 183: 373–377, 2005a.

McElduff A, Ross GP, Lagtrom JA, Champion B, Flack JR, Lau S-M, Moses RG, Seneratne S, McLean M, Cheung NW: Pregestational diabetes and pregnancy. An Australian experience. *Diabetes Care* 28:1260–1261, 2005b.

McElvy SS, Miodovnik M, Rosenn B, Khoury JC, Siddiqi T, Dignan PS, Tsang RC: A focused preconceptional and early pregnancy program in women with type 1 diabetes reduces perinatal mortality and malformation rates to general population levels. *J Matern-Fetal Med* 9:14–20, 2000.

McGill JB, Cole TG, Nowatzke W, Houghton S, Ammirati EB, Gautille T, Sarno MJ: Circulating 1,5-anhydroglucitol levels in adult patients with diabetes reflect longitudinal changes of glycemia. A U.S. trial of the GlycoMark assay. *Diabetes Care* 27:1859–1865, 2004.

McGivan JD, Pastor-Anglada M: Regulatory and molecular aspects of mammalian amino acid transport. *Biochem J* 299:321–334, 1994.

McGregor DO, Dellow WJ, Lever M, Bason PM, Robson RA, Chambers ST: Dimethylglycine accumulates in uremia and predicts elevated plasma homocysteine concentrations. *Kidney Int* 59:2267–2272, 2001.

McIntyre HD, Serek R, Crane DI, Veveris-Lowe T, Parry A, Johnson S, Leung KC, Ho KK, Bougoussa M, Hennen G, Igout A, Chan FY, Cowley D, Cotterill A, Barnard R: Placental growth hormone (GH), GH-binding protein, and insulin-like growth factor axis in normal, growth-retarded, and diabetic pregnancies: correlations with fetal growth. *J Clin Endocrinol Metab* 85:1143–1150, 2000.

McIntyre HD, Flack JR: Consensus statement on diabetes control in preparation for pregnancy. *Med J Aust* 181:326, 2004.

McKie AT, Barlow DJ: The SLC40 basolateral iron transporter family (IREG1/ferroportin/MTP1). *Pflugers Arch* 447:801–806, 2005.

McLachlan KA, O'Neal D, Jenkins A, Alford FP: Do adiponectin, TNFα, leptin and CRP relate to insulin resistance in pregnancy? Studies in women with and without gestational diabetes, during and after pregnancy. *Diabetes Metab Res Rev* 22:131–138, 2006.

McMahon SK, Ferreira LD, Ratnam N, Davey RJ, Youngs LM, Davis EA, Fournier PA, Jones TW: Glucose requirements to maintain euglycemia after moderate-intensity afternoon exercise in adolescents with type 1 diabetes are increased in a biphasic manner. *J Clin Endocrinol Metab* 92:963–968, 2007.

McManus R, Ryan EA: Insulin requirements in insulin-dependent and insulin-requiring gestational diabetic women during the final month of pregnancy. *Diabetes Care* 15:1323–1327, 1992.

McManus R, Kelleher D: Celiac disease-the villain unmasked? *N Engl J Med* 348:2573–2574, 2003.

McMillan-Price J, Petocz P, Atkinson F, O'Neill K, Samman S, Steinbeck K, Caterson I, Brand-Miller J: Comparison of 4 diets of varying glycemic load on weight loss and cardiovascular risk reduction in overweight and obese young adults. A randomized controlled trial. *Arch Intern Med* 166:1466–1475, 2006.

McMurray RG, Brabham VW, Hackney AC: Catecholamine responses in pregnant women: comparisons between low-impact aerobic dance and treadmill walking. *Biol Sport* 15:25–32, 1998.

McNair P, Kiilerich S, Christiansen C, Christensen MS, Madsbad S, Transbol I: Hyperzincuria in insulin treated diabetes mellitus—its relation to glucose homeostasis and insulin administration. *Clinica Chim Acta* 112:343–348, 1981.

Mecacci F, Carignani L, Cioni R Bartoli E, Parretti E, La Torre P, Scarselli G, Mello G: Maternal metabolic control and perinatal outcome in women with gestational diabetes treated with regular or lispro insulin: comparison with non-diabetic pregnant women. *Eur J Obstet Gynecol Reprod Biol* 111:19–24, 2003.

Meguro S, Funae O, Hosokawa K, Atsumi Y: Hypoglycemia detection rate differs among blood glucose monitoring sites. *Diabetes Care* 28:708–709, 2005.

Mehrabian M, Allayee H, Wong J, Shi W, Wang XP, Shaposhnik Z, Funk CD, Lusis AJ, Shih W: Identification of 5-lipoxygenase as a major gene contributing to atherosclerosis susceptibility in mice. *Circ Res* 91:120–126, 2002.

Meier JJ, Gallwitz B, Askenas M, Vollmer K, Deacon CF, Holst JJ, Schmidt WE, Nauck MA: Secretion of incretin hormones and the insulinotropic effect of gastric inhibitory polypeptide in women with a history of gestational diabetes. *Diabetologia* 48:1872–1881, 2005.

Melander A: Kinetics-effect relations of insulin-releasing drugs in patients with type 2 diabetes. Brief overview. *Diabetes* 53 (Suppl 3):S151–S155, 2004.

Mello G, Parretti E, Mecacci F, Pratesi M, Lucchetti R, Scarselli G: Excursion of daily glucose profiles in pregnant women with IDDM: relationship with perinatal outcome. *J Perinat Med* 25:488–497, 1997.

Mello G, Parretti E, Mecacci F, LaTorre P, Cioni R, Cianciulli D, Scarselli G: What degree of maternal metabolic control in women with type 1 diabetes is associated with normal body size and proportions in full-term infants? *Diabetes Care* 23:1494–1498, 2000.

Mello G, Parretti E, Cioni R, Lucchetti R, Carignani L, Martini E, Mecacci F, Lagazio C, Pratesi M: The 75-gram glucose load in pregnancy. Relation between glucose levels and anthropometric characteristics of infants born to women with normal glucose metabolism. *Diabetes Care* 26:1206–1210, 2003.

Melse-Boonstra A, Holm PI, Ueland PM, Olthof M, Clarke R, Verhoef P: Betaine concentration as a determinant of fasting total homocysteine concentrations and the effect of folic acid supplementation on betaine concentrations. *Am J Clin Nutr* 81:1378–1382, 2005.

Melvin CL, Gaffney C: Treating nicotine use and dependence of pregnant and parenting smokers: an update. *Nicotine Tob Res* 6S2:S107–124, 2004.

Mendez-Sanchez N, Gonzalez V, Chavez-Tapia N, Ramos MH, Uribe M: Weight reduction and ursodeoxycholic acid in subjects with nonalcoholic fatty liver disease. A double-blind, placebo-controlled trial. *Ann Hepatol* 3:108–112, 2004.

Mensing C, Boucher J, Cypress M, Weinger K, Mulcahy K, Barta P, Hosey G, Kppher W, Lasichak A, Lamb B, Mangan M, Norman J, Tanja J, Yauk L, Wisdom K, Adams C: National standards for diabetes self-management education. *Diabetes Care* 28 (Suppl 1):S72–S79, 2005.

Mention JJ, Ben Ahmed M, Begue B, Barbe U, Verkarre V, Asnafi V, Colombel JF, Cugnenc PH, Ruemmele FM, McIntyre E, Brousse N, Cellier C, Cerf-Bensussan N: Interleukin 15: a key to disrupted intraepithelial lymphocyte homeostasis and lymphomagensis in celiac disease. *Gastroenterology* 126: 1217–1218, 2003.

Merialdi M, Carroli G, Villar J, Abalos E, Gulmezoglu AM, Kulier R, de Onis M: Nutritional interventions during pregnancy for the prevention or treatment of impaired fetal growth: an overview of randomized controlled trials. *J Nutr* 133:1626S–1631S, 2003.

Merialdi M, Caulfield LE, Zavaleta N, Figueroa A, Costigan KA, Dominici F, Dipietro JA: Randomized controlled trial of prenatal zinc supplementation and fetal bone growth. *Am J Clin Nutr* 79:826–830, 2004.

Merimee T: Editorial: the interface between diabetic retinopathy, diabetes management, and insulin-like growth factors. *J Clin Endocrinol Metab* 82: 2808–2806, 1997.

Merlob P, Levitt O, Stahl B: Oral antihyperglycemic agents during pregnancy and lactation. A review. *Pediatr Drugs* 4:755–760, 2002.

Messina V, Melina V, Mangels AR: A new food guide for North American vegetarians. *J Am Diet Assoc* 103:771–775, 2003.

Metzger BE, Ravnikar V, Vileisis RA, Freinkel N: "Accelerated starvation" and the skipped breakfast in late normal pregnancy. *Lancet* 1:588–592, 1982.

Metzger M, Leibowitz G, Wainstein J, Glaser B, Raz I: Reproducibility of glucose measurements using the glucose sensor. *Diabetes Care* 25:1185–1191, 2002.

Midgley JP, Matthew AG, Greenwood CMT, Logan AG: Effect of reduced dietary sodium on blood pressure: a meta-analysis of randomized controlled trials. *JAMA* 275:1590–1597, 1996.

Miele C, Rochford JJ, Filippa N, Giorgetti-Reraldi S, Van Obberghen E: Insulin and insulin-like growth factor-I induce vascular endothelial growth factor mRNA expression via different signaling pathways. *J Biol Chem* 275:21695–21702, 2000.

Miettinen TA, Gylling H, Tuominen J, Simonen P, Koivisto V: Low synthesis and high absorption of cholesterol characterize type 1 diabetes. *Diabetes Care* 27: 53–58, 2004.

Mihailovic M, Cvetkovic M, Ljubic A, Kosanovic M, Nedeljkovic S, Jovanovic I, Pesut O: Selenium and malondialdehyde content and glutathione peroxidase activity in maternal and umbilical cord blood and amniotic fluid. *Biol Trace Elem Res* 73:47–54, 2000.

Mikhail MS, Anyaegbunam A, Garfinkel D, Palan PR, Basu J, Romney SL: Preeclampsia and antioxidant nutrients: decreased plasma levels of reduced ascorbic acid, α-tocopherol, and beta-carotene in women with preeclampsia. *Am J Obstet Gynecol* 171:150–157, 1994.

Milcali N, Simonoff E, Treasure J: Risk of major adverse perinatal outcomes in women with eating disorders. *Br J Psychiatry* 190:255–259, 2007.

Milczarek R, Sokolowska E, Hallmann A, Klimek J: The NADPH- and iron-dependent lipid peroxidation in human placental microsomes. *Mol Cell Biochem* 295:105–111, 2007.

Millard KN, Frazer DM, Wilkins SJ, Anderson GJ: Changes in the expression of intestinal iron transport and hepatic regulatory molecules explain the enhanced iron absorption associated with pregnancy in the rat. *Gut* 53:655–660, 2004.

Miller DI, Wishinsky H, Thompson G: Transfer of tolbutamide across the human placenta. *Diabetes* 11 (Suppl):93–97, 1962.

Miller EH: Metabolic management of diabetes in pregnancy. *Semin Perinatol* 18:414–431, 1994.

Miller ER III, Pastor-Barriuso R, Dalal D, Riemersma RA, Appel LJ, Guallar E: Meta-analysis: high-dosage vitamin E supplementation may increase all-cause mortality. *Ann Intern Med* 142:37–46, 2005.

Mills JL, McPartlin JM, Kirke PN, Lee YJ, Conley MR, Weir DG, Scott JM: Homocysteine metabolism in pregnancies complicated by neural-tube defects. *Lancet* 345:149–151, 1995.

Mills JL, Simpson JL, Cunningham GC, Conley MR, Rhoads GG: Vitamin A and birth defects. *Am J Obstet Gynecol* 177:31–36, 1996.

Mills JL, Jovanovic, L, Knopp R, Aarons J, Conley M, Park E, Lee YJ, Holmes L, Simpson JL, Metzger B: Physiological reduction in fasting blood glucose concentration in the first trimester of normal pregnancy: The Diabetes in Early Pregnancy Study. *Metabolism* 47:1140–1144, 1998.

Mills JL, Signore C: Neural tube defect rates before and after food fortification with folic acid. *Birth Defects Res A Clin Molec Teratol* 70:844–845, 2004.

Mills JL: Depressing observations on the use of selective serotonin-reuptake inhibitors during pregnancy. *N Engl J Med* 354:636–638, 2006.

Milman N, Bergholt T, Byg KE, Eriksen L, Graudal N: Iron status and iron balance during pregnancy. A critical reappraisal of iron supplementation. *Acta Obstet Gynecol Scand* 78:749–757, 1999.

Milman N, Bergholt T, Eriksen L, Byg K-E, Graudal N, Pedersen P, Hertz J: Iron prophylaxis during pregnancy—how much iron is needed? A randomized dose-response study of 20–80 mg ferrous iron daily in pregnant women. *Acta Obstet Gynecol Scand* 84:238–247, 2005.

Milman N: Iron and pregnancy—a delicate balance. *Ann Hematol* 85:559–565, 2006a.

Milman N, Byg KE, Bergholt T, Eriksen L, Hyas AM: Cobalamin status during normal pregnancy and postpartum: a longitudinal study comprising 406 Danish women. *Eur J Hematol* 76:521–525, 2006b.

Milman N, Byg KE, Hvas AM, Bergholt T, Eriksen L: Erythrocyte folate, plasma folate and plasma homocysteine during normal pregnancy and postpartum: a longitudinal study comprising 404 Danish women. *Eur J Hematol* 76:200–205, 2006c.

Mimouni F, Tsang RC, Hertzberg VS, Miodovnik M: Polycythemia, hypomagnesemia and hypocalcemia in infants of diabetic mothers. *Am J Dis Child* 140:798–800, 1986.

Mimouni F, Miodovnik M, Tsang RC, Holroyde J, Dignan PS, Siddiqi TA: Decreased maternal serum magnesium concentration and adverse fetal outcome in insulin-dependent diabetic women. *Obstet Gynecol* 70:85–88, 1987.

Mimouni F, Miodovnik M, Siddiqui TA, Khoury J, Tsang R: Perinatal asphyxia in infants of insulin-dependent diabetic mothers. *J Pediatr* 113:345–353, 1988b.

Mimouni F, Steichen JJ, Tsang RC, Hertzberg ZV, Miodovnik M: Decreased bone mineral content in infants of diabetic mothers. *Am J Perinatol* 5:339–343, 1988c.

Mimouni F, Tsang RC: Pregnancy outcome in insulin-dependent diabetes: temporal relationships with metabolic control during specific pregnancy periods. *Am J Perinatol* 5:334–338, 1988a.

Mimouni F, Tsang RC, Hertzberg VS, Neumann V, Ellis K: Parathyroid hormone and calcitriol changes in normal and insulin-dependent diabetic pregnancies. *Obstet Gynecol* 74:49–54, 1989.

Min Y, Ghebremeskel K, Thomas B, Offley-Shore B, Crawford M: Unfavorable effect of type 1 and type 2 diabetes on maternal and fetal essential fatty acid status: a potential marker of fetal insulin resistance. *Am J Clin Nutr* 82:1162–1168, 2005.

Miodovnik M, Rosenn BM, Khoury JC, Grigsby JL, Siddiqi TA: Does pregnancy increase the risk for progression of diabetic nephropathy? *Am J Obstet Gynecol* 174:1180–1191, 1996.

Mishra P, Younossi ZM: Abdominal ultrasound for diagnosis of nonalcoholic fatty liver disease (NAFLD). Editorial. *Am J Gastroenterol* 102:2716–2717, 2007.

Mitchell MD, Osepchook CC, Leung K-C, McMahon CD, Bass JJ: Myostatin is a human placental product that regulates glucose uptake. *J Clin Endocrinol Metab* 91:1434–1437, 2006.

Miyazaki Y, Mahankali A, Matsuda M, Glass L, Mahanlaki S, Ferrannini E, Cusi K, Mandarino LJ, DeFronzo RA: Improved glycemic control and enhanced insulin sensitivity in type 2 diabetic subjects treated with pioglitazone. *Diabetes Care* 24: 710–719, 2001.

Moat SJ, Doshi SN, Lang D, McDowell IFW, Lewis MJ, Goodfellow J: Treatment of coronary artery disease with folic acid: is there a future? *Am J Physiol* 287:H1–H7, 2004a.

Moat SJ, Lang D, McDowell IFW, Clarke ZL, Madhavan AK, Lewis MJ, Goodfellow J: Folate, homocysteine, endothelial function and cardiovascular disease. *J Nutr Biochem* 15:64–79, 2004b.

Moberg E. Lundblad S, Lins P-E, Adamson U: How accurate are home blood-glucose meters with special respect to the low glycemic range? *Diabetes Res Clin Pract* 19:239–243, 1993.

MOD—March of Dimes: Caffeine in pregnancy. Available at: www.MarchofDimes .com/professionals/14332_1148.asp. Accessed Jan 21, 2008.

Moe AJ: Placental amino acid transport. *Am J Physiol* 268:C1321–C1331, 1995.

Mohammed NH, Wolever TM: Effect of carbohydrate source on postprandial blood glucose in subjects with type 1 diabetes treated with insulin lispro. *Diabetes Res Clin Pract* 65:29–35, 2004.

Mohn A, Cerruto M, Lafusco D, Rrisco F, Tumini S, Stoppolini O, Chiarelli F: Celiac disease in children and adolescents with type 1 diabetes: importance of hypoglycemia. *J Pediatr Gastroenterol Nutr* 32:37–40, 2001.

Molberg O, Mcadam SN, Korner R, Quarsten H, Kristiansen C, Madsen L, Fugger L, Scott H, Noren O, Roepstorff P, Lundin KE, Sjostrom H, Sollid LM:

Tissue transglutaminase selectivity modifies gliadin peptides that are recognized by gut-derived T cells in celiac disease. *Nat Med* 4:713–717, 1998.

Molberg O, McAdam SN, Sollid LM: Role of tissue transglutaminase in celiac disease. *J Pediatr Gastroenterol Nutr* 30:232–240, 2000.

Molberg O, Solheim Flaete N, Jensen T, Lundin KE, Arentz-Hansen H, Anderson OD, Kjersti Uhlen A, Sollid LM. Intestinal T-cell responses to high-molecular-weight glutenins in celiac disease. *Gastroenterology* 125:337–344, 2003.

Moley KH: Hyperglycemia and apoptosis: mechanisms for congenital malformations and pregnancy loss in diabetic women. *Trends Endocrinol Metab* 12:78–82, 2001.

Molloy AM: Is impaired folate absorption a factor in neural tube defects? Editorial. *Am J Clin Nutr* 72:3–4, 2000.

Molloy AM, Mills JL, McPartlin J, Kirke PN, Scott JM, Daly S: Maternal and fetal plasma homocysteine concentrations at birth: the influence of folate, vitamin B12, and the 5,10-methylenetetrahydrofolate reductase 677C→T variant. *Am J Obstet Gynecol* 186:499–503, 2002.

Molloy AM, Mills JL, Cox C, Daly SF, Conley M, Brody LC, Kirke PN, Scott JM, Ueland PM: Choline and homocysteine interrelations in umbilical cord and maternal plasma at delivery. *Am J Clin Nutr* 82:836–842, 2005.

Molso M, Heikkinen T, Hakkola J, Hakala K, Wallerman O, Wadelius C, Laine K: Functional role of P-glycoprotein in the human blood-placental barrier. *Clin Pharmacol Ther* 78:123–131, 2005.

Molteni N, Bardella MT, Bianchi PA: Obstetric and gyncecological problems in women with untreated celiac sprue. *J Clin Gastroenterol* 12:37–39, 1990.

Mondestin MAJ, Ananth CV, Smulian JC, Vintzileos AM: Birth weight and fetal death in the United States: the effect of maternal diabetes during pregnancy. *Am J Obstet Gynecol* 187:922–926, 2002.

Monnier VM: Transition metals redux: reviving an old plot for diabetic vascular disease. *J Clin Invest* 107:799–801, 2001.

Monsen ALB, Ueland PM: Homocysteine and methylmalonic acid in diagnosis and risk assessment from infancy to adolescence. *Am J Clin Nutr* 78:7–21, 2003.

Montaner P, Dominguez R, Corcoy R: Self-monitored blood glucose in pregnant women without gestational diabetes. *Diabetes Care* 25:2104–2105, 2002.

Montelongo A, Lasuncion MA, Pallardo LF, Herrera E: Longitudinal study of plasma lipoproteins and hormones during pregnancy in normal and diabetic women. *Diabetes* 41:1651–1659, 1992.

Mooradian AD, Morley JE: Micronutrient status in diabetes mellitus. *Am J Clin Nutr* 45:877–895, 1987.

Mooradian AD, Failla M, Hoogwerf B, Maryniuk M, Wylie-Rosett: Selected vitamins and minerals in diabetes. *Diabetes Care* 17:464–479, 1994.

Mooradian AD, Bernbaum M, Albert SG: Narrative review: a rational approach to starting insulin therapy. *Ann Intern Med* 145:125–134, 2006.

Moore TR: A comparison of amniotic fluid fetal pulmonary phospholipids in normal and diabetic pregnancy. *Am J Obstet Gynecol* 186:641–650, 2002.

Moore LE, Briery CM, Clokey D, Martin RW, Williford NJ, Bofill JA, Morrison JC: Metformin and insulin in the management of gestational diabetes mellitus: preliminary results of a comparison. *J Reprod Med* 52:1011–1015, 2007.

Morales J: Defining the role of insulin detemir in basal insulin therapy. *Drugs* 67:2557–2584, 2007.

Morgan JF: Eating disorders and reproduction. *Aust N Z J Obstet Gynecol* 39: 167–173, 1999.

Morgan JF, Lacey JH, Chung E: Risk of postnatal depression, miscarriage, and preterm birth in bulimia nervosa: retrospective controlled study. *Psychosom Med* 68:487–492, 2006.

Morley R, Carlin JB, Pasco JA, Wark JD: Maternal 25-hydroxyvitamin D and parathyroid hormone concentrations and offspring birth size. *J Clin Endocrinol Metab* 91:906–912, 2006.

Moroz C, Traub L, Maymon R, Zahalka MA: PLIF, a novel human ferritin subunit from placenta with immunosuppressive activity. *J Biol Chem* 277:12901–12905, 2002.

Morris Buus R, Boockfor FR: Transferrin expression by placental trophoblast cells. *Placenta* 25:45–52, 2004.

Morris CD, Jacobson S-L, Anand R, Ewell MG, Hauth JC, Curet LB, Catalano PM, Sibai BM, Levine RJ: Nutrient intake and hypertensive disorders of pregnancy: evidence from a large prospective cohort. *Am J Obstet Gynecol* 184:643–651, 2001.

Morris SN, Johnson NR: Exercise during pregnancy. A critical appraisal of the literature. *J Reprod Med* 50:181–188, 2005.

Morrissette J, Takser L, St-Amour G, Smargiassi A, Lafond J, Mergler D: Temporal variation of blood and hair mercury levels in pregnancy in relation to fish consumption history in a population living along the St. Lawrence River. *Environ Res* 95:363–374, 2004.

Morse SA, Ciechanowski PS, Katon WJ, Hirsch IB: Isn't this just bedtime snacking? The potential adverse effects of night-eating symptoms on treatment adherence and outcomes in patients with diabetes. *Diabetes Care* 29:1800–1804, 2006.

Mosca A, Paleari R, Dalfra MG, Di Cianni G, Cuccuru I, Pellegrini G, Malloggi L, Bonomo M, Granata S, Ceriotti F, Castiglioni MT, Songini M, Tocco G, Masin M, Plebani M, Lapolla A: Reference intervals for hemoglobin A1C in pregnant women: data from an Italian multicenter study. *Clin Chem* 52:1138–1143, 2006.

Moses R, Schier G, Mathews J, Davis W: The accuracy of home glucose meters for the glucose range anticipated in pregnancy. *Aust N Z J Obstet Gynecol* 37: 282–286, 1997.

Moses RG, Luebcke M, Davis WS, Coleman KJ, Tapsell LC, Petocz P, Brand-Miller JC: Effect of a low-glycemic-index diet during pregnancy on obstetric outcomes. *Am J Clin Nutr* 84:807–812, 2006.

Moses–Kolko EL, Bogen D, Perel J, Bregar A, Uhl K, Levin B, Wisner KL: Neonatal signs after late in utero exposure to serotonin reuptake inhibitors: literature review and implications for clinical applications. *JAMA* 293:2372–2383, 2005.

Mosher PE, Nash MS, Perry AC, LaPerriere AR, Goldberg RB: Aerobic circuit exercise training: effect on adolescents with well-controlled insulin-dependent diabetes mellitus. *Arch Phys Med Rehabil* 79:652–657, 1998.

Mozaffarian D, Pischon T, Hankinson SE, Rifai N, Joshipura K, Willett WC, Rimm E: Dietary intake of *trans* fatty acids and systemic inflammation in women. *Am J Clin Nutr* 79:606–612, 2004.

Mozaffarian D, Katan MB, Ascherio A, Stampfer MJ, Willett WC: Trans fatty acids and cardiovascular disease. *N Engl J Med* 354:1601–1613, 2006a.

Mozaffarian D, Rimm EB: Fish intake, contaminants, and human health. *JAMA* 296:1885–1899, 2006b.

Mudaliar SR, Lindberg FA, Joyce M, Beerdsen P, Strange P, Lin A, Henry RR: Insulin aspart (B28 Asp-Insulin): a fast-acting analog of human insulin. Absorption kinetics and action profile compared with regular human insulin in healthy nondiabetic subjects. *Diabetes Care* 22:1501–1506, 1999.

Mueller CFH, Laude K, McNally S, Harrison DG: Redox mechanisms in blood vessels. *Arterioscler Thromb Vasc Biol* 25:274–278, 2005.

Mueller AS, Pallauf J: Compendium of the antidiabetic effects of supranutritional selenate doses. In vivo and in vitro investigations with type 1 db/db mice. *J Nutr Biochem* 17:548–560, 2006.

Murata K, Sakamoto M, Nakai K, Weihe P, Dakeishi M, Iwata T, Liu XJ, Ohno T, Kurasawa T, Kamiya K, Satoh H: Effects of methylmercury on neuro-development in Japanese children in relation to the Madeiran study. *Int Arch Occup Environ Health* 77:571–579, 2004.

Murphy JF, O'Riordan J, Newcombe RG, Coles EC, Pearson JF: Relation of hemoglobin levels in first and second trimesters to outcome of pregnancy. *Lancet* 1:992–995, 1986.

Murray D, Cox JL: Screening for depression during pregnancy with the Edinburgh depression scale (EPDS). *J Reprod Infant Psychol* 8:99–107, 1990.

Murray JA: The widening spectrum of celiac disease. *Am J Clin Nutr* 69:354–365, 1999.

Murray JA, Van Dyke C, Plevak MF, Dierkhising RA, Zinsmeister AR, Melton LJ 3rd: Trends in the identification and clinical features of celiac disease in a North American community. *Clin Gastroenterol Hepatol* 1:19–27, 2003.

Murray JA, Watson T, Clearman B, Mitros F: Effect of a gluten–free diet on gastrointestinal symptoms in celiac disease. *Am J Clin Nutr* 79:669–673, 2004.

Musi N, Hirshman MF, Nygren J, Svanfeldt M, Bavenholm P, Rooyackers O, Zhou G, Williamson JM, Ljunqvist O, Efendic S, Moller DE, Thorell A, Goodyear LJ: Metformin increases AMP-activated protein kinase activity in skeletal muscle of subjects with type 2 diabetes. *Diabetes* 51:2074–2081, 2002.

Mussell MP, Crosby RD, Crow SJ, Knopke AJ, Peterson CB, Wonderlich SA, Mitchell JE: Utilization of empirically supported psychotherapy treatments for individuals with eating disorders. A survey of psychologists. *Int J Eat Disord* 27:230–237, 2000.

Muthayya S, Kurpad AV, Duggan CP, Bosch RJ, Dwarkanath P, Mhaskar R, Thomas A, Vaz M, Bhat S, Fawzi WW: Low maternal vitamin B12 status is associated with intrauterine growth retardation in urban South Indians. *Eur J Clin Nutr* 60:791–801, 2006.

Mwanda OW, Dave P: Megaloblastic marrow in macrocytic anaemias at Kenyatta National and MP Shah Hospitals, Nairobi. *East Afr Med J* 76:610–614, 1999.

Myers GJ, Davidson PW, Cox C, Shamlaye CF, Palumbo D, Cernichiari E, Sloane-Reeves J, Wilding GE, Kost J, Huang LS, Clarkson TW: Prenatal methylmercury exposure from ocean fish consumption in the Seychelles Child Development Study. *Lancet* 361:1686–1692, 2003.

Nachum Z, Ben-Shlomo I, Weiner E, Shalev: Twice daily versus four times daily insulin dose regimens for diabetes in pregnancy: randomized controlled trial. *BMJ* 319:1223–1227, 1999.

Nadeau KJ, Klingensmith G, Zeitler P: Type 2 diabetes in children is frequently associated with elevated alanine aminotransferase. *J Pediatr Gastroenterol Nutr* 41:94–98, 2005.

Nader S: Thyroid disease and other endocrine disorders in pregnancy. *Obstet Gynecol Clin North Am* 31:257–285, 2004.

Nahum R, Brenner O, Zahalka MA, Traub L, Quintana F, Moroz C: Blocking of the placental immune-modulatory ferritin activates Th1 type cytokines and affects placenta development, fetal growth and the pregnancy outcome. *Hum Reprod* 19:715–722, 2004.

Nakahara R, Yoshiuchi K, Kumano H, Hara Y, Suematsu H, Kuboki T: Prospective study on influence of psychosocial factors on glycemic control in Japanese patients with type 2 diabetes. *Psychosomatics* 47:240–246, 2006.

Nakajima S, Saijo Y, Kato S, Sasaki S, Uno A, Kanagami N, Hirakawa H, Hori T, Tobiishi K, Todaka T, Nakamura Y, Yanagiva S, Sengoku Y, Iida T, Sata F, Kishi R: Effects of prenatal exposure to polychlorinated biphenyls and dioxins on mental and motor development in Japanese children at 6 months of age. *Environ Health Perspect* 114:773–778, 2006.

Nakamura Y, Ikeda S, Furukawa T, Sumizawa T, Tani A, Akiyama S, Nagata Y: Function of P-glycoprotein expressed in placenta and mole. *Biochem Biophys Res Comm* 235:849–853, 1997.

Nandakumaran M, al-Rayyes S, al-Yatama M, Sugathan TN: Effect of glucose load on the transport kinetics of palmitic acid in the human placenta: an in vitro study. *Clin Exp Pharmacol Physiol* 26:669–673, 1999.

Nandakumaran M, Al-Saleh E, Al-Shammari M, Harouny AK: Effect of hyperglycemic load on maternal-fetal transport of L-leucine in perfused human placental lobule: in vitro study. *Acta Diabetol* 42:16–22, 2002.

Nandakumaran M, Harouny AK, Al-Yatam M, Al-Azemi MK, Sugathan TN: Effect of increased glucose load on maternal-fetal transport of alpha-aminoisobutyric acid in the perfused human placenta: in vitro study. *Acta Diabetol* 39:75–81, 2005.

Nanovskaya TN, Nekhayeva IA, Patrikeeva SL, Hankins GDV, Ahmed MS: Transfer of metformin across the dually perfused human placental lobule. *Am J Obstet Gynecol* 195:1081–1085, 2006.

Napoli A, Ciampa F, Colatrella A, Fallucca F: Use of repaglinide during the first weeks of pregnancy in two type 2 diabetic women. *Diabetes Care* 29:2326–2327, 2006.

Natali A, Ferrannini E: Effects of metformin and thiazolidinediones on suppression of hepatic glucose production and stimulation of glucose uptake in type 2 diabetes: a systematic review. *Diabetologia* 49:434–441, 2006.

Navarro-Alarcon M, Lopez-G de la Serrana H, Perez-Valero V, Lopex-Martinez C: Serum and urine selenium concentrations as indicators of body status in patients with diabetes mellitus. *Sci Total Environ* 228:79–85, 1999.

Nazer Herrera J, Garcia Huidobro M, Cifuentes Ovalle L: Congenital malformations among offspring of diabetic women. *Rev Med Chile* 133:547–554, 2005.

NCEP - National Cholesterol Education Program Expert Panel: Executive summary of the Third Report of the National Cholesterol Education Program (NCEP) expert panel on detection, evaluation, and treatment of high blood cholesterol in adults (Adult Treatment Panel III). *JAMA* 285:2486–2497, 2001.

Ndrepepa G, Kastrati A, Braun S, Koch W, Kolling K, Mehilli J, Schomig A: A prospective cohort study of predictive value of homocysteine in patients with type 2 diabetes and coronary heart disease. *Clin Chem Acta* 373:70–76, 2006.

Neal J: Analysis of effectiveness of human U-500 insulin in patients unresponsive to conventional insulin therapy. *Endocr Pract* 11:305–307, 2005.

Nelen WL, Blom HJ, Steegers EA, den Heijer M, Thomas CM, Eskes TK: Homocysteine and folate levels as risk factors for recurrent early pregnancy loss. *Obstet Gynecol* 95:519–524, 2000.

Nemeth E, Tuttle MS, Powelson J, Vaughn MB, Donovan A, Ward DM, Ganz T, Kaplan J: Hepcidin regulates cellular iron efflux by binding to ferroportin and inducing its internalization. *Science* 306:2090–2093, 2004.

Nesbitt TS, Gilbert WM, Herrchen B: Shoulder dystocia and associated risk factors with macrosomic infants born in California. *Am J Obst Gynecol* 179:476–480, 1998.

Neufeld L, Hass J, Pelletier D: The timing of maternal weight gain during pregnancy and fetal growth. *Am J Hum Biol* 11:647–657, 1999.

Neufeld LM, Haas JD, Grajeda R, Martorell R: Changes in maternal weight from the first to second trimester of pregnancy are associated with fetal growth and infant length at birth. *Am J Clin Nutr* 79:646–652, 2004.

Neumark-Sztainer D, Patterson J, Mellin A, Ackard DM, Utter J, Story M, Sockalosky J: Weight control practices and disordered eating behaviors among adolescent females and males with type 1 diabetes. Associations with sociodemographics, weight concerns, familial factors, and metabolic outcomes. *Diabetes Care* 25:1289–1296, 2002.

Neuschwander-Tetri BA, Caldwell SH: Nonalcoholic steatohepatitis: summary of an AASLD Single Topic Conference. *Hepatology* 37:1202–1219, 2003.

Neuschwander-Tetri BA: Nonalcoholic steatohepatitis and the metabolic syndrome. *Am J Med Sci* 330:326–334, 2005.

Ney D, Hollingsworth DR: Nutritional management of pregnancy complicated by diabetes: historical perspective. *Diabetes Care* 4:647–655, 1981.

Ney D, Hollingsworth DR, Cousins L: Decreased insulin requirement and improved control of diabetes in pregnant women given a high-carbohydrate, high-fiber, low-fat diet. *Diabetes Care* 5:529–533, 1982.

Ng PC, Lam CW, Lee CH, Wong GW, Fok TF, Wong E, Ma KC, Chan IH: Leptin and metabolic hormones in infants of diabetic mothers. *Arch Dis Child Fetal Neonatal Med* 83:F193–F197, 2000.

Nichols GA, Brown JB: Unadjusted and adjusted prevalence of diagnosed depression in type 2 diabetes. *Diabetes Care* 26:744–749, 2003.

Nicholson WK, Fox HE, Cooper LA, Strobino D, Witter F, Powe NR: Maternal race, procedures, and infant birth weight in type 2 and gestational diabetes. *Obstet Gynecol* 108:626–634, 2006.

Nicolas G, Chauvet C, Viatte L, Danan JL, Bigard X, Devaux I, Beaumont C, Kahn A, Vaulont S: The gene encoding the iron regulatory peptide hepcidin is regulated by anemia, hypoxia, and inflammation. *J Clin Invest* 110:1037–1044, 2002.

Niculescu MD, Zeisel SH: Diet, methyl donors and DNA methylation: interactions between dietary folate, methionine and choline. *J Nutr* 132 (Suppl 8):2333S–2335S, 2002.

Nielsen GL, Sorensen HT, Nielsen PH, Sabroe S, Olsen J: Glycosylated hemoglobin as predictor of adverse fetal outcome in type 1 diabetic pregnancies. *Acta Diabetol* 34:217–222, 1997.

Nielsen LR, Ekbom P, Damm P, Glumer C, Frandsen MM, Jensen DM, Mathiesen ER: HbA1c levels are significantly lower in early and late pregnancy. *Diabetes Care* 27:1200–1201, 2004.

Nielsen GL, Norgard B, Puho E, Rothman KJ, Sorenson HT, Czeizel AE: Risk of specific congenital abnormalities in offspring of women with diabetes. *Diabet Med* 22:693–696, 2005.

Nielsen JN, O'Brien KO, Witter FR, Chang S-C, Mancini J, Nathanson MS, Caulfield LE: High gestational weight gain does not improve birth weight in a cohort of African American adolescents. *Am J Clin Nutr* 84:183–189, 2006.

Nielsen GL, Dethlefsen C, Moller M, Sorensen HT: Maternal glycated hemoglobin, pre-gestational weight, pregnancy weight gain and risk of large-for-gestational age babies: a Danish cohort study of 209 singleton type 1 diabetic pregnancies. *Diabet Med* 24:384–387, 2007.

Nieman KM, Rowling MJ, Garrow TA, Schalinske KL: Modulation of methyl group metabolism by streptozotocin-induced diabetes and all-*trans*-retinoic acid. *J Biol Chem* 279:45708–45712, 2004.

Niemi M, Cascorbi I, Timm R, Kroemer HK, Neuvonen PJ, Kivisto KT: Glyburide and glimepiride pharmacokinetics in subjects with different *CYP2C9* genotypes. *Clin Pharmacol Ther* 72:326, 2002.

NIH—National Institutes of Health, National Heart, Lung, and Blood Institute: Clinical guidelines on the identification, evaluation, and treatment of overweight and obesity in adults. The Evidence Report. *Obes Res* 6 (Suppl 2):51S–183S, 1998. Available at: www.nhlbi.nih.gov/guidelines/obesity. Accessed Mar 15, 2008.

NIH—National Institutes of Health, Consensus Development Conference Statement on Celiac Disease, June 28–30, 2005: Introduction. *Gastroenterology* 128 (4 Suppl 1):S1–9, 2005.

NIH—National Institutes of Health State-of-the-Science Panel: State-of-the-Science Conference Statement: multivitamin/mineral supplements and chronic disease prevention. *Ann Intern Med* 145:364–371, 2006.

Noordzij M, Uiterwaal CS, Arends LR, Kok FJ, Grobbee DE, Geleijnse JM: Blood pressure response to chronic intake of coffee and caffeine: a meta-analysis of randomized controlled trials. *J Hypertens* 23:921–928, 2005.

Nordstrom L, Spetz E, Wallstrom K, Walinder O: Metabolic control and pregnancy outcome among women with insulin-dependent diabetes mellitus. A twelve-year followup in the county of Jamtland, Sweden. *Acta Obstet Gynecol Scand* 77: 284–289, 1998.

Norgard B, Ffonager K, Sorenson HT, Olsen J: Birth outcomes of women with celiac disease: A nationwide historical cohort study. *Am J Gastroenterol* 94:2435–2439, 1999.

Noriega E, Peralta E, Rivera L, Saucedo S: Glycaemic and insulinaemic indices of Mexican foods high in complex carbohydrates in type 2 diabetic subjects. *Diabetes Nutr Metab* 14:43–50, 2001.

Norris SL, Engelgau MM, Naravan KM: Effectiveness of self-management training in type 2 diabetes: a systematic review of randomized controlled trials. *Diabetes Care* 24:561–587, 2001.

Not T, Tommasini A, Tonini G, Buratti E, Pocecco M, Tortul C, Valussi M, Crichiutti G, Berti I, Trevisol C, Azzoni E, Neri E, Torre G, Martelossi S, Soban M, Lenhardt A, Cattin L, Ventura A: Undiagnosed celiac disease and risk of autoimmune disorders in subjects with type 1 diabetes mellitus. *Diabetologia* 44: 151–155, 2001.

Notelovitz M: Sulphonylurea therapy in the treatment of the pregnant diabetic. *South Afr Med J* 45:226–229, 1971.

Nouwen A, Breton MC, Urquhart Law G, Descoteaux J: Stability of an empirical psychosocial taxonomy across type of diabetes and treatment. *Diabet Med* 24: 41–47, 2007.

NRC—National Research Council: *Toxicological Effects of Methylmercury.* Washington, DC: National Acadamies Press; 2000.

Nuttall FQ, Mooradian AD, DeMarais R, Parker S: The glycemic effect of different meals approximately isocaloric and similar in protein, carbohydrate, and fat content as calculated using the ADA exchange lists. *Diabetes Care* 6: 432–435, 1983.

O'Brien KO, Zavaletta N, Abrams SA, Caulfield LE: Maternal iron status influences iron transfer to the fetus during the third trimester of pregnancy. *Am J Clin Nutr* 77:924–930, 2003.

O'Brien KO, Donangelo CM, Vargas Zapata CL, Abrams SA, Spencer EM, King JC: Bone calcium turnover during pregnancy and lactation in women with low calcium diets is associated with calcium intake and circulating insulin-like growth factor-1 concentrations. *Am J Clin Nutr* 83:317–323, 2006.

O'Kane MJ, Lynch PLM, Moles KW, Magee SE: Determination of a Diabetes Control and Complications Trial-aligned HbA1c reference range in pregnancy. *Clin Chim Acta* 311:157–159, 2001.

O'Keane V, Marsh MS: Depression during pregnancy. *BMJ* 334:1003–1005, 2007.

O'Moore-Sullivan TM, Prins JB: Thiazolidinediones and type 2 diabetes: new drugs for an old disease. *Med J Aust* 176:381–386, 2002.

Obeid R, Munz W, Jager M, Schmidt W, Herrmann W: Biochemical indexes of the B vitamins in cord serum are predicted by maternal B vitamin status. *Am J Clin Nutr* 82:133–139, 2005.

Oberlander TF, Misri S, Fitzgerald CE, Kostaras X, Rurak D, Riggs W: Pharmacologic factors associated with transient neonatal symptoms following prenatal psychotropic medication exposure. *J Clin Psychiatry* 65:230–237, 2004.

Oberlander TF, Warburton W, Misri S, Aghajanian J, Hertzman C: Neonatal outcomes after prenatal exposure to selective serotonin reuptake inhibitor antidepressants and maternal depression using population-based linked health data. *Arch Gen Psychiatry* 63:898–906, 2006.

Oberlander TF, Warburton W, Misri S, Riggs W, Aghajanian J, Hertzman C: Major congenital malformations following prenatal exposure to serotonin reuptake inhibitors and benzodiazepines using population-based health data. *Birth Defects Res B Dev Reprod Toxicol* 83:68–76, 2008.

Ogburn AD: Pregnancy in patients with celiac disease. *Br J Obstet Gynecol* 82:293–294, 1975.

Ogunmodede F, Jones JL, Scheftel J, Kirkland E, Schulkin J, Lynfield R: Listerosis prevention knowledge among pregnant women in the USA. *Infect Dis Obstet Gynecol* 13:11–15, 2005.

Oken E, Wright RO, Kleinman KP, Bellinger D, Amarasiriwardena CJ, Hu H, Rich-Edwards JW, Gillman MW: Maternal fish consumption, hair mercury, and infant cognition in a U.S. cohort. *Environ Health Perspect* 113:1376–1380, 2005.

Okumura K, Aso Y: High plasma homocysteine concentrations are associated with plasma concentrations of thrombomodulin in patients with type 2 diabetes and link diabetic nephropathy to macroangiopathy. *Metabolism* 52:1517–1522, 2003.

Olafsdottir AS, Skuladottir AS GV, Thorsdottir I, Hauksson A, Thorgeirsdottir H, Steingrimsdottir L: Relationship between high consumption of marine fatty acids in early pregnancy and hypertensive disorders of pregnancy. *BJOG* 113:301–309, 2006.

Olefsky JM: Treatment of insulin resistance with peroxisome proliferator-activated receptor γ agonists. *J Clin Invest* 106:467–472, 2000.

Olney J, Faber N, Spitznagel E, Robins L: Increasing brain tumor rates: is there a link to aspartame? *J Neuropath Exp Neurol* 55:115–123, 1996.

Olson CM, Strawderman MS, Hinton PS, Pearson TA: Gestational weight gain and postpartum behaviors associated with weight change from early pregnancy to 1 year postpartum. *Int J Obes* 27:117–127, 2003.

Omori Y, Minei S, Testuo T, Nrmoto K, Shimuzu M, Sanaka M: Current status of pregnancy in diabetic women: a comparison of pregnancy in IDDM and NIDDM mothers. *Diabetes Res Clin Pract* 24 (Suppl): S273–S278, 1994.

Orhan H, Onderoglu L, Yucel A, Sahin G: Circulating biomarkers of oxidative stress in complicated pregnancies. *Arch Gynecol Obstet* 267:189–195, 2003.

Ornoy A, Ratzon N, Greenbaum C, Peretz E, Soriano D, Dulitzky M: Neurobehavior of school age children born to diabetic mothers. *Arch Dis Child* 79:94–99, 1998.

Ornoy A, Ratzon N, Greenbaum C, Wolf A, Dulitzky M: School-age children born to mothers with pregestational or gestational diabetes exhibit a high rate of inattention and fine and gross motor impairment. *J Pediatr Endocrinol Metab* 14:681–690, 2001.

Osius N, Karmaus W, Kruse H, Witten J: Exposure to polychlorinated biphenyls and levels of thyroid hormones in children. *Environ Health Perspect* 107:843–849, 1999.

Osterode W, Holler C, Ulberth F: Nutritional antioxidants, red cell membrane fluidity and blood viscosity in type 1 (insulin dependent) diabetes mellitus. *Diabet Med* 13:1044–1050, 1996.

Owen MR, Doran E, Halestrap AP: Evidence that metformin exerts its anti-diabetic effects through inhibition of complex 1 of the mitochondrial respiratory chain. *Biochem J* 348: 607–614, 2000.

Ozarda Ilcol Y, Uncu G, Ulus IH: Free and phospholipid-bound choline concentrations in serum during pregnancy, after delivery and in newborns. *Arch Physiol Biochem* 110:393–399, 2002.

Packer L, Kraemer K, Rimbach G: Molecular aspects of lipoic acid in the prevention of diabetes complications. *Nutrition* 17:888–895, 2001.

Page RCL, Kirk BA, Fay T, Wilcox M, Hosking DJ, Jeffcoate WJ: Is macrosomia associated with poor glycemic control in diabetic pregnancy? *Diabet Med* 13:170–174, 1996.

Pandini G, Frasca F, Mineo R, Sciacca L, Vigneri R, Belfiore A: Insulin/insulin-like growth factor I hybrid receptors have different biological characteristics depending on the insulin receptor isoform involved. *J Biol Chem* 277: 39684–39695, 2002.

Panlasigui LN, Thompson LU: Blood glucose lowering effects of brown rice in normal and diabetic subjects. *Int J Food Sci Nutr* 57:151–158, 2006.

Paradis V, Perlemuter G, Bonvoust F, Dargere D, Parfait B, Vidaud M, Conti M, Huet S, Ba N, Buffet C, Bedossa P: High glucose and hyperinsulinemia stimulate connective tissue growth factor expression: a potential mechanism involved in progression to fibrosis in nonalcoholic steatohepatitis. *Hepatology* 34:738–744, 2001.

Parentoni LS, de Faria EC, Bartelega MJLF, Moda VMS, Facin ACC, Castilho LN: Glycated hemoglobin reference limits obtained by high performance liquid chromatography in adults and pregnant women. *Clin Chim Acta* 274:105–109, 1998.

Parfitt VJ, Clark JDA, Turner GM, Hartog M: Maternal postprandial blood glucose levels influence infant birth weight in diabetic pregnancy. *Diabetes Res* 19: 133–135, 1992.

Parker JD, Abrams B: Prenatal weight gain advice: an examination of the recent prenatal weight gain recommendations of the Institute of Medicine. *Obstet Gynecol* 79:664–649, 1992.

Parkes JL, Slatin SL, Pardo S, Ginsberg BH: A new consensus error grid to evaluate the clinical significance of inaccuracies in the measurement of blood glucose. *Diabetes Care* 23:1143–1148, 2000.

Parretti E, Mecaci F, Papini M, Cioni R, Carignani L, Mignosa M, La Torre P, Mello G: Third-trimester maternal blood glucose levels from diurnal profiles in nondiabetic pregnancies. Correlation with sonographic parameters of fetal growth. *Diabetes Care* 24:1319–1323, 2001.

Parulkar AA, Pendergrass ML, Granda-Ayala R, Lee TR, Fonseca VA: Nonhypoglycemic effects of thiazolidinediones. *Ann Intern Med* 134:61–71, 2001.

Pastors JG, Warshaw H, Daly A, Franz M, Kulkarni K: The evidence for the effectiveness of medical nutrition therapy in diabetes management. *Diabetes Care* 25:608–613, 2002.

Patel N, Alsat E, Igout A, Baron F, Hennen G, Porquet D, Evain-Brion D: Glucose inhibits human placental GH secretion, in vitro. *J Clin Endocrinol Metab* 80:1743–1746, 1995.

Patrick TE, Powers RW, Daftary AR, Ness RB, Roberts JM: Homocysteine and folic acid are inversely related in black women with preeclampsia. *Hypertension* 43:1279–1282, 2004.

Patton HM, Sirlin C, Behling C, Middleton M, Schwimmer JB, Lavine JE: Pediatric nonalcoholic fatty liver disease: a critical appraisal of current data and implications for future research. *J Pediatr Gastroenterol Nutr* 43:413–427, 2006.

Pavia C, Ferrer I, Valls C, Artuch R, Colome C, Vilaseca MA: Total homocysteine in patients with type 1 diabetes. *Diabetes Care* 23:84–87, 2000.

Payen L, Courtois A, Campion JP, Guillouzo A, Fardel O: Characterization and inhibition by a wide range of xenobiotics of organic anion excretion by primary human hepatocytes. *Biochem Pharmacol* 60:1967–1975, 2000.

Payen L, Deligin L, Courtois A, Trinquart Y, Guillouzo A, Fardel O: The sulfonylurea glibenclamide inhibits multidrug resistance protein (MRP1) activity in human lung cancer cells. *Br J Pharmacol* 132:778–784, 2001.

Pearson KH, Nonacs RM, Viquers AC, Heller VL, Petrillo LF, Brandes M, Hennen J, Cohen LS: Birth outcomes following prenatal exposure to antidepressants. *J Clin Psychiatry* 68:1284–1289, 2007.

Peck RW, Price DE, Lang GD, MacVicar J, Hearnshaw JR: Birthweight of babies born to mothers with type 1 diabetes: is it related to blood glucose control in the first trimester? *Diabet Med* 8:258–262, 1991.

Pedersen J, Brandstrup E: Fetal mortality in pregnant diabetics. Strict control of diabetes with conservative management. *Lancet* 1:607–610, 1956.

Pedersen J, Osler M: Hyperglycemia as a cause of characteristic features of the fetus and newborn of diabetic mothers. *Danish Med Bull* 8:78–83, 1961.

Pena-Rosas JP, Nesheim mMC, Garcia-Casal MN, Crompton DWT, Sanjur D, Viteri FE, Frongillo EA, Lorenzana P: Intermittent iron supplementation regimens are able to maintain safe maternal hemoglobin concentrations during pregnancy in Venezuela. *J Nutr* 134:1099–1104, 2004.

Pengiran Tengah DSNA, Wills AJ, Holmes GKT: Neurological complications of celiac disease. *Postgrad Med J* 78:393–398, 2002.

Penney GC, Mair G, Pearson DWM: Outcomes of pregnancies in women with type 1 diabetes in Scotland: a national population-based study. *BJOG* 110:315–318, 2003a.

Penney GC, Mair G, Pearson DWM: The relationship between birth weight and maternal glycated hemoglobin (HbA1C) concentration in pregnancies complicated by type 1 diabetes. *Diabet Med* 20:162–166, 2003b.

Pennington JA: *Bowes and Church's Food Values of Portions Commonly Used.* 17th ed. Lippincott-Raven Publishers; 1998.

Pereira MA, Swain J, Goldfine AB, Rifai N, Ludwig DS: Effects of a low-glycemic load diet on resting energy expenditure and heart disease risk factors during weight loss. *JAMA* 292:2482–2490, 2004.

Peretti N, Bienvenu F, Bouvet C, Fabien N, Tixier F, Thivolet C, Levy E, Chatelain PG, Lachaux A, Nicolino M: The temporal relationship between the onset of type 1 diabetes and celiac disease: a study based on immunoglobulin A antitransglutaminase screening. *Pediatrics* 113:e418–e422, 2004.

Perez-Carreras M, Del Hoyo P, Martin MA, Rubio JC, Martin A, Castellano G, Colina F, Arenas J, solis-Herruzo JA: Defective hepatic mitochondrial respiratory chain in patients with nonalcoholic steatoheaptitis. *Hepatology* 38:999–1007, 2003.

Perriello G, Misericordia P, Volpi E, Santucci A, Santucci C, Ferrannini E, Ventura MM, Santeusanio F, Brunetti P, Bolli GB: Acute antihyperglycemic mechanisms of metformin in NIDDM. Evidence for suppression of lipid oxidation and hepatic glucose production. *Diabetes* 43:920–928, 1994.

Perros P, Singh RK, Ludlam CA, Frier BM: Prevalence of pernicious anemia in patients with type 1 diabetes mellitus and autoimmune thyroid disease. *Diabet Med* 17:749–751, 2000.

Perseghin G, Lattuada G, De Cobelli F, Esposito A, Costantino F, Canu T, Scifo P, De Taddeo F, Maffi P, Secchi A, Del Maschio A, Luzi L: Reduced intrahepatic fat content is associated with increased whole-body lipid oxidation in patients with type 1 diabetes. *Diabetologia* 48:2615–2621, 2005.

Persson B, Hanson U: Insulin dependent diabetes in pregnancy: impact of maternal blood glucose control on offspring. *J Paediatr Child Health* 29:20–23, 1993.

Persson B, Hanson U: Fetal size at birth in relation to quality of blood glucose control in pregnancies complicated by pregestational diabetes mellitus. *Brit J Obstet Gynecol* 103:427–433, 1996.

Persson B, Westgren M, Celsi G, Nord E, Ortqvist E: Leptin concentrations in cord blood in normal newborn infants and offspring of diabetic mothers. *Horm Metab Res* 31:467–471, 1999.

Persson B, Swahn M, Hjertberg R, Hanson U, Nord E, Nordlander E, Hansson L-O: Insulin lispro therapy in pregnancies complicated by type 1 diabetes mellitus. *Diabetes Res Clin Pract* 58:115–121, 2002.

Peter R, Luzio SD, Dunseath G, Miles A, Hare B, Backx K, Pauvaday V, Owens DR: Effects of exercise on the absorption of insulin glargine in patients with type 1 diabetes. *Diabetes Care* 28:560–565, 2005.

Peters U, Askling J, Gridley G, Ekbom A, Linet M: Causes of death in patients with celiac disease in a population-based Swedish cohort. *Arch Intern Med* 163:1566–1572, 2003.

Petersen KF, Dufour S, Befroy D, Lehrke M, Hendler RE, Shulman GI: Reversal of nonalcoholic hepatic steatosis, hepatic insulin resistance, and hyperglycemia by moderate weight reduction inpatients with type 2 diabetes. *Diabetes* 54:603–608, 2005.

Peterson CM, Jovanovic-Peterson L: Percentage of carbohydrate and glycemic response to breakfast, lunch, and dinner in women with gestational diabetes. *Diabetes* 40 (Suppl 2):172–174, 1991.

Petry CD, Eaton MA, Wobken JD, Mills MM, Johnson DE, Georgieff MK: Liver, heart, and brain iron deficiency in newborn infants of diabetic mothers. *J Pediatr* 121:109–114, 1992.

Petry CD, Wobken JD, McKay H, Eaton MA, Seybold VS, Johnson DE, Georgieff MK: Placental transferrin receptor in diabetic pregnancies with increased fetal iron demand. *Am J Physiol* 267:E507–E514, 1994.

Pettitt DJ, Baird HR, Aleck KA, Bennett PH, Knowler WC: Excessive obesity in offspring of Pima Indian women with diabetes during pregnancy. *N Engl J Med* 308:242–245, 1983.

Peuchant E, Brun JL, Rigalleau V, Dubourg L, Thomas MJ, Daniel JY, Leng JJ, Gin H: Oxidative and antioxidative status in pregnant women with either gestational or type 1 diabetes. *Clin Biochem* 37:293–298, 2004.

Peveler RC, Fairburn CG: The treatment of bulimia nervosa in patients with diabetes mellitus. *Int J Eat Disord* 11:45–53, 1992.

Peveler RC, Bryden KS, Neil HAW, Fairburn CG, Mayou RA, Dunger DB, Turner HM: The relationship of disordered eating habits and attitudes to clinical outcomes in young adult females with type 1 diabetes. *Diabetes Care* 28:84–88, 2005.

Peyrot M, Rubin RR, Lauritzen T, Snoek FJ, Matthews DR, Skovlund SE: Psychosocial problems and barriers to improved diabetes management: results of the Cross-National Diabetes Attitudes, Wishes and Needs (DAWN) Study. *Diabet Med* 22:1379–1385, 2005.

Peyrot M, Rubin RR, Siminerio LM; on behalf of the International DAWN Advisory Panel: Physician and nurse use of psychosocial strategies in diabetes care: results of the cross-national diabetes attitudes, wishes and needs (DAWN) study. *Diabetes Care* 29:1256–1262, 2006.

Peyrot M, Rubin RR: Behavioral and psychosocial interventions in diabetes: a conceptual review. *Diabetes Care* 30:2433–2440, 2007.

Pfeiffer CM, Caudill SP, Gunter EW, Bowman BA, Jacques PF, Selhub J, Johnson CL, Miller DT, Sampson EJ: Analysis of factors influencing the comparison of homocysteine values between the Third National Health and Nutrition Examination Survey (NHANES) and NHANES 1999+. *J Nutr* 130:2850–2854, 2000.

Phillipps AF, Dublin JW, Matty PJ, Raye J: Arterial hypoxemia and hyperinsulinemia in the chronically hyperglycemic fetal lamb. *Pediatr Res* 16:653–658, 1982.

Phillipps AF, Porte PJ, Stabinsky S, Rosenkrantz TS, Raye JR: Effects of chronic fetal hyperglycemia upon oxygen consumption in the ovine uterus and conceptus. *J Clin Invest* 74:279–286, 1984.

Piaquadio K, Hollingsworth DR, Murphy H: Effects of in-utero exposure to oral hypoglycemic drugs. *Lancet* 338:866–869, 1991.

Picarelli A, di Tola M, Sabbatella L, Mastracchio A, trecca A, Gabrielli F, di Cello T, Anania MC, Torsoli A: Identification of a new celiac disease subgroup: antiendomysial and anti-transglutaminase antibodies of IgG class in the absence of selective IgA deficiency. *J Intern Med* 249:181–188, 2001b.

Picarelli A, DiTola M, Sabbatella L, Gabrielli F, DiCello T, Anania MC, Mastracchio A, Silano M, De Vincenzi M: Immunologic evidence of no harmful effect of oats in celiac disease. *Am J Clin Nutr* 74:137–140, 2001a.

Picciano MF: Is homocysteine a biomarker for identifying women at risk of complications and adverse pregnancy outcomes? Editorial. *Am J Clin Nutr* 71:857–858, 2000.

Picciano MF: Pregnancy and lactation: physiological adjustments, nutritional requirements and the role of dietary supplements. *J Nutr* 133:1997S–2002S, 2003.

Pietrangelo A: Hereditary hemochromatosis—a new look at an old disease. *N Engl J Med* 350:2383–2397, 2004.

Pietzak MM: Follow-up of patients with celiac disease: achieving compliance with treatment. *Gastroenterology* 128 (Suppl 1):S135–S141, 2005.

Piper JM, Langer O: Does maternal diabetes delay fetal pulmonary maturity? *Am J Obstet Gynecol* 168:783–786, 1993.

Piper JM, Xenakis E, Langer O: Delayed appearance of pulmonary maturation markers is associated with poor glucose control in diabetes mellitus. *J Matern-Fetal Med* 7:148–153, 1998.

Piper JL, Gray GM, Khosla C: High selectivity of human tissue transglutaminase for immunoactive gliadin peptides: implications for celiac sprue. *Biochemistry* 41:386–393, 2002.

Pithova P, Kvapil M: Effect of using the electronic food-list on metabolic control in type 1 diabetes mellitus. *Diabetes* 55 (Suppl 1):A9, 2006.

Pitkin RM, Reynolds W, Filer LJ, Kling TG: Placental transmission and fetal distribution of saccharin. *Am J Obstet Gynecol* 111:280–286, 1971.

Pitkin RM: Calcium metabolism in pregnancy and the perinatal period: a review. *Am J Obstet Gynecol* 151:99–109, 1985.

Pitkin RM: Energy in pregnancy. Editorial. *Am J Clin Nutr* 69:583, 1999.

Pitsavos C, Panagiotakos DB, Tzima N, Chrysohoou C, Economou M, Zampelas A, Stefanadis C: Adherance to the Mediterranean diet is associated with total antioxidant capacity in healthy adults: the ATTICA study. *Am J Clin Nutr* 82:694–699, 2005.

Pivarnik JM, Stein AD, Rivera JM: Effect of pregnancy on heart rate/oxygen consumption calibration curves. *Med Sci Sports Exerc* 34:750–755, 2002.

Pizziol A, Tikhonoff V, Paleri CD, Russo E, Mazza A, Ginocchio G, Onesto C, Pavan L, Casiglia E, Pessina AC: Effects of coffee on glucose tolerance: a placebo-controlled study. *Eur J Clin Nutr* 52:846–849, 1998.

Plagemann A, Harder T, Kohloff R, Rohde W, Dorner G: Glucose tolerance and insulin secretion in children of mothers with pregestational IDDM or gestational diabetes. *Diabetologia* 40:1094–1100, 1997.

Plank J, Bodenlenz M, Sinner F, Magnes C, Gorzer E, Regittnig W, Endahl LA, Draeger E, Zdravkovic M, Pieber TR: A double-blind, randomized, dose-response study investigating the pharmacodynamic and pharmacokinetic properties of the long-acting insulin analog detemir. *Diabetes Care* 28:1107–1112, 2005a.

Plank J, Siebenhofer A, Berghold A, Jeitler K, Horvath K, Mrak P, Pieber TR: Systematic review and meta-analysis of short-acting insulin analogues in patients with diabetes mellitus. *Arch Intern Med* 165:1337–1344, 2005b.

Platt MJ, Stanisstreet M, Casson IF, Howard CV, Walkinshaw S, Pennycook S, McKendrick O: St Vincent's Declaration 10 years on: outcomes of diabetic pregnancies. *Diabet Med* 19:216–220, 2002.

Pofsay-Barbe KM, Wald ER: Listerosis. *Pediatr Rev* 25:151–159, 2004.

Polley BA, Wing RR, Sims CJ: Randomized controlled trial to prevent excessive weight gain in pregnant women. *Int J Obes Relat Metab Disord* 26:1494–1502, 2002.

Pollock-BarZiv SM, Davis C: Personality factors and disordered eating in young women with type 1 diabetes mellitus. *Psychosomatics* 46:11–18, 2005.

Polonsky WH, Fisher L, Earles J, Dudl RJ, Lees J, Mullan J, Jackson RA: Assessing psychosocial distress in diabetes. Development of the Diabetes Distress Scale. *Diabetes Care* 28:626–631, 2005.

Ponka P, Lok CN: The transferrin receptor: role in health and disease. *Int J Biochem Cell Biol* 31:1111–1137, 1999.

Ponka P: Recent advances in cellular iron metabolism. *J Trace Elem Exp Med* 16: 201–217, 2003.

Portela-Gomez GM, Johansson H, Olding L, Grimelius L: Co-localization of neuroendocrine hormones in the human fetal pancreas. *Eur J Endocrinol* 141:526–533, 1999.

Poston L, Raijmakers MYM: Trophoblast oxidative stress, antioxidants and pregnancy outcome—a review. *Placenta* 25 (Suppl A):S72–S78, 2004.

Poston L, Briley AL, Seed PT, Kelly FJ, Shennan AH; the Vitamins in Preeclampsia (VIP) Trial Consortium: Vitamin C and vitamin E in pregnant women at risk for preeclampsia (VIP trial): a randomized placebo-controlled trial. *Lancet* 367:1145–1154, 2006.

Potter JM, Reckless JPD, Cullen DR: The effect of continuous subcutaneous insulin infusion and conventional insulin regimes on 24-hour variations of blood glucose and intermediary metabolites in the third trimester of diabetic pregnancy. *Diabetologia* 21:534–539, 1981.

Poulaki V, Qin W, Joussen AM, Hurlbut P, Wiegand SJ, Rudge J, Yancopolous GD, Adamis AP: Acute intensive insulin therapy exacerbates diabetic blood-retinal barrier breakdown via hypoxia-inducible factor-1α and VEGF. *J Clin Invest* 109:805–815, 2002.

Poulaki V, Joussen AM, Mitsiades N, Mitsiades CS, Waki EF, Adamis AP: Insulin-like growth factor-I plays a pathogenetic role in diabetic retinopathy. *Am J Pathol* 165:457–469, 2004.

Powell EE, Jonsson JR, Clouston AD: Dangerous liaisons: the metabolic syndrome and nonalcoholic fatty liver disease. *Ann Intern Med* 143:753–754, 2005.

Powers RW, Majors AK, Kerchner LJ, Conrad KP: Renal handling of homocysteine during normal pregnancy and preeclampsia. *J Soc Gynecol Invest* 11:45–50, 2004.

Poyhoenen-Alho M, Roennemaa T, Saltevo J, Ekblad U, Kaaja RJ: Use of insulin glargine during pregnancy. *Acta Obstet Gynecol Scand* Aug 29, 2007 [Epub ahead of print].

PPP—Primary Prevention Project Collaborative Group: Low-dose aspirin and vitamin E in people at cardiovascular risk: a randomized trial in general practice. *Lancet* 357:89–95, 2001.

Prati D, Taioli E, Zanella A, Della Torre E, Butelli S, Del Vecchio E, Vianello L, Zanuso F, Mozzi F, Milani S, Conte D, Colombo M, Sirchia G: Updated definitions of health ranges for serum alanine aminotransferase levels. *Ann Intern Med* 137:1–9, 2002.

Prentice A, Spaaij C, Goldberg G, Poppitt SD, van Raaij JM, Totton M, Swann D, Black AE: Energy requirements of pregnant and lactating women. *Eur J Clin Nutr* 50 (Suppl):82S–111S, 1996.

Price N, Bartlett C, Gillmer MD: Use of insulin glargine during pregnancy: a case-control pilot study. *BJOG* 114:453–457, 2007.

Provenzale D, Reinhold RB, Golner B, Irwin V, Dallal GE, Papathanasopoulos N, Sahyoun N, Samloff IM, Russell RM: Evidence for diminished B12 absorption after gastric bypass: oral supplementation does not prevent low plasma B12 levels. *J Am Coll Nutr* 11:29–35, 1992.

PSTF—U.S. Preventative Services Task Force: Routine iron supplementation during pregnancy. *JAMA* 270:2848–2854, 1993.

PSTF—U.S. Preventative Services Task Force. Screening and behavior counseling interventions in primary care to reduce alcohol misuse. *Ann Intern Med* 140:555–557, 2004.

Punglia RS, Lu M, Hsu J, Kuroki M, Tolentino MJ, Keough K, Levy AP, Levy NS, Goldberg MA, D'Amato RJ, Adamis AP: Regulation of vascular endothelial growth factor expression by insulin-like growth factor-I. *Diabetes* 46:1619–1626, 1997.

Punnonen K, Irjala K, Rajamaki A: Serum transferrin receptor and its ratio to serum ferritin in the diagnosis of iron deficiency. *Blood* 89:1052–1057, 1997.

Qi L, Meigs JB, Liu S, Manson JE, Mantzoros C, Hu FB: Dietary fibers and glycemic load, obesity, and plasma adiponectin levels in women with type 2 diabetes. *Diabetes Care* 29:1501–1505, 2006a.

Qi L, van DamR, Liu S, Franz M, Mantzoros C, Hu FB: Whole-grain, bran, and cereal fiber intakes and markers of systemic inflammation in diabetic women. *Diabetes Care* 29:207–211, 2006b.

Quinlavan EP, Gregory JF 3rd: Effect of food fortification on folic acid intake in the United States. *Am J Clin Nutr* 77:221–225, 2003.

Raatz SK, Torkelson CJ, Redmon JB, Reck KP, Kwong CA, Swanson JE, Liu C, Thomas W, Bantle JP: Reduced glycemic index and glycemic load diets do not increase the effects of energy restriction on weight loss and insulin sensitivity in obese men and women. *J Nutr* 135:2387–2391, 2005.

Radaelli T, Varastehpour A, Catalano P, Hauguel-de Mouzon S: Gestational diabetes induces placental genes for chronic stress and inflammatory pathways. *Diabetes* 52:2951–2958, 2003.

Radaelli T, Uvena-Celebrezze J, Minium J, Huston-Presley L, Catalano P, Hauguel-de Mouzon S: Maternal interleukin-6, a marker of fetal growth and adiposity. *J Soc Gynecol Investig* 13:53–57, 2006.

Rae A, Bond D, Evans S, North F, Roberman B, Walters B: A randomized controlled trial of dietary energy restriction in the management of obese women with gestational diabetes. *Aust N Z J Obstet Gynecol* 40:416–422, 2000.

Raijmakers MT, Zusterzeel PL, Steegers EA, Hectors MP, Demacker PN, Peters WH: Plasma thiol status in preeclampsia. *Obstet Gynecol* 95:180–184, 2000.

Raijmakers MTM, Dechend R, Poston L: Oxidative stress and preeclampsia. Rationale for antioxidant clinical trials. *Hypertension* 44:374–380, 2004a.

Raijmakers MT, Roes EM, Zusterzeel PL, Steegers EA, Peters WH: Thiol status and antioxidant calacity in women with a history of severe preeclampsia. *Br J Obstet Gynecol* 111:207–212, 2004b.

Raipathak S, Rimm E, Morris JS, Hu F: Toenail selenium and cardiovascular disease in men with diabetes. *J Am Coll Nutr* 24:250–256, 2005.

Raiten DJ, Picciano MF: Vitamin D and health in the 21st century: bone and beyond. Executive summary. *Am J Clin Nutr* 80 (Suppl):1673S–1677S, 2004.

Rajdl D, Racek J, Steinerova A, Novotny Z, Stozicky F, Trefil L, Siala K: Markers of oxidative stress in diabetic mothers and their infants during delivery. *Physiol Res* 54:429–436, 2005.

Rajkovic A, Catalano PM, Malinow MR: Elevated homocysteine levels with preeclampsia. *Obstet Gynecol* 90:168–171, 1997.

Ramakrishna G, Rooke TW, Cooper LT: Iron and peripheral arterial disease: revisiting the iron hypothesis in a different light. *Vasc Med* 8:203–210, 2003.

Ramakrishnan U: Nutrition and low birth weight: from research to practice. *Am J Clin Nutr* 79:17–21, 2004.

Ramalho AC, deLourdes Lima M, Nunes F, Cambui Z, Barbosa C, Andrade A, Viana A, Martins M, Abrantes V, Aragao C, Temistocles M: The effect of resistance versus aerobic training on metabolic control in patients with type-1 diabetes mellitus. *Diabetes Res Clin Pract* 72:271–276, 2006.

Rami B, Sumnik Z, Schober E, Waldhor T, Battelino T, Bratanic N, Kurti K, Lebl J, Limbert C, Madacsy L, Odink RJ, Paskova M, Soltesz G: Screening detected celiac disease in children with type 1 diabetes mellitus: effect on the clinical course (a case control study). *J Pediatr Gastroenterol Nutr* 41:317–321, 2005.

Ramirez MM, Turrentine MA: Gastrointestinal hemorrhage during pregnancy in a patient with a history of vertical-banded gastroplasty. *Am J Obstet Gynecol* 173:1630–1631, 1995.

Ramirez GB, Cruz MC, Pagulayan O, Ostrea E, Dalisay C: The Tagum study I: analysis and clinical correlates of mercury in maternal and cord blood, breast milk, meconium, and infant's hair. *Pediatrics* 106:774–781, 2000.

Ramirez GB, Pagulayan O, Akagi H, Francisco RA, Lee LV, Berrova A, Vince Cruz MC, Casintahan D: Tagum study II: follow-up study after two years of age after prenatal exposure to mercury. *Pediatrics* 111:e289–295, 2003.

Ramos GA, Jacobson GF, Kirby RS, Ching JY, Field DR: Comparison of glyburide and insulin for the management of gestational diabetics with markedly elevated oral glucose challenge test and fasting hyperglycemia. *J Perinatol* 27:262–267, 2007.

Ramos-Arroyo MA, Rodriguez-Pinilla E, Cordero JF: Maternal diabetes: the risk for specific birth defects. *Eur J Epidemiol* 8:503–508, 1992.

Rampertab SD, Pooran N, Brar P, Singh P, Green PH: Trends in the presentation of celiac disease. *Am J Med* 119:355.e9–14, 2006.

Rand C, Macgregor A: Medical care and pregnancy outcome after gastric bypass surgery for obesity. *South Med J* 82:1319–1320, 1989.

Ransford RA, hayes M, Palmer M, Hall MJ: A controlled, prospective screening study of celiac disease presenting as iron deficiency anemia. *J Clin Gastroenterol* 35:228–233, 2002.

Rasmussen KM: Is there a causal relationship between iron deficiency or iron-deficiency anemia and weight at birth, length of gestation and perinatal mortality? *J Nutr* 131:590S–603S, 2001.

Rasmussen KM, Stoltzfus RJ: New evidence that iron supplementation during pregnancy improves birth weight: new scientific questions. Editorial. *Am J Clin Nutr* 78:673–674, 2003.

Ratnam S, Wijekoon EP, Hall B, Garrow TA, Brosnan ME, Brosnan JT: Effects of diabetes and insulin on betaine-homocysteine S-methyltransferase expression in the rat liver. *Am J Physiol* 290:E933–E939, 2006.

Ratner RE, Hirsch IB, Neifing JL, Garg SK, Mecca TE, Wilson CA; for the U.S. Study Group of Insulin Glargine in Type 1 Diabetes: Less hypoglycemia with insulin glargine in intensive insulin therapy for type 1 diabetes. *Diabetes Care* 23:639–643, 2000.

Ratzon N, Greenbaum C, Dulitzky M, Ornoy A: Comparison of the motor development of school-age children born to mothers with and without diabetes mellitus. *Phys Occup Ther Pediatr* 20:43–57, 2000.

Rauramo I, Andersson B, Laatikainen T: Stress hormones and placental steroids in physical exercise during pregnancy. *Br J Obstet Gynecol* 89:921–925, 1982.

Rave K, Bott S, Heinemann L, Sha S, Becker RHA, Willavize SA, Heise T: Time-action profile of inhaled insulin in comparison with subcutaneously injected insulin lispro and regular human insulin. *Diabetes Care* 28:1077–1082, 2005.

Rave K, Klein O, Frick AD, Becker RHA: Advantage of premeal-injected insulin glulisine compared with regular human insulin in subjects with type 1 diabetes. *Diabetes Care* 29:1812–1817, 2006.

Ravina A, Slezak L, Rubal A, Mirsky N: Clinical use of the trace element chromium (III) in the treatment of diabetes mellitus. *J Trace Elem Exp Med* 8:183–190, 1995.

Ravindran S, Zharikova OL, Hill RA, Nanovskaya TN, Hankins GD, Ahmed MS: Identification of glyburide metabolites formed by hepatic and placental microsomes of humans and baboons. *Biochem Pharmacol* 72:1730–1737, 2006.

Ray JG, Laskin CA: Folic acid and homocysteine metabolic defects and the risk of placental abruption, pre-eclampsia and spontaneous pregnancy loss: a systematic review. *Placenta* 20:519–529, 1999.

Ray JG, Vermeulen MJ, Shapiro JL, Kenshole AB: Maternal and neonatal outcomes in pregestational and gestational diabetes mellitus, and the influence of maternal obesity and weight gain: the DEPOSIT Study. *QJM* 94:347–356, 2001a.

Ray JG, O'Brien, TE, Chan, WS. Preconception care and the risk of congenital anomalies in the offspring of women with diabetes mellitus: a meta-analysis. *QJM* 94:435–444, 2001b.

Ray JG, Mamdoni M: Association between folic acid food fortification and hypertension or preeclampsia in pregnancy. *Arch Intern Med* 162:1776–1777, 2002.

Ray JG, Wyatt PR, Vermuelen MJ, Meier C, Cole DEC: Greater maternal weight and the ongoing risk of neural tube defects after folic acid flour fortification. *Obstet Gynecol* 105:261–265, 2005.

Rayburn W, Piehl E, Lewis E, Schork A, Sereika S, Zabrenskly K: Changes in insulin therapy during pregnancy. *Am J Perinatol* 2:271–275, 1985.

Rayburn W, Piehl E, Jacober S, Schork A, Ploughman L: Severe hypoglycemia during pregnancy: its frequency and predisposing factors in diabetic women. *Int J Gynecol Obstet* 24:263–268, 1986.

Raychaudhuri K, Maresh JA. Glycemic control throughout pregnancy and fetal growth in insulin-dependent diabetes. *Obstet Gynecol* 95:190–194, 2000.

Rayman MP, Bode P, Redman CWG: Low selenium status is associated with the occurrence of the pregnancy disease preeclampsia in women from the United Kingdom. *Am J Obstet Gynecol* 189:1343–1349, 2003.

Reader DM: Gestational diabetes. In: Mensing C, Cypress M, Halstensen C, McLaughlin S, Walker EA, eds. *The Art and Science of Diabetes Self-Management Education. A Desk Reference for Healthcare Professionals.* Chicago: American Association of Diabetes Educators; 2006:259–277.

Rebrin K, Steil GM, van Antwerp WP, Mastrototaro JJ: Subcutaneous glucose predicts plasma glucose independent of insulin: implications for continuous monitoring. *Am J Physiol* 277:E561–E571, 1999.

Redman CWG, Sargent IL: Pre-eclampsia, the placenta and the maternal systemic inflammatory response—a review. *Placenta* 24:S21–S27, 2003.

Reece EA, Coustan DR, Sherwin RS, Tuck S, Bates S, O'Connor T, Tamborlane WV: Does intensive glycemic control in diabetic pregnancies result in normalization of other metabolic fuels? *Am J Obstet Gynecol* 165:126–130, 1991.

Reece EA, Hagay Z, Gay LJ, O'Connor T, DeGennaro N, Homko CJ, Wiznitzer A: A randomized clinical trial of a fiber-enriched diabetic diet vs the standard ADA-recommended diet in the management of diabetes mellitus in pregnancy. *J Matern-Fetal Inv* 5:8–12, 1995.

Reece EA, Leguizamon G, Homko C: Stringent control in diabetic nephropathy associated with optimization of pregnancy outcomes. *J Matern-Fetal Med* 7:213–216, 1998.

Reece EA, Coustan DR, Gabbe SG, eds: *Diabetes in Women. Adolescence, Pregnancy, and Menopause.* 3rd ed. Philadelphia: Lippincott Williams & Wilkins; 2004a.

Reece EA, Eriksson UJ: Congenital malformations: epidemiology, pathogenesis, and experimental methods of induction and prevention. In: Reece EA, Coustan DR,

Gabbe SG, eds. *Diabetes in Women. Adolescence, Pregnancy, and Menopause.* 3rd ed. Philadelphia: Lippincott Williams & Wilkins; 2004b:169–204.

Refsum H, Yajnik CS, Gadkari M, Schneede J, Vollset SE, Orning L, Guttormsen AB, Joglekar A, Sayyad MG, Ulvik A, Ueland PM: Hyperhomocysteinemia and elevated methylmalonic acid indicate a high prevalence of cobalamin deficiency in Asian Indians. *Am J Clin Nutr* 74:233–241, 2001.

Refsum H, Smith AD, Ueland PM, Nexo E, Clarke R, McPartlin J, Johnston C, Engbaek F, Scheede J, McPartlin C, Scott JM: Facts and recommendations about total homocysteine determinations: an expert opinion. *Clin Chem* 50:3–32, 2004.

Refsum H, Nurk E, Smith AD, Ueland PM, Gjesdal CG, Bjelland I, Tverdal A, Tell GS, Nygard O, Vollset SE: The Hordaland Homocysteine Study: a community-based study of homocysteine, its determinants, and association with disease. *J Nutr* 136 (Suppl 6):1731S–1740S, 2006.

Reif DW: Ferritin as a source of iron for oxidative damage. *Free Rad Biol Med* 12:417–427, 1992.

Reiter CEN, Gardner TW: Retinal insulin and insulin signaling: implications for diabetic retinopathy. *Prog Ret Eye Res* 22:545–562, 2003.

Rembiasz K, Konturek PC, Karcz D, Konturek SJ, Ochmanski W, Bielanski W, Budzynski A, Stachura J: Biomarkers in various types of atrophic gastritis and their diagnostic usefulness. *Dig Dis Sci* 50:474–482, 2005.

Remillard RB, Bunce NJ: Linking dioxins to diabetes: epidemiology and biologic plausibility. *Environ Health Perspect* 110:853–858, 2002.

Rensch MJ, Merenich JA, Lieberman M, Long BD, Davis DR, McNally PR: Gluten-sensitive enteropathy in patients with insulin-dependent diabetes mellitus. *Ann Intern Med* 124:564–567, 1996.

Resnick LM, Barbagallo M, Bardicef M, Bardicef O, Sorokin Y, Evelhoch J, Dominguez LJ, Mason BA, Cotton DB: Cellular-free magnesium depletion in brain and muscle of normal and preeclamptic pregnancy. A nuclear magnetic resonance spectroscopic study. *Hypertension* 44:322–326, 2004.

Rettie AE, Jones JP: Clinical and toxicological relevance of CYP2C9: drug-drug interactions and pharmacogenetics. *Annu Rev Pharmacol Toxicol* 45:477–494, 2005.

Revelli A, Durando A, Massobrio M: Exercise and pregnancy: a review of maternal and fetal effects. *Obstet Gynecol Surv* 47:355–367, 1992.

Rey E, Attie C, Bonin A: The effects of first-trimester diabetes control on the incidence of macrosomia. *Am J Obstet Gynecol* 181:202–206, 1999.

Reyes H, Baez ME, Gonzalez MC, Hernandez I, Palma J, Ribalta J, Sandoval L, Zapata R: Selenium, zinc and copper plasma levels in intrahepatic cholestasis of pregnancy, in normal pregnancies and in healthy individuals, in Chile. *J Hepatol* 32:542–549, 2000.

Rhodes JC, Schoendorf KC, Parker JD: Contribution of excess weight gain during pregnancy and macrosomia to the cesarean delivery rate, 1990–2000. *Pediatrics* 111:1181–1185, 2003.

Rice DC: The US EPA reference dose for methylmercury: sources of uncertainty. *Environ Res* 95:406–413, 2004.

Rice DE, Schoeny R, Mahaffey K: Methods and rationale for derivation of a reference dose for methyl mercury by the US Environmental Protection Agency. *Risk Anal* 23:107–115, 2003.

Richardson T, Weiss M, Thomas P, Kerr D: Day after the night before. Influence of evening alcohol on risk of hypoglycemia in patients with type 1 diabetes. *Diabetes Care* 28:1801–1802, 2005.

Riddell LJ, Chisholm A, Williams S, Mann JI: Dietary strategies for lowering homocysteine concentrations. *Am J Clin Nutr* 71:1448–1454, 2000.

Riddle MC, Drucker DJ: Emerging therapies mimicking the effects of amylin and glucagon-like peptide 1. *Diabetes Care* 29:435–449, 2006.

Ridwan E, Schultink W, Dillon D, Gross R: Effects of weekly iron supplementation on pregnant Indonesian women are similar to those of daily supplementation. *Am J Clin Nutr* 63:884–890, 1996.

Rigg L, Cousins L, Hollinsworth D, Brink G, Yen SSC: Effects of exogenous insulin on excursions and diurnal rhythm of plasma glucose in pregnant diabetic patients with and without residual B-cell function. *Am J Obstet Gynecol* 136:537–543, 1980.

Riley WJ, Toskes PP, Maclaren NK, Silverstein J: Predictive value of gastric parietal cell autoantibodies as a marker for gastric and hematologic abnormalities associated with insulin dependent diabetes. *Diabetes* 31:1051–1055, 1982.

Rimm EB, Willett WC, Hu FB, Sampson L, Colditz GA, Manson JE, Hennekens C, Stampfer MJ: Folate and vitamin B6 from diet and supplements in relation to risk of coronary heart disease among women. *JAMA* 279:359–364, 1998.

Rizzo T, Metzger B, Burns WJ, Burns K: Correlations between antepartum maternal metabolism and intelligence of offspring. *N Engl J Med* 325:911–916, 1991.

Rizzo TA, Ogata ES, Dooley SL, Metzger BE, Cho NH: Perinatal complications and cognitive development in 2- to 5-year-old children of diabetic mothers. *Am J Obstet Gynecol* 171:706–713, 1994.

Rizzo T, Dooley S, Metzger B, Cho N, Ogata E, Silverman B: Prenatal and perinatal influences on long-term psychomotor development in offspring of diabetic mothers. *Am J Obstet Gynecol* 173:1753–1758, 1995.

Robb A, Wessling-Resnick M: Regulation of transferrin receptor 2 protein levels by transferrin. *Blood* 104:4294–4299, 2004.

Roberts PD, James H, Petrie A, Morgan JO, Hoffbrand AV: Vitamin B_{12} Status in pregnancy among immigrants to Britain. *Br Med J* 3:67–72, 1973.

Roberts JM, Hubel CA: Is oxidative stress the link in the two-stage model of pre-eclampsia? *Lancet* 354:788–789, 1999.

Roberts L, Jones TW, Fournier PA: Exercise training and glycemic control in adolescents with poorly controlled type 1 diabetes mellitus. *J Pediatr Endocrinol Metab* 15:621–627, 2002.

Roberts JM, Pearson G, Cutler J, Lindheimer M: Summary of the NHLBI Working Group on Research on Hypertension During Pregnancy. *Hypertension* 41:437–445, 2003.

Roberts EA, Yap J: Nonalcoholic fatty liver disease (NAFLD): approach in the adolescent patient. *Curr Treat Options Gastroenterol* 9:423–431, 2006.

Robertson D, Wade D, Workman R, Woolsley RL, Oates JA: Tolerance to the humoral and hemodynamic effects of caffeine in man. *J Clin Invest* 67: 1111–1117, 1981.

Robertson G, Leclercq I, Farrell GC: Nonalcoholic steatosis and steatohepatitis II. Cytochrome P-450 enzymes and oxidative stress. *Am J Physiol Gastrointest Liver Physiol* 281: G1135–G1139, 2001.

Robillard JE, Sessions C, Kennedy RL, Smith FG: Metabolic effect of constant hypertonic glucose infusion in well oxygenated fetuses. *Am J Obstet Gynecol* 130:199–203, 1978.

Robillon JF, Canivet B, Candito M, Sadoul JL, Julien D, Morand P, Chambon P, Freychet P: Type 1 diabetes mellitus and homocyst(e)ine. *Diabetes Metab* 20:494–496, 1994.

Robinson NJ, Glazier JD, Greenwood SL, Baker PN, Aplin JD: Tissue transglutaminase expression and activity in placenta. *Placenta* 27:148–157, 2006.

Rochon M, Rand L, Toth L, Gaddipatti S: Glyburide for the management of gestational diabetes: risk factors predictive of failure and associated pregnancy outcomes. *Am J Obstet Gynecol* 195:1090–1094, 2006.

Roden M: Mechanisms of disease: hepatic steatosis in type 2 diabetes—pathogenesis and clinical relevance. *Nat Clin Pract Endocrinol Metab* 2:335–348, 2006.

Rodin G, Olmsted MP, Rydall AC, Maharaj SI, Colton PA, Jones JM, Biancucci LA, Daneman D: Eating disorders in young women with type 1 diabetes mellitus. *J Psychosom Res* 53:943–949, 2002.

Rodrigues S, Ferris AM, Perez-Escamilla R, Backstrand JR: Obesity among offspring of women with type 1 diabetes. *Clin Invest Med* 21:258–266, 1998.

Roes EM, Hendricks JC, Raijmakers MT, Steegers-Theunissen RP, Groenen P, Peters WH, Steegers EA: A longitudinal study of antioxidant status during uncomplicated and hypertensive pregnancies. *Acta Obstet Gynecol Scand* 85:148–155, 2006.

Roessner S: Physical activity and prevention and treatment of weight gain associated with pregnancy: current evidence and research issues. *Med Sci Sports Exerc* 31 (Suppl):S560–S563, 1999.

Rohlfing CL, Wiedmeyer HM, Little RR, England JD, Tennill A, Goldstein DE: Defining the relationship between plasma glucose and HbA1c: analysis of glucose profiles and HbA1c in the Diabetes Control and Complications Trial. *Diabetes Care* 25:275–278, 2002.

Roland JM, Murphy HR, Ball V, Northcote-Wright J, Temple RC: The pregnancies of women with type 2 diabetes: poor outcomes but opportunities for improvement. *Diabet Med* 22:1774–1777, 2005.

Romon M, Nuttens M-C, Vambergue A, Verier-Mine O, Biausque S, Lemaire C, Fontaine P, Salomez J-L, Beuscart R: Higher carbohydrate intake is associated with decreased incidence of newborn macrosomia in women with gestational diabetes. *J Am Diet Assoc* 101:897–902, 2001.

Ronnenberg AG, Goldman MB, Chen D, Aitken IW, Willett WC, Selhub J, Xu X: Preconception homocysteine and B vitamin status and birth outcomes in Chinese women. *Am J Clin Nutr* 76:1385–1391, 2002.

Rooney BL, Schauberger CW: Excess pregnancy weight gain and long-term obesity: one decade later. *Obstet Gynecol* 100:245–252, 2002.

Rooney BL, Schauberger CW, Mathiason MA: Impact of perinatal weight change on long-term obesity and obesity-related illnesses. *Obstet Gynecol* 106:1349–1356, 2005.

Roseboom TJ, van der Meulen JK, van Montfrans GA, Ravelli AC, Osmond C, Barker DJ, Bleker OP: Maternal nutrition during gestation and blood pressure in later life. *J Hypertens* 19:29–34, 2001.

Rosenn B, Miodovnik M, Kranias G, Khoury J, Combs CA, Mimouni F, Siddiqi TA, Lipman MJ: Progression of diabetic retinopathy in pregnancy: association with hypertension in pregnancy. *Am J Obstet Gynecol* 166:1214–1218, 1992.

Rosenn B, Miodovnik M, Combs CA, Khoury J, Siddiqi TA: Poor glycemic control and antepartum obstetric complications in women with insulin-dependent diabetes. *Int J Obstet Gynecol* 43:21–28, 1993.

Rosenn BM, Miodovnik M, Hochberg G, Khoury JC, Siddiqui TA: Hypoglycemia: the price of intensive insulin therapy for pregnant women with insulin-dependent diabetes. *Obstet Gynecol* 85:417–422, 1995a.

Rosenn B, Siddiqi TA, Miodovnik M: Normalization of blood glucose in insulin-dependent pregnancies and the risks of hypoglycemia: a therapeutic dilemma. *Obstet Gynecol Surv* 50:56–61, 1995b.

Rosenn BM Miodovnik M: Glycemic control in the diabetic pregnancy: is tighter always better? *J Matern-Fetal Med* 9:29–34, 2000.

Rosenstock J, Park G, Zimmerman J; for the U.S. Insulin Glargine (HOE 901) Type 1 Diabetes Investigator Group: Basal insulin glargine (HOE 901) versus NPH insulin in patients with type 1 diabetes on multiple daily insulin regimens. *Diabetes Care* 23:1137–1142, 2000.

Rosenstock J, Dailey G, Massi-Benedetti M, Fritsche A, Lin Z, Salzman A: Reduced hypoglycemia risk with insulin glargine. A meta-analysis comparing insulin glargine with human NPH insulin in type 2 diabetes. *Diabetes Care* 28:950–955, 2005.

Ross LE, McLean LM: Anxiety disorders during pregnancy and the postpartum period: a systematic review. *J Clin Psychiatry* 67:1285–1298, 2006.

Rostom A, Dube C, Cranney A, Saloojee N, Sy R, Garritty C, Sampson M, Zhang L, Yazdi F, mamaladze V, Pan I, Macneil J, Mack D, Patel D, Moher D: The diagnostic accuracy of serologic tests for celiac disease: a systematic review. *Gastroenterology* 128:S38–S46, 2005.

Roth S, Abernathy MP, Lee WH, Pratt L, Denne S, Golichowski A, Pescovitz OH: Insulin-like growth factors I and II peptide and messenger RNA levels in macrosomic infants of diabetic pregnancies. *J Soc Gynecol Investig* 3:78–84, 1996.

Rothenberg SP, da Costa MP, Sequeira JM, Cracco J, Roberts JL, Weedon J, Quadros EV: Autoantibodies against folate receptors in women with a pregnancy complicated by a neural-tube defect. *N Engl J Med* 350:134–142, 2004.

Rothman KJ, Moore LL, Ringer MR, Nguyen UDT, Mannino S, Milunsky A: Teratogenicity of high vitamin A intake. *N Engl J Med* 333:1369–1373, 1995.

Roversi GD, Gargiulo M, Nicoloni U, Pedretti E, Marini A, Barbarini V, Peneff P: A new approach in the treatment of diabetic pregnant women. *Am J Obstet Gynecol* 135:567–576, 1979.

Rowan JA; the MIG Investigators: A trial in progress: gestational diabetes. Treatment with metformin compared with insulin (the Metformin in Gestational Diabetes Trial). *Diabetes Care* 30 (Suppl 2):S214–S219, 2007.

Ruberte J, Ayuso E, Navarro M, Carretero A, Nacher V, Haurigot V, George M, Llombart C, Casellas A, Costa C, Bosch A, Bosch F: Increased ocular levels of IGF-1 in transgenic mice lead to diabetes-like eye disease. *J Clin Invest* 113:1149–1157, 2004.

Rubin RR, Peyrot M: Psychological issues and treatments for people with diabetes. *J Clin Psychol* 57:457–478, 2001.

Ruchkin V, Martin A: SSRIs and the developing brain. Comment. *Lancet* 365: 451–453, 2005.

Rudolf MCH, Coustan DR, Sherwin RS, Bates SE, Felig P, Genel M, Tamborlane WV: Efficacy of the insulin pump in the home treatment of pregnant diabetics. *Diabetes* 30:891–895, 1981.

Ruiz C, Alegria A, Barbera R, Farre R, Lagarda J: Selenium, zinc and copper in plasma of patients with type 1 diabetes mellitus in different metabolic control states. *J Trace Elem Med Biol* 12:91–95, 1998.

Rumbold AR, Crowther CA, Haslam RR, Dekker GA, Robinson JS; the ACTS Study Group: Vitamins C and E and the risks of preeclampsia and perinatal complications. *N Engl J Med* 354:1796–1806, 2006.

Rusia U, Flowers C, Madan N, Agarwal N, Sood SK, Sikka M: Serum transferrin receptors in detection of iron deficiency in pregnancy. *Ann Hematol* 78:358–363, 1999.

Ryan EA, O'Sullivan MJ, Skyler JS: Insulin action during pregnancy. Studies with the euglycemic clamp technique. *Diabetes* 34:380–389, 1985.

Rydall AC, Rodin GM, Olmsted MP, Devenyi RG, Daneman D: Disordered eating behavior and microvascular complications in young women with insulin-dependent diabetes mellitus. *N Engl J Med* 336:1849–1854, 1997.

Saadah OI, Zacharin M, O'Callaghan A, Oliver MR, Catto-Smith AG: Effect of gluten-free diet and adherence on growth and diabetic control in diabetics with celiac disease. *Arch Dis Child* 89:871–879, 2004.

Saadeh S, Younossi ZM, Remer EM, Gramlich T, Ong JP, Hurley M, Mullen KD, Cooper JN, Sheridan MJ: The utility of radiological imaging in nonalcoholic fatty liver disease. *Gastroenterology* 123:745–750, 2002.

Sabate J: The contribution of vegetarian diets to health and disease: a paradigm shift? *Am J Clin Nutr* 78 (Suppl): 502S–507S, 2003.

Sachan A, Gupta R, Das V, Agarwal A, Awasthi PK, Bhatia V: High prevalence of vitamin D deficiency among pregnant women and their newborns in northern India. *Am J Clin Nutr* 81:1060–1064, 2005.

Sacks DA, Chen W, Greenspoon JS, Wolde-Tsadik G: Should the same glucose values be targeted for type 1 as for type 2 diabetic patients in pregnancy? *Am J Obstet Gynecol* 177:1113–1119, 1997.

Sacks DA, Liu AI, Wolde-Tsadik G, Amini SB, Huston-Presley L, Catalano PM: What proportion of birth weight is attributable to maternal glucose among infants of diabetic women? *Am J Obstet Gynecol* 194:501–507, 2006a.

Sacks DA, Feig DS, Liu IL, Wolde-Tsadik G: Managing type 1 diabetes in pregnancy: how near normal is necessary? *J Perinatol* 26:458–462, 2006b.

Sacks DB, Bruns DE, Goldstein DE, Maclaren NK, McDonald JM, Parrott M: Guidelines and recommendations for laboratory analysis in the diagnosis and management of diabetes mellitus. *Clin Chem* 48:436–472, 2002a.

Sacks DB, Bruns DE, Goldstein DE, Maclaren NK, McDonald JM, Parrott M: Guidelines and recommendations for laboratory analysis in the diagnosis and management of diabetes mellitus. Position statement (reprint). *Diabetes Care* 25:750–786, 2002b.

Sacks FM, Svetkey LP, Vollmer WM, Appel LJ, Bray GA, Harsha D, Obarzanek E, Conlin PR, Miller ER, Simons-Morton DG, Karanja N, Lin P-H; for the DASH-Sodium Collaborative Research Group: Effects on blood pressure of reduced dietary sodium and the dietary approach to stop hypertension (DASH) diet. *N Engl J Med* 344:3–10, 2001.

Sacks FM, Katan M: Randomized clinical trials on the effects of dietary fat and carbohydrate on plasma lipoproteins and cardiovascular disease. *Am J Med* 113(9B):13S–24S, 2002c.

Sagiv SK, Tolbert PE, Altshul LM, Korrick SA: Organochlorine exposures during pregnancy and infant size at birth. *Epidemiology* 18:120–129, 2007.

Sakai K, Clemmons DR: Glucosamine induces resistance to insulin-like growth factor I (IGF-I) and insulin in Hep G2 cell cultures: biological significance of IGF-I/insulin hybrid receptors. *Endocrinology* 144:2388–2395, 2003.

Sakamoto A, Nishimura Y, Ono H, Sakura N: Betaine and homocysteine concentrations in foods. *Pediatr Int* 44:409–413, 2002.

Sakamoto M, Kubota M, Liu XJ, Murata K, Nakai K, Satoh H: Maternal and fetal mercury and n-3 polyunsaturated fatty acids as a risk and benefit of fish consumption to fetus. *Environ Sci Technol* 38:3860–3863, 2004.

Sakamoto M, Kaneoka T, Murata K, Nakai K, Satoh H, Akagi H: Correlations between mercury concentrations in umbilical cord tissue and other biomarkers of fetal exposure to methylmercury in the Japanese population. *Environ Res* 103:106–111, 2007.

Salazar-Martinez E, Willett WC, Ascherio A, Manson JE, Leitzman MF, Stampfer MJ, Hu FB: Coffee consumption and risk of type 2 diabetes mellitus. *Ann Intern Med* 140:1–8, 2004.

Salmeron J, Manson JE, Stampfer MJ, Colditz GA, Wing AL, Willett WC: Dietary fiber, glycemic load and risk of non-insulin-dependent diabetes mellitus in women. *JAMA* 277:472–477, 1997.

Salvati VM, Mazzarella G, Giafrani C, Levings MK, Stefanile R, De Giulio B, Iaquinto G, Giardullo N, Auricchio S, Roncarolo MG, Troncone R: Recombinant human interleukin 10 suppresses gliadin dependent T cell activation in ex vivo cultured celiac intestinal mucosa. *Gut* 54:46–53, 2005.

Salvesen DR, Brudenell JM, Nicolaides KH: Fetal polycythemia and thrombocytopenia in pregnancies complicated by maternal diabetes mellitus. *Am J Obstet Gynecol* 166:1287–1292, 1992.

Salvesen DR, Brudenell JM, Nicolaides KH: Fetal plasma erythropoietin in pregnancies complicated by maternal diabetes. *Am J Obstet Gynecol* 168:88–94, 1993b.

Salvesen DR, Brudenell JM, Proudler AJ, Crook D, Nicolaides KH: Fetal pancreatic β-cell function in pregnancies complicated by maternal diabetes mellitus: relationship to fetal acidemia and macrosomia. *Am J Obstet Gynecol* 168: 1363–1369, 1993a.

Salvesen DR, Brudenell JM, Snijders R, Nicolaides KH: Effect of delivery on fetal erythropoietin and blood gases in pregnancies complicated by maternal diabetes. *Fetal Diagn Ther* 10:141–146, 1995.

Samsom M, Vermeijden JR, Smout AJPM, van Doorn E, Roelofs J, van Dam PS, Martens EP, Eelkman-Rooda SJ, van Berge-Henegouwen GP: Prevalence of delayed gastric emptying in diabetic patients and relationship to dyspeptic symptoms. A prospective study in unselected diabetic patients. *Diabetes Care* 26:3116–3122, 2003.

Sanchez-Albisua I, Wolf J, Neu A, Geiger H, Wascher I, Stern M: Celiac disease in children with type 1 diabetes mellitus: the effect of the gluten-free diet. *Diabet Med* 22:1079–1082, 2005.

Sanders TAB: Essential fatty acid requirements of vegetarians in pregnancy, lactation, and infancy. *Am J Clin Nutr* 70 (Suppl): 555S–559S, 1999.

Sanders DS, Carter MJ, Hurlstone DP, Pearce A, Ward AM, McAlindon ME, Lobo AJ: Association of adult celiac disease with irritable bowel syndrome: a case-control study in patients fulfilling ROME II criteria referred to secondary care. *Lancet* 358:1504–1508, 2001.

Sandoval DA, Aftab Guy DL, Richardson MA, Ertl AC, Davis SN: Effects of low and moderate antecedent exercise on counterregulatory responses to subsequent hypoglycemia in type 1 diabetes. *Diabetes* 53:1798–1806, 2004.

Sandoval DA, Guy DL, Richardson MA, Ertl AC, Davis SN: Acute, same-day effects of antecedent exercise on counterregulatory responses to subsequent hypoglycemia in type 1 diabetes mellitus. *Am J Physiol Endocrinol Metab* 290: E1331–E1338, 2006.

Sandstead HH, Smith J Jr: Deliberations and evaluations of approaches, endpoints, and paradigms for determining zinc dietary recommendations. *J Nutr* 126 (Suppl 9):2410S 2418S, 1996.

Sandstead HH, Egger NG: Is zinc nutriture a problem in persons with diabetes mellitus? Editorial. *Am J Clin Nutr* 66:681–682, 1997.

Santos VN, Lanzoni VP, Szejnfeld J, Shigueoka D, Parise ER: A randomized double-blind study of the short-time treatment of obese patients with nonalcoholic fatty liver disease with ursodeoxycholic acid. *Braz J Med Biol Res* 36:723–729, 2003.

Sanz EJ, De-las-Cuevas C, Kiuru A, Bate A, Edwards R: Selective serotonin reuptake inhibitors in pregnant women and neonatal withdrawal syndrome: a database analysis. *Lancet* 365:482–487, 2005.

Sategna-Guidetti C, Grosso S, Pulitano R, Benaduce E, Dani F, Carta Q: Celiac disease and insulin-dependent diabetes mellitus. Screening in an adult population. *Dig Dis Sci* 39:1633–1637, 1994.

Sategna-Guidetti C, Volta U, Ciacci C, Usai P, Carlino A, De Franceschi L, Camera A, Pelli A, Brossa C: Prevalence of thyroid disorders in untreated adult celiac disease patients and effect of gluten withdrawal: an Italian multicenter study. *Am J Gastroenterol* 96:751–757, 2001.

Sato RL, Li GG, Shaha S: Antepartum seafood consumption and mercury levels in newborn cord blood. *Am J Obstet Gynecol* 194:1683–1688, 2006.

Saukkonen T, Savilahti E, Reijonen H, Ilonen J, Tuomilehto-Wolf E, Akerblom HK; the Childhood Diabetes in Finland Study Group: Celiac disease: frequent occurrence after clinical onset of insulin dependent diabetes. *Diabet Med* 13:464–470, 1996.

Saverymutta SH, Joseph AEA, Maxwell JD: Ultrasound scanning in the detection of hepatic fibrosis and steatosis. *Br Med J* 292:13–15, 1986.

Scanlon KS, Yip R, Schieve LA, Cogswell ME: High and low hemoglobin levels during pregnancy: differential risks for preterm birth and small for gestational age. *Obstet Gynecol* 96:741–748, 2000.

Schaefer UM, Songster G, Xiang A, Berkowitz K, Buchanan TA, Kjos SL: Congenital malformations in offspring of women with hyperglycemia first detected during pregnancy. *Am J Obstet Gynecol* 177:1165–1171, 1997.

Schaefer-Graf UM, Buchanan TA, Xiang A, Songster G, Montoro M, Kjos SL: Patterns of congenital anomalies and relationship to initial maternal fasting glucose levels in pregnancies complicated by type 2 and gestational diabetes. *Am J Obst Gynecol* 182:313–320, 2000.

Schafer SA, Mussig K, Stefan N, haring HU, Fritsche A, Balletshofer BM: Plasma homocysteine concentrations in young individuals at increased risk of type 2 diabetes are associated with subtle differences in glomerular filtration rate but not insulin resistance. *Exp Clin Endocrinol Diabetes* 114:306–309, 2006.

Schaiff WT, Carlson MG, Smith SD, Levy R, Nelson DM, Sadovsky Y: Peroxisome proliferator-activated receptor-γ modulates differentiation of human trophoblast in a ligand-specific manner. *J Clin Endocrinol Metab* 85:3874–3881, 2000.

Schaiff WT, Bildirici I, Cheong M, Chern PL, Nelson DM, Sadovsky Y: Peroxisome proliferator-activated receptor-γ and retinoid X receptor signaling regulate fatty acid uptake by primary human placental trophoblasts. *J Clin Endocrinol Metab* 90:4267–4275, 2005.

Schatz H: Inhaled insulin and the dream of a needle-free insulin application. *Exp Clin Endocrinol Diabetes* 112:285–287, 2004.

Scheffler RM, Feuchtbaum LB, Phibbs CS: Prevention: the cost effectiveness of the California diabetes and pregnancy program. *Am J Public Health* 82:168–175, 1992.

Schenk S, Davidson CJ, Zderic TW, Byerley LO, Coyle EF: Different glycemic indexes of breakfast cereals are not due to glucose entry into blood but to glucose removal by tissue. *Am J Clin Nutr* 78:742–748, 2003.

Scherbaum WA, Lankisch MR, Pawlowski B, Somville T: Insulin Lispro in pregnancy—retrospective analysis of 33 cases and matched controls. *Exp Clin Endocrinol Diabetes* 110:6–9, 2002.

Schiff E, Friedman SA, Stampfer M, Kao L, Barrett PH, Sibai BM: Dietary consumption and plasma concentrations of vitamin E in pregnancies complicated by preeclampsia. *Am J Obstet Gynecol* 175:1024–1028, 1996.

Schiffman SS, Buckley C, Sampson H, Massey E, Baraniuk J, Follett J, Warwick Z: Aspartame and susceptibility to headache. *N Engl J Med* 317:1185–1187, 1987.

Schild RL, Schaiff WT, Carlson MG, Cronbach EJ, Nelson DM, Sadovsky Y: The activity of PPAR gamma in primary human trophoblasts is enhanced by oxidized lipids. *J Clin Endocrinol Metab* 87:1105–1110, 2002.

Schild RL, Sonnenberg-Hirche CM, Schaiff WT, Bildiricic I, Nelson DM, Sadovsky Y: The kinase p38 regulates peroxisome proliferators activated receptor. *Placenta* 27:191–199, 2006.

Schmitz O, Klebe J, Moller J, Arnfred J, Hermansen K, Orskov H, Beck-Nielsen H: In vivo insulin action in type 1 (insulin-dependent) diabetic pregnant women as assessed by the insulin clamp technique. *J Clin Endocrinol Metab* 61:877–881, 1985.

Schmon B, Hartmann M, Jones CJ, Desoye G: Insulin and glucose do not affect the glycogen content in isolated and cultured trophoblast cells of human term placenta. *J Clin Endocrinol Metab* 73:888–893, 1991.

Schneider JM, Curet LB, Olson RW, Shay G: Ambulatory care of the pregnant diabetic. *Obstet Gynecol* 56:144–149, 1980.

Schnyder G, Roffi M, Pin R, Flammer Y, Lange H, Eberli FR, Meier B, Turi ZG, Hess OM: Decreased rate of coronary restenosis after lowering of plasma homocysteine levels. *N Engl J Med* 345:1539–1600, 2001.

Schnyder G, Roffi M, Flammer Y, Pin R, Hess OM: Effect of homocysteine-lowering therapy with folic acid, vitamin B12, and vitamin B6 on clinical outcome after percutaneous coronary intervention: the Swiss Heart study: a randomized controlled trial. *JAMA* 288:973–979, 2002.

Schober SE, Sinks TH, Jones RL, Bolger PM, McDowell M, Osterloh J, Garrett ES, Canady RA, Dillon CF, Sun Y, Joseph CB, Mahaffey KR: Blood mercury levels in US children and women of childbearing age, 1999–2000. *JAMA* 289: 1667–1674, 2003.

Scholl TO, Hediger ML, Fischer RL, Shearer JW: Anemia vs iron deficiency: increased risk of preterm delivery in a prospective study. *Am J Clin Nutr* 55: 985–988, 1992.

Scholl TO, Hediger ML, Schall JI, Fischer RL, Khoo CS: Low zinc intake during pregnancy: its association with preterm and very preterm delivery. *Am J Epidemiol* 137:1115–1124, 1993.

Scholl T, Hediger M: Anemia and iron-deficiency anemia: compilation of data on pregnancy outcome. *Am J Clin Nutr* 59 (Suppl):492S–501S, 1994.

Scholl TO, Hediger ML, Schall JI, Khoo C-S, Fischer RL: Dietary and serum folate: their influence on the outcome of pregnancy. *Am J Clin Nutr* 63:520–525, 1996.

Scholl TO, Hediger ML, Bendich A, Schall JI, Smith WK, Krueger PM: Use of multivitamin/mineral prenatal supplements: influence on the outcome of pregnancy. *Am J Epidemiol* 146:134–141, 1997.

Scholl TO: High third-trimester ferritin concentration: association with very preterm delivery, infection, and maternal nutritional status. *Obstet Gynecol* 92:161–166, 1998.

Scholl TO, Sowers M, Chen X, Lenders C: Maternal glucose concentration influences fetal growth, gestation length, and pregnancy complications. *Am J Epidemiol* 154:514–520, 2001.

Scholl TO, Chen X, Khoo CS, Lenders C: The glycemic index during pregnancy: influence on infant birth weight, fetal growth, and biomarkers of carbohydrate metabolism. *Am J Epidemiol* 159:467–474, 2004.

Scholl TO: Iron status during pregnancy: setting the stage for mother and infant. *Am J Clin Nutr* 81 (Suppl):1218S–1222S, 2005.

Scholl TO, Chen X, Sims M, Stein TP: Vitamin E: maternal concentrations are associated with fetal growth. *Am J Clin Nutr* 84:1442–1448, 2006.

Schrezenmeir J, Tato F, Tato S, Kustner E, Krause U, Hommel G, Asp NG, Kasper H, Beyer J: Comparison of glycemic response and insulin requirements after mixed meals of equal carbohydrate content in healthy, type-1 and type-2 diabetic man. *Klin Wochenschr* 69:91, 1989.

Schuppan D: Current concepts of celiac disease pathogenesis. *Gastroenterology* 119:234–242, 2000.

Schuppan D, Hahn EG: Celiac disease and its link to type 1 diabetes mellitus. *J Pediatr Endocrinol Metab* 14 (Suppl 1):597–605, 2001.

Schwartz R, Gruppuso PA, Petzold K, Brambilla D, Hiilesmaa V, Teramo KA: Hyperinsulinemia and macrosomia in the fetus of the diabetic mother. *Diabetes Care* 17:640–648, 1994.

Schwarz JM, Neese RA, Turner S, Dare D, Hellertein MK: Short-term alterations in carbohydrate energy intake in humans. Striking effects on hepatic glucose production, de novo lipogenesis, lipolysis, and whole-body fuel selection. *J Clin Invest* 96:2735–2743, 1995.

Schwarz JM, Linfoot P, Dare D, Aghajanian K: Hepatic de novo lipogenesis in normoinsulinemic and hyperinsulinemic subjects consuming high-fat, low-carbohydrate and low-fat, high-carbohydrate isoenergetic diets. *Am J Clin Nutr* 77:43–50, 2003.

Sciullo E, Cardellini G, Baroni MG, Torresi P, Buongiorno A, Pozzilli P, Falluca F: Glucose transporter (Glut1, Glut3) mRNA in human placenta of diabetic and non-diabetic pregnancies. *Early Pregnancy* 3:172–182, 1997.

Scragg R, Holdaway I, Singh V, Metcalf P, baker J, Dryson E: Serum 25-hydroxyvitamin D3 levels are decreased in impaired glucose tolerance and diabetes mellitus. *Diabetes Res Clin Pract* 27:181–188, 1995.

See J, Murray JA: Gluten-free diet: the medical and nutrition management of celiac disease. *Nutr Clin Pract* 21:1–15, 2006.

Seeds JW, Peng TCC: Does augmented growth impose an increased risk of fetal death? *Am J Obstet Gynecol* 183:316–323, 2000.

Seely BL, Reichart DR, Takata Y, Yip C, Olefsky JM: A functional assessment of insulin/insulin-like growth factor-I hybrid receptors. *Endocrinology* 136:1635–1641, 1995.

Seissler J, Schott M, Boms S, Wohlrab U, Ostendorf B, Morgenthaler NG, Scherbaum WA: Autoantibodies to human tissue transglutaminase identify silent celiac disease in type 1 diabetes. *Diabetologia* 42:1440–1441, 1999.

Selhub J, Jacques PF, Rosenberg IH, Rogers G, Bowman BA, Gunter EW, Wright JD, Johnson CL: Serum total homocysteine concentrations in the third National Health and Nutrition Examination Survey (1991–1994): population reference ranges and contribution of vitamin status to high serum concentrations. *Ann Intern Med* 131:331–339, 1999.

Sells CJ, Robinson NM, Brown Z, Knopp RH: Long-term developmental follow-up of infants of diabetic mothers. *J Pediatr* 125:S9–S17, 1994.

Sermer M, Naylor CD, Gare DJ, Kenshole AB, Ritchie JWK, Farine D, Cohen HR, McArthur K, Holzapfel S, Biringer A, Chen E; for the Toronto Tri-Hospital Gestational Diabetes Investigators: Impact of increasing carbohydrate intolerance on maternal-fetal outcomes in 3637 women without gestational diabetes. *Am J Obstet Gynecol* 173:146–156, 1995.

Setji TL, Holland ND, Sanders LL, Pereira KC, Diehl AM, Brown AJ: Nonalcoholic steatohepatitis and nonalcoholic fatty liver disease in young women with polycystic ovary syndrome. *J Clin Endocrinol Metab* 91:1741–1747, 2006.

Sevillano J, Lopez-Perez IC, Herrera E, Ramos MD, Bocos C: Englitazone administration to late pregnant rats produces delayed body growth and insulin resistance on their fetuses and neonates. *Biochem J* 389:913–918, 2005.

Shaban MC, Fosbury J, Kerr D, Cavan DA: The prevalence of depression and anxiety in adults with type 1 diabetes. *Diabet Med* 23:1381–1384, 2006.

Shalom-Barak T, Nicholas JM, Wang Y, Zhang X, Ong ES, Young TH, Gendler SJ, Evans RM, Barak Y: Peroxisome proliferators-activated receptor gamma controls Muc1 transcription in trophoblasts. *Mol Cell Biol* 24:10661–10669, 2004.

Shan L, Molberg O, Parrot I, Hausch F, Filiz F, Gray GM, Sollid LM, Khosla C: Structural basis for gluten intolerance in celiac sprue. *Science* 297:2275–2279, 2002.

Sharpe PB, Chan A, Haan EA, Hiller JE: Maternal diabetes and congenital anomalies in South Australia 1986–2000: a population-based cohort study. *Birth Defects Res A Clin Mol Teratol* 73:605–611, 2005.

Shaw GM, Wasserman CR, O'Malley CD: Periconceptional vitamin use and reduced risk for conotruncal and limb defects in California. *Teratology* 49:372, 1994.

Shaw GM, Lammer EJ, Wasserman CR, O'Malley CD, Tolarova MM: Risks of orofacial clefts in children born to women using multivitamins containing folic acid periconceptionally. *Lancet* 345:393–396, 1995.

Shaw GM, Liberman RF, Todoroff K, Wasserman CR: Low birth weight, preterm delivery, and periconceptional vitamin use. *J Pediatr* 130:1013–1014, 1997.

Shaw AM, Escobar AJ, Davis CA: Reassessing the food guide pyramid: decision-making framework. *J Nutr Educ* 32:111–118, 2000.

Shaw GM, Carmichael SL, Yang W, Selvin S, Schaffer DM: Periconceptional dietary intake of choline and betaine and neural tube defects in offspring. *Am J Epidemiol* 160:102–109, 2004.

Shaw GM, Carmichael SL, Laurent C, Rasmussen SA: Maternal nutrient intakes and risk of orofacial clefts. *Epidemiology* 17:285–291, 2006.

Shaywitz B, Sullivan C, Anderson G, Gillespie S, Sullivan B, Shaywitz S: Aspartame, behavior, and cognitive function in children with attention deficit disorders. *Pediatrics* 93:70–75, 1994.

Sheard NF, Clark NG, Brand-Miller JC, Franz MJ, Pi-Sunyer FX, Mayer-Davis E, Kulkarni K, Geil P: Dietary carbohydrate (amount and type) in the prevention and management of diabetes. A statement by the American Diabetes Association. *Diabetes Care* 27:2266–2271, 2004.

Shearman DJC, Delamore JW, Gardner DL: Gastric function and structure in iron deficiency anemia. *Lancet* 1:845–848, 1996.

Sheetz MJ, King GL: Molecular understanding of hyperglycemia's adverse effects for diabetic complications. *JAMA* 288:2579–2588, 2002.

Shefali AK, Kavitha M, Deepa R, Mohan V: Pregnancy outcomes in pre-gestational and gestational diabetic women in comparison to nondiabetic women—a prospective study in Asian Indian mothers (CURES–35). *J Assoc Physicians India* 54:613–618, 2006.

Sheffield JS, Butler-Koster EL, Casey BM, McIntire DD, Leveno KJ: Maternal diabetes mellitus and infant malformations. *Obstet Gynecol* 100:925–930, 2002.

Sheiner E, Levy A, Silverberg D, Menes TS, Levy I, Katz M, Mazor M: Pregnancy after bariatric surgery is not associated with adverse perinatal outcome. *Am J Obstet Gynecol* 190:1335–1340, 2004.

Sheiner E, Peleg R, Levy A: Pregnancy outcome of patients with known celiac disease. *Eur J Obstet Gynecol Reprod Biol* 129:41–45, 2006.

Shekhawat PS, Garland JS, Shivpuri C, Mick GJ, Sasidharan P, Pelz CJ, McCormick KL: Neonatal cord blood leptin: its relationship to birth weight, body mass index, maternal diabetes, and steroids. *Pediatr Res* 43:338–343, 1998.

Sher KS, Mayberry JF: Female fertility, obstetric and gynecological history in celiac disease. A case control study. *Digestion* 55:243–246, 1994.

Sherwood KL, Houghton LA, Tarasuk V, O'Connor DL: One-third of pregnant and lactating women may not be meeting their folate requirements from diet alone based on mandated levels of folic acid fortification. *J Nutr* 136:2820–2826, 2006.

Shiell AW, Campbell-Brown M, Haselden S, Robinson S, Godfrey KM, Barker DJ: High-meat, low-carbohydrate diet in pregnancy: relation to adult blood pressure in the offspring. *Hypertension* 38:1282–1288, 2001.

Shimabukuro M, Higa N, Chinen, Yamakawa K, Takasu N: Effects of a single administration of acarbose on postprandial glucose excursion and endothelial dysfunction in type 2 diabetic patients: a randomized crossover study. *J Clin Endocrinol Metab* 91:837–842, 2006.

Siega-Riz AM, Bodnar LM, Savitz DA: What are pregnant women eating? Nutrient and food group differences by race. *Am J Obstet Gynecol* 186:480–486, 2002.

Siega-Riz AM, Savitz DA, Zeisel SH, Thorp JM, Herring A: Second trimester folate status and preterm birth. *Am J Obstet Gynecol* 191:1851–1857, 2004.

Sies H, Stahl W, Sevanian A: Nutritional, dietary and postprandial oxidative stress. *J Nutr* 135:969–972, 2005.

Sigal RJ, Kenny GP, Wasserman DH, Casteneda-Sceppa C: Physical activity/exercise and type 2 diabetes. ADA technical review. *Diabetes Care* 27:2518–2539, 2004.

Sigal RJ, Kenny GP, Wasserman DH, Castaneda-Sceppa C, White RD: Physical activity/exercise and type 2 diabetes. A consensus statement from the American Diabetes Association. *Diabetes Care* 29:1433–1438, 2006.

Sigman-Grant M, Morita J: Defining and interpreting intakes of sugars. *Am J Clin Nutr* 78 (Suppl):815S–826S, 2003.

Signore C, Mills JL, Cox C, Trumble AC: Effects of folic acid fortification on twin gestation rates. *Obstet Gynecol* 105:757–762, 2005.

Silva Idos S, Higgins C, Swerdlow AJ, Laing SP, Slater SD, Pearson DWM, Morris AD: Birthweight and other pregnancy outcomes in a cohort of women with pre-gestational insulin-treated diabetes mellitus, Scotland, 1979–95. *Diabet Med* 22:440–447, 2005.

Silver J, Kilav R, Naveh-Many T: Mechanisms of secondary hyperthyroidism. *Am J Physiol* 283:F367–F376, 2002.

Silverman BL, Landsberg L, Metzger BE: Fetal hyperinsulinism in offspring of diabetic mothers: association with the subsequent development of childhood obesity. *Ann N Y Acad Sci* 699:36–45, 1993.

Silverman BL, Rizzo TA, Cho NH, Metzger BE: Long-term effects of the intrauterine environment. *Diabetes Care* 21 (Suppl 2):B142–B149, 1998.

Silverstein J, Klingensmith G, Copeland K, Plotnick L, Kaufman F, Laffel L, Deeb L, Grey M, Anderson B, Holzmeister LA, Clark N: Care of children and adolescents with type 1 diabetes. A statement of the American Diabetes Association. *Diabetes Care* 28:186–212, 2005.

Simmons D, Thompson CF, Conroy C, Scott DJ: Use of insulin pumps in pregnancies complicated by type 2 diabetes and gestational diabetes in a multiethnic community. *Diabetes Care* 24:2078–2082, 2002.

Simmons D, Walters BNJ, Rowan JA, McIntyre HD: Metformin therapy and diabetes in pregnancy. *Med J Aust* 180:462–464, 2004.

Simo R, Lecube A, Segura RM, Arumi JG, Hernandez C: Free insulin growth factor-I and vascular endothelial growth factor in the vitreous fluid of patients with proliferative diabetic retinopathy. *Am J Ophthmol* 134:376–382, 2002.

Simonen PP, Gylling HK, Miettinen TA: Diabetes contributes to cholesterol metabolism regardless of obesity. *Diabetes Care* 25:1511–1515, 2002.

Sindhu SS: Serum levels of iron, folic acid and vitamin B$_{12}$ in the maternal and cord blood in the three major ethnic groups in Malaysia. *Indian Pediatr* 11:775–780, 1974.

Sivan E, Feldman B, Dolitzki M, Nevo N, Dekel N, Karasik A: Glyburide crosses the placenta in vivo in pregnant rats. *Diabetologia* 38:753–756, 1995.

Sivan E, Chen X, Homko CJ, Reece EA, Boden G: Longitudinal study of carbohydrate metabolism in healthy obese pregnant women. *Diabetes Care* 20:1470–1475, 1997.

Sivan E, Weisz B, Homko CJ, Reece EA, Schiff E: One or two hours postprandial glucose measurements: are they the same? *Am J Obstet Gynecol* 185:604–607, 2001.

Sjoberg K, Eriksson KF, Bredberg A, Wassmuth R, Eriksson S: Screening for celiac disease in adult insulin-dependent diabetes mellitus. *J Intern Med* 243:133–140, 1998.

Sjogren A, Floren C-H, Nilsson A: Magnesium deficiency in IDDM related to level of glycosylated hemoglobin. *Diabetes* 35:459–463, 1986.

Skikne BS, Flowers CH, Cook JD: Serum transferrin receptor: a quantitative measure of tissue iron deficiency. *Blood* 75:1870–1876, 1990.

Skyler JS, Skyler DL, Seigler DE, O'Sullivan MJ: Algorithms for adjustment of insulin dosage by patients who monitor blood glucose. *Diabetes Care* 4:311–318, 1981.

Skyler JS, Weinstock RS, Raskin P, Yale JF, Barrett E, Gerich JE, Gerstein HC; the Inhaled Insulin Phase III Type I Diabetes Study Group: Use of inhaled insulin in a basal/bolus insulin regimen in type 1 diabetic subjects. *Diabetes Care* 28: 1630–1635, 2005.

Slag MF, Ahmad M, Gannon MC, Nuttall FQ: Meal stimulation of cortisol secretion: a protein-induced effect. *Metabolism* 30:1104–1108, 1981.

Slow S, Donaggio M, Cressey PJ, Lever M, George PM, Chambers ST: The betaine content of New Zealand foods and estimated intake in the New Zealand diet. *J Food Comp Anal* 18:473–485, 2005.

Small M, Cameron A, Lunan CB, MacCuish AC: Macrosomia in pregnancy complicated by insulin-dependent diabetes mellitus. *Diabetes Care* 10:594–599, 1987.

Smecuol E, Maurino E, Vasquez H, Pedreira S, Niveloni S, Mazure R, Boerr L, Bai JC: Gynecological and obstetric disorders in celiac disease: frequent clinical onset during pregnancy or the puerperium. *Eur J Gastroenterol Hepatol* 8:63–89, 1996.

Smit JW, Huisman MT, van Tellingen O, Wiltshire HR, Schinkel AH: Absence or pharmacological blocking of placental P-glycoprotein profoundly increases fetal drug exposure. *J Clin Invest* 104:1441–1447, 1999.

Smith RG, Heise CC, King JC, Costa FM, Kitzmiller, JL: Serum and urinary magnesium, calcium and copper levels in insulin-dependent diabetic women. *J Trace Elem Electrolytes Health Dis* 2:239–243, 1988.

Smith LEH, Shen W, Perruzi C, Soker S, Kinose F, Xu X, Robinson G, Driver S, Bischoff J, Zhang B, Schaeffer JM, Senger DR: Regulation of vascular endothelial growth factor-dependent retinal neovascularization by insulin-like growth factor-1 receptor. *Nature Med* 5:1390–1395, 1999.

Smith JD, Terpening CM, Schmidt SO, Gums JG: Relief of fibromyalgia symptoms following discontinuation of dietary excitotoxins. *Ann Pharmacother* 35: 702–706, 2001.

Smith MA, Takeuchi K, Brackett RE, McClure HM, Raybourne RB, Williams KM, Babu US, Ware GO, Broderson JR, Doyle MP: Nonhuman primate model for Listeria monocytogenes-induced stillbirths. *Infect Immun* 71:1574–1579, 2003.

Smith B, Wingard DL, Smith TC, Kritz-Silverstein D, Barrett-Connor E: Does coffee consumption reduce the risk of type 2 diabetes in individuals with impaired glucose? *Diabetes Care* 29:2385–2390, 2006.

Smith MC, Moran P, Ward MK, Davison JM: Assessment of glomerular filtration rate during pregnancy using the MDRD formula. *BJOG* 115:109–112, 2008.

Smithberg M, Runner MN: Teratogenic effects of hypoglycemic treatments in inbred strains of mice. *Am J Anat* 113:479–489, 1963.

Smoak IW: Teratogenic effects of tolbutamide on early-somite mouse embryos in vitro. *Diabetes Res Clin Pract* 17:161–167, 1992.

Smoak IW: Embryopathic effects of the oral hypoglycemic agent chlorpropamide in cultured mouse embryos. *Am J Obstet Gynecol* 169:409–414, 1993.

Snoek FJ, Pouwer F, Welch GW, Polonsky WH: Diabetes-related emotional distress in Dutch and U.S. diabetic patients: cross-cultural validity of the Problem Areas in Diabetes Scale. *Diabetes Care* 23:1305–1309, 2000.

Sobande AA, Eskander M, Archibong EI: Complications of pregnancy and fetal outcomes in pregnant diabetic patients managed in Saudia Arabia. *West Afr J Med* 24:13–17, 2005.

Soedamah-Muthu SS, Chaturvedi N, Teerlink T, Idzior-Walus B, Fuller JH, Stehouwer CD; Eurodiab Prospective Complications Study Group: Plasma homocysteine and microvascular and macrovascular complications in type 1 diabetes: a cross-sectional nested case-control study. *J Intern Med* 258:450–459, 2005.

Sohlstrom A, Forsum E: Changes in adipose tissue volume and distribution during reproduction in Swedish women as assessed by magnetic resonance imaging. *Am J Clin Nutr* 61:287–295, 1995.

Soinio M, Marniemi J, Laakso M, Lehto S, Ronnemaa T: Elevated plasma homocysteine level is an independent predictor of coronary heart disease events in patients with type 2 diabetes mellitus. *Ann Intern Med* 140:94–100, 2004.

Soler NG, Walsh CH, Malins JM: Congenital malformations in infants of diabetic mothers. *Q J Med* 178:303–313, 1976.

Solini A, Santini E, Nannipieri M, Ferrannini E: High glucose and homocysteine synergistically affect the metalloproteinases-tissue inhibitors of metalloproteinases pattern, but not TGFβ expression, in human fibroblasts. *Diabetologia* 49: 2499–2506, 2006.

Sollid LM, Markussen G, Ek J, Gjerde H, Vartdal F, Thorsby E: Evidence for a primary association of celiac disease to a particular HLA-DQ alpha/beta heterodimer. *J Exp Med* 169:345–350, 1989.

Sollid CP, Wisborg K, Hjort J, Secher NJ: Eating disorder that was diagnosed before pregnancy and pregnancy outcome. *Am J Obstet Gynecol* 190:206–210, 2004.

Solomon F, Sompolinsky D, Langer R, Caspi E: A case of listerosis in pregnancy with fetal survival. *Eur J Obstet Gynecol Reprod Biol* 8:103–104, 1978.

Soos MA, Field CE, Siddle K: Purified hybrid insulin/insulin-like growth factor receptors bind insulin-like growth factor-I, but not insulin, with high affinity. *Biochem J* 290:419–426, 1993.

Sorbi D, Boynton J, Lindor KD: The ratio of aspartate aminotransferase to alanine aminotransferase: potential value in differentiating nonalacoholic steatohepatitis from alcoholic liver disease. *Am J Gastroenterol* 94:1018–1022, 1999.

Sorensen TK, Malinow MR, Williams MA, King IB, Luthy DA: Elevated second-trimester serum homocyst(e)ine levels and subsequent risk of preeclampsia. *Gynecol Obstet Invest* 48:98–103, 1999.

Sorrentino P, Tarantino G, Conca P, Perrella A, Terracciano ML, Vecchione R, Gargiulo G, Gennarelli N, Lobello R: Silent non-alcoholic fatty liver disease— a clinical-histological study. *J Hepatol* 41:751–757, 2004.

Sosenko IR, Kitzmiller JL, Loo SW, Blix P, Rubinstein AH, Gabbay KH: The infant of the diabetic mother. Correlation of increased cord blood C-peptide levels with macrosomia and hypoglycemia. *N Engl J Med* 301:859–862, 1979.

Sosenko JM, Kitzmiller JL, Fluckiger R, Loo SWH, Younger DM, Gabbay KH: Umbilical cord glycosylated hemoglobin in infants of diabetic mothers: relationships to neonatal hypoglycemia, macrosomia and cord serum C-peptide. *Diabetes Care* 5:566–570, 1982.

Soultanakis HN, Artal R, Wiswell RA: Prolonged exercise in pregnancy: glucose homeostasis, ventilatory and cardiovascular responses. *Semin Perinatol* 20: 315–327, 1996.

Specker B: Vitamin D requirements during pregnancy. *Am Clin Nutr* 80 (Suppl):1740S–1747S, 2004.

Spendlove D: Working in partnership. Commentary to Josse J et al. *Pract Diab Int* 20:293, 2003.

Spiegelman BM: PPAR-gamma: adipogenic regulator and thiazolidinedione receptor. *Diabetes* 47:507–514, 1998.

Spinnato JA 2nd, Freire S, Pinto E, Silva JL, Cunha Rudge MV, Martins-Costa S, Koch MA, Goco N, Santos CB, Cecatti JG, Costa R, Ramos JG, Moss N, Sibai BM: Antioxidant therapy to prevent preeclampsia: a randomized controlled trial. *Obstet Gynecol* 110:1311–1318, 2007.

Spinnewijn WE, Wallenburg HC, Struijk PC, Lotgering FK: Peak ventilatory responses during cycling and swimming in pregnant and nonpregnant women. *J Appl Physiol* 81:738–742, 1996.

Splaver A, Lamas GA, Hennekens CH: Homocysteine and cardiovascular disease: biological mechanisms, observational epidemiology, and the need for randomized trials. *Am Heart J* 148:34–40, 2004.

Spranger J, Buhnen J, Jansen V, Krieg M, Meyer-Schwickerath R, Blum WF, Schatz H, Pfeiffer AF: Systemic levels contribute significantly to increased intraocular IGF-I, IGF-II and IGF-BP3 in proliferative diabetic retinopathy. *Horm Metab Res* 32:196–200, 2000.

Spurgeon A: Prenatal methylmercury exposure and developmental outcomes: review of the evidence and discussion of future directions. *Environ Health Perspect* 114:307–312, 2006.

Stahl M, Berger W: Higher incidence of severe hypoglycemia leading to hospital admission in type 2 diabetic patients treated with long-acting versus short-acting sulphonylureas. *Diabet Med* 16:586–590, 1999.

Stanley K, Magides A, Arnot M, Bruce C, Reilly C, McFee A, Fraser R: Delayed gastric emptying as a factor in delayed postprandial glycemic response in pregnancy. *Brit J Obstet Gynecol* 102:288–291, 1995.

Stanner SA, Hughes J, Kelly CN, Butriss J: A review of the epidemiological evidence for the 'antioxidant hypothesis.' *Public Health Nutr* 7:407–422, 2004.

Stark KD, Pawlosky RJ, Beblo S, Murthy M, Flanagan VP, Janisse J, Buda-Abela M, Rockett H, Whitty JE, Sokol RJ, Hannigan JH, Salem N Jr: Status of plasma folate after folic acid fortification of the food supply in pregnant African American women and the influences of diet, smoking, and alcohol consumption. *Am J Clin Nutr* 81:669–677, 2005.

Steed L, Cooke D, Newman S: A systematic review of psychosocial outcomes following education, self-management and psychological interventions in diabetes mellitus. *Patient Educ Couns* 51:5–15, 2003.

Steel JM, Young RJ, Lloyd GG, Clarke BF: Clinically apparent eating disorders in young diabetic women: associations with painful neuropathy and other complications. *Br Med J* 294:859–862, 1987.

Steel JM, Johnstone FD, Hume R, Mao J-H: Insulin requirements during pregnancy in women with type 1 diabetes. *Obstet Gynecol* 83:253–258, 1994.

Steer P, Alam MA, Wadsworth J, Welch A: Relation between maternal hemoglobin concentration and birth weight in different ethnic groups. *BMJ* 310:489–491, 1995.

Steglink L, Pitkin R, Reynolds W, Brummel M, Filer LJ: Placental transfer of aspartate and its metabolites in the primate. *Metabolism* 28:669–676, 1979.

Stehouwer CDA, Gall M-A, Hougaard P, Jakobs C, Parving H-H: Plasma homocysteine concentration predicts mortality in non-insulin-dependent diabetic patients with and without albuminuria. *Kidney Int* 55:308–314, 1999.

Stein A, Ravelli A, Lumey L: Famine, third trimester pregnancy weight gain, and intrauterine growth: the Dutch famine birth cohort study. *Hum Biol* 67: 135–150, 1995.

Steinman D: *Diet for a Poisoned Planet. How to Choose Safe Foods for You and Your Family.* New York: Ballantine Books; 1990:173–174, 190–192, 283–284.

Stender S, Dyerberg J, Astrup A: High levels of industrially produced trans fat in popular fast foods. *N Engl J Med* 354:1650–1652, 2006.

Stenman S, Melander A, Groop P-H, Groop L: What is the benefit of increasing the sulphonylurea dose? *Arch Intern Med* 118:169–172, 1993.

Stephansson O, Dickman PW, Johansson A, Cnattingius S: Maternal hemoglobin concentration during pregnancy and risk of stillbirth. *JAMA* 284:2611–2617, 2000.

Stepniak D, Koning F: Celiac disease-sandwiched between innate and adaptive immunity. *Hum Immunol* 67:460–468, 2006.

Stern AH, Gochfeld M, Weisel C, Burger J: Mercury and methylmercury exposure in the New Jersey pregnant population. *Arch Environ Health* 56:4–10, 2001.

Stern AH: A revised probabilistic estimate of the maternal methyl mercury intake dose corresponding to a measured cord blood mercury concentration. *Environ Health Perspect* 113:155–163, 2005.

Stettler C, Jenni S, Allemann S, Steiner R, Hoppeler H, Trepp R, Christ ER, Zwahlen M, Diem P: Exercise capacity in subjects with type 1 diabetes mellitus in eu- and hyperglycemia. *Diabetes Metab Res Rev* 22:300–306, 2006.

Steuerwald U, Weihe P, Jorgensen PJ, Bjerve K, Brock J, Heinzow B, Budtz-Jorgensen E, Grandjean P: Maternal seafood diet, methylmercury exposure, and neonatal neurologic function. *J Pediatr* 136:599–605, 2000.

Stevens DL. The use of complementary alternative therapies in diabetes. *Clin Fam Pract* 4:191–xxx, 2002.

Stewart P, Darvill T, Lonky E, Reihman J, Pagano J, Bush B: Assessment of prenatal exposure to PCBs from maternal consumption of Great Lakes fish: an analysis of PCB pattern and concentration. *Environ Res* 80:S87–S96, 1999.

Stocker DJ: Management of the bariatric surgery patient. *Endocrinol Metab Clin North Am* 32:437–457, 2003.

Stotland NE, Caughey AB, Breed EM, Escobar GJ: Risk factors and obstetric complications associated with macrosomia. *Int J Gynecol Obstet* 87:220–226, 2004a.

Stotland NE, Hopkins LM, Caughey AB: Gestational weight gain, macrosomia, and risk of cesarian birth in nondiabetic nulliparas. *Obstet Gynecol* 104:671–677, 2004b.

Stotland NE, Haas JS, Brawarsky P, Jackson RA, Fuentes-Afflick E, Escobar GJ: Body mass index, provider advice, and target gestational weight gain. *Obstet Gynecol* 105:633–638, 2005.

Stotland NE, Cheng YW, Hopkins LM, Caughey AB: Gestational weight gain and adverse neonatal outcome among term infants. *Obstet Gynecol* 108:635–643, 2006.

Strachan MWJ, Frier BM: Optimal time of administration of insulin lispro. Importance of meal composition. *Diabetes Care* 21:26–31, 1998.

Strauss RS, Dietz WH: Low maternal weight gain in the second or third trimester increases the risk for intrauterine growth retardation. *J Nutr* 129:988–993, 1999.

Sturrock NDC, Fay TN, Pound N, Kirk BA, Danks LE: Analysis of 44,279 blood glucose estimations in relation to outcomes in 80 pregnant diabetic women. *J Obstet Gynecol* 21:253–257, 2001.

Sturtevant FM: Use of aspartame during pregnancy. Review. *Int J Fertil* 30:85–87, 1985.

Sugiyama M, Tang AC, Wakaki Y, Koyama W: Glycemic index of single and mixed foods among common Japanese foods with white rice as a reference food. *Eur J Clin Nutr* 57:743–52, 2003.

Suhonen L, Hiilesmaa V, Teramo K: Glycemic control during early pregnancy and fetal malformations in women with type 2 diabetes mellitus. *Diabetologia* 43: 79–82, 2000.

Sulieman M, Asleh R, Cabantchik ZI, Breuer W, Aronson D, Sulieman A, Miller-Lotan R, Hammerman H, Levy AP: Serum chelatable redox-active iron is an independent predictor of mortality after myocardial infarction in individuals with diabetes. *Diabetes Care* 27:2730–2732, 2004.

Sullivan JL: Stored iron and vascular reactivity. Editorial. *Arterioscler Thromb Vasc Biol* 25:1532–1535, 2005.

Sumnik Z, Cinek O, Bratanic N, Lebl J, Rozsai B, Limbert C, Paskova M, Schober E: Thyroid autoimmunity in children with coexisting type 1 diabetes mellitus and celiac disease: a multicenter study. *J Pediatr Endocrinol Metab* 19:517–522, 2006.

Suri R, Altshuler L, Hellemann G, Burt VK, Aquino A, Mintz J: Effects of antenatal depressant treatment on gestational age at birth and risk of preterm birth. *Am J Psychiatry* 164:1206–1213, 2007.

Surwit RS, van Tilburg MAL, Zucker N, McCaskill CC, Parekh P, Feinglos MN, Edwards CL, Williams P, Lane JD: Stress management improves long-term glycemic control in type 2 diabetes. *Diabetes Care* 25:30–34, 2002.

Susa JB, Schwartz R: Effects of hyperinsulinemia in the primate fetus. *Diabetes* 34: S36–S41, 1985.

Sutherland HW, Bewsher PD, Cormack JE, Hughes CRT, Reid A, Russell G, Stowers JM: Effect of moderate dosage of chlorpropamide in pregnancy on fetal outcome. *Arch Dis Child* 49:283–291, 1974.

Suwaki N, Masuyama H, Masumoto A, Takamoto N, Hiramatsu Y: Expression and potential role of peroxisome proliferator-activated receptor gamma in the placenta of diabetic pregnancy. *Placenta* 28:315–323, 2007.

Swanson CA, Reamer DC, Veillon C, King JC, Levander OA: Quantitative and qualitative aspects of selenium utilization in pregnant and nonpregnant women: an application of stable isotope methodology. *Am J Clin Nutr* 38:169–180, 1983.

Sweiry JH, Yudilevich DL: Characterization of choline transport at maternal and fetal interfaces of the perfused guinea-pig placenta. *J Physiol* 366:251–266, 1985.

Sweiry JH, Page KR, Dacke CG, Abramovich DR, Yudelivich DL: Evidence of saturable uptake mechanisms at maternal and fetal sides of the perfused human placenta by rapid paired-tracer dilution: studies with calcium and choline. *J Dev Physiol* 8:435–445, 1986.

Swensen AR, Harnack LJ, Ross JA: Nutritional assessment of pregnant women enrolled in the Special Supplemental Program for Women, Infants, and Children (WIC). *J Am Diet Assoc* 101:903–908, 2001.

Szabo AJ, Szabo O: Placental free-fatty-acid transfer and fetal adipose tissue development: an explanation of fetal adiposity in infants of diabetic mothers. *Lancet* 2:498–499, 1974.

Szajewska H, Horvath A, Koletzko B: Effect of n-3 long-chain polyunsaturated fatty acid supplementation of women with low-risk pregnancies on pregnancy outcomes and growth measures at birth: a meta-analysis of randomized controlled trials. *Am J Clin Nutr* 83:1337–1344, 2006.

Talal AH, Murray JA, Goeken JA, Sivitz WI: Celiac disease in an adult population with insulin-dependent diabetes mellitus: use of endomysial antibody testing. *Am J Gastroenterol* 92:1280–1284, 1997.

Talbot F, Nouwen A: A review of the relationship between depression and diabetes in adults: is there a link? *Diabetes Care* 23:1556–1562, 2000.

Tamura S, Shimomura L: Contribution of adipose tissue and de novo lipogenesis to nonalcoholic fatty liver disease. *J Clin Invest* 115:1139–1142, 2005.

Tamura T, Picciano MF: Folate and human reproduction. *Am J Clin Nutr* 83: 993–1016, 2006.

Tan M, Sheng L, Qian Y, Ge Y, Wang Y, Zhang H, Jiang M, Zhang G: Changes of serum selenium in pregnant women with gestational diabetes mellitus. *Biol Trace Elem Res* 83:231–237, 2001.

Taniguchi A, Fukushima M, Nakal Y, Ohgushi M, Kuroe A, Ohya M, Seino Y: Soluble tumor necrosis factor receptor 1 is strongly and independently associated with serum homocysteine in nonobese Japanese type 2 diabetic patients. *Diabetes Care* 29:949–950, 2006.

Tapanainen P, Leinonen E, Ruokonen A, Knip M: Leptin concentrations are elevated in newborn infants of diabetic mothers. *Horm Res* 55:185–190, 2001.

Tapsell LC, Gillen LJ, Patch CS, Batterham M, Owen A, Bare M, Kennedy M: Including walnuts in a low-fat/modified-fat diet improves HDL cholesterol-to-total cholesterol ratios in patients with type 2 diabetes. *Diabetes Care* 27:2777–2783, 2004.

Targher G, Bertolini L, Padovani R, Zenari L, Scala L, Cigolini M, Arcaro G: Serum 25-hydroxyvitamin D3 concentrations and carotid artery intima-media thickness among type 2 diabetic patients. *Clin Endocrinol (Oxf)* 65:593–597, 2006.

Tata LJ, Card TR, Logan RF, Hubbard RB, Smith CJ, West J: Fertility and pregnancy-related events in women with celiac disease: a population-based cohort study. *Gastroenterology* 128:849–855, 2005.

Taylor LM Jr, Moneta GL, Sexton GJ, Schuff RA, Porter JM: Prospective blinded study of the relationship between plasma homocysteine and progression of symptomatic peripheral arterial disease. *J Vasc Surg* 29:8–19, 1999.

Taylor R, Lee C, Kyne-Grzebalski D, Marshall SM, Davison JM: Clinical outcomes of pregnancy in women with type 1 diabetes. *Obstet Gynecol* 99:537–541, 2002.

Temple R, Aldridge V, Greenwood R, Heyburn P, Sampson M, Stanley K: Association between outcome of pregnancy and glycemic control in early pregnancy in type 1 diabetes. *BMJ* 325:1275–1276, 2002.

Temple RC, Aldridge VJ, Murphy HR: Prepregnancy care and pregnancy outcomes in women with type 1 diabetes. *Diabetes Care* 29:1744–1749, 2006a.

Temple RC, Aldridge V, Stanley K, Murphy HR: Glycemic control throughout pregnancy and risk of preeclampsia in women with type 1 diabetes. *BJOG* 113:1329–1332, 2006b.

ter Braak EW, Woodworth JR, Bianchi R, Cerimele B, Erkelens DW, Thijssen JHH, Kurtz D: Injection site effects on the pharmacokinetics and glucodynamics of insulin lispro and regular insulin. *Diabetes Care* 19:1437–1440, 1996.

ter Braak EWMT, Appelman AMMF, van der Tweel I, Erkelens DW, van Haeften TW: The sulfonylurea glyburide induces impairment of glucagon and growth hormone responses during mild insulin-induced hypoglycemia. *Diabetes Care* 25:107–112, 2002.

Tetsuo M, Hamada T, Yoshimatsu K, Ishimatsu J, Matsunaga T: Serum levels of 1,5-anhydro-D-glucitol during the normal and diabetic pregnancy and puerperium. *Acta Obstet Gynecol Scand* 69:479–485, 1990.

Tevaarwerk GJM, Harding PGR, Milne KJ, Jaco NT, Rodger NW, Hurst C: Pregnancy in diabetic women: outcome with a program aimed at normoglycemia before meals. *Can Med Assoc J* 125:435–440, 1981.

Thatcher SS, Jackson EM: Pregnancy outcome in infertile patients with polycysytic ovary syndrome who were treated with metformin. *Fertil Steril* 85:1002–1009, 2006.

Thomas AM, Gutierrez YM: *American Dietetic Association Guide to Gestational Diabetes Mellitus.* Chicago: American Dietetic Association; 2006b.

Thomas AM: Pregnancy with preexisting diabetes. In: Mensing C, Cypress M, Halstensen C, McLaughlin S, Walker EA, eds. *The Art and Science of Diabetes Self-Management Education. A Desk Reference for Healthcare Professionals.* Chicago: American Association of Diabetic Educators; 2006a:233–257.

Thomas B, Ghembremeskel K, Lowy C, Crawford M, Offley-Shore B: Nutrient intake of women with and without gestational diabetes with a specific focus on fatty acids. *Nutrition* 22:230–236, 2006c.

Thomas DE, Elliott EJ, Naughton GA: Exercise for type 2 diabetes mellitus. *Cochrane Database Syst Rev* 2006;(3):CD002968.

Thomas J, Jones G, Scarinci I, Brantley P: A descriptive and comparative study of the prevalence of depressive and anxiety disorders in low-income adults with type 2 diabetes and other chronic illnesses. *Diabetes Care* 26:2311–2317, 2003b.

Thomas MC, MacIsaac RJ, Tsalamandris C, Power D, Jerums G: Unrecognized anemia in patients with diabetes. A cross-sectional survey. *Diabetes Care* 26:1164–1169, 2003a.

Thomas M, Weisman SM: Calcium supplementation during pregnancy and lactation: effects on the mother and the fetus. *Am J Obstet Gynecol* 194: 937–945, 2006d.

Thorsdottir I, Torfadottir JE, Birgisdottir BE, Geirsson RT: Weight gain in women of normal weight before pregnancy: complications in pregnancy or delivery and birth outcome. *Obstet Gynecol* 99:799–806, 2002.

Tierney MJ, Tamada JA, Potts RO, Eastman RC, Pitzer K, Ackerman NR, Fermi SJ: The GlucoWatch Biographer: a frequent, automatic and noninvasive glucose monitor. *Ann Med* 32:632–641, 2000.

Toescu V, Nuttal SL, Martin U, Nightengale P, Kendall MJ, Brydon P, Dunne F: Changes in plasma lipids and markers of oxidative stress in normal pregnancy and pregnancies complicated by diabetes. *Clin Sci (Lond)* 106: 93–98, 2004.

Toh BH, Sentry JW, Alderuccio F: The causative H+/K+ ATPase in the pathogenesis of autoimmune gastritis. *Immunol Today* 21:348–354, 2000.

Toh BH, Alderuccio F: Pernicious anaemia. *Autoimmunity* 37:357–361, 2004.

Tolman KG, Fonseca V, Tan MH, Dalpiaz A: Narrative review: hepatobiliary disease in type 2 diabetes mellitus. *Ann Intern Med* 141:946–956, 2004.

Tommasini A, Not T, Kiren V, Baldas V, Santon D, Trevisiol C, Berti I, Neri E, Gerarduzzi T, Bruno I, Lenhardt A, Zamuner E, Spano A, Crovella S, Martellossi S, Torre G, Sblattero D, Marzari R, Bradbury A, Tamburlini G, Ventura A: Mass screening for celiac disease using antihuman transglutaminase antibody assay. *Arch Dis Child* 89:512–515, 2004.

Toole JF, Malinow MR, Chambless LE, Spence JD, Pettigrew LC, Howard VJ, Sides EG, Wang CH, Stampfer M: Lowering homocysteine in patients with ischemic stroke to prevent recurrent stroke, myocardial infarction, and death. The Vitamin Intervention for Stroke Prevention (VISP) randomized controlled trial. *JAMA* 291:565–575, 2004.

Torjman MC, Jahn L, Joseph JI, Crothall K, Goldstein BJ: Accuracy of the HemoCue portable glucose analyzer in a large nonhemogeneous population. *Diabetes Technol Therapeut* 3:591–600, 2001.

Torlone E, Gennarini A, Ricci NB, Bolli GB: Successful use of insulin glargine during entire pregnancy until delivery in six type 1 diabetic women. *Eur J Obstet Gynecol Reprod Biol* 132:238–239, 2007.

Tosiello L: Hypomagnesemia and diabetes mellitus: a review of clinical implications. *Arch Intern Med* 156:1143–1148, 1996.

Touger L, Looker HC, Krakoff J, Lindsay RS, Cook V, Knowler WC: Early growth in offspring of diabetic mothers. *Diabetes Care* 28:585–589, 2005.

Touyz RM: Reactive oxygen species, vascular oxidative stress, and redox signaling in hypertension: what is the clinical significance? *Hypertension* 44:248–252, 2004.

Towner D, Kjos SL, Leung B, Montoro MM, Xiang A, Mestman JH, Buchanan TA: Congenital malformations in pregnancies complicated by NIDDM. Increased risk from poor maternal metabolic control but not from exposure to sulfonylurea drugs. *Diabetes Care* 18:1446–1451, 1995.

Tracy TS, Venkataramanan R, Glover DD, Caritis SN; for the National Institute for Child Health and Human Development Network of Maternal-Fetal-Medicine Units: Temporal changes in drug metabolism (CYP1A2, CYP2D6 and CYP3A activity) during pregnancy. *Am J Obstet Gynecol* 192:633–639, 2005.

Trajanoski Z, Brunner GA, Gfrerer RJ, Wach P, Pieber TR: Accuracy of home blood glucose meters during hypoglycemia. *Diabetes Care* 19:1412–1415, 1996.

Tran ND, Hunter SK, Yankowitz J: Oral hypoglycemic agents in pregnancy. *Obstet Gynecol Surv* 59:456–463, 2004.

Trichopoulos D, Lagiou P: Mediterranean diet and overall mortality differences in the European Union. *Public Health Nutr* 7:949–951, 2004.

Trocho C, Pardo R, Rafecas I, Virgili J, Remesar X, Fernadez-Lopez JA, Alemany M: Formaldehyde derived from dietary aspartame binds to tissue components in vivo. *Life Sci* 63:337–349, 1998.

Troen AM, Lutgens E, Smith DE, Rosenberg IH, Selhub J: The atherogenic effect of excess methionine intake. *Proc Natl Acad Sci U S A* 100:15089–15094, 2000.

Trombetta M, Spiazzi G, Zoppini G, Muggeo M: Review article: type 2 diabetes and chronic liver disease in the Verona diabetes study. *Aliment Pharmacol Ther* 2 (Suppl):24–27, 2005.

Troncone R, Bhatnagar S, Butzner D, Cameron D, Hill I, Hoffnberg E, Maki M, Mendez V, de Jimenez MZ; European Society for Pediatric Gastroenterology, Hepatology and Nutrition: Celiac disease and other immunologically mediated disorders of the gastrointentinal tract: Working Group Report of the Second World Congress of Pediatric Gastroenterology, Hepatology, and Nutrition. *J Pediatr Gastroenterol Nutr* 39 (Suppl 2):S601–610, 2004.

Trumbo P, Yates AA, Schlicker S, Poos M: Dietary reference intakes: vitamin A, vitamin K, arsenic, boron, chromium, copper, iodine, iron, manganese, molybdemum, nickel, silicon, vanadium, and zinc. *J Am Diet Assoc* 101:294–301, 2001.

Trumbo P, Schlicker S, Yates AA, Poos M: Dietary reference intakes for energy, carbohydrate, fiber, fat, fatty acids, cholesterol, protein and amino acids. Commentary. *J Am Diet Assoc* 102:1621–1630, 2002.

Tsai JC, Perrella MA, Yoshizumi M, Hsieh CM, Haber E, Schlegel R, Lee ME: Promotion of vascular smooth muscle cell growth by homocysteine: a link to atherosclerosis. *Proc Natl Acad Sci U S A* 91:6369–6373, 1994.

Tsalikian E, Mauras N, Beck RW, Tamborlane WV, Janz KF, Chase HP, Wysocki T, Weinzimer SA, Buckingham BA, Kollman C, Xing D, Ruedy KJ; Diabetes Research in Children Network Direcnet Study Group: Impact of exercise on overnight glycemic control in children with type 1 diabetes mellitus. *J Pediatr* 147:528–534, 2005.

Tuomi T, Honkanen EH, Isomaa B, Sarelin L, Groop LC: Improved prandial glucose control with lower risk of hypoglycemia with nateglinide than with glibenclamide in patients with maturity-onset diabetes of the young type 3. *Diabetes Care* 29:189–194, 2006.

Tuomilehto J, Hu G, Bidel S, Lindstrom J, Jousilahti P: Coffee consumption and risk of type 2 diabetes mellitus among middle-aged Finnish men and women. *JAMA* 291:1213–1219, 2004.

Turner BC, Jenkins E, Kerr D, Sherwin RS, Cavan DA: The effect of evening alcohol consumption on next-morning glucose control in type 1 diabetes. *Diabetes Care* 24:1888–1893, 2001.

Turner RE, Langkamp-Henken B, Littell RC, Lutkowski MJ, Suarez MF: Comparing nutrient intake from food to the estimated average requirements shows middle- to upper-income pregnant women lack iron and possibly magnesium. *J Am Diet Assoc* 103:461–466, 2003.

Turnland JR: Human whole-body copper metabolism. *Am J Clin Nutr* 67:960S–964S, 1998.

Turyk M, Anderson HA, Hanrahan LP, Falk C, Steenport DN, Needham LL, Patterson DG Jr, Freels S, Persky V; Great Lakes Consortium: Relationship of serum levels of individual PCB, dioxin, and furan congeners and DDE with Great Lakes sport-caught fish consumption. *Environ Res* 100:173–183, 2006.

Twardowska-Saucha K, Greszczak W, Lacka B, Froelich J, Krywult D: Lipid peroxidation, antioxidant enzyme activity and trace element concentration in II and III trimester of pregnancy in pregnant women with diabetes. *Pol Arch Med Wewn* 92:313–321, 1994.

Tyrala EE: The infant of the diabetic mother. *Obstet Gynecol Clin North Am* 23: 221–241, 1996.

Ueland PM, Holm PI, Hustad S: Betaine: a key modulator of one-carbon metabolism and homocysteine status. *Clin Chem Lab Med* 43:1069–1075, 2005.

UKDH—UK Department of Health: *National Service Framework for Diabetes Standards.* London: Stationary Office; 2001; supplementary material published 15 March 2002. http://www.dh.gov.uk/PublicationsAndStatistics. Accessed Sept 23, 2006.

Ungar B, Stocks AE, Martin FI, Whittingham S, Mackay IR: Intrinsic-factor antibody, parietal-cell antibody, and latent pernicious anaemia in diabetes mellitus. *Lancet* 2:415–417, 1968.

USDA—U.S. Department of Agriculture, Agricultural Research Service: USDA national nutrient database for standard reference, release 17. Nutrient Data Laboratory home page; 2004. Available at: http://www.ars.usda.gov/main/site_main.htm?modecode=12354500. Accessed Mar 13, 2008.

Ushigome F, Takanaga H, Matsuo H, Yanai S, Tsukimori K, Nakano H, Uchiumi T, Nakamura T, Kuwano M, Ohtani H, Sawada Y: Human placental transport of vinblastine, vincristine, digoxin and progesterone: contribution of P-glycoprotein. *Eur J Pharmacol* 408:1–10, 2000.

Usta IM, Barton JR, Amon EA, Gonzalez A, Sibai BM: Acute fatty liver of pregnancy: an experience in the diagnosis and management of fourteen cases. *Am J Obstet Gynecol* 171:1342–1347, 1994.

Utzschneider KM, Kahn SE: The role of insulin resistance in nonalcoholic fatty liver disease. *J Clin Endocrinol Metab* 91:4753–4761, 2006.

Vaarasmaki M, Hartikainen A-L, Antilla M, Pirttiaho H: Out-patient management does not impair outcome of pregnancy in women with type 1 diabetes. *Diabetes Res Clin Pract* 47:111–117, 2000a.

Vaarasmaki MS, Hartikainen A-L, Anttila M, Pramila S, Koivisto M: Factors predicting peri- and neonatal outcome in diabetic pregnancy. *Early Hum Dev* 59:61–70, 2000b.

Vadachkoria S, Woelk GB, Mahomed K, Qiu C, Muy-Rivera M, Malinow MR, Williams MA: Elevated soluble vascular cell adhesion molecule-1, elevated homocyst(e)inemia, and hypertriglyceridemia in relation to preeclampsia risk. *Am J Hypertens* 19:235–242, 2006.

Vader LW, de Ru A, van der Wal Y, Kooy YM, Benckhuijsen W, Mearin ML, Drijfhout JW, van Veelen P, Koning F: Specificity of tissue transglutaminase explains cereal toxicity in celiac disease. *J Exp Med* 195:643–649, 2002.

Vahter M, Akesson A, Lind B, Bjors U, Schutz A, Berglund M: Longitudinal study of methylmercury and inorganic mercury in blood and urine of pregnant women, as well as in umbilical cord. *Environ Res* 84:186–194, 2000.

Valensise H, Liu YY, Federici M, Lauro D, Dell'anna D, Romanini C, Sesti G: Increased expression of low-affinity insulin receptor isoform and insulin/insulin-like growth factor-I hybrid receptors in term placenta from insulin-resistant women with gestational hypertension. *Diabetologia* 39:952–960, 1996.

Valerio G, Maiuri L, Troncone R, Buono P, Lombardi F, Palmieri R, Franzese A: Severe clinical onset of diabetes and increased prevalence of other autoimmune diseases in children with celiac disease diagnosed before diabetes mellitus. *Diabetologia* 45:1719–1722, 2002.

Valtuena S, Pellegrini N, Ardigo D, Del Rio D, Numersoso F, Scazzina F, Monti L, Zavaroni I, Brighenti F: Dietary glycemic index and liver steatosis. *Am J Clin Nutr* 84:136–142, 2006.

van Dam HA, van der Horst FG, Knoops L, Ryckman RM, Crebolder HF, van den Borne BH: Social support in diabetes: a systematic review of controlled intervention studies. *Patient Educ Couns* 59:1–12, 2005.

van de Laar FA, Lucassen PL, Akkermans RP, van de Lisdonk EH, Ruthen GE, van Weel C: α-Glucosidase inhibitors for patients with type 2 diabetes. Results from a Cochrane Systematic Review and meta-analysis. *Diabetes Care* 28:166–175, 2005.

van Wijngaarden E, Beck C, Shamlaye CF, Cernichiari E, Davidson PW, Myers GJ, Clarkson TW: Benchmark concentrations for methyl mercury obtained from the 9-year follow-up of the Seychelles Child Development Study. *Neurotoxicology* 27:702–709, 2006.

vanDam RM, Pasman WJ, Werhoef P: Effects of coffee consumption on fasting blood glucose and insulin concentrations. Randomized controlled trials in healthy volunteers. *Diabetes Care* 27:2990–2992, 2004.

vanDam RM, Willett WC, Manson JE, Hu FB: Coffee, caffeine, and risk of type 2 diabetes. A prospective cohort study in younger and middle-aged U.S. women. *Diabetes Care* 29:398–403, 2006.

vanderMeer IM, Karamali NS, Boeke AJP, Lips P, Middelkoop BJC, Verhoeven I, Wuistler JD: High prevalence of vitamin D deficiency in pregnant non-Western women in The Hague, Netherlands. *Am J Clin Nutr* 84:350–353, 2006.

Vangen S, Stoltenberg C, Holn S, Moe N, Magnus P, Harris JR, Stray-Pedersen B: Outcome of pregnancy among immigrant women with diabetes. *Diabetes Care* 26:327–332, 2003.

vanGuldener C, Donker AJ, Jakobs C, Teerlink T, de Meer K: No net renal extraction of homocysteine in fasting humans. *Kidney Int* 54:166–169, 1998.

Vanky E, Salvesen KA, Heimstad R, Fougner KJ, Romundstad P, Carlsen SM: Metformin reduces pregnancy complications without affecting androgen levels in pregnant polycystic ovary syndrome women: results of a randomized srudy. *Hum Reprod* 19:1734–1740, 2004.

Vanky E, Zahlsen K, Spigset O, Carlsen SM: Placental passage of metformin in women with polycystic ovary syndrome. *Fertil Steril* 83:1575–1578, 2005.

VanRooij IA, Swinkels DW, Blom HJ, Merkus HM, Steegers-Theunissen RP: Vitamin and homocysteine status of mothers and infants and the risk of nonsyndromic orofacial clefts. *Am J Obstet Gynecol* 189:1155–1160, 2003.

Varastehpour A, Radaelli T, Minium J, Ortega H, Herrera E, Catalano P, Hauguel-de Mouzon S: Activation of phospholipase A2 is associated with generation of placental lipid signals and fetal obesity. *J Clin Endocrinol Metab* 91:248–255, 2006.

Vargas-Zapata CL, Donangelo CM, Woodhouse LR, Abrams SA, Spencer EM, King JC: Calcium homeostasis during pregnancy and lactation in Brazilian women with low calcium intakes: a longitudinal study. *Am J Clin Nutr* 80:417–422, 2004.

Veith R, Cole D, Hawker G, Trang H, Rubin L: Wintertime vitamin D insufficiency is common in young Canadian women, and their vitamin D intake does not prevent it. *Eur J Clin Nutr* 55:1091–1097, 2001.

Veldman BAJ, Vervoort G, Blom H, Smits P: Reduced plasma total homocysteine concentrations in type 1 diabetes mellitus is determined by increased renal clearance. *Diabet Med* 22:301–305, 2005.

Vella A, Shah P, Basu R Basu A, Holst JJ, Rizza RA: Effect of glucagon-like peptide 1 (7–36) amide on glucose effectiveness and insulin action in people with type 2 diabetes. *Diabetes* 49:611–617, 2000.

Velzing-Aarts FV, Holm PI, Fokkema MR, van der Dijs FP, Ueland PM, Muskiet FA: Plasma choline and betaine and their relation to plasma homocysteine in normal pregnancy. *Am J Clin Nutr* 81:1383–1389, 2005.

Venn BJ, Walace AJ, Monro JA, Brown R, Frampton C, Green TJ: The glycemic load estimated from the glycemic index does not differ greatly from that measured using a standard curve in healthy volunteers. *J Nutr* 136:1377–1381, 2006.

Ventura A, Neri E, Ughi C, Leopaldi A, Citta A, Not T: Gluten-dependent diabetes-related and thyroid-related autoantibodies in patients with celiac disease. *J Pediatr* 137:263–265, 2000.

Verheijen ECJ, Critchley JA, Whitelaw DC, Tuffnell DJ: Outcomes of pregnancies in women with pre-existing type 1 or type 2 diabetes, in an ethnically mixed population. *BJOG* 112:1500–1503, 2005.

Verhoeff P, de Groot LC: Dietary determinants of plasma homocysteine concentrations. *Semin Vasc Med* 5:110–123, 2005.

Verkleij-Hagoort A, Verlinde M, Ursem N, Lindemans J, Helbing W, Ottenkamp J, Siebel F, Gittenberger-de Groot A, de Jonge R, Bartelings M, Steegers E, Steegers-Theunissen R: Maternal hyperhomocysteinemia is a risk factor for congenital heart disease. *BJOG* 113:1412–1418, 2006.

Ververs T, Kaasenbrood H, Visser G, Schobben F, deJong-van den Berg L, Egberts T: Prevalence and patterns of antidepressant drug use during pregnancy. *Eur J Clin Pharmacol* 62:863–870, 2006.

Vidal-Alaball J, Butler CC, Cannings-John R, Goringe A, Hood K, McCaddon A, McDowell I, Papaioannou A: Oral vitamin B_{12} versus intramuscular vitamin B_{12} deficiency. *Cochrane Database Syst Rev* 2005;(20):CD004655.

Viertel B, Guttner J: Effects of the oral antidiabetic repaglinide on the reproduction of rats. *Arzneimittelforschung* 50:425–440, 2000.

Vignini A, nanetti L, Bacchetti T, Ferretti G, Curatola G, Mazzanti L: Modification induced by homocysteine and low-density lipoprotein on human aortic endothelial cells. *J Clin Endocrinol Metab* 89:4558–4561, 2004.

Viguera AC, Whitfield T, Baldessarini RJ, Newport DJ, Stowe Z, Reminick A, Zurick A, Cohen LS: Risk of recurrence in women with bipolar disorder during pregnancy: prospective study of mood stabilizer discontinuation. *Am J Psychiatry* 164:1817–1824, 2007.

Vileikyte L, Leventhal H, Gonzalez JS, Peyrot M, Rubin RR, Ulbrecht JS, Garrow A, Waterman C, Cavanagh PR, Boulton AJ: Diabetic peripheral neuropathy and depressive symptoms: the association revisited. *Diabetes Care* 28:2378–2383, 2005.

Villar J, Merialdi M, Gulmezoglu AM, Abalos E, Carroli G, Kulier R, de Oni M: Nutritional interventions during pregnancy for the prevention or treatment of maternal morbidity and preterm delivery: an overview of randomized controlled trials. *J Nutr* 133:1606S–1625S, 2003.

Villar J, Abdel-Aleem H, Merialdi M, Mathai M, Ali MM, Zavaleta N, Purwar M, Hofmeyr J, Nguyen TN, Campódonico L, Landoulsi S, Carroli G, Lindheimer M; World Health Organizaton Calcium Supplementation for the Prevention of Preeclampsia Trial Group: World Health Organization randomized trial of calcium supplementation among low calcium intake pregnant women. *Am J Obstet Gynecol* 194:639–649, 2006.

Vinik AI, Maser RE, Mitchell BD, Freeman R: Diabetic autonomic neuropathy. ADA technical review. *Diabetes Care* 26:1553–1579, 2003.

Vinik A, Parson H, Ullal J: The role of PPARs in the microvascular dysfunction in diabetes. *Vascul Pharmacol* 45:54–64, 2006a.

Vinik AI, Ullal J, Parson HK, Barlow PM, Casellini CM: Pioglitazone treatment improves nitrosative stress in type 2 diabetes. *Diabetes Care* 29:869–876, 2006b.

Vohr BR, Lipsitt LP, Oh W: Somatic growth of children of diabetic mothers with reference to birth size. *J Pediatr* 97:196–199, 1980.

Vollset SE, Refsum H, Irgens LM, Emblem BM, Tverdal A, Gjessing HK, Monsen ALB, Ueland PM: Plasma total homocysteine, pregnancy complications, and adverse pregnancy outcomes: the Hordaland Homocysteine Study. *Am J Clin Nutr* 71:962–968, 2000.

Volta U, Molinaro N, de Franceschi L, Fratangelo D, Bianchi FB: IgA anti-endomysial antibodies on human umbilical cord tissue for celiac disease screening. Save both money and monkeys. *Dig Dis Sci* 40:1902–1905, 1995.

vonKries R, Kimmerle R, Schmidt JE, Hachmeister A, Bohm O, Wolf HG: Pregnancy outcomes in mothers with pregestational diabetes: a population-based study in North Rhine (Germany) from 1988 to 1993. *Eur J Pediatr* 156: 963–967, 1997.

Wafa WS, Khan MI: Use of U-500 regular insulin in type 2 diabetes. *Diabetes Care* 29:2175, 2006.

Wagner J, Tsimikas J, Abbott G, de Groot M, Heapy A: Racial and ethnic differences in diabetic patient-reported depression symptoms, diagnosis, and treatment. *Diabetes Res Clin Pract* 75:119–122, 2007.

Waite LL, Person EC, Zhou Y, Lim K, Scanlan TS, Taylor RN: Placental peroxisome proliferator-activated receptor-gamma is up-regulated by pregnancy serum. *J Clin Endocrinol Metab* 85:3808–3814, 2000.

Wald DS, Law M, Morris JK: Homocysteine and cardiovascular disease: evidence on causality from a meta-analysis. *BMJ* 325:1202, 2002.

Walker MC, Smith GN, Perkins SL, Keely EJ, Garner PR: Changes in homocysteine levels during normal pregnancy. *Am J Obstet Gynecol* 180:660–664, 1999.

Walkinshaw SA: Very tight versus tight control for diabetes in pregnancy. *Cochrane Database Syst Rev* 1996;(2):CD000226.

Walkinshaw SA: Pregnancy in women with preexisting diabetes: management issues. *Semin Fetal Neonatal Med* 10:307–315, 2005.

Wallace TM, Levy JC, Matthews DR: An increase in insulin sensitivity and basal beta-cell function in diabetic subjects treated with pioglitazone in a placebo-controlled randomized study. *Diabet Med* 21:568–576, 2004.

Wallberg-Henriksson H, Rincon J, Zierath JR: Exercise in the management of non-insulin dependent diabetes mellitus. *Sports Med* 25:25–35, 1998.

Walsh CH, Cooper BT, Wright AD, Malins JM, Cooke WT: Diabetes mellitus and celiac disease: a clinical study. *Q J Med* 47:89–100, 1978.

Walsh SW: Maternal-placental interactions of oxidative stress and antioxidants in preeclampsia. *Semin Reprod Endocrinol* 16:93–104, 1998.

Walter RM, Uriu-Hare JY, Lewis Olin K, Oster MH, Anawalt BD, Keen CL: Copper, zinc, manganese, and magnesium status and complications of diabetes mellitus. *Diabetes Care* 14:1050–1056, 1991.

Wang Y, Walsh SW, Guo J, Zhang J: The imbalance between thromboxane and prostacyclin in preeclampsia is associated with an imbalance between lipid peroxides and vitamin E in maternal blood. *Am J Obstet Gynecol* 165:1695–1700, 1991.

Wang D-S, Jonker JW, Kato Y, Kusuhara H, Schinkel AH, Sugiyama Y: Involvement of organic cation transporter 1 in hepatic and intestinal distribution of metformin. *J Pharmacol Exp Ther* 302:510–515, 2002.

Wang X, Demirtas H, Xu X: Homocysteine, B vitamins, and cardiovascular disease. Letter. *N Engl J Med* 355:208–209, 2006.

Wareham NJ, Swinn R, Fineman MS, Koda JE, Taylor K, Williams DE, Rahilly SO: Gestational diabetes mellitus is associated with an increase in the total concentration of amylin molecules. *Diabetes Care* 21:668–689, 1998.

Wasserman DH, Zinman B: Exercise in individuals with IDDM. ADA technical review. *Diabetes Care* 17:924–937, 1994.

Wassmann S, Wassmann K, Nickening G: Modulation of oxidant and antioxidant enzyme expression and function in vascular cells. *Hypertension* 44:381–386, 2004.

Waterman IJ, Emmison N, Dutta-Roy AK: Characterization of triacylglycerol hydrolase activities in human placenta. *Biochim Biophys Acta* 1394:169–176, 1998.

Watson JM, Jenkins EJ, Hamilton P, Lunt MJ, Kerr D: Influence of caffeine on the frequency and perception of hypoglycemia in free-living patients with type 1 diabetes. *Diabetes Care* 23:455–459, 2000.

Weickert MO, Mohlig M, Koebnick C, Holst JJ, Namsolleck P, Ristow M, Osterhoff M, Rochlitz H, Rudovich N, Spranger J, Pfeiffer AF: Impact of cereal fiber on glucose-regulating factors. *Diabetologia* 48:2343–2353, 2005.

Weinger K, Jacobson AM: Psychosocial and quality of life correlates of glycemic control during intensive treatment of type 1 diabetes. *Patient Educ Couns* 42:123–131, 2001.

Weinger K, Lee J: Psychosocial and psychiatric challenges of diabetes mellitus. *Nurs Clin North Am* 41:667–680, 2006.

Weiss PAM, Lichtenegger W, Winter R, Purstner P: Insulin levels in amniotic fluid. Management of pregnancy in diabetes. *Obstet Gynecol* 51:393–397, 1978.

Weiss PAM, Hofmann H: Intensified conventional insulin therapy for the pregnant diabetic patient. *Obstet Gynecol* 64:629–637, 1984.

Weiss PAM, Kainer F, Haas J: Cord blood insulin to assess the quality of treatment in diabetic pregnancies. *Early Hum Dev* 51:187–195, 1998.

Weisskopf MG, Anderson HA, Hanrahan LP, Kanarek MS, Falk CM, Steenport DM, Draheim LA; Great Lakes Consortium: Maternal exposure to Great Lakes sport-caught fish and dichlorodiphenyl dichlorethylene, but not polychlorinated bephenyls, is associated with reduced birth weight. *Environ Res* 97:149–162, 2005.

Welch GW, Jacobson AM, Polonsky WH: The Problem Areas in Diabetes Scale: an evaluation of its clinical utility. *Diabetes Care* 20:760–766, 1997.

Wen SW, Yang Q, Garner P, Fraser W, Olatunbosun O, Nimrod C, Walker M: Selective serotonin reuptake inhibitors and adverse pregnancy outcomes. *Am J Obstet Gynecol* 194:961–966, 2006.

Wender-Ozegowska E, Wroblewska K, Zawiejska A, Pietryga M, Szczapa J, Biczysko R: Threshold values of maternal blood glucose in early diabetic pregnancy—prediction of fetal malformations. *Acta Obstet Gynecol Scand* 84:17–25, 2005.

Weng X, Odouli R, Li D-K: Maternal caffeine consumption during pregnancy and the risk of miscarriage: a prospective cohort study. *Am J Obstet Gynecol* 198: 1–28–2008. DOI: 10.1016/j.ajog.2007.10.803.

Wentholt IM, Vollebregt MA, Hart AA, Hoekstra JB, Devries JH: Comparison of a needle-type and a microdialysis continuous glucose monitor in type 1 diabetic patients. *Diabetes Care* 28:2871–2876, 2005.

Wentholt IM, Hoekstra JB, De Vries JH: A critical appraisal of the continuous glucose-error grid analysis. *Diabetes Care* 29:1805–1811, 2006.

Wentzel P, Ejdesjo A, Ericksson UJ: Maternal diabetes in vivo and high glucose in vitro diminish GAPDH activity in rat embryos. *Diabetes* 52:1222–1228, 2003.

Werler MM, Lammer EJ, Rosenberg L, Mitchell AA: Maternal vitamin A supplementation in relation to certain birth defects. *Teratology* 42:497–503, 1990.

Wessling-Resnicke M: Iron imports. III. Transfer of iron from the mucosa into circulation. *Am J Physiol* 290:G1–G6, 2006.

Westgate JA, Lindsay RS, Beattie J, Pattison NS, Gamble G, Mildenhall LFJ, Breier BH, Johnstone FD: Hyperinsulinemia in cord blood in mothers with type 2 diabetes mellitus and gestational diabetes in New Zealand. *Diabetes Care* 29:1345–1350, 2006.

Wheeler ML. Nutrient database for the 2004 exchange lists for meal planning; *J Am Diet Assoc* 103:894–920, 2003.

Whiteman VE, Homko CJ, Reece EA: Management of hypoglycemia and diabetic ketoacidosis in pregnancy. *Obstet Gynecol Clin North Am* 23:87–107, 1996.

Whitlock EP, Polen MR, Green CA, Orleans T, Klein J: Behavioral counseling interventions in primary care to reduce risky/harmful alcohol use by adults: a summary of the evidence for the U.S. Preventive Services Task Force. *Ann Intern Med* 140:557–568, 2004.

Whittaker PG, Lee CH, Taylor R: Whole body protein kinetics in women: effect of pregnancy and IDDM during anabolic stimulation. *Am J Physiol* 279:E978–E988, 2000.

WHO—World Health Organization: Maternal anthropometry for prediction of pregnancy outcomes: memorandum from a USAID/WHO/PAHO/MotherCare meeting. *Bull World Health Organ* 69:523–532, 1991.

WHO—World Health Organization: *Obesity: Preventing and Managing the Global Epidemic.* Technical series # 894. Geneva: WHO; 1997:9.

Wibell L, Gebre-Medhin M, Lindmark G: Magnesium and zinc in diabetic pregnancy. *Acta Paediatr Scand* 320 (Suppl):100–106, 1985.

Widness JA, Teramo KA, Clemons GK, Voutilainen P, Stenman U-H, McKinlay SM, Schwartz R: Direct relationship of antepartum glucose control and fetal erythropoietin in human type 1 diabetic pregnancy. *Diabetologia* 33:378–383, 1990.

Wiesli P, Schmid C, Kerwer O, Nigg-Koch C, Klaghofer R, Seifert B, Spinas GA, Schwegler K: Acute psychological stress affects glucose concentrations in patients with type 1 diabetes following food intake but not in the fasting state. *Diabetes Care* 28:1910–1915, 2005.

Wijekoon EP, Hall B, Ratnam S, Brosnan ME, Zeisel SH, Brosnan JT: Homocysteine metabolism in ZDF (type 2) diabetic rats. *Diabetes* 54:3245–3251, 2005.

Wijendran V, Bendel RB, Couch SC, Philipson EH, Thomsen K, Zhang X, Lammi-Keefe CJ: Maternal plasma phospholipid polyunsaturated fatty acids in pregnancy with and without gestational diabetes mellitus: relations with maternal factors. *Am J Clin Nutr* 70:53–61, 1999.

Wijendran V, Hayes KC: Dietary *n*-6 and *n*-3 fatty acid balance and cardiovascular health. *Annu Rev Nutr* 24:597–615, 2004.

Wilkinson GR: The dynamics of drug absorption, distribution, and elimination. In: Hardman JG, Limbird LE, eds. *Goodman & Gilman's The Pharmacological Basis of Therapeutics.* 10th ed. New York: McGraw-Hill; 2002:3–29.

Wilkinson GR: Drug metabolism and variability among patients in drug response. *N Engl J Med* 352:2211–2221, 2005.

Willman S, Leveno K, Guzick D, Williams L, Whalley P: Glucose threshold for macrosomia in pregnancy complicated by diabetes. *Am J Obstet Gynecol* 154: 470–475, 1986.

Wilson JF: Balancing the risks and benefits of fish consumption. *Ann Intern Med* 141:977–980, 2004.

Wilson GT, Shafran R: Eating disorders guidelines from NICE. *Lancet* 365:79–81, 2005.

Wilson-Fritch L, Nicoloro S, Chouinard M, Lazar MA, Chui PC, Leszyk J, Straubhaar J, Czech MP, Corvera S: Mitochondrial remodeling in adipose tissue associated with obesity and treatment with rosiglitazone. *J Clin Invest* 114: 1281–1289, 2004.

Wiltshire E, Thomas DW, Baghurst P, Couper J: Reduced total plasma homocyst(e)ine in children and adolescents with type 1 diabetes. *J Pediatr* 138:888–893, 2001.

Winneke G, Bucholski A, Heinzow B, Kramer U, Schmidt E, Walkowiak J, Wiener JA, Steingruber HJ: Developmental neurotoxicity of polychlorinated biphenyls (PCBS): cognitive and psychomotor functions in 7-month old children. *Toxicol Lett* 102–103:423–428, 1998.

Wisborg K, Kesmodel U, Bech BH, Hedergaard M, Nenriksen TB: Maternal consumption of coffee during pregnancy and stillbirth and infant death in first year of life: prospective study. *BMJ* 326:420–423, 2003.

Wisner KL, Gelenberg AJ, Leonard H, Zarin D, Johanson R, Frank E: Pharmacologic treatment of depression during pregnancy. *JAMA* 282:1264–1269, 1999.

Wisser J, Florio I, Neff M, Konig V, Huch R, Huch A, von Mandach U: Changes in bone density and metabolism in pregnancy. *Acta Obstet Gynecol Scand* 84: 349–354, 2005.

Witt MF, White NH, Santiago JV: Role of site and timing of the morning insulin injection in type 1 diabetes. *J Pediatr* 103:528–533, 1983.

Wittgrove AC, Jester L, Wittgrove P, Clark GW: Pregnancy following gastric bypass for morbid obesity. *Obes Surg* 8:461–464, 1998.

Wolever TM, Nuttall FQ, Lee R, Wong GS, Josse RG, Csima A, Jenkins DJ: Prediction of the relative blood glucose response of mixed meals using the white bread glycemic index. *Diabetes Care* 8(5): 418–428, 1985.

Wolever TM, Jenkins DJ, Josse RG, Wong GS, Lee R: The glycemic index: similarity of values derived in insulin-dependent and non-insulin-dependent diabetic patients. *J Am Coll Nutr* 6:295–305, 1987.

Wolever TM, Nguyen PM, Chiasson JL, Hunt JA, Josse RG, Palmason C, Rodger NW, Ross SA, Ryan EA, Tan MH: Determinants of diet glycemic index calculated retrospectively from diet records of 342 individuals with non-insulin-dependent diabetes mellitus. *Am J Clin Nutr* 59:1265–1269, 1994.

Wolever TM, Bolognesi C: Prediction of glucose and insulin responses of normal subjects after consuming mixed meals varying in energy, protein, fat, carbohydrate and glycemic index. *J Nutr* 126:2807–2812, 1996.

Wolever TMS, Mehling C: High-carbohydrate/low-glycemic index dietary advice improves glucose disposition index in subjects with impaired glucose tolerance. *Br J Nutr* 87:477–487, 2002a.

Wolever TM, Mehling C: Long-term effect of varying the source or amount of dietary carbohydrate on postprandial plasma glucose, insulin, triacylglycerol, and free fatty acid concentrations in subjects with impaired glucose tolerance. *Am J Clin Nutr* 77:612–621, 2002b.

Wolever TM, Vorster HH, Bjorck I, Brand-Miller J, Brighenti F, Mann JI, Ramdath DD, Granfeldt Y, Holt S, Perry TL, Venter C, Xiaomei W: Determination of the glycemic index of foods: inter-laboratory study. *Eur J Clin Nutr* 57:475–482, 2003.

Wolever TM: Effect of blood sampling schedule and method of calculating the area under the curve on validity and precision of glycaemic index values. *Br J Nutr* 91:295–301, 2004.

Wolever TMS, Yang M, Zeng AY, Atkinson F, Brand-Miller JC: Food glycemic index, as given in glycemic index tables, is a significant determinant of glycemic responses elicited by composite breakfast meals. *Am J Clin Nutr* 83:1306–1312, 2006.

Wolfe HM, Zador IE, Gross TL, Martier SS, Sokol RJ: The clinical utility of maternal body mass index in pregnancy. *Am J Obstet Gynecol* 164:1306–1310, 1991.

Wolfe LA, Weissgerber TL: Clinical physiology of exercise in pregnancy: a literature review. *J Obstet Gynecol Can* 25:451–4533, 2003a.

Wolfe LA, Davies GAL: Canadian guidelines for exercise in pregnancy. *Clin Obstet Gynecol* 46:488–495, 2003b.

Wollesen F, Brattstrom L, Refsum H, Ueland PM, Berglund L, Berne C: Plasma total homocysteine and cysteine in relation to glomerular filtration rate in diabetes mellitus. *Kidney Int* 55:1028–1035, 1999.

Wong SF, Chan FY, Oats JJN, McIntyre DH: Fetal growth spurt and pregestational diabetic pregnancy. *Diabetes Care* 25:1681–1684, 2002.

Wood SL, Jick H, Sauve R: The risk of stillbirth in pregnancies before and after the onset of diabetes. *Diabet Med* 20:703–707, 2003.

Woolderink JM, vanLoon AJ, Storms F, deHeide L, Hoogenberg K: Use of insulin glargine during pregnancy in seven type 1 diabetic women. *Diabetes Care* 28:2594–2595, 2005.

Wortsman J, Matsuoka LY, Chen TC, Lu Z, Holick MF: Decreased bioavailability of vitamin D in obesity. *Am J Clin Nutr* 72:690–693, 2000.

Wu Z, Bidlingmaier M, Friess SC, Kirk SC, Buchinger P, Schiessel B, Strasburger CJ: A new nonisotopic, highly sensitive assay for the measurement of human placental growth hormone: development and clinical implications. *J Clin Endocrinol Metab* 88:804–811, 2003.

Wudel LJ Jr, Wright JK, Debelak JP, Allos TM, Shyr Y, Chapman WC: Prevention of gallstone formation in morbidly obese patients undergoing rapid weight loss: results of a randomized controlled pilot study. *J Surg Res* 102:50–56, 2002.

Wulffele MG, Kooy A, Lehert P, Bets D, Ogterop JC, Borger van der Burg B, Donker AJM, Stehouwer CDA: Effects of short-term treatment with metformin on serum concentrations of homocysteine, folate and vitamin B12 in type 2 diabetes mellitus: a randomized, placebo-controlled trial. *J Int Med* 254:455–463, 2003.

Wun Chan JC, Yu Liu HS, Sang Kho BC, Yin Sim JP, Lau TK, Luk YW, Chu RW, Fung Cheung FM, Tat Choi FP, Kwan Ma ES: Pernicious anemia in Chinese: a study of 181 patients in a Hong Kong hospital. *Medicine (Baltimore)* 85: 129–138, 2006.

Wyatt JW, Frias JL, Hoyme HE, Jovanovic L, Jovanovic L, Kaaja R, Brown F, Garg S, Lee-Paritz A, Seely EW, Kerr L, Mattoo V, tan M; the IONS Study Group: Congenital anomaly rate in offspring of mothers with type 1 diabetes treated with insulin lispro during pregnancy. *Diabet Med* 22:803–807, 2005.

Wylie BR, Kong J, Kozak SE, Marshall CJ, Yong SO, Thompson DM: Normal perinatal mortality in type 1 diabetes mellitus in a series of 300 consecutive pregnancy outcomes. *Am J Perinatol* 19:169–176, 2002.

Wylie-Rosett J, Albright AA, Apovian C, Clark NG, Delahanty L, Franz MJ, Hoogwerf B, Kulkarni K, Lichtenstein AH, Mayer-Davis E, Mooradian AD, Wheeler M: 2006–2007 American Diabetes Association nutrition recommendations: issues for practice translation. *J Am Diet Assoc* 107: 1296–1304, 2007.

Wyse LJ, Jones M, Mandel F: Relationship of glycosylated hemoglobin, fetal macrosomia, and birthweight macrosomia. *Am J Perinatol* 11:260–262, 1994.

Xing AY, Challier JC, Lepercq J, Cauzac M, Charron MJ, Girard J, Hauguel-de Mouzon S: Unexpected expression of glucose transporter 4 in villous stromal cells of human placenta. *J Clin Endocrinol Metab* 83:4097–4101, 1998.

Xu Y, Wang Q, Cook TJ, Knipp GT: Effect of placental fatty acid metabolism and regulation by peroxisome proliferator activated receptor on pregnancy and fetal outcomes. *J Pharm Sci* 96:2582–2606, 2007.

Yang LE, Leong PKK, Guzman JP, Rhee MS, McDonough AA: Modest K+ restriction provokes insulin resistance of cellular K+ uptake without decrease in plasma K+. *Ann N Y Acad Sci* 986:625–627, 2003.

Yang J, Cummings EA, O'Connell C, Jangaard K: Fetal and neonatal outcomes of diabetic pregnancies. *Obstet Gynecol* 108:644–650, 2006.

Yang QH, Carter HK, Mulinare J, Berry RJ, Friedman JM, Erickson JD: Race-ethnicity differences in folic acid intake in women of child-bearing age in the United States after folic acid fortification: findings from the National Health and Nutrition Examination Survey, 2001–2002. *Am J Clin Nutr* 85:1409–1416, 2007.

Yanigasawa K, Iwasaki N, Sanaka M, Minei S, Kanamori M, Omori Y, Iwamoto Y: Polymorphism of the beta3-adrenergic receptor gene and weight gain in pregnant diabetic women. *Diabetes Res Clin Pract* 44:41–47, 1999.

Yan-Jun L, Tsushima T, Minei S, Sanaka M, Nagashima T, Yanigisawa K, Omori Y: Insulin-like growth factors (IGFs) and IGF-binding proteins (IGFBP-1, -2 and -3) in diabetic pregnancy: relationship to macrosomia. *Endocr J* 43:221–231, 1996.

Yaris F, Yaris E, Kadioglu M, Ulku C, Kesim M, Kalyoncu NI: Normal pregnancy outcome following inadvertent exposure to rosiglitazone, glicazide, and atorvastatin in a diabetic and hypertensive woman. *Reprod Toxicol* 18:619–621, 2004.

Yavin E, Glozman S, Green P: Docohexaenoic acid accumulation in the prenatal brain. Prooxidant and antioxidant features. *J Molec Neurosci* 16:229–235, 2001.

Yeh GY, Eisenberg DM, Kaptchuk TJ, Phillips RS: Systematic review of herbs and dietary supplements for glycemic control in diabetes. *Diabetes Care* 26: 1277–1294, 2003.

Yi P, Melnyk S, Pogribna M, Pogribny IP, Hine RJ, James SJ: Increase in plasma homocysteine associated with parallel increases in S-adenosylhomocysteine and lymphocyte DNA hypomethylation. *J Biol Chem* 275:29318–29323, 2000.

Yi X, Maeda N: α-Lipoic acid prevents the increase in atherosclerosis induced by diabetes in apolipoprotein E-deficient mice fed high-fat/low-cholesterol diet. *Diabetes* 55:2238–2244, 2006.

Ylinen K: High maternal levels of hemoglobin A1C associated with delayed fetal lung maturation in insulin-dependent diabetic pregnancies. *Acta Obstet Gynecol Scand* 66:263–266, 1987.

Yogev Y, Ben-Haroush A, Chen R, Kaplan B, Phillip M, Hod M: Continuous glucose monitoring for treatment adjustment in diabetic pregnancies: a pilot study. *Diabet Med* 20:558–562, 2003a.

Yogev Y, Chen R, Ben-Haroush A, Phillip M, Jovanovic L, Hod, M: Continuous glucose monitoring for the evaluation of gravid women with type 1 diabetes mellitus. *Obstet Gynecol* 101:633–638, 2003b.

Yogev Y, Ben-Haroush A, Chen R, Rosenn B, Hod M, Langer O: Diurnal glycemic profile in obese and normal weight nondiabetic pregnant women. *Am J Obstet Gynecol* 191:949–953, 2004a.

Yogev Y, Ben-Haroush A, Chen R, Rosenn B, Hod M: Undiagnosed asymptomatic hypoglycemia: diet, insulin, and glyburide for gestational diabetic pregnancy. *Obstet Gynecol* 104:88–93, 2004b.

York R, Brown LP, Persily CA, Jacobsen BS: Affect in diabetic women during pregnancy and postpartum. *Nurs Res* 45:54–56, 1996.

Young DB, Ma G: Vascular protective effects of potassium. *Semin Nephrol* 19: 477–486, 1999.

Yusuf S, Dagenais G, Pogue J, Bosch J, Sleight P: Vitamin E supplementation and cardiovascular events in high-risk patients: the Heart Outcomes Prevention Evaluation Study. *N Engl J Med* 342:154–160, 2000.

Zachara BA, Wardak C, Didkowski W, Maciag A, Marchaluk E: Changes in blood selenium and glutathione concentrations and glutathione peroxidase activity in human pregnancy. *Gynecol Obstet Invest* 35:12–17, 1993.

Zander M, Madsbad S, Madsen JL, Holst JJ: Effect of 6-week course of glucagon-like peptide 1 on glycemic control, insulin sensitivity, and β-cell function in type 2 diabetes: a parallel-group study. *Lancet* 359:824–830, 2002.

Zarate A, Ochoa R, Hernandez M, Basurto L: Effectiveness of acarbose in the control of glucose tolerance worsening in pregnancy [Spanish]. *Ginecol Obstet Mex* 68:42–45, 2000.

Zeisel SH: Choline: an essential nutrient for humans. *Nutrition* 16:669–671, 2000.

Zeisel SH, Mar MH, Howe JC, Holden JM: Concentrations of choline-containing compounds and betaine in common foods. *J Nutr* 133:1302–1307, 2003.

Zeisel SH: Nutritional importance of choline for brain development. *J Am Coll Nutr* 23 (Suppl):621S–626S, 2004.

Zeisel SH: Choline, homocysteine, and pregnancy. Editorial. *Am J Clin Nutr* 82: 719–720, 2005.

Zeisel SH: Choline: critical role during fetal development and dietary requirements in adults. *Annu Rev Nutr* 26:229–250, 2006a.

Zeisel SH, Niculescu MD: Perinatal choline influences brain structure and function. *Nutr Rev* 64:197–203, 2006b.

Zenobi PD, Keller A, Jaeggi-Groisman SE, Glatz Y: Accuracy of devices for self-monitoring of blood glucose including hypoglycemic blood glucose levels. *Diabetes Care* 18:587–588, 1995.

Zeskind PS, Stephens LE: Maternal selective serotonin reuptake inhibitor use during pregnancy and newborn neurobehavior. *Pediatrics* 113:368–375, 2004.

Zgibor JC, Peyrot M, Ruppert K, Noullet W, Siminerio LM, Peeples M, McWilliams J, Koshinsky J, DeJesus C, Emerson S, Charron-Prochownik D; AADE/UPMC Diabetes Education Outcomes Project: Using the American Association of Diabetes Educators Outcomes System to identify patient behavior change goals and diabetes educator responses. *Diabetes Educ* 33:839–842, 2007.

Zhang L, Brett CM, Giacomini KM: Role of organic cation transporters in drug absorption and elimination. *Annu Rev Pharmacol Toxicol* 38:431–460, 1998.

Zhao W, Mosley BS, Cleves MA, Melnyk S, James SJ, Hobbs CA: Neural tube defects and maternal biomarkers of folate, homocysteine, and glutathione metabolism. *Birth Defects Res Clin Mol Teratol* 76:230–236, 2006a.

Zhao W, Chen Y, Lin M, Sigal RJ: Association between diabetes and depression: sex and age differences. *Public Health* 120:696–704, 2006b.

Zharikova OL, Ravindran S, Nanovskaya TN, Hill RA, Hankins GD, Ahmed MS: Kinetics of glyburide metabolism by hepatic and placental microsomes on human and baboon. *Biochem Pharmacol* 73:2012–2019, 2007.

Zheng H, Cable R, Spencer B, Votto N, Katz SD: Iron stores and vascular function in voluntary blood donors. *Arterioscler Thromb Vasc Biol* 25:1577–1583, 2005.

Zhu L, Nakabayashi M, Takeda Y: Statistical analysis of perinatal outcomes in pregnancy complicated with diabetes mellitus. *J Obstet Gynecol Res* 23:555–563, 1997.

Zib I, Raskin P: Novel insulin analogues and [their] mitogenic potential. *Diabetes Obes Metab* 8:611–620, 2006.

Ziegler D, Ametov A, Barinov A, Dyck PJ, Gurieva I, Low PA, Munzel U, Yakhno N, Raz I, Novosadova M, Maus J, Samigullin R: Oral treatment with a–lipoic acid improves symptomatic diabetic polyneuropathy. The SYDNEY 2 trial. *Diabetes Care* 29:2365–2370, 2006.

Zimran A, Hershko C: The changing pattern of megaloblastic anemia: megaloblastic anemia in Israel. *Am J Clin Nutr* 37:855–861, 1983.

Zucker P, Simon G: Prolonged symptomatic neonatal hypoglycemia associated with maternal chlorpropamide therapy. *Pediatrics* 42:824–825, 1968.

Management of Diabetic/ Medical Complications in Pregnancy

INTRODUCTION

This Technical Review presents evidence supporting management recommendations on diagnosis and treatment of the metabolic, macrovascular, microvascular, and neurological complications related to PDM and pregnancy, considering both type 1 and type 2 diabetes mellitus. The diabetes-linked problems of autoimmune gastritis/pernicious anemia, celiac disease, and fatty liver disease are discussed in Part I in the section titled "Medical Nutrition Therapy." Venous thromboembolism (VTE) is discussed in Part III in the section titled "Cesarean Delivery." Postpartum management is considered in Part IV.

Our primary focus is centered on evaluation and treatment of type 1 and type 2 diabetes both before pregnancy and throughout gestation, with the primary aim of delivering a healthy baby while preserving the health of the diabetic mother. We also emphasize the importance of continuity of multifaceted care for diabetes in the years before and after pregnancy to prevent long-term diabetic and cardiovascular complications. Although no doubt exists that prevention of hyperglycemia and severe hypoglycemia is necessary to achieve normal pregnancy outcome and continued maternal health, a glucocentric view does not suffice to prevent long-term complications of diabetes, especially CVD. Control of glucose, BP, lipids, nutrition, weight gain, smoking, and perhaps reduction of inflammation are needed to reduce CVD. Consideration of the many emerging biomarkers and pathogenic processes of cardiovascular, renal, retinal, and neurological disease are also important to understand the potential effects of treatment. Our recommendations to prevent complications or treat them when present are designed to encourage effective continuity of behaviors and pharmacotherapies through the reproductive years, as well as provide optimal care during pregnancy that is safe for the gravida and her fetus.

Fortunately, there is evidence that pregnancy is not a risk factor for long-term progression of diabetic microvascular complications, at least for women managed with the level of attention provided in research studies (Hemachandra 95, Kaaja 96, DCCT 00, Verier-Mine 05). Multivariate analysis of a small pair-matched case–control study demonstrated that having babies predicted the later incidence of neuropathy in Pittsburgh, but CHD and lower-extremity arterial disease did not increase after pregnancies (Hemachandra 95). In a cross-sectional analysis of 117 women with longstanding type 1 diabetes in Finland, there was no association between the number of pregnancies and the presence of cardiovascular autonomic dysfunction detected in 32% of the subjects (Airaksinen 93). In the larger European Diabetes (EURODIAB) Prospective Complications Study, giving birth was not significantly related to the later incidence of neuropathy, nephropathy, or retinopathy (Verier-Mine 05). However, we need additional studies of nutritional and pharmacological management of glucose, BP, lipids, albuminuria, and inflammation during pregnancy on long-term risk of CVD in diabetic women.

Data on complications in adolescents with type 1 and type 2 diabetes are useful to review with regard to understanding our patients before eventual pregnancy and gaining a view of pathogenic processes that are not influenced by aging. We are just beginning to understand the genetic and environmental factors that induce diabetic complications to cluster in families (DCCT 97a, Rogus 02, Purnell 03, Bowden 06). However, a negative family history does not mean that an individual patient need not participate in intensified, multifaceted care.

Abundant epidemiological (Adler 00, Stratton 00a, Fuller 01, Mattock 01, Orchard 01) and clinical trial data (DCCT 93,95a, Reichard 96, Haffner 98a,b, Purnell 98, UKPDS 98a,b, Gaede 99, Canga 00, Shichiri 00, Gaede 03, DCCT/EDIC 03a, ACCORD 04, BPT 05, DCCT/EDIC 05, Whelton 05, Cleary 06, Gaede 08) clearly support the need for excellent control of glucose, BP, lipids, weight, smoking, and perhaps the parallel processes of inflammation and oxidative stress to minimize complications and improve the quality of life of women with diabetes. Despite this widely published information, recent surveys indicate that translation of research results to management in the general diabetic population is far from sufficient to achieve these goals (Beckles 98, Haire-Joshu 99, George 01, Saadine 02, Charpentier 03, Gudbjornsdotter 03, Saydah 04, Comaschi 05, Eliasson 05, Jacobs 05a, Prevost 05, Wadwa 05, Zgibor 05, Kobayashi 06, Malik 06, Schwab 06, Shah 07). This is also true at academic medical centers and in managed care populations (McFarlane 02, Beaton 04). Much work remains to be done on the assessment of individual patient risk and barriers to care to achieve widespread application of effective treatment.

METABOLIC DISTURBANCES

—— Original contribution by William H. Herman MD, MPH
and John L. Kitzmiller MD

Diabetic Ketoacidosis in Pregnancy

Diabetic ketoacidosis (DKA) is a dangerous acute metabolic complication of diabetes associated with insulin deficiency, accelerated lipolysis, and hepatic glucose/ketone production with hyperglycemia and ketonemia, severe depletion of water and electrolytes from both the intracellular and ECF compartments, possible hyperosmolality in the extracellular space and mental obtundation, and increased anion gap metabolic acidosis (Kitzmiller 82, Hagay 94a, Kitabchi 01, Montoro 04, Carroll 05, Kitabchi 06). Diagnostic criteria for DKA are summarized in Table II.1. DKA may appear in diabetic patients of any age (Valabji 03, Wolfsdorf 06). It has been classically described in diabetic patients with β-cell autoimmunity and minimal to no insulin secretion

TABLE II.1 Diagnostic Criteria for Diabetic Ketoacidosis and Hyperosmolar Hyperglycemic State

Parameter	DKA Mild	DKA Moderate	DKA Severe	HHS
Plasma glucose (mg/dL)	>250*	>250*	>250*	>600
Arterial pH	7.25–7.30	7.00–7.24	<7.00	>7.30
Serum bicarbonate (mEq/L)	15–18	10–14.9	<10	>15
Urine ketones**	Positive	Positive	Positive	Small
Serum ketones**	Positive	Positive	Positive	Small
Effective serum osmolality (mOsm/kg)[a]	Variable	Variable	Variable	>320
Anion gap[b]	>10	>12	>12	Variable
Mental status	Alert	Alert/drowsy	Stupor/coma	Stupor/coma

DKA can occur with a lower plasma glucose concentration in pregnancy.
**Nitroprusside reaction method.*
[a]*Calculation: 2[measured Na(mEq/L)] + glucose (mg/dL)/18.*
[b]*Calculation: $(Na^+) - (Cl^- + HCO_3^-)$ (mEq/L).*

DKA, diabetic ketoacidosis; HHS, hyperosmoloar hyperglycemic state.
Modified from the 2001 Technical Review (Kitabchi 01), 2004 American Diabetes Association (ADA) Position Statement (ADA 04a), and 2006 ADA Consensus Statement (Kitabchi 06).

(type 1a), but there is a subset of ketosis-prone patients with permanent insulin deficiency and negative assays for β-cell autoimmunity (type 1b or "idiopathic" type 1 diabetes) (~21% of adult KTA patients; ~13% of new-onset diabetes with DKA) (Balasubramanyam 06). DKA can also complicate type 2 diabetes and is usually associated with cessation of medication, infection, pancreatitis, and/or obesity (Hother-Nielsen 88, Umpierez 99, Newton 04, Umpierrez 06a). Ketosis-prone type 2 diabetes is most common in the U.S. in African-American and Hispanic populations (Umpierrez 95, Westphal 96, Balasubramanyam 99, Kitabchi 03, Newton 04).

Ketosis-prone type 2 diabetes with newly diagnosed diabetes is recently characterized as β-cell autoantibody negative, β-cell function positive type 2 diabetes (A–β+; ~55% of adult DKA patients; ~74% of new-onset diabetes with DKA) or as β-cell autoantibody positive, β-cell function positive type 2 diabetes (A+β+; ~5% of adult DKA patients; ~7% of new-onset diabetes with DKA; about one-half have progressive deterioration of β-cell function) (Maldonado 03,05, Balasubramanyam 06, Umpierrez 06b). In these studies of patients with DKA, a fasting C-peptide concentration above or below 1.0 ng/mL correlated well with a C-peptide response above or below 1.5 ng/mL after intravenous glucagon stimulation (the standard test to assess endogenous insulin secretory reserve) and predicted long-term insulin secretion. The Aβ classification system yields very high predictive values >95% for long-term β-cell function and clinical phenotype in patients presenting with DKA and previous or newly diagnosed diabetes (Balasubramanyam 06, Umpierrez 06a), although these studies have not involved pregnant diabetic women. BMI lacks sensitivity and specificity as a marker for β-cell function in ketosis-prone patients (Yu 01, Maldonado 04, Mauvais-Jarvis 04, Balasubramanyam 06, Umpierrez 06).

DKA is graded as mild, moderate, or severe based on the degree of acidosis (Table II.1) (ADA 04a, Kitabchi 06). The even more dangerous syndrome of hyperosmolar hyperglycemic state (HHS) is not often diagnosed in pregnancy. The pathogenesis of DKA relates to "a reduction in the net effective action of circulating insulin coupled with a concomitant elevation of counterregulatory hormones, such as glucagon, catecholamines, cortisol, and growth hormone" (ADA 04a), and the risk is exacerbated in pregnancy. The "accelerated starvation," enhanced lipolysis and ketosis, and metabolic acidosis associated with normal pregnancy along with the increase in insulin resistance in the second and third trimesters account for much of the increased risk (Chauhan 95, Whiteman 96, Kamalkannan 03, Carroll 05). DKA develops more rapidly in pregnancy (Montoro 04), and the use of reagent strips to detect the presence of ketones in the urine is important when pregnant women feel unwell, blood glucose levels are high, or with intercurrent illness.

The prevalence of DKA in diabetic pregnancy has declined from 16.7% before 1960 (Kyle 63) to 7.8% from 1965 to 1985 (Cousins 87) to 1.2–4.1% in any trimester in recent decades (Kilvert 93, Montoro 93, Chauhan 96, Cullen 96, Schneider 03), probably as a result of SMBG and intensified insulin therapy (Whiteman 96). DKA in pregnancy has occurred more often in women with type 1 diabetes than in women with type 2 diabetes (Montoro 93), but data are limited for the latter group. One study reported a frequency of 3.3% in 61 pregnant women with type 2 diabetes (Clausen 05). In two recent series, 6 of 20 and 4 of 11 cases of DKA, respectively, occurred in pregnant women as the first sign of type 2 diabetes diagnosed during gestation (Montoro 93, Schneider 03). Predisposing factors for DKA during pregnancy include omission of insulin doses, insulin pump "failure" (usually patient related), infection, vomiting and dehydration, diabetic gastroparesis, and obstetrical use of beta-sympathomimetic drugs and glucocorticoids (Borberg 78, VanLierde 82, Berrnstein 90, Tibaldi 90, Rodgers 91, Kilvert 93, Montoro 93, Kamalkannan 03, Schneider 03).

In pregnancy, DKA jeopardizes both maternal and fetal survival. Although uncommon, maternal death due to DKA is still reported (Whiteman 96, Evers 04a), and fetal mortality ranges from 9% to 35% (Kilvert 93, Cullen 96, Carroll 05), mostly in cases presenting with a dead fetus on admission (Montoro 93, Schneider 03). The mechanisms of fetal death probably include impaired uterine blood flow with maternal dehydration and metabolic acidosis (Blechner 75), transfer of keto- and lactic acids across the placenta, decline in fetal oxygen content with severe hyperglycemia, possible impaired fetal oxygen delivery with phosphate deficiency, and possible fetal cardiac irregularities due to deficient potassium (Miodovnik 82a,b, Chauhan 95, Whiteman 96, Takahashi 00, Kamalakannan 03). It is reassuring that fetal death is unlikely once appropriate treatment for DKA is initiated in spite of poor fetal HR variability and late decelerations, which resolve with intensified management (LoBue 78, Rhodes 84, Hughes 87, Montoro 93, Hagay 94b, Greco 00).

Improved maternal and fetal outcomes of DKA require a high index of suspicion and prompt diagnosis. Classic symptoms of DKA include dry mouth, thirst, nausea, vomiting, abdominal pain, polyuria, weakness, change in mental status, and labored breathing (Chauhan 95, Cullen 96, Carroll 05). Classic signs include evidence of dehydration and intravascular volume depletion, fruity breath, and rapid deep respirations. Diagnosis of DKA is confirmed by laboratory documentation of hyperglycemia, anion gap acidosis, arterial pH <7.3, and ketonemia or ketonuria (Laffel 99). Initial clinical and laboratory evaluation of patients with suspected DKA is outlined in Table II.2 (Kitabchi 06, Bull 07). Anticipated deficits include total body water 6 L or 100 mL/kg, sodium 7–10 mEq/kg, chloride 3–5 mEq/kg, potassium 3–5 mEq/kg, phosphate

TABLE II.2 Initial Clinical and Laboratory Evaluation of Patients with Suspected Diabetic Ketoacidosis

- Assess volume status by checking mentation, BP and HR, core temperature, skin turgor, and urine output by in-dwelling catheter.
- Monitor fetal HR and uterine contractions continuously.
- Immediate measurement of plasma glucose, urine ketones by dipstick, urinalysis, plasma beta-hydroxybutyrate, arterial blood gases, serum ketones, complete blood count (leukocytosis proportional to blood ketone concentration; if WBC >25,000, suspect infection), blood urea nitrogen, creatinine (can be elevated by acetoacetate in colorimetric assay), electrolytes (with calculated anion gap; $[Na^+ - (Cl^- + HCO_3^-)]$; normal 7–9 mEq/L with current ion-specific electrode methodology; check local laboratory normal ranges for electrolytes; correct serum sodium for hyperglycemia: for each 100 mg/dL glucose >100 mg/dL, add 1.6 mEq to sodium value for corrected serum sodium value), calcium, magnesium, phosphate, and effective osmolality, ignoring freely permeable urea concentration (2[measured Na (mEq/L)] + [glucose (mg/dL)]/18).
- ECG, chest X-ray with abdomen shielded, urine, sputum, or blood cultures as clinically indicated.
- A1C allows interpretation of previously undiagnosed or poorly controlled diabetes or truly acute episode in an otherwise well-controlled patient.
- Serum amylase and lipase may be elevated in DKA without pancreatitis.

BP, blood pressure; DKA, diabetic ketoacidosis; ECG, electrocardiogram; HR, heart rate; WBC, white blood count.

Based on ADA 04a, Montoro 04, ACOG 05, Kitabchi 06, and Bull 07.

5–7 mEq/kg, calcium 1–2 mEq/kg, and magnesium 1–2 mEq/kg (Kitabchi 06). Low initial serum sodium reflects osmotic flux of water from the intracellular to the extracellular space with hyperglycemia; elevated sodium reflects a profound degree of water loss (Kitabchi 06). Elevated serum potassium is due to an extracellular shift of potassium caused by insulin deficiency, hypertonicity, and academia. "Patients with low normal or low serum potassium concentration on admission have severe total-body potassium deficiency and require very careful cardiac monitoring and more vigorous potassium replacement, because treatment lowers potassium further and can provoke cardiac dysrhythmia" (Kitabchi 06). In pregnancy, 10–30% of DKA cases have been reported to occur with moderately elevated glucose levels (<250 mg/dL) (Montoro 93, Cullen 96). For that reason, diabetic pregnant women with moderate hyperglycemia, nausea, vomiting, and poor oral intake should be evaluated for KTA.

DKA is best managed according to protocols in hospital critical care units with experience in monitoring high-risk pregnancies (Whiteman 96, Bull 07). All treatment protocols for DKA are based on correcting intra- and extravascular volume depletion; supplying insulin (after exclusion of hypokalemia) by infusion; carefully monitoring serum electrolytes, calcium, magnesium, phosphorous, and blood gases or venous pH, which should be repeated every 2–4 h in more severe cases; correcting electrolyte imbalances with sodium and potassium infusion; and identifying and treating precipitating factors. The basic steps in management are outlined in Table II.3 (Montoro 04, ACOG 05, Carroll 05, Kitabchi 06, Bull 07). This protocol is somewhat modified from the ADA Consensus Statement for DKA in adults due to the increased insulin resistance and blood volume of pregnancy. Controlled trials have shown no benefit from administration of bicarbonate or phosphate except in severe cases (Wilson 82, Becker 83, Fisher 83, Hale 84, Morris 86, Okuda 96, Green 98). The reader is referred to excellent reviews for the important details (Chauhan 95, Whiteman 96, Kitabchi 01, Carroll 05, Kitabchi 06).

TABLE II.3 Management of DKA During Pregnancy

IV Fluids: Isotonic sodium chloride; total replacement 4–6 L in first 12 h.
- Insert intravenous catheters. Maintain hourly flow sheet for fluids and electrolytes, potassium, insulin, laboratory results.
- Administer normal saline (0.9% NaCl) at 1.0–2.0 L/h for first hour.
- Infuse normal saline at 250–500 mL/h depending on hydration state × 8 h. If serum sodium is elevated, use half-normal saline (0.45% NaCl).
- When plasma or serum glucose reaches 200 mg/dL, change to 5% dextrose with 0.45% NaCl at 150–250 mL/h.
- After 8 h, use half-normal saline at 125 mL/h.

Potassium: Establish adequate renal function (urine output ~50 mL/h).
- If serum potassium is <3.3 mEq/L, hold insulin and give 20–30 mEq K$^+$/h until K$^+$ >3.3 mEq/L or is being corrected.
- If serum K$^+$ is >3.3 mEq/L but <5.3 mEq/L, give 20–30 mEq K$^+$ in each liter of i.v. fluid to keep serum K$^+$ between 4–5 mEq/L.
- If serum K$^+$ is >5.3 mEq/L, do not give K$^+$, but check serum K$^+$ every 2 h.

Insulin: Use Regular insulin intravenously.
- Loading dose: 0.1–0.2 units/kg i.v. bolus depending on plasma glucose 150–299 mg/dL or ≥300 mg/dL.
- Begin continuous insulin infusion at 0.1 units/kg/h.
- If plasma or serum glucose does not fall by 50–70 mg/dL in first hour, double insulin infusion every hour until a steady glucose decline is achieved.
- When plasma or serum glucose reaches 200 mg/dL, reduce insulin infusion to 0.05–0.1 units/kg/h.
- Keep plasma or serum glucose between 100 and 150 mg/dL until resolution of DKA.

Assess need for bicarbonate:
- pH >7.0: No HCO$_3$
- pH 6.9–7.0: Dilute NaHCO$_3$ (50 mmol) in 200 mL H$_2$O with 10 mEq KCl and infuse over 1 h. Repeat NaHCO$_3$ administration every 2 h until pH >7.0. Monitor serum K$^+$.
- pH <6.9: Dilute NaHCO$_3$ (100 mmol) in 400 mL H$_2$O with 20 mEq KCl and infuse for 2 h. Repeat NaHCO$_3$ administration every 2 h until pH >7.0. Monitor serum K$^+$.

DKA, diabetic ketoacidosis; i.v., intravenous.
Based on ADA 04a, Montoro 04, ACOG 05, Kitabchi 06, Bull 07.

Studies of DKA in pregnancy are observational, and thus guidelines are based on trials in nonpregnant patients and aggregate clinical experience. Continuous fetal HR monitoring and biophysical assessment are important to assess fetal well-being, but immediate delivery is usually not necessary for ominous patterns because many studies indicate that correction of DKA reverts the patterns to normal (Hagay 94, Chauhan 95, Whiteman 96). Immediate delivery carries the further risk of surgery in a metabolically compromised mother.

Prevention of DKA is paramount in pregnancy due to the possibility of fetal mortality. Patient education about sick day management, frequent blood glucose testing, increased insulin doses, and the significance of vomiting and dehydration is of utmost importance (Montoro 04). Use of reagent strips for urinary ketones when blood glucose levels are high or with intercurrent illness can help in the early identification of DKA when the occasional prior ketonuria associated with pregnancy has been absent (Kamalkannan 03). The opportunity for round-the-clock communication with clinical staff is vital.

Recommendations

- All women with type 1 diabetes who are planning pregnancy, all pregnant women with type 1 diabetes, and those with type 2 diabetes and GDM who are determined to be at risk for DKA should be educated about DKA, self monitoring of blood glucose and urine ketones, and DKA prevention with SMBG, MNT, appropriate insulin therapy, and sick day management. (A)

- Providers should maintain a high index of suspicion for DKA in diabetic pregnant women with nausea, vomiting, abdominal pain, fever, and poor oral intake. (A)

- Teach the pregnant patient to perform urine ketone measurements at times of illness or when persistent glucose levels are >200 mg/dL. Positive values should be reported promptly. (E)

- Protocols for management of DKA during pregnancy should include correction of volume depletion, insulin infusion, monitoring and correcting electrolyte imbalances, identifying and treating precipitating factors, and continuous fetal monitoring. (A)

- Initial DKA care is best given in intensive or special care units with experience in the monitoring of high-risk pregnancies. (E)

MATERNAL HYPOGLYCEMIA

—— Original contribution by William H. Herman MD, MPH and John L. Kitzmiller MD

Hypoglycemia is the most common and important adverse effect associated with intensive treatment of type 1 diabetes (DCCT 91, Cryer 03) and is a limiting factor in achieving optimal glycemic control in women with type 2 diabetes requiring insulin treatment (Gerich 00, Holstein 03, Zammit 05). As noted in Part I, all regimens of intensified insulin treatment produce periods of nonphysiological hyperinsulinemia. In a population-based study in Scotland, the frequency of self-reported hypoglycemia was 43 events/patient/year in type 1 diabetes compared with 16 events/patient/year in insulin-treated type 2 diabetes. The frequency of severe hypoglycemia requiring assistance was 1.2 events/patient/year in type 1 diabetes compared with 0.3 events/patient/year in insulin-treated type 2 diabetes (Donnelly 05). Similar frequencies were noted in patients with type 2 diabetes in Denmark (Akram 06) and in the U.K. (Henderson 03, Leese 03, UKHSG 07). Basal and prandial insulin-treated patients with type 2 diabetes self-reported hypoglycemic events at an annual rate of 5.3% during 6 years of management in the U.K. Prospective Diabetes Study Group (UKPDS) (Wright 06). In the DCCT, severe hypoglycemic episodes occurred in 216 of 817 subjects (26.4%) with type 1 diabetes recruited at ages 13–39 years, even though volunteers with a history of recurrent episodes of seizure or coma without warning symptoms of hypoglycemia were excluded (DCCT 91). The incidence of severe hypoglycemia in females was 58.7 events per 100 patient-years in the intensive treatment group and 23.3 events per 100 patient-years in the conventional treatment group. Nocturnal episodes were common in the DCCT: 43% of severe episodes occurred from midnight to 8 a.m., and

55% occurred during sleep at any time. In 51% of events while awake, symptoms of hypoglycemia were not recognized at the time of hypoglycemia. These episodes (including coma or seizures) were more common in the intensified treatment group (DCCT 91). Because intensified diabetes treatment is proven to reduce albuminuria, retinopathy, neuropathy, CVD, and fetal malformations (DCCT 93,95a, 96a, DCCT/EDIC 03a, 05), it is crucial to understand the pathophysiology of hypoglycemia and the means of prevention of this potentially fatal complication.

Symptoms of Hypoglycemia

Symptoms of hypoglycemia may be idiosyncratic, but they are generally grouped as neurogenic–autonomic (anxiety, nausea, palpitations, tremor, sweating, warmth), neuroglycopenic (difficulty in thinking, confusion, dizziness, headache, behavioral changes, seizure, coma), and nonspecific (blurred vision, hunger, weakness) (Hepburn 91, 92, Cox 93, Towler 93, Amiel 94, ADA 05). Evidence states that the adrenergic and cholinergic neurogenic symptoms are largely the result of sympathetic neural, rather than adrenomedullary, activation and that plasma norepinephine response and hemodynamic responses to hypoglycemia are largely the result of adrenomedullary activation (DeRosa 04). In normal subjects with insulin-induced hypoglycemia, activation of glucagon, epinephrine, norepinephrine, and growth hormone secretion began at arterialized venous plasma glucose concentrations of 65–68 mg/dL. Autonomic symptoms (anxiety, palpitations, sweating, irritability, tremor) began at 58 ± 2 (SEM) mg/dL, neuroglycopenic symptoms (dizziness, tingling, difficulty thinking, faintness) began at 51 ± 3 mg/dL, and deterioration in cognitive function tests began at 49 ± 2 mg/dL (Mitrakou 91). These results correspond with those of numerous other studies.

Pathophysiology

In type 1 diabetes and longstanding, insulin-treated type 2 diabetes, compromised physiological defenses against falling glucose concentrations are the result of the pathophysiology of glucose counterregulation and hypoglycemia-associated autonomic failure (Gerich 73, Amiel 87, Bischof 01, Cryer 04, ADA 05), which can have dramatic effects on the management of diabetes during pregnancy (Diamond 92, Rosenn 96, Bjorklund 98). The physiological and behavioral defenses against iatrogenic hypoglycemia in diabetes are illustrated in Figure II.1 (Cryer 06). The pathophysiology in insulin-deficient patients includes impairment of all three normal key defenses: (a) insulin levels do not decrease, (b) glucagon levels do not increase, and (c) the glycemic threshold for epinephrine secretion is shifted to a lower plasma glucose concentration (ADA 05). Failure of glucagon secretion to increase is likely due to a decrease in intraislet insulin and absence of the normal intra-islet decrease-of-insulin signal to the α-cell (Cryer 05, Gosmanov 05, Israelian 05, Raju 05). It is of interest that the glucagon response to exercise is preserved in type 1 diabetes, suggesting the stimulus-specific nature of the α-cell defect with repeated hypoglycemia (Galassetti 04).

Antecedent hypoglycemia shifts the glycemic thresholds for the sympathoadrenal, symptomatic, and cognitive dysfunction responses to lower plasma glucose concentrations (Dagogo-Jack 93, Veneman 93, Ovalle 98). The mechanisms of the hypoglycemia-induced downward shift of the glycemic thresholds that are sensed in the periphery (portal vein and carotid bodies) as well as the forebrain and hindbrain are not known. Current hypotheses (Cryer 05) include: (1) hypoglycemia-induced cortisol levels (or

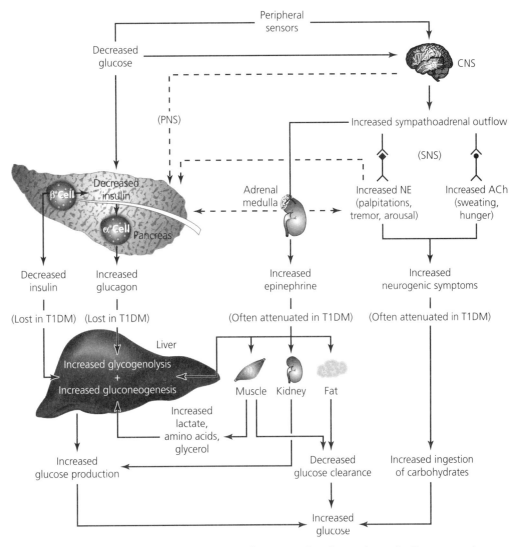

FIGURE II.1 Physiological and behavioral defenses against hypoglycemia. Decrements in insulin and increments in glucagon are lost, and increments in epinephrine and neurogenic symptoms are often attenuated in insulin-deficient diabetes (type 1 and longstanding type 2 diabetes). α-Cell, pancreatic islet α-cells; ACh, acetylcholine; β-Cell, pancreatic islet β-cells; CNS, central nervous system; NE, norepinephrine; PNS, parasympathetic nervous system; SNS, sympathetic nervous system. Modified from Cryer 06 and used with permission.

those of another systemic factor) that act on the brain to reduce sympathoadrenal responses to a given level of subsequent hypoglycemia (unlikely) (Davis 96, McGregor 02, Raju 03); (2) recent antecedent hypoglycemia upregulates blood–brain barrier transporters with increased fuel transport into the brain, which reduces responses to subsequent hypoglycemia (unlikely for glucose transport) (Brooks 86, Grill 90, Boyle 95, Segel 01, Mason 04); (3) recent antecedent hypoglycemia in some way alters brain metabolism and/or signaling, which ultimately results in reduced CNS-mediated responses to subsequent hypoglycemia (Borge 03, Evans 04, McCrimmon 04, Cryer 05); and (4) brain glycogen supercompensation after hypoglycemia, in which brain astrocyte glycogen rebounds to levels higher than before hypoglycemia and provides an expanded source of glycolytic and ultimately neuronal oxidative fuel, such as lactate, that reduces the sympathoadrenal response to a given level of subsequent hypoglycemia (Cryer 05). Recent evidence mentions altered neural insulin signaling (Fisher 05) or induction of hypothalamic genes by hypoglycemia (Mastaitis 05) as contributors to impaired sympathoadrenal counterregulation, but none of these approaches have been applied to study counterregulation in pregnancy. Clinical factors (imperfect insulin replacement, delayed or missed meals, increased physical activity, sleep, antecedent hypoglycemia) enhancing the reduced neuroendocrine responses to hypoglycemia are illustrated in Figure II.2 (Cryer 05).

Evidence also states that peripheral tissue responses to hypoglycemia may be abnormal in patients with insulin-deficient diabetes. Intensively treated patients with type 1 diabetes (mean AIC 6.7), without autonomic neuropathy or a history of hypoglycemia unawareness but with similar basal glucose, insulin, and epinephrine levels, had diminished effects of physiological levels of epinephrine on systolic BP, hepatic glucose production, glucose uptake, and lipolysis compared with conventionally treated patients (mean A1C 9.6) and nondiabetic controls (Guy 05a,b). The authors speculated that repetitive hypoglycemia and exposure to endogenous epinephrine might downregulate β1-adrenergic or β2-adrenergic receptors at the target organs, an idea for which there is conflicting

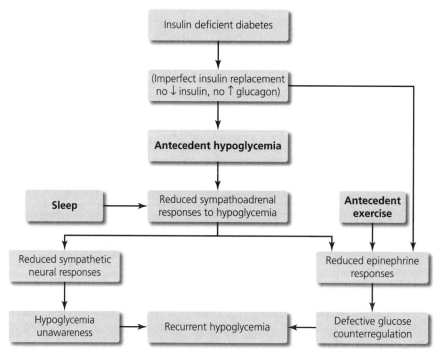

FIGURE II.2 Hypoglycemia-associated autonomic failure found in insulin-deficient diabetes mellitus. Lack of insulin decrement and glucagon increment refers to islet cell secretion. Based on Cryer 05 and used with permission.

evidence (Berlin 88, Trovik 94, Trovik 95, Fritsche 98, Korytskowski 98, Schwab 04, DeGalan 06). Hepatic glycogenolysis provides for endogenous glucose production during insulin-induced hypoglycemia in controls, but intensively treated patients with type 1 diabetes (mean A1C 6.5) and limited increases in plasma epinephrine and norepinephrine during hypoglycemia demonstrated no quantitative change in hepatic glycogen and no recovery of endogenous glucose production compared with controls after 90 min of blood glucose clamped at 60 mg/dL (Kishore 06). Catecholamine-stimulated lipolysis with delayed rise in plasma glycerol and FFAs contributes to protective stimulation of gluconeogenesis and suppression of glucose oxidation in healthy subjects with insulin-induced hypoglycemia (~54 mg/dL) (Fanelli 92,93a). However, the defective activation of skeletal muscle and adipose tissue lipolysis during experimental hypoglycemia in type 1 diabetes is thought to be due to deficient release of catecholamines rather than impaired adrenergic responsiveness (Enoksson 03, Bernroider 05).

Regarding type 2 diabetes, low-glucose thresholds for release of epinephrine and norepinephrine are higher in noninsulin-treated patients with type 2 compared with type 1 diabetes and glucagon secretion is usually preserved (Levy 98, Bischof 00, Spyer 00), but this comparison has not been made during early pregnancy in type 2 diabetes patients placed on insulin therapy. Poor glycemic control in type 2 diabetes leads to even higher glycemic thresholds for autonomic and symptomatic responses to hypoglycemia (Segel 02). With progressive insulin deficiency in type 2 diabetes, middle-aged patients exposed to hypoglycemia develop delayed and reduced decreases in insulin secretion, impaired increases of plasma glucagon and GH, and impaired symptomatic awareness similar to type 1 diabetes (Zammitt 05, Israelian 06). Recent antecedent hypoglycemia in longstanding type 2 diabetes also shifts glycemic thresholds for autonomic (including adrenomedullary epinephrine) and symptomatic responses to subsequent hypoglycemia to lower plasma glucose concentrations (Segel 02).

Gender differences are noted in the responses to hypoglycemia. Control and diabetic women have reduced neuroendocrine and autonomic nervous system responses to insulin-induced hypoglycemia compared with men (Amiel 93a, Davis 93, Diamond 93, Davis 00a,b). Estrogen blunted the neuroendocrine and metabolic responses to insulin-induced hypoglycemia in nondiabetic postmenopausal women (Sandoval 03). The differential gender responses to hypoglycemia may be related to lower muscle sympathetic nerve activity during hypoglycemia (altered CNS drive), but are not due to differential glycemic thresholds for responses in women and men (Davis 00c). There were no differences in reported autonomic or neuroglycopenic symptom scores during insulin-induced hypoglycemia in control or type 1 diabetic women compared with men (Geddes 06). In one study of healthy subjects, antecedent hypoglycemia produced less blunting of counterregulatory responses to subsequent hypoglycemia in women than in men (Davis 00a), and the authors speculated that could relate to the lack of difference in the frequency of hypoglycemia in men and women during the DCCT (DCCT 91). Antecedent hypoglycemia moderately reduces the expected glucagon response to subsequent exercise in women with type 1 diabetes, whereas the response is completely abolished in male patients (Galassetti 04). Regarding pregnancy, we lack sufficient data on the central or peripheral mechanisms of hypoglycemia counterregulation or modifications of hypoglycemia unawareness in women with diabetes.

Cardiac responses to hyperinsulinemic hypoglycemia (36–54 mg/dL; 2–3 mM) in type 1 diabetes include HR of 11 bpm, stroke volume of 9 mL, CO of 1.8 L/min, increased left volume ejection fraction of 11%, and peak filling rate of ~25%. This augmentation of systolic and diastolic left ventricular function was similar to that seen in hyperinsulinemic euglycemia in diabetic subjects, but of less intensity than that in hyperinsulinemic control subjects. The increases in cardiac function were thought to reflect both insulin-mediated sympathetic activation and peripheral vasodilation (Fisher 90, Russell 01). Another study of insulin-induced controlled hypoglycemia (54, then 36 mg/dL; 3, then 2 mM) produced an increase in supine HR of 8 bpm and progressive reductions of the high-frequency spectral component and beat-to-beat HR variability (reductions of cardiac vagal outflow) in type 1 diabetes and control subjects (Koivikko 05). These data raise the question whether cardiac autonomic irregularities exacerbated by hypoglycemia (Marques 97) contribute to unexplained deaths in patients with type 1 diabetes (dead-in-bed syndrome) (Tatterrsall 91, Sovik 99, Weston 99). Simultaneous 72-hour continuous glucose and cardiac monitoring in 19 insulin-treated patients with type 2 diabetes and CHD (mean age 50 years; duration 13 years) revealed 54 hypoglycemic episodes (<70 mg/dL), half of which were asymptomatic. Ten of the symptomatic episodes were accompanied by angina, including four with ECG abnormalities (Desouza 03).

Hypoglycemia Unawareness

The attenuated sympathetic neural activation found in intensively treated diabetes also causes the clinical syndrome of impaired awareness of hypoglycemia (degrees of unawareness), i.e., loss of the warning symptoms that previously allowed the patient to recognize developing hypoglycemia and take corrective action (Amiel 94, ADA 05, Cryer 05). This process is induced by recent antecedent iatrogenic hypoglycemia, which can cause a vicious cycle of recurrent hypoglycemia (Cryer 04, ADA 05). However, hypoglycemia unawareness is reversible in most affected patients by several weeks of meticulous avoidance of iatrogenic hypoglycemia, and the reduced epinephrine component of defective counterregulation can be variably improved (Fanelli 93b, Amiel 94, Cranston 94, Dagogo-Jack 94, Fanelli 94, ADA 05). It is presumed but not proven that such benefit can be obtained in pregnant patients with type 1 diabetes. The syndromes of defective glucose counterregulation and hypoglycemia without warning symptoms are forms of hypoglycemia-associated autonomic failure in patients with type 1 and advanced type 2 diabetes, and there is evidence that both syndromes are caused by recent episodes of hypoglycemia (Cryer 04). Additional forms of exercise-related and sleep-related hypoglycemia-associated autonomic failure are discussed in recent reviews (Cryer 03,04,05), as well as strategies to minimize the risk of hypoglycemia while improving glycemic control (Cryer 01).

Prevention of Hypoglycemia

There are limited studies of foods to prevent or correct hypoglycemia in patients with type 1 diabetes. Comparison of snacks of bread (15 gm carbohydrate, 85 kcal) versus bread plus boiled ham (205 kcal) given at a clamped glucose of 50 mg/dL (2.8 mM) in midmorning showed no difference in the ability to raise plasma glucose to 72 mg/dL (4 mM) in patients with type 1 diabetes (mean age 34 years, mean duration 11 years, mean glycohemoglobin 2.0% above upper limit of normal). Time to peak glucose was faster with the bread plus meat snack (30 ± 3 min vs. 54 ± 8 min), and the snack with protein did elicit an increase in plasma glucagon over 15–90 min. The subsequent decline in plasma glucose over 2 h did not differ between the two snacks (Gray 96).

The frequency of nocturnal hypoglycemia was assessed in a nonrandomized comparison of no bedtime snack versus a conventional snack at 2200 h (200 kcal, 26 gm carbohydrate, 6 gm fat, 11 gm protein) versus a cornstarch bar (194 kcal, 39 gm carbo-hydrate, 4 gm fat, 4 gm protein) versus 5 mg oral terbutaline in 21 patients with type 1 diabetes (mean age 26 years, mean duration 15 years, mean A1C 7.1) using a variety of insulin regimens (NPH, glargine, CSII). In the absence of a bedtime snack, mean plasma glucose (MPG) declined from 122 ± 11 mg/dL (7 ± 0.6 mM) at 2200 h to 99 ± 12 mg/dL (5.5 ± 0.7 mM) at 0230 h and 106 ± 14 mg/dL (5.9 ± 0.8 mM) at 0700 h; 43% of the patients had nocturnal glucose <60 mg/dL (3.3 mM). With the bedtime snack, MPG at 2200 h was ~108 mg/dL (~6 mM) (SD not provided), rose to ~130 mg/dL (7.2 mM) at 0230 h, and was ~105 mg/dL (~5.8 mM) at 0700 h; 33% of patients had nocturnal plasma glucose <60 mg/dL (3.3 mM) (NS). The cornstarch bar showed no advantage compared with the conventional bedtime snack, and terbuta-line reduced the frequency of nocturnal glucose at <60 mg/dL (3.3 mM) to 5% at the expense of MPG at 198 mg/dL (11 mM) at 0500 h (Raju 06). This study does not address the effect of a bedtime snack if overnight insulin is used to target the 0700-h plasma glucose at 60–99 mg/dL (3.3-5.5 mM), as recommended in pregnancy.

A randomized, placebo-controlled crossover trial compared no snack (aspartame placebo) with a bedtime snack (191 kcal, 30 gm carbohydrate, 3 gm fat, 11 gm protein) in 15 subjects with type 1 diabetes (mean age 41 years, mean duration 23 years, mean A1C 8.1) (Kalergis 03). If bedtime plasma glucose was <126 mg/dL (7 mM), mean overnight nadir glucose was 58 ± 9 mg/dL (3.2 ± 0.5 mM) with no snack and 122 ± 34 mg/dL (6.8 ± 1.9 mM) with the bedtime snack (p < 0.025). No overnight hypogly-cemic episodes (<72 mg/dL; <4 mM) occurred with the bedtime snack, but 11 epi-sodes occurred in 11 subjects taking placebo. At bedtime, glucose concentrations <126 mg/dL (<7 mM) and having no snack resulted in 67% of nights with ≥1 episode of hypoglycemia but no morning hyperglycemia (>180 mg/dL; >10 mM). At bedtime, glucose concentrations of 126–180 mg/dL (7–10 mM) and having no snack resulted in 33% of nights with nocturnal hypoglycemia and no morning hyperglycemia (Kalergis 03). Controlled studies of the effects of daytime or bedtime snacks on severe hypoglyc-emia are needed in pregnancies complicated by both type 1 and type 2 diabetes.

Classification of Hypoglycemia

The ADA Workgroup on Hypoglycemia recently defined and classified the following types of hypoglycemic episodes: (a) *severe hypoglycemia* is an event requiring the assist-ance of another person to administer carbohydrate or glucagon or to take other resusci-tative actions; (b) *documented symptomatic hypoglycemia* is an event during which typical symptoms of hypoglycemia are accompanied by a measured plasma glucose concentra-tion ≤70 mg/dL (3.9 mM); (c) *asymptomatic hypoglycemia* is an event not accompanied by typical symptoms but with a measured plasma glucose concentration ≤70 mg/dL; (d) *probable symptomatic hypoglycemia* (typical symptoms not accompanied by a plasma glucose measurement) (ADA 05). The glucose threshold of ≤70 mg/dL was chosen because antecedent plasma glucose concentrations at that level reduce sympathoadrenal responses to subsequent hypoglycemia, and the declining glycemic threshold for activa-tion of glucagon and epinephrine secretion is normally 65–70 mg/dL in nondiabetic nonpregnant individuals (ADA 05). The Workgroup also discussed the occurrence of relative symptomatic hypoglycemia accompanied by a measured plasma glucose con-centration >70 mg/dL, recognizing that "patients with chronically poor glycemic con-trol can experience symptoms of hypoglycemia as plasma glucose concentrations decline toward 70 mg/dL" (ADA 05).

Hypoglycemia in Pregnancy

There is strong evidence that normal postabsorptive plasma glucose declines by 10 mg/dL during early pregnancy (see Part I) and some evidence that the threshold for secretion of counterregulatory hormones is 48–57 mg/dL during normal gestation (Diamond 92, Bjorklund 98). Therefore, it is reasonable to use a threshold of <60 mg/dL (3.3 mM) to define documented symptomatic or asymptomatic hypoglycemia during pregnancy. In the following studies, different thresholds were used for definitions of these classes of hypoglycemia, yet all investigators used the standard definition for severe hypoglycemia of need for assistance. However, it is recognized that estimations of the frequency of severe hypoglycemia depend on patient or family recall in most clinical situations.

Of DCCT female subjects becoming pregnant, the percentage of women with a severe hypoglycemic event during gestation was 17.0% in 94 women in the original intensive therapy group and 19.8% in 86 women in the original conventional treatment group (of whom 26 converted to intensive therapy prior to conception; the rest converted after pregnancy was diagnosed). This compares with a frequency of severe hypoglycemia in 23–30% of subjects in the intensive treatment group in any given year of the DCCT study. Within both treatment groups throughout the DCCT, the strongest predictor of future risk of severe hypoglycemia was the number of prior episodes (DCCT 97b). Adolescents, subjects with totally deficient endogenous insulin secretion, and subjects with lower current A1C levels were also at increased risk, but a history of severe hypoglycemia and lower A1C levels accounted for only 9% of future episodes of severe hypoglycemia in the DCCT (DCCT 97b). During pregnancy, events occurred more than once in 5 of 16 women experiencing severe hypoglycemia in the original intensive therapy group and in 7 of 17 women in the original conventional therapy group. The event rate for severe hypoglycemia expressed per 100 pregnant months (no. events/total no. pregnancy months) was 2.8 in 135 pregnancies in the original intensive therapy group, 2.0 in 52 pregnancies converted to intensive therapy before conception, and 5.0 in 83 pregnancies of women converted after conception (p = 0.043) (DCCT 96). Two nonrandomized prospective studies of pregnancies in diabetic women using intensified preconception care reported low occurrences of severe hypoglycemic episodes in the first 8 weeks gestation (2 of 84 women and 2 of 25 women, respectively) but higher frequencies of documented symptomatic hypoglycemia (58% and 44%, respectively), with many women having more than two episodes per week (Steel 90, Kitzmiller 91).

Higher frequencies of severe hypoglycemia (29–45%) have been reported in other studies of pregnancy complicated by type 1 diabetes (Rayburn 86, Kimmerle 92, Rosenn 95a, Vaarasmaki 00b, Nielsen 08). In a recent prospective national survey of all type 1 diabetes pregnancies in 1 year in the Netherlands, 41% of 264 women were affected by severe hypoglycemia during the first trimester and 19% reported severe hypoglycemia when reassessed during the third trimester (Evers 04a). In a separate analysis of this study, 25% of the women reported severe hypoglycemia in the 4 months before conception, and the average occurrence of severe hypoglycemia was 0.9 episodes/last 4 months before gestation in 278 women with type 1 diabetes compared with 2.6 episodes/4 months in the first trimester (p < 0.001). The proportion of women with hypoglycemic coma prior to pregnancy was 9% compared with 19% in the first trimester, and the proportion with reduced hypoglycemia unawareness was 16% prior to pregnancy and 35% in the first trimester (Evers 02). The peak incidence of severe hypoglycemia in pregnancy occurs between 8 and 15 weeks gestation

(Kitzmiller 91,92, Rosenn 95, Nielsen 08), and asymptomatic documented nocturnal hypoglycemia is especially common (Hellmuth 00). Among pregnant women with type 1 diabetes, severe hypoglycemia is independently associated with history of severe hypoglycemia before gestation, slightly higher insulin dose, slightly lower A1C, and longer duration of diabetes (Evers 02, Nielsen 08). Using SMBG data of premeal and bedtime testing in a study comparing pregnant women with type 1 diabetes with pregnant women with type 2 diabetes, 19% of observation days had at least one value <50 mg/dL (2.8 mM) in 46 patients with type 1 diabetes compared with 2% of days in 113 patients with type 2 diabetes (Sacks 97).

Maternal hypoglycemia can be life threatening, and hypoglycemic deaths and deaths due to unintentional injuries associated with maternal hypoglycemia have been reported. Some evidence reports that recurrent severe hypoglycemia is associated with a decline in cognitive function in adults with type 1 diabetes (Wredling 90, Langan 91, Amiel 93b, Ryan 93), but specific studies of this outcome in pregnancy are lacking. Potential effects of maternal hypoglycemia on the fetus are less clear. Although studies of rat and mouse embryos have demonstrated an association between prolonged hypoglycemia and fetal malformations, human studies have not demonstrated any association between maternal hypoglycemic events and adverse fetal outcomes (Mills 88, Steel 90, Kitzmiller 91, Kimmerle 92, Rosenn 95, terBraak 02). Insulin-induced maternal hypoglycemia may result in decreased fetal HR variability without jeopardy to fetal well-being (Stangenberg 83). Two studies of induced hypoglycemia (40–45 mg/dL) in pregnant women with type 1 diabetes failed to demonstrate adverse effects on fetal HR, umbilical artery blood flow by Doppler studies, or fetal breathing or movements detected by US (Reece 95, Bjorklund 96). A single study of the relationship of maternal hypoglycemic events at intervals in the second and third trimesters in diabetic pregnant women did not find an association with measures of intellectual development in the young offspring (Rizzo 91).

Due to the potential for maternal harm from severe hypoglycemia, investigators of intensified glycemic control in pregnancy instituted protocols to minimize the occurrence of maternal hypoglycemia. The principles of care have been reviewed in Part I in the sections titled "Medical Nutrition Therapy," "Insulin Therapy," and "Physical Activity/Exercise and Management of Pregnant Women with Preexisting Diabetes." They include intensive education of patients and significant others, frequent SMBG, proper timing of adequate meals and snacks, correct administration of insulin doses, and careful management of physical activity. Even so, documented symptomatic hypoglycemia will occur four to twelve times per month on average in intensively treated pregnant patients (Mills 88, Steel 90, Kitzmiller 91, Kimmerle 92, Rosenn 95, terBraak 02), but severe hypoglycemia should be less frequent. Some evidence states that use of insulin analogs, especially with CSII by portable pumps, will reduce the frequency of maternal hypoglycemia (see the section titled "Insulin Therapy" in Part I).

Detailed strategies of how to ameliorate the problem of hypoglycemia in intensively treated pregnant patients have been published (Miller 94, Rosenn 95, Bolli 99, Jovanovic 00). Milk (8 oz) or 15 gm glucose tablets may be used to treat moderate symptomatic hypoglycemia with a plasma glucose concentration of 50–59 mg/dL to prevent marked rebound hyperglycemia from excess glucose consumption; the patient should remeasure the glucose concentration in 15–30 min to ensure that the problem is corrected (Miller 94, Whiteman 96). If plasma glucose is <50 mg/dL and the patient is able to swallow, 1 cup orange juice without added sugar will correct hypoglycemia more effectively; the patient should recheck blood glucose in 15 min to determine whether additional treatment is needed. With severe hypoglycemia and an uncooperative patient, a family member or coworker should inject 1 mg glucagon s.c. and call an emergency paramedic service for help with resuscitation. Glucagon injection for severe hypoglycemia in pregnancy was successful in reversing unconsciousness in 11 of 12 circumstances, with fingerstick glucose rising to 100–200 mg/dL within 30 mins of successful therapy. One patient remained stuporous after a single glucagon injection and was taken to the emergency room for glucose infusion before complete recovery (Rayburn 87). Once an unresponsive patient is alert and responsive, a snack or meal should be taken to prevent recurrent hypoglycemia.

Recommendations

- Educate and train all women with PDM who are planning pregnancy or who are already pregnant about the recognition and treatment of hypoglycemia, SMBG, and the need to carry glucose and a card indicating that the individual has insulin-treated diabetes. (E)

- Glucose (15–20 gm) is the preferred treatment for the conscious woman with hypoglycemia, although any measured form of carbohydrate that contains sugar may be used. If SMBG 15 min after treatment shows continued hypoglycemia, treatment should be repeated. Once SMBG glucose returns to normal, the woman should consume a meal or snack to prevent recurrence of hypoglycemia. (E)

- Advise women that the incidence of severe hypoglycemia is likely to increase during early pregnancy. Institution of intensified glycemic control prior to conception may result in a lower rate of severe hypoglycemic events during pregnancy and minimize the frequency of hypoglycemia unawareness. (A)

- Balance physical activity with the timing and amount of insulin doses and carbohydrate intake in meals and snacks to minimize iatrogenic hypoglycemia. (E)

- Teach patients to be aware of their glucose level prior to driving and to correct hypoglycemia before starting out. (E)

- Glucose targets should be raised for patients with hypoglycemia unawareness until the syndrome is reversed by meticulous prevention of hypoglycemic episodes. (E)

THYROID DISORDERS AND DIABETIC PREGNANCY

Original contribution by Martin N Montoro MD and John L. Kitzmiller MD

Definitions and General Prevalence of Hypothyroidism, Thyroid Autoimmunity, and Hyperthyroidism

Recent large population surveys in the U.S. (Canaris 00, Hollowell 02, Aoki 07) and elsewhere (Vanderpump 95, Bjoro 00, Carle 06, Hoogendoorn 06, O'Leary 06) define hypo- and hyperthyroidism according to serum TSH (chemiluminescence immunometric assay sensitive to 0.01 mU/L) and serum total thyroxine (T4) levels (enzyme immunoassay 4.5–13.2 µg/dL; 58–170 nmol/L) or free T4 levels (8–22 pmol/L). The

97.5th percentile for TSH in the female reference population (excluding risk factors) (NHANES III) rises after age 30: 3.59 at 12–19 years, 3.52 at 20–29 years, 3.70 at 30–39 years, 3.92 at 40–49 years, and 4.02 at 50–59 years (Hollowell 02). *Clinical hypothyroidism* defined as TSH >4.5 mU/L and T4 <4.5 µg/dL or report of current treatment was identified in 0.4% of white non-Hispanic individuals (Vanderpump 95, Canaris 02, Hollowell 02), in 0.1% of black non-Hispanic individuals, in 0.2% of Mexican-Americans, and in 0.2% of people of other races (Hollowell 02) In NHANES data collected during 1999 2002, hypothyroidism prevalence (TSH >4.5 mIU/L) was 3.1% in women of reproductive age (Aoki 07). Current debate surrounds the proper reference ranges for TSH and T4 (Andersen 02, Baloch 03, Surks 05, Wartofsky 05, Weiss 08). TSH upper reference limits are skewed upward by increased iodine intake, by inclusion of older or heavier subjects, and by people with occult autoimmune thyroid dysfunction (Bulow-Pedersen 05, Manji 06, DePergola 07, Spencer 07, Surks 07, Fox 08). The individual variation of circulating T4 is narrow and much smaller than the reference range (Andersen 02). *Subclinical hypothyroidism* defined as TSH >4.5 mU/L and T4 >4.5 µg/dL (U.S. disease-free population of 8 million people) was identified in 4.3% of white non-Hispanic individuals, in 1.4% of black non-Hispanic individuals, in 3.6% of Mexican-Americans, and in 3.4% of people of other races (Hollowell 02). TSH levels were measured at health fairs in Colorado (25,862 people, 94.4% white) and found to be elevated >5.1 mU/L in 4.1% of women at 18–24 years, 5.0% at 25–34 years, 6.1% at 35–44 years, and 9.2% at 45–54 years (Canaris 00).

In U.S. females in the NHANES III survey of almost 98 million women (1988–94), thyroid peroxidase antibodies (TPOAbs) were identified in 10.4–12.6% of disease-free women of reproductive age, with TgAb positivity found in 8.5–13.6%. Thyroid autoantibodies were equally common in non-Hispanic white women and Mexican-Americans and half as frequent in non-Hispanic black women. In this national survey, TPOAbs were significantly associated with TSH levels suggestive of hypo- or hyperthyroidism, but thyroglobulin antibodies (TgAbs) were not (Hollowell 02). *Clinical hyperthyroidism* defined as TSH <0.1 mU/L and T4 >13.2 µg/dL or report of current treatment was identified in 0.4–0.6% of white non-Hispanic individuals, in 0.5% of black non-Hispanic individuals, in 0.2% of Mexican-Americans, and in 0.4% of people of other races (Canaris 00, Hollowell 02). *Subclinical hyperthyroidism* defined as TSH <0.1 mU/L and T4 <13.2 µg/dL (U.S. disease-free population; NHANES III) was identified in 0.1% of white non-Hispanic individuals, in 0.4% of black non-Hispanic individuals, in 0.3% of Mexican-Americans, and in 0.3% of people of other races (Hollowell 02).

Thyroid Evaluation Prior to Pregnancy

In preconception screening of all women with type 1 or type 2 diabetes, if TSH is <0.1 mIU/mL or >4.5 mIU/mL, the patient should be evaluated for possible treatment of thyroid disease, which may improve pregnancy outcome (Col 04, Surks 04, Abalovich 07). If only the TPO titer is elevated, a TSH should be repeated during pregnancy at ~7–8, 12–14, and then at 20 weeks (Abalovich 07). The following evidence supports this position. Many young adult women with type 1 diabetes (30–60%) will eventually develop chronic autoimmune thyroid disease (more prevalent in women than men) (Betterle 84, Frasier 86, Cardoso 95, Fernandez-Casterner 99, Holl 99a, Kordonouri 02a, Umpierez 03, Barova 04, Gonzales 07). They should therefore all be screened for thyroid dysfunction with a TSH level and TPOAb titer, ideally before pregnancy.

TPOAbs were previously referred to as thyroid antimicrosomal antibodies. Analysis of a cohort of 125 women with type 1 diabetes (mean age 42 ± 5 years) followed from childhood showed 4% with Graves' disease and 41% with Hashimoto's thyroiditis (titers of TgAb or TPOAb >10 U/mL); 41% of the latter group were considered euthyroid with TSH <5.0 mU/L (McCanlies 98). In an early series of 311 women with type 1 diabetes not suspected of thyroid disease, 17% had elevated TSH levels, with increased risk in those with late-onset type 1 diabetes (Gray 80). Of the women with elevated TSH, 11% developed clinical hypothyroidism over a 4-year follow-up and most had thyroid autoimmunity at baseline (Gray 83). Female patients with type 1 diabetes who were followed annually elsewhere with screening examinations had a 12.3% annual risk of developing thyroid disease (Perros 95).

Both of the thyroid autoimmune disorders (Hashimoto's thyroiditis or Graves' disease) and type 1 diabetes have susceptibility genes in common (Sumnik 03, Badenhoop 04, Barker 06). A proportion of diabetic women with autoimmunity to TPO will also have antibodies against TgAbs; $\sim$60% of women with both autoantibodies will have hypoechogenicity of the thyroid on US examination. In young adults with type 1 diabetes, all patients with repeated positivity of both thyroid autoantibodies developed subclinical hypothyroidism within 4 years; the frequency was 11% in those with isolated anti-TPO positivity (Vondra 04). TSH levels were highest in young diabetic women with both thyroid autoantibodies positive (Kordonouri 02a,b). In a series of 301 girls with type 1 diabetes who were followed in Berlin, 19% developed autoimmune thyroiditis, with thyroid hormone replacement required in 67% of this group (Kordonouri 05). Female patients with type 1 diabetes and thyroid autoimmunity are also at increased risk for celiac disease (De Block 01, Jaeger 01, Collin 02, Kaspers 04, Glastras 05, Barker 06, Goodwin 06) and gastric PCAs (Riley 82, Perros 00) Celiac disease and autoimmune atrophic gastritis are discussed in Part I in the section titled "Medical Nutrition Therapy."

Hypothyroidism affects the metabolic management of diabetes and is associated with increased frequency of hypoglycemia in type 1 diabetes (Mohn 02, Vondra 05). Conversely, glucose uptake in muscle and adipose tissue is resistant to insulin in nondiabetic subjects with hypothyroidism (Rochon 03, Dimitriadis 06a). Subclinical hypothyroidism and insulin resistance are associated with reduced HDL-C and elevated total-C and TGs in diabetic and other women (Bakker 01, Chubb 05a). It is possible that treatment of subclinical hypothyroidism with levothyroxine will lower total-C and LDL-C based on data from small RCTs (Danese 00, Meier 01, Carracio 02, Monzani 04, Razvi 07).

Type 2 diabetes patients with or without GAD-antibodies can also develop thyroid autoantibodies (Gambelunghe 00, Vondra 05). Latent autoimmune diabetes mellitus (Davis 00d, Nabhan 05, Palmer 05, Beyan 06, Leslie 06, Reinehr 06) is increasingly recognized in young women with initial clinical appearance of type 2 diabetes but β-cell antibodies present, impaired β-cell function at diagnosis, and slow progression of β-cell failure. Autoimmune diabetes of slow onset is found in 25% of European individuals <35 years of age at diagnosis of diabetes (Stenstrom 05). In cross-sectional studies of newly diagnosed diabetic patients, young women with type 2 diabetes were as likely to have detectable TPOAbs (5–20%) and TgAbs (10–14%) as new type 1 diabetes patients of the same age (Landin-Olsson 92, Hathout 01). Numerous other cross-sectional or longitudinal studies demonstrate that 8.8–19% of women with type 2 diabetes have thyroid autoimmunity (Gambelunghe 00, Matejkova-Behanova 02, Radaideh 04, Chubb 05b) and 8.2–12.5% of subjects have hypothyroidism (subclinical hypothyroidism 4.1–8.6%) (Landin 92, Celani 94, Cardoso 95, Montoro 97, Fernandez-Soto 98, Smithson 98, Ortega-Gonzalez 00, Radaideh 04, Chubb 05b). Due to the increased prevalence of hypothyroidism compared with reference populations, all preconception or pregnant women with type 2 diabetes should be screened for thyroid dysfunction and autoimmunity. Thyroid US surveys of women with type 2 diabetes without overt thyroid disease showed an increased prevalence of thyroid nodules and parenchymatous goiter (Junik 06).

The prevalence of thyroid autoantibodies in U.S. reference populations is somewhat higher than the 6.5% thyroid autoimmunity found in a cohort of 1,660 consecutive pregnancies in Belgium (an area with restricted iodine intake) in 1990–1992: 1.0% had clinical hypothyroidism, 0.2% hyperthyroidism, and 5.3% were euthyroid with positive autoantibodies (3.9% TPOAb positive, 0.85% TgAb positive, 0.55% positive for both autoantibodies but with normal TSH). On sequential monitoring, the frequency of antibody positivity declined with advancing gestation. Of women without thyroid autoimmunity in this study, 20% had undetectable TSH values at the end of the first trimester due to high human chorionic gonadotropin (hCG) levels. Of pregnant women with thyroid autoimmunity, 10% had basal TSH levels at 11 weeks gestation between 3–4 mU/L, but 40% had serum TSH at this level late in the third trimester (16% >4 mU/L) (Glinoer 90,94). A large number of women with TPOAb positivity on screening at 17 weeks gestation developed postpartum thyroid dysfunction and later permanent clinical hypothyroidism (Premawardhana 00).

The current debate regarding screening for thyroid disease (Cooper 04) prior to or during the early pregnancy without diabetes is due to the widely identified association of subclinical hypothyroidism with cognitive deficits in the offspring of women with TSH elevations (Liu 94, Pop 95, Haddow 99, Allan 00, Badawi 00, Zoeller 03, LaFranchi 05). Other authors noted harmful effects of low maternal thyroxinemia at 12 weeks gestation, even with high normal TSH levels (Man 91, Pop 99, Morreale de Escobar 00a, Pop 03, Kooistra 06). Fetal brain development (neuronal multiplication, migration, architectural organization) is dependent on maternal thyroxine until the second trimester (Thorpe-Beeston 91, Fisher 00, Calvo 02, Lavado-Autric 03, Auso 04, Morreale de Escobar 04, Pop 05); later phases of fetal brain development (glial cell multiplication, migration, myelinazation) can also be affected by maternal hypothyroxinemia (Glinoer 00a, Morreale de Escobar 00b, Smallridge 01, Poppe 03). T4 and T3 cross the placenta, but TSH does not (Vulsma 89, Neale 04, Smallridge 05). Transthyretin, a high-affinity thyroid hormone-binding protein, has been identified in human trophoblast and localized to the subapical region of the cell (McKinnon 05). No RCT is available to prove the benefit of levothyroxine supplementation on infant development in the setting of maternal subclinical hypothyroidism. Because a pregnancy complicated by PDM is already a high-risk situation and multiple opportunities for harm exist that may impact the neonate, these provocative data further suggest the value of screening all diabetic women for thyroid dysfunction and autoimmunity, ideally before conception.

There is evidence for a significant association of thyroid autoimmunity with increased rates of spontaneous abortion in each of five unselected population studies, independent of TSH levels (total N 3,696 subjects; crude RR 1.9–4.4) (Stagnaro-Green 90, Glinoer 91, Lejeune 93, Iijima 97, Bagis 01), and in two of four smaller observational studies of women with recurrent early pregnancy loss (Pratt 93, Bussen 95, Esplin 98, Dendrinos 00). The only large study of the latter type observed a pregnancy loss rate of 22.5% in the thyroid autoantibody positive group (autoimmunity in 20.8% of total sample of 900 women with ≥2 consecutive miscarriages) compared with a loss rate of 14.5% in the antibody negative group (p 0.01) (Kutteh 99). A small Pittsburgh cohort of women with type 1 diabetes and euthyroid Hashimoto's thyroiditis reported a history of spontaneous abortion in 61.5% of patients (compared with 29.1% with no thyroid disease, p 0.05; 23.8% were reported with hypothyroid autoimmunity, but some patients were treated (McCanlies 98). Another series of 85 consecutive pregnant patients with type 1 diabetes in Denmark revealed 18.8% with TPOAbs, 2.4% with TgAbs, 50.6% with thyroid-stimulating antibodies, and 27.1% with PCAs. All patients with spontaneous abortions were positive for TPOAbs (Bech 91).

The etiology of increased early pregnancy loss with thyroid autoimmunity remains unknown. Thyroid autoimmunity could be a marker of an underlying generalized autoimmune imbalance leading to "rejection of the fetal graft" (Poppe 03), of reduced thyroid functional reserve with "subclinical" thyroiditis and inability to adapt to the needs of pregnancy (Glinoer 00b,06), or of advanced maternal age. The thyroid hormone hypothesis receives support from two intervention trials (1 small study, 1 large randomized study) in which supplementation with levothyroxine in apparently euthyroid women with thyroid autoimmunity and recurrent pregnancy loss significantly improved pregnancy outcome (Vaquero 00, Negro 06). These studies suggest the importance of preconception evaluation of thyroid status in diabetic women. If hypothyroidism has been diagnosed prior to pregnancy, an international panel (sponsored by the Endocrine Society and several thyroid associations) recommends adjustment of the preconception T4 dose to reach a TSH level ≤2.5 μU/mL before pregnancy (Abalovich 07).

Thyroid Function During Pregnancy

Thyroid balance during pregnancy is affected by hCG stimulation of the TSH receptors, increased free T4 in very early pregnancy, and the large progressive estrogen-induced increase in circulating thyroid binding globulin starting by 8 weeks gestation, with subsequent decline in the percentage of free T4 (Guillaume 85, Glinoer 99, Walker 05). Transition to the pregnancy steady-state requires an increased hormonal output by the maternal thyroid gland. If there is iodine restriction or overt iodine deficiency, the decrease in free thyroid hormone concentrations will be amplified during pregnancy (Glinoer 01). In later pregnancy, increased hormonal demands are maintained until term, "probably through transplacental passage of thyroid hormones and increased turnover of maternal thyroxin (T4), presumably under the influence of the placental (type III) deiodinase" (Glinoer 99). There is risk of hypothyroidism appearing as pregnancy advances because some diabetic women will be unable to compensate for the increased demands on the thyroid during pregnancy (Jovanovic-Peterson 88). In pregnant women who are known to be hypothyroid and dependent on exogenous levothyroxine, the increased (30–60%) thyroxine demand seems to start as early as 5 weeks and reaches a plateau at 16–20 weeks (Mandel 90, Tamaki 90, Alexander 04).

If there has been no preconception evaluation, screening for subclinical hypothyroidism during early pregnancy depends on measuring elevated TSH levels by using a sensitive assay. Evidence indicates that 97.5th-percentile TSH levels are lower during advancing gestation in an analysis of single-screening values in 10,568 singleton pregnancies in Texas (83% Hispanic, 12% black, 3% white, 2% other) (TSH 4.9 at 8 weeks, 3.3 at 12 weeks, 2.7 at 16 weeks, 3.2 at 20 weeks, 3.0 at 24 weeks) (Dashe 05). Controversy revolves around the use of free T4 assays in early pregnancy due to assay variations associated with serum protein changes in pregnancy. Free T4 levels decline in late pregnancy (Casey 06). Some are of the opinion that the total T4 reference range, adjusted by 1.5 for estrogen-induced increased protein binding in pregnancy, may be more effective in screening for hypothyroxinemia than free T4 (Demers 03, Mandel 05, Lebeau 06).

Hypothyroidism During Pregnancy

Hypothyroidism during pregnancy has been associated with increased rates of cardiac dysfunction, preeclampsia, prematurity/low BW, and fetal death (Montoro 81, Davis 88, Leung 93, Allan 00, Casey 05, Idris 05, Antolic 06). Adequate replacement of levothyroxine to render the patient euthyroid is thought to suppress the frequency of obstetrical complications (Montoro 81, Davis 88, Liu 94, Abalovich 02, Harborne 05, Wolfberg 05, Matalon 06, Tan 06). The T4 dosage usually needs to be incremented by 4–6 weeks gestation and may require a 30–50% increase in dosage (Mandel 90, Girling 92, Kaplan 92, Alexander 04, Abalovich 07). If hypothyroidism is diagnosed during pregnancy, the international thyroid panel recommends that the target TSH level for adjustment of thyroid replacement doses be ≤2.5 µU/mL in early pregnancy and <3.0 µU/mL later in gestation (Lebeau 06, Abalovich 07). Thyroid function tests should be remeasured every 30–40 days (Abalovich 07).

Most women with hypothyroidism (85%) will need more thyroxine as pregnancy advances (mean increase 47%), and surveillance of thyroid function is needed throughout gestation to make dose adjustments when needed; most adjustments will be needed during the first 16–20 weeks. However, bear in mind that increasing levothyroxine therapy at <4-to-6-week intervals may lead to overtreatment. Women with hypothyroidism taking exogenous levothyroxine need to know that ingesting ferrous sulfate and thyroxine simultaneously may lead to the formation of insoluble ferric–thyroxine complexes resulting in reduced absorption of thyroxine. Therefore, intake should be separated by at least 2 h (Campbell 92). Medications and chemicals that may interfere with the synthesis or intestinal absorption of thyroxine are listed in Table II.4. After delivery, thyroxine requirements return to prepregnancy levels; if the prepregnancy dose is unknown, recalculate it and make further adjustments to keep TSH within the normal range. It is safe to breast-feed while taking physiological doses of thyroxine.

Regarding screening for hypothyroidism, the Endocrine Society, the American Thyroid Association, and the American Association of Clinical Endocrinologists sponsored a consensus panel of 13 experts that concluded that "a TSH might be obtained in pregnant women or in women considering pregnancy who have a family or personal history of thyroid disease, signs and symptoms suggesting thyroid disease, or underlying autoimmune conditions," and that "aggressive case finding is appropriate in pregnant women" (Surks 04). In response, six other thyroid disease experts representing the leadership of the above organizations published an alternative opinion. This panel concluded that "TSH testing (followed by free T4 measurement when the TSH is abnormal) should be performed routinely during the prepregnancy evaluation or as soon as pregnancy is diagnosed" (Gharib 05). An analysis of thyroid function in 1,560 consecutive pregnant women in the U.K. in 2002–2003 (91.4% white, 4% South Asian, 4.6% other) revealed that 40 women (2.6%) had raised TSH >4.4 mU/L, 16 of whom also had low fT4 (1.0% clinical hypothyroidism), and that 33% of those with subclinical hypothyroidism were low risk in that they provided no personal or family history of

TABLE II.4 Screening for Hypothyroidism During Pregnancy

Highest Risk
- Previous therapy for hyperthyroidism or high-dose neck irradiation
- Previous postpartum thyroiditis (evidence of thyroid autoimmunity)
- Goiter (diffuse or nodular)
- Family history of thyroid disease
- Treatment with amiodarone: decreases T4 to T3 conversion and inhibits T3 action
- Type 1 diabetes mellitus or suspected hypopituitarism

Moderate Risk
- Any endocrinopathy and autoimmune disorder
- Hyperlipidemia
- Medications: Lithium, iodine, and antithyroid medications interfere with thyroid hormone synthesis and/or release. Carbamazepine, phenytoin, and rifampin increase thyroxine clearance. Aluminum hydroxide, calcium, cholestyramine, ferrous sulfate, sucralfate, and soy-containing products interfere with intestinal absorption of thyroxine.
- Exposure to certain industrial/chemical compounds, such as polybrominated biphenyl compounds

Based on Montoro 97 and used with permission.

thyroid disease or other autoimmune disorders. The authors concluded that "targeted thyroid function testing of only the high-risk group would miss about one third of pregnant women with overt/subclinical hypothyroidism" (Vaidya 07). Pending results of clinical trials of the effects of maternal treatment on long-term neurodevelopment in the offspring of pregnant women with subclinical hypothyroidism, the most recent Endocrine Society international panel recommends T4 replacement in women with overt hypothyroidism because the potential benefits outweigh the potential risks (Abalovich 07).

According to the ACOG, "There are insufficient data to warrant routine screening of asymptomatic women for hypothyroidism" (ACOG 02a). An early population survey in Maine of 2,000 consecutive pregnant women at 15–18 weeks gestation found serum TSH to be elevated >6 mU/L in 49 women (2.5%), with six being thyroxine deficient (0.3% of total); 58% of women with TSH >6 mU/L had positive titers for thyroid autoantibodies compared with 11% of controls (Klein 91). A prospective thyroid-screening study of 17,298 women (84% Hispanic) enrolling for prenatal care by 20 weeks gestation found subclinical hypothyroidism in 2.3% (serum TSH >97.5th percentile for gestational age; free T4 >0.68 ng/dL). These patients had significantly increased frequencies of placental abruption (1% vs. 0.3%; p 0.03) and preterm birth <34 weeks (4% vs. 2.5%; p 0.01) compared with women with normal TSH, but infant follow-up was not performed (Casey 05). A frequency of subclinical hypothyroidism >2% in pregnant women is at least 60-fold more common than congenital hypothyroidism (1:3,000) (Zoeller 03), for which neonatal screening has been mandatory. Of course, the severe clinical impact of untreated congenital hypothyroidism is undoubted. In the absence of adequate data on the frequency and meaning of subclinical hypothyroidism in pregnant women with type 2 diabetes, the clinician and patient must decide whether treatment is indicated. For clinicians wishing to use a risk factor approach rather than universal screening, indications for screening for hypothyroidism are presented in Table II.4.

Diabetes and hypothyroidism during pregnancy

A prospective multicenter study of 85 pregnant women with type 1 diabetes in the Netherlands (an iodine-sufficient country) found 18.3% to have subclinical hypothyroidism, 4.9% to have overt hypothyroidism, and 20.7% to have TPO autoimmunity. For the group of women, there was the expected trend for free T4 to decline during pregnancy and TSH to gradually rise, within normal limits. Surprisingly, no association was found between TPOab positivity in the first trimester and overt or subclinical hypothyroidism during pregnancy. It is important to note that of 31 diabetic women that were tested euthyroid prior to pregnancy, 12.9% developed subclinical hypothyroidism during gestation (Gallas 02). Other smaller studies of pregnant women with type 1 diabetes observed subclinical or overt hypothyroidism in 4.8%, 14.3%, and 16% of subjects, respectively, in New York City, Spain, and California (Jovanovic-Peterson 88, Alvarez-Marfany 94, Fernandez-Soto 97). Another survey of 85 women with type 1 diabetes in Denmark noted no overt hypothyroidism during pregnancy in spite of a 19% frequency of thyroid autoimmunity (Bech 91). Women with elevated thyroid antibodies are also at risk for postpartum thyroiditis and their newborns at risk for transient neonatal hypothyroidism. The latter, if undetected and untreated during the first 1–2 months after birth, may lead to various degrees of impaired cognitive development even if the antibodies eventually disappear and normal thyroid function returns at a later date.

Hyperthyroidism in Pregnancy

Clinical hyperthyroidism is found in 1.7% of patients with type 1 diabetes and 0.3% in type 2 diabetes (Mouradian 83, Perros 95) compared with 0.1–0.6% in the reference pregnant population (Glinoer 98, Mestman 98). Hyperthyroidism is associated with hepatic and adipose tissue insulin resistance (Dimitriadis 85,06b) and impairs glucose-stimulated insulin secretion in a pregnant animal model (Holness 05). Mild degrees of some classic symptoms and signs of hyperthyroidism (heat intolerance, anxiety, fatigue, tachycardia, palpitations, tremor, vomiting and weight loss in early pregnancy) are also found in euthyroid pregnancies (Mestman 98, Pearce 06). Clinicians should be aware of "falsely" reduced TSH during early pregnancy due to stimulation of TSH receptors by hCG with normal T3 and T4 levels (Kimura 90, Glinoer 93, Yamazaki 95, Yoshimura 95, Grun 97). There is structural homology in the hCG and TSH molecules and their receptors (Yoshimura 95). Approximately 10% of pregnant women with suppressed TSH levels will have a transient "gestational subclinical hyperthyroidism" often associated with vomiting (Glinoer 98), which does not require treatment.

Thyroid receptor antibodies are common in autoimmune diabetes and hyperthyroidism (Benker 89, Laurberg 98, Schott 00) and are risk factors for severity and outcome of Graves' ophthalmopathy (Eckstein 06). Some authorities recommend measurement of TSH receptor antibodies (TRAbs) (thyroid-stimulating immunoglobulins) at 26–28 weeks gestation to assess risk of fetal–neonatal hyperthyroidism, especially in women with hypothyroidism with a prior history of Graves' disease who are levothyroxine-treated for secondary hypothyroidism (Lebeau 06). The thyroid-stimulating immunoglobulins of Graves' disease cross the placenta and can cause transient neonatal hyperthyroidism (Skuza 96, Zimmerman 99).

Careful management of hyperthyroidism is important because thyrotoxicosis increases the risk for maternal and fetal complications (Mestman 98, Nader 04,

Pearce 06). The coexistence of hyperthyroidism and poorly controlled diabetes in pregnancy may increase the risk of poor perinatal outcome (Hare 78, Lowy 80, Mestman 98). Thyrotoxicosis can appear as hyperemesis (Goodwin 92, Nader 96), preeclampsia (Millar 94), or heart failure that is usually precipitated by clinical factors that increase cardiac workload (Davis 89, Easterling 91, Sheffield 04). The thionamide drugs carbimazol, methimazol, and propylthiouracil (PTU) cross the placenta and can result in fetal hypothyroidism and goiter (Cheron 81, Abuhamad 95, VanLoon 95, Momotani 97, Mortimer 97, Gallagher 01), which are minimized by targeting maternal T4 in the high normal-to-slightly elevated range (Momotani 86, Mestman 98, Pearce 06). PTU is the preferred drug because methimazole use has been associated with cutis aplasia and esophageal/choanal atresia (Wing 94, Cooper 05). The serum PTU profile after an oral dose in the third trimester was qualitatively similar to that in nonpregnant subjects, but serum PTU values were consistently lower in the late third trimester compared with postpartum values. Cord serum PTU levels were higher than simultaneous maternal serum levels, suggesting slower PTU clearance in the fetus. A strong inverse correlation was found between maternal serum PTU area under the curve in the third trimester and the cord serum free T4 index (Gardner 86). Long-term follow-up of children exposed to thionamides in utero has been reassuring (Messer 90, Eisenstein 92). Worthy of note is that many patients with Graves' disease describe an initial onset during the postpartum period (Nader 04). Small amounts of thionamides appear in breast milk, but thyroid function of nursing infants has not been affected (Azizi 00, Momotani 00).

Postpartum autoimmune thyroiditis is discussed in Part IV in the section titled "Postpartum Thyroiditis."

Recommendations

- Screen for thyroid dysfunction/autoimmunity with TSH and TPOAbs in women with types 1 and 2 diabetes before and during early pregnancy. Use gestation-specific TSH levels during pregnancy. (B)
- If there are normal TSH (<4.5 mIU/L before pregnancy, <2.5 mIU/L first trimester) and negative antibodies: no further action. (E)
- If there are normal TSH but elevated antibodies, measure TSH at 7–8, 14–16, and 26–30 weeks and follow closely postpartum (risk of hypothyroidism during pregnancy and postpartum thyroiditis after delivery). (E)
- During pregnancy, treat any TSH elevation ($\geq$2.5 μU/mL first half; $\geq$3.0 μU/mL second half). Follow closely during the first 20 weeks when the demands for thyroxine are highest, and readjust as needed to maintain euthyroidism (TSH <2.5 μU/mL first half; <3.0 μU/mL second half). (E)
- To assess thyroxine levels, consider measurement of adjusted total T4 in pregnancy due to assay variation for free T4 from gestational changes in plasma proteins. (E)
- If suppressed TSH (<0.03 μU/L) and raised T4 levels suggest clinical hyperthyroidism, consider measurement of TRAbs. (E)
- Treat clinical hyperthyroidism with moderate doses of propylthiouracil to maintain maternal T4 at or just above the upper range of normal to minimize drug-induced fetal hypothyroidism. (B)
- Alert the pediatrician about the newborn of a mother with elevated TRAb. (E)

MANAGEMENT OF CARDIOVASCULAR RISK FACTORS

To emphasize the role of diabetes as a major risk factor for CVD, the ADA, the NIH, the Juvenile Diabetes Foundation International, and the American Heart Association (AHA) published joint statements in 1999 (ADA 99, Grundy 99). The authors noted that the increase in CVD is "partly the result of pernicious effects of persistent hyperglycemia on the vasculature and partly due to the coexistence of other metabolic risk factors" (ADA 99). It was recognized that once diabetic patients develop clinical CHD, they have a particularly bad prognosis—which points to the importance of preventive therapies. These organizations support improved interventions for prevention of CVD by identifying and controlling the risk factors that lead to its development in people with diabetes. The ADA subsequently published Position Statements on "Hypertension Management" (ADA 04b), "Dyslipidemia Management" (ADA 04c), annual updates on standards of medical care (ADA 08a), and "Nutrition Recommendations and Interventions" (ADA 08b), that address the goals and methods of CVD prevention. The AHA published scientific statements on "Management of Risk Factors" (Grundy 02a), "Cardiovascular Disease Prevention in Women" (Mosca 04a,b), and dietary and lifestyle approaches to prevent and treat hypertension and dyslipidemia and to reduce the risk of CVD (see Table II.5) (Appel 06, Lichtenstein 06). Combined scientific statements from the AHA and ADA harmonized the previous sets of recommendations on primary prevention of CVD in people with diabetes mellitus (Eckel 06, Buse 07).

The recommendations parallel the 2005 Dietary Guidelines for Americans (DGA 05) and support current guidelines of the ADA (ADA 04b,c,08a,b), the National Cholesterol Education Program (NCEP) (NCEP 01,02, Grundy 04), the American College of Physicians (Snow 04), and Diabetes U.K. plus a consortium of British cardiovascular societies

TABLE II. 5 Diet and Lifestyle Recommendations for Cardiovascular Disease Risk Reduction*

- Balance calorie intake and physical activity to achieve or maintain a healthy body weight (achieve weight-gain goals for pregnancy, but avoid excessive weight gain).
- Consume a diet rich in vegetables and fruits.
- Choose whole-grain, high-fiber foods.
- Consume fish, especially oily fish, at least twice a week (choose species with low mercury content or consider supplementing with *n*-3 fatty acids).
- Limit your intake of saturated fat to <7% of energy, *trans* fats to <1% of energy, and cholesterol to <300 mg per day by:
  - choosing lean meats and vegetable alternatives
  - selecting fat-free (skim), 1%-fat, and low-fat dairy products
  - minimizing intake of partially hydrogenated fats
- Minimize your intake of beverages and foods with added sugar (for diabetes in pregnancy, use diet drinks in moderation and use fruit juices only to treat hypoglycemia).
- Choose and prepare foods with little or no salt.
- If you consume alcohol, do so in moderation (no alcohol intake recommended in pregnancy).
- When you eat food prepared outside of the home, follow these recommendations (and your individualized diabetes and pregnancy food plan).

Modified for diabetes and pregnancy.
Taken from Appel 06, Lichtenstein 06.

(Brit 05). These recommendations are based on clinical trial evidence demonstrating the effectiveness of the measures (Gaede 03, ACCORD 04, BPT 05, DCCT/EDIC 05, Whelton 05, Cleary 06, Gaede 08). If followed, the recommendations provide a solid base for MNT, physical activity, and drug therapy to achieve the comprehensive goals of the ADA/AHA for cardiovascular risk reduction in diabetic women.

Because the absolute and relative risks for CVD are dramatically increased in young adults with type 1 and type 2 diabetes compared with a nondiabetic population, CVD risk assessment and risk factor management should be vigorously applied in diabetic women of reproductive age (Colhoun 06, Wild 06). It has been recommended that office-based risk assessment should apply to all people with type 1 diabetes aged ≥16 years (Redberg 02). To date, the major concern for CVD in younger patients has been in women with type 1 diabetes. However, the rising tide of type 2 diabetes in the young (Pinhas-Hamiel 96,98, Dabelea 99, Rosenbloom 99, Fagot-Campagna 00, Grinstein 03, Pinhas-Hamiel 05, Duncan 06, Pinhas-Hamiel 07, Jones 08) may increase the prevalence of CVD in this group (Gungor 05) by the time they become pregnant, especially in those with biomarkers of insulin resistance or chronic inflammation (Cook 07, DeFerranti 07, Herder 07, Nandkeoliar 07, Shaibi 08). Indeed, a striking increased frequency of CVD (MI, stroke, peripheral vascular disease) was seen over a mean follow-up of 4 years after diagnosis of early-onset type 2 diabetes (age 18–44 years, mean age 37 years) in 1,600 female patients in Oregon compared with female controls (Hillier 03). Relevant to these increased risks, more research is needed on the role of central obesity and insulin resistance in amplifying the effects of hyperglycemia, hypertension, and dyslipidemia in young women with diabetes.

Management goals depend on a systematic program of CVD risk assessment with adequate follow-up (Wilson 98, Eddy 03, Buse 07). The goals for women with diabetes (ADA 08a) are to (1) aim for a near-normal plasma glucose level without significant hypoglycemia and A1C <6.3 in preparation for pregnancy; (2) aim for BP <130/80 mmHg (systolic BP <120 mmHg may yield the lowest rate of progression of coronary atherosclerosis) (Adler 00, Sipahi 06); (3) aim to keep LDL-C <100 mg/dL (2.6 mM), HDL-C >50 mg/dL (1.25 mM), and TGs <150 mg/dL (1.7 mM); (4) aim for weight control and specific reduction of central obesity; (5) be physically active at least 30 min daily 5 of 7 days, and (6) avoid use of and exposure to tobacco products (Lichtenstein 06). We can add (7) aim to prevent or reduce albuminuria (ADA 04d, de Zeeuw 06, ADA 08a). Most recommendations can be applied in pregnancy (refer to the sections titled "Glycemic Control and Perinatal Outcome," "Medical Nutrition Therapy," and "Physical Activity/Exercise and Management of Pregnant Women with Preexisting Diabetes" in Part I and to sections titled "Blood Pressure Control," "Management of Hyper/Dyslipidemias," and "Diabetic Nephropathy and Pregnancy" later in Part II).

CARDIOVASCULAR DISEASE IN DIABETIC WOMEN

—— *Original contribution by Pathmaja Paramsothy MD, MS and Robert H. Knopp MD*

The interrelated effects of postprandial hyperglycemia, hypertension, dyslipidemia, oxidative stress, and inflammation (Eckel 02, Saydah 04, Libby 05a, Dandona 07) contribute to the burden of CVD (Fox 04a): CHD, cardiovascular autonomic neuropathy (CAN), heart failure, and peripheral arteriosclerotic vascular disease, including ischemic stroke and lower-extremity arterial disease (LEAD). Changes in vascular structure and function occur early in the course of type 1 diabetes (Dahl-Jorgensen 05, Orchard 06), and the increasing duration of type 2 diabetes noted in young women becoming pregnant is also expected to increase CVD in this group. Summaries of new research on the pathophysiology of atherosclerosis, neuropathy, and myocardiopathy are presented in the appropriate sections. The general management of clinical CVD in patients with PDM has been reviewed (Jacoby 92, Simons 98, Herlitz 99, Beckman 02, Lavine 02, Creager 03, Luescher 03, Safley 05, Dzau 06) and is beyond the scope of this document. Our purpose is to help clinicians who are educating and caring for pregnant diabetic women to understand the importance of CVD in the life course of the woman with type 1 or type 2 diabetes (Legato 06) and to emphasize diagnostic tests and preventive risk factor management that can be maintained during gestation.

Coronary Heart Disease

Epidemiology of CHD in Diabetic Women

CHD risk in women with type 1 or type 2 diabetes, plus some evidence of atherosclerosis, is equivalent to risk in nondiabetic adults with established CHD (Barrett-Connor 91, Butler 98, Haffner 98a, Howard 02, Juutilainen 05, Whitely 05, Howard 06). Diabetes closes the gap in cardiovascular morbidity and mortality between men and women (Kanaya 02, Creager 03, Luescher 03, Natarajan 03, Mosca 04a, Larsson 05), and CVD is the leading cause of death in diabetic women aged ≥30 years (Laing 99, Hu 01, Barrett-Connor 04, Skrivarhaug 06, Soedamah-Muthu 06a). A population-based autopsy study in the central U.S. of 22 diabetic women aged 30–64 found evidence of any high-grade coronary atherosclerosis in 64% (RR 1.8 vs. 170 nondiabetic women); 50% had multivessel disease (RR 2.8) (Goraya 02). The WHO Multinational Study of Vascular Disease in Asia, Europe, and North America registered 1,266 patients with type 1 diabetes (mean age 44 years; mean duration 16 years) and 3,421 patients with type 2 diabetes (mean age 47 years; mean duration 8 years) in 1975–1977 and followed the subjects for 11–13 years. Dipstick-positive proteinuria was present at baseline in 27% of both groups, and 38% and 42% were smokers, respectively. Mortality from CHD was 8.1% in type 1 diabetes and 7.3% in type 2 diabetes compared with 5.4% and 2.4% mortality from renal disease, respectively. A 2.3-fold greater risk of CVD mortality was apparent in patients with heavy proteinuria (type 1 and type 2 diabetes; adjusted for age, duration of diabetes, systolic BP, cholesterol, and smoking); still, the majority of CVD deaths occurred in type 1 and type 2 diabetes patients without proteinura (Stephenson 95). Finally, the increment in lipids with insulin resistance and obesity is greater in women than in men (Knopp 03), as is the increment in CVD associated with diabetes (Barrett-Connor 04) by almost twofold (Juutilainen 08). The greater increment in CVD incidence with diabetes in women is explained by the greater risk factor severity (BP, HDL-C, TG) in diabetic women compared with men (Kanaya 02, Juutilainen 04). The hazard ratio (95% CI) of CHD mortality over an 18-year follow-up period was 16.9 (7.6–37.2) for women with type 1 diabetes (onset >30 years; duration ≥15 years) and 10.8 (5.9–19.7) for women with type 2 diabetes (onset >30 years; duration ≥15 years) compared with nondiabetic controls in Finland (Juutilainen 08).

"The risk of mortality from ischemic heart disease is exceptionally high in young adult women with type 1 diabetes" compared with nondiabetic women. Standardized mortality ratios were 44.8 in insulin-treated women aged 20–29 and 41.6 in women aged 30–39 (Laing 03a). The hazard ratio for new MI was 38X for diabetic women versus controls aged 20–34 in a large retrospective population study in Ontario. The 10-year risk of acute MI was ~2% in diabetic women (type unspecified) aged 31–40 and ~3% in diabetic women aged 41–45 (Booth 06). Myocardial ischemia is often "silent" or unrecognized by symptoms when testing is done in women with diabetes of both types (Koistinen 90, Rewers 92, MiSAD 97), which raises the question of whom and how to screen for evidence of CHD in diabetic women of reproductive age (Nesto 99, Rutter 07) and whether risk factors or risk indicators have sufficient power to predict the great majority of cases of myocardial ischemia. To be useful, the results of screening tests should lead to a change in management that will improve outcome (Grundy 02b).

In type 1 diabetes, the incidence of CHD is 1–2% per year among young, asymptomatic patients (Libby 05a). In the pioneering experience at the Joslin Diabetes Center in Boston, patients with juvenile-onset type 1 diabetes were followed for 20–40 years and examined in 1980–1981 (Krolewski 87). The prevalence of symptomatic CHD was zero when women were examined at ages 21–34 compared with 5.0% at ages 35–44. Asymptomatic CHD was detected by exercise ECG in 5.4% of women at ages 21–34 and in 10.8% at ages 35–44 years. After age 30, the mortality rate due to CHD increased rapidly and equally in both men and women, particularly among individuals with renal complications. Cumulative mortality due to CHD was 3.5% in women with type 1 diabetes by age 35, 6% by age 40, 13% by age 45, and 26% by age 50 (Figure 1 in Krolewski 87). In comparison, the cumulative mortality rate due to CHD by age 50 was ~2% for nondiabetic women in the Framingham Heart Study (Krolewski 87).

In 452 Wisconsin women with age at baseline of 10–45 years and type 1 diabetes of at least 5 years' duration, the 20-year age-adjusted cumulative incidence of MI was 13%. Predictive risk factors in multivariable analysis included hypertension, presence of neuropathy or retinopathy, age and duration of diabetes, and higher glyco-hemoglobin level (Klein 04). Of 312 female subjects with type 1 diabetes of onset before age 17 in Pittsburgh who were followed 6 years after baseline exams in 1986–1988, 8.7% developed CHD by a mean age of 40 ± 7 years (Forrest 00). About one-fourth of CHD-related events occurred in type 1 diabetes subjects <30 years of age. The annual major CHD event rate was 1.0% for women with diabetes durations of 20–30 years who had reached the ages of 28–38 years in an analysis extended to a 12-year follow-up (Pambianco 06). Independent risk factors associated with CHD in women in this database were systolic BP, duration of diabetes, TGs, depression, and lack of physical activity (Lloyd 96). CHD-associated morbidities included autonomic neuropathy (70%) based on an expiratory/inspiratory ratio <1.10 calculated from ECG R-R intervals according to an office-based method, distal symmetric polyneuropathy (64.5%), hypertension (55%), and LEAD (48%) based on a history of amputation or claudication or an ankle/brachial pressure index <0.8 for any of the 4 vessels (Olson 00).

CHD was strongly associated with the development of proteinuria in a landmark cohort study of young patients with type 1 diabetes who were followed during 1975–1981 at the Steno Memorial Hospital in Copenhagen (Jensen 87). Within the cohort, subjects in a case–control analysis were without signs of CHD or proteinuria at baseline, with a mean age of 33 years (range 15–48 years), mean diabetes duration of 19 years (range 6–42 years), and equal division between men and women. Fifty-nine cases were matched with 59 controls on the basis of development of proteinuria >500 mg/day over the 2–6 year follow-up; there was no gender influence on outcome. PDR was much more common at baseline (49.2% vs. 10.2%) in the subjects developing proteinuria. The cumulative incidence of CHD was 12% at 2 years after onset of proteinuria, 23.5% at 4 years, and 42% at 6 years compared with 2% at 2 years, 5% at 4 years, and 6% at 6 years in subjects without proteinuria. Among the proteinuric patients, those with CHD had higher BP at baseline (135/87 ± 16/9 vs. 128/82 ± 15/9; p < 0.05). Of 29 women developing proteinuria, 11 also developed CHD (38%) in this relatively short follow-up period (Jensen 87). The independent predictive value of albuminuria for arteriosclerotic vascular disease was maintained in an 11-year follow-up of this cohort (Deckert 96).

A multinational cross-sectional survey (EURODIAB) of 1,563 European women with type 1 diabetes aged 33 ±10 years found a CHD prevalence of 11.1% (1.5% MI, 1.8% angina, 0.1% coronary artery bypass graft [CABG], 7.7% abnormal ECG). Women with CHD had higher BMI and fasting TG and lower HDL-C; in multiple logistic regression analysis, significant persisting risk factors were age, BMI, and HDL-C (Koivisto 96). In further prospective analysis of 1,127 women with type 1 diabetes (mean age ~33 years, 14% smokers), 7.3% developed CHD over a 7-year follow-up. After adjustment, predictors included age, albuminuria, systolic BP, glucose level (Soedamah-Muthu 04), and ECG-left ventricular hypertrophy (LVH) (Giunti 05). The hazard ratio for major CVD events was 9.8 for women with type 1 diabetes aged <35 years compared with controls in a large U.K. population study and 15.4 for diabetic women aged 35–45 years. The absolute risk per 1,000 person-years was 0.5 for diabetic women <35 years and 3.5 for diabetic women aged 35–45 years. Women with type 1 diabetes were at a 10-year risk of >5% for developing a fatal CVD event by 50 years of age (Soedamah-Muthu 06b).

In a pooled analysis of the Pittsburgh and EURODIAB cross-sectional surveys of 888 women with type 1 diabetes at age 30 ± 11 years, 6.9% were found to have CHD. Hypertension and albuminuria were significant age-adjusted risk factors for CHD in this female population (Orchard 98). Considering all of the cited data, clinicians should expand their view to consider CHD risk in the relatively younger population of patients with type 1 diabetes.

Coronary artery calcification (CAC) measured by electron beam tomography is a marker for atherosclerosis (Sangiorgi 98) in type 1 diabetes (Orchard 06), and CAC correlates strongly with clinical CHD and other cardiovascular risk factors. Among 95 women with type 1 diabetes (mean age 37 years, mean duration of diabetes 23 years), the prevalence of CAC was 47% (adjusted OR 3.5 vs. controls well-matched for risk factors except 16% hypertension in type 1 diabetes vs. 6% in controls); other basic CVD risk factors did not explain this difference (Colhoun 00). In the Pittsburgh type 1 diabetes complications study, the prevalence of any CAC (minimum calcium threshold 1 mm area) in women without clinical CHD or ischemic ECG was 13% at age 18–29 years, 30% at age 30–39 years, and 61% at age 40–49 years. For type 1 diabetic women with CHD, the prevalence of any CAC was 40% at age 30–39 years and 68% at age 40–49 years (Figure 1 in Olson 00). Severe CAC (calcium score ≥400) had 73% sensitivity, 90% specificity, 35% positive predictive value (PPV), and 98% negative predictive value (NPV) for MI or < 49% for angiographic stenosis in women with type 1 diabetes (Olson 00). CAC was detected in 6.2% of 48 asymptomatic 17–28-year-old female subjects with type 1 diabetes of at least 5 years' duration (Starkman 03). These data support other studies providing evidence of coronary atherosclerosis at a relatively young age in women with type 1 diabetes beginning by 30 years of age (Crall 78, Valsania 91, Dabelea 03). In the DCCT/EDIC (Epidemiology of Diabetes Interventions and Complications) follow-up study (which excluded type 1 diabetes patients with hypertension and hypercholesterolemia on entry), extensive CAC was not present 7–9 years after the end of the trial in 34 women aged 20–29.

The prevalence of extensive calcification was 2.3% in 178 women aged 30–39 and 4.2% in 259 women aged 40–49. At these ages, prevalence figures did not differ according to previous treatment group. However, women ≥50 years of age who had been in the intensive treatment group had a lower prevalence of extensive calcification at 4.6% vs. 20.8% (Cleary 06).

Intravascular US is used as a research tool to identify coronary arteriosclerotic plaques that are not detected by angiography (Nissen 91, St Goar 92, Mintz 95, Erbel 99, Schartl 06). On a cross-section view of a coronary vessel, the percentage of the vessel area with stenosis is the plaque area divided by the vessel area × 100. In a sample of 29 asymptomatic nonpregnant Norwegian patients studied with intravascular US after 18 years of follow up for type 1 diabetes, 100% showed atherosclerotic plaques with >0.5-mm thickening of the intima in at least one of the main coronary arteries compared with 34% with >50% stenosis identified on angiography and only 15% with >1-mm ST-segment depression during an exercise ECG. Total-C and A1C over 18 years were independently related to coronary artery plaque formation as identified by US (Larsen 02).

Diabetic women with a clinical indication for coronary angiography are found to have a more severe, extensive, and distal type of CHD than individually matched nondiabetic control patients (Valsania 91, Pajunen 00). Coronary plaques have more inflammatory characteristics in diabetic patients than in nondiabetic coronary patients (Moreno 02, Burke 04), and acute events are more likely to be precipitated by endothelial erosion and superficial thrombus with diabetes than by disruption in the cap and thrombosis in the core of a lipid-rich plaque (Davies 96, Orchard 06).

Regarding type 2 diabetes, women aged 45–65 in the U.S. with diabetes duration >15 years and without a history of CHD have an eightfold risk of fatal CHD over 20 years compared with the reference population (Hu 01). Very similar data were obtained by following newly diagnosed patients with type 2 diabetes in Germany (Hanefeld 96) and the U.K. (Turner 98). Independent risk factors for CHD in type 2 diabetes are A1C, systolic BP, LDL-C, waist–hip ratio (Selvin 05), and ECG-LVH (Bruno 04). Once normotensive women with type 2 diabetes and microalbuminura reached their 50s, the univariate hazard ratio for a composite CVD end point was 3.2 compared with diabetic males and 8.2 when adjusted for age systolic BP, BMI, total-to-HDL cholesterol ratio, current smoking, and retinopathy. Women who had an event were not identified at baseline (Zandbergen 06).

Epidemiological data on CHD in younger women with type 2 diabetes are not as plentiful. In 832 women with type 2 diabetes of onset by age 18–44 years, the frequency of MI was 4.6% over a mean follow-up of 4 years after diagnosis, which represented an 11-fold RR of MI compared with matched control subjects. This was a much greater risk ratio than that found in women with type 2 diabetes of later onset and was greater than the RR of 3.9 found in males with early-onset type 2 diabetes (compared with control males) (Hillier 03). Competing hypotheses offer explanations regarding the relationship between type 2 diabetes and CVD (Bowden 06). One is that chronic hyperglycemia directly contributes to atherosclerosis independently of other risk factors (Andersson 95). Alternatively, type 2 diabetes worsens atherogenic risk factors, or CVD and type 2 diabetes share common genetic antecedents (Jarrett 84, Stern 95, Wagenknecht 01, Lange 02). At any rate, multifaceted intensified care has been shown to reduce CVD in patients with type 2 diabetes (Gaede 03,08).

Due to the accumulating mass of epidemiological data, diabetes is designated as a CHD risk equivalent to individuals having had a coronary event by many health organizations such as the ADA (ADA 04c,08a), the AHA (Mosca 04b), the American College of Physicians (Snow 04), and the National Cholesterol Education Program (NCEP 01,02, Grundy 04).

CHD and pregnancy

Active or previously treated CHD is reported to occur in 1 of 10,000 pregnant women, and with much greater frequency (1 in 350) in gestations complicated by diabetes (Leguizamon 04). The frequency of CHD in pregnancy is expected to increase further in light of the current epidemic of obesity and type 2 diabetes in the young (Rosenbloom 99, Marcovecchio 05). Acute MI occurred during or within 6 weeks after pregnancy in 1 of 35,700 deliveries in a California population study, and PDM was an important risk factor for MI (OR 4.3; CI 2.3–7.9), as was chronic hypertension (Ladner 05). In the U.S. Nationwide Inpatient Sample for the years 2000–2002 including 13.8 million pregnancy-related discharges, the rate of acute MI was 6.6 per 100,000 deliveries (in 859 cases, of which 27% were postpartum admissions). The case fatality rate was 5.1%. Location of the acute MI was reported in 85% of cases: 37% subendocardial, 25% anterior, 15% inferior, 5% lateral, and 3% posterior. Using multivariable logistic regression, significant risk factors and adjusted odds ratios associated with MI included diabetes (3.6), hypertension (21.7), thrombophilia (25.6), smoking (8.4), age 30–34 years (6.7), age 35–39 years (16.0), and age >40 years (15.2) (James 06). Of 10.0 million Canadian women admitted to the hospital for delivery between 1970 and 1998, 114 women had peripartum myocardial ischemia recorded as a discharge diagnosis, for a crude incidence rate of 1.1 per 100,000 deliveries; the case fatality rate was 1.8%. The RR was 8.1 for those aged >35 years, 60.4 for PDM (6 cases in 7,694 diabetic women; 0.08%), 8.7 for preexisting hypertension, 21.0 for renal disease, and 804.0 for dyslipidemia. Of 178 women reporting chronic CHD, 9 had recorded peripartum ischemia (5.1%) (Macarthur 06). These studies are limited by the disadvantages of retrospective use of administrative data. Increased awareness of a high degree of cardiovascular risk in diabetic women may allow detection of acute atherosclerotic complications in pregnancy and interventions for prevention of CVD in later life.

Accumulating case reports of CHD in pregnant women with PDM have been reviewed from time to time (Hare 77, Brown 95, Pombar 95, Gordon 96a, Bagg 99, Collins 02, Leguizmon 04). In the California population survey of acute MI associated with pregnancy, there were 14 cases in women with PDM: 11 in the antenatal period, 2 intrapartum, and 1 postpartum (Ladner 05). Of 34 previously reported cases of MI in PDM, 16 occurred before pregnancy, 8 in the first trimester (3 aborted), 3 in the second trimester, 3 in the third trimester, and 4 in the puerperium (Brown 95, Bagg 99, Darias 01, Collins 02, Leguizamon 04, Wilson 04, Salam 05). Maternal mortality was 73% before 1980, all occurring in cases with CHD diagnosed during pregnancy or postpartum. All but 1 of 23 cases reported from 1980 to 2005 survived. Troponin is effective in the diagnosis of acute MI during pregnancy because levels are not affected by gestation or delivery. In contrast, creatine kinase and myoglobin are present in the uterus and placenta (Krahenmann 00, Shade 02). Thus far, pregnancy has been successful in the few cases reported of CABG surgery prior to pregnancy (Brown 95, Dufour 97, Leguizamon 04); CABG has even been reported occasionally during pregnancy (Collins 02) as well as percutaneous coronary interventions (Ascarelli 96, Sebastian 98, Craig 99, Sullebarger 03, Dwyer 05). In the U.S. Inpatient Sample 2000–2002, cardiac procedures reported during pregnancy or postpartum included 45% heart catheterization, 16% angioplasty, 15% stent, 7% pulsation balloon, and 5% bypass graft (James 06).

Cardiovascular Autonomic Neuropathy

CAN is a common form of neuropathy in patients with type 1 and longstanding type 2 diabetes (Ewing 80, ADA 88, Ziegler 93, Spallone 97a, Valensi 97,03, Debono 07) and is independently associated with increased mortality (O'Brien 91, Rathmann 93a, Gerritsen 01, Maser 03). The imbalance of autonomic control (interplay of sympathetic and parasympathetic activity) is implicated in the pathophysiology of cardiac arrhythmias (Spallone 93, ESC 96). Reduction in variability of HR (measured by the R-R interval) is the earliest indicator of CAN (Genovely 88). HR variability during deep breathing decreases after age 20 in both control and diabetic groups by 4–5 beats per decade (Masaoka 85). Determination of the HR itself is not a reliable sign of diabetic CAN because patients "with parasympathetic dysfunction have a high resting HR most likely because of vagal neuropathy that results in unopposed increased sympathetic outflow. People with a combined parasympathetic/sympathetic dysfunction have slower HRs. With advanced nerve dysfunction, HR is fixed (Maser 05). HR may not be a good gauge of exercise capacity because HR_{max} is depressed in diabetic patients with CAN (Maser 05). Further discussion of the tests for cardioautonomic dysfunction can be found in the section titled "Clinical Assessment for CVD in Diabetic Women."

CAN is linked with CHD in women of reproductive age with type 1 diabetes (Olson 00, Kempler 02), and early signs of CAN can be detected in children and adolescents with a duration of diabetes >8 years and poor metabolic control (Piha 92, Donaghue 98, Tanaka 98, Chessa 02, Riihimaa 02, Javorka 05, Boysen 07). The clinical impact of CAN in adults relates to exercise intolerance, orthostatic hypotension, silent myocardial ischemia and painless infarction, intraoperative cardiovascular lability, and increased cardiac events (Kahn 86, Niakan 86, Burgos 89, Knuttgen 90, Murray 90, Ziegler 99, Kitamura 00, Valensi 01, Maser 05, Astrup 06). In type 1 diabetes patients, CAN is also associated with LVH and diastolic ventricular dysfunction (Taskiran 04, Debono 07), early-onset PDR (Krolewski 92, Spallone 97a), and DN (Sundkvist 93, Spallone 94).

The prevalence of altered respiratory HR ratio as the marker for CAN was 40% in a sample of 125 women with type 1 diabetes but without clinical CHD aged 22–52 years (mean age 37; diabetes duration 28 years) (Olson 00). In the EURODIAB assessment of 1,468 women with type 1 diabetes (mean age 33 ± 10 years), the prevalence of CAN (1 of 2 cardiovascular reflex responses abnormal) was 37%. A change in the ECG R-R ratio <1.04 on standing (mainly parasympathetic dysfunction) was abnormal in 24% of subjects, and 18% had orthostatic hypotension (mainly sympathetic dysfunction) defined as a fall in systolic BP >20 mmHg on standing. Both tests were abnormal in only 6% of women; it is therefore reasonable to perform more than one test. No gender differences were evident in this large cross-sectional study. In pooled data, the crude rate of CAN was 32% in patients aged 15–29 years and 35% in those aged 30–44 years. The variation in CAN prevalence with duration of type 1 diabetes was 26% in a duration <7 years, 35% in a duration of 8–14 years, and 43% at a duration ≥15 years. Other significant predictors of CAN were A1C, fasting TG, and AER (Kempler 02). In a 7-year follow-up of 956 EURODIAB type 1 diabetes patients without CAN at baseline (mean age 31 ± 9 years; duration 13 ± 8 years), clinical predictors of development of CAN in 17% of patients included A1C, systolic BP, retinopathy, and distal symmetrical polyneuropathy (Witte 05).

Adult groups with less hyperglycemia over time have reduced frequencies of CAN (Makimattila 00, Reichard 00, Larsen 04). Impairment of HR variability at baseline was found in 4.5% of 363 subjects randomized to intensified care in the secondary prevention cohort of the DCCT and in 7.8% in 352 subjects randomized to conventional care (both groups: mean age 27 ± 7 years). After 7–8 years of DCCT therapy, the prevalence of abnormal R-R variation <15 bpm was 11% in the intensive glycemic control group and 17% in the conventional treatment group (NS). In this trial, abnormal Valsalva ratios or confirmed orthostatic hypotension was uncommon in either treatment group (DCCT 98a). Some evidence exists that CAN is associated with positive tests for autoantibodies to autonomic nerve tissue (Granberg 05). Currently, there is no specific therapy for CAN except control of hyperglycemia and use of ACE inhibitors and beta-blockers (Vinik 03,06).

Cardiac autonomic function in pregnancy

There are surprisingly few recent studies of cardiac autonomic function in pregnancy with or without diabetes (review by Ekholm 96). Limited investigation showed that normal pregnant women had reduced HR variability in the second trimester, with facilitation of sympathetic regulation and attenuation of parasympathetic influence on HR (Ekholm 93,94, Brooks 97). Blunting of the tachycardic response to the Valsalva maneuver occurs during normal pregnancy (Souma 83, Ekholm 93). Alterations of HR responses are enhanced in preeclampsia (Airaksinen 95, Yang 00). Ingestion of glucose during pregnancy increased the low-frequency band (sympathetic activation) and decreased the high-frequency band (vagal activation) in power spectral analysis of HR variability (Weissman 06). A single study from Austria demonstrated that women with prior GDM and continued glucose intolerance had reduced HR variability (SD of R-R intervals) on continuous monitoring that was not related to insulin sensitivity (Gasic 07).

CAN in diabetic pregnancy

Few studies of CAN in pregnancies complicated by diabetes have been conducted. Case reports suggest that poor outcomes are associated with severe autonomic neuropathy in pregnancy (Hare 88, Steel 89, Hagay 96). HR variation in response to deep breathing diminished progressively during pregnancy in 10 nondiabetic pregnant women (23 bpm: first trimester; 15 bpm: third trimester; 22 bpm: 14 weeks postpartum), with similar values in 25 women with type 1 diabetes except for 19.5 bpm in the third trimester (NS). HR responses to standing up did not change during pregnancy in either group by any timepoint (mean 30:15, ratios 1.32–1.38). The pregnancy-induced increase in HR measured in a supine position (mean 71 bpm: first trimester; 82 bpm: third trimester; 67 bpm: 14 weeks postpartum) was less in diabetic women, but this group had a significantly higher supine HR than controls in the first trimester and postpartum (79 bpm: first trimester; 82 bpm: third trimeaster; 79 bpm: 14 weeks postpartum). The diabetic and control groups did not differ with respect to autonomic reflexes in the postpartum period (Airaksinen 87a). A similar temporary reduction in R-R interval variation with deep breathing, thought to be due to lowered ventilatory excursion at the end of pregnancy, was observed in 16 women with type 1 diabetes and 14 pregnant controls. In the first trimester, the diabetic group showed a larger 30:15 HR ratio in quick response to standing (1.35 ± 0.18 vs. 1.21 ± 0.11; p < 0.02), but mean values did not differ (1.25–1.26) in the third trimester (Lapolla 98). In a larger study of 94 diabetic women and 46 controls in each trimester, 8.5% of the patients were determined to have CAN, but no statement on progression was made in the abstract (original article written in Croatian) (Djelmis 03). There is one anecdotal observation of improvement of postural hypotension during diabetic pregnancy, perhaps associated with gestation-related fluid retention (Scott 88). Given the importance of CAN in long-term CVD outcomes, additional research is needed into measures of CAN in larger groups of diabetic pregnant women. As noted in the Introduction in Part II, little evidence suggests that pregnancy is a risk factor for subsequent deterioration of cardiovascular autonomic function (Airaksinen 93, Hemachandra 95, Verier-Mine 05).

Heart Failure

Heart failure occurs much more frequently in diabetic women than in female controls of equal age (Bell 03a, Sander 03, Piccini 04). The risk ratio for heart failure in 469 female and male patients with type 2 diabetes <45 years of age was 11.0 (95% CI 5.6–21.8) compared with nondiabetic controls in the same age range; the 6-year incidence for heart failure was 3.6%. Significant risk factors predicting higher rates of developing heart failure included presence of CHD, mean A1C, and proteinuria (Nichols 01,04). The majority of cases of heart failure in type 1 diabetes may be mediated by diffuse atherosclerosis and patchy myocardial ischemia (Picano 03a), but heart failure without coronary artery stenosis, valvular lesions, or hypertension (idiopathic or diabetic cardiomyopathy) is also more common in diabetic women than in controls (Zarich 89, Karnik 07).

Heart failure occurs with reduced systolic ventricular function and with preserved ejection fraction (left ventricular ejection fraction [LVEF] >50%), but diastolic ventricular dysfunction or with both echocardiographic characteristics present (Bell 03a,b, Zile 03, Piccini 04, Bursi 05, Aurigemma 06). Diastolic dysfunction refers to "mechanical and functional abnormalities present during relaxation and filling, whereas diastolic heart failure refers to clinical syndromes in which patients with heart failure have little or no ventricular dilation and significant, often dominant diastolic dysfunction" (Katz 06). Left ventricular (LV) myocardial structure and function may differ in systolic failure and diastolic failure due to distinct myocardiocyte abnormalities (vanHeerebeek 06). Conversely, worsening diastolic dysfunction in heart failure is associated with a progressive decline in systolic function measured in the long axis, with LVEF >50% (Yip 02, Vinereanu 05); some believe that diastolic and systolic heart failure are the extremes of a spectrum of different phenotypes of one and the same disease (Brutsaert 06).

Diabetic cardiomyopathy

Diabetic cardiomyopathy can be associated with either systolic or diastolic ventricular dysfunction or both (Fonorow 06). Early signs of diabetic cardiomyopathy (Picano 03a, Fang 04) are more frequent in younger females than in males with type 1 diabetes (Suys 04) and are three times more likely in those with microvascular complications (Bertoni 03, Andersen 05a). Morphological changes in the hearts of women with diabetes include myocyte hypertrophy, increased matrix collagen, interstitial fibrosis, and intramyocardial microangiopathy (Hardin 96). "These changes are probably consequences of altered myocardial glucose and fatty acid metabolism due to diabetes" (Picinni 04). LVH may or may not be present in patients with type 1 or type 2 diabetes who demonstrate ventricular dysfunction. When present, LVH is often associated with insulin resistance, hypertension, or nephropathy, but may also be found in normotensive patients without albuminuria (Galderisi 91, Sato 99, Bell 03b, Henry 04, Sato 05, Felicio 06). In the general population, LVH independently predicts higher rates of cardiac events, including sudden death due to ventricular arrhythmias (Kannel 91, Wolk 99,

Brown 00a). Improved glycemic control over 1 year (with stable BP) can induce regression of LVH in adults with type 1 diabetes as marked by decreases in interventricular septal thickness and LV mass (Coppelli 03, Aepfelbacher 04, Weinrauch 05).

At least 40% of heart failure is linked to predominant LV diastolic dysfunction, for which diabetes, hypertension, and microalbuminuria are major risk factors (Piccini 04, Zile 04, Bursi 06). The earliest presentation of diabetic cardiomyopathy is diastolic dysfunction with normal left atrial and ventricular dimensions and only mild systolic dysfunction parameters (Zarich 88, Bell 03b, Piccini 04). Diastolic dysfunction is diagnosed when the ejection fraction is preserved (>50%) and LV relaxation and compliance are impaired, resulting in an abnormal relationship between LV pressure and volume. Prolongation of isovolumetric relaxation times occurs, "which reflect the rate of active LV diastolic relaxation between aortic valve closure and the opening of the mitral valve. Relaxation of the myocardium is an energy-dependent process requiring calcium sequestration from the cytosol into the sarcoplasmic reticulum, and it is altered in diabetes" (Young 04). Early diastolic filling is impaired (Zile 02, Bell 03b), and there is exacerbation of the contribution of atrial contraction to diastolic filling (Young 04). Subsequently, higher filling pressures are needed to maintain normal LV end-diastolic volume (Piccini 04). LV diastolic dysfunction is associated with CAN (Ragonese 92, Lo 95, Rajan 02), correlates with A1C (Piccini 04), and improves over 1 year of better glycemic control (Iribarren 01, Grandi 06).

Diastolic dysfunction is more common in young diabetic female than male patients (Suys 04). It has been identified in 29–52% of asymptomatic young women (aged 20–39 years) and adolescents with type 1 diabetes of >5 years' duration (Airaksinen 84a,87b, Zarich 88, Ragonese 92, Borgia 99, Schannwell 02a, Adal 06). An echocardiographic study of 157 type 1 diabetes patients aged 12–39 years (mean age 26 years; mean diabetes duration 15 years; 100 males) excluded subjects with abnormal exercise ECG. The investigator found that 45 young patients had diastolic dysfunction (28.7%), 15 also had depressed systolic function, and only three patients had isolated systolic dysfunction (1.9%). Diastolic dysfunction was identified 8 years after diabetes diagnosis and systolic dysfunction after 18 years (Raev 94). Diastolic dysfunction was associated with microalbuminuria in many studies of young diabetic patients (Airaksinen 87b, Sampson 90, Ragonese 92, Watschinger 93, Raev 94, Guglielmi 95, Borgia 99), while others found increased ventricular contractility associated with increased CrCl (hyperfiltration) and microalbuminuria (Kimball 94) or decreased ventricular contractile function with exercise (Mildenberger 84, Borow 90). In addition to differences in cardiac parameters based on duration of diabetes and gender, ethnic differences need to taken into account during evaluations for diabetic cardiomyopathy (Carnethon 05, Bertoni 06).

The pathophysiology of diabetic diastolic dysfunction is related to several possible mechanisms: (1) augmented fatty acid utilization and decreased glucose consumption, (2) abnormalities in high-energy phosphate metabolism, (3) mitochondrial dysfunction with impaired depolarization and superoxide production, (4) impaired calcium transport, (5) cardiomyocyte hypertrophy and high resting tension (6) interstitial accumulation of advanced glycation end products (AGEs); (7) imbalance in collagen synthesis and degradation, (8) abnormal microvascular function, (9) activated cardiac renin–angiotensin system, and (10) decreased adiponectin levels (Taegtmeyer 02, Young 02, Diamant 03, Sam 05, Stevens 05, An 06a, Cesario 06, Hassouna 06, Katz 06, Poornima 06, Tsujino 06, vanHeerebeek 08). Experimental evidence suggests that hyperglycemia promotes myocyte apoptosis (Frustaci 00) mediated by activation of the transcription factor p53 and effector responses involving the local renin–angiotensin system (Fiordaliso 01).

Detection of diastolic dysfunction depends on standard echocardiography with pulsed-wave Doppler examinations during the second stage of the Valsalva maneuver or with tissue Doppler imaging. Due to the cost, it has been proposed to limit screening to patients with microalbuminuria (Bell 03b). Ventricular function measurements are discussed further in the section titled "Clinical Assessment for CVD in Diabetic Women." ACE inhibitors are used in diastolic heart failure (but not in pregnancy), and third-generation β-blockers, such as carvedilol, are of proven benefit in heart failure by providing the advantages of vasodilatation and decreased insulin resistance (Bell 03b, Piccini 04).

Systolic heart failure is essentially cardiac pump failure corresponding to an ejection fraction <50%. LV systolic dysfunction has multiple etiologies. In addition to diabetic cardiomyopathy, these etiologies include but are not limited to CHD, valvular heart disease, congenital heart disease, dilated cardio-myopathies, and restrictive cardiomyopathies. In young patients with type 1 diabetes and normal baseline LVEF, there is recent evidence of progressive contractile dysfunction associated with hyperglycemia, a functional impairment of cardiac sympathetic innervation, and limited myocardial perfusion with handgrip exercise (Scognamiglio 98,05a).

Observational studies have not emphasized clinically evident heart failure in diabetic pregnant women on more than an anecdotal basis unless there was severe preeclampsia (Leguizamon 04). LV systolic dysfunction is a key feature of peripartum cardiomyopathy (PPCM) (Pearson 00). It is unknown whether diabetes is a risk factor for this dangerous separate syndrome.

Assessment of cardiac function during pregnancy

This assessment must account for the physiological hemodynamic changes of pregnancy. The second trimester brings significant increases in total body water; blood volume by 45–50%; HR by 10 bpm; mitral, aortic, and pulmonary areas; mitral, aortic, and pulmonary stroke volume; mitral, aortic, and pulmonary CO by 43–48%; and cardiac index (CI). Slower progression occurs through the third trimester and is usually accompanied by an ~30% decrease in systemic vascular resistance (SVR) and decreased afterload (Robson 89, Duvekot 93,94, Mabie 94). A progressive increase of LV wall thickness and mass develops by the second trimester (Hunter 92, Schannwell 02b). Disagreement exists among studies as to whether end-diastolic and end-systolic LV dimensions increase and whether LVEFs increase, stay the same, or decrease during uncomplicated pregnancy (Katz 78, Laird-Meeter 79, Robson 89, Vered 91, Sadaniantz 92, Clapp 97, Mesa 99, Schannwell 03). Differences in measurements of LV dimensions may depend on use of preconception or postpartum measurements for nonpregnant control values because increased LV mass may persist for many months after delivery (Clapp 97). It is noted that interpretation of ejection phase indexes is difficult during pregnancy because they are affected by changes in ventricular mass, HR, venous return (preload), and afterload (Robson 89). Additional data are needed using load-independent measures.

Measurements of LV fractional shortening and LVEF did not differ in pregnant women with and without diabetes in the two available longitudinal studies (Airaksinen 86, Schannwell 03). However, the first study reported lower first-trimester stroke volume in 17 women with type 1 diabetes compared with controls and less increase in stroke volume and CO by the third trimester, especially in six women with microvascular complications. Only two diabetic women in this series had mild, controlled hypertension (Airaksinen 86). The second and larger study of 51 pregnant women with type 1 diabetes and 51 controls found similar values for stroke volume, CO, CI, and SVR in the first trimester in both groups, with the expected changes throughout pregnancy also similar in both groups. Investigators did report a decrease in LV fractional shortening in the third trimester in both groups, which returned to baseline by 8 weeks postpartum (Schannwell 03). Significant differences in LV fractional shortening were not observed between groups or between trimesters in the first study (Airaksinen 86). Additional investigations are needed about cardiac function in pregnant diabetic women.

Limited data can be found on the prevalence of diastolic ventricular dysfunction or diabetic cardiomyopathy in pregnancy. The natural gestational volume overload and atrial dilation are associated with a disturbed diastolic relaxation pattern late in uncomplicated pregnancy (reduction of peak early diastolic flow (E), increase of late filling with atrial contraction (A), and increased isovolumetric relaxation time) (Sadaniantz 92, Mesa 99, Schannwell 02). Women developing gestational hypertension evidenced delayed diastolic relaxation at the beginning of pregnancy, and one-half developed early signs of a restrictive diastolic filling pattern by 24 weeks gestation with increased relative wall thickness (Schannwell 01, Valensise 06). Patients with GDM showed a mild degree of diastolic abnormality (higher atrial filling wave, lower rapid filling wave) compared with controls in the third trimester with persistence at 8 weeks postpartum (Freire 06). Only one study investigated LV diastolic function using Doppler echocardiography in pregnant women with type 1 diabetes (Schannwell 03). As a group, the diabetic women showed signs of disturbed diastolic relaxation at the beginning of pregnancy. In 29 of 51 patients without albuminuria, there was deterioration of diastolic dysfunction with a restrictive filling pattern by the end of the second trimester. Ten of these 29 patients had complications before delivery: four with serious ventricular arrhythmia, three with ventricular tachycardia, and three with progressive dyspnea leading to induction of premature labor (Schannwell 03). Measures of ventricular function are discussed in more detail in the section titled "Clinical Assessment for CVD in Diabetic Women."

Ischemic Stroke

Ischemic stroke in young people aged 16–39 years is more common in women than men and was associated with hypertension and migraine, but not thrombophilia, in a U.K. population with a 44% frequency of smoking (Sastry 06). Ischemic stroke is much more common in relatively young diabetic women than female controls of similar age (Leys 02, Hillier 03, Mulnier 06, Sundquist 06), although the absolute risk is low (standardized mortality ratio 37.0; mortality rate 11.7 per 100,00 person-years at age 20–39 years (Laing 03b). The increased risk of ischemic stroke in diabetic versus nondiabetic women is independently associated with hyperglycemia; there was no increased risk in diabetic women reaching target fasting glucose levels (Boden-Albala 08).

Regarding stroke attributable to type 1 diabetes, stroke prevalence in the Pittsburgh cross-sectional survey of 281 women aged 29 ± 8 years was 1.4% (Orchard 92) compared with 0.6% in the EURODIAB cross-sectional survey of 1,582 women with type 1 diabetes aged 33 ± 10 years (29% smokers) (Koivisto 96). Young to middle-aged women with type 1 diabetes had a considerably higher risk of premature stroke than female controls in Sweden (standardized incidence ratio 26.1; 73.5 in the presence of DN) (Sundquist 06). A prospective study in the central U.S. found the 20-year age-adjusted cumulative incidence of stroke to be 4% in women with type 1 diabetes of at least 5 years' duration (aged 10–45 years at baseline) (Klein 04).

The increase in risk of stroke attributable to type 2 diabetes was highest among women aged 35–54 years in a population study in the U.K. (HR 8.2; 95% CI 4.3–15.5 compared with age- and sex-matched controls). The rate of stroke events per 10,000 person-years in nonpregnant women with type 2 diabetes was 15.3 at 35–44 years, 30.0 at 45–54 years, and 56.5 at 55–64 years. Independent risk factors for stroke in this type 2 diabetes cohort of 41,799 patients included duration of diabetes beyond 5 years, smoker at any time, BMI ≥35, hypertension, and atrial fibrillation (Mulnier 06). Early-onset type 2 diabetes in 1,600 patients aged 18–44 years yielded a 1.6% frequency of stroke over 4 years after diabetes diagnosis in Oregon, with a hazard ratio of 30.1 compared with matched controls (Hillier 03).

Carotid atherosclerosis marked by intima-media thickening (IMT) or plaque burden is also a predictor of CHD in young to middle-aged diabetic women (Wofford 91, Burke 95, Hodis 98, Larsen 05a). Suggestive evidence of carotid atherosclerosis is even found in children and adolescents with type 1 diabetes (Frost 02, Hayaishi-Okano 02, Jarvisalo 02, Yavuz 02). Independent significant correlates of carotid IMT in youth with type 1 diabetes include duration of diabetes, systolic BP, weight, and height (Schwab 07).

In 2006, two national working groups (AHA/American Stroke Association and the National Institute of Neurological Disorders and Stroke [NINDS]) released recommendations on primary prevention of ischemic stroke and on future research (Bushnell 06, Goldstein 06). The groups reviewed evidence that tight control of hypertension and appropriate use of statins will reduce the risk of strokes in diabetic patients and that tight glycemic control will reduce the risk of CVD. They confirmed other CVD guidelines in setting targets for control of weight, BP, glucose, and lipids.

We have few data on the risk of ischemic stroke in diabetic pregnant women. In a large U.S. population survey of >9 million pregnancies using hospital discharge data, the risk of ischemic stroke was 9.2 per 100,000. Ischemic stroke represented 27% of pregnancy-associated strokes of all types. Of 766 ischemic strokes, 29% were associated with an antepartum discharge code, 31% with intrapartum (delivery) codes, and 45% with postpartum codes. Risk of pregnancy-related strokes of all types was more likely with maternal diabetes in univariate analysis (OR 2.5; 95% CI 1.3–4.6), but this association was probably weakened by inclusion of the code for GDM as well as PDM (James 05). Other risk factors in this and another large U.S. study included age ≥35 years, migraine, thrombophilia, systemic lupus erythematosus, chronic hypertension, gestational hypertension–preeclampsia, and smoking (Lanska 98,00, James 05). The risk of pregnancy-related stroke (all types) was 49.8 per 100,000 in a population-based cohort of 654,957 pregnant women in Sweden in 1987–1995 (Birth and Inpatient Registers). Crude RR was 1.7 (0.7–3.7) for an association with maternal diabetes (both PDM and GDM) (Ros 02).

Lower Extremity Arterial Disease

LEAD, also known as peripheral arterial disease (PAD), contributes to serious morbidity and excess mortality in both type1 and type 2 diabetes via occlusive arterial disease in the lower extremities and the association of LEAD with CHD and ischemic stroke (Marso 06). Diabetes is most strongly associated with below-the-knee LEAD (femoral–popliteal, tibial); hypertension and smoking are more associated with proximal PAD in the aorto-ilio-femoral vessels (ADA 03). Intermittent claudication is the most common symptom of LEAD, "defined as pain, cramping, or aching in the calves, thighs, or buttocks that appears reproducibly with walking exercise and is relieved by rest" (ADA 03). The limb-threatening manifestations of PAD, such as rest pain, non-healing wounds, tissue loss, or gangrene, are collectively termed critical limb ischemia (ADA 03). One-fourth of patients will demonstrate progression of LEAD symptoms over a 5-year period, with limb loss in ~4%; >20% will experience major cardiovascular events (Weitz 96).

More than one-half of diabetic patients with abnormal lower extremity arterial tests do not report claudication (Weitz 96, Wang 05a), possibly related to the association of LEAD with peripheral neuropathy. The absence of peripheral pulses also suffers from insensitivity as a predictor of LEAD; estimation of the prevalence of LEAD should rely upon a validated and reproducible test, such as the ABI, which is a noninvasive, quantitative measurement of the patency of the lower extremity arterial system (ADA 03). The ABI test involves using a BP cuff and handheld Doppler device to estimate systolic pressure in the dorsalis pedis and posterior tibial arteries compared with the brachial artery pressure, expressed as a ratio. The ABI has been validated against angiographically confirmed disease, and a ratio <0.9 was found to be 95% sensitive and almost 100% specific (Bernstein 82, Belch 03). A more conservative ratio of <0.8 has been used in some studies of diabetic women in their 30s and 40s (DCCT 86, Klein 03). A widely quoted survey using ABI in diabetic patients of both types who were >40 years of age reported a prevalence of LEAD of 20% (Elhadd 97). One limitation of the ABI is the possibility of abnormally elevated values due to calcified, poorly compressible vessels, but this problem is mainly found in older patients and is less likely in women (Forrest 00, ADA 03). An ABI ratio >1.30 suggests noncompressible arteries (Hiatt 01). Use of the ABI test and other diagnostic tests performed in the vascular clinic are discussed in greater detail in the section titled "Clinical Assessment for CVD in Diabetic Women."

The pathophysiology of atherosclerosis is relevant to the pathogenisis of LEAD in diabetes. The abnormal metabolic state of diabetes results in the pathogenic processes of (1) oxidative stress, (2) inflammation, (3) endothelial cell dysfunction with decreased bioavailability of endothelium-derived NO, (4) increased production of vasoconstrictors with increased vascular tone and vascular smooth muscle growth and migration, and (5) enhanced platelet aggregation and thrombosis coupled with impaired fibrinolysis (Olson 02, Marso 06). Risk factors for development of LEAD in diabetes include smoking, chronic or intermittent hyperglycemia, duration of diabetes, mixed hyperlipidemia (especially TGs), hypertension, hyperhomocysteinemia (MacGregor 99, Selvin 04a, Smith 04, Wildman 05, Cassar 06, Marso 06, Gonzalez-Clementi 08), and elevated BMI and fibrinogen in women (Klein 03). Ethnicity studies reveal a twofold higher risk of PAD in African-American people and equivalent risks in Asians, Hispanics, and non-Hispanic whites (Kullo 03, Pasternak 04).

Data are limited on the prevalence of LEAD in women of reproductive age with type 1 diabetes. Using only questionnaire data reporting intermittent claudication, peripheral artery bypass surgery, or lower limb amputation, LEAD developed in 2.7% of 259 patients with type 1 diabetes (mean age 35 years; duration 18 years) followed for 10 years in Denmark (Deckert 96). However, in the Pittsburgh population of 636 patients with type 1 diabetes (men and women; mean age 28 years; mean duration 20 years), 12.4% had evidence of LEAD defined by an ABI ratio <0.9, claudication, or amputation for a vascular cause at the baseline examination in 1986–1988. In this study, 278 women without LEAD at baseline (mean age 30 ± 8 years) were followed for 6 years, and 13.7% developed an abnormal ABI or claudication. Independent predictors of development of LEAD in multivariable analysis were smoking, duration of diabetes, glycohemoglobin, and LDL-C (Forrest 00). In the DCCT follow-up study of relatively healthy diabetic patients at intake into the trial, an average of four ABI tests <0.90 was detected in 2.0% of 405 women (mean age 39 ± 7 years; mean duration 18 years) with type 1 diabetes several years after conclusion of the trial. No relationship was found between average ABI and prior DCCT treatment group (Klein 03). The frequency of peripheral vascular disease codes in the medical records of patients with early-onset type 2 diabetes (aged 18–44 years) was 1.6% over a mean of 4 years after diagnosis of diabetes; the hazard ratio was 3.6 for increased risk compared with matched controls (Hillier 03). We have only anecdotal reports of LEAD complicating diabetes and pregnancy.

Early diagnosis of LEAD depends on the awareness of primary care physicians employing complete physical examination and simple testing with appropriate referrals to a vascular clinic or specialist (Hirsch 01, Dolan 02, Belch 03, Gonzalez-Clemente 08). Management of diabetic patients with early LEAD depends on prevention of hyperglycemia, reduction of CVD risk factors, cessation of smoking, supervised treadmill exercise therapy, use of cilostazol in the absence of heart failure (inadequate studies in human pregnancy; causes malformations and stillbirths in rodent pregnancy), and antithrombotic therapy (Weitz 96, Hiatt 01, ADA 03).

Risk Factors for Cardiovascular Disease in Women with PDM

The risk factors for CHD are very similar in pregnancy as well as in other diabetic women of reproductive age and older women (Table II.6) (Hare 77, Pombar 95, Gordon 96a, Collins 02, Knopp 02, Orchard 03, Sullebarger 03, Barrett-Conner 04). Recent evidence confirms that hyperglycemia is an important risk factor and that intensified glycemic control is beneficial. Many studies show that CHD is more frequent with a history of poor glycemic control and that mortality during CVD events is worsened by ongoing hyperglycemia (Jensen-Urstad 96, Haffner 98b, Lawson 99, Lehto 99, Stratton 00, Larsen 02, Luescher 03, Snell-Bergeon 03, Barrett-Connor 04, Juttilainen 04, Selvin 04b, Meier 05, Scognamiglio 05b, Stettler 06, Boden-Albala 08, Juutilainen 08).

The DCCT type 1 intensive diabetes management group had a 57% reduction in serious CVD events (p = 0.02) in long-term follow-up after the trial, proving that tight control of diabetes reduces CVD. CVD benefits were independently related to decline in A1C values during the 6–7-year intensive treatment trial, even though A1C levels rose during the 11-year follow-up in which similar cardioprotective drug therapy was used in both study groups. These and other DCCT results support the concept of imprinting some kind of biochemical or tissue benefit by a prior period of improved glycemic control. The mean age of DCCT subjects at baseline was 27 years, with mean duration of diabetes of 6 years and mean age of 45 years at the end of the EDIC (DCCT/EDIC 05). Therefore, these results are quite relevant to diabetic women who might or do become pregnant. CVD benefit occurred even though ~25% of subjects (with the highest baseline BMI) gained an excess amount of weight and showed small increases in BP, cholesterol, and TGs during intensive treatment (Purnell 98). These obesity traits may be heritable in this subset (Purnell 03). After the DCCT trial, progression of carotid artery IMT over 6 years was also significantly less in women in the original intensive therapy group. Besides the treatment group, modifiable risk factors for IMT progression in multivariate analysis included smoking and systolic BP

TABLE II.6 CHD Risk Factors or Indicators Probably Applicable to Diabetic Pregnant Women*

Established Risk Factors
- Older age
- Long duration of diabetes
- Insulin resistance factors, central obesity, and inflammation
- Hypertension
- Renal disease including microalbuminuria
- Smoking
- Hypercholesterolemia
- Combined hyperlipidemia (elevated LDL-C and triglycerides)
- Low HDL-C levels
- Family history of premature arteriosclerotic vascular disease in first-degree relatives (<55 in males; <65 in females)
- Oral contraceptive use at age ≥35 prior to pregnancy

Emerging Risk Factors or Indicators
- Poor glycemic control; as a determinant of other factors
- Cardiac autonomic dysfunction
- Prolonged QT interval
- Left ventricular hypertrophy measured by electrocardiography or echocardiography
- Carotid intima-media thickening
- Low adiponectin
- Elevated B-type natriuretic peptide
- Elevated C-reactive protein by high-sensitive assay (hsCRP)
- Elevated total homocysteine levels
- Elevated Lp(a)
- Elevated serum uric acid

Inflammatory Conditions Aggravating Risk Factors (examples)
- Chronic periodontal disease; lupus erythematosis

Best assessed prior to gestation.

CHD, coronary heart disease.

(DCCT/EDIC 03). Extensive CAC on follow-up was also independently related to A1C levels during the trial, with a lower prevalence in women ≥50 years of age who had been in the intensive treatment group (Cleary 06).

Combinations of risk factors are worse than single risk factors alone and increase risk of CVD exponentially. It is fair to state that CHD in pregnancy almost always occurs with combinations of risk factors that might include diabetes of long duration or heterozygous familial hypercholesterolemia; other risk factors include smoking and oral contraceptive use after age 35. The risk factors are comprised of those that are well established, those that are emerging, and concomitant inflammatory factors that amplify both (Table II.6). Despite ample evidence of benefit, we must emphasize that management of basic, well-established risk factors in diabetic women often has been inadequate during usual medical care (Soedamah-Muthu 02, Pyorala 04, Mosca 05, Wadwa 05, Zgibor 05, Wang 07). There is considerable debate about the role of new biomarkers for CVD in clinical practice (deLemos 06, Rothenbacher 06, Tang 06, Wang 06a, St Clair 07). Inflammation is now understood to be an important part of the pathogenesis of atherosclerosis (Ross 99, Hansson 05), and markers of inflammation strongly predict onset and progression of atherosclerosis in diabetic women of reproductive age (Costacou 05a, Schram 05, Wadwa 06). The effect of intensified glycemic control on markers of inflammation is complex; 3 years of DCCT therapy reduced levels of soluble intracellular adhesion molecule type 1 and increased levels of soluble TNF-α receptor-1 and hsCRP among those who gained weight (Schaumberg 05). A diagram of the sources of inflammatory markers and cytokines that may be involved in the pathophysiology of CVD is presented in Figure II.3 (Rader 00).

DN and microalbuminuria are well-known risk factors for CHD in asymptomatic diabetic patients (Earle 96, Rutter 99, Kim 07). However, algorithms to detect low risk of abnormal coronary angiography among diabetic candidates for kidney (Manske 93, Koch 97, Ramanathan 05, Witczak 06) or islet transplants (Senior 05) fail to reach consensus.

In a 1987–1990 Minneapolis survey of coronary angiograms in 110 azotemic renal transplant candidates (45% women) with onset of type 1 diabetes by age 30, coronary stenosis >50% of diameter was observed in 1 of 5 patients aged ≤25 years, 14 of 47 (29.8%) aged 25.1–35.0 years, 22 of 42 (52.4%) aged 35.1–45.0 years, and in 100% of 16 patients aged >45 years (Manske 92a). In a multivariate comparison of risks for coronary stenosis in the 52 renal failure patients aged 20–35 years, relative odds with 95% CI were 26.0 (1.4–496) for family history of a first-degree relative with an MI before age 55 years, 8.6 (1.0–77.2) for hypertension treated for >5 years, and 2.3 (1.1–5.1) for A1C. In the multivariate comparison in the group of 42 azotemic patients aged 35.1–45 years, the risks were somewhat different: 7.9 (1.0–6.1) for >5 pack/years smoking, 2.2 (1.2–3.3) for diabetes duration, and 1.8 (1.0–3.3) for A1C. In spite of the increased risk with smoking, 36% of renal failure patients who never smoked had significant coronary artery stenoses. Of 34 renal failure patients with diabetes duration <20 years, 32.4% had CHD (Manske 92a). In a subset of 14 female renal transplant candidates with type 1 diabetes found to have significant coronary stenosis on angiography, age-groups at randomization (prior to renal transplant) to medical therapy or coronary revascularization (which showed better posttransplant survival) were 3 aged 25–34 years, 5 aged 35–39 years, and 6 aged 40–49 years (Manske 92b). Therefore, CHD seems to be common in relatively young diabetic women with renal failure.

In a contemporaneous analysis of 125 asymptomatic type 1 diabetes patients with CrCl <25 mL/min from the same hospital and authors, the prevalence of coronary artery stenosis >50% was 31% in 27 patients aged <30 years, 29% in 34 patients aged 30–34.9 years, and >50% in the 35–40 and 40–45-year-old age-groups (Manske 93). In this analysis, independent, significant (p < 0.05) risk factors for coronary stenosis in 90 patients <45 years of age were abnormal ST T-segments on ECG at rest (RR 5.7; CI 1.5–21.5) and duration of diabetes (RR 1.6; CI 1.2–2.0). The authors tested a clinical algorithm to predict the presence of coronary artery stenosis >50% of diameter in 70 patients <45 years of age: abnormal ST T-segments on ECG, smoking ≥5 pack-years, or diabetes for at least 25 years. Coronary stenosis was present in 33 of 47 of those predicted and in 1 of 23 of those not predicted. Sensitivity was 97%, PPV 70%, specificity 61%, and NPV 96%. The authors recommended that pretransplant coronary angiography can be avoided in patients <45 years of age without a smoking history, ST T wave changes on ECG, or diabetes duration >25 years (Manske 93).

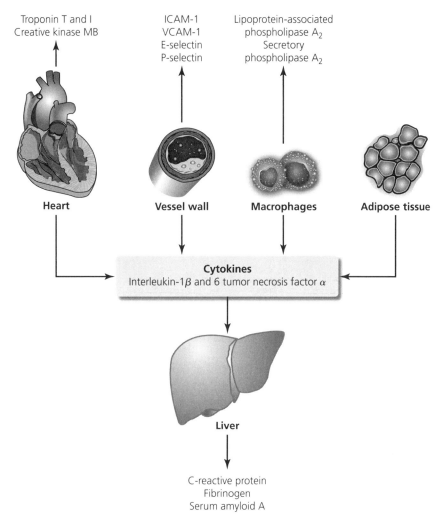

Troponin T and I
Creative kinase MB

ICAM-1
VCAM-1
E-selectin
P-selectin

Lipoprotein-associated
phospholipase A_2
Secretory
phospholipase A_2

Heart   **Vessel wall**   **Macrophages**   **Adipose tissue**

Cytokines
Interleukin-1β and 6 tumor necrosis factor α

Liver

C-reactive protein
Fibrinogen
Serum amyloid A

FIGURE II.3 Sources of inflammatory markers and cytokines related to cardiovascular disease. Markers (e.g., C-reactive protein, fibrinogen, serum amyloid A) originate in the liver, and their production is stimulated by systemic cytokines (e.g., interleukin-1β, interleukin-6, tumor necrosis factor-α). Cytokines are produced at several extrahepatic sites (e.g., heart, vascular endothelium and smooth muscle cells, macrophages, adipose tissue, placenta) that can also produce other types of inflammatory markers. The heart secretes troponin T and I, creatine kinase MB, and B-type natriuretic peptide (BNP not pictured) in response to injury and stress. The atherosclerotic vessel wall produces soluble adhesion molecules in response to cytokines (e.g., intercellular adhesion molecule 1 (ICAM-1), vascular cell adhesion molecule 1 (VCAM-1), E-selectin, P-selectin). Macrophages secrete phospholipases in response to inflammation. Lipoprotein-associated phospholipase A_2 (LpPLA2; also known as platelet-activating factor acetylhydrolase) predicts morbidity and mortality from CVD and may enhance atherogenesis by hydrolyzing oxidized phospholipids.
Modified from Rader 2000 and used with permission. CVD, cardiovascular disease.

Other analyses of CHD in patients with diabetic renal failure yield different interpretations. Coronary angiography was performed during the first 6 months of dialysis treatment in 105 consecutive patients evaluated for renal transplantation in Germany (77 type 1 diabetes, 28 type 2 diabetes). Clinical symptoms and ECG ST-segment depression assessed at rest did not distinguish between patients with or without CAD. CAD was detected by angiography in 4 of 14 (29%) patients aged <30 years and in 13 of 43 (30%) patients aged 30–45 years inclusive. Because diabetic patients with end-stage renal disease have a poor effort tolerance, noninvasive diagnostic procedures coupled with exercise were considered to be of limited value. Therefore, the authors recommended coronary angiography in all diabetic patients with renal failure prior to renal transplantation for purposes of risk stratification and to determine which patients might benefit from coronary revascularization (Koch 97). Authors conducting a retrospective analysis of 97 renal transplant candidates in Tennessee of coronary stenosis >70% of diameter were unable to identify a suitable age threshold to predict severe CAD, but they did state that "invasive tests may not be necessary in young, African American diabetic patients who have no smoking history and a BMI <25" (Ramanathan 05). In a population study of 155 asymptomatic diabetic renal transplant candidates undergoing routine pretransplant coronary angiography in Norway during 1999–2004, no coronary stenosis was detected in 11 patients aged <35 years; sensitivity and NPV was 100% and specificity was 14% for this cut-off value, but this was a post hoc analysis (Witczak 06).

In a prospective cohort study in Alberta, Canada, 60 consecutive patients with type 1 diabetes who were candidates for islet transplant (mean age 46 ± 10 years; 62% female; 47% smoked at any time; 35% on antihypertensive drugs; 70% normoalbuminuric) underwent coronary angiography, stress ECG, and myocardial perfusion imaging (MPI). Of 53 patients without coronary symptoms, 43% had coronary stenoses >50% of diameter. Stress ECG and MPI had low sensitivity as predictors of hemodynamically relevant abnormal angiography. Only 8 of 60 patients met the Minneapolis pre-renal transplant criteria for low risk of CAD, and none had coronary stenosis (Senior 05).

Pathogenesis of atherosclerosis in diabetes

Related probable contributors to pathogenesis of atherosclerosis in diabetes include (1) insulin resistance with flux of FFA to macrovascular endothelial cells, mitochondrial oxidation of FFA, and production of reactive oxygen species (Dabelea 03, Orchard 03, Perseghin 03, Brownlee 05); (2) oxidative and nitrosative stress (autoxidation of glucose) (Wolff 87), mitochondrial electron-chain generation of superoxide, activation of the DNA repair enzyme poly(ADP-ribose) polymerase (PARP), and decrease of glyceraldehyde-3-phosphate dehydrogenase (GAPDH) (Brownlee 01,05, Leopold 05); (3) superoxide interaction with NO, forming the vasculotoxic peroxynitrite, with overactivation of PARP (Pieper 95, Dominguez 98, Keaney 99, Orchard 99, Valabhji 01, Maara 02, Maritim 03, Brandes 05, Mabley 05, Pacher 06); (4) lipid peroxidation (marked by F2-isoprostanes, the nonenzymatic oxidation products of arachidonic acid formed in situ on esterified phospholipids and released in free form by the action of phospholipases) (Roberts 97, Davi 99); and (5) advanced AGE products formed by the glycoxidation of fructoselysine (Vlassara 88, Yan 94, Kislinger 99, Cipollone 03, Yan 03, Ahmed 05, Basta 06). Abundant evidence indicates that hyperglycemia enhances these pathogenic processes (Morigi 98, Williams 98, Du 01, Algensiaedt 03, Brownlee 05, Nieuwdorp 06). Figure II.4 diagrams the vascular pathways of oxidative and nitrosative

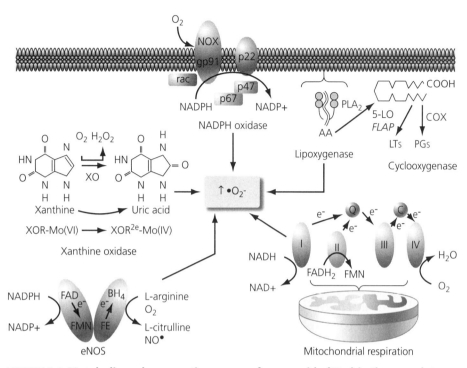

FIGURE II.4 Metabolic and enzymatic sources of superoxide ($\cdot O_{2-}$) in the vasculature.
(1) NADPH oxidase is comprised of multiple membrane-bound and cytoplasmic subunits. The enzyme is activated when the cytoplasmic subunits p67 and p47 and the small G-protein *rac* assemble with the membrane-bound NOX and p22^{phox}. NADPH oxidase uses NADPH as a substrate and, in vascular cells, is considered an important source of reactive oxygen species (ROS) generation. (2) The lipoxygenases and cyclooxygenases (COX) generate ROS indirectly by promoting formation of inflammatory mediators. Arachidonic acid (AA) that is cleaved from the membrane by phospolipase A$_2$ (PLA$_2$) is then metabolized by 5-lipoxygenase (5-LO) in the presence of its accessory protein (FLAP) to form leukotrienes (LTs). AA is also metabolized by COX to form members of another family of inflammatory mediators, the prostaglandins (PGs). (3) Mitochondria also generate superoxide as electrons are transferred from complex I to complex IV during cellular respiration. (4) Xanthine oxidase (XO), which converts hypoxanthine and xanthine to uric acid, is an additional source of ROS. As xanthine is converted to uric acid, two electrons are donated to molybdenum (Mo) at the active site of the enzyme, thereby reducing it from Mo(VI) to Mo(IV). (5) Endothelial nitric oxide synthase (eNOS), when substrate or cofactors are not replete, uncouples to generate superoxide in preference to NO. Although ambient ROS production is involved in basal cellular homeostatic function, vascular disease ensues when there is increased ROS generation and/or decreased antioxidant defense. There is evidence that hyperglycemia stimulates these processes. When superoxide anions accumulate in the vessel wall, they react and form a number of pathogenic ROS: (a) peroxynitrites and peroxynitrous acids from NO, (b) H$_2$O$_2$ via superoxide dysmutase, (c) lipid peroxides, and (d) hypochlorite and hypochlorous acid from H$_2$O$_2$ and Cl$^-$ via myeloperoxidase.
Q, coenzyme Q; C, cytochrome C; FAD, flavin adenine dinucleotide; FMN, flavin mononucleotide; FE, heme iron; BH$_4$, tetrahydrobiopterin. Modified from Leopold 05 and used with permission.

stress as well as the several sources of superoxide anion within the cell (Leopold 05). Increasing attention is given to gender-specific differences in the pathophysiology of atherosclerosis (Quyyumi 06).

The high-risk HLA genotype DQ2/8 may be associated with atherogenic vascular and lipid phenotypes in young patients with type 1 diabetes (Odermarsky 07). Type 2 diabetic patients with the null genotype for glutathione *S*-transferase (important in modulation of inflammation and oxidation) have excess premature vascular morbidity and death (Doney 05). Studies with endothelial cells show that oscillating high glucose is more effective in triggering the generation of nitrotyrosine and inducing the expression of adhesion molecules and IL-6 than stable high glucose (Piconi 04). Intervention trials are contemplated to prevent CVD by pharmacological reduction of oxidative stress (Cai 03, Ceriello 03, Pacher 05), blockade of receptors for AGE (RAGE) activation (Jandeleit-Dahm 05), or metabolic therapy to inhibit cardiac mitochondrial oxidation of FFA (Rosano 06). It is fascinating to learn that common antihypertensive drugs, such as ACE inhibitors and calcium channel blockers (CCBs), have strong antioxidant potential at the intracellular level (Steinhauff 04, Ceriello 06, Sudano 06, Yoshi 06).

Adiponectin, a product of adipocytes and placenta, is another risk factor circulating in fairly high concentrations that accumulates in damaged vascular walls and modulates the endothelial inflammatory response and production of ROS (Ouchi 99, Okamoto 00, Kubota 02, Ouedraogo 06). Low adiponectin levels in type 1 diabetes female subjects may be associated with elevated risk for CHD (Costacou 05b, Maahs 05a). Increased levels of adiponectin are positively associated with abnormal renal function (macroalbuminuria, rising creatinine) and duration of type 2 diabetes (Looker 04).

Clinical Assessment for CVD in Diabetic Women

In addition to assessment of risk factors, further evidence to suspect CVD in pregnancy can be obtained from the symptom history, physical examination, laboratory testing, and noninvasive testing of cardiovascular function.

Screening for CHD

It is increasingly recognized that CHD presents differently in women than in men, which may impact early diagnosis and treatment (Barrett-Connor 04, Bairey-Merz 06). Atypical or absence of chest pain is more common in diabetic women with myocardial ischemia (Douglas 96, Nesto 99, Knopp 02), probably due to cardiac neuropathy (Faerman 77). Should suspicion arise of CHD on historical or clinical grounds in pregnant women with PDM, noninterventional, nonradiological testing of cardiac function can be ordered.

The ADA/American College of Cardiology (ACC) Consensus Development Conference on the diagnosis of CHD in people with diabetes (ADA 98) emphasized the importance of early identification of CHD so that therapies proven to reduce the incidence of CVD events can be applied (Gaede 03, Hurst 03, Gaede 08). A similar conclusion was reached by a diabetes and CVD prevention conference organized by the AHA (Grundy 02b). CHD can present as early as the third and fourth decade of life in type 1 diabetes, and CHD may already be present at the time of diagnosis of type 2 diabetes. The conferences concluded that the coronary arteries are involved more diffusely and that disease may extend more distally in multiple arteries in diabetes. Diabetic women are also at increased risk of developing congestive heart failure. The ADA/ACC conference recommended using the indications for cardiac testing in diabetic patients listed in Table II.7 and

TABLE II.7 Conditions Warranting Testing for Coronary Heart Disease in Diabetic Women

1. Typical or atypical cardiac symptoms
2. Resting electrocardiograph suggestive of ischemia or infarction
3. Peripheral or carotid occlusive arterial disease
4. Sedentary lifestyle, age >35 years, and plans to begin a vigorous exercise program
5. Two or more of the risk factors listed below (a-e) in addition to diabetes [controversial]
    a. Total cholesterol >200 mg/dL, LDL-C >100 mg/dL, HDL-C <50 mg/dL, or triglycerides > 150 mg/dL*
    b. BP >140/90
    c. Smoking history
    d. Family history of premature CHD (males aged <55, females aged <65)
    e. Positive micro/macroalbuminuria test

Based on the Consensus Development Conference on the Diagnosis of Coronary Heart Disease in People with Diabetes (ADA 98). Section 5 remains controversial because diabetic women >45 years of age may have CHD in the absence of these factors (Wackers 04), but there is evidence that these factors do increase the risk of CVD in diabetic women of reproductive age.
*Lipid thresholds are adapted to 2007 diabetes-linked CVD risk factor reduction guidelines (ADA 07, Buse 07).

CHD, coronary heart disease; CVD, cardiovascular disease.

presented flow diagrams for cardiac testing in asymptomatic and symptomatic diabetic patients. For the symptomatic group or those with an abnormal resting electrocardiogram, cardiac testing is mandatory. Evidence of peripheral or carotid occlusive arterial disease also increases the risk substantially. The AHA considers symptomatic diabetic women to be at the same risk level as patients with an abnormal resting or treadmill ECG and recommends stress cardiac imaging as the initial noninvasive technique. The AHA also recommends that local expertise and availability should guide the selection of cardiac imaging techniques (stress echo or stress perfusion imaging) in women with known or suspected CAD who are candidates for cardiac testing (Micres 05). If the imaging test is normal or mildly abnormal with normal LV function, the woman can be referred for further aggressive risk factor modification and/or anti-ischemic treatment. If the test is moderately or severely abnormal or the LVEF is reduced, the patient should proceed to coronary angiography or intravascular US. The latter technique can reveal pathological findings in angiographically normal arteries (Mintz 95, Erbel 99, Larsen 02, Schartl 06).

Controversy surrounds cardiac testing of asymptomatic women with diabetes (Grundy 02b, DiCarli 05, DeLuca 06, Bax 07). The Framingham Heart Study demonstrated that preclinical signs of a compromised coronary circulation include silent ischemia, ECG-LVH, blocked intraventricular conduction, and repolarization abnormalities. The impact of diabetes on CHD is greatest for women and varies with the basic BP, LDL-C, and HDL-C risk factors (Kannel 86). An algorithm based on the Framingham dataset assigns points based on these risk factors. Assuming the presence of hypertension, LDL-C >160 mg/dL, HDL-C <45 mg/dL, and no smoking history, the 10-year CHD risk would be 2% for diabetic women aged 30–34 years, 6% at 35–39 years, 11% at 40–44 years, and 17% at 45–49 years (Wilson 98). The 1998 ADA/ACC consensus panel concluded that asymptomatic patients with diabetes with ≤1 risk factors and a normal resting 12-lead ECG do not require cardiac testing (ADA 98), but this recommendation undergoes continuing study (Earle 96, Janand-Delenne 99, Rutter 02, Sultan 04, Chico 05, Faglia 05, Sorajja 05, Anand 06, Bax 06, Miller 06, Sejil 06, Sibal 06, Beller 07, Johansen 07, Kim 07, Zeina 08).

An international consortium of investigators recommended that patients at increased risk for CHD (such as women aged ≥35 years with diabetes duration >10 years) be screened directly for the presence and severity of atherosclerosis by structure and function testing as opposed to the traditional approach of estimating the likelihood of atherosclerotic disease indirectly by evaluating the multiplicity of risk factors for the disease (Naghavi 06). Recent studies show that using the 1998 guidelines fails to detect a significant percentage of patients with silent ischemia who have few risk factors, at least in older patients with type 2 diabetes (Wackers 04, Rajagopalan 05, Valensi 05, Fornengo 06, Scognamiglio 06, Zgibor 06). Coronary evaluation of asymptomatic patients with type 2 diabetes (aged ≤60 years) with or without two or more risk factors demonstrated that the former group (1,121 patients) had a higher prevalence of three-vessel disease (33% vs. 7.6%), diffuse disease (54.9% vs. 18.0%), and vessel occlusion (31.2% vs. 3.8%) as well as a lower frequency of one-vessel disease (46.3% vs 70.6%); 55% of this group had coronary anatomy allowing a revascularization procedure. The authors concluded that the criterion of two or more risk factors did not help to identify asymptomatic patients with a higher prevalence of CHD (64.6% vs. 65.5%), yet an aggressive coronary evaluation approach in asymptomatic patients without risk factors identified patients with a more favorable angiographic anatomy (Scognamiglio 06). Alternatively, a large prospective study of 521 consecutive asymptomatic diabetic outpatients found a high negative predictive value (0.98) of first-line bioclinical stratification for the occurrence of coronary events over a 1–3-year follow-up (Vanzetto 07).

The 2007 ADA Standards of Medical Care in Diabetes states (paraphrasing): "To identify the presence of CHD in diabetic patients without clear or suggestive symptoms of coronary artery disease, a risk factor-based approach to the initial diagnostic evaluation and subsequent follow-up is recommended… Abnormal risk factors should be treated as described elsewhere in these guidelines, irrespective of coronary artery disease status…Candidates for a screening cardiac stress test include those with (1) an abnormal resting ECG, (2) a history of peripheral or carotid occlusive disease, and (3) sedentary life style, age >35 years, and plans to begin a vigorous exercise program… [it is unknown whether beginning a pregnancy is the equivalent of a vigorous exercise program]…evidence suggests that non-invasive tests can improve assessment of future CHD risk. There is, however, no current evidence that such testing in asymptomatic patients with risk factors improves outcomes or leads to better utilization of treatments…the optimal therapeutic approach to the diabetic patient with silent myocardial ischemia is unknown. Certainly if major coronary artery disease is identified, aggressive intervention appears justified. If minor stenoses are detected, however, it is unknown whether there is any benefit to further invasive evaluation and/or therapy. There are no well-conducted prospective trials with adequate control groups to shed light on this subject. Accordingly, there are no evidence-based guidelines for screening the asymptomatic diabetic patient for coronary artery disease" (ADA 07).

The 2008 revision of the ADA Standards eliminates this language and proposes that risk factors should be evaluated to stratify asymptomatic patients by 10-year risk (by Framingham criteria) and that risk factors be treated accordingly. In patients >40 years of age with another cardiovascular risk factor (hypertension, family history, dyslipidemia, microalbuminuria, CAN, smoking), ACE inhibitor, aspirin, and statin therapy (if not contraindicated, as in pregnancy) should be used to reduce the risk of cardiovascular events (ADA 08a). This position on screening reflects the failure of the risk factor–based approach to identify which older patients will have silent ischemia on cardiac testing (Wackers 04) and evidence that silent myocardial ischemia may reverse over time (Wackers 07). There also is evidence that intensive medical therapy may provide equal outcomes (25% death from any cause or nonfatal MI over 5 years) as percutaneous interventions in 766 diabetic and 1,521 nondiabetic patients (only 15% female; mean age 62 ± 10 years) with objective evidence of stable myocardial ischemia and significant coronary artery disease (Boden 07).

Candidates for further cardiac testing in the 2008 Statement include those with (a) typical or atypical cardiac symptoms and (b) an abnormal resting electrocardiogram (ADA 08a). Other investigators state that "early identification of diabetic patients with silent myocardial ischemia is very important because a significant reduction of mortality and morbidity for cardiovascular diseases can be achieved by the early identification of patients with coronary artery disease, for whom revascularization is important" (Sultan 04). Controlled prospective trials are needed to determine the benefit of identifying relatively younger asymptomatic diabetic women with coronary ischemia and whether interventions beyond aggressive basic risk factor management will reduce the clinical burden of CVD. Further investigation is needed about application of some of the novel risk indicators listed in Table II.6 in the testing algorithm in Table II.7.

No prospective studies have been conducted of screening for CHD before or during diabetic pregnancy. The question of threshold age or duration of diabetes for screening asymptomatic women with a negative resting ECG but two or more additional risk factors (BP, lipids, albuminuria, smoking, family history) remains open. Epidemiological studies of CHD in diabetic women reviewed in the section titled "Coronary Heart Disease" indicate significant risk by age 30–35 with diabetes duration of $\geq$10 years. This population is perhaps an ideal group of patients to screen for silent myocardial ischemia because they will be going through 9–12 months of highly motivated behavior modification to achieve optimal glycemic control for pregnancy and then will face many years of productive life in which CVD prevention provides a big payoff. It is interesting that screening for CVD prior to renal or pancreatic transplantion is well accepted, but screening before a possibly problematic pregnancy is not. The screening ideally would be done in anticipation of pregnancy. If screening of asymptomatic women with risk factors is performed, the simplest approach is stress electrocardiography with hemodynamic assessment. Patients with abnormal stress ECG and patients unable to perform exercise require additional or alternative testing. Stress nuclear perfusion and stress echocardiography are valuable next-level diagnostic procedures, and consultation with a cardiologist is suggested (ADA 07).

The elements of clinical assessment are briefly reviewed in the following sections, with comments on applications in pregnancy where appropriate.

Risk factor history

The classical risk factors listed in the preceding section should be reviewed. Ongoing research is focused on possible gender-specific differences in traditional and novel risk markers (Nicholson 99, Shaw 06a). The family history is particularly important because it serves as a guide to high familial risk even if the risk factor is not known or identifiable. To obtain the best family history, a family tree should be constructed consisting of second-degree relatives (grandparents, uncles, aunts), as well as first-degree relatives (parents, siblings). Recording information about second-degree relatives provides a clue to familial risk factors when first-degree relatives are still young and as yet asymptomatic from CHD. Noncoronary arteriosclerotic disease also signifies increased CHD risk. Such conditions include stroke, transient ischemic attack, intermittent claudication, or arteriosclerotic renal artery stenosis.

Symptom history

The Rose angina questionnaire is a standardized instrument that is widely used for assessment of typical exertional angina (Rose 62, Sorlie 96, May 97, Nicholson 99) and is largely free of biases due to ethnic differences in women (LaCroix 89) or the diagnostic practices of physicians (Hemingway 08):

1. Have you ever had any pain or discomfort? (yes)
2. Do you get it when you walk uphill or hurry?
3. Do you get it when you walk at an ordinary pace on the level?   [If yes to 2. or 3., go on to question 4.]
4. What do you do if you get it while walking? (stop or slow down)
5. If you stand still, what happens? (relieved)
6. How soon? (10 minutes or less)
7. Location? (typical is chest or left arm; women describe more throat, neck, or jaw pain than men)

Persistent angina with nonobstructive CAD remains a serious health matter in women (Hemingway 06, Shaw 06b) and predicts an increased rate of cardiovascular events over 5 years (Johnson 06). The original Rose questionnaire (Rose 62) "included an optional section that asked about other precipitants of discomfort and discomfort other than pain, pressure, or heaviness" (Bittner 08). Angina precipitated by stimuli, such as emotional stress and mental upset, or occurring at rest or during sleep may be important among women (Pepine 94, Krantz 06, Bittner 08). Assessment for depression is needed in the evaluation of risk for CHD progression in women (Rutledge 06). Typical or atypical anginal pain may more likely be associated with microvascular disease in women (Cannon 88, Pepine 06) "that limits the coronary microcirculation during stress" (Johnson 06).

It is problematic that CHD is often "silent" and not always accompanied by angina in patients with diabetes (Nesto 88, Zarich 94, Nesto 99). CAD symptoms can be very subtle in women (Phillpott 01, Kimble 03, Mosca 04, Bittner 08). Unexplained fatigue can antedate abnormalities in exercise tolerance testing. Other atypical symptoms can be aching or pressure in nontypical parts of the chest or neck or even symptoms masquerading as gastroesophageal reflux. Similarly, women having an MI are more likely than men to have jaw, neck, or shoulder pain, nausea, vomiting, fatigue, or dyspnea (Wilcosky 87, Philpott 01, Barrett-Connor 04). Symptoms such as dyspnea, diaphoresis, or nausea are typical anginal equivalents in diabetic patients (Jacoby 92). In addition, sudden death from MI is more common in women than in men and is said to be due to lack of collateral arterial blood flow associated with chronic ischemia (Knopp 02).

Physical examination

Physical signs of arteriosclerotic vascular disease can be easily overlooked or even reasonably omitted from the physical examination of healthy pregnant women. However, in the presence of the subtle symptoms mentioned earlier or a history of the aforementioned CVD risk factors, the examination should search for simple physical signs:

- *Corneal arcus* is a CVD risk factor in its own right in people <50 years of age (Chambless 90). Arcus "senilis" is a crescentic deposit of cholesterol ester at the margin of the iris, seen first superiorly, then inferiorly, and then circumferentially.

- *Carotid bruits* not transmitted from the heart almost always signify arteriosclerotic disease, even if they do not signify operable vascular lesions.

- *Aortic ejection murmur sclerosis.* When the murmur is isolated over the area of the aortic valve without stenosis, it can signify aortic sclerosis, which is related to the injury of vascular endothelium, a process akin to atherosclerosis itself. Thus, calcific aortic sclerosis of the aortic valve is highly correlated with CAD (O'Brien 96, Jaffer 02). Both conditions have the common etiology of injury of vascular endothelium from the classical CVD risk factors resulting in inflammation, scarring, and eventual calcium deposition. Murmurs of aortic sclerosis typically do not signify hemodynamically significant valvular stenosis. The incidence of aortic sclerosis in diabetic pregnancy is unknown. Echocardiography may be necessary to distinguish other anatomical lesions.

- *Abdominal or femoral bruits* may also signify proximal arteriosclerotic vascular disease, in which intermittent claudication can be felt in the buttock or thigh. Bruits can often be heard over the aortic bifurcation, the common iliac arteries, and the femoral arteries (Carter 81).

- *Foot pulses* that are asymmetric or absent suggest the presence of distal arteriosclerotic peripheral vascular disease, which in turn is highly associated with coronary and carotid artery disease (Burke 95, McDermott 05). Only 0.7% of normal extremities are missing both the dorsalis and posterior tibial pulses, at least as detected by a handheld Doppler device (McGee 98).

Laboratory assessment

Early identification of vascular risk "is a cornerstone of diabetes management and facilitates tailored intervention at an early stage of disease when a more useful response is likely to be obtained" (Groop 05). "It is difficult to evaluate the cardiovascular status of patients with diabetes because of complex symptomology, evidence of silent ischemia, and subclinical cardiac disease" (Kragelund 06). Thus, research goes forward to identify early predictors or biomarkers of CVD (Vasan 06) "that will identify end-organ pathology and facilitate its repair" (Groop 05). A recent review notes previous proposals correlating the various biomarkers with stages of coronary plaque development: stable plaque > unstable plaque > plaque rupture > thrombosis > ischemia > necrosis > LV remodeling (Vasan 06).

- *Lipid profile.* The lipid profile is constituted by fasting TG, cholesterol, HDL-C, and calculated LDL-C. See the section titled "Dyslipidemias in Preexisting Diabetes and Pregnancy" for further discussion of testing and interpretation of results.

- *Lp(a).* This test can be obtained from most commercial laboratories. Samples should be analyzed immediately or frozen at –70° if stored for long periods because the protein can degrade at conventional –20° freezer storage. An elevation in Lp(a) is often found in younger women with early-onset CAD or stroke without major elevations in the standard lipid profile. An elevation might also be expected if family members have had early-onset CAD without major hyperlipidemia. Lp(a) levels are independent predictors of risk of future CHD (Bennet 08).

- *Homocysteine.* This test is now commonly performed in hospital and commercial laboratories and can be very elevated in young people with homocysteinemia or homocysteinuria. It predicts mortality in type 2 diabetes (Stehouwer 99), especially in conjunction with early nephropathy (Lanfredini 98, Davies 00). Homocysteinemia is associated with venous thrombosis, accelerated arteriosclerotic disease, and impaired coronary circulation (Tawakol 02, Coppola 04). However, therapeutic trials on the effect of lowering homocysteine levels by folate and B-vitamin intake have been disappointing (Loscalzo 06). Homocysteine levels are lower in uncomplicated pregnancy, probably due to the lower level of methionine substrate and to estrogen enhancement of the remethylation of Hcy (see the sections titled "Medical Nutrition Therapy," "B-Complex Vitamins," and "Folate" in Part I). Effects of hyperhomocysteinemia in diabetic pregnant women are poorly characterized.

- *C-reactive protein (CRP).* This protein is classically elevated in conditions such as rheumatic fever and is increased in any inflammatory condition, including arteriosclerosis (Hansson 05, Schwedler 05). Elevations of CRP also correlate with insulin resistance and abdominal obesity and are found in poorly controlled type 2 diabetes (Visser 99, King 03). Cholesterol feeding elevates CRP in otherwise healthy, lean subjects, but not in the obese (Tannock 03). CRP is generated in the liver in response to the cytokine IL-6 released from distant sites of inflammation as well as abdominal fat stores. High-sensitivity assays for CRP in diabetic patients without acute infection are used as an inconsistent predictor of CVD risk in diabetic women (Ridker 00, Colhoun 02a, Danesh 04, Best 05, Bowden 05). There is recent evidence for vascular or renal production of CRP, especially with atherosclerosis or transplant rejection (Jabs 03a,b, Wilson 06). In addition to its role as a downstream marker of inflammation, CRP is studied for its direct pathological effects on endothelial (Wang 05b) and phagocytic cells (Fu 02). Estrogen enhances the plasma level of CRP, which is an effect of uncertain significance. This being the case, it is not surprising that CRP is elevated as early as 4 weeks gestation (Sacks 04). Further CRP elevations in pregnancy are associated with smoking, preeclampsia, GDM, hypercholesterolemia, and independently with aortic atherosclerosis in young offspring (Retnakaran 03, Tjoa 03, Wolf 03, Ligouri 08). A single study has shown third-trimester CRP to not differ in 39 pregnant women with type 1 diabetes compared with 8 controls, but CRP did correlate with elevated A1C and progression of retinopathy in the diabetic group (Loukovaara 05a).

- *B-type natriuretic peptide (initially called Brain NP).* Cardiac BNP is synthesized in and released by ventricular myocytes as a prohormone in response to volume expansion and ventricular wall stress and is then released into the circulation following cleavage into active BNP and an [inactive] NH_2-terminal pro-BNP (NT-pro-NP) fragment, which has a longer half-life than active BNP (Groop 05). Either can be easily assayed. BNP and pro-BNP concentrations are closely related and increased in cardiac (and peripheral) venous blood from failing hearts (Goetze 05). BNP (as well as atrial NP and C-type NP released by endothelial cells in response to shear stress) augments urinary volume and sodium excretion, suppresses the renin-angiotensin-aldosterone system and endothelin, inhibits the sympathetic nervous system, and relaxes vascular smooth muscle (Mark 04). "All three types of responsible cells (atrial, ventricular, and endothelial) respond to hemodynamic stress by activating transcription of the genes encoding the natriuretic peptides in order to manufacture peptides that are not normally produced in those cells. In each of these anatomical areas, the higher the stress, the greater the level of natriuretic peptide produced and released into the bloodstream" (Baughman 02).

Rapid assays of BNP or its inactive *N*-terminal fragment correlate with systolic and diastolic dysfunction in patients with CVD (Maeda 98, Sagnella 98, Doust 04, Silver 04, Yamaguchi 04, Bursi 06, Richards 06, Vanderheyden 06, Grewal 08), and the assays are used in the emergency diagnosis of dyspnea and heart failure in diabetic and other patients (DTCHF 01, Mueller 04, Mueller 06). Diabetes does not appear to confound BNP levels in the emergency department diagnosis of heart failure (Wu 04, O'Donoghue 07). In a large multicenter study, the diagnostic accuracy of BNP in diagnosing congestive heart failure was 83% at a cutoff of 100 pg/mL. The NPV of BNP at levels <50 pg/mL was 96% (Maisel 02). For patients without acute dyspnea but needing cardiac evaluation, the NPV of BNP <20 pg/mL was 96% for LV systolic dysfunction and 100% for systolic plus diastolic dysfunction. The authors stated that such a low value might preclude the need for echocardiography (Atisha 04). Assays also predict CVD events and death in prospective studies of patients without heart failure at baseline (Wang 04, Gaede 05, Tarnow 05, Rana 06, Rothenbacher 06, Tarnow 06, Bibbins-Domingo 07). BNP or NT-proNP may be promising screening markers for left venticular dysfunction in female patients with diabetes (Epshteyn 03, Bhalla 04, Magnusson 04a, Andersen 05b, Costello-Boerrigter 06, Valle 06), and the peptides were independent risk factors for mortality in diabetic patients with stable CAD (Kragelund 06). Excessive secretion of NT-proBNP was independently associated with CHD and overt nephropathy in middle-aged patients with type 2 diabetes (Beer 05).

A rapid serum assay for BNP may be a useful screening test for pregnant women with acute-onset dyspnea, suggesting either systolic or diastolic ventricular dysfunction from volume overload, increased afterload from vasoconstrictive preeclampsia, or inherent cardiomyopathy (Folk 05). In preliminary studies, serum NT-pro-NP levels were higher in hypertensive pregnant women than controls (Fleming 01, Kale 05). BNP levels remained stable throughout uncomplicated pregnancy, and levels <40 pg/mL at term had a negative predictive value of 92% for excluding preeclampsia (Resnik 05). A single prospective study of BNP in pregnant women with type 1 diabetes found unchanged levels compared with nondiabetic pregnant controls (Loukovaara 05b).

- *Uric acid.* Elevated serum uric acid is associated with hypertension, renal disorders, and the syndrome of insulin resistance/hyperinsulinemia (Johnson 04, Yang 05, Lee 06, Nakagawa 06). Insulin decreases the renal excretion of uric acid (Galvan 95, Muscelli 96, TerMaaten 97), and uric acid clearance decreases with impaired insulin-mediated glucose disposal (Facchini 91); however, hyperuricemia precedes development of hyperinsulinemia in the metabolic syndrome (Niskanen 06). Recent systematic reviews demonstrated that elevated serum uric acid is an independent risk factor for cardiovascular outcomes in high-risk patients, especially in women (Alderman 04, Baker 05), including those with diabetes (Rathmann 93b, Lehto 98, Newman 06, Ioachimescu 07). A genome-wide association study identified a gene associated with hyperuricemia in a hypertensive population linked to a gene regulating a glucose transporter (Wallace 08).

Uric acid may also be a mediator of endothelial dysfunction, inflammation, and vascular disease via several mechanisms (Rao 91, Sanchez-Lozada 02, Johnson 03, Mercuro 04, Kanellis 05, Sanchez-Lozada 06). Allopurinol treatment improves cardiovascular function, but the postulated mechanism is inhibition of xanthine oxidase activity and its contribution to oxidative stress (Butler 00, Cappola 01, Struthers 02, Weimert 03). At lower physiological concentrations, urate is a major antioxidant in plasma (Maxwell 97, Nieto 00, Waring 01). Uric acid preferentially reacts with peroxynitrite (Kuzkaya 05) and stimulates the expression of extracellular superoxide dismutase (Hink 02). However, at higher concentrations, uric acid paradoxically can act as a pro-oxidant (Hayden 04).

The role of hyperuricemia in the development of CVD in diabetes is problematic (Moriarity 00) because serum uric acid is often lower in diabetic patients without nephropathy than in controls (Golik 93, Golembiewska 05), perhaps as a marker of oxidative stress linked to overproduction of nitric oxide in young diabetic women (Pitocco 08). Hyperglycemia and glucosuria with insulin deficiency may increase renal excretion of uric acid (Herman 82, Gotoh 05). Serum uric acid rises slightly during pregnancy in healthy women until there is a larger increase before delivery (Lain 05). Long known as a marker for preeclampsia (Lam 05, Seow 05, Powers 06), current controversy revolves around whether serum uric acid predicts the severity of the dangerous pregnancy syndrome (Lim 98, Williams 02, Weerasekera 03, Roberts 05, Cnossen 06, Deruelle 06, Thangaratinam 06) or has a pathogenetic role (Many 96, Kang 04, Lam 05). It will be difficult to sort out the role of serum uric acid as a contributor to CVD in diabetic pregnant women due to multiple interrelated risk factors.

Assessment of cardiac function and anatomy

Many studies illustrate the lack of recognition (Mosca 05) and difficulty of diagnosis of CHD in diabetic women (Kamalesh 04, Nasir 04, Wackers 04, Heller 05). Women manifest CVD in ways different from men (Chung 06). To increase awareness of evaluating CVD in women (Jacobs 05b), the AHA recently published Position Statements about noninvasive testing (Mieres 05) and interventional procedures (Lansky 05) in women with CHD.

ECG. Physiological changes of pregnancy can affect interpretation of the ECG. The increase in resting HR of ~10 bpm may result in decreased P-R, QRS, and QT intervals, and minimal changes in QRS voltage; inferior ST-segment depression may also occur (Carruth 81, Stein 99, Connolly 02, Elkayam 05). Premature atrial and ventricular depolarizations are often seen in pregnancy (Gowda 03), which somewhat increases the susceptibility to cardiac arrhythmias (Shotan 97, Elkayam 05). Rotation of the heart due to enlargement of the gravid uterus can cause a left (or right) shift of the electrical axis (Wenger 64, Elkayam 98), but true axis deviation (−30 degrees) implies heart disease (McAnulty 04).

ECG evidence of LVH is a predictor of CHD morbidity and mortality (Lonn 03). LVH causes electrical heterogeneity in the heart and is associated with sudden cardiac death secondary to ventricular arrhythmias (Schouten 91, Wolk 99, Festa 00). ECG-LVH is more common in female compared with male patients with diabetes, and there are ethnic differences in the QRS voltage-duration measures (Okin 02, Bruno 04, Giunti 05). ECG-LVH does not predict echo-LVH well in diabetic patients (Dawson 04). Regression of ECG-LVH is less useful as a surrogate marker of treatment outcomes in hypertensive patients with diabetes (Okin 06). Little work has been done on the electro-cardiographic diagnosis of LVH in pregnancy and whether it is affected by diabetes.

Resting 12-lead ECG is used to detect evidence of previously unrecognized ischemic events (Scheidt-Nave 90) and cardiac conduction defects (Movahed 07). Although the yield is low, an ECG is indicated for maximum protection in pregnant women ≥35 years of age with duration of type 1 diabetes ≥10 years or duration of type 2 diabetes ≥5 years because silent ischemia is common in diabetes (Nesto 99, Kharlip 06). The ECG is primarily a record of previous transmural MI or an indication of an acute MI. One cannot reliably infer imminence of a heart attack from an ECG. Abnormal findings include S-T wave abnormalities, Q waves, QRS voltage-duration markers of LVH, and prolonged QT duration as an indicator of repolarization problems.

Various screening methods have been used to detect asymptomatic CAD in women with diabetes (Janand-Delenne 99, Greenland 01, Tavel 01). Continuous 24-hour heart monitoring with the Holter technique is considered insensitive. Exercise ECG (treadmill test) is widely used, but has low specificity to be cost-effective when screening low-risk populations and lacks the sensitivity to be consistently predictive of CAD in high-risk groups (Inzucchi 01, Johansen 07). MPI is a more expensive alternative prior to pregnancy if exercise ECG is not feasible (Janand-Delenne 99, Giri 02). However, interpretation of these tests is made difficult by diabetes-related factors such as exercise intolerance, LVH, nonischemic diabetic cardiomyopathy, and CAN (Nesto 99). Typical or atypical chest pain or other vague upper body symptoms related to exercise are additional indications for a stress ECG. Recall that atypical symptoms are common in women with myocardial ischemia (Douglas 96, Nesto 99). Limiting or nonlimiting chest pain during exercise ECG is of limited predictive value in women (Mieres 05). Peak treadmill HR, functional capacity, and HR recovery 1–2 min after exercise are important predictors of subsequent development of clinical CAD (Gerson 88, Mieres 05). We are not aware of systematic studies of exercise ECG in pregnancies complicated by diabetes.

In an early observational study of exercise ECG in 40 asymptomatic young patients with type 1 diabetes, ST-segment changes were abnormal in 11.6% of patients age 20–30 years and in 35.7% of patients aged 31–40 years (Levitas 72). HR_{max} was lower in women with a diabetes duration of 6–29 years in a later study of 50 women with type 1 diabetes aged 15–40 years compared with nondiabetic controls (173 ± 16 vs. 187 ± 11; $p < 0.05$). Only 2 of 50 women had 1-mm ST depressions during the test (Airaksinen 85). Exercise ECG was compared with coronary angiography in an early multicenter analysis of experience using a registry of 113 diabetic patients with documented CAD, with most <60 years of age. Silent ischemic changes with or without exercise-induced angina predicted mortality of 50% and 41% over 6 years in diabetic patients, respectively, compared with 7% in patients without ischemic changes. Thirty-one patients had "negative" exercise ECGs (27% of the diabetic group) and 1–3 coronary arteries narrowed ≥70% (Weiner 91). Subsequent studies confirmed that 18–34% of high-risk patients have false negative exercise ECGs (Ditchburn 01, Bacci 02), although the ECG stress test had a good NPV for cardiac events (Cosson 04). In diabetic women with a low pretest probability of CAD, the exercise ECG has a high NPV. In asymptomatic diabetic women of higher risk due to the presence of standard risk factors, a normal resting ECG, and capable of exercise, current guidelines propose that the stress exercise ECG test is an alternative for the initial test (Mieres 05). During late pregnancy, ST depression was more common during exercise ECG at 37 weeks (6 of 15) compared with 29 weeks (2 of 15) or 6 weeks postpartum (1 of 15) in asymptomatic healthy volunteers (Asher 93).

New research has explored the relation of ECG QT interval to cardiac mortality in patients with diabetes (Linnemann 03, Stettler 07). The QT interval corrected for HR (previous cardiac cycle length) is known as QTc; >440 ms is considered abnormally prolonged (Veglio 02), but recent data suggest values are ~20 ms longer in 50-year-old women than in men (Festa 00). Using the Fridericia formula to correct QT for HR (Fridericia 20) in a U.S. survey of 8,367 subjects >39 years of age, the 95th percentile of QTc for women was 9 ms above that for men. The 95th percentile for QTc was 455 ms in women aged 40–49 years (Benoit 05). QT-prolonging drugs that are in use with diabetes include erythromycin and antidepressants (Curtis 03). QT interval dispersion (QTd) is calculated by using the difference between the maximum and minimum QTc in any thoracic lead; a QTd >80 ms is considered abnormally increased (Cowan 88, Schouten 91, Zaidi 96, Elming 98). LVH causes electrical heterogeneity in the heart associated with prolongation of QTd (Wolk 99).

Age-adjusted QTd intervals were not significantly different among controls and patients with type 1 or type 2 diabetes, but QTd was independently associated with duration of type 1 diabetes and microalbuminuria in type 2 diabeters (Psallas 06). In large surveys of type 1 diabetes patients whose mean age was 33 years, QTd values were similar in men and women. Some women with normal QTd still have abnormally prolonged QTc; the prevalence of prolonged QTc in diabetic women was 6–20% (Airaksinen 84, Veglio 02) and 23% in diabetic children and adolescents with diabetes (Suys 02). QTc >440–550 ms on the 12-lead ECG may be associated with increased risk of ventricular arrhythmias and primary cardiac arrest in adult patients with type 1 (Veglio 99, Veglio 00, Rossing 01, Veglio 02, Stettler 07) and type 2 diabetes (Christensen 00, Festa 00, Cardoso 03, Takebayashi 04, Rana 05, Salles 05, Whitsel 05), even in young (10–20 years of age) patients with type 1 diabetes (Suys 06). In these studies QT prolongation is related to diastolic BP, LVH, and low glucose values, plus CAN in men but not women.

Speculation exists that prolonged QT interval could explain cases of fatal nocturnal hypoglycemia in type 1 diabetes (Campbell 91, Weston 97, Veglio 00) because evidence suggests that insulin-induced hypoglycemia or its adrenergic response can produce abnormal cardiac repolarization (Robinson 03,04, Murphy 04). Slight prolongation of QTc can be seen in nondiabetic women with abdominal obesity (Park 97). Consumption of fatty fish with *n*-3 dietary fatty acids >1 gm/day reduced the likelihood of prolonged QT interval in a large population-based study (Mozaffarian 06). Treatment with β-adrenergic blockers decreases QTc interval, but not QTd (Ebbehoj 04, Lee 05), and reduces the risk for cardiac events (Rashba 98, Moss 00).

A study of healthy, nonobese women in late pregnancy showed slight prolongation of the QT interval normalized for HR and changes in ventricular depolarization and repolarization patterns (Lechmanova 02a,b). In pregnant mice, downregulation of cardiac Kv4.3 gene expression and remodeling of Kv4.3 channels is accompanied by a reduction in transient outward K+ currents, a longer action potential, and prolongation of the QT interval (Eghbali 05). Patients with severe preeclampsia had longer QTc intervals than pregnant controls in two studies (470 vs. 436; 452 vs. 376 ms, respectively) (Isezuo 04, Sen 06). We are not aware of studies of QT interval prolongation in diabetes with pregnancy.

The congenital long QT syndrome (a result of several mutations in six genes encoding subunits of cardiac potassium and sodium channels) has a particular risk of life-threatening tachycardia in women, especially in the postpartum period (Engelstein 03). Women with hereditary long QT syndrome (QTc >440 ms) had a frequency of cardiac events (aborted cardiac arrest, syncope) of 0.9% before pregnancy, 4.5% during pregnancy, and 9.1% during 40 weeks postpartum. First-degree female relatives of these women who themselves had QTc >470 ms did not have increased events during or after pregnancy (Rashba 98). There is some evidence for an increased risk of fetal hydrops and death (Miller 04, Schwartz 04) or sudden infant death (Schwartz 98, Tester 05, Arnestad 07) in offspring of women with unsuspected mosaicism for LQTS-associated mutations.

Tests for CAN. Fairly simple, clinically available tests for evaluating cardiovascular autonomic function that have been in use for >20 years are presented in Table II.8. Office ECG or a fetal heart monitor can be used to monitor HR responses to autonomic stimuli. The evolution of CAN involves early changes in tests of parasympathetic function, with later signs of sympathetic damage (Ewing 82,85, ADA 92). Tests of cardiovascular autonomic function are influenced by age, weight, and position, but not by gender (Ziegler 92a). Testing should be standardized as much as possible as to time of day, time from meal, insulin injection and hypoglycemia, avoidance of caffeine and tobacco, and cognizance of use of cardio-reactive medications (Spallone 97b). Autonomic dysfunction may be suggested by a supine resting HR >100, yet there are problems with assessing basal HR in diabetes (see section titled "Cardiovascular Autonomic Neuropathy"), and physiologic increases in HR occur in pregnancy.

TABLE II.8 Standard Tests of Cardiovascular Autonomic Function in the Clinic or Office for Patients with Diabetes

Parameter	Normal	Borderline	Abnormal	Comment
Tests Reflecting Mainly Parasympathetic Function				
HR response to Valsalva manuever (Valsalva ratio)	≥1/21	1/11 to 1/20	≤1/10	Ratio of longest to shortest R-R interval (1st tachycardia; 2nd bradycardia) or HR min/max
HR (R-R interval) variation during deep breathing (maximum/minimum HR)	≥15 bpm	11–14 bpm	≤10 bpm	Six breaths over 1 min (5 sec in, 5 sec out)
Immediate HR response to standing (30th beat:15th beat ratio)	≥1.04	1.01–1.03	≤1.00	Shortest R-R, fastest HR @ 15; longest R-R, slowest HR @ 30
Tests Reflecting Mainly Sympathetic Function				
BP response to standing (fall in systolic BP)	≤10 mmHg	11–29 mmHg	≥30 mmHg	CAN: BP falls with no vasoconstrictive correction
BP response to sustained handgrip (highest diastolic BP vs. mean of 3 pre-grip diastolic BPs)	≥16 mmHg	11–15 mmHg	≤10 mmHg	Maintain near-maximal handgrip up to 5 min; BP q 1 min

BP, blood pressure; bpm, beats per min; HR, heart rate; Hg, mercury; CAN, cardiovascular autonomic neuropathy. Modified from Ewing 1982 and used with permission.

During the strain period of the Valsalva maneuver, BP drops and HR rises; after release, BP rises to more than basal level and HR decreases (Ewing 82). HR responses are blocked by atropine but are unaffected by propranolol. The patient blows into a mouthpiece and holds pressure of 40 mmHg for 15 seconds, repeated three times. Avoid the test in patients with active proliferative retinopathy. In patients with autonomic damage, BP slowly falls during strain and slowly returns to normal after release, with no overshoot rise in BP and no change in HR. Results are expressed as the ratio of the longest R-R interval (overshoot bradycardia) to the shortest R-R interval (tachycardia during strain) (Ewing 82).

Abnormal expiratory–inspiratory RR-interval variation (another measure of the parasympathetic nervous system) is an objective early indicator of CAN in diabetic patients (Genovely 88, ADA 92, Maser 05). Eliciting HR variation by deep breathing at six breaths per min is the most convenient technique (Ewing 81). An ECG is recorded throughout the period of deep breathing, with a marker used to indicate the onset of each inspiration and expiration. The mean of the difference in bpm between the maximum and minimum HRs for the six measured cycles is calculated or is expressed as a ratio of the mean HR at expiration over inspiration (Ewing 82).

On arising, the vagal nerve mediates an increase in HR that is maximal about the 15th beat, with a relative overshoot bradycardia by the 30th beat. Patients with CAN show only a gradual or no increase in HR after standing (Ewing 78). The HR response is expressed by the 30:15 ratio (Ewing 82), but more sophisticated analyses of HR variability suggest that the 30:15 test is not useful in diabetes (Ziegler 92a). Supine resting R-R variation of 0–6% may also be used as an indicator of CAN (Airaksinen 85). Excess diastolic BP response to handgrip exercise and postural hypotension (fall in systolic >20 or >30 mmHg) (Kempler 01) are usually found with extensive peripheral sympathetic damage (Ewing 82). Of the standard tests for cardiac autonomic function, the Valsalva effect and the lying-to-standing effect, both on RR-interval, have the best coefficients of variation (9.2% and 6.4%, respectively) (Valensi 93, 03). With positive findings on these simple tests, consider an electrophysiological study or cardiology referral.

Continuous HR variation on 24-h Holter monitoring is also used to study alterations of cardiac autonomic function and provides data on the circadian rhythm of sympathovagal activity (Furlan 90), "which can be affected earlier than and differently from cardiovascular reflex tests" (Spallone 97b). Time domain analysis reports the standard deviation of normal-to-normal (sinus rhythm) R-R intervals (SDNN) is more readily available and can be used for screening (range 10–55 ms). Frequency domain analysis shows both low (energy in the power spectrum between 0.12 and 0.12 Hz) and high frequency (energy in the power spectrum between 0.12 and 0.40 Hz) components of power spectral density and has a greater ability to differentiate vagal and sympathetic modulation of HR (Ziegler 92b, Spallone 97b, Ducher 99). Sympathetic activation reduces total power of R-R interval variability, and vagal activation increases the high frequency component (ESC 96). The high frequency component is reduced in diabetic patients with predominantly vagal dysfunction, and the low frequency components are decreased with sympathetic dysfunction (Ziegler 92b, Chessa 02, Javorka 05, Kudat 06). Frequency domain analysis can be used in short-term recording (3 min supine during spontaneous breathing); abnormal results associate with elevated A1C (Makimattila 00) and predict a higher risk of CVD mortality in patients with diabetes, hypertension, or prior history of heart disease (Gerritsen 01).

Exercise echocardiography. This testing is the best of the noninvasive evaluations for coronary artery disease in diabetic pregnant women (Bossone 99, Bigi 01, Picano 03b,

Raggi 05). According to an AHA Consensus Statement, for women, "stress echocardiography with exercise or dobutamine is an effective and highly accurate noninvasive means of detecting nonischemic heart disease" and "provides incremental value over the exercise ECG and clinical variables in women with suspected or known coronary heart disease" (Mieres 05). It also detects abnormalities in LV wall motion by US, comparing postexercise LV contraction to LV wall motion assessed previously at rest (also suggesting cardiomyopathy). This testing is appropriate for pregnancy because it does not involve radiation exposure and is indicated if there is concern about the diagnosis of CHD. Unstable symptoms, possibility of coronary dissection, and new-onset chest pain require admission and cardiology consultation.

Transthoracic echocardiography. This test evaluates cardiac structure and function. It is important in the evaluation of symptoms of heart failure and in identification of patients with LV dysfunction whose condition can improve with treatment (Colonna 05). Two-dimensional echocardiography is used to measure LV dimensions, volume, mass, ejection fraction, and atrial size (Fraser 95, Otto 04). LVEFs are higher in women than in men, independent of differences in LV volume. Gender-specific thresholds for a low LVEF defined at the 2.5th percentile from a healthy nonpregnant reference population aged 30–65 years old are <61% in women and <55% in men (earlier studies and current data noted in Chung 06). A limitation of LV fractional shortening and echocardiography-derived ejection fraction is that they are sensitive to loading conditions, and increased preload and decreased afterload occur during normal pregnancy (Robson 89, Duvekot 93, Mone 96, Desai 04). Load-independent measures include LV velocity of circumferential fiber shortening and LV systolic wall stress (Poppas 97). Other cardiac abnormalities involving congenital defects, valvular function, pericardial effusion, atria, aortic root, pulmonary artery pressure, right ventricular systolic function, and so forth can also be evaluated. Abnormal echocardiographic findings warrant further follow-up during pregnancy and postpartum.

LVH is common with hypertension and exacerbated by diabetes (Galderisi 91, Henry 04, Sato 05, Felicio 06). LVH is also common in obese adolescent patients with type 2 diabetes (Daniels 95, Ettinger 05). In adults with either type 1 or type 2 diabetes, LVH is a risk factor for CHD, repolarization defects (prolonged QTc), and cardiovascular mortality (Wolk 99, Brown 00a, Veglio 02). However, several studies of type 1 diabetic women of reproductive age revealed normal LV dimensions and function, but increased atrial size (Lo 95).

Minimal risk to mother and fetus results from repeated echocardiography; it can therefore be used for serial assessment during gestation. Two-dimensional echocardiographic studies of normal pregnant women usually reveal no change in LV volumes or LVEF in spite of increased LV mass proportional to increased maternal weight and enlarged LV outflow area, which contributes to increased stroke volume. There is a progressive increase in left atrial area reflective of increased preload (Vered 91, Sadaniantz 92, Mendelson 00, Schannwell 02, Simmons 02). One detailed report of 37 healthy pregnant women aged 26–41 years presented the 95% CI for second-trimester left atrial size at 2.4–4.0 cm, LV fractional shortening at 25–45%, LVEF at 58–70%, and LV mass index at 49–81 gm/m^2 (Mesa 99). Blood volume can increase up to 70% during normal pregnancy. The normal volume-overload state of pregnancy is associated with 10–30% increases in LV wall thickness (Robson 89, Poppas 97, Mesa 99, Desai 04). Although LV mass and left atrial size increase in normotensive nondiabetic pregnancies, levels that define the presence of echocardiographic LVH (LV mass index 110 g/m^2) do not occur in most women (Mabie 94, Desai 04).

Doppler echocardiography. Doppler echocardiography (aortic, apical, suprasternal) is used to measure diastolic flow velocities to estimate diastolic dysfunction (Nishimura 89). LV diastolic dysfunction often precedes systolic dysfunction in diabetes. Examination of nonpregnant patients with type 1 diabetes with normal LV dimensions and LVEFs (mean ages: 18, 26, 27, and 32 years in the study groups, respectively) showed that 30–50% had at least two abnormal variables of mitral inflow velocity (reduced early filling velocity [E], increased atrial filling velocity [A] for atrial contraction), and decreased ratio of peak E/A <1.6 (Zarich 88, Ragonese 92, Lo 95, Borgia 99). The "mitral inflow profile is affected by a complex interaction of many factors, including myocardial relaxation, ventricular compliance, pericardial restraint, preload and afterload, and myocardial contractility" (Mesa 99). Isometric exercise magnified the diastolic abnormalities, suggesting a contribution by autonomic dysfunction (Ragonese 92, Borgia 99). Thus, type 1 diabetic women of reproductive age may have evidence of disturbed diastolic performance, especially with longer diabetes duration (Lo 95) or if complicated by microvascular disease (Ragonese 92, Borgia 99).

No standardized guidelines exist for the assessment of diastolic function in diabetic pregnant women. Doppler studies of normal pregnant women in the third trimester show that the ratio of early to late diastolic flow velocity is decreased in pregnancy (Sadaniantz 92, Schannwell 02, Desai 04), with the decreased values (E/A max 1.3 vs. 1.9) being similar to those in some nonpregnant diabetic women, as noted earlier. The E/A ratio progressively declines from 1.6 to 1.3 throughout normal pregnancy (Mesa 99). Disturbed diastolic relaxation patterns return to normal by 8 weeks postpartum (Sadaniantz 92, Mesa 99, Schannwell 02) and are not abnormal after nondiabetic women have multiple pregnancies (Sadaniantz 96). Abnormal diastolic parameters have been demonstrated in hypertensive pregnant women (Valensise 01). As noted in the section titled "Heart Failure," only one study of diastolic ventricular dysfunction using Doppler echocardiography in pregnant women with type 1 diabetes has been conducted, and it showed abnormal results in 57% of subjects (Schannwell 03). We need further studies of diastolic dysfunction in pregnancies complicated by PDM.

Because mitral inflow velocity is dependent on filling pressure as well as LV relaxation and compliance, new quantitative tissue Doppler imaging (TDI) parameters (Garcia 98, Yu 03a, Colonna 05) are studied as more sensitive and load-independent indicators of early asymptomatic LV dysfunction (Fang 03a, Suys 04, Young 04, Fang 05a,b, Shivalkar 06) in the hope that early intervention with ACE inhibitor or β-blocker therapy can prevent progression to heart failure. TDI parameters of systolic or diastolic ventricular dysfunction may be identified before the appearance of abnormalities using conventional two-dimensional and Doppler echocardiography (von Bibra 05, Palmieri 06, Di Cori 07). TDI may also discriminate between the myocardial effects of diabetes and hypertension (Kosmala 04, Colonna 05). The technique is applied to quantitation of segments of the myocardium, and parameters include peak systolic velocity, peak early diastolic velocity of the mitral annulus (E_m), isovolumic relaxation time (IRT), end systolic strain (ESS) and strain rate, and measures of LV asynchrony (Korosoglou 06). Investigators are determining the usefulness of TDI in the staging of diabetic cardiomyopathy (Picano 03b, Colonna 05, Di Bonito 05). First, a reduction in contractility can be observed in the blunting of backscatter cyclic variations in either the entire myocardial wall or limited to the subendothelial layer (Naito 01). Next, myocardial tissue fibrosis, which corresponds to microvascular damage, is visible as increased echo density at tissue characterization (Fang 03a) when TDI contractile indexes begin to decline (Colonna 05). At a more advanced stage, a reduced inotropic reserve (Colonna 05) can be observed during exercise (Fang 03b, Scognamiglio 05). Finally, "wall motion abnormalities at rest and a global reduction in EF can occur along with clinical signs of diabetic chronic heart failure" (Colonna 05).

TDI is currently used in the diagnosis of fetal cardiac disease (Paladini 00, Barnett 01, Rein 02, Chan 05). A prospective study of spectral TDI in 35 healthy pregnant women showed that peak myocardial velocities during early diastole increased during the second trimester and decreased during the third trimester. Peak myocardial velocities during atrial contraction increased with advancing gestational age (Fok 06). TDI detected asynchrony and abnormal strain rate of the maternal LV myocardium in a pregnant woman with palpitations and left heart failure (Williams 03). A single study using TDI in women with GDM showed a mild degree of diastolic abnormality, with a significant decrease in E_m and persistent increase in A_m (late mitral annulus velocity) (Freire 06). To our knowledge, TDI techniques have not been applied to the study of cardiomyopathy in pregnant women with PDM.

Carotid Ultrasound. Carotid artery assessments are increasingly used as an indicator of atherosclerosis, and several approaches to assessment are possible. One is by determining the impairment of blood flow by measuring turbulence in the common carotid artery by Doppler US. Scant literature exists on this subject in diabetic pregnancy. The logic of the test is that it is a routine test done on an accessible artery. Unpublished Doppler US examinations done in the first trimester of diabetic pregnancy showed no flow abnormalities in ~50 studied subjects. Therefore, use of this test to detect peripheral artery atherosclerosis would most logically be used in the highest-risk patients, such as older diabetic smokers, in whom the ascertainment of peripheral vascular disease would further increase the likelihood of CAD.

Other approaches to carotid artery assessment by US are measurements of IMT (Fernandes 06, Markus 06) or plaque burden (Held 01, Charvat 06) by high-resolution B-mode US. Although reference values have been published in nonpregnant people (Salonen 90, Folsom 94, D'Agostino 96, Espeland 96), standardization is difficult and the technique is still used primarily in research. Nonetheless, carotid artery IMT >0.90–1.1 mm is correlated to CVD risk in many populations (Hodis 98, Graner 06, Wang 06b), including 2,436 subjects <50 years of age (Lorenz 06). Women have lower IMT values than men unless CHD is present (Kablak-Ziembicka 05). In a community population study (n = 3,383; mean age: 52), mean IMT of the common carotid was 0.74 ± 0.15 mm (range 0.36–2.13), mean IMT of the bifurcation was 0.92 ± 0.84 mm (range 0.34–3.6), and mean IMT of the internal carotid was 0.77 ± 0.31 mm (range 0.32–3.7). Progression rates over 3 years at the internal carotid rather than the common carotid yielded much greater absolute changes in IMT and better correlations with atherosclerotic risk factors, probably reflecting the predilection of the bifurcation and internal carotid artery for atherosclerotic plaques (Mackinnon 04). A local IMT thickness >140 mm is considered to be a plaque.

For type 1 diabetes, the DCCT/EDIC investigators found that baseline reproducibility analyses of replicate measures resulted in absolute mean differences of 0.04 mm for both the common carotid and the internal carotid measured just beyond the bifurcation. Visualization of the internal carotid was less uniform than the common carotid. Mean IMT was not greater in 278 women with type 1 diabetes aged 30–39 years at the common carotid (0.66 ± 0.08 mm) or the internal carotid (0.63 ± 0.14) after the trial than in 27 age-matched controls, and values were within the error of measurement compared with the diabetic men (EDIC 99). The absence of difference between diabetic subjects and controls may be due to the exclusion of diabetic subjects with hypertension or dyslipidemia at baseline (EDIC 99) because other studies of relatively young patients with diabetes reported IMT values that were higher than controls (Yamasaki 94, Bonora 97). After 6 years further follow-up, IMT was significantly greater in DCCT diabetic subjects than in controls, even though progression was less in the women that had been in the intensive treatment group (Δ 0.032 vs. 0.046 mm in the original conventional therapy group; p = 0.02). Predictors of progression of IMT included mean A1C during the trial and end-of-trial systolic BP, urinary AER, and ratio of LDL-C to HDL-C (Nathan 03).

Median common carotid IMT was 0.62 mm (range 0.44–1.23) in 148 type 1 diabetes patients (median age: 48 years; diabetes duration: 26 years) in South Africa (Distiller 06) compared with a mean common carotid IMT of 0.83 ± 0.13 in 195 type 1 diabetes patients (mean age: 55 years) in France. Diabetic subjects in the latter group had no history of cardiovascular events, but carotid plaques were noted in 48% (Bernard 05). In 45 children with type 1 diabetes aged 7–14 years, maximum carotid IMT was 0.55 vs. 0.51 mm in controls (p < 0.01) and correlated inversely with brachial artery flow-mediated dilation responses (Jarvisalo 04). IMT was associated with A1C over 18 years in diabetic women (mean age: 25–43 years) and predicted percentage of coronary vessel area stenosis and myocardial infarction (Larsen 05a), in addition to the risk predicted by other established factors (Bernard 05). In a meta-analysis of 20 cross-sectional studies, carotid artery IMT values were 0.13 (95% CI 0.12–0.14) mm greater in adult type 2 diabetic subjects than in controls (Brohall 06). Progression of carotid IMT over 3 years related to slight deterioration of A1C in patients with type 2 diabetes (Kawasumi 06).

One study of the layers of the left common carotid artery by high-resolution US at term normal pregnancy demonstrated that pregnant subjects had a thinner intima layer (0.25 vs. 0.27 mm) and a thicker media layer (0.31 vs. 0.29 mm) compared with fertile nonpregnant controls (Sator 99). Measurement of carotid IMT measurements after pregnancy showed increased values compared with those in nulliparous fertile women (Blaauw 06). We are not aware of studies of carotid IMT in diabetic pregnancy. Additional research is required of this promising technique in the area of pregnancy to bring it to the clinical level.

Ankle arm index (ankle/brachial index [ABI]). This test provides a ratio of BP in the ankle compared with the arm and defines PAD at a value of <0.9 (Hiatt 95, Soffers 96, Hiatt 01, ADA 03, Mohler 04). According to an AHA Scientific Statement based on an AHA/ADA workshop, the ABI measurement is recommended for any diabetic patient with leg pain of unknown etiology or newly detected to have decreased pulses, femoral bruits, or a foot ulcer; for baseline examination of a woman with type 1 diabetes aged ≥35 years or with ≥20 years' duration of diabetes; and for baseline examination of a woman with type 2 diabetes aged ≥40 years (Orchard 93). According to an ADA Consensus Development Conference, a diagnostic ABI should be performed in any patient with symptoms of PAD and "should be considered in diabetic patients <50 years of age who have other PAD risk factors (e.g., smoking, hypertension, hyperlipidemia, or duration of diabetes >10 years)" (ADA 03).

The patient should rest supine for 5 min, and then an inflatable BP cuff and a handheld Doppler probe used at an angle of 60° should measure systolic BP in the right brachial artery, right dorsalis pedis and posterior tibial arteries, left dorsalis pedis and posterior tibial arteries, and left brachial artery; the measurements are then repeated in reverse order. An appropriately sized BP cuff is placed just above the ankle. By using the highest brachial systolic pressure as the denominator and the average of the pedal artery pressures (on the same side) as the numerator, the ABI yielded ratios most predictive of walking endurance and velocity in LEAD (McDermott 00,01). The ADA Consensus Guidelines recommend using the highest brachial pressure as the denominator of the ABI and the highest pedal pressure as the numerator for the ABI ratio in each leg (ADA 03). A normal ratio is considered to be 0.90–1.30; values >1.30 suggest poorly compressible arteries at the ankle level due to the presence of medial artery calcification, which makes the diagnosis of LEAD by ABI difficult. Moderate occlusive disease is suggested by an ABI of 0.40–0.69 and severe disease with an ABI <0.40 (ADA 03). Congenital absence of the dorsalis pedis artery is noted in only 2% of extremities compared with 0.1% for the posterior tibial artery. If one artery is small, the other will usually be prominent, which explains why physicians use whichever pedal pulse has the highest pressure to calculate the ABI and why only 0.7% of normal extremities are missing both pedal pulses (McGee 98).

A value <0.9 is a fairly extreme impairment for someone who is healthy enough to become pregnant, but 7.4% of 125 women with type 1 diabetes (aged 22–52 years) but without clinical CHD in Pittsburgh in 1996–1998 had an ABI <0.8 (Olson 00). Lesser levels of impairment relative to the mean value of a ~ 1.2 might provide a clue to impaired blood flow in the lower extremity or disclose asymmetry in blood flow to the lower extremities. This test is of interest in diabetes with pregnancy, smokers, those with combined hyperlipidemia (both TG and LDL-C elevated), or renal disease. Each of these risk factors predisposes to peripheral vascular disease. Abdominal or femoral artery bruits or missing or asymmetrical foot pulses would also be an indication for assessment of ankle-arm testing.

Patients with LEAD will usually need vascular laboratory assessment of the location and severity of the obstruction (ADA 03). Tests may include segmental pressures and pulse volume recordings, treadmill functional testing, systolic toe pressures, duplex sonography, or a magnetic resonance angiogram (Hiatt 01, ADA 03). Contrast X-ray angiography is used for anatomical evaluation of the patient in whom a revascularization procedure is intended (Faglia 98, ADA 03).

Cardiovascular Disease Risk Factor Management in Diabetic Pregnancy

The ADA, AHA, and ACC (Mosca 04, Appel 06, Lichtenstein 06, Smith 06, Buse 07, ADA 08a) provide evidence-based guidelines on primary and secondary prevention of CVD in diabetic women; they are adapted for pregnancy in this and other appropriate sections of these Technical Reviews. Much improvement in clinical application is needed because there is evidence of poor risk factor control in most populations of women with type 1 or type 2 diabetes (Soedamah-Muthu 02, Pyorala 04, Mosca 05, Wadwa 05, Zgibor 05).

- *Glycemic control.* A 7-year period of intensified diabetes management for type 1 diabetes reduced the risk of serious CVD events over an 18-year follow-up (DCCT/EDIC 06). The goal of therapy is to maintain A1C as close to normal as possible without significant hypoglycemia. Management of diabetes during pregnancy is discussed in detail in Part I.

- *Physical activity.* The goal is 30 min of brisk walking or its equivalent 7 days per week (minimum 5 days/week). Assess risk with a physical activity history and/or exercise test.

- *Smoking.* Smoking abatement programs are described in Part I in the section titled "Behavioral Therapy." In brief, pregnancy provides one of the better opportunities to attempt smoking cessation in women who still smoke. Advice from the physician is an essential start. Combining an antismoking program, use of nicotine patches with the physicians' endorsement, and education about the health benefits to the fetus offers a realistic chance to stop smoking. Patients with CVD are advised to have no exposure to environmental tobacco smoke.

- *Hypertension and cardiovascular management.* The goal is to maintain BP <130/80 and >109/64 during pregnancy with agents that are safe for the fetus. Beta-blockers are used for LV dysfunction with or without heart failure symptoms unless contraindicated. Refer to the following section titled "Blood Pressure Control."

- *Renal disease management.* The goal is to reduce albuminuria. ACE inhibitors and angiotensin-receptor blockers (ARBs) must not be used in pregnancy. Studies are needed on the effect of glycemic control and antihypertensive treatment on albuminuria during pregnancy. Refer to the section titled "Diabetic Nephropathy and Pregnancy" later in Part II.

- *Lipid management.* The primary goal is to maintain LDL-C <130 mg/dL for primary CVD prevention and <100 mg/dL for secondary CVD prevention. If TGs are >200 mg/dL, the secondary goal is to maintain total-C minus HDL-C at <130 mg/dL. During pregnancy, emphasis is placed on (1) MNT to lower cholesterol and reduce saturated fats and *trans* fats, or on (2)nutritional supplements, most notably fish oil, for the treatment of hypertriglyceridemia to prevent or treat pancreatitis. Ingestion of medium-chain triglycerides (MCTs) as a nonchylomicron-absorbed alternative to conventional fat is a second alternative. Fibrates and niacin (anecdotal reports) are medication alternatives for lowering TG. Refer to the section titled "Management of Dyslipidemias in Pregnant Women with PDM" for more details.

- *Lp(a) treatment.* Lp(a) levels are not altered in pregnancy. Consistently reliable methods to treat Lp(a) are not available. Niacin can lower Lp(a) as much as 30%, but there is no published experience with this agent in pregnancy nor any proof that Lp(a) reduction prevents CAD in any setting. Paradoxically, an antiatherogenic diet with a reduced amount of total and saturated fat and either low or high in vegetables increased plasma Lp(a) by 7–9% in nondiabetic women and also increased oxidized LDL 19–27% (Silaste 04). We are not aware of studies of this effect in pregnant women with PDM.

- *Homocysteine reduction treatment.* Folic acid in high doses of 4 mg/day with or without pyridoxine (B6) and vitamin B12 supplementation is associated with the best Hcy reductions on the order of 30%. Low-dose folic acid (400 mcg/d) improves vascular function through effects on endothelial nitric oxide synthase and vascular oxidative stress (Shirodaria 07). Population-wide reductions in Hcy may have already occurred with the supplementation of flour into the food supply to increase folate intake by ~400 micrograms daily. In nonpregnant adults, the success of high-dose folate supplementation in preventing heart disease or stroke is uncertain (Schnyder 02, Liem 03, Toole 04, HOPE 06). To our knowledge, the safety of high-dose B-vitamin administration in pregnancy is not known.

- *Vasospasm and antiarrhythmia therapy.* Fish oil has been associated with almost immediate reductions in CHD independent of effects on cholesterol levels (Mosca 04b). In addition, two major observational studies have shown fewer sudden deaths in association with ingesting two fish meals per week (Hu 02,03, He 04) (equivalent to two 1-g fish oil capsules daily containing 30% omega-3 fatty acids). Although untested in pregnancy, such treatment could provide an immediate prophylactic benefit.

- *Antianginals, aspirin, and clopidogrel.* Should patients be having bona fide angina, nitroglycerin in various forms can be considered. Nitroglycerin has been used in oral, skin patch, or intravenous formulations in pregnancy to achieve uterine muscle relaxation (Bujold 03, Bisits 04, Bullarbo 05, Gill 06). Daily low-dose aspirin is recommended in diabetic women >40 years of age with another CVD risk factor (hypertension, family history, dyslipidemia, microalbuminuria, CAN, smoking) to reduce the risk of cardiovascular events (ADA 08a). Use of aspirin and clopidogrel before and during pregnancy is discussed in the following paragraphs.

Aspirin therapy

A putative preventive treatment in pregnancy would be the irreversible COX 1 and 2 inhibitor aspirin (Colwell 97), low doses of which (40–80 mg) inhibit platelet thromboxane production but not aortic or venous production of prostacyclin (Weksler 83). A systematic review of 11 clinical studies comparing aspirin dosage for the prevention of CVD concluded that data did not support the routine, long-term use of doses > 75–81 mg/day. "Higher doses, which may be commonly prescribed, do not better prevent events but are associated with increased risks of gastrointestinal bleeding" (Campbell 07). The authors made the caveat that patients with diabetes might need higher dosages and that there is a wide range of individual dose responses on ex vivo measures of platelet responsiveness (Campbell 07). Gender differences that might affect aspirin dosing and efficacy include slower clearance of acetylsalicylic acid in women (Jochmann 05) and conflicting results on aspirin effects on agonist-induced platelet aggregation in women (Becker 06). Clinically, women are known to have much less protection against MI than men, but greater protection against stroke (Berger 06). The AHA/ADA Consensus Statement on primary prevention of CVD states that "aspirin therapy (75–162 mg/day) should be recommended as a primary prevention strategy in those with diabetes at increased cardiovascular risk, including those who are >40 years of age or who have additional risk factors (family history of CVD, hypertension, smoking, dyslipidemia, or albuminuria)" (Buse 07). A dose of 81 mg/day in diabetic males is associated with a ~30% reduction in recurrent MI (ETDRS 92, ATC 02), and primary prevention of MI in all males is well established (Berger 06); controversy surrounds whether as much protection occurs in women (Manson 91, Sacco 03, ADA 04e, Levin 05). A dose of 100 mg every other day (Ridker 96) failed to reduce ischemic stroke (OR 0.8; 95% CI 0.6–1.1; p = 0.21) or MI (OR 1.2; 95% CI 0.9–1.8; p = 0.25) in 24,025 female health professionals aged 45–54 years, of whom only 3% had diabetes. In the total study of 39,876 women aged 45 to >65 years, the risk of ischemic stroke was reduced (OR 0.8; 95% CI 0.6–0.9), but MI was not reduced; gastrointestinal bleeding episodes requiring transfusion were increased (OR 1.4; 95% CI 1.1–1.8). Interestingly, in 1,027 diabetic women of aged ≥45 years in this trial, aspirin reduced ischemic stroke but not MI (Ridker 05). Two other RCTs including women also demonstrated that aspirin reduced stroke but not MI and increased bleeding episodes, but diabetic women were not analyzed separately (Hansson 98, CGPPP 01). Prospective controlled studies of aspirin prophylaxis are inadequate in diabetic women of reproductive age. Although a recent meta-analysis confirmed a twofold increase in risk of any major bleeding with low-dose aspirin versus placebo in trials of primary or secondary prevention of athero-thrombotic disease, the absolute increased risk attributable to aspirin is small at 0.13% per year (McQuaid 06).

Platelets are more sensitive to aggregation in diabetes, but are less sensitive to the inhibiting effects of aspirin and clopidogrel (Bhatt 02, Colwell 03, Watala 04, Angiolillo 05). Several studies suggested a reduced pharmacological effect of aspirin in women compared with men (Harrison 83, Escolar 86, Spranger 89). The most recent and largest study found higher baseline platelet aggregation in response to agonists in women compared with men and greater persistence of platelet reactivity after aspirin therapy, at least in aggregation assays that were only indirectly dependent on COX-1. Complete suppression of the direct COX-1 platelet activation pathway was seen in women. The authors caution that the extent to which ex vivo tests of platelet function represent in vivo activity is unknown (Becker 06). The proportion of subjects with aspirin resistance is greater in women (Gum 01). The frequency of aspirin nonrespond-ers (Gum 03) has not been determined in diabetic pregnant women.

Use of aspirin during pregnancy

A systematic review of eight studies revealed no evidence for an overall increase in the risk of congenital malformations that could be associated with aspirin. However, a significantly increased risk of gastroschisis (OR 2.4; 95% CI 1.4–3.9) was reported (Kozer 02). Subsequent population-based case–control studies of aspirin use in early pregnancy reported an increased risk of vascular disruptions such as gastroschisis (OR 2.7; 95% CI 1.2–5.9) (Werler 02, James 08) and renal anomalies (adjusted OR 3.5; 95% CI 1.4–8.8) (Abe 03), but one showed no increased risk of gastroschisis, cleft lip, or NTDs (Norgard 05). Experimental studies show that aspirin produces cardiovascular and midline abdominal defects in rats but not rabbits (Cappon 03, Gupta 03, Burdan 06). Six large RCTs of low-dose aspirin after the first trimester to prevent preeclampsia showed no benefit in pregnant women, even those considered at high risk (CLASP 94, ECPPA 96, Caritis 98, Rotchell 98, Subtil 03, Yu 03b), including diabetic women (Sibai 00). Some of the trials showed a slight increase in maternal bleeding with aspirin use, but no increase in neonatal bleeding. Maternal low-dose aspirin therapy has mild antiplatelet effects in the fetus and newborn because cord serum levels of thromboxane B2 are reduced (Parker 00); platelet thromboxane A2 formation in newborn infants was suppressed, but recovered within 2–3 days after delivery (Leonhardt 03). In a small randomized trial, maternal aspirin 100 mg/day throughout the second and third trimesters was not associated with differences in uterine, umbilical, aor-tic, middle cerebral, or ductus arteriosus Doppler blood flow compared with the placebo group. Diabetic women were excluded from this study (Grab 00).

Clopidogrel

An RCT in >6,000 patients with LEAD determined that the platelet ADP-blocker clopidogrel (75 mg once daily) was more effective than aspirin (75 mg once daily) in reducing risk of a composite end point of MI, ischemic stroke, and vascular death. The greater benefit applied to diabetic patients, and clopidogrel was as well tolerated as aspirin. Gastrointestinal hemorrhage was reported by 2.0% of subjects using clopidog-rel and 2.7% of subjects using aspirin (CAPRIE 96, Bhatt 02). Only anecdotal reports refer to the use of clopidogrel during pregnancy (Klinzing 01).

Recommendations

- Evaluation of risk for CVD is best performed prior to pregnancy. (E)
- Screen for standard cardiovascular risk factors in all diabetic women (hypertension; dyslipidemia; albuminuria; smoking; family history of premature CHD). Construct a family tree of first- and second-degree relatives for the presence of risk factors and CHD or stroke. (A)
- Screen for evidence of CVD by simple physical examination for carotid bruits, aortic ejection murmur, abdominal and femoral bruits, and absent or asymmetrical foot pulses. (E)
- Obtain information on symptoms of CVD and CAN. Consider carotid US testing, ABI, HR variability with deep breathing, and orthostatic BP in patients at high risk. (E)
- Obtain resting ECG before or during pregnancy in patients with diabetes aged ≥35 years. (E)
- Patients with atypical pain, possible angina or anginal equivalent, or other reasons to suspect active CHD, including significant dyspnea or abnormal resting ECG, should have cardiology consultation for consideration of stress ECG, stress echocardiography, or other testing. (E)
- Patients aged >35 years with duration of type 1 diabetes ≥15 years or duration of type 2 diabetes ≥10 years with excess cardiovascular risk, especially with signs of CAN or carotid/lower extremity vascular disease, should be considered for stress ECG or stress echocardiogram or other tests for CHD. (E)
- Consider use of BNP plus 2-D and/or Doppler echocardiography or TDI to detect systolic or diastolic ventricular dysfunction for excessive dyspnea or suggestive physical examination findings. Obtain cardiology consultation if there is evidence of cardiomyopathy. (E)
- Treat CVD risk factors, such as hyperglycemia, hypertension, and dyslipidemia (see specific recommendations adapted for pregnancy in relevant sections), and initiate a coordinated smoking cessation program. (A)
- Reduce risk for CVD in diabetic women with two oily-fish meals per week (of low-risk for excess mercury; fish oil 1 gm/day may be substituted). (A)
- Consider anesthesia and mode of delivery in light of evidence of CVD. (E)

BLOOD PRESSURE CONTROL

—— Original contribution by John L. Kitzmiller MD, MS and Florence M. Brown MD

Hypertension and Diabetes

In adults aged ≥18 years, BP is now classified as normal, prehypertension, stage 1 hypertension, or stage 2 hypertension in the Joint National Committee Seventh Report; BP criteria are shown in Table II.9 (Chobanian 03a,b). The classification is based on the mean of two or more seated BP readings with a cuff of appropriate size on a validated instrument at each of two or more office visits. "Because of the clear synergistic risks of

TABLE II.9 JNC 7 Classification of Office Blood Pressure for Adults ≥18 years with or without Diabetes

BP Classification	Systolic BP (mmHg)	Diastolic BP (mmHg)	Comment
Normal	<120	<80	Both S and D required for normal.
Prehypertension *Diabetes*	120–139 *120–129*	80–89	Either S or D or both S/D indicate need for lifestyle modification to prevent further rise in BP and possible CVD; if BP remains ≥130/80 in DM after 3 months, add drug treatment
Hypertension, stage 1 *Diabetes*	140–159 *130–159*	90–99 *80–99*	Either S or D strongly predicts CKD and CVD in DM. Either S or D requires drug treatment in DM.
Hypertension, stage 2	≥160	≥100	Either S or D can impair perinatal outcome.

Taken from Chobanian 03b and modified according to ADA 08a.

BP, blood pressure; CKD, chronic kidney disease; CVD, cardiovascular disease; D, diastolic; DM, diabetes mellitus; JNC, Joint National Committee; S, systolic.

hypertension and diabetes, the diagnostic cut-off for a diagnosis of hypertension is lower in people with diabetes (BP ≥130/80) than in those without diabetes (BP ≥140/90)" (ADA 08a). Joint statements of cardiovascular societies in the U.K. (Brit 05, Williams 06) and Canada (Myers 05, Khan 06) present a somewhat different classification of hypertension, but the treatment guidelines are quite similar. Unfortunately, publication of the guidelines has not resulted in adequate hypertension control for patients with type 1 diabetes in Europe (Soedamah-Muthu 02) or the U.S. (Ong 07, Wang 07).

Systolic BP is the point at which the first of two or more sounds is heard (phase 1), and diastolic BP is the point before the disappearance of sounds (phase 5) (Pickering 05, Safar 06). No compelling evidence states that the measurement technique should be different in women with diabetes or pregnancy (NBP 00, Arauz-Pacheco 02, Chobanian 03b). An important new modification encountered with diabetes guidelines is that, with repeated BPs 130–139 mmHg systolic *or* 80 and 89 mmHg diastolic after 3 months of behavioral therapy (Svetkey 05), drug therapy should be added to maintain BP<130/80. This is the target BP for hypertensive diabetic patients based on level A, RCT-derived evidence (Chobanian 03b, Khan 06, ADA 07). Recent epidemiologic evidence suggests that enhanced CVD and renal outcomes may be obtained with systolic BP <120 mmHg (Orchard 01, Sipahi 06, Shankar 07), and current RCTs are testing that hypothesis in diabetic patients.

Epidemiology of hypertension with diabetes

Studies of the prevalence of hypertension unfortunately used different criteria to diagnose the condition. Hypertension of at least stage 1 in the U.S. (≥140/90) was 3% at 18–39 years of age in non-Hispanic white women compared with 8% in non-Hispanic black women in the 1999–2004 NHANES database; at 40–59 years of age, the prevalence was 29% in non-Hispanic white women compared with 49% in non-Hispanic black women and 30% in Mexican-American females (Ong 07). Ethnic variation in the prevalence of hypertension in 3,292 U.S. community-based premenopausal women (aged 42–52 years) is noted in the Study of Women's Health Across the Nation (SWAN) (Table II.10). Among black and Hispanic women, only 35.4% and 16.8%, respectively, had normal BP. Among 720 hypertensive participants, only 53.9% were receiving

TABLE II.10 Prevalence of Hypertension (Treated vs. Untreated) and Prehypertension in Ethnic Groups of Premenopausal Women in the U.S.

Ethnic Group	Number	Hypertension, Treated (%)	BP (<140/<90) (%) (treatment to goal)	Hypertension, Untreated (%)	Prehypertension (%)	Normal BP (<120/<80)
Black	932	22.4	51.2	15.7	26.5	35.4
White	1,543	8.0	77.9	6.6	25.7	59.9
Chinese	250	4.4	72.7	8.4	20.0	67.2
Hispanic	286	10.5	30.0	17.1	55.6	16.8
Japanese	281	5.4	80.0	5.7	25.3	63.7

Study of Women's Health Across the Nation (SWAN).

BP criteria according to JNC 7 (Chobanian 03b). Data based on Lloyd-Jones 05.

treatment, and only 32.2% were controlled to goal levels (<140/<90 mmHg). The prevalence of treatment to goal BP was highest among whites, Chinese-Americans, and Japanese-Americans; significantly lower in African-Americans; and dramatically lower in Hispanic women (Lloyd-Jones 05).

Women with diabetes have more risk of hypertension than do males (Legato 06). The prevalence of hypertension in young patients with type 1 diabetes (threshold 140/90 or history of treatment) varied from 3.3% to 13.3% in data gathered from 11 centers in 10 countries (median 9.0%; 605 patients of mean age 17.8 years, duration 9.4 years, 51% female). For 271 slightly older patients with longer duration of type 1 diabetes (mean age 29 years; duration 20.6 years; 49.2% female), variation in hypertension prevalence was 17.3% for Israel, 24.4% for Pittsburgh, 40.7% for Finland, and 32.4% for Sweden (Walsh 04). In a larger database from the same WHO-sponsored population-based DiaComp study, the prevalence of self-reported hypertension varied from 1.2% (Japan) to 15.1% (Chicago) among 1,833 type 1 diabetes patients from 15 countries (mean age 17.3 years; duration 9.4 years; 54% female). The prevalence varied from 13.5% (Japan) to 50.0% (Brazil) among 824 patients with type 1 diabetes of longer duration (19.9 years; mean age 28.7 years; 54.1% female). Hypertension showed a strong and significant association with all diabetic and macrovascular complications in this global study, which seeks to determine the basis for regional variation in hypertension and other complications (Walsh 06). In a community-based study during the year 2000 in the U.K., 26% of 220 type 1 diabetes patients (mean age 38.2 ± 12.2 years; mean duration 12.4 ± 8.5 years) had hypertension (BP ≥140/90), and 60% of the hypertensive diabetic patients did not have micro – or macroalbuminuria (Joseph 03). Hypertension prevalence in a community-based study of type 1 diabetes was 28% in 1996–1998 in Pittsburgh (mean age 28 years; mean diabetes duration 20 years) (Zgibor 01). In Colorado, 43% of 652 patients with type 1 diabetes (mean age 37 ± 9 years; mean diabetes duration 23.2 ± 8.9 years) were noted to have hypertension during 2000–2002 compared with 15% in 764 nondiabetic controls of similar age. Although hypertension is strongly associated with diabetic renal damage, one-half of the hypertensive diabetic patients in this study did not have albuminuria >30 mg/day (Maahs 05b).

Surveys of hypertension in patients with type 2 diabetes in the U.S. (71%) and in Australia (69%) are skewed by the inclusion of much older patients (Donnelly 97, Geiss 02). The prevalence of hypertension in Germany at 16–60 years of age is 79% for type 2 diabetes compared with 47% for type 1 diabetes, but the majority of treated cases are in those >40 years of age (Schiel 06). In the original WHO Multinational Study of Vascular Disease in Diabetes, hypertension (>160/95 or on treatment) was detected in 38.5% of 1,812 women with type 2 diabetes (mean age 47 years; range 35–55 years), of whom one-fifth had isolated systolic BP >160 mmHg (Fuller 89). By the age of 45, ~40% of patients with type 2 diabetes become hypertensive in the U.K. (UKPDS 98). Hypertension (160/90) was noted to be already present (48% untreated) at the diagnosis of type 2 diabetes in 46.5% of 1,512 female patients recruited for the UKPDS (mean age 52 ± 9 years) (HDSG 93). In this landmark study of type 2 diabetes and treatment with antihyperglycemic and antihypertensive agents, the lower the achieved systolic BP (from >170 down to <120 mmHg), the lower the risk of all complications (fatal and nonfatal MI, heart failure, fatal and nonfatal stroke, amputation or death from peripheral vascular disease, microvascular end points) (Adler 00). In the Hypertension Optimal Treatment trial, 499 patients with type 2 diabetes and baseline diastolic BP of 100–115 mmHg were randomized to a target diastolic BP <80 mmHg (mean achieved systolic 140 ± 12 mmHg); this group had significantly fewer major cardiovascular events over a 3–5 year follow-up (Hansson 98).

Data are limited on the prevalence of hypertension in diabetic women in their reproductive years. The EURODIAB IDDM Complications cross-sectional study examined randomly selected women with type 1 diabetes from diabetes clinics in 18 countries in 1989–1990. The prevalence of hypertension (BP ≥140/90) in 707 females aged 15–29 years was 12.3% compared with 22.2% in 631 women aged 30–44 years. Only 44% of women in the latter group were aware of hypertension, and 39% were treated. The prevalence of near-stage 2 hypertension (BP ≥ 160/95) was 7.7% at age 15–29 years and 12.5% at age 30–44 years (Collado-Mesa 99). In patients with type 1 diabetes onset before age 35 at the Steno Clinic in Denmark, 764 women aged 16–59 years were identified in 1988. Hypertension was defined as systolic BP ≥160 mmHg or diastolic BP ≥95 at three timepoints or ongoing antihypertensive treatment. Thus, the degree of hypertension was close to stage 2 by current criteria. The prevalence of hypertension in diabetic and control women in different age-groups according to level of albuminuria from this study is presented in Table II.11. The increased prevalence with albuminuria

TABLE II.11 Prevalence (%) of Hypertension* in Nonpregnant Women with Type 1 Diabetes and in Nondiabetic Controls

Number	Albuminuria	16–19 Years	20–29 Years	30–39 Years	40–49 Years	50–59 Years
579 DM1	<30 mg/24 h	0.0	0.7	2.2	8.6	14.1
95 DM1	30–300 mg/24 h	0.0	7.4	26.7	33.3	33.3
90 DM1	>300 mg/24 h	50.0	78.3	86.5	100.0	80.0
>5,000 controls	Unknown	0.4	1.4	1.7	7.6	13.1

*Hypertension, ≥160/95.

DM1, type 1 diabetes.

Taken from Norgaard 90; used with permission.

is apparent (incipient or clinical DN), and so-called "essential hypertension" was not more common in diabetic women without albuminuria than in age-matched controls. Unfortunately, the number of subjects in each of the cells was not presented, and one suspects that small numbers is a limitation of the study (Norgaard 90). Hypertension prevalence in type 2 diabetic women in a community-based population study in Minnesota was 16.7% at 30–39 years of age and 43.8% at 40–49 years of age, but the number of patients in the cells was small (Sprafka 88). Perhaps we can conclude that 15–35% of women with type 1 diabetes entering pregnancy will be hypertensive (unless women with albuminuria and/or hypertension select out of pregnancy) and that we need additional data on younger patients with type 2 diabetes.

Adolescent females with diabetes may soon enough become pregnant, and epidemiological data are available for this population (Tarn 86, Knerr 08). In 10–19-year-old females in the U.S. with diabetes (91% type 1 diabetes), 28% were recorded as having high BP or taking BP medication (>90th percentile for age and height) (Rodriguez 06). National BP percentiles for age and height for all youth have been published in a readily available journal (NBP 04). For example, >120/84 is the 90th percentile at age 16 at the 50th percentile for height. Stage 1 hypertension in female adolescents with diabetes is defined as an average systolic or diastolic BP ≥95th percentile for age and height measured on at least three separate days (e.g., ≥129/84 at age 17, 50th percentile for height). Pharmacotherapy is recommended for stage 2 hypertension in nondiabetic adolescents (NBP 04) (e.g., ≥149/95 at age 16; at ≥18 years of age, use adult JNC 7 BP standards) (Chobanian 03). However, the ADA Consensus Panel for diabetes care in children and adolescents recommends pharmacological therapy for BPs consistently >130/80, in addition to dietary intervention and exercise (Silverstein 05).

In the largest data set of 27,358 young patients with type 1 diabetes in Germany, 13% of those aged 17–26 years had hypertension. Most had raised systolic BP; only 4.8% received BP-lowering therapy (Schwab 06). Elevated systolic and diastolic BP was slightly more frequent in females compared with males (Dost 08). In Australia, the frequency of hypertension was 16% in 1,393 patients aged 14–17 years with type 1 diabetes compared with 36% in 58 patients with type 2 diabetes in the same age range (Eppens 06). Ambulatory BP monitoring revealed that systolic BP burden (percent of time above 95th percentile) was 19% in the daytime and 1.4% in the nighttime in 63 Greek type 1 diabetes patients aged 7–18 years compared with an 11.5% daytime diastolic burden and 0.8% nighttime diastolic burden (Theochari 96). In a small multiethnic sample of adolescents with type 2 diabetes in New York City (mean BMI: 35 ± 7), office hypertension was detected in 58% of the group (BP ≥95th percentile for age, sex, and height). Systolic pressures were significantly higher than in obese controls, and systolic nocturnal non-dipping was present in 56% (Ettinger 05).

Other studies confirm that slightly higher daytime or nighttime systolic BP is related to overweight and insulin dose in young patients with diabetes and that glycemic control is related to daytime or nighttime diastolic BP (Holl 99b, Darcan 06). Elevated nocturnal BP and reduced nocturnal "dipping" might reflect subclinical autonomic neuropathy (Holder 97) and was associated with development of incipient nephropathy (microalbuminuria) (Lurbe 02, Darcan 06, Dost 08). Ambulatory daytime systolic and diastolic BP load is also associated with microalbuminuria and glomerulopathy in adolescents with type 1 (Lurbe 93, Mortensen 94, Torbjornsdotter 01,04, Darcan 06, Eppens 06) and type 2 diabetes (Ettinger 05). It may be difficult to reliably detect mild hypertension in adolescent patients due to the prominence of the "white coat" effect on BP that is prevalent in this group (Harshfield 94, Nishibata 95, Waeber 06). Ambulatory or BP self-monitoring is useful to rule out or establish the diagnosis of hypertension (Holl 99b).

Hypertension-associated general morbidity

In a meta-analysis of >1 million individual patients in 61 studies around the globe, absolute risks for death from ischemic heart disease or stroke began to rise significantly at usual systolic BP>130 and usual diastolic BP >80 mmHg in women aged 50–59 years without a history of vascular disease at baseline (PSC 02). An eightfold increased mortality risk was seen from ischemic heart disease at systolic BP ≥172 and diastolic BP ≥108 as well as an eightfold mortality risk from stroke at systolic BP ≥162 and diastolic BP ≥97 mmHg. For women in their 40s, the "hazard" ratio for decreased mortality from ischemic heart disease was 0.40 (95% CI 0.32–0.49) with a 20-mmHg reduction in systolic BP <172 and 0.41 (95% CI 0.34–0.49) for decreased mortality from stroke with a 20-mmHg reduction in systolic BP <162 (PSC 02). In the Pittsburgh Epidemiology of Diabetes Complications 10-year prospective study of 589 patients with onset of type 1 diabetes before age 17 and mean age at baseline of 29 years, the RR for mortality was 3.0 for systolic BP of 120–129 (reference value <110) and 7.2 for systolic BP >130; the RR for mortality was 2.4 for diastolic BP >80 and 4.0 for diastolic BP >90 (reference value <80) (Orchard 01). These values obtained from epidemiological data parallel the observed benefits of relatively short-term RCTs of BP-lowering treatments (Gueyffier 97, BPL 00); as noted in trials, the benefits are greatest in those at high risk of vascular disease, such as diabetic women.

The coexistence of chronic hypertension in young and older nonpregnant patients with diabetes also substantially increases the risk of micro- and macrovascular complications including progression of retinopathy, worsening of albuminuria, and cardiovascular events (Arauz-Pacheco 02, Chobanian 03b, JBS 05). RCTs of antihypertensive treatment that reduced these complications (Hansson 98, Arauz-Pacheco 02, Berlowitz 03, Black 03, Bakris 04a, BPT 05) are the basis of current guidelines that target the maintenance of BP at <130/80 mmHg in nonpregnant patients with diabetes and hypertension if it can be safely achieved (Choban 03a, ADA 04,07). Combinations of two or more drugs are usually needed to achieve the target BP goal (Bakris 00,03a, Choban 03b, Fox 04b, Whelton 05). However, only 58% of 1,565 diabetic hypertensive patients were treated in the U.S. NHANES conducted in 1999–2000; 47% of those treated had BP controlled to <140/90, and only 25% had BP controlled to <130/85 (Hajjar 03). Only 31% of diabetic patients (75% type 2 diabetes) in a random sample from 30 managed care organizations across the U.S. were at BP <130/80; of 3,647 patients treated with antihypertensive drugs, only 20.6% were at goal (Andros 06). The inadequacy of BP-lowering treatment for diabetic women is similar in other populations (Collado-Mesa 99, Soedamah-Muthu 02, Joseph 03, Nilsson 03, Comaschi 05, Eliasson 05, Prevost 05, Schiel 06).

Self-monitoring or ambulatory monitoring of BP

This monitoring is recommended by European and North American consensus groups to be used by trained patients under medical supervision (O'Brien 03, Stergiou 04, Pickering 06). Self-monitoring has reasonable accuracy and predicts CVD and nephropathy better than office BP (Ohkubo 98, Nordmann 99, Masding 01, Kamoi 02, Bobrie 04, Andersen 05c, Agarwal 06). Self-monitoring has lower cost and wider availability than ambulatory monitoring, but self-monitoring devices available on the market may be poorly standardized. Wrist and finger devices are not recommended

(Stergiou 04). Ambulatory monitoring allows measurements over a full 24-h period, and the effect of nocturnal BP can be evaluated. Ambulatory monitoring also allows evaluation of the pulsatile component (pulse pressure) and the steady component (mean arterial pressure [MAP]) of the repetitive continuous wave of BP (Hermida 04). Controlled trials of both systems reveal that home BP values are usually lower than office values, predict cardiovascular events, and are useful for monitoring the effects of treatment (Kurtz 03, Cappucio 04, Mancia 04, Staessen 04, Pickering 06). However, home BP monitoring occasionally reveals "masked hypertension," with high values seen at home and normal values in the office (Pickering 02, Andersen 05c, Stergiou 05). Self-monitoring BP can be used as a screening test to detect just the opposite: lower values at home, signifying "white coat hypertension" that requires confirmation with ambulatory monitoring (Verdecchia 05).

As noted in the JNC 7 report, continuous "ambulatory monitoring provides information about BP during daily activities and sleep," and the level of BP using ambulatory monitoring correlates better than office measurements with target organ injury (Chobanian 03). "Blood pressure self-measurements may benefit patients by providing information on response to antihypertensive medication, improving patient adherance to therapy, and in evaluating white-coat hypertension. Individuals with a mean BP of more than 135/85 mm Hg measured at home are generally considered to be hypertensive" (Chobanian 03). Ambulatory BP ≥135/85 was accepted as confirmation of hypertension (defined as >140/90 in the office) (Verdecchia 03,05). Average self-monitored morning and evening BP ≥130/80 mmHg suggests high BP that requires further evaluation and treatment in diabetic women (Stergiou 04, Pickering 05). The Standards of Medical Care in Diabetes—2008 states that home or 24-hour ambulatory BP monitoring may provide additional evidence of "white coat" and masked hypertension and other discrepancies between office and "true" blood pressure. "However, the preponderance of the clear evidence of benefits of treatment of hypertension in people with diabetes is based on office measurements" (ADA 08a).

Hypertensive Disorders in Pregnancy

Hypertensive disorders are defined as indicated in Table II.12 based on guidelines recently published by consensus groups (Helewa 97, Moutquin 97, Rey 97, Brown 00b, Gifford 00, NBP 00, ACOG 01, Chobanian 03a,b, Oakley 03). All categories are more common in diabetic than in nondiabetic women (Leguizamon 06). Chronic hypertension can occur with or without preexisting albuminuria and is a risk factor for midtrimester abortion, premature birth, FGR, placental abruption, and neonatal morbidity (Silverstone 80, McCowan 96, Haelterman 97, Jain 97, Sibai 98, Sibai 00a, Ray 01a,b, Magee 03a, Roberts 03, Zetterstrom 05,06), especially in black and Asian-Indian women (Lydakis 98, Samadi 98). Chronic hypertension was independently associated with an increased risk of acute MI during or within 6 weeks after pregnancy (OR 24.9; 95% CI 14.8–40.3) in a population-based study of 151 cases of MI among 5.5 million deliveries in 1991–2000 (Ladner 05). Preeclampsia is a potentially dangerous multifaceted syndrome with new hypertension and proteinuria >300 mg/24 h (ACOG 02b). Edema is not included in the diagnosis due to its nonspecificity. Preeclampsia superimposed on chronic hypertension occurs in 14–34% of nondiabetic women with preexisting hypertension (Rey 94, McCowan 96, Sibai 98, Ray 01a, August 04). This can be a difficult diagnosis with a sudden increase in BP, sudden change in proteinuria, or evidence of end-organ dysfunction such as hemolysis, thrombocytopenia, intravascular coagulation, elevation in hepatic

TABLE II.12 Categories of Hypertensive Disorders in Pregnancy

Categories	Definition	Comment
Chronic hypertension	BP ≥140 S or ≥90 D prior to pregnancy or before 20 weeks gestation; BP ≥130/80 in diabetes	Persists >12 weeks postpartum
Preeclampsia	BP ≥140 S or ≥90 D with proteinuria (≥300 mg/24 h) after 20 weeks gestation	More frequent in DM with baseline albuminuria, even if normotensive; can progress to eclampsia (seizures or coma)
Chronic hypertension with superimposed preeclampsia	New-onset proteinuria after 20 weeks; in a woman with hypertension and proteinuria prior to 20 weeks: sudden two- to threefold increase in proteinuria, sudden increase in BP, thrombocytopenia, or elevated plasma transaminase	Often occurs preterm, with increased frequency of fetal growth restriction or perinatal mortality
Gestational hypertension	New hypertension without proteinuria after 20 weeks gestation; BP normal by 12 weeks postpartum	May represent preproteinuric phase of preeclampsia or recurrence of chronic hypertension abated in midpregnancy

NBP Working Group, 2000. Modified from Chobanian 03b, ADA 08b.
Blood pressure (BP) in mmHg.

D, diastolic; DM, diabetes mellitus; S, systolic.

transaminases, or pulmonary edema (Gifford 00). Predictors of increased risk of superimposed preeclampsia include higher BMI, systolic BP >140 mmHg at 20 weeks, or serum uric acid >3.6 mg/dL at 12–20 weeks gestation (Masse 93, Sibai 98, Lee 00, Stamilio 00, Chappell 02, August 04). In this category, the prognosis for mother or fetus is worse than with either condition alone.

Gestational hypertension

Gestational hypertension is a nonspecific diagnosis in that it includes women with apparently new hypertension "who have not yet manifested proteinuria" (Gifford 00). A substantial proportion (10–50%) will be diagnosed with preeclampsia before or after delivery (Magee 03a), with greater risk if hypertension is identified <34 weeks (Saudan 98, Barton 01) or cardiac remodeling has already occurred (Novelli 03). Recent evidence suggests that nondiabetic women with stage 2 gestational hypertension who never develop preeclampsia have increased risks of premature delivery, FGR, and neonatal morbidity independent of obesity (Xiong 99, Hauth 00, Waugh 00, Buchbinder 02, Magee 03a). The prevalence, pathogenesis, and outcomes of gestational hypertension are inadequately studied in women with PDM. Nondiabetic women with gestational hypertension often have signs of insulin resistance or metabolic syndrome as well as risk factors for later CVD (Caruso 99, Thadhani 99, Martin 01, Bartha 02, Ness 03, Novelli 03, Seely 03). However, gestational hypertension without proteinuria in women with type 1 diabetes did not predict diabetic nephropathy an average of 11 years after pregnancy, as did preeclampsia (Gordin 07).

Normative blood pressure in pregnancy

Knowledge of BP levels in normal pregnancy may be relevant to setting targets for treatment of hypertensive diabetic pregnant women. BP levels are influenced by the hemodynamic and vascular changes of pregnancy related to effects of hormones, cytokines, and GFs. From a large cross-sectional survey of 3,234 white pregnant women in Switzerland (Ochsenbein-Kolble 04) and a prospective multicenter study of 326 healthy pregnant women in the U.S. (Peterson 92), the 5th, 50th, and 95th percentiles or mean ± SD values for systolic and diastolic BPs in each trimester are presented in Table II.13. Ambulatory BP thresholds of diurnal mean systolic (115 mmHg) and diastolic BP (68 mmHg) that have good sensitivities and specificities in discriminating risk of development of gestational hypertension or preeclampsia are lower than the 95th percentile or two SD values using conventional measurements at 20 weeks (Napoli 03, Hermida 05). In the entire group of pregnant women, both systolic and diastolic BP levels decline slightly from early pregnancy, reaching a trough in mid-pregnancy and then rising to end ~4 mmHg higher than in early pregnancy. In women developing gestational hypertension or preeclampsia, BP remains stable during the first half of gestation and then continuously increases until delivery (Hermida 05). In the Swiss survey, Asians and blacks had consistently lower systolic and diastolic BP values than white women, but only 5.5 mmHg had to be subtracted from systolic values and 2 mmHg from diastolic values to apply Caucasian norms to Asians. For blacks, the adjusted values would be 4.5 mmHg systolic and 2.5 mmHg diastolic BP (Ochsenbein 04).

TABLE II.13 Office BP Levels in Groups of Normal Pregnant Women,[a,b] BP Levels by Daytime Ambulatory Monitoring in Women with Type 1 Diabetes, and Controls Who Were Normotensive at Baseline (<130/80)[c]

Weeks Gestation	Group (no.)	2.5th–5th Percentile	50th Percentile or Mean	95th–98.5th Percentile
10	145 controls[a]	91/48	108/60	128/74
12	315 controls[b]	84/49	106/66	129/82
12–14	71 DM1[c]	85/54	118//1	130/80
12–14	48 controls[c]	88/48	114/68	130/80
20	39 controls[a]	89/48	107/59	128/73
20	295 controls[b]	82/46	105/63	128/81
18–22	69 DM1[c]	100/57	116/72	132/86
18–22	40 controls[c]	93/45	117/69	141/93
36	179 controls[a]	94/52	111/63	131/78
36	281 controls[b]	86/49	116/67	133/85
30–35	66 DM1[c]	90/56	115/71	141/86
30–35	48 controls[c]	96/53	114/69	132/84

[a]*Ochsenbein-Kolble 2004, percentiles.*
[b]*Peterson 1992, mean ± 2 SD.*
[c]*Napoli 2003, mean ± 2 SD.*

BP systolic/diastolic, mmHg.
BP, blood pressure; DM1, type 1 diabetes.

Large epidemiological surveys revealed a U-shaped relationship between BP and pregnancy outcome. An analysis of outcomes in 14,833 singleton gestations in Northern California showed that midtrimester MAP >90 mmHg (110/80, 120/75, 130/70, and so forth) was related to significantly increased rates of stillbirth, subsequent preeclampsia, and FGR. BP is a continuum in the population; with each 5-mmHg rise in midtrimester MAP, there was a progressive increase in the perinatal mortality rate. Midtrimester MAP <75 mmHg was associated with increased frequency of FGR, but not with stillbirth (Page 76a). Further analysis showed that subjects labeled with "chronic hypertension" (midtrimester MAP ≥90; third trimester MAP ≥105, without proteinuria) had increased rates of stillbirth and FGR in both black and white populations (Page 76b). The Collaborative Perinatal Project collected data from 38,636 pregnant women and showed increased fetal mortality with maximum observed diastolic BP in pregnancy <65 mmHg or >85 mmHg (Friedman 78, Zhang 01). In a survey of 22,255 consecutive births in England, the frequency of infants <10th percentile of weight for gestational age was 3.65% if maximum diastolic BP was ≤60 mmHg, 2.63% at 61–70 mmHg, 3.22% at 71–89 mmHg, and 6.87% at ≥90 mmHg (Steer 97). A larger study of 210,814 nulliparous mothers and their singleton births from 1988–2000 showed that BW was maximal with the highest diastolic BP (adjusted for maternal height and weight) at 70–80 mmHg, with a slight decline in BW in the group with the highest diastolic BP at 60 or 90 mmHg. Crude perinatal mortality was least (~0.4%) with the highest diastolic pressure at 80 mmHg and increased by ~0.1% in the group with the highest diastolic pressure at 60 or 90 mmHg (Steer 04).

Investigators using ambulatory BP monitoring to improve the precision and relevance of BP measurements found strong, independent inverse associations between mean (Churchill 97) or daytime diastolic BP and indexes of fetal growth across a range of diastolic BP levels of 65–100 mmHg (Waugh 00). From the epidemiological–statistical perspective, the apparent U-shaped relationship of BP to perinatal outcome (Iwasaki 02) supports the targeting of maternal systolic BP between 110 and 130 mmHg and between 65 and 80 mmHg diastolic in chronically hypertensive pregnant women with PDM. Thus, lower-range targets are at the midzone of normal distribution and upper-range targets are >95th percentiles of normal, thereby being equivalent to treatment thresholds recommended for nonpregnant diabetic women to reduce risk of CKD and CVD.

Prevalence of hypertension in diabetic pregnant women

The prevalence of chronic hypertension (using older criteria of >140/90) is 10–17% in pregnancies of women with type 1 diabetes, increases with age and duration of diabetes (Vaarasmaki 02), and predicts increased rates of prematurity and neonatal morbidity; much of the latter is associated with superimposed preeclampsia (Diamond 85, Cousins 87, Greene 89, Hanson 98, McElvy 00, Cundy 02, Heard 04, Vreeburg 04, Gonzalez-Gonzalez 08). In a large prospective multicenter study of women using insulin prior to pregnancy, preeclampsia was diagnosed in 18% of diabetic women without hypertension or proteinuria at baseline, in 22% with hypertension, in 29% with proteinuria (>300 mg/24 h), and in 26% with both hypertension and proteinuria at baseline (Sibai 00b). In the N.Y. state hospital discharge database for 1993–2002, 10.7% of 6,772 pregnant women with type 1 diabetes were identified with "essential" hypertension (also denoted as preexisting hypertension) compared with 1.4% in >2 million pregnant women without hypertension (crude RR 7.6). Of the 725 type 1 diabetic women with "essential" hypertension, 24% had superimposed preeclampsia. The rate of gestational hypertension in women with type 1 diabetes was 3.5% (crude RR 2.3) and total preeclampsia was 14.1% (crude RR 4.15), of whom 26% were identified with severe preeclampsia or eclampsia (Tanaka 07).

Chronic hypertension is more common in pregnant women with type 2 rather than type 1 diabetes (GDFSG 91, Sacks 97, Cundy 02). In the N.Y. state hospital discharge database for 1993–2002, 12.3% of 3,509 pregnant women with type 2 diabetes were identified with "essential" hypertension (crude RR 8.8). Of the 432 type 2 diabetic women with "essential" hypertension, 22% had superimposed preeclampsia. The rate of gestational hypertension in women with type 2 diabetes was 2.7% and total preeclampsia was 10.2% (crude RR 3.0), of whom 21% were identified with severe preeclampsia or eclampsia (Tanaka 07). Baseline factors predicting development of new hypertension (gestational or preeclampsia) in both types of diabetic pregnancy include nulliparity, duration of diabetes, A1C >9.0 %, systolic BP >120 mmHg, or diastolic BP >80 mmHg; also included are signs of microvascular disease, such as albuminuria >30 mg/24 h and DR (Hanson 98, Hiilesmaa 00, Cundy 02). However, studies of gestational hypertension in diabetic women are inadequate to determine perinatal outcome or to provide any basis for treatment.

Close monitoring of BP is important throughout pregnancy (Lauszus 07). Twenty-four-h continuous ambulatory monitoring or self-measurement of BP at home can identify white-coat hypertension in women with apparent essential hypertension based on sitting BP ≥140/90 in the office, but no history of antihypertensive treatment prior to pregnancy and normal BP at home (Brown 05). Several studies of ambulatory BP monitoring during pregnancy in nondiabetic (Halligan 93, Benedetto 97, Brown 98, Bellomo 99, Brown 99, Waugh 00, Brown 01, Walker 02, Hermida 03a,b, Brown 04, Hermida 05, Rey 07) and diabetic women (Flores 99, Lauszus 01, Napoli 03) and of self-monitoring BP at home (Zuspan 91, Ross-McGill 00, Waugh 03) during pregnancy generally support these principles. However, no RCTs have been conducted in diabetic pregnant women to prove benefit as have been conducted for older patients with chronic hypertension (Mancia 04, Staessen 04). Hypertension monitoring guidelines (Pickering 05, Verdecchia 05) recommend sequential use of self-monitoring and ambulatory monitoring of BP during pregnancy with validated instruments in trained patients to identify white-coat hypertension, which is important "so that pregnant women are not admitted to hospital or given antihypertensive drugs unnecessarily or excessively" (O'Brien 03). The role of self or ambulatory BP monitoring in assessment of antihypertensive therapy in pregnancies with diabetes needs to be clarified.

BP targets for the management of chronic hypertension in pregnancy in the nondiabetic population are debatable. Based on small RCTs in which most subjects had gestational hypertension, previous consensus guidelines suggested withholding drug treatment until systolic BP is >150–160 mmHg or diastolic BP is >100–110 mmHg unless there is evidence of target organ damage (NBP 00, ACOG 01, Choban 03b, Oakley 03). This suggestion is based on inconsistent evidence of neonatal benefit from treatment to lower targets and the belief that nondiabetic women with stage 1 hypertension would be at low risk of cardiovascular complications within the short time frame of pregnancy. Although hypertension–preeclampsia during nondiabetic pregnancy is linked to later CVD events (Jonsdottir 95, Seeley 99, Kestenbaum 03, Wilson 03, Arnadottir 05), no trials have evaluated whether treatment during and after pregnancy will reduce CVD risk. The Canadian Hypertension Society Consensus Conference (Rey 97) and the Australasian Hypertension Society (Brown 00b) recommended the initiation of drug treatment at thresholds >140/90 for preexisting

TABLE II.14 Randomized, Controlled Trials of Antihypertensive Drug Therapy Prior to 28 Weeks Gestation in Pregnant Women with Chronic Hypertension[a]

Author (year)[b]	Study group (N)	Comparison Group (N)	Significant Treatment: Maternal	Effects: Infant
Leather, 1968	Methyldopa and bendrofluazide, 23	No drug, 24	Diastolic BP lowered 10 mmHg	Gestation 10 days longer; fetal loss 0 of 23 vs. 5 of 24
Redman, 1976,77 Mutch, 1977a,b Cockburn, 1982	Methyldopa, 101	No drug, 107	S/D BP lowered 10/6 mmHg; threefold less signs of late severe hypertension	Reduced midpregnancy loss; BW, SGA NS; infant development NS
Arias, 1979	Thiazide plus methyldopa or hydralazine, 29	No drug, 29	Less late-pregnancy aggravation of hypertension	BW, SGA NS
Sibai, 1984	Thiazide continued, 10	Thiazide stopped by 14 weeks, 10	Much less gain in plasma volume at 26–32 weeks; MAP NS	Perinatal outcome NS
Weitz, 1987	Methyldopa, 13	Placebo, 12	MAP lowered from 108 to 96 mmHg	Gestation 10 days longer; BW NS; SGA 0 of 13 vs. 3 of 12
Butters, 1990	Atenolol, 15	Placebo, 14	Mean diastolic BP 74 vs. 81 in control group	Reduced placental weight and BW; atenolol 10/15 SGA; infant weight NS at 1 year
Sibai, 1990	Methyldopa, 87; labetalol, 86	No drug, 90	Mean systolic BP* 126 vs. 122 vs. 133; mean diastolic BP* 78 vs. 76 vs. 82	Perinatal outcome NS

[a]*Mostly stage 1 hypertension.*
[b]*All are English-language publications.*
**At 27–29 weeks after ~16 weeks of treatment; percentage of subjects who were African-American not stated.*

BP, blood pressure; BW, birth weight; MAP, mean arterial pressure; N, number; NS, no significant difference; S/D, systolic/diastolic; SGA, small for gestational age (<10th percentile)

hypertension in pregnancy. No trials have been conducted on the treatment of isolated systolic hypertension during pregnancy despite the fact that systolic hypertension is the best predictor of superimposed preeclampsia (Stone 94, Odegard 00, Duckitt 05, Martin 05) and maternal complications (Cunningham 05).

A Cochrane Review (Abalos 04,07) evaluated 46 studies of antihypertensive drug therapy for mild to moderate systolic (140–169 mmHg) and diastolic hypertension (85, 90, or 95 up to 109 mmHg) during pregnancy (28 were placebo-controlled or had no treatment), but only eight trials analyzed results in women with chronic hypertension (some trials with multiple publications) (Table II.14) (Leather 68, Redman 76, Mutch 77a,b, Redman 77, Arias 79, Cockburn 82, Sibai 84,

Weitz 87, Butters 90, Sibai 90). One of the studies was published in Portuguese only (Kahhale 85). The Cochrane reviewers found a significant halving (95% CI 0.41 to 0.64 for RR) of the risk of developing severe hypertension (>170/110 mmHg) associated with the use of antihypertensive drugs, but little evidence of effect on the risk of developing preeclampsia (95% CI 0.84 to 1.18 for RR) (Abalos 04). There was also no clear effect on FGR or perinatal death (95% CI 0.46 to 1.09 for RR), but the point estimate was a 29% reduction in fetal or neonatal death with antihypertensive drug treatment. Six trials evaluated the effects of treatment on miscarriage, thereby implying hypertension early in pregnancy, and a significant reduction was found RR 0.27 (95% CI 0.09 to 0.80). The Cochrane reviewers concluded that it "remains unclear whether antihypertensive drug therapy for mild-moderate hypertension during pregnancy is worthwhile" (Abalos 04,07). A Cochrane Review on the use of oral β-blockers for mild to moderate hypertension during pregnancy found that β-blockers reduced the frequency of subsequent severe hypertension and antepartum admissions to the hospital (Magee 04).

Examination of Table II.14 indicates that none of the RCTs concerning treatment of chronic hypertension in nondiabetic pregnant women were large trials, and none have been published since 1990. One of the moderately sized trials showed perinatal benefit from treatment with methyldopa (Redman 77) and the other did not (Sibai 90), but they both studied very different populations before and during the era of applied perinatal/medical technology. It is apparent that the evidence is inadequate to conclude whether antihypertensive therapy benefits, harms, or is neutral toward the fetus of the chronically hypertensive woman, and adequately powered RCTs are urgently needed.

The JNC 7 authors stated that antihypertensive medication should be continued as needed to control BP "for pregnant women with target organ damage or a prior requirement for multiple antihypertensive agents for BP control" (Chobanian 03b). In two recent reports, the NHLBI Working Group on High Blood Pressure in Pregnancy was silent on whether chronically hypertensive diabetic women are considered as having "target organ damage" (NBP 00, Roberts 03). Many clinicians and investigators do consider it on the basis of high rates of endothelial dysfunction and oxidative stress (Wolff 97, Savvidou 02, Wender 04), hypertrophic remodeling of small arteries (Endemann 04), LVH (Liu 03, Suys 04), and microalbuminuria (Ekbom 01, Clausen 05, Leitao 05, Strain 05) in this population. Diabetic women of reproductive age with hypertension are certainly considered at increased risk of heart disease, as discussed in Part II in the section titled "Cardiovascular Disease in Diabetic Women." Due to these maternal risk factors, we believe that continued pharmacotherapy of diabetic women with chronic hypertension is justified during pregnancy.

The widely quoted meta-analysis of randomized trials in nondiabetic pregnant women with hypertensive disorders suggested that producing a fall in MAP of 10 mmHg would reduce BW by 145 grams, yet it included only four trials in pregnant women with chronic hypertension among 15 trials that provided data on FGR (vonDadelszen 00,02). One of the four trials used atenolol versus placebo and observed significantly lower placental and fetal weight with atenolol treatment (Butters 90), an effect confirmed by other studies when this β-blocker is used from early pregnancy (Lip 97a, Easterling 99, Lydakis 99, Easterling 01, Bayliss 02). Other chronic hypertension trials used methyldopa or labetalol and showed no treatment effect in reducing BW despite lowered BP (Arias 79, Weitz 87, Sibai 90). The Cochrane Review of the use of oral β-blockers for mild to moderate hypertension during pregnancy determined that β-blockers appear to increase the incidence of SGA infants (RR 1.36; 95th CI 1.02–1.82) in 12 trials comparing β-blockers with placebo/no β-blocker; the analysis did not account for differing hemodynamic effects of various β-blockers (Magee 04). As noted, few of these trials studied women with chronic hypertension; when β-blockers were compared with methyldopa, drug safety seemed to be equivalent (Magee 04).

No RCTs have evaluated the maternal or fetal risks and benefits of treating chronic hypertension in women with PDM during their pregnancies. Nevertheless, strong evidence for aggressive treatment in the nonpregnant diabetic female population gives support to recommendations for stricter control of BP in the pregnant diabetic woman as well. In the absence of pregnancy, diabetic women are considered to be at high risk for CVD because they may have beginning target organ damage. We conclude that prevention of severe hypertension in late pregnancy would be a valuable benefit for diabetic women with chronic hypertension. RCTs are needed to evaluate the effect of treatment of hypertension in women with PDM during pregnancy as well as the short- and long-term risk of progression of DR, development of macular edema, worsening albuminuria and renal function, myocardial dysfunction, and carotid intimal and medial thickness as a measure of atherosclerosis. Effects on perinatal outcome also need evaluation. Until such studies, we recommend treatment to keep BP <130/80 but >109/64 in diabetic pregnant women with chronic hypertension.

Treatment of hypertension in pregnancy

Behavior modification is very important in the management of hypertension. Although salt restriction is receiving renewed attention in the treatment of nonpregnant diabetic women (Law 91, He 05, Weinberger 05), restriction of sodium intake below 1.5 gm/day is not recommended during pregnancy (IOM 04). On the other hand, prevention of frequently observed excess sodium intake above 2.3 gm/day may be wise, but has not been prospectively studied in pregnant women with PDM. Based on studies in nonpregnant women with and without diabetes (Dietary Approach to Stop Hypertension [DASH]) (ADA 04), dietary enhancement of potassium intake to 4.7 gm/day is considered beneficial in the management of hypertension during pregnancy (IOM 04). MNT is discussed in detail of Part I. Other behavioral modifications may be helpful in the management of stage 1 hypertension during pregnancy, such as relaxation training and prescribed physical activity or rest at home (Moutquin 97, Sorensen 03, Svetkey 05). Pending more data, the recommendation of the NHLBI Working Group on High Blood Pressure in Pregnancy "is to discourage aerobic exercise by pregnant women with hypertension" due to concern with maintenance of adequate placental blood flow (NBP 00).

Medication choices

Medications are similar to those used in pregnancies uncomplicated by diabetes including methyldopa, long-acting CCBs, β-blockers that decrease vascular resistance but not CO, and clonidine or prazosin as fourth-line agents (Table II.15) (Ferrari 97, Conway 00, Ferrer 00, NBP 00, Rosenthal 02, Montan 04, Duley 05). Multiple drug therapy (≥2 agents at maximal doses) is often needed to achieve BP targets in diabetes (ADA 08a). ACE inhibitors and ARBs must not be used in any stage of pregnancy due to the possibility of fetal damage (Cooper 06). Despite a black box warning by the FDA in 1992, first-trimester ACE inhibitor use actually increased in one state after 1996 (Bowen 08). Diuretics are not often used for hypertension in pregnancy due to concern about reduced plasma volume and uteroplacental blood flow with chronic or acute use (Sibai 84). An overview of randomized trials of diuretics in nearly 7,000 pregnant

TABLE II.15 Antihypertensive Agents Used During Pregnancy

Class	Name	Group and Tissue Selectivity; Mechanism of Action	Clinical Comment
Central sympathoplegic	Methyldopa	α2-agonist; decreased peripheral–renal vascular resistance	Mental lassitude; normal long-term infant follow-up
	Clonidine	α2A- and imidazoline agonist; decreased vascular resistance, including capacitance vessels; decreased CO	Transdermal; not used with depression
Calcium channel blocker, long-acting preferable	Verapamil	Phenylalkylamine; arteriole ≤ cardiac effects	Used in SVT
	Diltiazem	Benzothiazepine; arteriole = cardiac; decreased vascular resistance	Decreases albuminuria; antioxidant
	Nifedipine, nicardipine	Dihydropyridine; arteriole > cardiac; reflex symptom activation	Short-acting agents may increase cardiac morbidity
	Isradipine, nisoldipine, nitrendipine, amlodipine	Second- and third-generation dihydropyridine; decreased vasular resistance	Antioxidant effects
α-Antagonist	Prazosin	α1A > α2B,C; relaxes both arterioles and venules	Retention of salt and water
β-Blocker, nonselective	Propranolol	β1 = β2-antagonist; decreased CO and perhaps decreased renin	Lipid soluble; potentiates antidepressants
	Pindolol	β1 = β2-antagonist; partial β agonist; decreased vascular resistance	
β-Blocker, cardioselective	Atenolol	β1 selective; decreased HR and CO	Not metabolized; excreted in urine
	Metoprolol	β1 selective; decreased HR and CO	CYP286 variation; poor metabolizers
	Acebutolol	β1 selective, partial β agonist; decreased vascular resistance; less decreased CO	
β-Blocker, mixture of nonselective antagonists	Labetalol, 4 isomers	β1 = β2 > α1 > α2-antagonist; partial β2 agonist; decreased vascular resistance; no decreased HR or CO	No apparent decrease in uterine blood flow
	Carvedilol, 2 isomers	Nonselective β-antagonist, α1-antagonist; decreased vascular resistance	Fewer metabolic effects; antioxidant

Data from Luescher 98, Smith 98, Hoffman 04, Benowitz 04, and Jacob 04.
CO, cardiac output; HR, heart rate; SVT, supraventricular tachycardia.

women concluded that increases in maternal BP and edema are reduced and direct toxic effects on the neonate are not increased, but perinatal survival is not improved (Collins 85).

Methyldopa is commonly used as first-step therapy in pregnancy based on the early landmark RCT in chronic hypertension that demonstrated reduced fetal loss and no long-term adverse effects on 101 infants exposed in utero (Redman 76, Cockburn 82), in spite of placental transfer of methyldopa (Jones 78), transiently lower systolic BP in newborn infants (Whitelaw 81), and temporarily reduced head circumference (HC) in male infants (Mutch 77a,b, Moar 78). The Cochrane Review of 14 studies of mostly gestational hypertension and preeclampsia (Abalos 04) reported that any antihypertensive drug compared with methyldopa yielded a 51% reduced risk of the baby dying (RR 0.49; 95% CI 0.24–0.99), perhaps because methyldopa is sometimes neither well tolerated nor effective with stage 2 hypertension. Compared with 26 historical controls of whom 9 received antihypertensive therapy later in pregnancy, methyldopa prescribed by 17 weeks gestation to 10 microalbuminuric pregnant women with type 1 diabetes who required antihypertensive treatment prior to pregnancy or had early pregnancy BP >140/90 reduced preterm delivery prior to 34 weeks (0% vs. 23%, p < 0.02) without significant effect on preeclampsia (20% vs. 42%, NS). In this observational study, an unknown number of the 10 subjects were supplemented with labetalol or nifedipine, and some were allowed to continue furosemide initiated before pregnancy (Nielsen 06). Methyldopa had no influence on umbilical artery resistance in human Doppler and in vitro (Houlihan 04) studies, but lowered uterine or placental artery resistance in two of three reports (Rey 92, Montan 93, Gunenc 02). Methyldopa also reduced vascular resistance and increased mean flow velocity in the right central retinal artery if the drug lowered diastolic BP in a single study of preeclamptic gravidae (Hung 00). Possible benefit or harm from this effect in hypertensive diabetic pregnant women with retinopathy is unknown. In experimental models of renal disease in pregnant rats, methyldopa improved the impaired GFR without effect on proteinuria in adriamycin nephrosis (Podjarny 95); it also normalized systolic BP and improved GFR and proteinuria in a hypertensive pregnancy model induced by NO synthase inhibition (Podjarny 01). If therapeutic lifestyle modifications and methyldopa do not control BP <130/80 in diabetic pregnant women with chronic hypertension, second-step pharmacological agents should be considered.

Calcium-channel blockers

Nondihydropyridine L-type CCBs (Kuga 90, Luescher 98) may be preferred over the dihydropyridine group (L− + T-type) (Table II.15) for hypertension in diabetic women because of their tendency to reduce renal albumin excretion and partially preserve renal autoregulation; dihydropyridine CCBs may increase albuminuria and obliterate renal autoregulation in diabetic women (Andren 88, Demarie 90, Hayashi 96, Bakris 97, Smith 98, Griffin 99,01, Hayashi 03, Bakris 04b, Gashti 04, Griffin 04). In an RCT studying hypertensive type 2 diabetes patients with persistent microalbuminuria despite ACE inhibitor treatment, diltiazem reduced progression of albuminuria over 2 years compared with captopril (Perez-Maraver 05). CCBs may improve vascular health in ways beyond their BP-lowering effects. As an example, amlodipine and nifedipine inhibited in vitro LDL oxidation and glycation (Chen 97, Sobal 01, Toba 06), and amlodipine and manidipine normalized eNOS expression and attenuated the overexpression of molecules associated with inflammation and oxidative stress in aortas from rats with chronic

L-*N*ᴳ-nitro-L-arginine methyl ester (L-NAME)–induced inhibition of NO synthesis (Turgan 03, Toba 05). Evidence also suggests that diltiazem has antioxidant effects in experimental models (Obata 02, Kaymaz 04, Anjeneyulu 05). In a retrospective analysis of a small group of pregnant women with chronic renal disease, diltiazem use was associated with diminution of proteinura across gestation when the expectation was for large gestational increases in proteinuria (Khandewal 02). RCTs on the use of diltiazem in diabetic pregnant women with chronic hypertension or microalbuminuria are needed (Reece 02).

Diltiazem is subjected to complex and almost complete metabolism by enzymes with possible induced activity during pregnancy: desacetylation (esterases) and demethylation (polymorphic enzyme cytochrome P450, CYP2D6, CYP3A4) (Pichard 90, Molden 00,02), but effects on diltiazem pharmacokinetics in pregnancy are unclear (Bregante 00). There is uptake of diltiazem by protein-binding sites in many tissues (Weir 95, Bregante 00). Placental transfer of diltiazem and its active metabolites was demonstrated in rabbits (Bregante 00, Fraile 01). Diltiazem had no apparent untoward effects on the fetus or infant in a small study comparing it with oral nifedipine for premature labor (El-Sayed 98).

Dihydropyridine CCBs are metabolically eliminated to a high degree during first pass through the liver; during pregnancy, clearance of oral nifedipine is enhanced, half-life is shortened, and peak blood levels are lower. Umbilical cord blood concentrations approach those of the mother (Barton 91, Prevost 92). Perhaps due to its short half-life, placental transfer of intravenous nicardipine appears to be more limited (umbilical/maternal concentration ratio 0.1–0.23) (Bartels 07). Nifedipine infusion in normotensive pregnant ewes reduced fetal O_2 content and pH, but no deleterious fetoplacental blood flow changes were witnessed (Blea 97). Nicardipine infusion in normotensive pregnant Rhesus monkeys (Ducsay 87) and angiotensin-treated pregnant sheep (Parisi 89a,b) reduced fetal pO_2 and pH, but direct infusion into the chronically catheterized ovine fetus produced little hemodynamic change and no asphyxia (Holbrook 89). In chronically instrumented pregnant goats, nicardipine infusion transiently reduced uterine blood flow without causing fetal acidosis (Matsuda 93, Sakamoto 96).

Human studies with nifedipine showed improvement of elevated uteroplacental blood flow resistance in some, but not all, hypertensive pregnant subjects and no changes in fetal vascular flow indexes (Lindow 88, Pirhonen 90a,b, Puzey 91, Cobellis 06). Controlled comparisons of isradipine, nicardipine, or nifedipine versus placebo or other agents in gestational hypertension or preeclampsia have not produced obvious deleterious effects on the human fetus (Moretti 90, Wide-Swensson 91, Grunewald 92, Sibai 92, Carbonne 93, Jannet 94, Wide-Swensson 95, GSIG 98, Scardo 99, Hall 00, Borghi 02, Brown 02, Elatrous 02, Seki 02). Increased CI and selective renal arteriolar dilation with natriuresis and increased urinary output may be important characteristics of nifedipine use in the setting of acute severe hypertension in pregnancy (Vidaeff 05). Intravenous nicardipine can produce severe tachycardia in preeclamptic women (Aya 99, Hanff 05). Analysis of the limited use of CCBs in the first trimester did not demonstrate a teratogenic effect, but there are indications that too tight of a control over maternal BP can cause fetal limb defects (Magee 96, Sorensen 98,01). Follow-up of 94 children 18 months after in utero exposure to nifedipine for maternal hypertension revealed no differences in indicators of development or health of the infants compared with 65 infants of untreated hypertensive mothers (Bortolus 00).

Beta-blockers

Consideration of β-blockers for hypertension in diabetic women depends on their α- and β-adrenergic/tissue selectivity, lipophilicity, pharmacodynamics, hemodynamic effects in pregnancy, and possibility of drug interactions with other agents. Cardiovascular and metabolic effects of sympathetic nervous system stimulation are mediated through the adrenoceptors α1A, α1B, α1D, α2A, α2B, α2C, β1, β2, and β3, and the selectivity of adrenoceptor agonists and antagonists relates to the strength and specificity of their binding to receptors (Table II-15). Effects of sympathomimetic drugs on BP are mainly based on effects on the heart (α1 and β1, increased force and rate of contraction), peripheral vascular resistance, and capacitance vessels influencing venous return (α1, α2, vascular smooth muscle contraction; β2, vascular smooth muscle relaxation) (Hoffman 04). α2-Agonists also inhibit lipolysis, and β3 stimulation enhances lipolysis; β2-receptor agonists cause bronchodilation, decreased glucose utilization, and activation of hepatic glycogenolysis; combined α1 and β2 stimulation may enhance glucose disposal (Hoffman 04, Jacob 04).

Propranolol is the prototype nonselective β1- and β2-receptor antagonist. It lowers BP primarily as a result of decreasing CO, but it also inhibits the β1 stimulation of renin production by catecholamines and may act on peripheral presynaptic β-receptors to reduce sympathetic vasoconstrictor nerve activity (Benowitz 04). Original cardioselective β1-receptor antagonists (atenolol, metoprolol) were developed to avoid untoward effects of β2 blockade in the bronchioles and periphery. They lower BP by decreasing CO without permitting a reflex increase in vascular resistance, but other blockers with partial β-agonist activity (acebutolol, carvedilol, labetalol, pindolol) decrease peripheral resistance directly without much effect on HR or CO (ManVeld 82, Benowitz 04). Compared with the older β1/β2-nonselectives propranolol, oxprenolol and timolol, and the β1-selectives atenolol and metoprolol, β-blockers with vasodilating activity (carvedilol, labetalol, pindolol, others) cause less increase in insulin resistance, plasma glucose, cholesterol, and TGs in type 2 diabetes (Dornhorst 85, Albergati 92, Holzgreve 03, Bakris 04c, Jacob 04). The high incidence of hypoglycemia unawareness in pregnancies complicated by type 1 diabetes might potentially be exacerbated by use of adrenoceptor antagonists; however, in hypertensive type 2 diabetes patients, carvedilol was associated with less hypoglycemia and bradycardia than was metoprolol (Bakris 04c). Carvedilol is prominently used to treat heart failure and cardiomyopathy. In addition to its hemodynamic benefits, carvedilol has anti-inflammatory activity, inhibits lipid peroxidation of cell membranes, and protects cells from oxygen radical-mediated activity (Feuerstein 97, Dandona 00, Lysko 00, Cheng 03, Fahlbusch 04, Yang 04, Yuan 04). Studies are needed concerning the possible indications and benefits of treatment with carvedilol in pregnancies complicated by diabetes.

As previously noted, use of the β1-selective β-blocker atenolol in early pregnancy may disproportionately limit fetal growth, an effect apparently greater in occurrence than with other β-blockers (Magee 04). Oxprenolol treatment yielded equivalent results to methyldopa in two small early studies (Fidler 83, Gallery 85). Compared with nicardipine, metoprolol was less effective in controlling maternal BP, creatinine, and uric acid and in decreasing umbilical artery resistance in one randomized trial in nondiabetic women with gestational hypertension in the second half of pregnancy (Jannet 94). Labetalol compared favorably with hydralazine (Walker 83, Ashe 87, Mabie 87, Cruikshank 91, Hjertberg 93, Magee 03b, Vigil-DeGrazia 06) and was equal to nifedipine (Scardo 99, Vermillion 99) in controlling severe hypertension in pregnancy, without apparent unwanted effects on the mother or fetus. In this setting, bolus infusion of labetalol (20-mg initial dose) reduces BP without reflex tachycardia, bradycardia, increased intracranial pressure, or reduced cerebral, renal, and coronary blood flow (Vidaeff 05). Intravenous labetalol (50 mg) induced only minor changes in plasma glucose, insulin, C-peptide, and lipid metabolism in hypertensive women in the third trimester of pregnancy (Lunell 81). When oral labetalol was compared with bed rest (Lang 84), placebo (Pickles 89,92), or methyldopa (Plouin 88) for stage 1 gestational hypertension in pregnancy, labetalol significantly reduced BP without increasing the frequency of FGR.

The renal clearance of atenolol parallels CrCl during pregnancy, but without effect on apparent oral clearance, which is possibly related to high variance in bioavailability (Hebert 05). In comparison, greater metoprolol clearance and reduced peak plasma concentrations during pregnancy result from increased hepatic metabolism of the drug (Hogstedt 85). One investigator found no alteration in the clearance or volume of distribution of intravenous labetalol with pregnancy (Rubin 83a), but another group noted the terminal elimination half-life of oral labetalol to be considerably shortened to 1.7 ± 0.3 h in pregnant women with hypertension compared with 6–8 h in normotensive volunteers or nonpregnant hypertensive patients. The mean apparent oral elimination clearance was 22 mL/min/kg. Food delayed the time to peak serum concentration from 20 to 60 min after oral dosing (Rogers 90). Substantial interindividual variability of elimination half-lives (4.3–6.9 h), oral clearance (32–73 mL/min/kg), and pharmacodynamic parameters of oral labetalol (150–450 mg twice daily) was described in hospitalized women with average diastolic BP of 100–120 mmHg in the third trimester (Saotome 93). We are not aware of studies on the pharmacokinetics of carvedilol during pregnancy.

Regarding placental and fetal hemodynamics, atenolol seems to increase uteroplacental and fetal vascular resistance estimated by Doppler flow studies compared with pindolol (Montan 87,92, Rasanen 95). Labetalol did not decrease uteroplacental blood flow indexes despite reduction in maternal BP in human studies (Lunell 82, Nylund 84, Jouppila 86) and produced little change in umbilical artery pulsatility in most fetuses (Harper 91, Pirhonen 91). Infusion of labetalol (0.5 mg/kg) in chronically instrumented pregnant goats reduced maternal BP and uterine blood flow without change in fetal HR, BP, or acid–base status (Sakamoto 96). All β-blockers cross the placenta into the fetal circulation in spite of their differences in lipophilicity (Melander 78, Dumez 81, Lindeberg 84, Nylund 84) and transiently reduce newborn HR and BP, but are not associated with neonatal hypo- or hyperglycemia (Eliahou 78, Dumez 81).

Limited information exists on the efficacy and safety of clonidine or prazosin as fourth-line treatment for chronic hypertension in pregnancy. Maternal and neonatal effects of clonidine were equivalent to methyldopa in a randomized trial in the third trimester of 95 subjects with chronic or gestational hypertension or preeclampsia (Horvath 85). A small randomized trial of clonidine plus hydralazine versus placebo for third-trimester hypertension showed less aggravated hypertension, less development of proteinuria, and reduced preterm delivery in the active treatment group (Phippard 91). Clonidine binds to linked α2-adrenoceptors–imidazoline binding sites in the human placenta (Bagamery 98,99), crosses the term placenta (Ala-Kokko 97), and is concentrated in AF (Hartikainen-Sorri 87); however, data are inadequate to determine the effect on neonates. Currently, controversy surrounds the use of clonidine to enhance intrathecal–epidural anesthesia during labor (Paech 02, Missant 04, Roelants 05) as well as whether clonidine, an α2A-agonist, would be neuroprotective on perinatal excitotoxic brain injury as demonstrated in murine experiments (Laudenbach 02).

Prazosin also crosses the human placenta (Bourget 95), and the mean elimination half-life is somewhat prolonged during pregnancy (171 min) (Rubin 83b). A small trial comparing nifedipine with prazosin to control severe hypertension in the third trimester showed that both agents allowed 12–15 days to be gained without difference in maternal or neonatal characteristics except that fetal death occurred in 5 of 71 pregnancies in the prazosin group and 1 of 74 pregnancies in the nifedipine group (Hall 00). Two earlier uncontrolled studies showed no excess perinatal mortality when prazosin was used to treat 41 pregnant women with hypertension without proteinuria, but FGR was observed in 24% of infants. When prazosin plus oxprenolol was used to treat 22 women with early preeclampsia, fetal loss occurred in 32% (Lubbe 81, Dommisse 83).

ACE inhibitors should not be used in any stage of pregnancy due to their association with fetopathy including renal tubular dysplasia, intrauterine growth restriction, hypocalvaria, patent ductus arteriosus, fetal anuria, and neonatal death when used in the second and third trimesters (Rosa 89, Hulton 90, Barr 91, Brent 91, Hanssens 91, Martin 92, Bhatt-Mehta 93, Pryde 93, Lavoratti 97, NBP 00, Tabacova 03). Although postmarketing surveillance of ACE inhibitors suggested that first-trimester use did not pose a risk to the fetus (CDC 97), a recent analysis of a cohort of 29,507 infants of nondiabetic mothers found that 209 infants exposed to ACE inhibitors in the first trimester alone had an increased risk of major congenital malformations of various types (RR 2.71; 95% CI 1.7–4.3). Thankfully, there was no increased risk of malformations in 202 infants exposed to other antihypertensive drugs in early pregnancy (Cooper 06). This large study followed several reports of small, uncontrolled series in which ACE inhibitor–embryopathy was thought dependent on the presence of fetal kidneys after 12 weeks gestation (Barr 94, Lip 97b, Steffenson 98, Yip 98); however, angiotensin receptors are widely expressed in fetal tissues (Grady 91, Everett 97, Forhead 97, Norwood 97, Lamparter 99, Burrell 01, Hu 04). ACE inhibitors should be stopped when pregnancy is anticipated. Similar concerns surround the safety of *angiotensin II-receptor blockers* in any trimester of pregnancy. Case reports have shown second- and third-trimester fetopathy similar to the defects that occur with ACE inhibitors (Briggs 01, Chung 01, Lambot 01, Martinovic 01, Saji 01, Cox 03, Nayar 03, Pietrement 03, Schaefer 03). ARBs must not be used during pregnancy, and they should be stopped preconception because little is known about their potential teratogenicity (Alwan 05). As noted earlier, patients with albuminuria may be switched to diltiazem.

Recommendations

- BP should be measured at every clinical visit. Patients found to have systolic BP ≥130 mmHg or diastolic BP ≥80 mmHg should have BP confirmed on a separate day. Repeat systolic BP >130 mmHg or diastolic BP >80 mmHg confirms a diagnosis of hypertension in diabetic women. (C)

- Women with diabetes in the preconception period should be treated to a systolic BP <130 mmHg and to a diastolic BP <80 mmHg. (B)

- Patients with systolic BP >140 mmHg or diastolic blood pressure >90 mmHg should receive pharmacological therapy that is safe for anticipated pregnancy in addition to lifestyle and behavioral therapy. Multiple drug therapy (≥2 agents at maximal doses) is generally required to achieve BP targets. (A)

- Although diabetic women with a systolic BP of 130–139 mmHg or a diastolic BP of 80–89 may be given lifestyle therapy alone for a maximum of

3 months, the urge to try for pregnancy may suggest the addition of pharmacological agents that are safe for pregnancy to achieve target goals prior to conception. (E)

- During pregnancy in diabetic women with chronic hypertension, pharmacological therapy should be added as needed to achieve BP target goals of 110–129 mmHg systolic and 65–79 mmHg diastolic in the interests of long-term maternal health and minimization of impaired fetal growth. (E)

- ACE inhibitors and ARBs are contraindicated in gestation and should be stopped when pregnancy is anticipated. Effective contraception should be used by diabetic women treated with these agents. (A)

- BP medications that are safe for pregnancy should be added sequentially until target BP levels are achieved. These agents include methyldopa, long-acting CCBs, and selected beta-adrenergic blockers. (E)

- Hypertensive diabetic pregnant patients may be instructed to avoid excess salt intake but should not be severely salt restricted. Adequate potassium intake should be encouraged. (E)

- Home BP self-monitoring and 24-h ambulatory BP monitoring may provide additional evidence of "white coat" and masked hypertension and other discrepancies between office and "true" BP. However, the preponderance of the clear evidence regarding the benefits of treatment of hypertension in women with diabetes is based on office measurements. (E)

- Patients not achieving target BP despite multiple drug therapy should be referred to a physician experienced in the care of diabetic pregnant patients with hypertension. (E)

- Insufficient data prevent making a recommendation for or against treatment of diabetic women with stage 1 gestational hypertension. Diabetic patients with stage 2 gestational hypertension should be treated to prevent acute maternal vascular complications. (E)

- All diabetic pregnant women, especially those with hypertension, should be closely monitored for development of preeclampsia. (E)

MANAGEMENT OF HYPER/DYSLIPIDEMIAS

—— *Original contribution by Robert H. Knopp MD and Pathmaja Paramsothy MD, MS*

Lipids, Lipoproteins, Apolipoproteins, and Roles in Atherothrombosis

Plasma lipoproteins are noncovalent complexes of lipids with proteins, known as apolipoproteins, which are genetically and structurally distinct. The major apolipoproteins in human plasma are classified A-I, A-II, A-III, A-IV, B, C-I, C-II, C-III, D, and E (Havel 01). Lipoprotein particles transport insoluble cholesterol and TGs (triacylglycerols) in plasma, providing them for cell structure and metabolism (Brunzell 08). Lipoproteins of different densities (VLDL, intermediate-density lipoprotein [IDL], LDL, HDL) were first characterized by using ultracentrifugation and then electrophoresis of plasma; density (gm/mL) is related to protein content and inversely related to lipid content, molecular weight, and particle diameter. The percent composition of the lipid fraction (phospholipids, esterified cholesterol, unesterified cholesterol, triacylglycerols) varies in different plasma lipoprotein classes. Cholesterol is present in the highest concentration within LDL particles, and triacylglycerols (TGs) are mainly found within the larger but less dense VLDL particles. VLDLs are produced by the liver, supply FFAs to tissues, and predominate in carriage of TGs. "LDLs are byproducts of VLDL metabolism and, in the normal state, are the primary carriers of cholesterol. . . . HDL particles are produced by the liver and intestine and then become mature and enriched with other apolipoproteins and lipids by exchanges with chylomicrons and VLDL" (Brunzell 08). The most prominent apolipoprotein in LDL, IDL, and VLDL is apoB, while apoA-I is most prominent in HDL_2 and HDL_3. The apoC family and apoE are mainly found in IDL and VLDL (Havel 01).

The plasma level of LDL-C is commonly estimated by the Friedewald formula (Friedewald 72) after measurement of fasting total plasma cholesterol and TGs along with HDL-C. However, this value includes variable amounts of IDL-C and lipoprotein(a) [Lp(a)] and underestimates LDL as TG levels rise. Measurement of LDL-C within the particles "may not accurately reflect the true burden of atherogenic LDL particles" because cholesterol content varies individually and is affected by insulin resistance and hyperglycemia (Brunzell 08). Measurements of LDL particle number and size may eventually provide better discrimination of cardiovascular risk. Many investigators and clinicians use the estimate of non–HDL-C (total-C minus HDL-C) for assessment of risk and results of therapy because this method includes all of the cholesterol present in lipoprotein particles considered to be atherogenic [VLDL, IDL, LDL, Lp(a)] (Frost 98, Lu 03, Liu 05, Ridker 05, Liu 06). Others recommend additional measurement of total apoB or the apoB/apoA-I ratio as a reflection of the total number of atherogenic particles (Walldius 01, Grundy 02c, Sniderman 03, Ridker 05, Sniderman 06, Walldius 06a,b), but the proposal is not unanimous (Ingelsson 07).

The much larger but least dense chylomicrons of enterocyte/lymph origin (87% triacylglycerol, 9% phospholipids, 3% cholesterol, 1% apoB) are present in plasma in the postabsorptive period (Havel 01). Most chylomicrons are removed from circulating blood by adipose and hepatic capillary endothelial LPL. In the liver, chylomicron and large VLDL remnants pass through endothelial cell fenestrae to the space of Disse and hepatocyte microvilli where they bind initially to heparan sulfate proteoglycans (HSPG), HSPG-bound apoE, and HSPG-bound hepatic lipase, followed by transfer to the endocytic receptors LDL-R and LDL receptor-related protein (LRP1). Hepatic lipase hydrolysis of the remnant lipids increases exposure of the endocytic receptor-binding domain of apoE, which increases the affinity of the remnant particles for LRP1. Surface apoE is a high-affinity ligand to LDL-R and LRP1 (Havel 04). "The endocytic receptors migrate with their cargo to coated pits at the microvillar bases where they undergo endocytosis to form primary endosomes. . . . The extent to which proteoglycans, hepatic lipase, and surface apoE themselves undergo endocytosis with the remnant particles is unknown" (Havel 04).

Lipids, lipoproteins, and apolipoproteins are complexly involved in atherothrombotic diseases. As an example, alleles of apoE associated with elevated LDL are risk factors for CAD, but other alleles of apoE may have a cardioprotective effect (Curtiss 00, Song 04, Davignon 05). Hepatic apoB lipoproteins form a spectrum of particle densities, and a single large apoB-100 protein molecule is a permanent constituent of the phospholipid monolayer covering each spherical particle in the circulation (Sniderman 01). ApoB-100 is responsible for recognition and uptake of LDL by the LDL receptor. Oxidized LDL particles are taken up by scavenger receptors on vascular smooth muscle cells and macrophages; with excess cholesteryl esters, the latter transform into foam cells (Kwan 07).

Insulin deficiency or resistance results in hepatic overproduction of apoB and VLDL (Taskinen 03) and impaired LDL-R–mediated removal of LDL (Chait 79). Increased plasma levels of LDL result in increased transport into the intima and binding to proteoglycans, where a variety of atherogenic modifications occur (Skalen 02, Brunzell 08). LDL-C levels >70 mg/dL strongly predict CHD in type 2 diabetes (Turner 98, Howard 00), and "interventions that reduce LDL cholesterol are associated with stabilization and regression of atherosclerosis in proportion to the cholesterol lowering achieved" (Brunzell 08). However, many cardiometabolic-risk patients with near-normal LDL-C levels have an "atherogenic lipid triad" of high TGs, low HDL-C, and a preponderance of small, dense LDL particles (Nesto 05, Farmer 08) that have increased endothelial permeability, enhanced binding to proteoglycans, and easier oxidation/glycation (Brunzell 08). Insulin resistance without obesity results in elevated TG, total-C, LDL-C, apoB, and non–HDL as well as decreased HDL; abdominal obesity exacerbates elevated TG and low HDL-C (Knopp 03a, Nieves 03). Lp(a) is a particularly atherogenic LDL with apolipoprotein(a) bound to apoB-100 by a disulfide bond (Utermann 89, Tsimakis 05, Kollerits 06). Lp(a) levels independently predict future CHD in general populations (Bennet 08), but "there is little evidence that insulin resistance or diabetes influences Lp(a) concentrations" (Brunzell 08). Oxidized phospholipids in plasma are predominantly localized on Lp(a) (Edelstein 03, Tsimakis 05). Elevated apoC-III concentrations are associated with increased macrovascular disease risk, albuminuria, and retinopathy, and correlate with increased levels of TGs, total-C, LDL-C, apoA-I, and apoB in patients with type 1 diabetes (Klein 05).

As noted, increased plasma levels of LDL-C (>70–160 mg/dL) are predictive of increased CVD events in women with risk factors (Pridker 05) and provide increased substrate for atherogenic lipoprotein modification (oxidation, glycosylation, autoantibody-immune complex formation) in diabetes (Yla-Herttuala 89, Lopez-Virella 96, Turner 98, Orchard 99, Howard 00, Miranova 00, Virella 03, Lopez-Virella 07) and obesity (Knopp 06b, Weinbrenner 06). Small/dense LDL-C particles are more atherogenic than large, buoyant particles (Mcnuct 05). Aggregated LDL particles (Llorente-Cortes 02) and increased insulin (Misra 99) upregulate the LDL LRP1 in vascular smooth muscle cells, which mediates LDL internalization, and binds a wide variety of lipoprotein ligands (apoE-enriched VLDL, LPL-TG–rich lipoprotein complexes, lipoprotein(a); chylomicron remnants in macrophages) involved in foam cell formation (Fujioka 98, Llorente-Cortes 05).

Two forms of A_2 phospholipase that hydrolyze oxidized phospholipids to generate lysophospholipids and fatty acids may interlink LDL, atherogenesis, and inflammation (Kugiyama 99, Caslake 00). Type II secretory phospholipase A_2 is found in the media of normal and diseased arteries; by modifying LDL, it forms small, high-density particles (Sartipy 99). Lipoprotein-associated phospholipase A_2 (Lp-PLA2), also known as platelet-activating factor acetylhydrolase, circulates bound to LDL and is also a marker of small, dense LDL particles (Gazi 05). Its products seem to promote atherogenesis in that Lp-PLA2 activity is an independent predictor of CAD and ischemic stroke (Oei 05, Elkind 06, May 06, Wooton 06). Lp-PLA2–released lysophosphatidylcholine has proinflammatory properties (MacPhee 99). Research continues on the role of these enzymes in the complication of diabetes by atherosclerosis (Noto 06, Iwase 08).

The complex biosynthesis of HDL-C involves the synthesis and secretion of its major protein components (apoA-I in liver and intestine; apoA-II liver only); followed by the mostly extracellular acquisition of phospholipids and cholesterol via the ABCA1 pathway; further acquisition of lipids from peripheral tissue cells and TG-rich lipoproteins, and the assembly and generation of mature HDL particles with cholesteryl ester (CE) via LCAT (Rader 06). Catabolism of mature HDL-C is also affected by multiple processes: (1) remodeling to smaller particles and generation by hepatic and endothelial lipases of lipid-poor apoA-I that can be filtered through the glomerulus and degraded in renal tubular cells via the cubulin-megalin pathway; (2) direct selective hepatic uptake of HDL free cholesterol and HDL-CE by the scavenger receptor class BI (SR-BI) without mediating degradation of apo-lipoproteins; (3) back-transfer of HDL2 via cholesteryl ester transfer protein (CETP) to apoB-containing VLDL/LDL lipoproteins, which can then be taken up by the hepatocyte via the LDL receptor, with hydrolysis to free cholesterol and excretion directly into bile or by conversion to bile acids (Rader 06).

The antiatherogenic effectiveness of HDL-C is proportional to its size and density; larger and more buoyant particles with a greater concentration of apoA proteins on the particle surface are more cardio-protective. These HDL particles are thought to participate in reverse cholesterol transport, "removing free cholesterol from cells and atherosclerotic plaque and incorporating it into its structure" (Menuet 05). In vitro assays show that HDL may have anti-inflammatory, antioxidant and antithrombotic effects that could contribute to CVD protection (Barter 04, Mineo 06, Barter 07).

Gender Differences in Lipoprotein Metabolism in Women With and Without Obesity and Insulin Resistance

Estrogen increases the formation of hepatic lipoproteins and apoproteins, serving to provide lipid and apoB for the ovum, and enhanced lipid transport to the placenta (Knopp 06a). There is a greater adipose store and heightened FFA (NEFA) mobilization by peripheral lipolysis during fasting in women than men (Merimee 73, Jensen 95, Nielsen 03), resulting in greater delivery to the liver and oxidation of substrate FFA (Kushlan 81). These differences are enhanced with obesity, insulin resistance and diabetes (Masding 03). In the hepatocytes there is estrogen-driven increased FFA uptake and esterification to triacylglycerol (TG) and VLDL secretion. The net effect is a twofold greater rate of VLDL entry (phospholipids, triacylglycerols, free cholesterol, apolipoproteins B, C, and E) into the circulation in women compared with men (Mittendorfer 03, Knopp 06a).

Plasma levels of TG and VLDL cholesterol are not increased in women compared with men because the rates of VLDL transport and removal are greater in women than men, perhaps due to higher lipoprotein lipase activity in women (Maehira 90, Mittendorfer 03, Knopp 06a). However, plasma TGs are increased more with obesity and diabetes in women than men, and the clearance of TG is reduced in obesity and diabetes (Masding 03). TGs are stronger mediators of cardiovascular disease (CVD) risk in women than men (Hokanson 96, Knopp 06a, Sarwar 07). The main pathways of cholesterol traffic through the lipoprotein cascade in women are illustrated in Figure II.5 (Knopp 06a). Increased formation of LDL-C is expected from increased entry of VLDL-C and VLDL remnants (apoB and cholesterol) into the circulation in women (Knopp 06). Estrogen upregulation of the LDL receptor (Ma 86) and increased rate of LDL removal is the probable reason that LDL-C levels are not usually greater in women compared with men. LDL removal via binding of its ligand apoB to hepatic

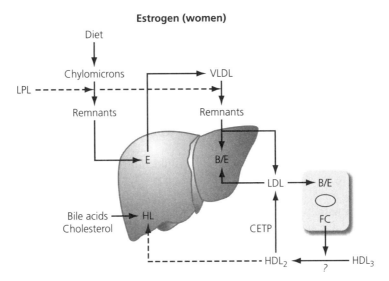

FIGURE II.5 Cholesterol traffic through the lipoprotein cascade in women. Solid arrows indicate increased traffic, and dashed arrows indicate less traffic compared with men.
B/E, apolipoproteins B and E; CETP, cholesterol ester transfer protein; FC, free cholesterol; HDL, high-density lipoprotein; HL, hepatic lipase; LDL, low-density lipoprotein; LPL, lipoprotein lipase; VLDL, very low-density lipoprotein. Adapted from Knopp 2006a and used with permission.

LDL receptors largely determines plasma levels of LDL. With hepatocyte depletion of cholesterol (as with decreased intake of saturated fat and cholesterol), SREBPs are activated, inducing synthesis of the LDL receptor. Concurrently, expression of the protease PCSK9 is turned on, providing a counterregulatory mechanism that degrades the hepatic LDL receptor to prevent excessive uptake of cholesterol (Cohen 06, Tall 06). Due to the greater rate of triacylglycerol production and equivalent impairment of VLDL or LDL removal caused by obesity and insulin resistance results in greater extent of abnormality in each lipid fraction in diabetic women than men (Walden 84).

Average HDL-C plasma levels are 55 mg/dL in healthy women compared with 45 mg/dL in men. The higher levels in women may be due to (1) estrogen stimulus to apoA-I synthesis in the liver; (2) estrogen-mediated generation of surface remnants from the twofold increased rate of VLDL metabolism (phospholipids, free cholesterol, apoC, apoE), which should lead to greater HDL_2-C formation; and (3) estrogen-mediated reduction in hepatic lipase activity and decreased TG removal from HDL with slower conversion to a smaller, more dense form (mixture of apoAI and apoAII; HDL_3) (Knopp 06). Women with lower concentrations of plasma HDL-C have an increased risk of future CVD events (Ridker 05), and low HDL is more predictive of CVD in women than in men (Knopp 06). As plasma TGs rise with insulin resistance and obesity, CETP facilitates the exchange of cholesterol ester in the HDL core lipoprotein for TGs, causing the HDL particle to become smaller (Murakami 95, Menuet 05). There is also a conformational change of apoA-I, with functional alteration of the HDL particles in type 2 diabetes (Kontush 08). Insulin resistance–increased CETP activity is linked to decreased activity of LPL and elevated activity of hepatic lipase, which further reduces the size of HDL by hydrolyzing phospholipids and TGs (Menuet 05). The smaller HDL particle is metabolized and cleared at an abnormally high rate, resulting in low HDL levels (Eckel 95).

Lipid Disorders Associated with Type 1 Diabetes

No characteristic lipid profile exists in type 1 diabetes, but individual nonpregnant women (n = 154; mean age 31 ± 10 years) may suffer from hypertriglyceridemia >200 mg/dL (>2.25 mM) (1.3%), hypercholesterolemia (15.6%), LDL-C >160 mg/dL (>4.1 mM) (16%), and low HDL-C <45 mg/dL (<1.1 mM) (20%). Improvement of glycemic control lowered the frequencies of dyslipidemia to be similar to those of nondiabetic control women (Perez 00). Optimization of glyccmic control with intensified insulin therapy for 3–6 months also reduced the proportion of small/dense LDL particles in women with type 1 diabetes (Caixas 97a), but not Lp(a) levels (Perez 98). As a group, type 1 diabetes patients may have increased cholesterol absorption but decreased hepatic synthesis of cholesterol compared with nondiabetic adults (Gylling 04, Miettinen 04). Prior to pregnancy, many young female patients with type 1 diabetes already have elevated LDL-C, Lp(a), and apoB as well as reduced HDL-C levels compared with controls (Willems 96, Attia 97, Gunczler 02, Adal 06, Gunczler 06, Kershnar 06, Rodriguez 06, Schwab 06). In 151 children in the U.K. with type 1 diabetes of 3 years' duration, total-C was elevated in 15.3% of the population and TG in 17.9%; both lipids were abnormal in 5.6%. Total-C, TG, and VLDL-C were significantly correlated to A1C (Abraha 99). Over the course of 6 months of treatment of type 1 diabetes in 104 patients aged 7–19 years in France, TG, LDL-C, and apoB varied in parallel with A1C, suggesting a tight association with the quality of glycemic control (Attia 97).

The prevalence of dyslipidemia was 28–51% in large cross-sectional surveys of type 1 diabetes subjects in Europe (Perez 00, Idzior-Walus 01) and the U.S. (Wadwa 05). In the observational prospective study of 589 young patients with type 1 diabetes who were followed for 10 years in Pittsburgh, TG >150 mg/dL (>1.7 mM), LDL-C >100 mg/dL (>2.6 mM), and HDL-C <55 mg/dL (<1.4 mM) had strong relationships (RR 1.8–12.1) with CHD (RR 0.4 for HDL-C), LEAD, and mortality (Orchard 01). At conclusion of the DCCT study of subjects with type 1 diabetes, levels of TG and LDL-C were reduced by intensive diabetes treatment (DCCT 95b). In addition, the conventional treatment group of type 1 diabetes subjects had significantly elevated Lp(a) and apoB compared with the intensive treatment group, as well as increased cholesterol in the atherogenic, denser LDL-C fractions (Purnell 95).

In the DCCT/EDIC follow-up study, differences between the groups in glycemic control and lipoproteins faded, but 23% of women had elevated LDL-C >130 mg/dL (>3.4 mM), 49% had high-risk levels of LDL particle concentrations measured by nuclear magnetic resonance spectroscopy, 16% had small/dense LDL particles, 12% had elevated apoB levels ≥110 mg/dL, and 33% had elevated Lp(a) levels ≥25 mg/dL (Jenkins 03a). Concurrent glycemic control measured by A1C independently correlated with conventional total TG, small VLDL subclass TG, small HDL-C subclass, LDL particle concentration, and apoB in 428 women (mean age 39 ± 7 years). The A1C threshold for abnormal lipoproteins seemed to be 8.0% (Jenkins 03a). Lipoprotein subclass measurements by proton nuclear magnetic resonance spectroscopy in three studies of type 1 diabetes cohorts revealed that small LDL particles were more common in women than in men (Colhoun 02b) and predicted CHD (Soedamah-Muthu 03) and carotid IMT (Lyons 06). Albuminuria in type 1 diabetes is associated with elevated TG, small/dense LDL, IDL, and apoB (Lahdenpera 94, Groop 96, Sibley 99, Jenkins 03b).

In other studies, renal dysfunction in type 1 diabetes is associated with increased Lp(a) (Jenkins 91, Jerums 93).

Lipid Disorders Associated with Type 2 Diabetes

Type 2 diabetes has atherogenic hyperlipidemia as a hallmark. It is designated as a CHD risk equivalent by the NHLBI (NCEP 01,02, Grundy 04), the AHA (Mosca 04), the ADA (ADA 04), and the American College of Physicians (Snow 04) because CHD risk is equivalent to nondiabetic adults with established CHD (10-year absolute CHD risk >20%). The RRs for CHD mortality with elevated lipid parameters were ~200% higher than that for individuals without diabetes in corresponding lipid levels in a pooled post-hoc analysis of four publicly available datasets containing 18,363 subjects without diabetes and 1,018 subjects with type 2 diabetes (Liu 05). Diabetic dyslipidemia is characterized by an elevated total TG level >150 mg/dL (>1.7 mM), elevated levels of TG-rich lipoproteins (VLDL-C, IDL-C), low levels of cardioprotective HDL-C <50 mg/dL (<1.25 mM) in women, smaller/denser particles of LDL (Goldberg 01, Blake 02, Vakkilainen 03), and, more controversially, increases in LDL-C >100 mg/dL (>2.6 mM) and non–HDL-C levels (total-C minus HDL-C) >130 mg/dL (Knopp 03b, Schulze 04, Liu 05, Legato 06). Inflammation and diabetes reduce HDL concentrations by a variety of mechanisms (Rohrer 04). The categorical cutoff point for non–HDL-C (>130 mg/dL) may be a stronger predictor than the estimated LDL-C cutoff point (>100 mg/dL) of risk for CHD death among patients with diabetes (Lehto 97, Grundy 02, Liu 05). In the Framingham Offspring Study, the proportion of diabetic women with markedly dyslipidemic values exceeded proportions in the control group: TG >250 mg/dL (>2.8 mM), 29% vs. 3%; total-C >240 mg/dL (>6.2 mM), 41% vs. 23%; LDL-C >160 mg/dL (>4.2 mM), 35% vs. 22%; and small/dense LDL particles, 40% vs. 11% (Siegel 96). Intensified glycemic control reduces TG, VLDL-C, and small/dense LDL and improves HDL-C levels in women with type 2 diabetes, but doesn't change Lp(a) (Caxias 97a,b).

Ethnic differences can be found in lipid levels in adult type 2 diabetes patients. Baseline levels of total-C were highest in white subjects, LDL-C was lowest in Asian-Indians, HDL-C was highest in Afro-Caribbeans, and TG was lowest in Afro-Caribbeans in the UKPDS (Davis 01). Insulin resistance, excess abdominal adiposity, hyperglycemia, and chronic elevations of FFAs contribute to the altered metabolism of TG, TG-rich lipoproteins, and small/dense LDL-C particles (Nieves 03, Boden 04, Krauss 04). Patients with both types of diabetes demonstrate an increased fractional escape rate of LDL-C from the intravascular compartment, especially if systolic hypertension or albuminuria is present (Jensen 05). Postprandial hypertriglyceridemia may also contribute to early atherosclerosis in type 2 diabetes (Teno 00). Dyslipidemia is already found in 30–60% of young people with type 2 diabetes (Ettinger 05, Kershnar 06).

All patients with type 1 or type 2 diabetes should have an annual fasting lipid profile that measures TC, HDL-C, LDL-C, and TG (ADA 08a); patients should be tested more frequently if lipid treatment is ongoing. Continuing research focuses on the role of atherogenic apoB lipoproteins of hepatic origin (Wagner 99, Sniderman 01,02, Taskinen 03, Wagner 03), the total-to-HDL cholesterol ratio in the CHD risk of diabetic dyslipidemia (Gimeno-Orna 04, Drexel 05, Holman 05, Wagner 05), and the possible role of the defective metabolism of oxidized phospholipids by HDL from people with type 2 diabetes (Boemi 01, Mastorikou 06). Albuminuria and nephropathy are associated with elevated Lp(a) (Song 05) and the hypertriglyceridemic/hyper-apoB phenotype (Tseng 05) in type 2 diabetes.

Clinical trial results support LDL-C as the primary target of therapy in diabetic dyslipidemia with a goal of <100 mg/dL (NCEP 01, ADA 04c, Grundy 04, Mosca 04) in patients with no other CVD risk factors, but <70 mg/dL if there is a history of smoking, hypertension, or premature CHD in first-degree relatives (Brunzell 08). There is evidence that using the more aggressive target is beneficial as long as it is part of the global treatment of cardiometabolic risks, especially hypertension (Gaede 08, Howard 08). When TG levels are ≥200 mg/dL, non–HDL-C becomes a secondary target (<130 mg/dL) of cholesterol-lowering therapy (NCEP 01, ADA 04c). The 2008 ADA/ACC consensus panel recommended targeting non–HDL-C <100 mg/dL and apoB <80 mg/dL in the highest-risk diabetic patients with at least one other major CVD risk factor in addition to dyslipoproteinemia (Brunzell 08). As part of case finding for individuals at risk for CHD, discovering elevated plasma TG and cholesterol as well as low HDL-C levels in diabetic pregnancy provides a rationale for aggressive attention to lipid and other cardiovascular risk factor prevention in the postpartum period and following years.

Physiological Lipid Changes in Normal Pregnancy

There are remarkable progressive hyperlipidemic changes in normal pregnancy (Knopp 82, Desoye 87, Herrera 88, Knopp 92a, Silliman 93, Iglesias 94, Alvarez 96, Knopp 97,98, Brizzi 99, Herrera 00, De Vriese 01, Herrera 04). Beyond the physiological changes, lipid profile abnormalities in pregnancy identify enhanced CVD risk during the pregnancy and beyond. Such a condition may be termed gestational lipemia (Montes 84), analogous to gestational diabetes. Both conditions are detected during gestation and both

TABLE II.16 Upper Limits of Normal for Plasma Total Triglyceride, Total Cholesterol, and LDL-C in Normal Pregnancy

| Gestational Week | Triglyceride | 90th Percentile | | 10th Percentile |
		Cholesterol	LDL-C	HDL-C
0	115	225	140	40
10	140	230	143	50
20	210	275	165	62
27	265	290	180	61
30	300	295	186	58
33	315	300	192	52
36	340	300	200	46
39	370	300	204	45

Data based on 90th-percentile values of triglyceride and cholesterol in 1,329 nonpregnant (0 week; 181 for LDL-C and HDL-C), nonhormone-using women aged 25–29 years from the Lipid Research Clinics Prevalence Study (Knopp 80). Data based on 90th-percentile values in 553 pregnant nondiabetic women at 36 weeks gestation (Knopp 82) with mean values of plasma lipoprotein levels measured serially at 10, 20, 27, 30, 33, 36, and 39 weeks gestation (N range 8–20) (Knopp 98). These data allowed a continuous plot of the 90th-percentile values to be drawn in Figure II.7 for triglyceride as well as total and LDL-C throughout gestation. The same approach is used for the 10th-percentile values of HDL-C.
Data based on Knopp 82.
HDL-C, high-density lipoprotein cholesterol; LDL-C, low-density lipoprotein cholesterol.

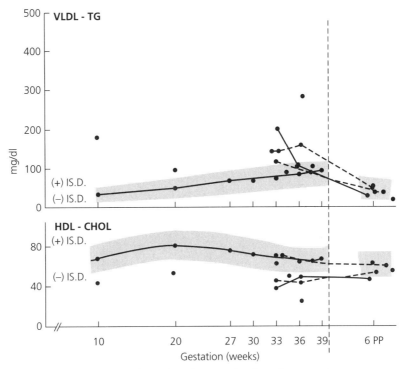

FIGURE II.6 Gestational lipemia: abnormal values in gestation return to normal postpartum. The shaded area is 1 ± SD from the mean for VLDL–TG and HDL-C in normal pregnancy. Three subjects with multiple measurements before and after delivery are shown by connected lines (dashed or solid). Individual data points are for single-subject observations of VLDL–TG and HDL-C. All subjects had type 2 diabetes.
Reproduced with permission from Knopp 80. HDL-C, high-density lipoprotein cholesterol; TG, triglyceride; VLDL, very low-density lipoprotein.

identify "prelipemia" or "pre-diabetes," respectively. It is usually inapparent postpartum, but is eventually overt in subsequent years (there is the expected congruence between both conditions in pregnancy (Butte 00), but many women with "gestational lipemia" have normal glucose tolerance). Table II.16 shows the change in the upper limits for TG, total-C, and LDL-C and the lower limits for HDL-C in normal pregnancy (Knopp 80, LRC 80, Knopp 82,98). Figure II.6 illustrates how elevated VLDL–TG and low HDL-C levels in gestation return to normal postpartum in such individuals (Knopp 80). Gestational lipemia may signify risk for subsequent development of overt dyslipidemia and premature CVD (Montes 84). Indeed, apparently healthy pregnancy is also characterized by progressive increases in apoA-I, apoB, apoC-III, apoE, and Lp(a) in some, but not all, studies (Mazurkiewicz 94, Alvarez 96, Winkler 00). Long-term research is needed to determine the actual postpartum predictive importance of gestational lipemia for CVD risk factors in women with diabetes.

Regarding cholesterol levels in normal pregnancy, total plasma levels increase 25–50% by term (Figure II.7) (Knopp 98); corresponding LDL-C levels increase by an average of 50% by term. There is some evidence for an accumulation of more buoyant LDL with advancing gestation (Silliman 94, Winkler 00). HDL$_2$ increases from the

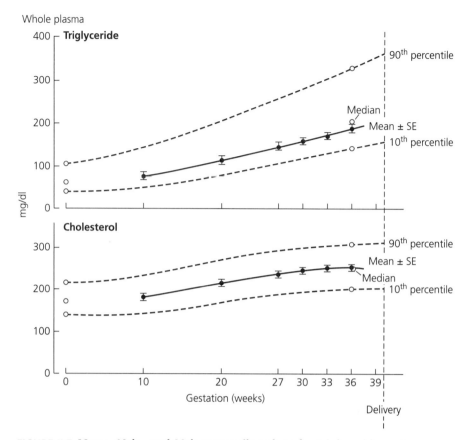

FIGURE II.7 Mean, 10th-, and 90th-percentile values for triglyceride and cholesterol in normal pregnancy.

nonpregnant average of 55 mg/dL to ~80 mg/dL as a maximum in midgestation; the smaller HDL_3 actually decreases in pregnancy (Alvarez 96). Thereafter, HDL-C declines somewhat until term, but not to nonpregnant levels (Figures II.6 and II.8) (Knopp 98). Mean and ± SD and percentile reference values for lipid and lipoprotein levels in pregnancy have been published (Knopp 82). Based on these data and measurements in nonpregnant individuals, the mean, 10th-, and 90th-percentile values for TG and cholesterol have been calculated and are shown in Figure II.7 (Knopp 98). Corresponding mean changes in VLDL, LDL, and HDL-C levels throughout gestation are depicted in Figure II-8 (Knopp 98).

Cholesterol is taken up by placental trophoblasts in the form of lipoproteins (Woolett 05) through receptor-mediated as well as receptor-independent transport, and there is a concentration-dependent efflux of cholesterol from the basolateral surface of the trophoblast (Wyne 98, Schmid 03). In the first half of pregnancy, fetal plasma cholesterol concentrations correlate strongly with maternal levels, but the relationship is lost in the last 3 months of pregnancy as fetal concentration declines. High non–HDL-C concentrations in the second trimester were independently associated with increased risk of fetal macrosomia in a population-based cohort study of 2,500 pregnancies (Clausen 05). Eight types of lipoprotein receptors are expressed in the

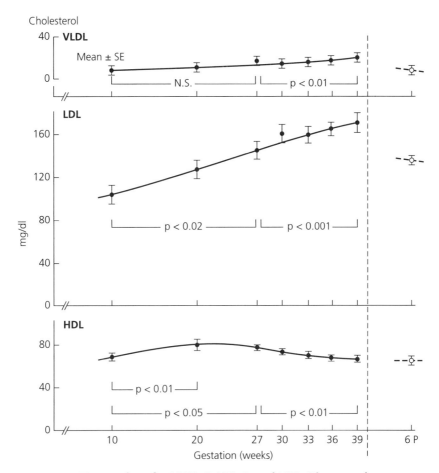

FIGURE II.8 Mean values for VLDL-C, LDL-C, and HDL-C in normal pregnancy. HDL-C, high-density lipoprotein cholesterol; LDL-C, low-density lipoprotein cholesterol; VLDL-C, very low-density lipoprotein cholesterol.

placenta or trophoblast (Woolett 05). Human term placental tissue expresses apoB and microsomal TG transfer protein (MTP), which are mandatory for assembly and secretion of apoB-containing lipoproteins, as in enterocytes and hepatocytes. ApoB-100 was recovered in particles of similar density to LDL by immunoprecipitation studies of the media around placental explants. The authors speculated that placental lipoprotein formation constitutes a novel pathway of lipid transfer from the mother to the developing fetus (Madsen 04). Human trophoblast cells also express phospholipid transfer protein (PLTP) with high activity, which normally has the important function of transferring phospholipids from VLDL to HDL, thereby leading to HDL generation and remodeling (Albers 95, Tall 00). LDLs suppressed the PLTP secretion in trophoblast cells through an LDL receptor–independent MAPK signaling pathway (Tu 04). The role of this placental system in pregnancies complicated by diabetes is unknown. The role of placental TG hydrolases (lipases) in the transfer of NEFAs to the fetus of diabetic mothers is reviewed in Part I in the section titled "Medical Nutrition Therapy" (Goldstein 85, Kuhn 90, Kaminsky 91, Merzouk 03, Magnusson 04b, Min 05).

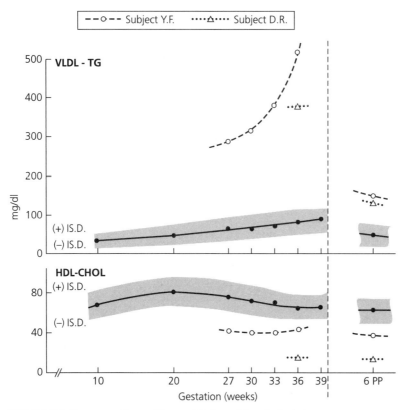

FIGURE II.9 Exaggeration of hypertriglyceridemia in late pregnancy.
Serial observations were made in two hypertriglyceridemic, nondiabetic
women in late gestation and postpartum compared with mean ± 1 SD
reference values for VLDL–TG and HDL-C. HDL-C, high-density lipoprotein
cholesterol; VLDL–TG, very low-density lipoprotein–triglyceride.

Maternal hypercholesterolemia (250–450 mg/dL) is associated with enhanced intimal accumulation of oxidized LDL and fatty streak formation in the fetal aorta (Napoli
97), which persisted in children aged 2–15 years (Napoli 99). Weight-adjusted abdominal aortic IMT is increased in macrosomic IDM and associated with increased cholesterol, VLDL, and TG concentrations in cord blood compared with macrosomic and
normal-weight controls (Akcakus 07, Koklu 07). We lack other data on the possible
contribution of maternal diabetes to the risk of early atherogenesis in the offspring.

Effects of Hypertriglyceridemia in Pregnancy
The physiological hyperlipidemia of normal pregnancy is associated with a two- to
fourfold TG increase by term (Figure II.7) (Herrera 88, Knopp 98). TG levels may
increase many times that amount in type 2 diabetic pregnancies or with prior
hypertriglyceridemia, so both pregnancy and diabetes will exaggerate this condition.
Figure II.9 illustrates this effect in two hypertriglyceridemic, nondiabetic women. The
result is a seriously increased risk for pancreatitis in hyperlipidemia-prone diabetic
pregnancy, especially in type 2 diabetes. Prevention of pancreatitis requires anticipatory
lipid screening and monitoring. TG levels >2,000 mg/dL are serious elevations

associated with acute pancreatitis, occurring typically in the third trimester with an incidence of 1 in 1,000 pregnancies (Nies 90). Because the TG level can rise rapidly from 1,000 to 2,000 mg/dL, treatment is initiated at the 1,000-mg/dL level. The same could occur in a type 1 diabetic pregnancy if the patient also has genetic hypertriglyceridemia.

Hypertriglyceridemia in pregnancy (>90th percentile for gestational age) is associated with a decrease in LDL particle size and the predominance of small/dense particles in many women (Silliman 94, Sattar 97, Hubel 98, Brizzi 99, Martin 99). Hypertri-glyceridemia is also a risk factor for the development of preeclampsia, which has enhanced oxidation of LDL as one of its components (Hubel 96). The hyperlipidemia phenotype of type 2 diabetes also involves a propensity to enhanced LDL oxidation, and enhanced oxidative stress may be an underlying element in the vasculopathy of preeclampsia. Elevated plasma TG levels predict increased BW with the same degree of statistical power as postprandial glucose levels in a setting of late second-trimester glycemic testing for gestational diabetes and, by extension, type 2 diabetes in pregnancy (Knopp 92b, Kitajima 01, Di Cianni 05). Placental TG concentrations and mRNA expression of endothelial lipase and hormone-sensitive lipase (but not placental lipoprotein lipase) were increased in type 1 diabetes, especially with suboptimal glycemic control. The authors thought the findings supported the possibility of enhanced maternal–fetal transport of FFAs (Lindegaard 06). We are not aware of studies of interventions to lower TGs in pregnancies of women with PDM beyond those of glycemic control.

Effects of Diabetes on Plasma Lipids in Pregnancy

Diabetic pregnancy may unmask a hyperlipidemia trait not yet apparent in the nonpregnant state (Knopp 86). A lipid profile in pregnancy aids the assessment of CVD risk in the individual diabetic gravida and prompts preventive cardiology measures in the postpartum period. Groups of women with type 1 diabetes in pregnancy are typically not dyslipidemic compared with similar populations of nondiabetic pregnant controls using conventional lipid profiles (Knopp 73,80,81, Hollingsworth 82, Montelongo 92, Pekelharing 95, Kilby 98, Toescu 04, Wender-Ozegowska 08). As an example of type 1 diabetes, a cohort of ~90 pregnant subjects with type 1 diabetes followed prospectively through pregnancy compared with a nondiabetic control group had identical plasma TG levels throughout gestation (Figure II.10) (Knopp 93). Plasma cholesterol levels were slightly lower in the pregnant diabetic group after 20 weeks gestation (Figure II.10) due to a lower HDL-C level (Figure II.11). HDL reduction was due to a decrease in the HDL_3-C subfraction, the smallest and densest of the HDL subfractions (Knopp 93). Consistent with this observation were reductions in the HDL apolipoproteins A-I and A-II, both present in HDL_3. In this study, the VLDL-C plus LDL-C levels (non–HDL-C) were identical to nondiabetic control levels throughout gestation (Figure II.9) (Knopp 93). It may be that the physiological hyperlipidemia of pregnancy obscures the degree of dyslipidemia seen in many young women with type 1 diabetes prior to pregnancy.

Other investigators found that women with poorly controlled type 1 diabetes in late pregnancy (mean A1C 8.9) had increased apoB-100 concentrations in maternal and umbilical cord blood, reduced apoA-I levels in HDL_3, and elevated TG levels in the maternal VLDL, HDL_2, and HDL_3 fractions compared with well-controlled diabetic women (mean A1C 6.1) and nondiabetic pregnant controls (mean A1C 5.8). LDL-C levels and LCAT activities were not significantly different in the three groups (Merzouk 00a). Macrosomic infants of poorly controlled diabetic mothers had higher lipoprotein profiles at birth (Merzouk 00b), as did nonmacrosomic IDMs in another

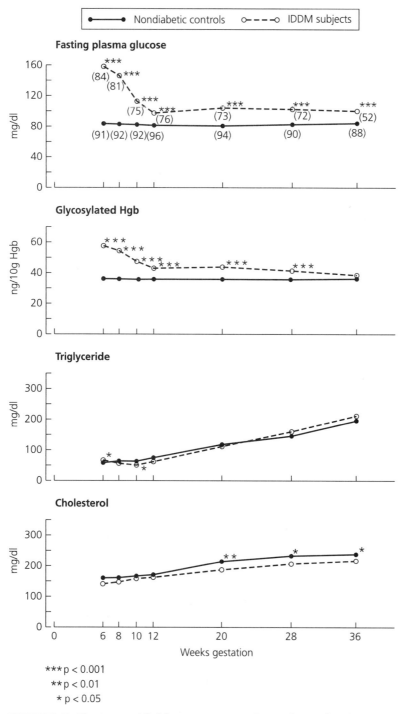

FIGURE II.10 Glucose and lipid measurements in a cohort of type 1 diabetes and normal pregnant subjects. Reproduced with permission from Knopp 93.

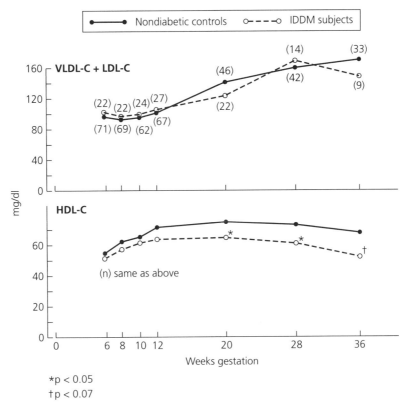

**FIGURE II.11 VLDL + LDL and HDL-C levels in type 1 diabetes and
normal pregnant subjects.** Reproduced with permission from Knopp 93.
HDL-C, high-density lipoprotein cholesterol; LDL, low-density lipoprotein;
VLDL, very low-density lipoprotein.

study (Kilby 98). Additional research is needed on the role of maternal–placental lipoproteins and apolipoproteins in fetal growth in diabetic pregnancies and on atherogenesis in placental and offspring blood vessels.

Regarding type 1 diabetic pregnant patients with proteinuria, there is a greater gestational rise in total-C and LDL-C and a decline in HDL-C compared with diabetic
pregnant women without proteinuria. Women with nephropathy had higher baseline
and progressive total TG elevations, but the percentage of increase during pregnancy
was equivalent in both groups (Biesenbach 94a).

The lipid profile of pregnant women with type 2 diabetes more closely resembles
the dyslipidemia of type 2 diabetes in nonpregnant people with elevated TG and
depressed HDL-C levels, as shown in Figure II.9 (Knopp 80, Hollingsworth 82). Such
patients are at risk for developing a severe exaggeration of hypertriglyceridemia in late
gestation, as illustrated in Figure II.6. As noted earlier, cases of hypertriglyceridemic
pancreatitis are reported in nondiabetic pregnant women (Lykkesfeldt 81), but are only
anecdotally known with type 2 diabetes and are reported in gestational diabetes
(Bar-David 96).

Assessment and Evaluation

What Lipids to Test? A standard overnight fasting lipid profile should generally be suffi-cient. The standard lipid profile consists of direct measurements of TG, cholesterol, and HDL-C as well as estimated LDL-C or calculation of non–HDL-C.

Specialized Lipid Testing. Should a question of enhanced cardiovascular risk exist during the pregnancy, additional information may be obtained from measurements of Lp(a) and apolipoproteins B and A-I.

- Lp(a) consists of a glycoprotein denoted as (a) that is attached to apolipoprotein B. Lp(a) enhances binding of LDL to the arterial wall and also inhibits throm-bolysis because the structure of (a) resembles plasminogen and inhibits its thrombolytic effect (Scanu 03). Lp(a) seems to be especially associated with enhanced cardiovascular and cerebrovascular risk in women (Foody 00). Values are not altered by pregnancy (Mazurkiewicz 94).

- ApoB is the main protein of VLDL and LDL and is responsible for the binding of LDL to its receptor. ApoB is useful in judging the atherosclerotic significance of combined hyperlipidemia when TG and cholesterol values are both elevated. Levels increase in gestation until week 33 in parallel with cholesterol (Desoye 87). ApoB may be more predictive of CVD than other lipid predictors (Walldius 01).

- ApoA-I is the major protein of HDL and can help explain why HDL-C levels are low in hypertriglyceridemic people. If apoA-I is normal, then the HDL-C should also be normal if the TG is reduced to normal. If the apoA-I level is low, then the HDL-C level will not likely improve regardless of any decrease in TGs, which is a higher risk condition. An average apoA-I level in late gestation is ~190 mg/dL (Desoye 87).

When to Test? The lipoprotein profile can be obtained at any time in gestation and com-pared with norms for total plasma TG and cholesterol, as shown in Table II.16 and Figures II.6 through II.8. To anticipate whether a primary hyperlipidemia exists and whether it may develop into a serious elevation as gestation proceeds, a lipid profile should be obtained as part of the initial clinical and laboratory evaluation. If a patient has had a recent lipid profile prior to pregnancy and is normal, initial testing may not be necessary. If hypertriglyceridemia is detected or known previously, a repeat fasting lipid profile should be obtained no later than the end of the second trimester, which is the time of greatest TG elevations in pregnant women with type 2 diabetes (Knopp 80). Subsequent testing depends on what is found and whether therapy is initiated. Refer to the following section on the management of dyslipidemias in PDM.

Management of Dyslipidemias in Pregnant Women with PDM

Medical Nutrition Therapy

Food plan. The main goal should be to follow the recommendations proposed for high risk-for-CHD patients in multiple guidelines (Haffner 98, Krauss 00, NCEP 02, ADA 04c, Mosca 04, Brunzell 08) to limit saturated fat to <7% of calories, limit cho-lesterol to <200 mg/day, and replace *trans* fatty acid–containing foods with MUFA or PUFA sources. This should minimize the influence of diet on the physiological rise of LDL-C in pregnancy. Relative amounts of carbohydrate and fat are not crucial to lipid regulation in pregnancy because the induction of hypertriglyceridemia with high carbohydrate intake is progressively blunted as gestation proceeds (Warth 77). Use of an antiatherogenic diet in normal pregnant controls was effective in reducing the rise in total-C and LDL-C during pregnancy without effect on maternal TG or apoB or on lipid levels in cord blood and neonates (Khoury 05). A very low cholesterol diet reduced elevated total-C levels during pregnancy by 20%, and an added cholesterol diet increased total-C by 19%, most of which was seen in the LDL-C fraction (McMurry 81). MNT is not well studied for dyslipidemias during pregnancies complicated by PDM.

Dietary supplements.   If the plasma TG level becomes >1,000 mg/dL, TG-lowering therapy should be initiated. Therapy should consist of fish oil supplementation and, if not fully effective or not tolerated, by the addition of MCTs. Restriction of fat calories to <10% of total calories and TPN have also been tested (Hsia 95). Intensified glycemic control is also an important element in the management of the hypertriglyceridemia of pregnancy.

Omega-3 fatty acids consisting of EPA and DHA together in fish oil can be administered at 3–9 g/day. A typical 1-g fish oil capsule contains between 30% and 70% of omega-3 fatty acids, with the more concentrated forms being more expensive but minimizing the number of capsules needed. A 90% EPA/DHA formulation is now available by prescription as Omacor at a maximum dosage of 4 g/day. Clinical experience indicates that plasma TG levels and the abdominal pain of recurrent pancreatitis can be reduced with fish oil even in late gestation when plasma TG levels otherwise rise to their highest levels in pregnancy (see Figure II.6). A potential side effect of omega-3 fatty acid supplementation in pregnancy is prolongation of labor due to the tocolytic effect of prostacyclins generated from omega-3 fatty acids.

Direct arterial wall and antiarrhythmic benefits of omega-3 fatty acids are attained at much lower doses of fish oil and are equivalent to two fatty fish meals per week or two 1-g fish oil capsules containing 30% omega-3 fatty acids. Contraindicated in pregnancy are raw fish, swordfish, tile fish, and large game fish. The TG-lowering effect of α-linolenic acid, an 18 carbon-long omega-3 fatty acid (18:3) found in walnuts and flaxseed oil, appears to be less effective than the omega-3 fatty acids of fish oil, EPA (20:5), and DHA (22:6), which may result from the poor conversion of 18:3 to 20:5 and 22:6.

Soy isoflavones in soy protein had a modest LDL-C–lowering effect in trials in nondiabetic, hypercholesterolemic subjects (Taku 07).

Medium-chain triglycerides.   MCTs are TG emulsions comprised of fatty acids of medium length that are typically 8 and 10 carbons long (caprylic and capric acids, respectively). MCTs are directly absorbed into the portal circulation and delivered directly to the liver; they do not enter the systemic circulation in the form of chylomicrons. MCTs provide an alternate source of calories to dietary long-chain fatty acids, which are absorbed in the form of chylomicrons. The advice of an RD is required to obtain the MCT and determine the amount and form in which it is given. MCTs are typically used in severely hypertriglyceridemic children who are intolerant to dietary fat, but they may be applied in pregnancy.

Physical activity.   Walking during the postprandial period decreased alimentary lipemia in healthy nonpregnant subjects (Hardman 95). During pregnancy, bouts of aerobic exercise temporarily raised plasma TG levels over 20 min postexertion (McMurray 88). Pregnant women with type 1 diabetes randomized to walk 20 min (1 mile) after each meal compared with no added exercise showed significantly lower fasting total-C and TG levels (Hollingsworth 87). Because walking is used to help control postprandial glucose excursions and weight gain during diabetic pregnancy, it is of interest to learn more about the probable interrelated effects of glycemia, insulin action, and exercise on lipids and apolipoproteins.

Lipid-Lowering Medications in Diabetic Pregnancy

Statins. Statins are contraindicated for use in pregnancy because they are teratogenic in animal models and are therefore labeled category X. As noted above, hypercholesterolemia can be lowered somewhat by dietary therapy in pregnancy. It is unknown whether long-term reduction of CHD in high-risk diabetic women will be materially altered by hypercholesterolemia over the duration of gestation. The only conceivable indication for statin treatment in pregnancy would be overt CHD in the last two trimesters, in which the mother experiences unstable angina or an acute MI, because statin treatment has been shown to have short-term benefit in such conditions (Pitt 99, Knopp 06b).

Fibric acids. Because severe hypertriglyceridemia is the most clinically important lipid elevation in pregnancy, treatment with medication focuses on this condition (i.e., plasma TG levels >1,000 mg/dL). Anecdotally, PPAR α-agonists of the fibric acid class, such as gemfibrozil, have been used in pregnant women with severe hypertriglyceridemia with clinical benefit in amelioration of hypertriglyceridemia and symptoms of pancreatitis. Drugs in this class work by enhancing the oxidation of fatty acids in the liver and peripheral tissues (Knopp 99, Kreisberg 03). Of the two fibric acid derivatives available in the U.S., gemfibrozil (Lopid) and fenofibrate (Tricor), the latter has the better record of not interacting with other drugs that are not used in pregnancy, notably the statin class. Fenofibrate and gemfibrozil are labeled as category C (unproved) for use in pregnancy. Clofibrate crosses the rat placenta and induces CYP-4504a in fetal tissues and intestinal peroxisomes (Laclide-Drouin 95, Simpson 96). Bezafibrate inhibited differentiation of human trophoblast cells in culture and reduced fatty acid-binding protein expression (Daoud 05). Fenofibrate use in pregnant rats exerted expected molecular effects in the maternal liver (induction of fatty acid and lipoprotein catabolism, reduction of TG-rich lipoprotein secretion), but was unable to reverse the typical hypertriglyceridemia of gestation (Soria 05) and increased fetal plasma and liver triacylglycerol and cholesterol concentrations (Soria 02).

Niacin. A conceivable alternative to the fibrate class is low-dose (1,000 or 1,500 mg) extended-release niacin (McKenney 04), which inhibits fatty acid mobilization from fat stores and leads to the lowering of TG and LDL-C and elevation of HDL-C. However, niacin is not as effective as the fibrate class in lowering TGs in severe hypertriglyceridemia. In comparison with gemfibrozil in patients with low HDL-C, extended-release niacin raised HDL-C by 26% vs. 13%, raised apoA-I by 11% vs. 4%, reduced Lp(a) by 20% vs. 0%, reduced TG by 29% vs. 40%, and had no adverse effect on LDL-C (no change vs. +9%) (Guyton 00). Extended-release niacin can be used once daily at bedtime, resulting in a lower rate of skin flushing and no additional rate of hepatoxicity compared with immediate-acting niacin, which is given three times daily (McKenney 04). Skin flushing may be minimized by using aspirin 325 mg prior to niacin (Pejic 06). No formal studies of niacin use in pregnancy have been conducted to our knowledge, although there are anecdotal reports. Use of standard niacin in diabetic pregnancy has been limited by the tendency of niacin products to raise plasma glucose (Goldberg 08), thereby requiring an increase in glucose-lowering treatment. However, two RCTs of extended-release niacin or crystalline nicotinic acid versus placebo in subjects with type 2 diabetes showed no significant change in A1C levels during 16–48 weeks of therapy, with the expected favorable lipoprotein changes (Elam 00, Grundy 02d). Nicotinic acid and extended-release niacin are listed as category C during pregnancy.

Bile acid–binding resins. The only nonabsorbed lipid-lowering agents are the bile acid–binding resins (category B). These are of limited effectiveness when used alone, yielding a 10–20% reduction in LDL. The best tolerated and effective agent of the class is colesevelam (Welchol), given as two or three 0.625-mg capsules b.i.d. with meals.

Inhibitors of cholesterol absorption. Ezetimibe is the only currently available drug in this class and may be useful; it has been found to lower LDL-C levels by an average of 18% and considerably more in some cases. It is listed as category C and has not been studied in pregnancy.

Plant sterols. These sterols, such as sitosterol and sitostanol, are found in nature and normally are minimally absorbed from the intestine. They inhibit dietary and biliary cholesterol absorption and can lower LDL-C by 10–15%. They are found in margarine products, such as Benecol and Take Control. However, no formal studies of plant sterols in pregnancy have been conducted to our knowledge.

Postpartum lipid assessment and management is discussed in Part IV in the section titled "Treating Dyslipidemias in the Postpartum Period."

Recommendations

- Measure fasting lipid profile at least annually in women with type 1 or type 2 diabetes and more often if needed to achieve goals. In women with low-risk lipid values (LDL-C <100 mg/dL, <2.6 mM; HDL-C >50 mg/dL, >1.25 mM; and TGs <150 mg/dL, <1.7 mM), lipid assessments may be repeated every 2 years. (E)
- For women with dyslipidemia and overt CVD, prior to conception, perform a risk/benefit assessment of global medical management and the expectations for pregnancy. (E)
- Prior to pregnancy, follow current guidelines for nutrition and pharmacotherapy along with exercise and weight control for diabetic women with dyslipidemia. The primary treatment goal is an LDL-C <100 mg/dL (2.6 mM) in women without overt CVD and an LDL-C <70 mg/dL (1.8 mM) in women with overt CVD, hypertension, smoking, or a family history of premature CHD. (A)
- The secondary treatment goal for women with diabetes is TG levels <150 mg/dL (1.7 mM) and HDL-C >50 mg/dL (1.3 mM). (C)
- Lifestyle modification focusing on the reduction of saturated fat (<7% of energy), *trans* fat (as little as possible), and cholesterol intake (<200 mg/day); weight control; and increased physical activity has been shown to improve the lipid profile in women with diabetes. (A). These treatment principles can be maintained during pregnancy, although the lipid profile will show a physiological change. (E)
- Statin therapy is contraindicated in any stage of gestation and should be discontinued in anticipation of pregnancy. (E)
- Obtain a standard lipid profile in all pregnant diabetic patients at registration if one has not been obtained prior to pregnancy. The purpose of the profile is risk

assessment; correlation with indexes of cardiovascular, renal, and thyroid disease; and education and preparation of patients with dyslipidemia for continuing lifestyle modification and later pharmacological treatment to sustain long-term health protection. (E)

- Measurement of apolipoproteins or lipoprotein subfractions to help with risk assessment or guide therapy may best be done before or after pregnancy because evidence-based guidelines cannot be established for their use in pregnancy. (E)

- Sequential measurements of the TG level during pregnancy are important in patients with hypertriglyceridemia. (E)

- Cholesterol-lowering drugs are unapproved for use in pregnancy except for bile acid–binding resins. MNT may be helpful in reducing hypercholesterolemia in pregnancy. Plant sterol–containing margarines could be useful as a dietary approach for cholesterol lowering. (E)

- For diabetic pregnant women with TG levels ≥1,000 mg/dL, treatment is indicated to reduce the risk of pancreatitis. Add fish oil capsules to attain omega-3 fatty intakes of 3–9 g/day. (B) Secondary strategies include a low-fat diet, MCTs, TPN, fibric acids, and niacin. (E)

DIABETIC NEPHROPATHY AND PREGNANCY

—— Original contribution by John L. Kitzmiller MD, MS and Martin N. Montoro MD

Characteristics of Diabetic Nephropathy

DN usually occurs in stages (Mogensen 88) and is characterized by early renal hypertrophy and hyperfiltration, progressive albuminuria, tubulointerstitial disease, and eventual decline in glomerular filtration to glomerulosclerosis and end-stage renal disease (ESRD), when renal replacement therapy becomes necessary (Tsalamandris 94, Gall 97, Ritz 99, ADA 04d, Thomson 04, Amin 05, Gross 05, Remuzzi 06, Zerbini 06). GFR may decline in the absence of albuminuria in a minority of cases (Caramori 03, Kramer 03). Stages of albuminuria as well as GFR levels in DN and chronic kidney disease (CKD) are listed in Table II.17. Criteria are supported by the National Kidney Foundation, the ADA, and the AHA (NKF 02, Eknoyan 03, Levey 03, Sarnak 03, ADA 04d, Levey 05, Vassalotti 07). In the absence of interventions, microalbuminuria may increase by 10–20% per year and progress to macroalbuminuria (overt DN) over 10–15 years (Viberti 82, Mogensen 84, Warram 96, Rossing 02a, Adler 03, Giorgino 04). Microalbuminuria is also a marker for increased risk of CVD (deZeeuw 06, Zandbergen 07, Cirillo 08). Microalbuminuria may regress in the setting of improved glucose, BP, and lipid levels (Perkins 03, Giorgino 04, Araki 05). Progression of microalbuminuria is associated with early decline of GFR, elevated A1C, central obesity, and excretion of markers of inflammation from the kidneys (Hovind 04, Amin 05, deBoer 07, Perkins 07, Wolkow 08). Hypertension (Krolewski 88, Norgaard 90, Sowers 01, Thomas 01, Lurbe 02), anemia (Bosman 02, Thomas 97, McFarlane 06), dyslipidemia (Biesenbach 94a, Jenkins 03, Knopp 03, Kwan 07), and increased risk for CVD (Fuller 01, Gerstein 01, Sarnak 03, Zandbergen 06, Kim 07, Lajer 08) are other important characteristics of DN (Whaley-Connell 08). Familial clustering of DN suggests the importance of genetic susceptibilities and possible perinatal transmission of risk factors

TABLE II.17 Stages of the Evolution of Diabetic Nephropathy and Common Effects on Pregnancy

Stages	GFR	Albuminuria	Pregnancy Effect
Hyperfiltration	≥150	<30 mg/day	Unknown
Microalbuminuria	≥90	30–299 mg/day	Increased preeclampsia
Macroalbuminuria	≥90	≥300 mg/day	Increased preeclampsia
Early nephropathy	60–89	TPE ≥500 mg/day	Increased fetal growth restriction
Moderate CKD	30–59	Massive proteinuria	Poor perinatal outcome
Severe CKD	15–29	Less proteinuria	Delay pregnancy to post transplant
Kidney failure	<15		Dialysis

There may be overlap between groupings. Some patients with hyperfiltration may already have albuminuria. Some patients with early diabetic nephropathy may not yet have albuminuria, and some with proteinuria may have estimated GFR >90 mL/min/m³.

Table modified from Mogensen 88, NKF 02, Eknoyan 03, Levey 03, and Sarnak-American Heart Association 03.

CKD, chronic kidney disease; GFR, glomerular filtration rate, quantified as mL/min/m², or estimated from adjusted serum creatinine or cystatin C in non-pregnant subjects or by creatinine clearance during pregnancy; TPE, urinary total protein excretion.

(Quinn 96, Rudberg 98, Canani 99, Harjutsalo 04), but the major genes are yet to be identified despite much investigation.

Multiple interventions have been shown to prevent the development and to slow or arrest the progression of nephropathy, with the most important being intensified glycemic control (DCCT 95c, UKPDS 98a, Shichiri 00) and reduction of BP (UKPDS 98b, Bakris 00,03b, Whaley-Connell 05, ADA 08a) as well as albuminuria/proteinuria (Keane 03a, DeZeeuw 04, Araki 07, Eijkelkamp 07, Bakris 08). Prior intensive treatment of type 1 diabetes in the DCCT had a sustained effect on reducing new cases of microalbuminuria by 59% and macroalbuminuria by 84% over the 7–8 years after conclusion of the trial (DCCT/EDIC 03). Waist circumference was an additional predictor of development of albuminuria (deBoer 07). During this follow-up, the decline rate in 4–h CrCl was 0.34 mL/min/m² (deBoer 07). Significantly fewer participants in the original intensive treatment group reached a serum creatinine (sCr) level ≥2 mg/dL (0.7% vs. 2.8%; p = 0.04), and development of hypertension was also less frequent (30% vs. 40%; p < 0.001) (DCCT/EDIC 03). Regarding BP control, some antihypertensive agents (such as ACE inhibitors [Lewis 93, Laffel 95], ARBs [Brenner 01, Lewis 01, Parving 01a, Herman 03], nondihydropyridine CCBs [Bakris 00], and the β-blocker carvedilol [Bakris 05, Hart 07]) seem to have specific renoprotective activity in addition to BP control, perhaps due to their antioxidant or anti-inflammatory properties.

Although the prevalence of overt DN has been 20–35% after 20 years of type 1 diabetes (Krolewski 96, Tryggvason 05, Pambianco 06), the incidence has diminished in recent years in settings with intensified multifactorial care (Gaede 99, Hovind 03, Nordwall 04). The prevalence of ESRD has declined to 1–5% (Keane 03b, Nishimura 03, Finne 05), and the survival rate of DN has increased (Hovind 04, Astrup 05, Rossing 05). Patients and clinicians should be educated that primary and secondary prevention efforts are effective. In 33 patients with ESRD due to DN in a Swedish database of 4,414 individuals with onset of type 1 diabetes at 0–14 years of age, age of onset of renal failure was 25–36 years with duration of diabetes 15–23 years (Svensson 06).

Fewer data exist on the prevalence of stages of DN in women of reproductive age with type 2 diabetes. In a 6–12-year follow-up of 43 patients with type 2 diabetes onset at age 15–34 years in Sweden, 23% developed micro/macroalbuminuria compared with 5.6% in 426 patients with type 1 diabetes (Svensson 03). Among subjects aged 25–65 years with new-onset type 2 diabetes recruited to the UKPDS, 23% had developed microalbuminuria by the 10-year follow-up and 7% had macroalbuminuria; estimated CrCl was reduced in 24%. In multivariate models, plasma TGs, LDL-C, A1C, systolic BP, and waist circumference were independently associated with progression to macroalbuminuria; female sex was a risk factor for reduced CrCl (Retnakaran 06). In Japan, the incidence of overt nephropathy after a mean follow-up of 6.8 years was 14% in patients with type 2 diabetes onset prior to age 30 (Yokoyama 98). Among minority patients with youth-onset type 2 diabetes, microalbuminuria was present in 40% in New York (Ettinger 05) and 44% in New Zealand (Scott 06). The frequency of overt DN was 20% in youth-onset type 2 diabetes after 25 years of diabetes in Pima Indians (Krakoff 03), and the incidence rate of ESRD was five times higher with youth-onset compared with adult-onset type 2 diabetes (Pavkov 06).

The development of DN in female adolescents with type 1 diabetes has been widely investigated; it is of interest because many of these patients will eventually become pregnant. Glycemic control and nighttime BP affected glomerular indexes on renal biopsies repeated after 6 years in normotensive and normoalbuminuric patients (Perrin 04). Recent cross-sectional analyses revealed a prevalence of microalbuminuria of 5–10% in 1992–1998 (Holl 99c, Olsen 00, Rihimaa 00) and 3% in 2001 (Mohsin 05). The probability of microalbuminuria was strongly related to A1C (Rudberg 93, Olsen 00, Rihimaa 00). The 6-year incidence of microalbuminuria was 4.6% and macro-albuminuria was 0.6% in a large longitudinal study in Australia (Stone 06). In multivariate analysis, factors associated with persistent microalbuminuria in this population include duration of diabetes >10 years, A1C, obesity, cholesterol >200 mg/dL (>5.2 mM), and BP >95th percentile (Stone 06). Elevated albumin excretion ($\geq$30 mg/gm creat) was more common in youth with type 2 diabetes compared with type 1 diabetes (prevalence 22.2% vs. 9.2%; p < 0.0001) in a multicenter observational study. Female sex, A1C, hypertension, and TG levels were independently associated with albumin excretion, even when controlling for obesity (Maahs 07).

Assessment of Renal Function and Albuminuria Before Pregnancy

Evaluation of renal function and albuminuria (Kramer 05, Kong 06) is essential before or early in pregnancy in all women with type 1 or type 2 diabetes. Current guidelines recommend annual evaluation of estimated GFR in all adults with diabetes because decreased GFR is found in a proportion of patients without increased albumin excretion (ADA 08a). Standard reference methods (clearance of inulin, p-aminohippurate, ^{51}Cr-EDTA, iohexol and ^{125}I-iothalamate) to measure GFR are difficult to use clinically. To avoid possible errors in cumbersome 24-h urine collections in ambulatory patients, GFR has been estimated by calculations based on inverse sCr and more popularly with sCr adjusted for age, gender, race, body weight, mass, and surface area (Cockcroft–Gault formula, MDRD equation) (Gault 92, Perrone 92, Sampson 92, Levey 99, Hallan 04, Levey 07). Controversy surrounds the determination of which formula is best in women of different ages, body mass, diet, and degree of renal function (Lewis 04, Rule 04, Ibrahim 05, Rigalleau 05, Stevens 06).

The difficulties are partially due to problems with inter- and intralaboratory calibration of sCr measurement (Coresh 02, Miller 05, Murthy 05, Myers 06, Stevens 07a). With obesity, no formula is reliable (Verhave 05), and if GFR is >80 mL/min, calculated estimations based on sCr can be 30–50 units above or below the true GFR (Sampson 92, Froissart 05, Ibrahim 05, Rossing 06, Stevens 07b). In type 2 diabetes patients with overt DN who were followed for 6 years, both equations underestimated the decline in GFR measured by ^{51}Cr-EDTA (Rossing 06). Even in hospitalized patients with a GFR <40 mL/min/1.73m^2, estimation equations were not reliable measures of the actual level of renal function (Poggio 05).

Cystatin C is a cationic, nonglycosylated, low-molecular-weight cysteine proteinase that is produced by all nucleated cells at a stable rate, freely filtered by glomeruli, and completely degraded in the tubular cells (Grubb 00, Tan 02). The concentration of serum cystatin C inversely reflects GFR more closely than estimators based on sCr in most studies of nonpregnant subjects (Bostom 00, Dharnidharka 02, Strevens 02, Fricker 03, Knight 04, Rule 06, Stevens 08). Measurement of serum cystatin C is a good reciprocal indicator of GFR in diabetes and is useful in sequential analysis of patients with normal or elevated GFR (Mussap 02, Tan 02, Perkins 05a,b, MacIsaac 06, Perkins 07). A serum cystatin C level cutoff of >1.10 mg/L (>82.1 nM) had better screening characteristics than sCr-based methods for moderate CKD (reference GFR <60 mL/min/1.73 m^2) in diabetic subjects, but the tests had similar characteristics with GFR 60–89 mL/min/1.73 m^2) (MacIsacc 07). Controversy surrounds whether cystatin C is affected by skeletal body mass (Vinge 99, Finney 00, Macdonald 06), but most investigators think that it is not (Stevens 08).

Assessment of albuminuria is another essential feature of evaluation of diabetic women prior to conception (ADA 04d,08a) and during early pregnancy (ACOG 05). The pathogenesis of albuminuria in diabetes is unresolved (Russo 02). Uncertainty exists concerning the relative contributions of the glomerular endothelial fenestrations (D'Amico 03, Singh 07), glomerular shunt pores with macroalbuminuria (Andersen 00, Oberbauer 01, Harvey 07), podocyte foot process/slit diaphragm injury (Wolf 05, Kalluri 06), and impaired receptor-mediated tubular reabsorption (Brunskill 01, Russo 02, Gekle 05, Birn 06). A sequential study of size selectivity of the glomerulus in patients with type 2 diabetes showed no difference in pore or shunt size in patients with microalbuminuria compared with normoalbuminuric patients, but did confirm that patients developing macroalbuminuria (>2,000 mg/gm Cr) had an excess number of large pores that served as a macromolecular "shunt" and correlated with the extent of podocyte foot process broadening (Lemley 00). Podocyte foot processes in microalbuminuric patients were no different than those found in controls. The authors concluded that microalbuminuria must be a result of changes in glomerular charge selectivity and/or tubular handling of filtered proteins (Lemley 00). Current studies on the mechanisms of albuminuria in diabetic and other people have not been applied to pregnant women with PDM.

Due to the postural/diurnal and activity- and diet-induced variance in albumin excretion (greater in daytime) (Eshoj 87, Tomaselli 89, Stehouwer 90, Wiegmann 90, Mogensen 95a), measurement of albumin in well-collected 24-h urine samples has been the standard for most studies of albuminuria. Compared with assessments of albumin concentration or ratio to creatinine (uACR) in random or first-morning urine samples (Warram 98, NKF 02) or of dipstick measurements of albumin in urine samples (Higby 95, Waugh 05), 24-h collections provide more complete information. However, due to the ease of collecting random urine samples and the presumed difficulty of 24-h collections, current guidelines suggest the use of uACR as a screening test for albuminuria in most patients (Bakris 00, Levey 03, ADA 04d,08a). Optimal sensitivity for a screening test should be >95% (Sacks 02). When used in female non-pregnant diabetic patients, sensitivity of the ACR at >22, 25, 31, and 33 mg/gm (>2.5, 2.8, 3.5, 3.7 g/mol) to identify UAE at >30 mg/day was 93%, 93.5%, 96.1%, and 97.4%, respectively, with PPVs of 81.3%, 77.3%, 68.9%, and 81% (Bakker 99, Houlihan 02, Lepore 02, Incerti 05). The 95th percentile for random ACR in a normal female population was 25 mg/gm (Warram 96). In one large study, the intraindividual coefficient of variation for urinary creatinine measurement was 34.8% in random urine samples and 11% in 24-h collections (Incerti 05). Due to the false positive rates (low PPV) in the abovementioned studies, a positive screening test may be confirmed with a timed urine collection (Lepore 02, Incerti 05).

"Because of variability in urinary albumin excretion, two of three specimens collected within a 3- to 6-month period should be abnormal before considering a patient to have crossed a diagnostic threshold. Exercise within 24 hours, infection, fever, congestive heart failure, marked hyperglycemia and marked hypertension may elevate urinary albumin excretion over baseline values" (ADA 08a). Measurement of a spot urine sample for albumin only, whether by immunoassay or a dipstick method specific for albumin, is susceptible to false-negative and false-positive determinations as a result of variation in urine concentration due to dehydration and other factors (ADA 08a). Current definitions of clinical albuminuria or proteinuria in nonpregnant women are ≥300 mg/day urine albumin excretion (UAE); >199 μg/min AER; and ≥500 mg/day total protein excretion (TPE) (Eknoyan 03, Levey 03, ADA 04d, Gross 05). The National Kidney Foundation (NKF 02) and the Global Kidney Initiative (Levy 05) accept measurements of albuminuria ≥30 mcg/mg Cr in two of three spot urine samples as an indicator of kidney damage, and the ADA defines microalbuminuria as 30–299 mcg/mg Cr and macroalbuminuria as ≥300 mcg/mg Cr (ADA 08a).

In Europe and elsewhere, an upper normal limit of 42 μcg/mg (3.5 mg/mmol) is proposed to define microalbuminuria in females due to lower muscle mass and uCr excretion (Mogensen 95b, Mortensen 04, Warram 04). If microalbuminuria is suspected on the basis of a random urine ACR screening test, it may be quantified with timed urine collections so that more accurate assessment can be used to monitor its course and the effects of treatment. Persistent microalbuminuria is an early, reversable stage of DN in type 1 diabetes (Giorgino 04, Araki 05, Perkins 07) and is a marker for development of nephropathy or macrovascular disease in type 2 diabetes (ADA 08a). Microalbuminuria may return to normal "spontaneously" (Steinke 05) and certainly can with intensified glycemic control (DCCT 95,02,03) and antihypertensive or reno-protective therapy (Bakris 00, Parving 01b, ADA 04d). In both type 1 and type 2 diabetes (as in essential hypertension in nonpregnant patients without diabetes), microalbuminuria is also linked to vascular dysfunction and increased CVD risk (Deckert 89, Jensen 00, Gerstein 01, Stehouwer 02, Liu 03, Ritz 03, Cirillo 04, Leitao 05, Strain 05, Kim 07, Lajer 08).

Macroalbuminuria (≤300 mg/24 h; ≤200 mcg/min; ≤300 mcg/mg Cr) or TPE ≤500 mg/24 h associated with dipstick positive proteinuria indicates clinical or overt DN in the absence of other causes of albuminuria/proteinuria (ADA 04d). Proteinuria is more than a marker of DN, for an increasing degree of proteinuria contributes to the tubulo-interstitial pathology of advancing CKD (Remuzzi 99, Walls 01, Eddy 04, Abbate 06), and treatment to reduce proteinuria may be beneficial (Wilmer 99, Hovind 01, de Zeeuw 04, Hovind 04).

Assessment of Renal Function and Albuminuria During Pregnancy

Comparison of estimated GFR by the MDRD equation (sCr adjusted for age, gender, and race) with measured insulin clearance demonstrated that eGFR significantly underestimated true GFR in early and late normal gestation and also in pregnancies complicated by preeclampsia or CKD (Smith 08). The lower sCr levels observed in pregnancy reflect hemodilution due to increased plasma volume as well as hyperfiltration. Thus, the association between sCr and renal function during pregnancy is weakened, and the use of the MDRD equation in pregnant women with renal complications is not recommended (Smith 08). Calculated GFR based on sCr and prepregnancy weight has been compared with creatinine clearance (CrCl) during pregnancy. At CrCl >80 mL/min, the Cockcroft–Gault formula overestimated CrCl in pregnant women with proteinuria, with an *r* value of 0.83 for 26 women in the first trimester (Quadri 94). CrCl calibrated for body size as an estimate of GFR and tubular secretion can be quantified with a well-instructed 24-h urine collection, which is also useful to assess the degree of albuminuria. Autoanalyzers measuring sCr concentration tend to overestimate sCr by 20–30% due to "noncreatinine chromogens" that are not found in urine, but some balance of error is achieved with CrCl in healthy adults because of tubular secretion of urinary creatinine (uCr) of $\sim$12 $\pm$ 10% (Lemann 90, Coresh 02). The tubular secretion and extrarenal clearance of creatinine increase with a decline in renal function (Levey 89, Rossing 06). The major problem with use of CrCl is incomplete timed urine collections.

Cystatin C as an inverse indicator of GFR is inadequately evaluated during pregnancy, with conflicting results (Cataldi 99, Strevens 02,03, Moodley 04, Akbari 05, Babay 05). It is problematic that serum cystatin C is higher during pregnancy than after pregnancy, but GFR is known to be higher during pregnancy. Cystatin C did not increase until the third trimester in a large prospective study with sequential measurements in uncomplicated singleton pregnancies (Kristensen 07a). Maternal levels are increased with preeclampsia (Strevens 03, Kristensen 07b, Franceschini 08). The fetal, placental, and decidual tissue contribution to serum cystatin C is unclear (Kristensen 07c, Malamitsi-Puchner 07, Song 07). We lack careful studies of all of these techniques compared with reference methods of measuring GFR in large numbers of pregnancies complicated by diabetes (Sims 61, Krutzen 92, Olafsson 96).

Proteinuria increases substantially during normal pregnancy up to 300 mg/day (Cheung 89, Higby 94, Roberts 96), perhaps due to increased renal blood flow and decreased tubular absorption or increased tubular secretion of proteins (Pedersen 81, Bernard 92, Cavallone 92). UAE shows a more modest increase up to 30 mg/day (Pedersen 81, Lopez-Espinoza 86, Wright 87, Misiani 91, Bernard 92, Higby 94, Taylor 97) or a random urine sample albumin-to-creatinine ratio (uACR) up to 22 μg/mg (22 mg/gm) (Konstantin-Hansen 92, Waugh 03b). Assessment of albuminuria during normal pregnancy shows that timed overnight collections produce much less albuminuria than during the daytime (Douma 95). A simple method to increase the accuracy of a positive uACR screening test is to test a second sample after 2–3 months; if the results are discordant, conduct a third test to distinguish persistent from transient elevations of UAE (Warram 98). However, this method is not practical in the compressed time frame of pregnancy. uACR showed good correlation with 24-h urine albumin measurements <10 mg/day in early pregnancy (Pearson correlation test *r* = 0.964) in 43 women without later hypertension (Risberg 04). Random urine ACR values of 238 mg/gm (27 mg/mmol) had the following predictive values for detecting albuminuria

>300 mg/day in 54 hypertensive pregnant women: sensitivity 95%, specificity 100%, PPV 100%, NPV 86% (Nisell 06). However, another study from Sweden found poor correlation between random urine ACR and 24-h albuminuria in 31 women with preeclampsia (Wikstrom 06). Random urine ACR >2.0–8.0 mg/mmol predicted 24-h proteinuria with only fair accuracy in two small studies (Waugh 05a, Kyle 08). Random spot urine albumin concentrations also showed a weak association with 24-h proteinuria in women with preeclampsia (Kieler 03).

The criterion for urinary TPE as a marker for preeclampsia in pregnancy has long been set at >300 mg/day (ACOG 02, Roberts 03), but there are no widely accepted criteria for UAE to define preeclampsia. Diagnostic limits for proteinuria in urine collections are influenced by the method of laboratory assay (Waugh 05b). Screening for proteinuria during pregnancy by a urinary dipstick protein test is a poor predictor of absent or severe proteinuria (Kuo 92, Lindow 92, Meyer 94). The urine total protein/creatinine ratio (PCR) as a predictor of TPE in pregnancies with preeclampsia was somewhat better in some but not all studies, with excessive variance in successive hourly to 8-hourly samples in preeclamptic women (Chesley 39, Lindow 92, Quadri 94, Young 96, Robert 97, Saudan 97, Ramos 99, Rodriguez-Thompson 01, Neithardt 02, Durnwald 03, Gonsales-Valerio 05, Schubert 06). The urine PCR is inadequately studied at the low end of the proteinuria spectrum. A Cochrane analysis of nine studies of the spot urine PCR discussed the predictive power of cutoff points of 0.15–0.50 mg/mg (17–57 mg/mmol) for 24-h TPE >300 mg/day. The authors recalculated a cutoff of 265 gm/gm (30 mg/mmol) and reported sensitivity of 84%, specificity of 76%, positive likelihood ratio of 3.53 (95% CI 2.83–4.49), and negative likelihood ratio of 0.21 (95% CI 0.13-0.31) using pooled data from 1,003 women. They concluded that the spot PCR is a reasonable "rule-out" test for proteinuria in hypertensive pregnancies (Cote 08). However, use of random PCR for screening in diabetic pregnant women would not detect microalbuminuria (Combs 91, Rodby 95). The 24-h urine collection remains the standard for quantifying proteinuria in women with preeclampsia, overt DN, or other nephropathies with dipstick positive urinalysis, and it can also be used for CrCl to estimate the GFR.

Microalbuminuria During Diabetic Pregnancy

Normotensive diabetic women with uncomplicated pregnancies may or may not have larger increases in TPE and UAE than controls by the second half of gestation (Biesenbach 89, McCance 89, Combs 91,93, Biesenbach 94b, MacRury 95, Ekbom 00, Schroeder 00). For diabetic pregnant women, there is a single study of ACR in repetitive random urine samples compared with 24-h UAE in 110 women without macroalbuminuria. The sensitivity of ACR ≥22 mg/g (≥2.5 g/mol) to predict UAE at 30–299 mg/day (7 cases) was 85.7%, with both a specificity and a PPV of 100% in this small study (Justesen 06). The sensitivity was lower if the upper limit of normal ACR was assigned to be 31 mg/g (3.5 g/mol). The authors agreed that repetitive measurements are needed because the day-to-day coefficient of variation was 40% for 24-h urine collections and 49% for random urine samples (Justesen 06). Confirming studies are needed on the precision of urinary ACR to predict albuminuria in larger numbers of diabetic pregnant women. If repeated screening tests are positive, albuminuria should be quantified by 24-h collection. It is important to note that filtered albumin is excreted as a complex mixture of modified albumin products (immunoreactive and unreactive total albumin, albumin complexed with fatty acids, lysosomal protease-modified albumin fragments) that are not completely detected by current radioimmunoassays for urinary albumin in the UAE 30–299-mg/day range in diabetic subjects

(Curry 98, Osicka 00, Comper 03). These analyses have not been applied to urine samples of diabetic pregnant women.

The prevalence of microalbuminuria during pregnancy in diabetic women is poorly characterized. Two prospective studies serving large regions of Denmark yielded frequencies of 11% and 12% for microalbuminuria in a total of 391 pregnant women with type 1 diabetes (Ekbom 01, Lauszuz 02) compared with 14.3% in 56 patients in Germany (Schroder 00). Another study in Denmark counted 8 cases (13%) of baseline microalbuminuria in 61 pregnant women with type 2 diabetes (Clausen 05). In New Zealand, 22% of pregnancies with type 1 diabetes had baseline microalbuminuria compared with 33% with type 2 diabetes (Cundy 02). Diabetic women with microalbuminuria who are not intensively managed can have large increases in both UAE and TPE by the third trimester, and patients with clinical albuminuria can reach nephrotic levels of heavy proteinuria (3–20 gm/day) (McCance 89, Winocour 89, Biesenbach 94b, MacRury 95). It is uncertain whether increases in albuminuria and proteinuria are due to glomerular–tubular changes of pregnancy coupled with diabetic pathology or whether they are superimposed renal changes of preeclampsia. Albuminuria/proteinuria usually decreases postpartum.

Of 180 women with type 1 diabetes becoming pregnant in the DCCT, 8.3% were classified as having microalbuminuria on prior entry to the study (4-h timed urine ≥40 mg/24 h), and only 5.6% developed microalbuminuria during pregnancy. Of the original 12 subjects with microalbuminuria, only two had microalbuminuria at the end of the study, which was well after pregnancy (DCCT 00). Microalbuminuria during early diabetic pregnancy indicates an increased risk of development of preeclampsia, with the largest studies expressing rates of 35–60% (Winocour 89, Biesenbach 94b, Schroeder 00, Ekbom 01, Lauszus 01, Cundy 02). It is not clear whether this relationship reflects common pathogenic features, such as peripheral vascular dysfunction and sensitivity to placental angiogenic factors marked by microalbuminuria, or whether it is due to early renal pathology. One small study suggested that treatment of 10 microalbuminuric hypertensive diabetic women with methyldopa earlier in pregnancy reduced preterm delivery before 34 weeks by reducing preeclampsia compared with 9 historical controls with onset of treatment at 20–33 weeks (Nielsen 06). In a retrospective analysis of a small group of pregnant women with chronic renal disease, diltiazem use was associated with diminution of proteinuria across gestation, in which the expectation was for large gestational increases in proteinuria (Khandelwal 02). We need RCTs of renoprotective interventions designed to reduce microalbuminuria that are safe for the fetus (e.g., nondihydropyridine CCBs) with reduction of preeclampsia as an end point (Bar 95, Reece 02).

Diabetic Nephropathy During Pregnancy

Diagnosis and prevalence. The diagnosis of clinical (overt) DN is presumed if there is persistent macroalbuminuria or proteinuria (dipstick positive) before 20 weeks gestation in the absence of bacteriuria or evidence of other renal or urinary tract disorders in a woman with PDM (Kitzmiller 81a, Reece 88). Nephrolithiasis is more common with diabetes (especially urate in type 2 diabetes) (Cameron 06, Daudon 06) and might explain abnormal urinalysis (Taylor 05, Lieske 06). Renal biopsies (Kuller 01, Day 08) have not typically been performed to confirm the diagnosis of DN in pregnancy unless done prior to gestation. Most investigators have used the nonpregnant definitions to define clinical nephropathy or microalbuminuria, respectively. Low levels of macroalbuminuria (300–499 mg/day) during pregnancy may reflect gestational changes in the nephrons rather than a definite diagnosis of overt DN because this degree of albuminuria usually returns to subclinical levels after pregnancy. Controversy surrounds the determination of whether early pregnancy proteinuria of 199–499 mg/day is a risk factor for preeclampsia in diabetic women (Combs 93, How 04), which is probably due to the vagaries of gestational increases in proteinuria.

Some retrospective observational studies of diabetic pregnant women with proteinuria have used baseline TPE at ≥300 mg/day, so these series probably include women with preclinical DN (microproteinuria or microalbuminuria) prior to pregnancy. Based on a baseline TPE >300–500 mg/day, the prevalence of DN in recent large surveys of diabetic pregnant women is 5.3–6.4% in type 1 diabetes (FDSG 91, Hanson 93, Jensen 04) compared with 1–4% in type 2 diabetes (Nordstrom 98, Cundy 00, Gunton 00, Lauszus 01, Wylie 02, DPGF 03). Even if uncommon, DN plays a large role in contributing to maternal and perinatal morbidity (Reece 98a, Sibai 00, Rosenn 00, Lauenborg 03, Kitzmiller 04a, Carr 06, Landon 07). Two multi-center studies of 127 diabetic pregnant women with baseline TPE >500 mg/day yielded rates of PDR of 37%, chronic hypertension of 46%, preeclampsia of 39%, and delivery before 34 weeks gestation of 26% (Combs 93, How 04). BP levels >130/80 (mean arterial pressure >100 mmHg) in the first half of pregnancy in patients with both type 1 and type 2 diabetes and UAE >300 mg/day were associated with increased risks of superimposed preeclampsia, preterm birth <32 weeks, and a tendency to FGR (Carr 06). Although we lack RCTs in pregnancy, plentiful observational data suggest that excellent control of maternal hyperglycemia and hypertension and coordinated multispecialty care are important to reduce perinatal complications and prevent decline in renal function during and after pregnancy.

Course of renal function during and after pregnancy. In pooled data from 11 observational studies of 225 cases of DN during pregnancy in 1981–1996, TPE exceeded 5 gm/day in 26% by the third trimester (Kitzmiller 04b). It is unclear whether these cases of heavy proteinuria had greater risks of impaired renal function or accelerated hypertension (presumed preeclampsia) because no series was large enough for multivariate analysis to clarify these relationships. No controlled trials are available to determine whether intensified glycemic control or antihypertensive therapy can reduce the frequency of heavy proteinuria during pregnancy, and two small uncontrolled studies of intensified care were inconclusive (Jovanovic 84, Bar 99). It is also unknown whether heavy proteinuria during pregnancy contributes to subsequent renal tubulo-interstitial damage (Remuzzi 99, Walls 01, Eddy 04) in diabetic women, but concern for that may play a role in the decision to deliver the baby.

Due to the expected increase in CO and renal blood flow during the first half of pregnancy, it is difficult to assess glomerular hyperfiltration (CrCl >150 mL/min/kg) in women with PDM as a sign of glomerular hypertension or a hyperdynamic cardiac state. Hyperfiltration of this degree was observed in only 3 of 48 women with DN before 20 weeks gestation in two detailed clinical audits (Kitzmiller 81a, Reece 88). Renal volume as measured by US increased significantly in pregnant women with type 1 diabetes independently of duration of diabetes or presence of microvascular disease. A weak correlation existed between third-trimester renal volume and CrCl (Lauszus 95). One study of iohexol clearance assessed GFR in 44 diabetic pregnant women (8 with macroalbuminuria) at various stages of gestation, 11 of whom had GDM. Iohexol clearance was <100 mL/min/1.73 m^2 in seven women, which predicted only two of seven women with sCr >1.05 mg/dL (>80 μM); one of four women with preeclampsia had low clearance (Olofsson 96). Further observational studies of women with DN show that well-controlled patients without impaired renal function at baseline can demonstrate the rise in CrCl observed in normal pregnancy (Jovanovic 84, Kimmerle 95, Bar 99). During pregnancy, CrCl remains stable in three-quarters of DN patients with initial preserved renal function and declines in two-thirds of patients with azotemia in early pregnancy (Kitzmiller 81a, Grenfell 86b, Reece 88, Kimmerle 95, Gordon 96b, Kaaja 96, Mackie 96, Purdy 96, Bar 99, Dunne 99, Irfan 04). Investigators state that decline in GFR during and after gestation is associated with accelerated hypertension in pregnancy (Biesenbach 92,99), but others note the difficulty to ascertain whether hypertension worsens renal function or whether worsening renal function exacerbates hypertension (Irfan 04). We lack controlled studies on the effect of renoprotective therapies during pregnancy on the progression of DN.

Progression to renal failure during pregnancy is uncommon, but only eight completed pregnancies with initial sCr >2.0 mg/dL (>177 μM) are recorded in the aggregate patient series. GFR declined during pregnancy in three studies, and five needed renal replacement therapy within 4 years after pregnancy. In the aggregate series, 45% of women with mildly impaired renal function in early pregnancy progressed to renal failure 12 years postpartum (Table II.18) (Kitzmiller 81a, Grenfell 86b, Reece 88, Kimmerle 95, Gordon 96b, Kaaja 96, Mackie 96, Miodovnik 96, Purdie 96, Bar 99, Dinnc 99, Bagg 03, Irfan 04). The question remains as to whether pregnancy exacerbates subsequent progression of nephropathy. Limited case–control studies of previously pregnant women with DN compared with patients who were never pregnant did not demonstrate that pregnancy increases the risk of renal failure over the next 10 years (Hemachandra 95, Kaaja 96, Purdy 96, Rossing 02b). Observational follow-up studies demonstrate that the rate of decline of GFR after pregnancy is similar to that expected in nonparous women with DN (Kitzmiller 81a, Reece 90, Kimmerle 95, Gordon 96b, Mackie 96, Miodovnik 96, Dunne 99). A large type 1 diabetes population survey found that age- and duration-adjusted prevalence of macroalbuminuria was not as common in 582 women that had been pregnant as in 776 nulliparous women who had never

TABLE II.18 Course of Renal Function During and After Pregnancy in Women with Diabetic Nephropathy Comparing Patients with Preserved versus Impaired Renal Function in Early Pregnancy

	Initial Renal Function	
Number	**150 Preserved**	**103 Impaired***
Accelerated hypertension**	21 of 49 (42.9%)	41 of 70 (58.6%)
Progression of proteinuria >3 gm/day**	20 of 49 (40.8%)	52 of 70 (74.3%)
Chronic anemia	2 of 51 (3.9%)	51 of 80 (63.8%)
GFR decline >15% during pregnancy	40 of 150 (26.7%)	69 of 103 (67.0%)
Renal failure after pregnancy***	7 of 150 (4.7%)	46 of 103 (44.7%)
Death	1 of 150 (0.7%)	5 of 68 (7.4%)

Denominators differ due to variable analysis by authors.
*sCr >1.2–1.4 mg/dL (>106–125 μM) or CrCl <80 mL/min.
**Difficult to distinguish from superimposed preeclampsia.
***Need for renal replacement therapy 1–12 years after pregnancy.
Data based on Kitzmiller 81a, Grenfell 86a, Reece 88, Kimmerle 95, Gordon 96b, Kaaja 96, Mackie 96, Purdy 96, Bar 99, Dunne 99, Irfan 04.

TABLE II.19 Perinatal Outcome in 188 Women with DN Whose Pregnancies Advanced to >20 Weeks Gestation, Grouped by Preserved or Impaired Renal Function in Early Pregnancy

	Preserved Initial Renal Function (123)	Impaired Initial Renal Function (65)*
Delivery <34 weeks	17 (13.8%)	29 (44.6%)
Fetal growth restriction (<10th %)	17 (13.8%)	18 (27.7%)
Major congenital malformation	8 (6.5%)	5 (7.7%)
Stillbirth	2 (1.6%)	2 (3.1%)
Neonatal death	0	2 (3.1%)
Perinatal survival	121 (98.4%)	61 (93.8%)

*sCr >1.2–1.4 mg/dL (>106–125 μM) or CrCl <80 mL/min.
Data based on Kitzmiller 81a, Jovanovic 84, Dicker 86, Reece 88, Kimmerle 95, Mackie 96, Purdy 96, Bar 99, Khoury 02.

DN, diabetic nephropathy.

been pregnant, even after controlling for better glycemic control in the parous group (Chaturvedi 95).

Perinatal outcome. FGR and premature delivery, most often induced due to preeclampsia or signs of fetal distress, are both common in DN and more so with baseline-impaired renal function (Table II.19) and stage 2 hypertension (Kitzmiller 81a, Jovanovic 84, Dicker 86, Reece 88, Kimmerle 95, Mackie 96, Purdy 96, Bar 99, Khoury 02). Perinatal outcomes are similar in other series that did not present data based on initial maternal renal function (Grenfell 86a, Reece 90, Combs 93, Gordon 96b, Holley 96, Miodovnik 96, Dunne 99, Bagg 03, Carr 06). Analysis of a limited number of cases shows the major determinants of low BW to be midpregnancy height of BP and depth of CrCl (Kitzmiller 81a, Reece 88, Greene 89, Kimmerle 95, Bar 00) as well as the degree of proteinuria in some studies (Main 84, Gordon 96b). With preserved renal function and controlled hypertension, maternal hyperglycemia leads to fetal macrosomia in DN, as with other classes of diabetes in pregnancy (Kitzmiller 81a, Reece 88, Bar 99). CrCl <60 mL/min/kg or sCr >1.5 mg/dL (>132 mM) in early pregnancy is usually associated with severe hypertension and predicts the greatest risk of impaired fetal growth, fetal hypoxia, and preterm delivery (Grenfell 86a, Kimmerle 95, Mackie 96, Purdy 96, Reece 98b, Biesenbach 00, Khoury 02). In spite of this morbidity, perinatal survival is 94% with baseline-impaired renal function and near normal in DN when renal function is preserved.

A few investigators performed follow-up studies of 115 infants of mothers with DN (Kitzmiller 81a, Reece 88, Kimmerle 95, Bar 00, Biesenbach 00). Child growth delay at 2–3 years of age was observed in 16% of infants, most of whom were SGA at birth. Mild to severe developmental delay was found in 12%, which was associated with major congenital malformations, birth trauma, or severe perinatal asphyxia. Data on immediate and long-term perinatal outcome and maternal renal function are useful for counseling women with DN prior to pregnancy. The possibility that being SGA is associated with small kidneys and reduced nephron number at birth, impaired childhood kidney growth, and renal dysfunction later in life (Hinchcliffe 92, Brenner 94, Manalich 00, Ingelfinger 02, Schmidt 05) has not been studied in offspring of women with DN, but it could contribute to the familial clustering of diabetic renal complications (Pettitt 90, McCance 95, McAllister 99).

Renal transplants and subsequent pregnancy. A low rate of graft dysfunction has been recorded during pregnancy in a limited number of diabetic women with renal transplants in the cyclosporine era, but hypertension, preeclampsia, and preterm delivery are very common (Grenfell 86b, Ogburn 86, First 95, Armenti 97, Cruz-Lemini 07). Similar rates of these complications are seen in pregnancies after combined kidney–pancreas transplants (Skannal 96, Armenti 97, Barrou 98, Karaitis 99, McGrory 99, Wilson 01). With either situation, the course of renal function during pregnancy depends on baseline GFR and control of hypertension (Sturgiss 92, Cararach 93, Salmela 93, Armenti 94,00,06). Diagnosis and treatment of urinary tract infection (UTI) is important (Hou 99). By analyzing the larger body of data on pregnant women with kidney transplants due to other renal diseases, a review of 3,382 pregnancies showed a 96% perinatal survival rate if sCr is <1.5 mg/dL (<132 μM), but only a 75% survival rate if sCr is >1.4 mg/dL (Davison 94). Although the immunosuppressants azathioprine and cyclosporine cross the placenta, they are not thought to be teratogenic, and reports of fetal growth delay associated with cyclosporine therapy are inconclusive (Sturgiss 91, Armenti 95, Stanley 99, Bar-Oz 01, Armenti 02, McKay 05). Preliminary studies of the effects on pregnancy of tacrolimus suggest a possible problem with neonatal hyperkalemia (Eisenberg 97, Armenti 00, Kainz 00, Pergola 01, Hou 03a). Mycophenolate mofetil (MMF) is apparently associated with fetal structural defects, but no defects have been reported with sirolimus exposure (Sifontis 06, Perez-Aytes 08). Fortunately, azathioprine may be as effective as MMF when used in combination with cyclosporine in preventing acute and chronic allograft dysfunction (Remuzzi 07), without as much risk to the fetus. Published guidelines on preconception counseling of women with renal transplants emphasize waiting for 2 years of stable graft function with sCr <1.5–2.0 mg/dL (133–177 μM) and TPE <500 mg/day, with good control of blood glucose and BP (Lindheimer 92, Hou 99, Hou 03).

Renal dialysis in pregnancy. Data on diabetic pregnant women on dialysis are only available from observational studies of all forms of renal disease. The risk of death for a dialysis patient is not increased by pregnancy, but severe hypertension, oligo- or polyhydramnios, and preterm labor are common, and perinatal survival is only 60–78% (Kioko 83, Hou 94, Bagon 98, Chan 98, Hou 98, Okundaye 98, Romao 98, Chao 02, Holley 03, Kazancioglu 03, Haase 06, Reddy 07). Therapeutic abortion usually fails to rescue renal function in women with new-onset ESRD (Jones 96). In patients using dialysis prior to pregnancy, treatment of chronic anemia with erythropoietin or blood transfusions is usually required (Hou 93).

Therapeutic interventions. Therapeutic interventions are important in diabetic women with incipient or overt DN (Landon 07). No RCTs of intensified glycemic control, antihypertensive treatment, or specific dietary or pharmacological regimens have been conducted in diabetic women with microalbuminuria, macroalbuminuria, or heavy proteinuria during pregnancy. Observational data suggest that prevention of hyperglycemia and hypertension in these patients is associated with the best maternal–fetal outcomes (Reece 98a,b, Kitzmiller 04a,b, Carr 06, Nielsen 06), which support the evidence-based guidelines for management of these women before and after pregnancy (Bakris 00, ADA 04d,08a). Use of ACE inhibitors or ARBs should be discontinued before pregnancy due to fetal risks, and patients should be changed to other antihypertensive agents if treatment is indicated (refer to the section titled "Blood

Pressure Control"). Controlled trials of diltiazem are needed in pregnant women with micro- or macroalbuminuria to determine whether this nondyhydropyridine CCB will improve perinatal outcome or decrease superimposed preeclampsia based on its ability to reduce albuminuria and improve renal function in nonpregnant diabetic subjects (Smith 98, Bakris 04, Gashti 04). Restriction of dietary protein intake may be effective in slowing the decline in renal function in nonpregnant women with DN (ADA 04d); however, minimal protein ingestion during gestation should be 1.1 gm/kg/day due to fetal needs (see the section titled "Medical Nutrition Therapy" in Part I). Severe anemia may be treated successfully with erythropoietin during pregnancy (McGregor 91, Yankowitz 92, Hou 93, Braga 96, Hou 03). Diuretic therapy may be needed in nephrotic patients with severe, debilitating edema. Diabetic women with moderate to severe microvascular disease may also have uterine vascular lesions (Kitzmiller 81b), and resting in the lateral position may improve renal and uteroplacental blood flow by enhanced venous return and CO. Treatment of diabetic women with renal transplants is based on published clinical experience in nondiabetic renal diseases (Lindheimer 92, Hou 99,03). Guidelines for the management of dialysis and pregnancy have been published (Hou 02).

Recommendations

- Determine the level of albuminuria and estimate GFR with sCr before pregnancy in all women with PDM. (E)
- During early pregnancy, assess UAE with a random urine/creatinine ratio. (E)
- In pregnant patients with micro- or macroalbuminuria, measure properly instructed 24-h CrCl because estimated GFR by the MDRD equation is not accurate in gestation. (E)
- To reduce the risk and/or slow the progression of nephropathy and to improve perinatal outcome, optimize glucose and BP control. (A)
- Discontinue ACE inhibitors and ARBs in anticipation of pregnancy, and use agents as discussed in the section on hypertension in pregnancy titled "Blood Pressure Control." (E)
- In women with overt nephropathy, consult an RD and restrict protein intake to ~1.1 gm/kg body weight/day (~10% of daily calories = current adult RDA for protein), but not <60 gm/day. (E)
- Consider referral to a center experienced in the care of diabetic renal disease and pregnancy when either the GFR has fallen to <60 mL/min per 1.73 m^2 or difficulties have occurred in the management of hypertension. (E)

DIABETIC RETINOPATHY AND PREGNANCY

—— Original contribution by Florence M. Brown MD
and Lois B. Jovanovic MD

Classification and Pathogenesis

Diabetic retinopathy (DR) has been classified according to the complex Early Treatment Diabetic Retinopathy Study (ETDRS) severity scale to grade fundus photographs in clinical trials (ETDRS 91). In 2002, an international consensus group developed a new

TABLE II.20 International Clinical Diabetic Retinopathy Disease Severity Scale

Disease Severity Level	Findings Based upon Dilated Ophthalmoscopy	Frequency of Examinations
No apparent retinopathy	No abnormalities	First and third trimester
Mild NPDR	Microaneurysms only	First and third trimester
Moderate NPDR	More than just microaneurysms, but less than severe NPDR	Each trimester
Severe NPDR	Any of the following, but no proliferative changes: >20 intraretinal hemorrhages in each of 4 quadrants; definite venous beading in ≥2 quadrants; prominent intraretinal vascular/microvascular abnormalities in ≥1 quadrant	Monthly
PDR	≥1 of the following: neovascularization; vitreous/preretinal hemorrhage	Monthly if active; each trimester if previously treated

Based upon Wilkinson 03 and Fong 04b.

NPDR, nonproliferative diabetic retinopathy; PDR, proliferative diabetic retinopathy.

severity scale as a more practical measure in routine clinical use based upon dilated ophthalmoscopy (Table II.20) (Wilkinson 03); this severity scale has been presented in the latest ADA Technical Review and Position Statement on DR (Fong 04a,b). Classification of retinopathy during pregnancy is the same as classification in nonpregnant diabetic patients. The first two of five levels (no apparent retinopathy; mild NPDR: microaneurysms only) have low risk of clinically significant progression over several years (Fong 04b). The third level is moderate NPDR, which includes findings of limited intraretinal hemorrhages, hard or soft exudates (SEs), and venous beading in only one quadrant (ETDRS 91). The third level has moderate risk of progression and was formerly called mild or moderate background DR. Severe NPDR presents an ominous risk of progression at the fourth level. The fifth level is PDR, which is characterized by the growth of new vessels on the surface of the retina and posterior surface of the vitreous (Fong 04b).

An international disease severity scale was also presented for diabetic macular edema (DME), which is defined as retinal thickening from leaky blood vessels, or hard exudates (lipids) in the posterior pole. DME can develop at all stages of retinopathy (Fong 04b). Severity is based on distance from the center of the macula (distant, mild DME; approaching the macula, moderate DME; involving the center of the macula, severe DME) (Wilkinson 03). Determination of the severity of retinal thickening requires a three-dimensional assessment that is best performed by a dilated examination using slit-lamp biomicroscopy and/or stereo fundus photography (Fong 04b).

Vision loss due to DR results from several mechanisms, as presented in Table II.21.

Intensified glycemic control reduces long-term progression of DR in both type 1 (DCCT 95d,e) and type 2 diabetes (UKPDS 98a, Stratton 00b). The DCCT investigators concluded that the greatest long-term protective effect of tight glycemic control occurred when A1C was brought down to normal (DCCT 95f,96b). The benefit of reducing DR continued over 7 years after conclusion of the trial, even when A1C no longer differed in the original treatment groups (DCCT 02). Strict control of BP was

TABLE II.21 Causes of Visual Loss in Diabetic Retinopathy

Central vision impaired by macular edema or capillary nonperfusion

New vessels and contraction of accompanying fibrous tissue distort the retina and lead to tractional retinal detachment

Preretinal or vitreous hemorrhage

Neovascular glaucoma

Macular nonperfusion

Based on Fong 04a,b.

also shown to reduce DR in patients with type 2 diabetes in some (UKPDS 98b,c), but not all, studies (Estacio 00).

In the first year of intensified diabetes management, there may be a transient increase of retinopathy, known as "early worsening" (Lauritzen 83, KROC 84, Dahl-Jorgensen 85, Chantelau 97, Henricsson 97). The largest and most detailed analysis of early worsening was evaluated as part of the DCCT investigation (DCCT 98b). Early worsening was defined as progression of three or more steps on the ETDRS final scale, development of SEs (cotton-wool spots) and dilated tortuous intraretinal vessels (intraretinal microvascular abnormalities; IRMA), or clinically important retinopathy (severe NPDR, PDR, level 3 DME) observed at the 6- or 12-month visit. Of 348 type 1 diabetes patients randomized to intensive care with no retinopathy at baseline, 3.7% had progressed ≥3 steps, 1.1% developed SE and/or IRMA, and none developed serious early worsening. The respective percentages were 7.6%, 15.3%, and 0.8% in 249 patients with microaneurysms only at baseline. All of these percentages were approximately double those found in patients in the conventional care group. The frequency of early worsening was somewhat greater in the small group of subjects with moderate/severe NPDR at baseline, in whom development of serious early worsening was 19% in both treatment groups. Most importantly, patients with early worsening reaped the long-term benefit of intensified management in that their cumulative incidence of sustained 3-step or more progression at 5 years' follow-up was 20% in the intensified care group compared with 58% in the conventional care group (DCCT 98b).

The pathogenesis of DR is complex, involving hyperglycemia, increased hexosamine flux, overproduction of mitochondrial superoxide and cytosolic NADH, polyol accumulation, AGEs, diacylglycerol–protein kinase C (PKC) activation, oxidative damage, inflammation, hypoxia, apoptotic death of pericytes and endothelial cells, and production and signaling of angiogenic or growth factors such as erythropoieten, VEGF, GH, insulin-like GF-1, transforming GF-β, and low pigment epithelium-derived growth factor (PEDF) (Aiello 98, Brownlee 01, Lorenzi 01, Scheetz 02, Fong 04b, Frank 04, Nyengaard 04, Aiello 05, Brownlee 05,Watanabe 05). The interacting effects of IGF-1 and VEGF (Smith 99, Kondo 03, Poulaki 04, Ruberte 04) may be enhanced by hyperinsulinemia (King 85, Poulaki 02, Bronson 03, Reiter 03).

All of these processes/factors may be in play during pregnancy (Jovanovic 04). The growth factors IGF-1 and VEGF as well as placental growth hormone are produced by the placenta (DiSalvo 95, Khaliq 98) and may act in the retina (Lauszus 03). Blood levels of hormones such as estrogen, progesterone, and human placental lactogen (hPL) increase dramatically in pregnancy and may accelerate retinopathy (Larinkari 02), possibly through their effects on VEGF (Aiello 98, Mitamura 02). In addition, pregnant women with type 1 diabetes have higher perimacular capillary blood flow than pregnant controls (Chen 94, Loukovaara 03a), although one study found decreased volumetric blood flow in seven diabetic patients during pregnancy (Schocket 99), perhaps due to differences in methodology or patient selection (Sheth 02). The retinal venous diameter seems to decrease from the first to the third trimester in both healthy and diabetic women except for those who smoke (Schocket 99, Larsen 05b). Attempts to correlate angiogenic, vasoactive, inflammatory, or IGF factors with these hemodynamic changes or the development and progression of DR in pregnancy were unsuccessful (Loukovaara 04,05a,b,c).

Course of Retinopathy During Pregnancy

Most of the recent population-based studies of type 1 diabetic pregnancies have not reported data on DR because they focused on perinatal outcome. In two studies, the prevalence of PDR was 6.8% in Denmark (Jensen 04) and 7% in France (GDFSG 91). In a subsequent French survey in 2000–2001, the frequency of DR of any type was reported to be 34% in 289 pregnant women with type 1 diabetes and 2.7% in 146 pregnant women with type 2 diabetes (DPGF 03). In Copenhagen, the prevalence of PDR was 10.4% in 240 pregnant women with type 1 diabetes in 1996–2001 compared with no cases in 61 women with type 2 diabetes (Clausen 05). A large referral center for British Columbia reported a 15% frequency of PDR in 247 pregnant women with type 1 diabetes (Wylie 02), but this frequency may be biased by the referral of more complicated patients. Single-center audits of type 2 diabetes in pregnancy yield prevalence rates of 2.0–28.1% NPDR and 0–4.3% PDR (Omori 94, Sacks 97); anecdotal cases of florid PDR in type 2 diabetes during pregnancy have been reported (Hagay 94c, Kitzmiller 99).

Levels of severity of DR were reported as none, background DR, or PDR in16 studies (1980–2001) of >1,000 pregnant women with type 1 diabetes who had dilated ophthalmoscopic examinations by specialists (Horvat 80, Johnston 80, Dibble 82, Moloney 82, Jovanovic 84, Ohrt 84, Price 84, Phelps 86, Serup 86, Laatikainen 87, Rosenn 92, Reece 94, Lovestam-Adrian 97, Lapolla 98, McElvy 01, Temple 01). The aggregate results are presented in Table II.22, along with the frequency of progression

TABLE II.22 Grade of Diabetic Retinopathy at Baseline Dilated Ophthalmoscopic Examination and Progression of Diabetic Retinopathy During Pregnancy

Change During Pregnancy	Grade of Retinopathy at Initial Examination			
	None	**Background**	**PDR (previously untreated)***	**Photocoagulation Before Pregnancy**
Pregnancies (N)	669	566	55	42
No change or improved	579 (86.5%)	329 (58.1%)	15 (27.3%)	33 (78.6%)
Progressed to or in NPDR	89 (13.3%)	196 (34.6%)	NA	NA
Progressed to or in PDR*	1 (0.15%)	41 (7.2%)	40 (72.7%)	9 (21.4%)

1,332 pregnancies in 16 observational studies reported in 1980–2001; almost all patients had type 1 diabetes.
*Many cases treated soon after diagnosis in pregnancy.
Data based on Horvat 80, Johnston 80, Dibble 82, Moloney 82, Jovanovic 84, Price 84, Ohrt 86, Phelps 86, Serup 86, Laatikainen 87, Rosenn 92, Reece 94, Lovestam-Adrian 97, Lapolla 98, McElvy 01, Temple 01.

NPDR, nonproliferative diabetic retinopathy; PDR, proliferative diabetic retinopathy; NA, not applicable.

during pregnancy. From three prospective investigations of 353 women with type 1 diabetes using stereoscopic retinal fundus photographs early in pregnancy, the combined distribution of levels of severity are presented in Table II.23 (Klein 90, Chew 95, Axer-Siegel 96). From both sets of data, it is apparent that the risk of progression to NPDR or within NPDR is common and that the risk of developing PDR during pregnancy varies from 1.3% to 29.4% according to baseline severity of NPDR. Progression often occurs in the second trimester. In 784 cases of no apparent retinopathy at baseline in the combined studies (47% of diabetic women), one developed PDR during pregnancy (Lovestam-Adrian 97). A few anecdotal cases of PDR occurring de novo by the end of pregnancy have been reported (Cassar 78, Kitzmiller 93, Hagay 94c, Bastion 05), but it is very uncommon. The risk of progression of untreated PDR in pregnancy is very high (unless there was prior laser photocoagulation), which is another argument for careful preconception evaluation and management of diabetic women (Rahman 07). Other unusual cases are reported of the development of PDR in pregnancy from microaneurysms only seen at the basal examination (Sinclair 84, Laatikainen 87, Klein 90, Temple 01, Chatterjee 03). In a careful longitudinal retinal study using red-free photographs, both the rate of microaneurysm formation and rate of disappearance increased during pregnancy in women with type 1 diabetes, with the disappearance rate exceeding the formation rate 6 months postpartum. The temporary flare-up of microaneurysms was associated with the greatest decrease in A1C (Hellstedt 97).

The course of DME is not as well characterized during pregnancy. In the literature since 1978, only six groups have reported a total of 21 cases developing DME during pregnancy among 304 patients with DR (6.9%) (Cassar 78, Sinclair 84, Laatikainen 87, Axer-Siegel 96, Lovestam-Adrian 97, Temple 01). Baseline examinations in these cases revealed microaneurysms only in six cases, moderate NPDR in four, severe NPDR in two, PDR in four, and prior photocoagulation in five. At the time of diagnosis during pregnancy, DME was associated with new PDR in seven cases. In a series of seven cases of severe macular edema during pregnancy (Sinclair 84), baseline proteinuria and nerve fiber layer infarcts were associated with DME in five women. Of nine pregnant women with

TABLE II.23 Grading Diabetic Retinopathy from Stereoscopic Color Fundus Photographs at Baseline in 353 Pregnancies of Women with Type 1 Diabetes

Level of Retinopathy	Distribution in Early Pregnancy	Progression During Pregnancy	Developed PDR
No apparent retinopathy	115 (32.6%)	24 (20.9% of level 1)	None
Microaneurysms or blot hemorrhages only	80 (22.7%)	36 (45% of level 2)	1 (1.3%)
Moderate NPDR	47 (13.3%)	14 (29.8% of level 3)	3 (6.4%)
Severe NPDR	68 (19.3%)	36 (52.9% of level 4)	20 (29.4%)
Proliferative diabetic retinopathy	43 (12.2%)	Most progress if not treated	NA

Level of severity in the studies was based on the ETDRS grading system (ETDRS 1991), but is presented here according to the International Clinical Severity Scale (Wilkinson 03, Fong 04a) except for blot hemorrhages in level 2. Progression is ≥1 step in at least one eye.

Data from Klein 90, Chew 95, and Axer-Siegel 96. Phelps 86 also used fundus photographs at entry and after delivery, but did not stratify patients with NPDR.

NA, not applicable; NPDR, nonproliferative diabetic retinopathy; PDR, proliferative diabetic retinopathy.

maculopathy and PDR in Denmark, six also had nephropathy (Lauszus 98). In a study of DN in pregnancy, macular edema was noted in 6 of 35 patients (17.1%) (Irfan 04). DME seems to cluster with PDR, DN, and superimposed preeclampsia during gestation.

Macular surface topography was prospectively examined in 41 pregnant women with type 1 diabetes; macular volume above the reference plane was slightly increased compared with nondiabetic controls and was seen to the greatest extent in patients with clear progression of DR during pregnancy (Loukovaara 03b). Macular capillary blood flow velocity was progressively increased during pregnancy in 46 women with type 1 diabetes compared with controls and was greatest in patients with more severe retinopathy (Loukovaara 02). Evidence of progressively increased perimacular capillary blood flow was also obtained. The authors speculated that retinal capillary hyperperfusion may play a role in the development of DR and DME during pregnancy (Loukovaara 03a).

The question remains whether the short-term risk of progression of DR in pregnancy is greater than the risk found in nonpregnant women with similar diabetes characteristics followed for 9–12 months (Sheth 02). In one prospective study using a pregnant case subject versus a nonpregnant control approach, pregnancy itself was an independent risk factor for ≥2-step progression (adjusted OR 2.3), and factors for nonprogression were in the lowest quartiles for A1C (OR 1.7) and diastolic BP (OR 1.7) (Klein 90). In a smaller retrospective study, controls were matched by age and duration of diabetes, and no differences were found regarding incidences of any type of DR or sight-threatening deterioration over a 2-year period, including before and after pregnancy (Lovestam-Adrian 97). Regarding 86 initial pregnancies in the intensive treatment group of the DCCT who had undergone retinal examinations, progression of DR to any extent was observed in 31% of visits while pregnant compared with 23% while not pregnant (OR adjusted for recent change in A1C, 1.63; p < 0.05) (DCCT 00). The pregnancy effect was more pronounced in the 79 initial pregnancies in women who were previously in the conventional treatment group (adjusted OR 2.48; p < 0.001), who had a greater decline in A1c values from nonpregnant levels than women in the intensive treatment group (64% dropped >1.7% vs. 26% dropped >1.3%). More clinically meaningful, in the intensive treatment group, DR that was worse than baseline level by ≥3 steps was observed in 6.1% of visits during pregnancy compared with 5.7% among visits while not pregnant. In the conventional treatment group, progression ≥3 steps was observed in 17% of visits during pregnancy vs. 13.3% for visits while not pregnant. Overall, in both treatment groups, only three patients (1.8%) required laser photocoagulation during pregnancy (DCCT 00).

Risk Factors for Progression of Retinopathy in Pregnancy
Several factors increase the risk for progression of retinopathy during pregnancy: (1) retinal status at conception, (2) duration and earlier onset of diabetes, (3) elevated first-trimester A1C and persisting poor glycemic control *or* rapid normalization of blood glucose, and (4) hypertension (Soubrane 98, Lauszus 00, Rosenn 00, Sheth 02, Dinn 03, Jovanovic 04, Loukovaara 05, Kaaja 07, Rahman 07). Duration of diabetes is an independent risk factor for the progression of retinopathy in pregnancy (Chew 95, Temple 01). The risk of ≥2-step progression for women with type 1 diabetes increases after 5 years' duration of diabetes and peaks at 15–20 years' duration. The Diabetes in Early Pregnancy Study demonstrated risks of progression of 5%, 14%, 34%, 45%, and 36% for women with diabetes duration of 0–5 years, 6–10 years, 11–15 years, 16–20 years, and >20 years, respectively (Chew 95).

Elevated first-trimester A1C followed by rapid improvement of maternal glucose is reported to accelerate DR in pregnancy (Larinkari 82, Phelps 86, Latikainen 87, Klein 90, Rosenn 92, Lovestam 95, Axer-Siegel 96, Kitzmiller 99, Temple 01). The prospective study with the least progression of retinopathy reported the lowest A1C levels at conception and thus the least drop in levels during gestation (Temple 01). The Diabetes in Early Pregnancy Study demonstrated that baseline A1C >6 standard deviations above the mean is associated with progression of retinopathy, but the rate of decline of A1C was not greater in women with progression than without progression of retinopathy (Chew 95). It is difficult to determine the independent effect of initial poor glycemic control and abrupt institution of strict control on the progression of retinopathy (Lovestam 97, Rosenn 00, Dinn 03). Best results will probably be achieved when glycemia is optimized prior to conception. Whether any form of insulin treatment is related to development of neovascularization in poorly controlled patients during pregnancy is discussed in the section titled "Insulin Therapy" in Part I.

Diastolic (Klein 90) or systolic (Axer-Siegel 96) chronic hypertension is an additional risk factor for progression of retinopathy in pregnant women in some studies (Rosenn 92), but no controlled trials of antihypertensive therapy with retinopathy as primary or secondary end points have been conducted. Progression of DR also occurs more often in women who later develop preeclampsia (but not gestational hypertension) during pregnancy. Of 414 diabetic women showing no progression of DR during pregnancy in a pooled analysis of five studies (Price 84, Laatikainen 87, Lovestam-Adrian 97, Mcelvy 01, Temple 01), preeclampsia was detected in 11.8% compared with 27.8% in 90 women who did have progression of DR ($X^2 = 15.0$; $p = 0.001$); however, three other investigators reported no association of DR progression with preeclampsia (Ohrt 86, Axer-Siegel 96, Lauszus 00). PDR is strongly associated with DN in pregnant and nonpregnant women (Kitzmiller 81, Jovanovic 84, Phelps 86, Reece 88, Lauszus 98, Temple 01), which probably implicates common pathogenic factors for progression of widespread microvascular pathology in these patients. It is unknown whether the hypertension commonly found with DN in pregnancy accelerates progression of NPDR to PDR. In 52 cases of DN in pregnancy from three reports with individual patient data, 34 women also had PDR (65.4%) and 29 were hypertensive (56%). Of the group with PDR, 62% were hypertensive compared with a 44% rate of hypertension in nephropathic patients without PDR (Kitzmiller 81, Jovanovic 84, Reece 88). The association of hypertension with PDR in these pregnant women with nephropathy is not significant, which is probably due to a β-error with small numbers ($X^2 = 1.43$; $p = 0.37$).

Retinopathy After Pregnancy

In the DCCT, the frequency of visits with any further retinopathy progression observed at 6–12 months after pregnancy was 7.6% in the intensive treatment group vs. 19.1% in the conventional treatment group. Some patients required laser photocoagulation postpartum (DCCT 00). In an observational study of 27 type 1 diabetes patients in whom NPDR had progressed during pregnancy, 22% persisted at the same level when examined 12 months postpartum and the rest regressed (Axer-Siegel 96). These findings plus other reports of postpartum progression of PDR (Conway 91, Reece 94, Lauszus 00) support the need for careful ophthalmological evaluation some months after gestation.

Regarding pregnancy effects on long-term DR, at the end of the DCCT study, neither the existence of ≥3-step progression over baseline nor severe NPDR were more common in women who had pregnancies than those who did not in either treatment group (DCCT 00). The prevalence of PDR was the same (35% vs. 36%) over a 10-year period between 80 women with type 1 diabetes who had a successful pregnancy and 80 never-pregnant patients matched for age, duration of diabetes, race, and marital history (Hemachandra 95). In a large survey of European nulliparous compared with parous women with type 1 diabetes, the prevalence of all retinopathy or PDR was significantly lower in parous women, even after adjusting for glycemic control (Chaturvedi 95). This result is similar to the lower rate of progression of DR after pregnancy compared with matched controls who were never pregnant that was witnessed in a smaller study (Kaaja 96). The prevalence of any retinopathy or PDR was not lessened in diabetic women having one versus two pregnancies (Vaarasmaki 02). Therefore, in spite of the approximately doubled risk of temporary short-term progression of retinopathy during pregnancy, the long-term risk of progression does not appear to differ from that of women who have never been pregnant.

A few investigators have studied the association of PDR and pregnancy outcome (Klein 88, Reece 94). Three studies of PDR found that the perinatal complications that did occur were attributable to DN (Reece 96, Lauszus 98, Mcelvy 01). In one investigation, FGR was related to progression of all levels of DR and to chronic hypertension in multivariate analysis, controlling for nephropathy and preeclampsia (Mcelvy 01). When the vascular complications of diabetes are so closely linked, it is difficult to ascribe outcomes to any single factor in small retrospective studies.

Evaluation of the Retina

All patients with diabetes need an annual dilated and comprehensive eye examination by an ophthlamologist or optometrist (ADA 08a). This examination should be a mainstay of preconception care (Kitzmiller 96, Aiello 98, Fong 04). In addition, baseline retinal photographs should be taken to document the status of the retina when pathology is present so as to compare them with the status of the retina as pregnancy progresses. A dilated eye examination is superior to a nondilated evaluation because it has been well documented that 50% of patients may actually have DR when a direct ophthalmoscopic examination is reported as normal (Moss 85). Proper examination of the retina requires the equipment and expertise of an eye care provider experienced with DR who has the capability to detect retinal thickening in the posterior pole (DME) (Fong 04a). The frequency of eye examinations during pregnancy should be determined based on the levels and risk factors noted earlier (see Table II.20). At a minimum, patients should be evaluated in the first trimester (unless seen within 3 months of preconception) and again in the third trimester of pregnancy if they have no or mild NPDR. For patients with moderate NPDR, dilated eye examinations should be performed each trimester and 3 months postpartum. For patients with severe NPDR, monthly examinations may be necessary as determined by the eye care provider. Patients with any level of macular edema, severe NPDR, or any PDR should be promptly referred to an ophthalmologist experienced in the evaluation and treatment of DR (ADA 08a).

When to Treat Diabetic Pregnant Women with Laser Photocoagulation

No randomized trials of pregnant women with DR have been conducted in which photocoagulation therapy has been the study variable. Nevertheless, there are extensive trials reported in nonpregnant patients, and thousands of pregnant patients have received laser therapy (Kohner 96, Sheth 02). Current treatment guidelines for nonpregnant individuals generally recommend prompt laser photocoagulation for significant neovascularization of the optic nerve head or any neovascularization in the presence of vitreous hemorrhage. In addition, laser photocoagulation should be considered with any retinal neovascularization or with severe or very severe NPDR, especially in patients with type 2 diabetes. Macular edema that is threatening vision may not respond well to laser photocoagulation, and diuretics or corticosteroids may be used (Sinclair 85, Kohner 96). Macular edema usually regresses in the postpartum period (Kohner 96, Sheth 02).

Vitrectomy can be performed as needed for vitreous hemorrhage or retinal detachment, even during the second or third trimesters, with the assistance of an anesthetist experienced with pregnancy (Kohner 96).

In general, a proactive treatment approach is recommended in pregnant patients with advanced DR because retinopathy progression can be rapid in the setting of gestation. However, such treatment must be tempered by the fact that retinopathy progression can cease and may regress postpartum. Some experts believe that new vessels occurring late in pregnancy should not be left untreated in the expectation of postpartum reversal because the new vessels may bleed or form fibrous proliferation, making treatment more difficult (Kohner 96). Regardless, very careful follow-up by ophthalmologists skilled in the treatment of DR is essential for the pregnant patient with advanced retinopathy (Fong 04a), including care after delivery (Kohner 96).

Many patients with retinal neovascularization are encouraged to avoid the Valsalva maneuver to reduce the risk of serious hemorrhage. In that situation, it makes sense to avoid maternal bearing-down efforts in the second stage of labor by using epidural anesthesia or CS. No controlled studies on the route of delivery have been conducted regarding the risk of serious hemorrhage in women with active PDR.

Medical management of DR based on new insights into pathogenesis is under investigation to avoid the destructive nature of laser photocoagulation. Current trials involve inhibition of VEGF (van Wijngaarden 05) and blockade of angiotensin receptors, the β-isoform of PKC, and growth hormone using somatostatin (Porta 04). It is unclear whether these approaches would be safe during pregnancy. Approaches that were not successful include inhibition of platelet aggregation, aldose reductase inhibition, and attempted blockage of the formation of AGEs (Porta 04).

Recommendations

- Preconception care for all type 1 and type 2 diabetic women should include a dilated and comprehensive eye examination by an opthalmologist or optometrist. Women should be counseled on the risk of development and/or progression of DR. (B)
- To reduce the risk or slow the progression of retinopathy, optimize glycemic and BP control. (A)
- Promptly refer patients with any level of macular edema, severe NPDR, or any PDR to an ophthalmologist who is knowledgeable and experienced in the management and treatment of DR. (A)
- Blood glucose levels should be lowered to normal over a 6-month period in the subgroup of preconception patients with severe NPDR or PDR before pregnancy is attempted. (A)
- Blood glucose levels should be normalized rapidly in all pregnant women regardless of retinal status or first-trimester A1C. (E)

- Eye examination with dilated pupils should occur in the first trimester with close follow-up throughout pregnancy and for 1 year postpartum. (B)

- Follow-up dilated eye examinations should be based on the presence or absence of risk factors. Patients who have no or minimal retinopathy should be evaluated in the first and third trimesters. Patients with mild retinopathy should be evaluated every trimester. Patients with moderate to severe NPDR or PDR should be evaluated monthly at the discretion of the eye care provider. (E)

- Laser photocoagulation therapy is indicated to reduce the risk of vision loss in preconception and pregnant patients with high-risk PDR, clinically significant macular edema, and in some cases of severe NPDR. (A)

- In women with untreated PDR, vaginal delivery with the associated Valsalva maneuver during labor has been associated with retinal and vitreous hemorrhage. Assisted second-stage delivery or cesarean delivery should be considered in consultation with an obstetrician and ophthalmologist. (E)

DIABETIC NEUROPATHIES

—— Original contribution by Barak Rosenn MD

Classification and Testing for Diabetic Neuropathies

Diabetic neuropathies are heterogenous and affect different parts of the nervous system, with focal or diffuse manifestations. They can be grouped as sensory, focal/multifocal, and autonomic; the diagnostic criteria are listed in Table II.24 (Thomas 97, Boulton 05). Some neuropathic symptoms are difficult to distinguish from complaints of pregnancy. Diabetic neuropathies are common complications (15–40%) that affect people with both type 1 (Mohsin 05, Nordwall 06, Orchard 06) and type 2 diabetes (Davies 06), but accurate estimates of their prevalence in pregnancy are unavailable due to the paucity of reliable data. In one regional study, 37% of all patients with type 1 diabetes >18 years of age were affected by peripheral neuropathy (Maser 89), as were nearly one-third of young type 1 diabetes patients in a large European study (Tesfaye 05). In distal sensorimotor polyneuropathy, loss of functional sensory nerves predisposes the patient to the development of ulcers that subsequently become infected and ultimately lead to limb amputation. CAN causes substantial morbidity and increased mortality (Vinik 03). The DCCT (DCCT 95g, Martin 06) and other studies (Amthor 94, Larsen 03) clearly demonstrated that improved blood glucose control reduces the risk of distal sensorimotor and autonomic neuropathies in type 1 diabetes.

Chronic sensorimotor distal symmetric polyneuropathy (DPN) is the most common form of diabetic neuropathy. Diffuse damage is found in all peripheral nerve fibers: motor, sensory, and autonomic (Perkins 05c). This insidious disorder typically involves the longest axons first and slowly progresses from the feet to the hands. The accepted clinical definition of DPN is "the presence of symptoms and/or signs of peripheral nerve dysfunction in people with diabetes after the exclusion of other causes" (Boulton 04). Sensory loss usually occurs first, followed by loss of motor function, in a stocking-and-glove distribution (Perkins 05c). Because up to 50% of cases of DPN may be asymptomatic, careful physical examination of the lower limbs is essential, with confirmation with quantitative electrophysiology as well as sensory and autonomic function

TABLE II.24 Diagnostic Criteria, Clinical, and Some Laboratory Findings in Diabetic Neuropathies

Type of neuropathy	Symptoms	Signs and tests
Acute sensory neuropathy	Acute pain in legs with change in glycemic control	Few neurological signs
Chronic sensorimotor distal symmetric polyneuropathy (DPN)	Burning pain, stabbing sensations, para- or hyperasthesiae, deep aching pain in feet and hands; worse at night	Loss of vibration, pressure, pain, and temperature perception; absent ankle reflexes; warm or cold foot; dry skin
Mononeuropathies of median, ulnar, radial, and common peoneal nerves (cranial rare)	Weakness or pain in nerve distribution (palsies of peroneal or third cranial nerve)	Reduction in both nerve conduction and amplitude
Entrapment of ulnar, median, peroneal, and medial plantar nerves	Weakness or pain in nerve distribution; carpal tunnel syndrome	Electrophysiological studies show blocks in conduction at entrapment site
Proximal motor amyotrophy	Severe neuropathic pain and uni- or bilateral muscle weakness	Atrophy in proximal thigh muscles; rule out CIDP and spinal stenosis
Cardiovascular autonomic neuropathy (CAN)	Early fatigue and weakness with exercise; postural dizziness, lightheadedness, weakness, syncope	Resting HR >100 bpm, lack of HR variability <10 bpm, inspiration/ expiration R-R interval <1.10–1.17 depending on age; BP supine and standing (fall in systolic >20 torr without HR response); resting and stress thallium myocardial scintigraphy if nonpregnant
Gastrointestinal autonomic dysfunction; gastroparesis	Postprandial upper abdominal discomfort, early satiety, nausea, vomiting, belching, bloating; constipation alternating with diarrhea	Gastric emptying or barium study, endoscopy, electrogastrogram
Genitourinary tract dysfunction	Urinary retention, frequency, nocturia, incontinence; vaginal dryness	Cystometrogram, postvoiding sonography

Based on Thomas 97 and Boulton 05.

BP, blood pressure, CAN, cardiovascular autonomic neuropathy; CIDP, chronic inflammatory demyelinating polyneuropathy; DPN, distal symmetric polyneuropathy; HR, heart rate; R wave on ECG.

testing (Boulton 98, Perkins 01, Boulton 05). Neuropathic pain can be very severe. Focal or multifocal neuropathy affects cranial nerves or other asymmetric loci in the trunk or limbs (Ayyar 04, Boulton 04). The spinal cord can be involved, as assessed by MRI (Selvarajah 06). Guidelines on standardized measures of diabetic neuropathy have been published (Asbury 92, Thomas 97, Boulton 05), and the 128-Hz tuning fork at the hallux of the foot produces acceptable results (Meijer 05).

The pathogenesis of DPN is complex and similar to that of diabetic microvascular complications (Sheetz 02), with contributions from increased polyol pathway, decreased myoinositol, oxidative stress, nerve hypoxia, increased PKC, increased nonenzymatic glycation, decreased long-chain fatty acid metabolism, and decreased neurotrophism by insulin and GFs (Feldman 03, Vinik 03, Boulton 04, Brusee 04, Boulton 05). It is presumed these processes are operative in pregnancies with poor glycemic control, but there has been little research on this.

Diabetic autonomic neuropathy (DAN) usually affects the long vagus nerves initially and progresses to affect the shorter nerves of the autonomic sympathetic system. Autonomic dysfunctions can be detected in ~40% of patients with type 1 and ~65% of patients with type 2 diabetes (Freccero 04, Low 04). DAN can develop early in the disease process and may involve any system in the body, either clinically or subclinically. Manifestations of DAN include resting tachycardia with exercise intolerance, postural hypotension, impaired cutaneous blood flow regulation (Vinik 03), gastroparesis (Camilleri 07), diarrhea, constipation (Bytzer 01, De Block 02, Samsom 03), genitourinary dysfunction, hypoglycemia unawareness, and diminished counterregulatory responses to hypoglycemia (Boulton 05). These complications are associated with significant morbidity; once CAN becomes symptomatic, the mortality rate may be as high as 50% within 5 years (Vinik 03). The pooled RR for subsequent mortality for studies that defined CAN with at least two abnormalities was 3.45 (95% CI 2.66–4.47; $p < 0.001$) in a recent meta-analysis (Maser 03). CAN and predominance of sympathetic activity are associated with blunted nocturnal fall in diastolic BP (nondipper phenomenon), which is linked to a higher degree of target organ damage in normotensive and hypertensive subjects (Palatini 92, Spallone 93, Pecis 00). CAN is discussed further in the section titled "Cardiovascular Disease in Diabetic Women."

Diabetic Neuropathies and Pregnancy

Very little is known about the effects of pregnancy on the natural course of neuropathies or their effects on the course and outcome of pregnancy. In asymptomatic patients, specific tests are required to diagnose autonomic neuropathy involving the cardiovascular system. Although these tests are not routinely performed during pregnancy, they should be considered, especially when risk factors for CVD are evident. Autonomic neuropathy involving the gastrointestinal system may also be difficult to determine during pregnancy because nausea, vomiting, and constipation are common symptoms of normal pregnancy. Thus, the reported prevalence of diabetic neuropathy in pregnancy varies widely between 8.5–32% (Airaksinen 93, Djelmis 03, Lapolla 03).

In the absence of prospective studies on the effect of pregnancy on the natural history of diabetic neuropathy, information has been derived mainly from retrospective and cohort studies with all of their inherent biases. In a nested study comparing nulliparous and parous women with type 1 diabetes, the incidence of DPN was almost ten times higher in the group of women who completed a pregnancy within the previous 2 years compared with control subjects who did not complete a pregnancy during that time (Hemachandra 95); however, no difference occurred between the groups after a 4-year follow-up period. These findings suggest that a short-term increase in the incidence of polyneuropathy may occur in association with pregnancy, but that pregnancy is not associated with an increase in the prevalence of this complication in the long term. In contrast, a smaller study from Italy suggested that pregnancy is not associated with short-term worsening of peripheral neuropathy and that motor conduction velocity actually improves progressively during the course of pregnancy (Lapolla 98).

Female gender has been found to be an independent risk factor for autonomic neuropathy in type 1 diabetes, but the contribution of pregnancy to this increased risk was not singled out (Maser 90). In contrast, a cross-sectional study in 117 women with type 1 diabetes showed that previous pregnancy is not a risk factor for development or deterioration of DAN (Airaksinen 93). Similarly, a cross-sectional study comparing 776 nulliparous and 582 parous women with type 1 diabetes found that the orthostatic decrease in systolic BP, a measure of autonomic neuropathy, was significantly less pronounced in parous than in nulliparous women (Chaturvedi 95).

Only limited information can be found on whether symptoms of autonomic neuropathy worsen during pregnancy, and much of the information is derived from isolated case reports. Exacerbation of autonomic neuropathy during pregnancy has been reported by some authors (Steele 89, Macleod 90, Hare 91,94), whereas others have noticed transient improvement in symptoms during pregnancy (Scott 88). Of particular importance is the association of autonomic neuropathy with an increased risk of severe hypoglycemia. Blunted counterregulatory responses to hypoglycemia in women with diabetic neuropathy appear to diminish even further during pregnancy (Diamond 92, Rosenn 96). Indeed, more than two-thirds of pregnant women with type 1 diabetes have at least one episode of severe hypoglycemia, particularly during the first half of pregnancy (Rosenn 95).

The effect of diabetic neuropathy on the outcome of pregnancy is often difficult to separate from other known risk factors for poor pregnancy outcome, such as poor metabolic control and coexisting microvascular disease. However, in a prospective study of 100 women with type 1 diabetes, 23 women were identified with autonomic dysfunction. A complication of pregnancy was more than two times as likely to occur in this group compared with the group with no autonomic dysfunction (Airaksinen 90). Additional limited information on this issue comes from case reports, suggesting an increased risk of poor perinatal outcome (Steele 89, Macleod 90, Hare 91,94). The presence of gastroparesis is particularly relevant in that, with the hyperemesis of pregnancy, it results in exacerbation of nausea and vomiting (Steel 89, Macleod 90, vanStuijvenberg 95, Dodds 06, Fell 06). The result is irregular absorption of nutrients, inadequate nutrition, and aberrant glucose control.

In summary, from the few reports of pregnancy in women with autonomic neuropathies, it seems that pregnancy does not alter the natural course of DAN except for diabetic gastroparesis. Although a successful outcome of the pregnancy is possible in the presence of symptomatic diabetic neuropathy, significant maternal and perinatal morbidity may occur.

Treatment of Diabetic Neuropathies in Pregnancy

Practically no data exist on treatment of diabetic neuropathies during pregnancy. Treatment depends on manifestations of the disease, as is well reviewed in ADA Position Statements and Technical Reviews of diabetic neuropathies (Vinik 03, Boulton 04,05). Two types of pain are associated with DPN: C-fiber pain is characterized by hyperesthesia and burning, and these can be treated by topical application of capsaicin (considered safe in pregnancy) or treatment with clonidine, a category C drug that has not been reported to cause harm in pregnancy. The second type of pain, A-fiber pain, is a more deeply seated ache that does not usually respond to the aforementioned treatments. This pain may respond to treatment with tricyclic antidepressants, such as amitriptyline or nortriptyline. Both are category D drugs because of the possible risk of teratogenicity, but both appear to be relatively safe for use after the first trimester, with some evidence of minimal effects on newborn behavior (Altshuler 96, Heikkinen 01, Gentile 05). Antiepileptic drugs, such as carbamazepine and gabapentin, have also been used effectively in the management of neuropathic pain (Backonja 98, Raja 05); however, as with any antiepileptic drug, use of these medications during pregnancy must take into account their teratogenic potential (McAuley 02, Wilton 02, Montouris 03). In severe cases of DPN, methadone may be useful (Hays 05).

Consultation with cardiology and diabetology specialists should be arranged for comanagement of the unusual pregnant diabetic patient with symptomatic CAN. Management of the more commonly symptomatic gastroparesis consists of adjusting food intake to multiple small feedings and decreasing the amount of fat in the diet. Many patients benefit from treatment with prokinetic agents such as metoclopramide (Reglan), a category B drug that is considered safe for use throughout pregnancy, and domperidone (Boulton 05). Erythromycin, another category B drug considered safe in pregnancy (except for the estolate form), may also be helpful in the treatment of gastroparesis due to its action on the motilin receptor and by shortening gastric emptying time. Severe cases may require chronic TPN.

Recommendations

- All patients should be screened for DPN and autonomic neuropathy at least annually, using simple clinical tests. (B)
- Educate all patients about self-care of the feet. For those with DPN, facilitate enhanced foot care education and refer for special footware. Counsel women with diabetes that pregnancy does not appear to increase the risk for development or progression of distal sensorimotor or DANs except for transient but possible severe effects on gastroparesis. (B)
- Advise women with gastroparesis that this complication is associated with a high risk of morbidity and a risk of poor perinatal outcome. Apply standard medications for hyperemesis and nutritional support as needed. (C)
- Advise women with chronic sensorimotor DPN or CAN that these conditions may be associated with an increased risk of perinatal complications and will require cautious management. (B)
- Assess the presence of clinically diminished counterregulatory responses to hypoglycemia, and educate patients to minimize its occurrence. (E)
- Treat symptomatic diabetic women with DPN, CAN, or gastrointestinal autonomic neuropathies as appropriate for pregnancy. (E)

Part 2 Reference

Abalos E, Duley L, Steyn DW, Henderson-Smart DJ: Antihypertensive drug therapy for mild to moderate hypertension during pregnancy (Cochrane Review). In: *The Cochrane Library*, Issue 2. Chichester, UK: John Wiley & Sons, Ltd.; 2004.

Abalos E, Duley L, Steyn D, Henderson-Smart DJ: Antihypertensive drug therapy for mild to moderate hypertension during pregnancy. *Cochrane Database Syst Rev* 2007 Jan 24;(1):CD002252.

Abalovich M, Guttierrez S, Alcaraz G, Maccallini G, Garcia A, Levalle O: Overt and subclinical hypothyroidism complicating pregnancy. *Thyroid* 12:63–68, 2002.

Abalovich M, Amino N, Barbour LA, Cobin RH, De Groot LJ, Glinoer D, Mandel SJ, Stagnaro-Green A: Management of thyroid dysfunction during pregnancy and postpartum: an Endocrine Society Clinical Practice Guideline. *J Clin Endocrinol Metab* 92:(Suppl 8):S1–S47, 2007.

Abbate M, Zoja C, Remuzzi G: How does proteinuria cause progressive renal damage? *J Am Soc Nephrol* 17:2974–2984, 2006.

Abe K, Honein MA, Moore CA: Maternal febrile illnesses, medication use, and the risk of congenital renal anomalies. *Birth Defects Res A Clin Mol Teratol* 67: 911–918, 2003.

Abraha A, Schiltz C, Konopelska-Bahu T, James T, Watts A, Stratton IM, Matthews DR, Dunger DB: Glycemic control and familial factors determine hyperlipidemia in early childhood diabetes. Oxford Regional Prospective Study of Childhood Diabetes. *Diabet Med* 16:598–604, 1999.

Abuhamad AZ, Fisher DA, Warsof SL, Slotnick RN, Pyle PG, Wu SY, Evans AT: Antenatal diagnosis and treatment of fetal goitrous hypothyroidism: case report and review of the literature. *Ultrasound Obstet Gynecol* 6:368–371, 1995.

ACCORD Study Group: The ACCORD trial: a multidisciplinary approach to control cardiovascular risk in type 2 diabetes mellitus. *Pract Diabetol* 23:6–11, 2004.

ACOG—American College of Obstetricians and Gynecologists: Chronic hypertension in pregnancy. Practice Bulletin # 29. *Obstet Gynecol* 98:177–185, 2001.

ACOG—American College of Obstetrics and Gynecology: Clinical management guidelines for obstetrician-gynecologists. ACOG Practice Bulletin # 37. *Obstet Gynecol* 100:387–396, 2002a.

ACOG—American College of Obstetricians and Gynecologists: Diagnosis and management of preeclampsia and eclampsia. Practice Bulletin # 33. *Obstet Gynecol* 99:159–166, 2002b.

ACOG—American College of Obstetricians and Gynecologists: Pregestational diabetes mellitus. Clinical management guidelines for obstetrician-gynecologists. ACOG Practice Bulletin # 60. *Obstet Gynecol* 105:675–683, 2005.

ADA—American Diabetes Association/American Academy of Neurology: Report and recommendations of the San Antonio conference on diabetic neuropathy. Consensus statement. *Diabetes Care* 11:592–597, 1988.

ADA—American Diabetes Association; Asbury AK, Porte D Jr, Griffin J, Ward JD, Sima AAF, Albers JW, Kimura J, Arezzo KJ, Rendell M, Vinik A, de Tejada IS (chairs); Kahn R (staff): Proceedings of a consensus development conference on standardized measures in diabetic neuropathy. *Diabetes Care* 15 (Suppl 3):1080–1107, 1992.

ADA—American Diabetes Association: Consensus development conference on the diagnosis of coronary heart disease in people with diabetes: 10–11 February 1998, Miami, Florida. *Diabetes Care* 21:1551–1559, 1998.

ADA—American Diabetes Association; National Heart, Lung, and Blood Institute; Juvenile Diabetes Foundation International; National Institute of Diabetes and Digestive and Kidney Diseases; American Heart Association: Diabetes mellitus: a major risk factor for cardiovascular disease. A joint editorial statement. *Circulation* 100:1132–1133, 1999.

ADA—American Diabetes Association Consensus Panel; Sheehan P, Edmonds M, Januzzi JL, Regensteiner J, Sanders L, Sykes M: Peripheral arterial disease in people with diabetes. Consensus statement. *Diabetes Care* 26:3333–3341, 2003.

ADA—American Diabetes Association: Hyperglycemic crises in diabetes. Position statement. *Diabetes Care* 27:S94–S102, 2004a.

ADA—American Diabetes Association: Hypertension management in adults with diabetes. Position statement. *Diabetes Care* 27:S65–S67, 2004b.

ADA—American Diabetes Association: Dyslipidemia management in adults with diabetes. Position statement. *Diabetes Care* 27 (Suppl 1):S68–S71, 2004c.

ADA—American Diabetes Association: Nephropathy in diabetes. Position statement. *Diabetes Care* 27 (Suppl 1):S79–S83, 2004d.

ADA—American Diabetes Association: Aspirin therapy in diabetes. Position statement. *Diabetes Care* 27 (Suppl 1):S72–S73, 2004e.

ADA—American Diabetes Association Workgroup on Hypoglycemia: Defining and reporting hypoglycemia in diabetes. *Diabetes Care* 28:1245–1249, 2005.

ADA—American Diabetes Association: Standards of medical care in diabetes—2007. Position statement. *Diabetes Care* 30 (Suppl 1):S4–S36, 2007.

ADA—American Diabetes Association: Standards of medical care in diabetes—2008. Position statement. *Diabetes Care* 31 (Suppl 1):S12–S54, 2008a.

ADA—American Diabetes Association: Nutrition recommendations and interventions for diabetes. A position statement of the American Diabetes Association. *Diabetes Care* 31 (Suppl 1):S61–S78, 2008b.

Adal E, Koyuncu G, Aydin A, Celebi A, Kavunoglu G, Cam H: Asymptomatic cardiomyopathy in children and adolescents with type 1 diabetes mellitus: association of echocardiographic indicators with duration of diabetes mellitus and metabolic parameters. *J Pediatr Endocrinol Metab* 19:713–726, 2006.

Adler AI, Stratton IM, Neil HAW, Yudkin JS, Matthews DR, Cull CA, Wright AD, Turner RC, Holman RR; UK Prospective Diabetes Study Group: Association of systolic blood pressure with macrovascular and microvascular complications of type 2 diabetes (UKPDS 36): prospective observational study. *BMJ* 321:421–419, 2000.

Adler AI, Stevens RJ, Manley SE, Bilous RW, Cull CA, Holman RR; UKPDS Group: Development and progression of nephropathy in type 2 diabetes: the United Kingdom Prospective Diabetes Study (UKPDS 64). *Kidney Int* 63:225–232, 2003.

Aepfelbacher FC, Yeon SB, Weinrauch LA, D'Elia J, Burger AJ: Improved glycemic control induces regression of left ventricular mass in patients with type 1 diabetes mellitus. *Int J Cardiol* 94:47–51, 2004.

Agarwal R, Andersen MJ: Prognostic importance of clinic and home blood pressure recordings in patients with chronic kidney disease. *Kidney Int* 69:406–411, 2006.

Ahmed N, Babaei-Jadidi R, Howell SK, Thornalley PJ, Beisswenger PJ: Glycated and oxidized protein degradation products are indicators of fasting and postprandial hyperglycemia in diabetes. *Diabetes Care* 28:2465–2471, 2005.

Aiello LP, Gardner TW, King GL, Blankenship G, Cavallerano JD, Ferris FL, Klein R: Diabetic retinopathy. Technical review. *Diabetes Care* 21:143–156, 1998.

Aiello LP: Angiogenic pathways in diabetic retinopathy. Editorial. *N Engl J Med* 353:839–841, 2005.

Airaksinen J, Ikaheimo M, Kaila J, Linnaluoto M, Takkunen J: Impaired left ventricular filling in young female diabetics. An echocardiographic study. *Acta Med Scand* 216:509–516, 1984a.

Airaksinen J, Ikaheimo M, Kaila J, Linnaluoto M, Takkunen J: Systolic time intervals and the QT-QS2 interval in young female diabetics. *Ann Clin Res* 16:188–191, 1984b.

Airaksinen KE: Electrocardiogram of young diabetic subjects. *Ann Clin Res* 17: 135–138, 1985.

Airaksinen KE, Ikaheimo MJ, Salmela PI, Kirkinen P, Linnaluoto MK, Takkunen JT: Impaired cardiac adjustment to pregnancy in type 1 diabetes. *Diabetes Care* 9:376–383, 1986.

Airaksinen KE, Salmela PI, Ikaheimo MJ, Kirkinen P, Linnaluoto MK, Takkunen JT: Effect of pregnancy on autonomic nerve function and heart rate in diabetic and nondiabetic women. *Diabetes Care* 10:748–751, 1987a.

Airaksinen KE, Ikaheimo MJ, Linnaluoto MK, Huikuri HV, Takkunen JT: Increased left atrial size relative to left ventricular size in young women with insulin-dependent diabetes: a pre-clinical sign of the specific heart disease of diabetes? *Diabetes Res* 6:37–41, 1987b.

Airaksinen KE, Anttila LM, Linnaluoto MK, Jouppila PI, Takkunen JT, Salmela PI: Autonomic influence on pregnancy outcome in IDDM. *Diabetes Care* 13:756–761, 1990.

Airaksinen KE, Salmela PI: Pregnancy is not a risk factor for a deterioration of autonomic nervous function in diabetic women. *Diabet Med* 10:540–542, 1993.

Airaksinen KE, Kirkinen P, Takkunen JT: Autonomic nervous dysfunction in severe pre-eclampsia. *Eur J Obstet Gynecol Reprod Biol* 19:269–276, 1995.

Akbari A, Lepage N, Keely E, Clark HD, Jaffey J, MacKinnon M, Filler G: Cystatin-C and beta trace protein as markers of renal function in pregnancy. *BJOG* 112:575–578, 2005.

Akcakus M, Kokiu E, Baykan A, Yikilmaz A, Coskun A, Gunes T, Kurtoglu S, Narin N: Macrosomic newborns of diabetic mothers are associated with increased aortic intima-media thickness and lipid concentrations. *Horm Res* 67:277–283, 2007.

Akram K, Pedersen-Bjergaard U, Carstensen B, Borch-Johnsen K, Thorsteinsson B: Frequency and risk factors of severe hypoglycemia in insulin-treated type 2 diabetes: a cross-sectional survey. *Diabet Med* 23:750–756, 2006.

Ala-Kokko TI, Pienimaki P, Lampela E, Hollmen AI, Pelkonen O, Vahakangas K: Transfer of clonidine and dexmedetomidine across the isolated perfused human placenta. *Acta Anaesthesiol Scand* 41:313–319, 1997.

Albergati F, Paterno E, Venuti RP, Lombardo I, Semino S, Viviani GL, Adezati L: Comparison of the effects of carvedilol and nifedipine in patients with essential hypertension and non-insulin-dependent diabetes mellitus. *J Cardiovasc Pharmacol* 19 (Suppl 1):S86–S89, 1992.

Albers JJ, Wolfbauer G, Cheung MC, Day JR, Ching AFT, Lok S, Tu A-Y: Functional expression of human and mouse plasma phospholipid transfer protein: effect of recombinant and plasma PLTP on HDL subspecies. *Biochim Biophys Acta* 1258:27–34, 1995.

Alderman M, Aiyer KJ: Uric acid: role in cardiovascular disease and effects of losartan. *Curr Med Res Opin* 20:369–379, 2004.

Alexander EK, Marqusee E, Lawrence J, Jarolim P, Fischer GA, Larsen PR: Timing and magnitude of increases in levothyroxine requirements during pregnancy in women with hypothyroidism. *N Engl J Med* 351:241–249, 2004.

Algenstaedt P, Schaefer C, Biermann T, Hamann A, Schwarzloh B, Greten H, Ruther W, Hansen-Algenstaedt N: Microvascular alterations in diabetic mice correlate with level of hyperglycemia. *Diabetes* 52:542–549, 2003.

Allan WC, Haddow JE, Palomaki GE, Williams JR, Mitchell ML, Hermos RJ, Faix JD, Klein RZ: Maternal thyroid deficiency and pregnancy complications: implications for population screening. *J Med Screen* 7:127–130, 2000.

Altshuler LL, Cohen L, Szuba MP, Burt VK, Gitlin M, Mintz J: Pharmacologic management of psychiatric illness during pregnancy: dilemmas and guidelines. *Am J Psychiatry* 153:592–606, 1996.

Alvarez JJ, Montelongo A, Iglesias A, Lasuncion MA, Herrera E: Longitudinal study on lipoprotein profile, high density lipoprotein subclass, and postheparin lipases during gestation in women. *J Lipid Res* 37:299–308, 1996.

Alvarez-Marfany M, Roman SH, Drexler AJ, Robertson C, Stagnaro-Green A: Long-term prospective study of postpartum thyroid dysfunction in women with insulin-dependent diabetes mellitus. *J Clin Endocrinol Metab* 79:10–16, 1994.

Alwan S, Polifka JE, Friedman JM: Angiotensin II receptor antagonist treatment during pregnancy. *Birth Defects Res A Clin Mol Teratol* 73:123–130, 2005.

Amiel SA, Tamborlane WV, Simonson DC, Sherwin RS: Defective glucose counterregulation after strict control of insulin-dependent diabetes mellitus. *N Engl J Med* 316:1376–1383, 1987.

Amiel S, Maran A, Powne J, Umpleby A, Macdonald L: Gender differences in counterregulation to hypoglycemia. *Diabetologia* 36:460–464, 1993a.

Amiel SA, Gale E: Physiological responses to hypoglycemia. Counterregulation and cognitive function. *Diabetes Care* 16 (Suppl 3):48–55, 1993b.

Amiel SA: Limits of normality: the mechanisms of hypoglycemia unawareness. R.D. Lawrence Lecture 1994. *Diabet Med* 11:918–924, 1994.

Amin R, Turner C, van Aken S, Bahu TK, Watts A, Lindsell DR, Dalton RN, Dunger DB: The relationship between microalbuminuria and glomerular filtration rate in young type 1 diabetic subjects: the Oxford Regional Prospective Study. *Kidney Int* 68:1740–1749, 2005.

Amthor KF, Dahl-Jorgensen K, Berg TJ, Heier MS, Sandvik L, Aagenaes O, Hanssen KF: The effect of 8 years of strict glycemic control on peripheral nerve function in IDDM patients: the Oslo Study. *Diabetologia* 37:579–584, 1994.

An D, Rodrigues B: Role of changes in cardiac metabolism in development of diabetic cardiomyopathy. *Am J Physiol* 291:H1489–H1506, 2006.

Anand DV, Lim E, Hopkins D, Corder R, Shaw LJ, Sharp P, Lipkin D, Lahiri A: Risk stratification in uncomplicated type 2 diabetes: prospective evaluation of the combined use of coronary artery calcium imaging and selective myocardial perfusion scintigraphy. *Eur Heart J* 27:713–721, 2006.

Andersen S, Blouch K, Bialek J, Deckert M, Parving H-H, Myers BD: Glomerular permselectivity in early stages of overt diabetic nephropathy. *Kidney Int* 58:2129–2137, 2000.

Andersen S, Pedersen KM, Bruun NH, Laurberg P: Narrow individual variations in serum T(4) and T(3) in normal subjects: a clue to the understanding of subclinical thyroid disease. *J Clin Endocrinol Metab* 87:1068–1072, 2002.

Andersen NH, Poulsen SH, Poulsen PL, Knudsen ST, Helleberg K, Hansen KW, Berg TJ, Flyvbjerg A, Mogensen CE: Left ventricular dysfunction in hypertensive patients with type 2 diabetes mellitus. *Diabet Med* 22:1218–1225, 2005a.

Andersen NH, Poulsen SH, Knudsen ST, Heickendorff L, Mogensen CE: NT-proBNP in normalbuminuric patients with type 2 diabetes mellitus. *Diabet Med* 22:188–195, 2005b.

Andersen MJ, Khawandi W, Agarwal R: Home blood pressure monitoring in CKD. *Am J Kidney Dis* 45:994–1001, 2005c.

Andersson DKG, Svardsudd K: Long-term glycemic control relates to mortality in type II diabetes. *Diabetes Care* 18:1534–1543, 1995.

Andren L, Hoglund P, Dotevall A, Eggertsen R, Svensson A, Olson S-O, Wadenvik H: Diltiazem in hypertensive patients with type II diabetes mellitus. *Am J Cardiol* 62:114G–120G, 1988.

Andros V, Egger A, Dua U: Blood pressure goal attainment according to JNC 7 guidelines and utilization of antihypertensive drug therapy in MCO patients with type 1 or 2 diabetes. *J Manag Care Pharm* 12:303–309, 2006.

Angiolillo DJ, Fernandez-Ortiz A, Bernardo E, Ramirez C, Sabate M, Jimenez-Quevedo P, Hernandez R, Moreno R, Escaned J, Alfonso F, Banuelos C, Costa MA, Bass TA, Macaya C: Platelet function profiles in patients with type 2 diabetes and coronary artery disease on combined aspirin and clopidogrel treatment. *Diabetes* 54:2430–2435, 2005.

Anjeneyulu M, Chopra K: Diltiazem attenuates oxidative stress in diabetic rats. *Ren Fail* 27:335–344, 2005.

Aoki Y, Belin RM, Clickner R, Jeffries R, Phillips L, Mahaffey KR: Serum TSH and total T4 in the United States population and their association with participant characteristics: National Health and Nutrition Examination Survey (NHANES 1999–2002). *Thyroid* 17:1211–1223, 2007.

Antolic B, Gersak K, Verdenik I, Novak-Antolic Z: Adverse effects of thyroid dysfunction on pregnancy and pregnancy outcome: epidemiologic study in Slovenia. *J Matern Fetal Neonatal Med* 19:651–654, 2006.

Appel LJ, Brands MW, Daniels SR, Karanja N, Elmer PJ, Sacks FM: Dietary approaches to prevent and treat hypertension. A scientific statement from the American Heart Association. *Hypertension* 47:296–308, 2006.

Araki S, Haneda M, Sugimoto T, Isono M, Isshiki K, Kashiwagi A, Koya D: Factors associated with frequent remission of microalbuminuria in patients with type 2 diabetes. *Diabetes* 54:2983–2987, 2005.

Araki S, Haneda M, Koya D, Hidaka H, Sugimoto T, Isono M, Isshiki K, Chin-Kanasaki M, Uzu T, Kashiwagi A: Reduction in microalbuminuria as an integrated indicator for renal and cardiovascular risk reduction in patients with type 2 diabetes. *Diabetes* 56:1727–1730, 2007.

Arauz-Pacheco C, Parrott MA, Raskin P: The treatment of hypertension in patients with diabetes. Technical review. *Diabetes Care* 25: 134–147, 2002.

Arias F, Zamora J: Antihypertensive treatment and pregnancy outcome in patients with mild chronic hypertension. *Obstet Gynecol* 53:489–494, 1979.

Armenti VT, Ahlswede KM, Ahlswede BA, Jarrell BE, Moritz MJ, Burke JF: National Transplantation Pregnancy Registry—outcomes of 154 pregnancies in cyclosporine-treated female kidney transplant recipients. *Transplantation* 57:502–506, 1994.

Armenti VT, Ahlswede KM, Ahlswede BA, Cater JR, Jarrell BE, Mortiz MJ, Burke JF Jr: Variables affecting birthweight and graft survival in 197 pregnancies in cyclosporine-treated female kidney transplant recipients. *Transplantation* 59: 476–479, 1995.

Armenti VT, McGrory CH, Cater J, Radomski JS, Jarrell BE, Moritz MJ: The National Transplantation Pregnancy Registry: comparison between pregnancy outcomes in diabetic cyclosporine-treated female kidney recipients and CyA-treated female pancreas-kidney recipients. *Transplant Proc* 29:669–670, 1997.

Armenti VT, Radomski JS, Moritz MJ, Phillips LZ, McGrory CH, Coscia LA: Report from the National Transplantation Pregnancy Registry (NTPR): outcomes of pregnancy after transplantation. *Clin Transpl* 123–134, 2000.

Armenti VT, Moritz MJ, Cardonick EH, Davison JM: Immunosuppression in pregnancy: choices for infant and maternal health. *Drugs* 62:2361–2375, 2002.

Armenti VT, Daller JA, Constantinescu S, Silva P, Radomski JS, Moritz MJ, Gaughan WJ, McGrory CH, Coscia LA: Report from the National Transplantation Pregnancy Registry: outcomes of pregnancy after transplantation. *Clin Transpl* 57–70, 2006.

Arnadottir GA, Geirsson RT, Arngrisson R, Jonsdottir LS, Olafsson O: Cardiovascular death in women who had hypertension in pregnancy: a case-control study. *BJOG* 112:286–292, 2005.

Arnestad M, Crotti L, Rognum TO, Insolia R, Pedrazzini M, Ferrandi C, Vege A, Wang DW, Rhodes TE, George AL Jr, Schwartz PJ: Prevalence of long-QT syndrome gene variants in sudden infant death syndrome. *Circulation* 115:361–367, 2007.

Ascarelli MH, Grider AR, Hsu HW: Acute myocardial infarction during pregnancy managed with immediate percutaneous transluminal coronary angioplasty. *Obstet Gynecol* 88:655–657, 1996.

Ashe RG, Moodley, Richards AM, Philpott RH: Comparison of labetalol and dihydralazine in hypertensive emergencies of pregnancy. *S Afr Med J* 71: 354–356, 1987.

Asher UA, Ben-Shlomo I, Said M, Nabil H: The effects of exercise induced tachycardia on the maternal electrocardiogram. *Br J Obstet Gynecol* 100:41–45, 1993.

Astrup AS, Tarnow L, Rossing P, Pietraszek L, Riis Hansen P, Parving HH: Improved prognosis in type 1 diabetic patients with nephropathy: a prospective follow-up study. *Kidney Int* 68:1250–1257, 2005.

Astrup AS, Tarnow L, Rossing P, Hansen BV, Hilsted J, Parving HH: Cardiac autonomic neuropathy predicts cardiovascular morbidity and mortality in type 1 diabetic patients with diabetic nephropathy. *Diabetes Care* 29:334–336, 2006.

ATC—Antithrombotic Trialists' Collaboration: Collaboration meta-analysis of randomized trials of anti-platelet therapy for prevention of death, myocardial infarction, and stroke in high risk patients. *BMJ* 324:71–86, 2002.

Atisha D, Bhalla MA, Morrison LK, Felicio L, Clopton P, Gardetto N, Kazanegra R, Chiu A, Maisel AS: A prospective study in search of an optimal B-natriuretic peptide level to screen patients for cardiac dysfunction. *Am Heart J* 148:518–523, 2004.

Attia N, Touzani A, Lahrichi M, Balafrej A, Kabbaj O, Girard-Globa A: Response of apoprotein A-IV and lipoproteins to glycemic control in young people with insulin-dependent diabetes mellitus. *Diabet Med* 14:242–247, 1997.

August P, Helseth G, Cook EF, Sison C: A prediction model for superimposed preeclampsia in women with chronic hypertension during pregnancy. *Am J Obstet Gynecol* 191:1666–1672, 2004.

Aurigemma GP: Diastolic heart failure—a common and lethal condition by any name. Editorial. *N Engl J Med* 355:308–310, 2006.

Auso E, Lavado-Autric R, Cuevas E, Excobar del Rey F: A moderate and transient deficiency of maternal thyroid function at the beginning of fetal neocorticogenesis alters neuronal migration. *Endocrinology* 145:4037–4047, 2004.

Axer-Siegel R, Hod M, Fink-Cohen S, Kramer M, Weinberger D, Schindel B, Yassur Y: Diabetic retinopathy during pregnancy. *Ophthalmology* 103:1815–1819, 1996.

Aya AG, Mangin R, Hoffet M, Eledjam JJ: Intravenous nicardipine for severe hypertension in pre-eclampsia—effects of an acute treatment on mother and foetus. *Intensive Care Med* 25:1277–1281, 1999.

Ayyar DR, Sharma KR: Chronic demyelinating polyradiculoneuropathy in diabetes. *Curr Diab Rep* 4:409–412, 2004.

Azizi F, Khoshniat M, Bahrainian M, Hedayani M: Thyroid function and intellectual development of infants nursed by mothers taking methimazole. *J Clin Endocrinol Metab* 85:3233–3238, 2000.

Babay Z, Wakeel JA, Addar M, Mittwalli A, Tariff N, Hammad D, Askar AA, Choudhary AR: Serum cystatin C in pregnant women: reference values, reliable and superior diagnostic accuracy. *Clin Exp Obstet Gynecol* 32:175–179, 2005.

Bacci S, Villella M, Villella A, Langialonga T, Grili M, Rauseo A, Mastroianno S, De Cosmo S, Fanelli R, Trischitta V: Screening for silent myocardial ischaemia in type 2 diabetic patients with additional atherogenic risk factors: applicability and accuracy of the exercise stress test. *Eur J Endocrinol* 147:649–654, 2002.

Backonja M, Beydoun A, Edwards KR, Schwartz SL, Fonseca V, Hes M, LaMoreaux L, Garofalo E; for the Gabapentin Diabetic Neuropathy Study Group: Gabapentin for the symptomatic treatment of painful neuropathy in patients with diabetes mellitus. A randomized controlled trial. *JAMA* 280:1831–1836, 1998.

Badawi N, Kurinczuk JJ, Mackenzie CL, Keogh JM, Burton PR, Pemberton PJ, Stanley FJ: Maternal thyroid disease: a risk factor for newborn encephalopathy in term infants. *Br J Obstet Gynecol* 107:798–801, 2000.

Badenhoop K, Boehm BO: Genetic susceptibility and immunological synapse in type 1 diabetes and thyroid autoimmune disease. *Exp Clin Endocrinol Diabetes* 112:407–415, 2004.

Bagamery K, Kovacs L, Nyari T, Falkay G: Do α2–adrenergic receptors and imidazoline binding sites coexist in the human term placenta? Evidence from direct binding studies. *Mol Hum Reprod* 4:384–391, 1998.

Bagamery K, Kovacs L, Viski S, Nyari T, Falkay G: Ontogeny of imidazoline binding sites in the human placenta. *Acta Obstet Gynecol Scand* 78:89–92, 1999.

Bagg W, Henley PG, Macpherson P, Cundy TP: Pregnancy in women with diabetes and ischemic heart disease. *Aust NZ J Obstet Gynecol* 39:99–102, 1999.

Bagg W, Neale L, Henley P, MacPherson P, Cundy T: Long-term maternal outcome after pregnancy in women with diabetic nephropathy. *N Z Med J* 116:U566, 2003.

Bagis T, Gokcel A, Saygili ES: Autoimmune thyroid disease in pregnancy and the postpartum period: relationship to spontaneous abortion. *Thyroid* 11:1049–1053, 2001.

Bagon JA, Vernaeve H, De Muylder X, Lafontaine JJ, Martens J, Van Roost G: Pregnancy and dialysis. *Am J Kidney Dis* 31:756–765, 1998.

Bairey-Merz CN, Shaw LJ, Reis SE, Bittner V, Kelsey SF, Olson M, Johnson BD, Pepine CJ, Mankad S, Sharaf BL, Rogers WJ, Pohost GM, Lerman A, Quyyumi AA, Sopko G: WISE Investigators: insights from the NHLBI-sponsored Women's Ischemia Syndrome Evaluation (WISE) study. Part II: gender differences in presentation, diagnosis, and outcome with regard to gender-based pathophysiology of atherosclerosis and macrovascular and microvascular coronary disease. *J Am Coll Cardiol* 47 (Suppl 3):S21–S29, 2006.

Baker JF, Krishnan E, Chen L, Schumacher HR: Serum uric acid and cardiovascular disease: recent developments, and where do they leave us? *Am J Med* 118: 816–826, 2005.

Bakker AJ: Detection of microalbuminuria. Receiver operating characteristic curve analysis favors albumin-to-creatinine ratio over albumin concentration. *Diabetes Care* 22:307–313, 1999.

Bakker SJL, ter Maaten JC, Popp-Snijders C, Slaets JPJ, Heine RJ, Gans ROB: The relationship between thyrotropin and low density lipoprotein cholesterol is modified by insulin sensitivity in healthy euthyroid subjects. *J Clin Endocrinol Metab* 86:1206–1211, 2001.

Bakris GL, Mangrum A, Copley JB, Vicknair N, Sadler R: Effect of calcium channel or beta-blockade on the progression of diabetic nephropathy in African-Americans. *Hypertension* 29:744–750, 1997.

Bakris GL, Williams M, Dworkin L, Elliott WJ, Epstein M, Toto R, Tuttle K, Douglas J, Hsueh W, Sowers J; for the National Kidney Foundation Hypertension and Diabetes Executive Committees Working Group: Preserving renal function in adults with hypertension and diabetes: a consensus approach. Position statement. *Am J Kidney Dis* 36:646–661, 2000.

Bakris GL, Weir MR: Achieving goal blood pressure in participants with type 2 diabetes: conventional versus fixed-dose combination approaches. *J Clin Hypertens* 5:202–209, 2003a.

Bakris GL, Weir MR, Shahinfar S, Zhang Z, Douglas J, van Dijk DJ, Brenner BM; RENAAL Study Group: Effects of blood pressure level on progression of diabetic nephropathy: results from the RENAAL study. *Arch Intern Med* 163:1555–1565, 2003b.

Bakris GL, Bakris G, Efrain-Messerli FH, Mancia G, Erdine S, Cooper-Dehoff R, Pepine CJ: Clinical outcomes in the diabetes cohort of the INVEST. *Hypertension* 44:637–642, 2004a.

Bakris GL, Weir MR, Secic M, Campbell B, Weis-McNulty A: Differential effects of calcium antagonist subclasses on markers of nephropathy progression. *Kidney Int* 65:1991–2002, 2004b.

Bakris GL, Fonseca V, Katholi RE, McGill JB, Messerli FH, Phillips RA, Raskin P, Wright JT Jr, Oakes R, Lukas MA, Anderson KM, Bell DSH; for the GEMINI Investigators: Metabolic effects of carvedilol vs metoprolol in patients with type 2 diabetes mellitus and hypertension. A randomized controlled trial. *JAMA* 292:2227–2236, 2004c.

Bakris GL, Fonseca V, Katholi RE, McGill JB, Messerli F, Phillips RA, Raskin P, Wright JT Jr, Waterhouse B, Likas MA, Anderson KM, Bell DSH; the GEMINI

Investigators: Differential effects of β-blockers on albuminuria in patients with type 2 diabetes. *Hypertension* 46:1309–1315, 2005.

Bakris GL: Slowing nephropathy progression: focus on proteinuria reduction. *Clin J Am Soc Nephrol* 3:S3–S10, 2008.

Balasubramanyam A, Zern JW, Hyman DJ, Pavlik V: New profiles of diabetic ketoacidosis: type 1 and type 2 diabetes and the effect of ethnicity. *Arch Intern Med* 159:2317–2322, 1999.

Balasubramanyam A, Garza G, Rodriguez L, Hampe CS, Gaur L, Lernmark A, Maldonado MR: Accuracy and predictive value of classification schemes for ketosis-prone diabetes. *Diabetes Care* 29:2575–2579, 2006.

Baloch Z, Carayon P, Conte-Devolx B, Demers LM, Feldt-Rasmussen U, Henry JF, LiVosli VA, Niccoli-Sire P, John R, Ruf J, Smyth PP, Spencer CA, Stockigt JR: Laboratory support for the diagnosis and monitoring of thyroid disease. Laboratory medicine practice guidelines. *Thyroid* 13:3–126, 2003.

Bar J, Hod M, Erman A, Friedman S, Ovadia Y: Microalbuminuria: prognostic and therapeutic implications in diabetic and hypertensive pregnancy. *Diabet Med* 48:649–656, 1995.

Bar J, Chen R, Schoenfeld A, Orvieto R, Yahav J, Ben-Rafael Z, Hod M: Pregnancy outcome in patients with insulin dependent diabetes mellitus and diabetic nephropathy treated with ACE inhibitors before pregnancy. *J Ped Endocrinol Metab* 12:659–665, 1999.

Bar J, Ben-Rafael Z, Padoa A, Orvieto R, Boner G, Hod M: Prediction of pregnancy outcome in subgroups of women with renal disease. *Clin Nephrol* 53:437–444, 2000.

Bar-David J, Mazor M, Leiberman JR, Ielig I, Maislos M: Gestational diabetes complicated by severe hypertriglyceridemia and acute pancreatitis. *Arch Gynecol Obstet* 258:101–104, 1996.

Barker JM: Clinical review: type 1 diabetes-associated autoimmunity: natural history, genetic associations, and screening. *J Clin Endocrinol Metab* 91:1210–1217, 2006.

Barnett SB, Maulik D; International Perinatal Doppler Society: Guidelines and recommendations for safe use of Doppler ultrasound in perinatal applications. *J Matern-Fetal Med* 10:75–84, 2001.

Barova H, Perusicova J, Hill M, Sterzl I, Vondra K, Masek Z: Anti-GAD-positive patients with type 1 diabetes mellitus have higher prevalence of autoimmune thyroiditis than anti-GAD-negative patients with type 1 and type 2 diabetes mellitus. *Physiol Res* 53:279–286, 2004.

Bar-Oz B, Hackman R, Einarson T, Koren G: Pregnancy outcome after cyclosporine therapy during pregnancy: a meta-analysis. *Transplantation* 71:1051–1055, 2001.

Barr M, Cohen MM: ACE inhibitor fetopathy and hypocalvaria: the kidney-skull connection. *Teratology* 44:485–495, 1991.

Barr M: Teratogen update: angiotensin-converting enzyme inhibitors. *Teratology* 50:399–409, 1994.

Barrett-Connor EL, Cohn BA, Wingard DL, Cohn BA, Edelstein SL: Why is diabetes mellitus a stronger risk factor for fatal ischemic heart disease in women than men? The Rancho Bernardo Study. *JAMA* 265:627–631, 1991.

Barrett-Connor E, Giardina E-G V, Gitt A, Gudat U, Steinberg HO, Tschoepe D: Women and heart disease. The role of diabetes and hyperglycemia. *Arch Intern Med* 164:934–942, 2004.

Barrou BM, Gruessner AC, Sutherland DE, Gruessner RW: Pregnancy after pancreas transplantation in the cyclosporine era: report from the International Pancreas Transplant Registry. *Transplantation* 65:524–527, 1998.

Bartels PA, Hanff LM, Mathot RAA, Steegers EAP, Vulto AG, Visser W: Nicardipine in pre-eclamptic patients: placental transfer and disposition in breast milk. *BJOG* 114:230–233, 2007.

Barter PJ, Nicholls S, Rye KA, Anantharamaiah GM, Navab M, Fogelman AM: Antiinflammatory properties of HDL. *Circ Res* 95:764–772, 2004.

Barter PJ, Puranik R, Rye KA: New insights into the role of HDL as an anti-inflammatory agent in the prevention of cardiovascular disease. *Curr Cardiol Rep* 9:493–498, 2007.

Bartha JL, Romero-Carmona R, Torrejon-Cardoso R, Comino-Delgado R: Insulin, insulin-like growth factor-1, and insulin resistance in women with pregnancy-induced hypertension. *Am J Obstet Gynecol* 187:735–740, 2002.

Barton JR, Prevost RR, Wilson DA, Whybrew WD, Sibai BM: Nifedipine pharmacokinetics and pharmacodynamics during the immediate postpartum period in patients with preeclampsia. *Am J Obstet Gynecol* 165:951–954, 1991.

Barton JR, O'Brien JM, Bergauer NK, Jacques DL, Sibai BM: Mild gestational hypertension remote from term: progression and outcome. *Am J Obstet Gynecol* 184:979–983, 2001.

Basta G, Sironi AM, Lazzerini G, Del Turco S, Buzzigoli E, Casolaro A, Natali A, Ferrannini E, Gastaldelli A: Circulating soluble receptor for advanced glycation end products is inversely associated with glycemic control and S100A12 protein. *J Clin Endocrinol Metab* 91:4628–4634, 2006.

Bastion ML, Barkeh HJ, Muhaya M: Accelerated diabetic retinopathy in pregnancy—a real and present danger. *Med J Malaysia* 60:502–504, 2005.

Baughman KL: B-type natriuretic peptide—a window to the heart. Perspective. *N Engl J Med* 347:158–159, 2002.

Bax JJ, Bonow RO, Tschope D, Inzucchi SE, Barrett E; Global Dialogue Group for the Evaluation of Cardiovascular Risk in Patients with Diabetes: The potential of myocardial perfusion scintigraphy for risk stratification of asymptomatic patients with type 2 diabetes. *J Am Coll Cardiol* 15:754–760, 2006.

Bax JJ, Young LH, Frye RL, Bonow RO, Steinberg HO, Barrett EJ: Screening for coronary artery disease in patients with diabetes. *Diabetes Care* 30:2729–2736, 2007.

Bayliss H, Churchill D, Beevers M, Beevers DG: Anti-hypertensive drugs in pregnancy and fetal growth: evidence for "pharmacological programming" in the first trimester. *Hypertens Preg* 21:161–174, 2002.

Beaton SJ, Nag SS, Gunter MJ, Gleeson JM, Sajjan SS, Alexander CM: Adequacy of glycemic, lipid, and blood pressure management for patients with diabetes in a managed care setting. *Diabetes Care* 27:694–698, 2004.

Bech K, Hoier-Madsen M, Feldt-Rasmussen, Jensen BM, Molsted-Pedersen L, Kuhl C: Thyroid function and autoimmune manifestations in insulin-dependent diabetes mellitus during and after pregnancy. *Acta Endocrinol* 124:534–539, 1991.

Becker DJ, Brown DR, Steranka BH, Drash AL: Phosphate replacement during treatment of diabetic ketosis: effects on calcium and phosphorus homeostasis. *Am J Dis Child* 137:241–246, 1983.

Becker DM, Segal J, Vaidya D, Yanek LR, Herrera-Galeano JE, Bray PF, Moy TF, Becker LC, Faraday N: Sex differences in platelet reactivity and response to low-dose aspirin therapy. *JAMA* 295:1420–1427, 2006.

Beckles GL, Engelgau MM, Narayan KM, Herman WH, Aubert RE, Williamson DF: Population-based assessment of the level of care among adults with diabetes in the U.S. *Diabetes Care* 21:1432–1438, 1998.

Beckman JA, Creager MA, Libby P: Diabetes and atherosclerosis. Epidemiology, pathophysiology, and management. *JAMA* 287:2570–2581, 2002.

Beer S, Golay S, Bardy D, Feihl F, Gaillard RC, Bachmann C, Waeber B, Ruiz J: Increased plasma levels of N-terminal brain natriuretic peptide (NT-proBNP) in type 2 diabetic patients with vascular complications. *Diabetes Metab* 31:567–573, 2005.

Belch JJF, Topol EJ, Agnelli G, Bertrand M, Califf RM, Clement DL, Creager MA, Easton JD, Gavin JR III, Greenland P, Hankey G, Hanrath P, Hirsch AT, Meyer J, Smith SC, Sullivan F, Weber MA; the Prevention of Atherothrombotic Disease Network: Critical issues in peripheral arterial disease detection and management. A call to action. *Arch Intern Med* 163:884–892, 2003.

Bell DSH: Heart failure. The frequent, forgotten, and often fatal complication of diabetes. *Diabetes Care* 26:2433–2441, 2003a.

Bell DSH: Diabetic cardiomyopathy. *Diabetes Care* 26:2949–2951, 2003b.

Beller GA: Noninvasive screening for coronary atherosclerosis and silent ischemia in asymptomatic type 2 diabetic patients: is it appropriate and cost-effective? *J Am Coll Cardiol* 49:1918–1923, 2007.

Bellomo G, Narducci PL, Rondoni F, Pastorelli G, Stangoni G, Angeli G, Verdecchia P: Prognostic value of 24-hour blood pressure in pregnancy. *JAMA* 282: 1447–1452, 1999.

Benedetto C, Zonoca M, Giarola M, Maula V, Chiarolini L, Carandente F: 24-hour blood pressure monitoring to evaluate the effects of nifedipine in pre-eclampsia and in chronic hypertension in pregnancy. *Br J Obstet Gynecol* 104:682–688, 1997.

Benker G, Kotulla P, Kendall-Taylor P, Emrich D, Reinwein D: TSH binding-inhibiting antibodies in hyperthyroidism: relationship to clinical signs and hormone levels. *Clin Endocrinol* 30:19–28, 1989.

Bennet A, Di Angelantonio E, Erqou S, Eiriksdottir G, Sigurdsson G, Woodward M, Rumley A, Lowe GDO, Danesh J, Gudnason V: Lipoprotein(a) levels and risk of future coronary heart disease. *Arch Intern Med* 168:598–608, 2008.

Benoit SR, Mendelsohn AB, Nourjah P, Staffa JA, Graham DJ: Risk factors for prolonged QTc among U.S. adults: Third National Health and Nutrition Examination Survey. *Eur J Cardiovasc Prev Rehabil* 12:363–368, 2005.

Benowitz NL: Antihypertensive agents. In: Katzung BG, ed. *Basic and Clinical Pharmacology.* 9th ed. New York: Lange Medical Books/McGraw-Hill; 2004:160–183.

Berger JS, Roncaglioni MC, Avanzini F, Pangrazzi I, Tognoni G, Brown DL: Aspirin for the primary prevention of cardiovascular events in women and men. A sex-specific meta-analysis of randomized controlled trials. *JAMA* 295:306–313, 2006.

Berlin I, Grimaldi A, Landault C, Zoghbi F, Thervet F, Puech AJ, Legrand JC: Lack of hypoglycemic symptoms and decreased β-adrenergic sensitivity in insulin-dependent diabetic patients. *J Clin Endocrinol Metab* 66:273–278, 1988.

Berlowitz DR, Ash AS, Hickey EC, Glickman M, Friedman R, Kader B: Hypertension management in patients with diabetes: the need for more aggressive therapy. *Diabetes Care* 26:355–359, 2003.

Bernard A, Thielemans N, Lauwerys R, Van M: Selective increase in the urinary excretion of protein 1 (Clara cell protein) and other low molecular weight proteins during normal pregnancy. *Scand J Lab Invest* 52:871–878, 1992.

Bernard S, Serusclat A, Targe F, Charriere S, Roth O, Beaune J, Berthezene F, Moulin P: Incremental predictive value of carotid ultrasonography in the assessment of coronary risk in a cohort of asymptomatic type 2 diabetic subjects. *Diabetes Care* 28:1158–1162, 2005.

Bernroider E, Brehm A, Krssak M, Anderwald C, Trajanoski Z, Cline G, Shulman GI, Roden M: The role of intramyocellular lipids during hypoglycemia in patients with intensively treated type 1 diabetes. *J Clin Endocrinol Metab* 90:5559–5565, 2005.

Bernstein EF, Fronek A: Current status of non-invasive tests in the diagnosis of peripheral arterial disease. *Surg Clin North Am* 62:473–487, 1982.

Bernstein IM, Catalano PM: Ketoacidosis in pregnancy associated with the parenteral administration of terbutaline and betamethasone. A case report. *J Reprod Med* 35:818–820, 1990.

Bertoni AG, Tsai A, Kasper EK, Brancati FL: Diabetes and idiopathic cardiomyopathy. A nation-wide case control study. *Diabetes Care* 26:2791–2795, 2003.

Bertoni AG, Goff DC, D'Agostino RB, Liu K, Hundley WG, Lima JA, Polak JF, Saad MF, Szklo M, Tracy RP, Siscovik DS: Diabetic cardiomyopathy and subclinical cardiovascular disease. The Multi-Ethnic Study of Atherosclerosis (MESA). *Diabetes Care* 29:588–594, 2006.

Best LG, Zhang Y, Lee ET, Yeh J-L, Cowan L, Palmieri V, Roman M, Devereux RB, Fabsitz RR, Tracy RP, Robbins D, Davidson M, Ahmed A, Howard BV: C-reactive protein as a predictor of cardiovascular risk in a population with a high prevalence of diabetes. The Strong Heart Study. *Circulation* 112:1289–1295, 2005.

Betterle C, Zanette F, Pedini B, Presotto F, Rapp LB, Monciotti CM, Rigon F: Clinical and sub-clinical organ-specific autoimmune manifestations in type 1 (insulin-dependent) diabetic patients and their first-degree relatives. *Diabetologia* 26:431–436, 1984.

Beyan H, Ola T, David R, Leslie G: Progression of autoimmune diabetes: slowly progressive insulin-dependent diabetes mellitus or latent autoimmune diabetes of adult. *Ann N Y Acad Sci* 1079:81–89, 2006.

Bhalla MA, Chiang A, Epshteyn VA, Kazanegra R, Bhalla V, Clopton P, Krishnaswamy P, Morrison LK, Chiu A, Gardetto N, Mudaliar S, Edelman SV,

Henry RR, Maisel AS: Prognostic role of B-type natriuretic peptide levels in patients with type 2 diabetes mellitus. *J Am Coll Cardiol* 44:1047–1052, 2004.

Bhatt DL, Marso SP, Hirsch AT, Ringleb RA, Hacke W, Topol EJ: Ampified benefit of clopidogrel versus aspirin in patients with diabetes mellitus. *Am J Cardiol* 90:625–628, 2002.

Bhatt-Mehta V, Deluga KS: Fetal exposure to lisinopril: neonatal manifestations and management. *Pharmacotherapy* 13:515–518, 1993.

Bibbins-Domingo K, Gupta R, Na B, Wu AH, Schiller NB, Whooley MA: N-terminal fragment of the prohormone brain-type natriuretic peptide (NT-proBNP), cardiovascular events, and mortality in patients with stable coronary heart disease. *JAMA* 297:169–176, 2007.

Biesenbach G, Zasgornik J: Incidence of transient nephrotic syndrome during pregnancy in diabetic women with and without pre-existing microalbuminuria. *Br Med J* 299:366–367, 1989.

Biesenbach G, Stoeger H, Zasgornik J: Influence of pregnancy on progression of diabetic nephropathy and subsequent requirement of renal replacement therapy in female type 1 diabetic patients with impaired renal function. *Nephrol Dial Transplant* 7:105–109, 1992.

Biesenbach G, Janko O, Stoeger H, Zasgornik J: Increases in serum lipids during pregnancy in type 1 diabetic women with nephropathy. *Diabet Med* 11:262–267, 1994a.

Biesenbach G, Zasgornik J, Stoeger H, Grafinger P, Hubmann R, Kaiser W, Janko O, Stuby U: Abnormal increases in urinary albumin excretion during pregnancy in IDDM women with pre-existing microalbuminuria. *Diabetologia* 37:905–910, 1994b.

Biesenbach G, Grafinger P, Stoeger H, Zarzgornik J 2nd: How pregnancy influences renal function in nephropathic type 1 diabetic women depends on their pre-conceptional creatinine clearance. *J Nephrol* 12:41–46, 1999.

Biesenbach G, Grafinger P, Zasgornik J, Stoeger H: Perinatal complications and three-year followup of infants of diabetic mothers with diabetic nephropathy stage IV. *Ren Fail* 22:573–580, 2000.

Bigi R, Desideri A, Cortigiani L, Bax JJ, Celegon L, Fiorentini C: Stress echocardiography for risk stratification of diabetic patients with known or suspected coronary artery disease. *Diabetes Care* 24:1596–1601, 2001.

Birn H, Christensen EI: Renal albumin absorption in physiology and pathology. *Kidney Int* 69:440–449, 2006.

Bischof MG, Ludwig C, Hofer A, Kletter K, Krebs M, Stingl H, Nowotny P, Waldhausel W, Roden M: Hormonal and metabolic counterregulation during and after high-dose insulin-induced hypoglycemia in diabetes mellitus type 2. *Horm Metab Res* 32:417–423, 2000.

Bischof MG, Bernroider E, Ludwig C, Kurzemann S, Kletter K, Waldhausl W, Roden M: Effect of near physiologic insulin therapy on hypoglycemia counterregulation in type-1 diabetes. *Horm Res* 56:151–158, 2001.

Bisits A, Madsen G, Knox M, Gill P, Smith R, Yeo G, Kwek K, Daniel M, Leung TN, Cheung K, Chung T, Jones I, Toohill J, Tudehope D, Giles W: The Randomized

Nitric Oxide Tocolysis Trial (RNOTT) for the treatment of preterm labor. *Am J Obstet Gynecol* 191:683–690, 2004.

Bittner V: Angina pectoris. Reversal of the gender gap. Editorial. *Circulation* 117:1505–1507, 2008.

Bjorklund AO, Adamson UK, Almstrom NH, Enocksson EA, Gennser GM, Lins P-ES, Westgren LMR: Effects of hypoglycemia on fetal heart activity and umbilical artery Doppler waveforms in pregnant women with insulin-dependent diabetes mellitus. *Br J Obstet Gynecol* 103:413–420, 1996.

Bjorklund A, Adamson U, Andreasson K, Carlstrom K, Hennen G, Igout A, Lins PE, Westgren M: Hormonal counterregulation and subjective symptoms during induced hypoglycemia in insulin-dependent diabetes mellitus patients during and after pregnancy. *Acta Obstet Gynecol Scand* 77:625–634, 1998.

Bjoro T, Holmen J, Kruger O, Midthjell K, Hunstad K, Schreiner T, Sandnes L, Brochmann H: Prevalence of thyroid disease, thyroid dysfunction and thyroid peroxidase antibodies in a large, unselected population. The Health Study of Nord-Trondelag (HUNT). *Eur J Endocrinol* 143:639–647, 2000.

Blaauw J, van Pampus MG, Van Doormaal JJ, Fokkema MR, Fidier V, Smit AJ, Aarnoudse JG: Increased intima-media thickness after early-onset preeeclampsia. *Obstet Gynecol* 107:1345–1351, 2006.

Black HR, Elliott WJ, Grandits G, Grambsch P, Lucente T, White WB, Neaton JD, Grimm RH Jr, Hansson L, Lacourciere Y, Muller J, Sleight P, Weber MA, Williams G, Wittes J, Zanchetti A, Anders RJ: Principal results of the Controlled Onset Verapamil Investigation of Cardiovascular End Points (CONVINCE) trial. *JAMA* 289:2073–2082, 2003.

Blake GJ, Otvos JD, Rifai N, Ridker PM: Low-density lipoprotein particle concentration and size as determined by nuclear magnetic resonance spectroscopy as predictors of cardiovascular disease in women. *Circulation* 106:193–1937, 2002.

Blea CW, Barnard JM, Magness RR, Phernetton TM, Hendricks SK: Effect of nifedipine on fetal and maternal hemodynamics and blood gases in the pregnant ewe. *Am J Obstet Gynecol* 176:922–930, 1997.

Blechner JN, Stenger VG, Prystowsky H: Blood flow to the human uterus during maternal metabolic acidosis. *Am J Obstet Gynecol* 121:789–794, 1975.

Bobrie G, Chatellier G, Genes N, Clerson P, Vaur L, Vaisse B, Menard J, Mallion J-M: Cardiovascular prognosis of "masked hypertension" detected by blood pressure self-measurement in elderly treated hypertensive patients. *JAMA* 291:1342–1349, 2004.

Boden G, Laakso M: Lipids and glucose in type 2 diabetes. What is the cause and effect? *Diabetes Care* 27:2253–2259, 2004.

Boden WE, O'Rourke RA, Teo KK, Hartigan PM, Maron DJ, Kostuk WJ, Knudtson M, Dada M, Casperson P, Harris CL, Chaitman BR, Shaw L, Gosselin G, Nawaz S, Title LM, Gau G, Blaustein AS, Booth DC, Bates ER, Spertus JA, Berman DS, Mancini GB, Weintraub WS; the COURAGE Trial Research Group: Optimal medical therapy with or without PCI for stable coronary disease. *N Engl J Med* 356:1503–1516, 2007.

Boden-Albala B, Cammack S, Chong J, Wang C, Wright C, Rundek T, Elkind MS, Paik MC, Sacco RL: Diabetes, fasting glucose levels, and the risk of ischemic stroke and vascular events: findings from the Northern Manhattan study (NOMAS). *Diabetes Care* Mar 13 2008 (Epub ahead of print).

Boemi M, Leviev I, Sirolla C, Pieri C, Marra M, James RW: Serum paraoxonase is reduced in type 1 diabetic patients compared to non-diabetic, first degree relatives: influence on the ability of HDL to protect LDL from oxidation. *Atherosclerosis* 155:229–235, 2001.

Bolli GB: How to ameliorate the problem of hypoglycemia in intensive as well as nonintensive treatment of type 1 diabetes. *Diabetes Care* 22 (Suppl 2):B43–B52, 1999.

Bonora E, Tessari R, Micciolo R, Zenere M, Targher G, Padovani R, Falezza G, Muggeo M: Intimal-medial thickness of the carotid artery in nondiabetic and type 1 diabetes patients. *Diabetes Care* 20:627–631, 1997.

Booth GL, Kapral MK, Fung K, Tu JV: Relation between age and cardiovascular disease in men and women with diabetes compared with non-diabetic people: a population-based retrospective study. *Lancet* 368:29–36, 2006.

Borberg C, Gillmer MDG, Beard RW, Oakley NW: Metabolic effects of beta-sympathomimetic drugs and dexamethasone in normal and diabetic pregnancy. *Br J Obstet Gynecol* 85:184–189, 1978.

Borge MA, Tamborlane WV, Shulman GI, Sherwin RS: Local lactate perfusion of the ventromedial hypothalamus suppresses hypoglycemic counterregulation. *Diabetes* 52:663–666, 2003.

Borghi C, Esposti DD, Cassani A, Immordino V, Bovicelli L, Ambrosioni E: The treatment of hypertension in pregnancy. *J Hypertens* 20 (Suppl 2):S52–S56, 2002.

Borgia MV, Pellicelli AM, Medici F, Barbo Cosial J, Cabanero J, Huelmos A, De Paola G, Lionetti M: Left ventricular filling in young patients affected by insulin dependent diabetes mellitus: a stress Doppler echocardiography study. *Minerva Endocrinol* 24:97–102, 1999.

Borow KM, Jaspan JB, Williams KA, Neumann A, Wolinski-Walley P, Lang RM: Myocardial mechanics in young adult patients with diabetes mellitus: effects of altered load, inotropic state and dynamic exercise. *J Am Coll Cardiol* 15:1508–1517, 1990.

Bortolus R, Ricci E, Chatenoud L, Parazzini F: Nifedipine administered in pregnancy: effect on the development of children at 18 months. *Br J Obstet Gynecol* 107:792–794, 2000.

Bosman DR, Winker AS, Marsden JT, MacDougall IC, Watkins PJ: Anemia with erythropoietin deficiency occurs early in diabetic nephropathy. *Diabetes Care* 24:495–499, 2002.

Bossone E, Armstrong WF: Exercise echocardiography: principles, methods and clinical use. *Cardiol Clin North Am* 17:447–460, 1999.

Bostom AG, Dworkin LD: Cystatin C measurement: improved detection of mild decrements in glomerular filtration rate versus creatinine-based measurements? *Am J Kidney Dis* 36:205–207, 2000.

Boulton AJM, Gries FA, Jervell JA: Guidelines for the diagnosis and outpatient management of diabetic peripheral neuropathy. *Diabet Med* 15:508–514, 1998.

Boulton AJM, Malik RA, Arezzo JC, Sosenko JM: Diabetic somatic neuropathies. Technical review. *Diabetes Care* 27:1458–1486, 2004.

Boulton AJM, Vinik AI, Arezzo JC, Bril V, Feldman EL, Freeman R, Malik RA, Maser RE, Sosenko JM, Ziegler D: Diabetic neuropathies. A statement by the American Diabetes Association. *Diabetes Care* 28:956–962, 2005.

Bourget P, Fernandez H, Edouard D, Lesne-Hulin A, Ribou F, Baton-Saint-Mleux C, Lelaider C: Disposition of a new rate controlled formulation of prazosin in the treatment of hypertension during pregnancy: transplacental passage of prazosin. *Eur J Drug Metab Pharmacokinet* 20:233–241, 1995.

Bowden DW, Lange LA, Langefeld CD, Brosnihan KB, Freedman BI, Carr JJ, Wagenknecht LE, Herrington DM: The relationship between C-reactive protein and subclinical cardiovascular disease in the Diabetes Heart Study (DHS). *Am Heart J* 150:1032–1038, 2005.

Bowden DW, Rudock M, Ziegler J, Lehtinen AB, Xu J, Wagenknecht LE, Herrington D, Rich SS, Freedman BI, Carr JJ, Langefeld CD: Coincident linkage of type 2 diabetes, metabolic syndrome, and measures of cardiovascular disease in a genome scan of the Diabetes Heart Study. *Diabetes* 55:1985–1994, 2006.

Bowen ME, Ray WA, Arbogast PG, Ding H, Cooper WO: Increasing exposure to angiotensin-converting enzyme inhibitors in pregnancy. *Am J Obstet Gynecol* 198:291.e1–291.e5, 2008.

Boyle PJ, Kempers SF, O'Connor AM, Nagy RJ: Brain glucose uptake and unawareness of hypoglycemia in patients with insulin-dependent diabetes mellitus. *N Engl J Med* 333:1726–1731, 1995.

Boysen A, Lewin MA, Hecker W, Leichter HE, Uhlemann F: Autonomic function testing in children and adolescents with diabetes mellitus. *Pediatr Diabetes* 8:261–264, 2007.

BPL—Blood Pressure Lowering Treatment Trialists' Collaboration: Effects of ACE inhibitors, calcium antagonists, and other blood pressure-lowering drugs: results of prospectively designed overviews of randomized trials. *Lancet* 355:1955–1964, 2000.

BPL—Blood Pressure Lowering Treatment Trialists' Collaboration: Effects of different blood pressure-lowering regimens on major cardiovascular events in individuals with and without diabetes mellitus. Results of prospectively designed overviews of randomized trials. *Arch Intern Med* 165:1410–1419, 2005.

Braga J, Marques R, Branco A, Goncalves J, Lobato L, Pimentel JP, Flores MM, Goncalves E, Jorge CS: Maternal and perinatal implications of the use of human recombinant erythropoietin. *Acta Obstet Gynecol Scand* 75:449–453, 1996.

Brandes RP: Triggering mitochondrial radical release. A new function for NADPH oxidases. Editorial commentary. *Hypertension* 45:847–849, 2005.

Bregante MA, Aramayona JJ, Fraile LJ, Garcia MA, Solans C: Diltiazem blood pharmacokinetics in the pregnant and non-pregnant rabbit: maternal and fetal tissue levels. *Xenobiotica* 8:831–841, 2000.

Brenner BM, Chertow GM: Congenital oligonephropathy and the etiology of adult hypertension and progressive renal injury. *Am J Kidney Dis* 23:1171–1175, 1994.

Brenner BM, Cooper ME, de Zeeuw D, Keane WF, Mitch WE, Parving HH, Remuzzi G, Snapinn SM, Zhang Z, Shahinfar S: Effects of losartan on renal and cardiovascular outcomes in patients with type 2 diabetes and nephropathy. *N Engl J Med* 345:870–878, 2001.

Brent RL, Beckman DA: Angiotensin-converting enzyme inhibitors, an embryopathic class of drugs with unique properties: information for clinical teratology counselors. *Teratology* 43:543–546, 1991.

Briggs GG, Nageotte MP: Fatal fetal outcome with the combined use of valsartan and atenolol. *Ann Pharmacother* 35:859–861, 2001.

Brit—British Cardiac Society, British Hypertension Society, Diabetes UK, HEART UK, Primary Care Cardiovascular Society, Stroke Association: JBS 2: Joint British Societies guidelines on prevention of cardiovascular disease in clinical practice. *Heart* 91 (Suppl V):v1–v52, 2005.

Brizzi P, Tonolo G, Esposito F, Puddu L, Dessole S, Maioli M, Milia S: Lipoprotein metabolism during normal pregnancy. *Am J Obstet Gynecol* 181:430–434, 1999.

Brohall G, Oden A, Fagerberg B: Carotid artery intima-media thickness in patients with type 2 diabetes mellitus and impaired glucose tolerance: a systematic review. *Diabet Med* 23:609–616, 2006.

Bronson SK, Reiter CEN, Gardner TW: An eye on insulin. Commentary. *J Clin Invest* 111:1817–1819, 2003.

Brooks DJ, Gibbs JSR, Sharp P, Herold S, Turton DR, Luthra SK, Kohner EM, Bloom SR, Jones TW: Regional cerebral glucose transport in insulin-dependent diabetic patients studied using [11C]3–o-methyl-d-glucose and positron emission tomography. *J Cereb Blood Flow Metab* 6:240–244, 1986.

Brooks VL, Kane CM, Van Winkle DM: Altered heart rate baroflex during pregnancy: role of sympathetic and parasympathetic nervous systems. *Am J Physiol* 273:R960–R966, 1997.

Brown FM, Hare JW: Diabetic neuropathy and coronary heart disease. In: Reece EA, Coustan DR, eds. *Diabetes Mellitus in Pregnancy.* 3rd ed. New York: Churchill Livingstone; 1995.

Brown MA, Robinson A, Bowyer L, Buddle ML, Martin A, Hargood JL, Cario CM: Ambulatory blood pressure monitoring in pregnancy: what is normal? *Am J Obstet Gynecol* 178:836–842, 1998.

Brown MA, Robinson A, Jones M: The white coat effect in hypertensive pregnancy: much ado about nothing? *Br J Obstet Gynecol* 106:474–480, 1999.

Brown DW, Giles WH, Croft JB: Left ventricular hypertrophy as a predictor of coronary heart disease mortality and the effect of hypertension. *Am Heart J* 140:848–856, 2000a.

Brown MA, Higgins J, Lowe S, McCowan L, Oats J, Peek MJ, Rowan JA, Walters BNJ: The detection, investigation and management of hypertension in pregnancy: full consensus statement. *Aust N Z J Obstet Gynecol* 40:139–155, 2000b.

Brown MA, Davis GK, McHugh L: The prevalence and clinical significance of nocturnal hypertension in pregnancy. *J Hypertens* 19:1437–1444, 2001.

Brown MA, Buddle ML, Farrel T, Davis GK: Efficacy and safety of nifedipine tablets for the acute treatment of severe hypertension in pregnancy. *Am J Obstet Gynecol* 187:1046–1050, 2002.

Brown MA, McHugh L, Mangos G, Davis G: Automated self-initiated blood pressure or 24-hour ambulatory blood pressure monitoring in pregnancy? *BJOG* 111: 38–41, 2004.

Brown MA, Mangos G, Davis G, Homer C: The natural history of white coat hypertension during pregnancy. *BJOG* 112:601–606, 2005.

Brownlee M: Biochemistry and molecular cell biology of diabetic complications. *Nature* 414:813–820, 2001.

Brownlee M: The pathobiology of diabetic complications. A unifying mechanism. Banting Lecture 2004. *Diabetes* 54:1615–1625, 2005.

Bruno G, Giunti S, Bargero G, Ferrero S, Pagano G, Perin PC: Sex-differences in prevalence of electrocardiographic left ventricular hypertrophy in type 2 diabetes: the Casale Monferrato Study. *Diabet Med* 21:823–828, 2004.

Brunskill NJ: Mechanisms of albumin uptake by proximal tubular cells. *Am J Kidney Dis* 37 (Suppl 2):S17–S20, 2001.

Brunzell JD, Davidson M, Furberg CD, Goldberg RB, Howard BV, Stein JH, Witztum JL: Lipoprotein management in patients with cardiometabolic risk. Consensus statement from the American Diabetes Association and the American College of Cardiology Foundation. *Diabetes Care* 31:811–822, 2008.

Brussee V, Cunningham FA, Zochodne DW: Direct insulin signaling of neurons reverses diabetic neuropathy. *Diabetes* 53:1824–1830, 2004.

Brutsaert DL, DeKeulenaer GW: Diastolic heart failure: a myth. *Curr Opin Cardiol* 21:240–248, 2006.

Buchbinder A, Sibai BM, Caritis S, MacPherson C, Hauth J, Lindheimer MD, Klebanoff M, VanDorsten P, Landon M, Paul R, Miodovnik M, Meis P, Thurnau G; for the NICHHD Network of Maternal-Fetal Medicine Units, Bethesda, Maryland: Adverse perinatal outcomes are significantly higher in severe gestational hypertension than in mild preeclampsia. *Am J Obstet Gynecol* 186: 66–71, 2002.

Bujold E, Marquette GP, Ferreira E, Gauthier RJ, Boucher M: Sublingual nitroglycerin versus intravenous ritodrine as tocolytic for external cephalic version: a double-blinded randomized trial. *Am J Obstet Gynecol* 188:1454–1459, 2003.

Bull SV, Douglas IS, Foster M, Albert RK: Mandatory protocol for treating adult patients with diabetic ketoacidosis decreases intensive care unit and hospital lengths of stay: results of a nonrandomized trial. *Crit Care Med* 35:41–47, 2007.

Bullarbo M, Tjugum J, Ekerhovd E: Sublingual nitroglycerin for management of retained placenta. *Int J Gynaecol Obstet* 91:228–232, 2005.

Bulow-Pedersen I, Laurberg P, Knudsen N, Joergensen T, Perrild H, Ovesen L, Rasmussen LB: A population study of the association between thyroid autoantibodies in serum and abnormalities in thyroid function and structure. *Clin Endocrinol (Oxfd)* 62:713–720, 2005.

Burdan F, Szumilo J, Dudka J, Korobowicz A, Klepacz R: Congenital ventricular septal defects and prenatal exposure to cyclooxygenase inhibitors. *Braz J Med Biol Res* 39:925–934, 2006.

Burgos LG, Ebert TJ, Asiddao C, Turner LA, Pattison CZ, Wang-Cheng R, Kampine JP: Increased intraoperative cardiovascular morbidity in diabetics with autonomic neuropathy. *Anesthesiology* 70:591–597, 1989.

Burke GL, Evans GW, Riley WA, Sharrett AR, Howard G, Barnes RW, Rosamond W, Crow RS, Rautaharju PM, Heiss G: Arterial wall thickness is associated with prevalent cardiovascular disease in middle-aged adults: the Atherosclerosis Risk in Communities (ARJC) Study. *Stroke* 26:386–391, 1995.

Burke AP, Kolodgie FD, Zieske A, Fowler DR, Weber DK, Varghese PJ, Farb A, Virmani R: Morphologic findings of coronary atherosclerotic plaques in diabetics: a postmortem study. *Arterioscler Thromb Vasc Biol* 24:1266–1271, 2004.

Burrell JH, Hegarty BD, McMullen JR, Lumbers ER: Effects of gestation on ovine fetal and maternal angiotensin receptor subtypes in the heart and major blood vessels. *Exp Physiol* 86:71–82, 2001.

Bursi F, Weston SA, Redfield MM, Jacobsen SJ, Pakhomov S, Nkomo VT, Meverden RA, Roger VL: Systolic and diastolic heart failure in the community. *JAMA* 296:2209–2216, 2005.

Buse JB, Ginsberg HN, Bakris GL, Clark NG, Costa F, Eckel R, Fonseca V, Gerstein HC, Grundy S, Nesto RW, Pignone MP, Plutzky J, Porte D, Redberg R, Stitzel KF, Stone NJ: Primary prevention of cardiovascular diseases in people with diabetes mellitus. A scientific statement from the American Heart Association and the American Diabetes Association. Dual publication in *Diabetes Care* 30:162–172, 2007; *Circulation* 115:114–126, 2007.

Bushnell CD, Hurn P, Colton C, Miller VM, del Zoppo G, Elkind MS, Stern B, Herrington D, Ford-Lynch G, Gorelick P, James A, Brown CM, Choi E, Bray P, Newby LK, Goldstein LB, Simpkons J: Advancing the study of stroke in women: summary and recommendations for future research from an NINDS-sponsored multidisciplinary working group. *Stroke* 37:2387–2399, 2006.

Bussen S, Steck T: Thyroid autoantibodies in euthyroid nonpregnant women with recurrent spontaneous abortions. *Hum Reprod* 10:2938–2940, 1995.

Butler R, MacDonald TM, Struthers AD, Morris AD: The clinical implications of diabetic heart disease. *Eur Heart J* 19:1617–1627, 1998.

Butler R, Morris AD, Beich JJ, Hill A, Struthers AD: Allopurinol normalized endothelial dysfunction in type 2 diabetics with mild hypertension. *Hypertension* 35:746–751, 2000.

Butte NF: Carbohydrate and lipid metabolism in pregnancy: normal compared with gestational diabetes mellitus. *Am J Clin Nutr* 71 (Suppl):1256S-1261S, 2000.

Butters L, Kennedy S, Rubin PC: Atenolol in essential hypertension during pregnancy. *BMJ* 301:587–589, 1990.

Bytzer P, Talley NJ, Leemon M, Young LJ, Jones MP, Horowitz M: Prevalence of gastrointestinal symptoms associated with diabetes mellitus: a population-based survey of 15,000 adults. *Arch Intern Med* 161:1989–1996, 2001.

Cai H, Griendling KK, Harrison DG: The vascular NAD(P)H oxidases as therapeutic targets in cardiovascular diseases. *Trends Pharmacol Sci* 24:471–478, 2003.

Caixas A, Ordonez-Llanos J, de Leiva A, Payes A, Homs R, Perez A: Optimization of glycemic control by insulin therapy decreases the proportion of small dense LDL particles in diabetic patients. *Diabetes* 46:1207–1213, 1997a.

Caixas A, Perez A, Ordonez-Llanos J, Bonet R, Rigla M, Castellvi A, Bayen L, de Leiva A: Lack of change of lipoprotein(a) levels by the optimization of glycemic control with insulin therapy in NIDDM patients. *Diabetes Care* 20:1459–1461, 1997b.

Calvo RM, Jauniaux E, Gulbis B, Asuncion M, Gervy C, Contempre B, Morreale de Escobar G: Fetal tissues are exposed to biologically relevant free thyroxine concentrations during early phases of development. *J Clin Endocrinol Metab* 87:1768–1777, 2002.

Cameron MA, Maalouf NM, Adams-Huet B, Moe OW, Sakhaee K: Urine composition in type 2 diabetes: predisposition to uric acid nephrolithiasis. *J Am Soc Nephrol* 17:1422–1428, 2006.

Camilleri M: Diabetic gastroparesis. *N Engl J Med* 356:820–829, 2007.

Campbell IW: Dead in bed syndrome: a new manifestation of nocturnal hypoglycemia? *Diabet Med* 8:3–4, 1991.

Campbell NRC, Hasinoff BB, Stalts H, Rao B, Wong NCW: Ferrous sulfate reduces thyroxine efficacy in patients with hypothyroidism. *Ann Intern Med* 117: 1010–1013, 1992.

Campbell CL, Smyth S, Montalescot G, Steinhubl SR: Aspirin dose for the prevention of cardiovascular disease. A systematic review. *JAMA* 297:2018–2024, 2007.

Canani LH, Gerchman F, Gross JL: Familial clustering of diabetic nephropathy in Brazilian type 2 diabetic patients. *Diabetes* 48:909–913, 1999.

Canaris GJ, Manowitz NR, Mayor G, Ridgway C: The Colorado Thyroid Disease Prevalence Study. *Arch Intern Med* 160:526–534, 2000.

Canga N, de Irala J, Vara E, Duaso MJ, Ferrer A, Martinez-Gonzales MA: Intervention study for smoking cessation in diabetic patients: a randomized controlled trial in both clinical and primary health care settings. *Diabetes Care* 23:1455–1460, 2000.

Cannon RO III, Epstein SE: "Microvascular angina" as a cause of chest pain with angiographically normal coronary arteries. *Am J Cardiol* 61:1138–1343, 1988.

Cappola TP, Kass DA, Nelson GS, Berger RD, Rosas GO, Kobeissi ZA, Marban E, Hare JM: Allopurinol improves myocardial efficiency in patients with idiopathic dilated cardiomyopathy. *Circulation* 104:2407–2411, 2001.

Cappon GD, Gupta U, Cook JC, Tassinari MS, Hurtt ME: Comparison of the developmental toxicity of aspirin in rabbits when administered throughout organogenesis or during sensitive windows of development. *Birth Defects Res B Dev Reprod Toxicol* 68:38–46, 2003.

Cappuccio FP, Kerry SM, Forbes L, Donald A: Blood pressure control by home monitoring: meta-analysis of randomized trials. *BMJ* 329:145–148, 2004.

CAPRIE Steering Committee: A randomized, blinded, trial of clopidogrel versus aspirin in patients at risk of ischemic events (CAPRIE). *Lancet* 348:1329–1339, 1996.

Caramori ML, Fioretto P, Mauer M: Low glomerular filtration rate in normoalbuminuric type 1 diabetic patients: an indicator of more advanced glomerular lesions. *Diabetes* 52:1036–1040, 2003.

Cararach V, Carmona F, Monleon FJ, Andreu JL: Pregnancy after renal transplantation: 25 years experience in Spain. *Br J Obstet Gynecol* 100:122–125, 1993.

Carbonne B, Jannet D, Touboul C, Khelifati Y, Milliez J: Nicardipine treatment of hypertension during pregnancy. *Obstet Gynecol* 81:908–914, 1993.

Cardoso C, Ohwovoriole AE, KuKu SF: A study of thyroid function and prevalence of thyroid autoantibodies in an African diabetic population. *J Diabetes Complications* 9:37–41, 1995.

Cardoso CR, Salles GF, Deccache W: Prognostic value of QT interval parameters in type 2 diabetes mellitus: results of a long-term follow-up prospective study. *J Diabetes Complications* 17:169–178, 2003.

Caritis S, Sibai B, Hauth J, Lindheimer MD, Klebanoff M, Thom E, VanDorsten P, Landon M, Paul R, Miodovnik M, Meis P, Thurnau G: Low-dose aspirin to prevent preeclampsia in women at high risk. *N Engl J Med* 338:701–705, 1998.

Carle A, Laurberg P, Pedersen IB, Knudsen N, Perrild H, Ovesen L, Rasmussen LB, Jorgensen T: Epidemiology of subtypes of hypothyroidism in Denmark. *Eur J Endocrinol* 154:21–28, 2006.

Carnethon MR, Bertoni AG, Shea S, Greenland P, Ni H, Jacob DR Jr, Saad M, Liu K: Racial/ethnic differences in subclinical atherosclerosis among adults with diabetes: the Multi-Ethnic Study of Atherosclerosis. *Diabetes Care* 28: 2768–2770, 2005.

Carr DB, Koontz GL, Gardella C, Holing EV, Brateng DA, Brown ZA, Easterling TR: Diabetic nephropathy in pregnancy: suboptimal hypertensive control associated with preterm delivery. *Am J Hypertens* 19:513–519, 2006.

Carracio N, Ferrannini E, Monzani F: Lipoprotein profile in subclinical hypothyroidism: response to levothyroxine replacement; a randomized placebo-controlled study. *J Clin Endocrinol Metab* 87:1533–1538, 2002.

Carroll MA, Yeomans ER: Diabetic ketoacidosis in pregnancy. *Crit Care Med* 33 (Suppl):S347–S353, 2005.

Carruth JE, Mivis SB, Brogan DR, Wenger NK: The electrocardiogram in normal pregnancy. *Am Heart J* 102:1075–1078, 1981.

Carter SA: Arterial auscultation in peripheral vascular disease. *JAMA* 246:1682–1686, 1981.

Caruso A, Ferrazani S, De Carolis S, Lucchese A, Lanzone A, De Santis L, Paradisi G: Gestational hypertension but not preeclampsia is associated with insulin resistance syndrome characteristics. *Hum Reprod* 14:219–223, 1999.

Casey BM, Dashe JS, Wells CE, McIntire DD, Byrd W, Leveno KJ, Cunningham FG: Subclinical hypothyroidism and pregnancy outcomes. *Obstet Gynecol* 105:239–245, 2005.

Casey BM, Leveno KJ: Thyroid disease in pregnancy. *Obstet Gynecol* 108:1283–1292, 2006.

Caslake MJ, Packard CJ, Suckling KE, Holmes SD, Chamberlain P, Macphee CH: Lipoprotein-associated phospholipase A_2, platelet-activating factor acetylhydrolase: a potential new risk factor for coronary artery disease. *Atherosclerosis* 150:413–419, 2000.

Cassar J, Kohner EM, Hamilton AM, Gordon H, Joplin GF: Diabetic retinopathy and pregnancy. *Diabetologia* 15:105–111, 1978.

Cassar K: Intermittent claudication. *BMJ* 333:1002–1005, 2006.

Cataldi L, Mussap M, Bertelli L, Ruzzante N, Farnos V, Plebani M: Cystatin C in healthy women at term pregnancy and in their infant newborns: relationship between maternal and neonatal serum levels and reference values. *Am J Perinatol* 16:287–295, 1999.

Cavallone D, Malagolini N, Frasca G-M, Stefoni S, Serafini-Cessi F: Salt-precipitation method does not isolate to homogeneity Tamm-Horsfall glycoprotein from urine of proteinuric patients and pregnant women. *Clin Biochem* 35:405–410, 2002.

CDC—Centers for Disease Control and Prevention: Postmarketing surveillance for angiotensin converting enzyme inhibitor use during the first trimester of pregnancy—United States, Canada and Israel, 1987–1995. *MMWR Morb Mortal Wkly Rep* 46:240–242, 1997.

Celani MF, Bonati ME, Stucci N: Prevalence of abnormal thyrotropin concentrations measured by a sensitive assay in patients with type 2 diabetes mellitus. *Diabetes Res* 27:15–25, 1994.

Ceriello A: New insights on oxidative stress and diabetic complications may lead to a "causal" antioxidant therapy. *Diabetes Care* 26:1589–1596, 2003.

Ceriello A: Controlling oxidative stress as a novel molecular approach to protecting the vascular wall in diabetes. *Curr Opin Lipidol* 17:510–518, 2006.

Cesario DA, Brar R, Shivkumar K: Alterations in ion channel physiology in diabetic cardiomyopathy. *Endocrinol Metab Clin North Am* 35:601–610, 2006.

Chait A, Bierman EL, Albers JJ: Low-density lipoprotein receptor activity in cultured human skin fibroblasts: mechanism of insulin-induced stimulation. *J Clin Invest* 64:1309–1319, 1979.

Chambless LE, Fuchs FD, Linn S, Kritchevsky SB, Larosa JC, Segal P, Rifkind BM: The association of corneal arcus with coronary heart disease and cardiovascular disease mortality in the Lipid Research Clinics Mortality Follow-up Study. *Am J Public Health* 80:1200–1204, 1990.

Chan WS, Okun N, Kjellstrand CM: Pregnancy in chronic dialysis: a review and analysis of the literature. *Int J Artif Organs* 21:259–268, 1998.

Chan LY, Fok WY, Wong JT, Yu CM, Leung TN, Lau TK: Reference charts of gestation-specific tissue Doppler imaging indices of systolic and diastolic functions in the normal fetal heart. *Am Heart J* 150:750–755, 2005.

Chantelau E, Kohner EM: Why some cases of retinopathy worsen when diabetic control improves. Worsening retinopathy is not a reason to withhold intensive insulin treatment. Commentary. *BMJ* 315:1105–1106, 1997.

Chao A-S, Huang J-Y, Lien R, Kung F-T, Chen P-J, Hsieh PCC: Pregnancy in women who undergo long-term hemodialysis. *Am J Obstet Gynecol* 187:152–156, 2002.

Chappell LC, Seed PT, Briley A, Kelly FJ, Hunt BJ, Charnock-Jones I, Mallet AI, Poston L: A longitudinal study of biochemical variables in women at risk for preeclampsia. *Am J Obstet Gynecol* 187:127–136, 2002.

Charpentier G, Genes N, Vaur L, Amar J, Clerson P, Cambou JP, Gueret P; the ESPOIR Diabetes Study investigators: Control of diabetes and cardiovascular risk factors in patients with type 2 diabetes: a nationwide French survey. *Diabetes Metab* 29:152–158, 2003.

Charvat J, Michalova K, Chiumsky J, Horackova M, Valenta Z, Zdarska D: The significance of carotid artery disease in asymptomatic type 2 diabetic patients. *J Int Med Res* 34:13–20, 2006.

Chatterjee S, Tsaloumas MD, Geet H, Lipkin G, Dunne FP: From minimal background diabetic retinopathy to profuse sight threatening vitreoretinal hemorrhage: management issues in a case of pregestational diabetes and pregnancy. *Diabet Med* 20:683–685, 2003.

Chauhan SP, Perry KG Jr: Management of diabetic ketoacidosis in the obstetric patient. *Obstet Gynecol Clin North Am* 22:143–155, 1995.

Chauhan SP, Perry KG, McLaughlin BN, Roberts WE, Sullivan CA, Morrison JC: Diabetic ketoacidosis complicating pregnancy. *J Perinatol* 16:173–175, 1996.

Chen HC, Newsom RS, Patel V, Cassar J, Mather H, Kohner EM: Retinal blood flow changes during pregnancy in women with diabetes. *Invest Ophthalmol Vis Sci* 35:3199–3208, 1994.

Chen L, Haught WH, Yang B, Saldeen TG, Parathasarathy S, Mehta JL: Preservation of endogenous antioxidant activity and inhibition of lipid peroxidation as common mechanisms of antiatherosclerotic effects of vitamin E, lovasatin and amlodipine. *J Am Coll Cardiol* 30:569–575, 1997.

Cheng SM, Yang SP, Ho LJ, Tsao TP, Chang DM, Lai JH: Carvedilol modulates in-vitro granulocyte-macrophage colony-stimulating factor-induced interleukin-10 production in U937 cells and human monocytes. *Immunol Invest* 32:43–58, 2003.

Cheron RG, Kaplan MM, Larsen PR, Selenkow HA, Crigler JF: Neonatal thyroid function after propylthiouracil therapy for maternal Graves' disease. *N Engl J Med* 304:525–528, 1981.

Chesley LC: The variability of proteinuria in the hypertensive complications of pregnancy. *J Clin Invest* 18:617–620, 1939.

Chessa M, Butera G, Lanza GA, Bossone E, Delogu A, De Rosa G, Marietti G, Rosti L, Carminati M: Role of heart rate variability in the early diagnosis of diabetic autonomic neuropathy in children. *Herz* 27:785–790, 2002.

Cheung CK, Lao T, Swaminathan R: Urinary excretion of some proteins and enzymes during normal pregnancy. *Clin Chem* 35:1978–1980, 1989.

Chew EY, Mills JL, Metzger BE, Remaley NA, Jovanovic-Peterson L, Knopp RH, Conley M, Rand L, Simpson JL, Holmes LB, Aarons JH; National Institute of Child Health and Human Development Diabetes in Early Pregnancy Study: Metabolic control and progression of retinopathy. *Diabetes Care* 18:631–637, 1995.

Chico A, Tomas A, Novials A: Silent myocardial ischemia is associated with autonomic neuropathy and other cardiovascular risk factors in type 1 and type 2 diabetic subjects, especially in those with microalbuminuria. *Endocrine* 27: 213–217, 2005.

Chobanian AV, Bakris GL, Black HR, Cushman WC, Green LA, Izzo JL Jr, Jones DW, Materson BJ, Oparil S, Wright JT Jr, Roccella EJ; National High Blood Pressure Education Program Coordinating Committee: The seventh report of the Joint National Committee on Prevention, Detection, Evaluation, and Treatment of High Blood Pressure. Executive summary. *JAMA* 289: 2560–2572, 2003a.

Chobanian AV, Bakris GL, Black HR, Cushman WC, Green LA, Izzo JL Jr, Jones DW, Materson BJ, Oparil S, Wright JT Jr, Roccella EJ; National High Blood Pressure

Education Program Coordinating Committee: Seventh Report of the Joint National Committee on Prevention, Detection, Evaluation, and Treatment of High Blood Pressure. JNC 7—Complete Version. *Hypertension* 42:1206–1252, 2003b.

Christensen PK, Gall MA, Major-Pedersen A, Sato A, Rossing P, Breum L, Pietersen A, Kastrup J, Parving HH: QTc interval length and QT dispersion as predictor of mortality in patients with non-insulin-dependent diabetes. *Scand J Clin Lab Invest* 60:323–332, 2000.

Chubb SAP, Davis WA, Davis TME: Interactions among thyroid function, insulin sensitivity, and serum lipid concentrations: the Freemantle Diabetes Study. *J Clin Endocrinol Metab* 90:5317–5320, 2005a.

Chubb SAP, Davis WA, Inman Z, Davis TME: Prevalence and progression of subclinical hypothyroidism in women with type 2 diabetes: the Freemantle Diabetes Study. *Clin Endocrinol* 62:480–486, 2005b.

Chung NA, Lip GYH, Beevers DG, Beevers DG: Angiotensin-II-receptor inhibitors in pregnancy. *Lancet* 357:1620, 2001.

Chung AK, Das SR, Leonard D, Peshock RM, Kazi F, Abdullah SM, Canham RM, Levine BD, Drazner MH: Women have higher left ventricular ejection fractions than men independent of differences in left ventricular volume. The Dallas Heart Study. *Circulation* 113:1597–1604, 2006.

Churchill D, Perry IJ, Beevers MD: Ambulatory blood pressure in pregnancy and fetal growth. *Lancet* 349:7–10, 1997.

Cipollone F, Iezzi A, Fazia M, Zuchelli M, Pini B, Cuccurullo C, De Cesare D, De Blasis G, Muraro R, Bei R, Chiarelli F, Schmidt AM, Cuccurullo F, Messetti A: The receptor RAGE as a progression factor amplifying arachidonate-dependent inflammatory and proteolytic response in human atherosclerotic plaques: role of glycemic control. *Circulation* 108:1070–1077, 2003.

Cirillo M, Laurenzi M, Panarelli P, Mancini M, Zanchetti A, De Santo NG: Relation of urinary albumin excretion to coronary heart disease and low renal function: role of blood pressure. *Kidney Int* 65:2290–2297, 2004.

Cirillo M, Lanti MP, Menotti A, Laurenzi M, Mancini M, Zanchetti A, De Santo NG: Definition of kidney dysfunction as a cardiovascular risk factor. Use of urinary albumin excretion and estimated glomerular filtration rate. *Arch Intern Med* 168:617–624, 2008.

Clapp JF III, Capeless E: Cardiovascular function before, during and after the first and subsequent pregnancies. *Am J Cardiol* 80:1469–1473, 1997.

CLASP—Collaborative Low-dose Aspirin Study in Pregnancy Collaborative Group: A randomized trial of low-dose aspirin for the prevention and treatment of preeclampsia among 9364 pregnant women. *Lancet* 343:619–629, 1994.

Clausen TD, Mathiesen E, Ekbom P, Hellmuth E, Mandrup-Poulsen T, Damm P: Poor pregnancy outcome in women with type 2 diabetes. *Diabetes Care* 28: 323–328, 2005a.

Clausen T, Burski TK, Oyen N, Godang K, Bollerslev J, Henriksen T: Maternal anthropometric and metabolic factors in the first half of pregnancy and risk of neonatal macrosomia in term pregnancies. A prospective study. *Eur J Endocrinol* 153:887–894, 2005b.

Cleary PA, Orchard TJ, Genuth S, Wong ND, Detrano R, Backlund J-YC, Zinman B, Jacobson A, Sun W, Lachin JM, Nathan DM; the DCCT/EDIC Research Group: The effect of intensive glycemic treatment on coronary artery calcification in type 1 diabetic participants of the Diabetes Control and Complications Trial/Epidemiology of Diabetes Interventions and Complications (DCCT/EDIC) Study. *Diabetes* 55:3556–3565, 2006.

Cnossen JS, de Ruyter-Hanhijarvi H, van der Post JA, Mol BW, Khan KS, ter Riet G: Accuracy of serum uric acid determination in predicting preeclampsia: a systematic review. *Acta Obstet Gynecol Scand* 85:519–525, 2006.

Cobellis L, De Luca A, Pecori E, Mastrogiacomo A, Di Pietro L, Iannella I, Fornaro F, Scaffa C, Cobellis G, Colacurci N: Mid-trimester fetal-placental velocimetry response to nifedipine may predict early the onset of preeclampsia. *In Vivo* 20:183–186, 2006.

Cockburn J, Moar VA, Ounsted M, Redman CW: Final report of study on hypertension during pregnancy: the effects of specific treatment on the growth and development of the children. *Lancet* 1: 647–649, 1982.

Cohen JC, Boerwinkle E, Mosley TH Jr, Hobbs HH: Sequence variation in *PCSK9*, low LDL, and protection against coronary heart disease. *N Engl J Med* 354:1264–1272, 2006.

Col NF, Surks MI, Daniels GH: Subclinical thyroid disease. Clinical applications. *JAMA* 291:239–243, 2004.

Colhoun HM, Rubens MB, Underwood SR, Fuller JH: The effect of type 1 diabetes mellitus on the gender difference in coronary artery calcification. *J Am Coll Cardiol* 36:2160–2167, 2000.

Colhoun HM, Schalkwijk C, Rubens MB, Stehouwer CDA: C-reactive protein in type 1 diabetes and its relationship to coronary artery calcification. *Diabetes Care* 25:1813–1817, 2002a.

Colhoun HM, Otvos JD, Rubens MB, Taskinen MR, Underwood SR, Fuller JH: Lipoprotein subclasses and particle sizes and their relationship with coronary artery calcification in men and women with and without type 1 diabetes. *Diabetes* 51:1949–1956, 2002b.

Colhoun H: Coronary heart disease in women: why the disproportionate risk? *Curr Diab Rep* 6:22–28, 2006.

Collado-Mesa F, Colhoun HM, Stevens LK, Boavida J, Ferriss JB, Karamanos B, Kempler P, Michel G, Roglic G, Fuller JH; the EURODIAB IDDM Complications Study Group: Prevalence and management of hypertension in type 1 diabetes mellitus in Europe: the EURODIAB IDDM Complications Study. *Diabet Med* 16:41–49, 1999.

Collin P, Kaukinen K, Valimaki M, Salmi J: Endocrinological disorders and celiac disease. *Endocr Rev* 23:464–483, 2002.

Collins R, Yusuf S, Peto R: Overview of randomized trials of diuretics in pregnancy. *Br Med J* 290:17–23, 1985.

Collins JS, Bossone Eagle KA, Mehta RH: Asymptomatic coronary artery disease in a pregnant patient. A case report and review of the literature. *Herz* 27:548–554, 2002.

Colonna P, Pinto FJ, Sorino M, Bovenzi F, D'Agostino C, de Luca I: The emerging role of echocardiography in the screening of patients at risk of heart failure. *Am J Cardiol* 96:42L-51L, 2005.

Colwell JA: Aspirin therapy in diabetes. Technical review. *Diabetes Care* 20: 1767–1771, 1997.

Colwell JA, Nesto RW: The platelet in diabetes. Focus on prevention of ischemic events. *Diabetes Care* 26:2181–2188, 2003.

Comaschi M, Coscelli C, Cucinotta D, Malini P, Manzato E, Nicolucci A; SFIDA Study Group—Italian Association of Diabetologists (AMD): Cardiovascular risk factors and metabolic control in type 2 diabetic subjects attending outpatient clinics in Italy: the SFIDA (survey of risk factors in Italian diabetic subjects by AMD) study. *Nutr Metab Cardiovasc Dis* 15:204–211, 2005.

Combs CA, Wheeler BC, Kitzmiller JL: Urinary protein/creatinine ratio before and during pregnancy in women with diabetes mellitus. *Am J Obstet Gynecol* 165:920–923, 1991.

Combs CA, Rosenn B, Kitzmiller JL, Khoury JC, Wheeler BC, Miodovnik M: Early-pregnancy proteinuria in diabetes related to preeclampsia. *Obstet Gynecol* 82:802–807, 1993.

Comper WD, Osivka TM, Jerums G: High prevalence of immuno-unreactive intact albumin in urine of diabetic patients. *Am J Kidney Dis* 41:336–342, 2003.

Connolly HM: Cardiovascular diagnostic and therapeutic options during pregnancy. In: Douglas PS, ed. *Cardiovascular Health and Disease in Women.* 2nd ed. Philadelphia: WB Saunders Co; 2002:510–523.

Conway M, Baldwin J, Kohner EM, Schulenburg WE, Cassar J: Postpartum progression of diabetic retinopathy. *Diabetes Care* 14:1110–1111, 1991.

Conway DL, Langer O: Selecting antihypertensive therapy in the pregnant woman with diabetes mellitus. *J Matern-Fetal Med* 9:66–69, 2000.

Cook S, Gidding SS: Modifying cardiovascular risk in adolescent obesity. Editorial. *Circulation* 115:2251–2253, 2007.

Cooper DS: Subclinical thyroid disease: consensus or conundrum? Commentary. *Clin Endocrinol* 60:410–412, 2004.

Cooper DS: Antithyroid drugs. *N Engl J Med* 352:907–917, 2005.

Cooper WO, Hernandez-Diaz S, Arbogast PG, Dudley JA, Dyer S, Gideon PS, Hall K, Ray WA: Major congenital malformations after first-trimester exposure to ACE inhibitors. *N Engl J Med* 354:2443–2451, 2006.

Coppelli A, Giannarelli R, Mariotti R, Rondinini L, Fossati N, Vistoli F, Aragona M, Rizzo G, Boggi U, Mosca F, DelPrato S, Marchetti P: Pancreas transplant alone determines early improvemnt of cardiovascular risk factors and cardiac function in type 1 diabetic patients. *Transplantation* 76:974–976, 2003.

Coppola A, Astarita C, Oliviero M, Fontana D, Picardi G, Esposito K, Marfella R, Coppola L, Giugliano D: Impairment of coronary circulation by acute hyper-homocysteinemia in type 2 diabetic patients. *Diabetes Care* 27:2055–2056, 2004.

Coresh J, Astor BC, McQuillan G, Kusek J, Greene T, Van Lente F, Levey AS: Calibration and random variation of the serum creatinine assay as critical elements of using equations to estimate glomerular filtration rate. *Am J Kidney Dis* 39:920–929, 2002.

Cosson E, Paycha F, Paries J, Cattan S, Ramadan A, Meddah D, Attali JR, Valensi P: Detecting silent coronary stenoses and stratifying cardiac risk in patients with diabetes: ECG stress test or exercise myocardial scintigraphy? *Diabet Med* 21:342–348, 2004.

Costacou T, Lopes-Virella MF, Zgibor J, Virella G, Otvos J, Walsh M, Orchard TJ: Markers of endothelial dysfunction in the prediction of coronary artery disease in type 1 diabetes: the Pittsburgh Epidemiology of Diabetes Complications Study. *J Diabetes Complications* 19:183–193, 2005a.

Costacou T, Zgibor JC, Evans RW, Otvos J, Lopes-Virella MF, Tracy RP, Orchard TJ: The prospective association between adiponectin and coronary artery disease among individuals with type 1 diabetes. The Pittsburgh Epidemiology of Diabetes Complications Study. *Diabetologia* 48:41–48, 2005b.

Costello-Boerrigter LC, Boerrigter G, Redfield MM, Rodehaffer RJ, Urban LH, Mahoney DW, Jacobsen SJ, Heublein DM, Burnett JC Jr: Amino-terminal pro-B-type natriuretic peptide and B-type natriuretic peptide in the general community: determinants and detection of left ventricular dysfunction. *J Am Coll Cardiol* 47:345–353, 2006.

Cote AM, Brown MA, Lam E, Dadelszen PV, Firoz T, Liston RM, Magee LA: Diagnostic accuracy of urinary spot protein:creatinine ratio for proteinuria in hypertensive pregnant women: systematic review. *BMJ* Apr 10, 2008. doi:10.1136/bmj.39532.543947.BE (Epub ahead of print).

Cousins L: Pregnancy complications among diabetic women: review 1965–1985. *Obstet Gynecol Surv* 42:140–149, 1987.

Cowan JC, Hilton CJ, Griffiths CJ: Sequence of epicardial repolarization and configuration of the T wave. *Br Heart J* 60:424–433, 1988.

Cox DJ, Gonder-Frederick L, Antoun B, Cryer PE, Clarke WL: Perceived symptoms in the recognition of hypoglycemia. *Diabetes Care* 16:519–527, 1993.

Cox RM, Anderson JM, Cox P: Defective embryogenesis with angiotensin II receptor antagonists in pregnancy. *BJOG* 110:1038–1040, 2003.

Craig S, Ilton M: Treatment of acute myocardial infarction with coronary artery balloon angioplasty and stenting. *Aust N Z J Obstet Gynecol* 39:194–196, 1999.

Crall F, Roberts W: The extramural and intramural coronary arteries in juvenile diabetes mellitus. Analysis of nine necropsy patients aged 19 to 38 years with onset of diabetes before age 15 years. *Am J Med* 64:221–230, 1978.

Cranston I, Lomas J, Maran A, Macdonald I, Amiel SA: Restoration of hypoglycemia awareness in patients with long-duration insulin-dependent diabetes. *Lancet* 344:283–287, 1994.

Creager MA, Luescher TF, Cosentino F, Beckman JA: Diabetes and vascular disease. Pathophysiology, clinical consequences, and medical therapy: part I. *Circulation* 108:1527–1532, 2003.

Cruickshank DJ, Robertson AA, Campbell DM, MacGillivray I: Maternal obstetric outcome measures in a randomized controlled study of labetalol in the treatment of hypertension in pregnancy. *Clin Exp Hypertens Preg* B10:333–344, 1991.

Cruz-Lemini MC, Ibarguengoita-Ochoa F, Villanueva-Gonzalez MA: Perinatal outcome following renal transplantation. *Int J Gynecol Obstet* 96:76–79, 2007.

Cryer PE: Hypoglycemia risk reduction in type 1 diabetes. *Exp Clin Endocrinol Diabetes* 109 (Suppl 2):S412–S423, 2001.

Cryer PE, Davis SN, Shamoon H: Hypoglycemia in diabetes. Technical review. *Diabetes Care* 26:1902–1912, 2003.

Cryer PE: Diverse causes of hypoglycemia-associated autonomic failure in diabetes. *N Engl J Med* 350:2272–2279, 2004.

Cryer PE: Mechanisms of hypoglycemia-associated autonomic failure and its component syndromes in diabetes. *Diabetes* 54:3592–3601, 2005.

Cryer PE: Mechanisms of sympathoadrenal failure and hypoglycemia in diabetes. *J Clin Invest* 116:1470–1473, 2006.

Cullen MT, Reece EA, Homko CJ, Sivan E. The changing presentations of diabetic ketoacidosis during pregnancy. *Am J Perinatol* 13:449–451, 1996.

Cundy T, Gamble G, Townend K, Henley PG, MacPherson P, Roberts AB: Perinatal mortality in type 2 diabetes mellitus. *Diabet Med* 17:33–39, 2000.

Cundy T, Slee F, Gamble G, Neale L: Hypertensive disorders of pregnancy in women with type 1 and type 2 diabetes. *Diabet Med* 19:482–489, 2002.

Cunningham FG: Severe preeclampsia and eclampsia: systolic hypertension is also important. Editorial. *Obstet Gynecol* 105:237–238, 2005.

Curry S, Mandelkow H, Franks N: Crystal structure of human serum albumin complexed with fatty acid reveals an asymmetric distribution of binding sites. *Nat Struct Biol* 5:827–835, 1998.

Curtis LH, Ostbye T, Sendersky V, Hutchison S, Allen LaPointe NM, Al-Khatib SM, Yasuda SU, Dans PE, Wright A, Califf RM, Woosley RL, Schulman KA: Prescription of QT-prolonging drugs in a cohort of about 5 million outpatients. *Am J Med* 114:135–141, 2003.

Curtiss LK: ApoE in atherosclerosis: a protein with multiple hats. Editorial. *Arterioscler Thromb Vasc Biol* 20:1852–1853, 2000.

D'Agostino RB, Burke G, O'Leary D, Rewers M, Selby J, Savage PJ, Saad MF, Bergman RN, Howard G, Wagenknecht L, Haffner SM: Ethnic differences in carotid wall thickness: the Insulin Resistance Atherosclerosis Study. *Stroke* 27:1744–1749, 1996.

D'Amico G, Bazzi C: Pathophysiology of proteinuria. *Kidney Int* 63:809–825, 2003.

Dabelea D, Pettitt DJ, Jones KL, Arslanian SA: Type 2 diabetes mellitus in minority children and adolescents: an emerging problem. *Endocrinol Metab Clin North Am* 28:709–729, 1999.

Dabelea D, Kinney G, Snell-Bergeon JK, Hokanson JE, Eckel RH, Ehrlich J, Garg S, Hamman RF, Rewers M: Effect of type 1 diabetes on the gender difference in coronary artery calcification: a role for insulin resistance? The Coronary Artery Calcification in Type 1 Diabetes (CACTI) Study. *Diabetes* 52:2833–2839, 2003.

Dagogo-Jack SE, Craft S, Cryer PE: Hypoglycemia-associated autonomic failure in insulin-dependent diabetes mellitus. *J Clin Invest* 91:819–828, 1993.

Dagogo-Jack S, Rattarasarn C, Cryer PE: Reversal of hypoglycemia unawareness, but not defective glucose counterregulation, in IDDM. *Diabetes* 43:1426–1434, 1994.

Dahl-Jorgensen K, Brinchmann-Hansen O, Hanssen KF, Sandvik L, Aagenaes O; Aker Diabetes Group: Rapid tightening of blood glucose control leads to transient deterioration of diabetic retinopathy in insulin-dependent diabetes mellitus: the Oslo Study. *Br Med J* 290:811–815, 1985.

Dahl-Jorgensen K, Larsen JR, Hanssen KF: Atherosclerosis in childhood and adolescent type 1 diabetes: early disease, early treatment? *Diabetologia* 48: 1445–1453, 2005.

Dandona P, Karne R, Ghanim H, Hamouda W, Aljada A, Magsino CH: Carvedilol inhibits reactive oxygen species generation by leukocytes and oxidative damage to amino acids. *Circulation* 101:122–124, 2000.

Dandona P, Chaudhuri A, Ghanim H, Mohanty P: Proinflammatory effects of glucose and anti-inflammatory effect of insulin: relevance to cardiovascular disease. *Am J Cardiol* 99 (Suppl):15B–26B, 2007.

Danese MD, Ladenson PW, Meinert CL, Powe NR: Effect of thyroxine therapy on serum lipoproteins in patients with mild thyroid failure: a quantitative review of the literature. *J Clin Endocrinol Metab* 85:2993–3001, 2000.

Danesh J, Wheeler JG, Hirschfield GM, Eda S, Eiriksdottir G, Rumley A, Lowe GDO, Pepys MB, Gudnason V: C-reactive protein and other circulating markers of inflammation in the prediction of coronary artery disease. *N Engl J Med* 350:1387–1397, 2004.

Daniels SR, Kimball TR, Morrison JA, Khoury P, Meyer RA: Indexing left ventricular mass to account for differences in body size in children and adolescents without cardiovascular disease. *Am J Cardiol* 76:699–701, 1995.

Daoud G, Simoneau L, Masse A, Rassart E, Lafond J: Expression of cFABP and PPAR in trophoblast cells: effect of PPAR ligands on linoleic acid uptake and differentiation. *Biochim Biophys Acta* 1687:181–194, 2005.

Darcan S, Goksen D, Serdaroglu E, Buyukinan M, Coker M, Berdeli A, Kose T, Cura A: Alterations of blood pressure in type 1 diabetic children and adolescents. *Pediatr Nephrol* 21:672–676, 2006.

Darias R, Herranz L, Garcia-Inglemo MT, Pallardo LF: Pregnancy in a patient with type 1 diabetes mellitus and prior heart disease. *Eur J Endocrinol* 144:309–310, 2001.

Dashe J, Casey BM, Wells CE, McIntire DD, Byrd EW, Leveno KJ, Cunningham FG: Thyroid-stimulating hormone in singleton and twin pregnancy: importance of gestional age-specific reference ranges. *Obstet Gynecol* 106:753–757, 2005.

Daudon M, Traxer O, Conort P, Lacour B, Jungers P: Type 2 diabetes increases the risk for uric acid stones. *J Am Soc Nephrol* 17:2026–2033, 2006.

Davi G, Ciabottoni G, Consoli A, Messetti A, Falco A, Santarone S, Pennese E, Vitacolonna E, Bucciarelli T, Costantini F, Capani F, Patrono C: In vivo formation of 8-iso-prostaglandin $F_{2\alpha}$ and platelet activation in diabetes mellitus. Effects of improved metabolic control. *Circulation* 99:224–229, 1999.

Davies MJ: Stability and instability: two faces of coronary atherosclerosis. The Paul Dudley White Lecture 1995. *Circulation* 94:2013–2020, 1996.

Davies L, Wilmshurst EG, McElduff A, Gunyon J, Clifton-Bligh P, Fulcher GR: The relationship among homocysteine, creatinine clearance, and albuminuria in patients with type 2 diabetes. *Diabetes Care* 24:1805–1809, 2000.

Davies M, Brophy S, Williams R, Taylor A: The prevalence, severity, and impact of painful diabetic peripheral neuropathy in type 2 diabetes. *Diabetes Care* 29:1518–1522, 2006.

Davignon J: Apolipoprotein E and atherosclerosis. Beyond lipid effect. Editorial. *Arterioscler Thromb Vasc Biol* 25:267–269, 2005.

Davis LE, Leveno KJ, Cunningham FG: Hypothyroidism complicating pregnancy. *Obstet Gynecol* 72:108–112, 1988.

Davis LE, Lucas MJ, Hankins GDV, Roark ML, Cunningham FG: Thyrotoxicosis complicating pregnancy. *Am J Obstet Gynecol* 160:63–70, 1989.

Davis SN, Cherrington AD, Goldstein R, Jacobs J, Price L: Effects of insulin on the counterregulatory responses to equivalent hypoglycemia in normal females. *Am J Physiol* 265:E680–E689, 1993.

Davis SN, Shavers C, Costa F, Mosqueda-Garcia R: Role of cortisol in the pathogenesis of deficient counterregulation after antecedent hypoglycemia in normal humans. *J Clin Invest* 98:680–691, 1996.

Davis SN, Shavers C, Costa F: Gender-related differences in counterregulatory responses to antecedent hypoglycemia in normal humans. *J Clin Endocrinol Metab* 85:2148–2157, 2000a.

Davis SN, Fowler S, Costa F: Hypoglycemia counterregulatory responses differ between men and women with type 1 diabetes. *Diabetes* 49:65–72, 2000b.

Davis SN, Shavers C, Costa F: Differential gender responses to hypoglycemia are due to alterations in CNS drive and not glycemic thresholds. *Am J Physiol* 279: E1054–E1063, 2000c.

Davis TM, Zimmet P, Davis WA, Bruce DG, Fida S, Mackay IR: Autoantibodies to glutamic acid decarboxylase in diabetic patients from a multi-ethnic Australian community: the Freemantle Diabetes Study. *Diabet Med* 17:667–674, 2000d.

Davis TME, Cull CA, Holman RR; U.K. Prospective Diabetes Study (UKPDS) Group: Relationship between ethnicity and glycemic control, lipid profiles, and blood pressure during the first 9 years of type 2 diabetes. U.K. Prospective Diabetes Study (UKPDS 55). *Diabetes Care* 24:1167–1174, 2001.

Davison JM: Pregnancy in renal allograft recipients: prognosis and management. *Clin Obstet Gynecol (Bailliere's)* 8:501–525, 1994.

Dawson A, Rana BS, Pringle SD, Donnelly LA, Morris AD, Struthers AD: How much echo left ventricular hypertrophy would be missed in diabetics by applying the Losartan Intervention for Endpoint Reduction electrocardiogram criteria to select patients for angiotensin receptor blockade? *J Hypertens* 22:1403–1408, 2004.

Day C, Hawkins P, Hildebrand S, Sheikh L, Taylor G, Kilby M, Lipkin G: The role of renal biopsy in women with kidney disease identified in pregnancy. *Nephrol Dial Transplant* 23:201–206, 2008.

DCCT—Diabetes Control and Complications Trial Research Group: Design and methodologic considerations for the feasibility phase. *Diabetes* 35:530–545, 1986.

DCCT—Diabetes Control and Complications Trial Research Group: Epidemiology of severe hypoglycemia in the Diabetes Control and Complications Trial. *Am J Med* 90:450–459, 1991.

DCCT—Diabetes Conrol and Complications Trial Research Group: The effect of intensive treatment of diabetes on the development and progression of long-term complications in insulin-dependent diabetes mellitus. *N Engl J Med* 329:977–986, 1993.

DCCT—Diabetes Control and Complications Trial Research Group: The effect of intensive diabetes therapy on the development and progression of neuropathy. *Ann Intern Med* 122:561–568, 1995a.

DCCT—Diabetes Control and Complications Trial Research Group: Effect of intensive diabetes management on macrovascular events and risk factors in the Diabetes Control and Complications Trial. *Am J Cardiol* 75:894–903, 1995b.

DCCT—Diabetes Control and Complications Trial Research Group: Effect of intensive therapy on the development and progression of diabetic nephropathy in the Diabetes Control and Complications Trial. *Kidney Int* 47:1703–1720, 1995c.

DCCT—Diabetes Control and Complications Trial Research Group: The effect of intensified diabetes treatment on the progression of diabetic retinopathy in insulin-dependent diabetes mellitus. *Arch Ophthalmol* 113:36–51, 1995d.

DCCT—Diabetes Control and Complications Trial Research Group: Progression of retinopathy with intensive versus conventional treatment in the Diabetes Control and Complications Trial. *Ophthalmology* 102:647–661, 1995e.

DCCT—Diabetes Control and Complications Trial Research Group: The relationship of glycemic exposure (HbA1C) to the risk of development and progression of retinopathy in the Diabetes Control and Complications Trial. *Diabetes* 44:968–983, 1995f.

DCCT—Diabetes Control and Complications Trial Research Group: Effect of intensive diabetes treatment on nerve conduction in the Diabetes Control and Complications Trial. *Ann Neurol* 38:869–880, 1995g.

DCCT—Diabetes Control and Complications Trial Research Group: Pregnancy outcomes in the Diabetes Control and Complications Trial. *Am J Obstet Gynecol* 174:1343–1353, 1996a.

DCCT—Diabetes Control and Complications Trial Research Group: The absence of a glycemic threshold for the development of long-term complications: the perspective of the Diabetes Control and Complications Trial. *Diabetes* 45:1289–1298, 1996b.

DCCT—Diabetes Control and Complications Trial Research Group: Clustering of long-term complications in families with diabetes in the Diabetes Control and Complications Trial. *Diabetes* 46:1829–1839, 1997a.

DCCT—Diabetes Control and Complications Trial Research Group: Hypoglycemia in the Diabetes Control and Complications Trial. *Diabetes* 46:271–286, 1997b.

DCCT—Diabetes Control and Complications Trial Research Group: The effect of intensive diabetes therapy on measures of autonomic nervous system function in the Diabetes Control and Complications Trial (DCCT). *Diabetologia* 41: 416–423, 1998a.

DCCT—Diabetes Control and Complications Trial Research Group: Early worsening of diabetic retinopathy in the Diabetes Control and Complications Trial. *Arch Ophthalmol* 116:874–886, 1998b.

DCCT—Diabetes Control and Complications Trial Research Group: Effect of pregnancy on microvascular complications in the Diabetes Control and Complications Trial. *Diabetes Care* 23:1084–1091, 2000.

DCCT/EDIC—Diabetes Control and Complications Trial/Epidemiology of Diabetes Interventions and Complications Research Group: Intensive diabetes therapy and carotid intima-media thickness in type 1 diabetes mellitus. *N Engl J Med* 348:2294–2303, 2003a.

DCCT/EDIC—Diabetes Control and Complications Trial/Epidemiology of Diabetes Interventions and Complications Research Group, Writing Team: Sustained effect of intensive treatment of type 1 diabetes mellitus on development and progression of diabetic nephropathy. *JAMA* 290:2159–2167, 2003b.

DCCT/EDIC—Diabetes Control and Complications Trial/Epidemiology of Diabetes Interventions and Complications Study Research Group: Intensive diabetes treatment and cardiovascular disease in patients with type 1 diabetes. *N Engl J Med* 353:2643–2653, 2005.

De Block CE, De Leeuw IH, Vertommen JJ, Rooman RP, Du Caju MV, Van Campenhout CM, Weyler JJ, Winnock F, Van Autreve J, Gorus FK; Belgian Diabetes Registry: Beta-cell, thyroid, gastric, adrenal and celiac autoimmunity and HLA-DQ types in type 1 diabetes. *Clin Exp Immunol* 126:236–241, 2001.

De Block CEM, De Leeuw IH, Pelckmans PA, Callens D, Maday E, Van Gall LF: Delayed gastric emptying and gastric autoimmunity in type 1 diabetes. *Diabetes Care* 25:912–917, 2002.

De Vriese SR, Dhont M, Christophe AB: Oxidative stability of low density lipoproteins and vitamin E levels increase in maternal blood during normal pregnancy. *Lipids* 36:361–366, 2001.

de Zeeuw D, Remuzzi G, Parving H-H, Keane WF, Zhang Z, Shahinfar S, Snapinn S, Cooper ME, Mitch WE, Brenner B: Albuminuria, a therapeutic target for cardiovascular protection in type 2 diabetic patients with nephropathy. *Circulation* 110:921–927, 2004a.

de Zeeuw D, Remuzzi G, Parving HH, Keane WF, Zhang Z, Shahinfar S, Snapinn S, Cooper ME, Mitch WE, Brenner BM: Proteinuria, a target for renoprotection in patients with type 2 diabetic nephropathy: lessons from RENAAL. *Kidney Int* 65:2309–2320, 2004b.

de Zeeuw D, Parving H-H, Henning RH: Microalbuminuria as an early marker for cardiovascular disease. *J Am Soc Nephrol* 17:2100–2105, 2006.

deBoer IH, Sibley SD, Kestenbaum B, Sampson JN, Young B, Cleary PA, Steffes MW, Weiss NS, Brunzell JD; Diabetes Control and Complications Trial/ Epidemiology of Diabetes Interventions and Complications Study Research Group: Central obesity, incident microalbuminuria, and change in creatinine clearance in the Epidemiology of Diabetes Interventions and Complications Study. *J Am Soc Nephrol* 18:235–243, 2007a.

deBoer IH, Steffes MW: Glomerular filtration rate and albuminuria: twin manifestations of nephropathy in diabetes. *J Am Soc Nephrol* 18:1036–1037, 2007b.

Deckert T, Feldt-Rasmussen B, Borch-Johnson K, Jensen T, Kofoed-Enevolsen A: Albuminuria reflects widespread vascular damage: the Steno hypothesis. *Diabetologia* 32:219–226, 1989.

Deckert T, Yokoyama H, Mathiesen E, Ronn B, Jensen T, Feldt-Rasmussen B, Borch-Johnsen K, Jensen JS: Cohort study of predictive value of urinary albumin excretion for atherosclerotic vascular disease in patients with insulin dependent diabetes. *BMJ* 312:871–874, 1996.

DeFerranti SD, Osganian SK: Epidemiology of pediatric metabolic syndrome and type 2 diabetes mellitus. *Diab Vasc Dis Res* 4:285–296, 2007.

DeGalan BE, De Mol P, Wennekes L, Schouwenberg BJJ, Smits P: Preserved sensitivity to β_2-adrenergic receptor agonists in patients with type 1 diabetes mellitus and hypoglycemia unawareness. *J Clin Endocrinol Metab* 91:2878–2881, 2006.

deLemos JA: The latest and greatest new biomarkers. Which ones should we measure for risk prediction in our practice? Editorial. *Arch Intern Med* 166:2428–2430, 2006.

DeLuca AJ, Kaplan S, Aronow WS, Sandhu R, Butt A, Akoybyan A, Weiss MB: Comparison of prevalence of unrecognized myocardial infarction and of silent myocardial ischemia detected by a treadmill exercise test and myocardial perfusion stress test in patients with or without diabetes. *Am J Cardiol* 98: 1045–1046, 2006.

Demarie BK, Bakris GL: Effects of different calcium antagonists on proteinuria associated with diabetes mellitus. *Ann Intern Med* 113:987–988, 1990.

Demers L, Spencer CA: Laboratory medicine practice guidelines: laboratory support for the diagnosis and monitoring of thyroid disease. *Thyroid* 13:6–20, 2003.

Dendrinos S, Papasteriades C, Tarassi K, Christodoulakos G, Prasinos G, Creatsas G: Thyroid autoimmunity in patients with recurrent spontaneous miscarriages. *Gynecol Endocrinol* 14:270–274, 2000.

DePergola G, Ciampolillo A, Paolotti S, Tretotoli P, Giorgino R: Free triodothyronine and thyroid stimulating hormone are directly associated with waist circumference, independently of insulin resistance, metabolic parameters and blood pressure in overweight and obese women. *Clin Endocrinol (Oxfd)* 67: 265–269, 2007.

DeRosa MA, Cryer PE: Hypoglycemia and the sympathoadrenal system: neurogenic symptoms are largely the result of sympathetic neural, rather than adrenomedullary, activation. *Am J Physiol* 287:E32–E41, 2004.

Deruelle P, Coudoux E, Ego A, Houfflin-Debarge V, Codaccioni X, Subtil D: Risk factors for post-partum complications occurring after preeclampsia and HELLP syndrome. A study in 453 consecutive pregnancies. *Eur J Obstet Gynecol Reprod Biol* 125:59–65, 2006.

Desai DK, Moodley J, Naidoo DP: Echocardiographic assessment of cardiovascular hemodynamics in normal pregnancy. *Obstet Gynecol* 104:20–29, 2004.

Desouza C, Salazar H, Cheong B, Murgo J, Fonseca V: Association of hypoglycemia and cardiac ischemia. A study based on continuous monitoring. *Diabetes Care* 26:1485–1489, 2003.

Desoye GM, Schweditsch MO, Pfeiffer KP, Zechner R, Kostner GM: Correlation of hormones with lipid and lipoprotein levels during normal pregnancy and postpartum. *J Clin Endocrinol Metab* 64: 704–712, 1987.

DGA—U.S. Department of Agriculture, U.S. Department of Health and Human Services: *Dietary Guidelines for Americans, 2005*. 6th ed. Washington, DC: U.S. Government Printing Office; 2005.

Dharnidharka VR, Kwon C, Stevens G: Serum cystatin C is superior to serum creatinine as a marker of kidney function: a meta-analysis. *Am J Kidney Dis* 40:221–226, 2002.

Di Bonito P, Moio N, Cavuto L, Covino G, Murena E, Scilla C, Turco S, Capaldo B, Sibilio G: Early detection of diabetic cardiomyopathy: usefulness of tissue Doppler imaging. *Diabet Med* 22:1720–1725, 2005.

Di Carli MF, Hachamovitch R: Should we screen for occult coronary artery disease among asymptomatic patients with diabetes? *J Am Coll Cardiol* 45:50–53, 2005.

Di Cianni G, Miccoli R, Volpe L, Lencioni C, Ghio A, Giovannitti G, Cuccuru I, Pellegrini G, Chatzianagnostou K, Boldrini A, Del Prato S: Maternal triglyceride levels and newborn weight in pregnant women with normal glucose tolerance. *Diabet Med* 22:21–25, 2005.

Di Cori A, Di Bello V, Miccoli R, Talini E, Palagi C, Donne MGD, Penno G, Nardi C, Bianchi C, Mariani M, Del Prato S, Balbarini A: Left ventricular function in normotensive young adults with well-controlled type 1 diabetes mellitus. *Am J Cardiol* 99:84–90, 2007.

Diamant M, Lamb HJ, Groeneveld Y, Endert EL, Smit JWA, Bax JJ, Romijn JA, de Roos A, Raddar JK: Diastolic dysfunction is associated with altered myocardial metabolism in asymptomatic patients with well-controlled type 2 diabetes mellitus. *J Am Coll Cardiol* 42:328–335, 2003.

Diamond MP, Shah DM, Hester RA, Vaughn WK, Cotton RB, Boehm FH: Complication of insulin-dependent diabetic pregnancies by preeclampsia and/or chronic hypertension: analysis of outcome. *Am J Perinatol* 2:263–267, 1985.

Diamond MP, Reece EA, Caprio S, Jones TW, Amiel S, DeGennaro N, Laudano A, Addabbo M, Sherwin RS, Tamborlane WV: Impairment of counterregulatory hormone responses to hypoglycemia in pregnant women with insulin-dependent diabetes mellitus. *Am J Obstet Gynecol* 166:70–77, 1992.

Diamond M, Jones T, Caprio S, Hallarman L, Meredith-Diamond M, Addabbo M, Tamborlane W, Sherwin R: Gender influences counterregulatory hormone responses to hypoglycemia. *Metabolism* 42:1568–1572, 1993.

Dibble CM, Kochenour NK, Worley RJ, Tyler FH, Swartz M: Effect of pregnancy on diabetic retinopathy. *Obstet Gynecol* 58:699–704, 1982.

Dicker D, Feldberg D, Peleg D, Karp M, Goldman JA: Pregnancy complicated by diabetic nephropathy. *J Perinat Med* 14:299–306, 1986.

Dimitriadis G, Baker B, Marsh H, Mandarino L, Rizza R, Bergman R, Haymond M, Gerich J: Effect of thyroid hormone excess on action, secretion, and metabolism of insulin in humans. *Am J Physiol* 248:E593–E601, 1985.

Dimitriadis G, Mitrou P, Lambadiari V, Boutati E, Maratou E, Panagiotakos DB, Koukkou E, Tzanela M, Thalassinos N, Raptis SA: Insulin action in adipose tissue and muscle in hypothyroidism. *J Clin Endocrinol Metab* 91:4930–4937, 2006a.

Dimitriadis G, Mitrou P, Lambadiari V, Boutati E, Maratou E, Koukkou E, Tzanela M, Thalassinos N, Raptis SA: Glucose and lipid fluxes in the adipose tissue after meal ingestion in hyperthyroidism. *J Clin Endocrinol Metab* 91:1112–1118, 2006b.

Dinn RB, Harris A, Marcus PS: Ocular changes in pregnancy. *Obstet Gynecol Surv* 58:137–144, 2003.

DiSalvo J, Bayne ML, Conn G, Kwok PW, Trivedi PG, Soderman DD, Palisi TM, Sullivan KA, Thomas KA: Purification and characterization of a naturally occurring vascular endothelial growth factor—placenta growth factor heterodimer. *J Biol Chem* 270:7717–7723, 1995.

Distiller LA, Joffe BI, Melville V, Welman T, Distiller GB: Carotid artery intima-media complex thickening in patients with relatively long-surviving type 1 diabetes mellitus. *J Diabetes Complications* 20:280–284, 2006.

Ditchburn CJ, Hall JA, de Belder M, Davies A, Kelly W, Bilous R: Silent myocardial ischaemia in patients with proved coronary artery disease: a comparison of diabetic and non-diabetic patients. *Postgrad Med J* 77:395–398, 2001.

Djelmis J, Ivanisevic M, Reljanovic M, Ilijic M, Bljajic D, Tuzovic L: Cardiovascular neuropathy in pregnant women with type 1 diabetes. *Acta Med Croatica* 57: 275–280, 2003.

Dodds L, Fell DB, Joseph KS, Allen VM, Butler B: Outcomes of pregnancies complicated by hyperemesis gravidarum. *Obstet Gynecol* 107:285–292, 2006.

Dolan NC, Liu K, Criqui MH, Greenland P, Guralnik JM, Chan C, Schneider JR, Mandapat AL, Martin G, McDermott MM: Peripheral artery disease, diabetes, and reduced lower extremity functioning. *Diabetes Care* 25:113–120, 2002.

Dominguez C, Ruiz E, Gussinye M, Carrascosa A: Oxidative stress at onset and in early stages of type 1 diabetes in children and adolescents. *Diabetes Care* 21:1736–1742, 1998.

Dommisse J, Davey DA, Roos PJ: Prazosin and oxprenolol therapy in pregnancy hypertension. *S Afr Med J* 64:231–233, 1983.

Donaghue KC: Autonomic neuropathy: diagnosis and impact on health in adolescents with diabetes. *Horm Res* 50 (Suppl 1):33–37, 1998.

Doney ASF, Lee S, Leese GP, Morris AD, Palmer CAN: Increased cardiovascular morbidity and mortality in type 2 diabetes is associated with the glutathione S transferase theta-null genotype. A Go-DARTS Study. *Circulation* 111: 2927–2934, 2005.

Donnelly R, Molyneaux L, McGill M, Yue DK: Detection and treatment of hypertension in patients with non-insulin-dependent diabetes mellitus: does the "rule of halves" apply to a diabetic population? *Diabetes Res Clin Pract* 37:35–40, 1997.

Donnelly LA, Morris AD, Frier BM, Ellis JD, Donnan PT, Durrant R, Band MM, Reekie G, Leese GP; DARTS/MEMO Collaboration: Frequency and predictors of hypoglycemia in type 1 and insulin-treated type 2 diabetes: a population-based study. *Diabet Med* 22:749–755, 2005.

Dornhorst A, Powell SH, Pensky J: Aggravation by propranolol of hyperglycemic effect of hydrochlorothiazide in type II diabetes without alteration of insulin secretion. *Lancet* 1:123–126, 1985.

Dost A, Klinkert C, Kapellen T, Lemmer A, Naeke A, Grabert M, Kreuder J, Holl RW; the DPV Science Initiative: Arterial hypertension determined by ambulatory blood pressure profiles. Contribution to microalbuminuria risk in a multicenter investigation in 2,105 children and adolescents with type 1 diabetes. *Diabetes Care* 31:720–725, 2008.

Douglas PS, Ginsburg GS: The evaluation of chest pain in women. *N Engl J Med* 334:1311–1315, 1996.

Douma CE, van der Posy JAM, Van Acker BAC, Boer K, Koopman MG: Circadian variation of urinary albumin excretion in pregnancy. *Br J Obstet Gynecol* 102:107–110, 1995.

Doust JA, Glaziou PP, Pietrzak E, Dobson AJ: A systematic review of the diagnostic accuracy of natriuretic peptides for heart failure. *Arch Intern Med* 164:1978–1984, 2004.

DPGF—Diabetes and Pregnancy Group, France: French multicentric survey of outcome of pregnancy in women with pregestational diabetes. Diabetes Care 26:2990–2993, 2003.

Drexel H, Aczel S, Marte T, Benzer W, Langer P, Moll W, Saely CH: Is atherosclerosis in diabetes and impaired fasting glucose driven by elevated LDL cholesterol or by decreased HDL cholesterol? *Diabetes Care* 28:108–114, 2005.

DTCHF—Diagnosis and Treatment of Chronic Heart Failure Task Force, European Society of Cardiology: Guidelines for the diagnosis and treatment of chronic heart failure. *Eur Heart J* 22:1527–1560, 2001.

Du XL, Edelstein D, Dimmeler S, Ju Q, Sui C, Brownlee M: Hyperglycemia inhibits endothelial nitric oxide synthase activity by posttranslational modification of the Akt site. *J Clin Invest* 108:1341–1348, 2001.

Ducher M, Cerutti C, Gustin MP, Abou-Amara S, Thivolet C, Lavulle M, Paultre CZ, Fauvel JP: Noninvasive exploration of cardiac autonomic neuropathy. Four reliable methods for diabetes? *Diabetes Care* 22:388–393, 1999.

Duckitt K, Harrington D: Risk factors for pre-eclampsia at antenatal booking: systematic review of controlled studies. *BMJ* 330:565, 2005.

Ducsay CA, Thompson JS, Wu AT, Novy MJ: Effects of calcium entry blocker (nicardipine) tocolysis in rhesus macaques: fetal plasma concentrations and cardiorespiratory changes. *Am J Obstet Gynecol* 157:1482–1486, 1987.

Dufour P, Berard J, Vinatier D, Subtil D, Guinet B, Bourzoufi P: Pregnancy after myocardial infarction and a coronary artery bypass graft. *Arch Gynecol Obstet* 259:209–213, 1997.

Dumez Y, Tchobroutsky C, Hornych H, Amiet-Tyson C: Neonatal effects of maternal administration of acebutolol. *Br Med J* 283:1077–1079, 1981.

Duncan GE: Prevalence of diabetes and impaired fasting glucose among U.S. adolescents: National Health and Nutrition Examination Survey, 1999–2002. *Arch Pediatr Adolesc Med* 160:523–528, 2006.

Dunne FP, Chowdhury TA, Hartland A, Smith T, Brydon PA, McConkey C, Nicholson HO: Pregnancy outcome in women with insulin-dependent diabetes mellitus complicated by nephropathy. *QJM* 92:451–454, 1999.

Durnwald C, Mercer B: A prospective comparison of total protein/creatinine ratio versus 24-hour urine protein in women with suspected preeclampsia. *Am J Obstet Gynecol* 189:848–852, 2003.

Duvekot JJ, Cheriex EC, Pieters FA, Menheere PP, Peeters LH: Early pregnancy changes in hemodynamics and volume homeostasis are consecutive adjustments triggered by a primary fall in systemic vascular tone. *Am J Obstet Gynecol* 169:1382–1392, 1993.

Duvekot JJ, Peeters LH: Maternal cardiovascular hemodynamic adaptation to pregnancy. *Obstet Gynecol Surv* 49 (Suppl 12):S1–S14, 1994.

Dwyer BK, Taylor L, Fuller A, Brummel C, Lyell DJ: Percutaneous transluminal coronary angioplasty and stent placement in pregnancy. *Obstet Gynecol* 106:1162–1164, 2005.

Dzau VJ, Antman EM, Black HR, Hayes DL, Manson JE, Plitzky J, Popma JJ, Stevenson W: The cardiovascular disease continuum validated: clinical evidence of improved patient outcomes. Part I: pathophysiology and clinical trial evidence (risk factors through stable coronary heart disease). *Circulation* 114:2850–2870, 2006.

Earle KA, Mishra M, Morocutti A, Barnes D, Stephens E, Chambers J, Viberti GC: Microalbuminuria as a marker of silent myocardial ischemia in IDDM patients. *Diabetologia* 39:854–856, 1996.

Easterling TR, Schmucker BC, Carlson KL, Millard SP, Benedetti TJ: Maternal hemodynamics in pregnancies complicated by hyperthyroidism. *Obstet Gynecol* 78:348–352, 1991.

Easterling T, Brateng D, Schmucker B, Brown Z, Millard S: Prevention of preeclampsia: a randomized trial of atenolol in hyperdynamic patients prior to the onset of hypertension. *Obstet Gynecol* 93:725–733, 1999.

Easterling TR, Carr DB, Brateng D, Diederichs C, Schmucker B: Treatment of hypertension in pregnancy: effect of atenolol on maternal disease, preterm delivery, and fetal growth. *Obstet Gynecol* 98:427–433, 2001.

Ebbehoj E, Arildsen H, Hansen KW, Mogensen CE, Molgaard H, Poulsen PL: Effects of metoprolol on QT interval and QT dispersion in type 1 diabetic patients with abnormal albuminuria. *Diabetologia* 47:1009–1015, 2004.

Eckel RH, Yost Jensen DR: Alterations in lipoprotein lipase in insulin resistance. *Int J Obes Relat Metab Disord* 19:S16–S21, 1995.

Eckel RH, Wassef M, Chait A, Sobel B, Barrett E, King G, Lopes-Virella M, Reusch J, Ruderman N, Steiner G, Vlassara H; Writing Group II: Diabetes and cardiovascular disease. Pathogenesis of arteriosclerosis in diabetes. AHA Prevention Conference VI. *Circulation* 105:e138–e143, 2002.

Eckel RH, Kahn R, Robertson RM, Rizza RA: Preventing cardiovascular disease and diabetes: a call to action from the American Diabetes Association and the

American Heart Association. Dual publication in *Circulation* 113:2943–2946, 2006 and *Diabetes Care* 29:1697–1699, 2006.

Eckstein AK, Plicht M, Lax H, Neuhauser M, Mann K, Lederbogen S, Heckmann C, Esser J, Morgenthaler NG: Thyrotropin receptor antibodies are independent risk factors for Graves' ophthalmopathy and help to predict severity and outcome of the disease. *J Clin Endocrinol Metab* 91:3464–3470, 2006.

ECPPA—Estudo Colaborativo para Prevencao da Pre-eclampsia com Aspirina Collaborative Group: Randomized trial of low dose aspirin for the prevention of maternal and fetal complications in high-risk pregnant women. *Br J Obstet Gynecol* 103:39–47, 1996.

Eddy DM, Schlessinger L: Archimedes: a trial-validated model of diabetes. *Diabetes Care* 26:3093–3101, 2003.

Eddy AA: Proteinuria and interstitial injury. *Nephrol Dial Transplant* 19:277–281, 2004.

Edelstein C, Pfaffinger D, Hinman J, Miller E, Lipkind G, Tsimikas S, Bergmark C, Getz GS, Witztum JL, Scanu AM: Lysine-phosphatidylcholine adducts in Kringle V impart unique immunological and potential pro-inflammatory properties to human apolipoprotein(a). *J Biol Chem* 278:52841–52847, 2003.

EDIC—Epidemiology of Diabetes Interventions and Complications Research Group: Effect of intensive diabetes treatment on carotid artery wall thickness in the epidemiology of diabetes interventions and complications. *Diabetes* 48:383–390, 1999.

Eghbali M, Deva R, Alioua A, Minosyan TY, Ruan H, Wang Y, Toro L, Stefani E: Molecular and functional signature of heart hypertrophy during pregnancy. *Circ Res* 96:1208–1216, 2005.

Eijkelkamp WBA, Zhang Z, Remuzzi G, Parving H-H, Cooper ME, Keane WF, Shahinfar S, Gleim GW, Weir MR, Brenner BM, de Zeeuw, D: Albuminuria is a target for renoprotective therapy independent from blood pressure in patients with type 2 diabetic nephropathy: post hoc analysis from the Reduction in Endpoints in NIDDM with the Angiotensin II Antagonist Losartin (RENAAL) Trial. *J Am Soc Nephrol* 18:1540–1546, 2007.

Eisenberg JA, Armenti VT, McGrory CH, et al: National Transplantation Pregnancy Registry (NTPR): use of muromonab-CD3(OKT3) during pregnancy in female transplant recipients. *Am Soc Transpl Phys* 20:1997.

Eisenstein Z, Weiss M, Katz Y, Bank H: Intellectual capacity of subjects exposed to methimazole or propylthiouracil in utero. *Eur J Pediatr* 151:558–589, 1992.

Ekbom P, Damm P, Norgaard K, Clausen P, Feldt-Rasmussen U, Feldt-Rasmussen B, Nielsen LH, Moelsted-Pedersen L, Mathiesen ER: Urinary albumin excretion and 24-hour blood pressure as predictors of pre-eclampsia in type 1 diabetes. *Diabetologia* 43:927–931, 2000.

Ekbom P, Damm P, Feldt-Rasmussen B, Feldt-Rasmussen U, Molvig J, Mathiesen ER: Pregnancy outcome in type 1 diabetic women with microalbuminuria. *Diabetes Care* 24:1739–1744, 2001.

Ekholm EM, Piha SJ, Antila KJ, Erkkola RU: Cardiovascular autonomic reflexes in mid-pregnancy. *Br J Obstet Gynecol* 100:177–182, 1993.

Ekholm EM, Piha Erkkola RU, Antila KJ: Autonomic cardiovascular reflexes in pregnancy. A longitudinal study. *Clin Auton Res* 4:161–165, 1994.

Ekholm EM, Erkkola RU: Autonomic cardiovascular control in pregnancy. *Eur J Obstet Gynecol Reprod Biol* 64:29–36, 1996.

Eknoyan G, Hostetter T, Bakris GL, Hebert GL, Levey AS, Parving HH, Steffes MW, Toto R: Proteinuria and other markers of chronic kidney disease: a position statement of the National Kidney Foundation (NKF) and the National Institute of Diabetes, Digestive and Kidney Diseases (NIDDK). *Am J Kidney Dis* 42: 617–622, 2003.

Elam MB, Hunninghake DB, Davis KB, Garg R, Johnson C, Egan D, Kostis JB, Sheps DS, Brinton EA: Effect of niacin on lipid and lipoprotein levels and glycemic control in patients with diabetes and peripheral arterial disease: the ADMIT study: a randomized study. The Arterial Disease Multiple Intervention Trial. *JAMA* 284:1263–1270, 2000.

Elatrous S, Nouira S, Ounes Besbes L, Marghli S, Boussarssar M, Sakkouhi M, Abroug F: Short-term treatment of severe hypertension in pregnancy: prospective comparison of nicardipine and labetalol. *Intens Care Med* 28:1281–1286, 2002.

Eliahou HE, Silverberg ZDS, Reisin E, Romem I, Mashiach S, Serr DM: Propranolol for the treatment of hypertension in pregnancy. *Br J Obstet Gynecol* 85:431–436, 1978.

Eliasson B, Cederholm J, Nilsson P, Gudbjornsdottir S; Steering Committee of the Swedish National Diabetes Register: The gap between guidelines and reality: type 2 diabetes in a National Diabetes Register 1996–2003. *Diabet Med* 22:1420–1426, 2005.

Elkayam U: Cardiac evaluation during pregnancy. In: Elkayam U, Gleicher N, eds. *Cardiac Problems in Pregnancy.* 3rd ed. New York: Wiley-Liss; 1998:23–32.

Elkayam U: Pregnancy and cardiovascular disease. In: *Braunwald's Heart Disease. A Textbook of Cardiovascular Medicine.* 7th ed. Philadelphia: Elsevier Saunders; 2005:1965–1984.

Elkind MS, Tai W, Coates K, Paik MC, Sacco RL: High-sensitivity C-reactive protein, lipoprotein-associated phospholipase A_2, and outcome after ischemic stroke. *Arch Intern Med* 166:2073–2080, 2006.

Ellhadd TA, Jung RT, Newton RW, Stonebridge PA, Belch JJ: Incidence of asymptomatic peripheral arterial occlusive disease in diabetic patients attending a hospital clinic. *Adv Exp Med Biol* 428:45–48, 1997.

Elming H, Holm E, Jun L, Torp-Pedersen C, Kober L, Kircshoff M, Malik M, Camm J: The prognostic value of the QT interval and QT interval dispersion in all-cause and cardiac mortality and morbidity in a population of Danish citizens. *Eur Heart J* 19:1391–1400, 1998.

El-Sayed YY, Holbrook RH Jr, Gibson R, Chitkara U, Druzin ML, Baba D: Diltiazem for maintenance tocolysis of preterm labor: comparison to nifedipine in a randomized trial. *J Matern-Fetal Med* 7:217–221, 1998.

Endemann DH, Pu Q, De Ciuceis C, Savoia C, Virdis A, Neves MF, Touyz RM, Schiffrin EL: Persistent remodeling of resistance arteries in type 2 diabetic patients on antihypertensive treatment. *Hypertension* 43:399–404, 2004.

Engelstein ED: Long QT syndrome: a preventable cause of sudden death in women. *Curr Women's Health Rep* 3:126–134, 2003.

Enoksson S, Caprio SK, Rife F, Shulman GI, Tamborlane WV, Sherwin RS: Defective activation of skeletal muscle and adipose tissue lipolysis in type 1 diabetes mellitus during hypoglycemia. *J Clin Endocrinol Metab* 88:1503–1511, 2003.

Eppens MC, Craig ME, Cusumano J, Hing S, Chan AKF, Howard NJ, Silink M, Donaghue KC: Prevalence of diabetes complications in adolescents with type 2 compared with type 1 diabetes. *Diabetes Care* 29:1300–1306, 2006.

Epshteyn V, Morrison K, Krishnaswamy P, Kazanegra R, Clopton P, Mudaliar S, Edelman S, Henry R, Maisel A: Utility of B-type natriuretic peptide (BNP) as a screen for left ventricular dysfunction in patients with diabetes. *Diabetes Care* 26:2081–2087, 2003.

Erbel R, Ge J, Gorge G, Baumgart D, Haude M, Jeremias A, von Birgelen C, Jollet N, Schwedtmann J: Intravascular ultrasound classification of atherosclerotic lesions according to American Heart Association recommendation. *Coron Artery Dis* 10:489–499, 1999.

ESC—European Society of Cardiology Task Force and the North American Society of Pacing and Electrophysiology: Heart rate variability: standards of measurement, physiological interpretation and clinical use. *Circulation* 93:1043–1065, 1996.

Escolar G, Bastida E, Garrido M, Rodriguez-Gomez J, Castillo R, Ordinas A: Sex-related differences in the effects of aspirin on the interaction of platelets with endothelium. *Thromb Res* 44:837–847, 1986.

Eshoj O, Feldt-Rasmussen B, Larsen ML, Mogensen EF: Comparison of overnight, morning and 24-hour urine collections in the assessment of diabetic albuminuria. *Diabet Med* 4:531–533, 1987.

Espeland MA, Craven TE, Riley WA, Corson J, Romont A, Furberg CD: Reliability of longitudinal ultrasonographic measurements of carotid intimal-medial thickness. *Stroke* 27:480–485, 1996.

Esplin MS, Branch DW, Silver R, Stagnaro-Green A: Thyroid autoantibodies are not associated with recurrent pregnancy loss. *Am J Obstet Gynecol* 179:1583–1586, 1998.

Estacio RO, Jeffers BW, Gifford N, Schrier RW: Effect of blood pressure control on diabetic microvascular complications in patients with hypertension and type 2 diabetes. *Diabetes Care* 23:B54–B64, 2000.

ETDRS—Early Treatment Diabetic Retinopathy Study Research Group: Grading diabetic retinopathy from stereoscopic color fundus photographs: an extension of the modified Airlie House classification. *Ophthalmology* 98:786–806, 1991.

ETDRS—Early Treatment Diabetic Retinopathy Study Investigators: Aspirin effects on mortality and morbidity in patients with diabetes mellitus: Early Treatment Diabetic Retinopathy Study report # 14. *JAMA* 268:1292–1300, 1992.

Ettinger LM, Freeman K, DiMartino-Nardi JR, Flynn JT: Microalbuminuria and normal ambulatory blood pressure in adolescents with type 2 diabetes mellitus. *J Pediatr* 147:67–73, 2005.

Evans ML, McCrimmon RJ, Flanagan DE, Keshavarz T, Fan X, McNay EC, Jacob RJ, Sherwin RS: Hypothalamic ATP-sensitive K+ channels play a key role in sensing hypoglycemia and triggering counterregulatory epinephrine and glucagon responses. *Diabetes* 53:2542–2551, 2004.

Everett AD, Fisher A, Tufro-McReddie A, Harris M: Developmental regulation of angiotensin type 1 and type 2 receptor gene expression and heart growth. *J Moll Cell Cardiol* 29:141–149, 1997.

Evers IM, ter Braak EWMT, de Valk HW, van der Schoot B, Janssen N, Visser GHA: Risk indicators predictive for severe hypoglycemia during the first trimester of type 1 diabetic pregnancy. *Diabetes Care* 25:554–559, 2002.

Evers IM, de Valk HW, Visser GHA: Risk of complications of pregnancy in women with type 1 diabetes: nationwide prospective study in the Netherlands. *BMJ* 328:915–918, 2004.

Ewing DJ, Campbell IW, Murray A, Neilson JMM, Clarke BF: Immediate heart-rate response to standing: simple test for autonomic neuropathy in diabetes. *Br Med J* i:145–147, 1978.

Ewing DJ, Campbell IW, Clarke BF: Assessment of cardiovascular effects in diabetic autonomic neuropathy and prognostic implications. *Ann Intern Med* 92: 308–311, 1980.

Ewing DJ, Borsey DQ, Bellavere F, Clarke BF: Cardiac autonomic neuropathy in diabetes—comparison of measures of R-R interval variation. *Diabetologia* 21: 18–24, 1981.

Ewing DJ, Clarke BF: Diagnosis and management of diabetic autonomic neuropathy. *Br Med J* 285:916–918, 1982.

Ewing DJ, Martyn CN, Young RJ, Clarke BF: The value of cardiovascular autonomic function tests: 10 years' experience in diabetes. *Diabetes Care* 8:491–498, 1985.

Facchini F, Chen YD, Hollenbeck CB, Reaven GM: Relationship between resistance to insulin-mediated glucose uptake, urinary uric acid clearance, and plasma uric acid concentration. *JAMA* 266:3008–3011, 1991.

Faerman I, Faccio E, Milei J, Nunez R, Jadzinski M, Fox D, Rapaport M: Autonomic neuropathy and painless myocardial infarction in diabetic patients. Histologic evidence of their relationship. *Diabetes* 26:1147–1158, 1977.

Faglia E, Favales F, Quarantiello A, Calia P, Clelia P, Brambilla G, Rampoldi A, Morabito A: Angiographic evaluation of peripheralarterial occlusive disease and its role as a prognostic determinanat for major amputation in diabetic patients with foot ulcers. *Diabetes Care* 21:625–630, 1998.

Faglia E, Manuela M, Antonella Q, Michela G, Vincenzo C, Maurizio C, Roberto M, Alberto M: Risk reduction of cardiac events by screening of unknown asymptomatic coronary artery disease in subjects with type 2 diabetes mellitus at high cardiovascular risk: an open-label randomized pilot study. *Am Heart J* 149;e1–e6, 2005.

Fagot-Campagna A, Pettitt DJ, Engelgau MM, Burrows NR, Geiss LS, Valdez R, Beckles GL, Saaddine J, Gregg EW, Williamson DF, Narayan KM: Type 2 diabetes among North American children and adolescents: an epidemiologic review and a public health perspective. *J Pediatr* 136:664–672, 2000.

Fahlbusch SA, Tsikas D, Mehls C, Gutszi FM, Boger RH, Frolich JC, Stichtenoth DO: Effects of carvedilol on oxidative stress in human endothelial cells and healthy volunteers. *Eur J Clin Pharmacol* 60:83–88, 2004.

Fanelli C, De Feo P, Porcellati F, Perriello G, Torlone E, Santeusanio F, Brunetti P, Bolli GB: Adrenergic mechanisms contribute to the late phase of hypoglycemic glucose counterregulation in humans by stimulating lipolysis. *J Clin Invest* 89:2005–2013, 1992.

Fanelli C, Calderone S, Epifano L, De Vincenzo A, Modarelli F, Pampanelli S, Perriello G, De Feo P, Brunetti P, Gerich JE, Bolli GB: Demonstration of a critical role for free fatty acids in mediating counterregulatory stimulation of gluconeogenesis and suppression of glucose utilization in humans. *J Clin Invest* 92:1617–1622, 1993a.

Fanelli CG, Epifano L, Rambotti AM, Pampanelli S, Di Vicenzo A, Modarelli F, Lepore M, Annibale B, Clofetta M, Bottini P, Porcellati F, Scionti L, Santeusanio F, Brunetti P, Bolli GB: Meticulous prevention of hypoglycemia normalizes the glycemic thresholds and magnitude of most neuroendocrine responses to, symptoms of, and cognitive function during hypoglycemia in intensively treated patients with short-term IDDM. *Diabetes* 42:1683–1689, 1993b.

Fanelli C, Pampanelli S, Epifano L, Rambotti AM, Di Vincenzo A, Modarelli F, Ciofetta M, Lepore M, Annibale B, Torlone E, Perriello G, De Feo P, Santeusanio F, Brunetti P, Bolli GB: Long-term recovery from unawareness, deficient counterregulation and lack of cognitive dysfunction during hypoglycemia, following institution of rational, intensive insulin therapy in IDDM. *Diabetologia* 37:1265–1276, 1994.

Fang ZY, Yuda S, Anderson V, Short L, Case C, Marwick TH: Echocardiographic detection of early diabetic myocardial disease. *J Am Coll Cardiol* 41:611–617, 2003a.

Fang ZY, Najos-Valencia O, Leano R, Marwick TH: Patients with early diabetic heart disease demonstrate a normal myocardial response to dobutamine. *J Am Coll Cardiol* 42:446–453, 2003b.

Fang ZY, Prins JB, Marwick TH: Diabetic cardiomyopathy: evidence, mechanisms, and therapeutic implications. *Endocrine Rev* 25:543–567, 2004.

Fang ZY, Schull-Meade R, Leano R, Mottram PM, Prins JB, Marwick TH: Screening for heart disease in diabetic subjects. *Am Heart J* 149:349–354, 2005a.

Fang ZY, Schull-Meade R, Downey M, Prins JB, Marwick TH: Determinants of subclinical diabetic heart disease. *Diabetologia* 48:394–402, 2005b.

Farmer JA: Diabetic dyslipidemia and atherosclerosis: evidence from clinical trials. *Curr Diab Rep* 8:71–77, 2008.

Feldman EL: Oxidative stress and diabetic neuropathy: a new understanding of an old problem. Commentary. *J Clin Invest* 111:431–433, 2003.

Felicio JS, Pacheco JT, Ferreira SR, Plavnik F, Moises VA, Kohlmann Jr, Ribeiro AB, Zanella MT: Hyperglycemia and nocturnal systolic blood pressure are associated with left ventricular hypertrophy and diastolic dysfunction in hypertensive diabetic patients. *Cardiovasc Diabetol* 5:19, 2006.

Fell DB, Dodd L, Joseph KS, Allen VM, Butler B: Risk factors for hyperemesis gravidarum requiring hospital admission during pregnancy. *Obstet Gynecol* 107:277–284, 2006.

Fernandes VR, Polak JF, Edvardsen T, Carvalho B, Gomes A, Bluemke DA, Nasir K, O'Leary DH, Lima JA: Subclinical atherosclerosis and incipient regional myocardial dysfunction in asymptomatic individuals: the Multi-Ethnic Study of Atherosclerosis (MESA). *J Am Coll Cardiol* 47(12): 2420–2428, 2006.

Fernandez-Casterner M, Molina A, Lopez-Jimenez L, Gomez JM, Soler J: Clinical presentation and early course of type 1 diabetes in patients with and without thyroid autoimmunity. *Diabetes Care* 22:377–381, 1999.

Fernandez-Soto L, Gonzalez A, Lobon JA, Lopez JA, Peterson CM, Escobar-Jimenez F: Thyroid peroxidase autoantibodies predict poor metabolic control and need for thyroid treatment in pregnant IDDM women. *Diabetes Care* 20:1524–1528, 1997.

Fernandez-Soto ML, Jovanovic LG, Gonzalez-Jimenez A, Lobon-Hernandez JA, Escobar-Jimenez F, Lopez-Cozar LN, Barredo-Acedo F, Campos-Pastor MM, Lopez-Medina JA: Thyroid function during pregnancy and the postpartum period: iodine metabolism and disease states. *Endocr Pract* 4: 87–105, 1998.

Ferrari R: Major differences among the three classes of calcium antagonists. *Eur Heart J* 18 (Suppl A):A56–A70, 1997.

Ferrer RL, Sibai BM, Mulrow CD, Chiquette E, Stevens KR, Cornell J: Management of mild chronic hypertension during pregnancy: a review. *Obstet Gynecol* 96: 849–860, 2000.

Festa A, D'Agostino R Jr, Rautaharju P, Mykkaenen L, Haffner SM: Relation of systemic blood pressure, left ventricular mass, insulin sensitivity, and coronary artery disease to QT interval duration in nondiabetic and type 2 diabetic subjects. *Am J Cardiol* 86:1117–1122, 2000.

Feuerstein G, Shusterman NH, Ruffolo RR Jr: Carvedilol update IV: prevention of oxidative stess, cardiac remodeling and progression of congestive cardiac failure. *Drugs Today* 33:453–473, 1997.

Fidler J, Smith V, Fayers P, De Swiet M: Randomized controlled comparative study of methyldopa and oxprenolol in treatment of hypertension in pregnancy. *Br Med J* 286:1927–1930, 1983.

Finne P, Reunanen A, Stenman S, Groop PH, Gronhagen-Riska C: Incidence of end-stage renal disease in patients with type 1 diabetes. *JAMA* 294:1782–1787, 2005.

Finney H, Newman DJ, Price CP: Adult reference ranges for serum cystatin C, creatinine and predicted creatinine clearance. *Ann Clin Biochem* 37:49–59, 2000.

Fiordaliso F, Leri A, Cesselli D, Limana F, Safai B, Nadal-Ginard B, Anversa P, Kajstura J: Hyperglycemia activates p53 and p53–regulated genes leading to myocyte cell death. *Diabetes* 50:2363–2375, 2001.

First MR, Combs CA, Weiskittel P, Miodovnik M: Lack of effect of pregnancy on renal allograft survival or function. *Transplantation* 59:472–476 1995.

Fisher JN, Kitabchi AE: A randomized study of phosphate therapy in the treatment of diabetic ketoacidosis. *J Clin Endocrinol Metab* 57:177–180, 1983.

Fisher BM, Gillen G, Hepburn DA, Dargie HJ, Frier BM: Cardiac responses to acute insulin-induced hypoglycemia in humans. *Am J Physiol* 258:H1775–H1779, 1990.

Fisher DA, Nelson JC, Carlton EI, Wilcox RB: Maturation of human hypothalamic-pituitary-thyroid function and control. *Thyroid* 10:229–234, 2000.

Fisher SJ, Bruning JC, Lannon S, Kahn CR: Insulin signaling in the central nervous system is critical for the normal sympathoadrenal response to hypoglycemia. *Diabetes* 54:1447–1451, 2005.

Fleming SM, O'Byrne L, Grimes H, Daly KM, Morrison JJ: Amino-terminal pro-brain natriuretic peptide in normal and hypertensive pregnancy. *Hypertens Preg* 20:169–175, 2001.

Flores L, Levy I, Aguilera E, Martinez S, Gomis R, Esmatjes E: Usefulness of ambulatory blood pressure monitoring in pregnant women with type 1 diabetes. *Diabetes Care* 22:1507–1511, 1999.

Fok WY, Chan LY, Wong JT, Yu CM, Lau TK: Left ventricular diastolic function during normal pregnancy assessment by spectral tissue Doppler imaging. *Ultrasound Obstet Gynecol* 28:789–793, 2006.

Folk JJ, Lipari CW, Nosovitch JT, Silverman RK, Carlson RJ, Navone AJ: Evaluating ventricular function with B-type natriuretic peptide in obstetric patients. *J Reprod Med* 50:147–154, 2005.

Folsom AR, Eckfeldt JH, Weitzman S, Ma J, Chambless LE, Barnes RW, Cram KB, Hutchinson RG: Relation of carotid artery wall thickness to diabetes mellitus, fasting glucose and insulin, body size and physical activity. *Stroke* 25:666–673, 1994.

Fong DS, Aiello L, Gardner TW, King GL, Blankenship G, Cavallerano JD, Ferris FL III, Klein R; for the American Diabetes Association: Retinopathy in diabetes. Position statement. *Diabetes Care* 27:S84–S87, 2004a.

Fong DS, Aiello LP, Ferris FL III, Klein R: Diabetic retinopathy. Technical review. *Diabetes Care* 27:2540–2553, 2004b.

Fonorow GC, Srikanthan P: Diabetic cardiomyopathy. *Endocrinol Metab Clin North Am* 35:575–599, 2006.

Foody JM, Milberg JA, Robinson K, Pearce GL, Jacobsen DW, Sprecher DL: Homocysteine and lipoprotein(a) interact to increase CAD risk in young men and women. *Arterioscler Thromb Vasc Biol* 20:493–499, 2000.

Forhead AJ, Pipkin FB, Sutherland MF, Fowden AL: Changes in the maternal and fetal renin-angiotensin systems in response to angiotensin II type 1 receptor blockade and angiotensin-converting enzyme inhibition in pregnant sheep during late gestation. *Exp Physiol* 82:761–776, 1997.

Fornengo P, Bosio A, Epifani G, Pallisco O, Mancuso A, Pascale C: Prevalence of silent myocardial ischaemia in new-onset middle-aged type 2 diabetic patients without other cardiovascular risk factors. *Diabet Med* 23:775–779, 2006.

Forrest K YZ, Becker DJ, Kuller LH, Wolfson SK, Orchard TJ: Are predictors of coronary heart disease and lower-extremity arterial disease in type 1 diabetes the same? A prospective study. *Atherosclerosis* 148:159–169, 2000.

Fox CS, Coady S, Sorlie PD, Levy D, Meigs JB, D'Agostino RB Sr, Wilson PW, Savage PJ: Trends in cardiovascular complications of diabetes. *JAMA* 292: 2495–2499, 2004a.

Fox JC, Leight K, Sutradar SC, Demopoulos LA, Gleim GW, Lewin AJ, Bakris GL: The JNC 7 approach compared to conventional treatment in diabetic patients with hypertension: a double-blind trial of initial monotherapy vs. combination therapy. *J Clin Hypertens* 6:437–444, 2004b.

Fox CS, Pencina MJ, D'Agostino RB, Murabito JM, Seely EW, Pearce EN, Vasan RS: Relations of thyroid function to body weight. Cross-sectional and longitudinal observations in a community-based sample. *Arch Intern Med* 168:587–592, 2008.

Fraile LJ, Bregante MA, Garcia MA, Solans C: Altered diltiazem metabolism in the neonatal rabbit following intra-uterine chronic exposure to diltiazem. *Xenobiotica* 31:177–185, 2001.

Franceschini N, Qiu C, Barrow DA, Williams MA: Cystatin C and preeclampsia: a case control study. *Ren Fail* 30:89–95, 2008.

Frank RN: Diabetic retinopathy. *N Engl J Med* 350:48–58, 2004.

Fraser GE, Luke R, Thompson S, Smith H, Carter S, Sharpe N: Comparison of echocardiographic variables between type 1 diabetics and normal controls. *Am J Cardiol* 75:141–145, 1995.

Frasier SD, Penny R, Snyder R, Goldstein I, Graves D: Antithyroid antibodies in Hispanic patients with type 1 diabetes mellitus. *AJDC* 140:1278–1280, 1986.

Freccero C, Svensson H, Bornmyr S, Wollmer P, Sundkvist G: Sympathetic and parasympathetic neuropathy are frequent in both type 1 and type 2 diabetic patients. *Diabetes Care* 27:2936–2941, 2004.

Freire CM, Nunes Mdo C, Barbosa MM, Longo JR, Nogueira AI, Diniz SS, Machado LJ, de Oliveira AR Jr: Gestational diabetes: a condition of early diastolic abnormalities in young women. *J Am Soc Echocardiogr* 19:1251–1256, 2006.

Fricker M, Wiesli P, Brandle M, Schwegler B, Schmid C: Impact of thyroid dysfunction on serum cystatin C. *Kidney Int* 63:1944–1947, 2003.

Fridericia LS: EKG systolic duration in normal subjects and heart disease patients. *Acta Med Scand* 53:469–488, 1920.

Friedewald WT, Levy RI, Fredrickson DS: Estimation of the concentration of low-density lipoprotein cholesterol in plasma, without use of the preparative ultracentrifuge. *Clin Chem* 18:499–502, 1972.

Friedman EA, Neff RK: Hypertension-hypotension in pregnancy. Correlation with fetal outcome. *JAMA* 239:2249–2251, 1978.

Fritsche A, Stumvoll M, Grub M, Sieslack S, Renn W, Schmulling R-M, Haring H-U, Gerich JE: Effect of hypoglycemia on β-adrenergic sensitivity in normal and type 1 diabetic subjects. *Diabetes Care* 21:1505–1510, 1998.

Froissart M, Rossert J, Jacqot C, Paillard M, Houillier P: Predictive performance of the Modification of Diet in Renal Disease and Cockcroft-Gault equations for estimating renal function. *J Am Soc Nephrol* 16:763–773, 2005.

Frost PH, Havel RJ: Rationale for use of non-high-density lipoprotein cholesterol rather than low-density lipoprotein cholesterol as a tool for lipocholesterol screening and assessment of risk and therapy. *Am J Cardiol* 81:26B–31B, 1998.

Frost D, Friedl A, Beischer W: Determinants of early carotid atherosclerosis progression in young patients with type 1 diabetes mellitus. *Exp Clin Endocrinol Diabetes* 110:92–94, 2002.

Frustaci A, Kajstura J, Chimenti C, Jakoniuk I, Leri A, Maseri A, Nadal-Ginard B, Anversa P: Myocardial cell death in human diabetes. *Circ Res* 87:1123–1132, 2000.

Fu T, Borensztajn J: Macrophage uptake of low-density lipoprotein bound to aggregated C-reactive protein: possible mechanism of foam-cell formation in atherosclerotic lesions. *Biochem J* 366:195–201, 2002.

Fujioka Y, Cooper AD, Fong LG: Multiple processes are involved in the uptake of chylomicron remnants by mouse peritoneal macrophages. *J Lipid Res* 39: 2339–2349, 1998.

Fuller JH, Head J; WHO Multinational Study Group: Blood pressure, proteinuria and their relationship with circulatory mortality: the WHO Multinational Study of Vascular Disease in Diabetes. *Diabete Metab* (Paris) 15:273–277, 1989.

Fuller JH, Stevens LK, Wang SL: Risk factors for cardiovascular mortality and morbidity: the WHO Multinational Study of Vascular Disease in Diabetes. *Diabetologia* 44 (Suppl 2):S54–S64, 2001.

Furlan R, Guzzetti S, Crivellaro W, Dassi S, Tinelli M, Baselli G, Cerutti S, Lombardi F, Pagani M, Malliani A: Continuous 24-hour assessment of the neural regulation of systemic arterial pressure and RR variabilities in ambulant subjects. *Circulation* 81:537–547, 1990.

Gaede P, Vedel P, Parving HH, Pedersen O: Intensified multifactorial intervention in patients with type 2 diabetes mellitus and microalbuminuria: the Steno type 2 randomized study. *Lancet* 353:617–622, 1999.

Gaede P, Vedel P, Larsen N, Jensen GV, Parving H-H, Pedersen O: Multifactorial intervention and cardiovascular disease in patients with type 2 diabetes. *N Engl J Med* 348:383–393, 2003.

Gaede P, Hildebrandt P, Hess G, Parving H-H, Pedersen O: Plasma NT-pro-brain natriuretic peptide as a risk marker for cardiovascular disease in patients with type 2 diabetes and microalbuminuria. *Diabetologia* 48:156–163, 2005.

Gaede P, Lund-Anderson II, Parving H-H, Pedersen O: Effect of a multifactorial intervention on mortality in type 2 diabetes. *N Engl J Med* 358:580–591, 2008.

Galassetti P, Tate D, Neill RA, Morrey S, Wasserman DH, Davis SN: Effect of sex on counterregulatory responses to exercise after antecedent hypoglycemia in type 1 diabetes. *Am J Physiol* 287:E16–E24, 2004.

Galderisi M, Anderson KM, Wilson PWF, Levy D: Echocardiographic evidence for the existence of a distinct diabetic cardiomyopathy (the Framingham Heart Study). *Am J Cardiol* 68:85–89, 1991.

Gall MA, Hougaard P, Borch-Johnsen K, Parving HH: Risk factors for development of incipient and overt diabetic nephropathy in patients with non-insulin dependent diabetes mellitus: prospective, observational study. *BMJ* 314: 783–788, 1997.

Gallagher MP, Schachner HC, Levine LS, Fisher DA, Berdon WE, Oberfield SE: Neonatal thyroid enlargement associated with propylthiouracil therapy of Graves' disease during pregnancy: a problem revisited. *J Pediatr* 139:896–900, 2001.

Gallas PRJ, Stolk RP, Bakker K, Endert E, Wiersinga WM: Thyroid dysfunction during pregnancy and in the first postpartum year in women with diabetes mellitus type 1. *Eur J Endocrinol* 147:443–451, 2002.

Gallery EDM, Ross MR, Gyory AZ: Antihypertensive treatment in pregnancy: analysis of different responses to oxprenolol and methyldopa. *Br Med J* 291: 563–566, 1985.

Galvan AQ, Natali A, Baldi S, Frascerra S, Sanna G, Ciociaro D, Ferrannini E: Effect of insulin on uric acid excretion in humans. *Am J Physiol* 268:E1–E5, 1995.

Gambelunghe G, Forini F, Laureti S, Murdolo G, Toraldo G, Santeusanio F, Brunetti P, Sanjeevi CB, Falorni A: Increased risk for endocrine autoimmunity in Italian type 2 diabetic patients with GAD65 autoantibodies. *Clin Endocrinol (Oxf)* 52:565–573, 2000.

Garcia MJ, Thomas JD, Klein AL: New Doppler echocardiographic applications for the study of diastolic function. *J Am Coll Cardiol* 32:865–875, 1998.

Gardner DF, Cruikshank DP, Hays PM, Cooper DS: Pharmacology of propylthiouracil (PTU) in pregnant hyperthyroid women: correlation of maternal PTU concentrations with cord serum thyroid function tests. *J Clin Endocrinol Metab* 62:217–220, 1986.

Gashti CN, Bakris GL: The role of calcium antagonists in chronic kidney disease. *Curr Opin Nephrol Hypertens* 13:155–161, 2004.

Gasic S, Winzer C, Bayerle-Eder M, Roden A, Pacini G, Kautzky-Willer A: Impaired cardiac autonomic function in women with prior gestational diabetes mellitus. *Eur J Clin Invest* 37:42–47, 2007.

Gault MH, Longerich LL, Harnett JD, Wesolowski C: Predicting glomerular function from adjusted serum creatinine. *Nephron* 62:249–256, 1992.

Gazi I, Lourida ES, Filippatos T, Tsimihodimos V, Elisaf M, Tselepis AD: Lipoprotein-associated phospholipase A2 activity is a marker of small, dense LDL particles in human plasma. *Clin Chem* 51:2264–2273, 2005.

GDFSG—Gestation and Diabetes in France Study Group: Multicenter survey of diabetic pregnancy in France. *Diabetes Care* 14:994–1000, 1991.

Geddes J, Warren RE, Sommerfield AJ, McAulay V, Strachan MWJ, Allen KV, Deary IJ, Frier BM: Absence of sexual dimorphism in the symptomatic responses to hypoglycemia in adults with and without type 1 diabetes. *Diabetes Care* 29:1667–1669, 2006.

Geiss LS, Rolka DB, Englegau MM: Elevated blood pressure among U.S. adults with diabetes, 1988–1994. *Am J Prev Med* 22:42–48, 2002.

Gekle M: Renal tubule albumin transport. *Annu Rev Physiol* 67:573–594, 2005.

Genovely H, Pfeifer MA: RR-variation: the autonomic test of choice in diabetes. *Diabetes Metab Rev* 4:255–271, 1988.

Gentile S: The safety of newer antidepressants in pregnancy and breastfeeding. *Drug Saf* 28:137–152, 2005.

George PB, Tobin KJ, Corpus RA, Devlin WH, O'Neill WW: Treatment of cardiac risk factors in diabetic patients: how well do we follow the guidelines? *Am Heart J* 142:857–863, 2001.

Gerich JE, Langlois M, Noacco C, Karam J, Forsham PH: Lack of a glucagon response to hypoglycemia in diabetes: evidence for an intrinsic pancreatic alpha-cell defect. *Science* 182:171–173, 1973.

Gerich JE: Hypoglycemia and counterregulation in type 2 diabetes. Commentary. *Lancet* 356:1946–1947, 2000.

Gerritsen J, Dekker JM, TenVoorde BJ, Kostense PJ, Heine RJ, Bouter LM, Heethaar RM, Stehouwer CDA: Impaired autonomic function is associated with increased mortality, especially in subjects with diabetes, hypertension, or a history of cardiovascular disease. The Hoorn Study. *Diabetes Care* 24:1793–1798, 2001.

Gerson MC, Khoury JC, Hertzberg VS, Fischer EE, Scott RC: Prediction of coronary artery disease in a population of insulin-requiring diabetic patients: results of an 8-year follow-up study. *Am Heart J* 116:820–826, 1988.

Gerstein HC, Mann JFE, Yi Q, Zinman B, Dinneen SF, Hoogwerf B, Halle JP, Young J, Rashkow A, Joyce C, Nawaz S, Yusuf S; for the HOPE Study Investigators: Albuminuria and risk of cardiovascular events, death, and heart failure in diabetic and nondiabetic individuals. *JAMA* 286:421–426, 2001.

Gharib H, Tuttle RM, Baskin HJ, Fish LH, Singer PA, McDermott MT: Consensus statement: Subclinical thyroid dysfunction: a joint statement on management from the American Association of Clinical Endocrinologists, the American Thyroid Association, and the Endocrine Society. *J Clin Endocrinol Metab* 90:581–585, 2005.

Gill A, Madsen G, Knox M, Bisits A, Giles W, Tudehope D, Rogers Y, Smith R: Neonatal neurodevelopmental outcomes following tocolysis with glycerol trinitrate patches. *Am J Obstet Gynecol* 195:484–487, 2006.

Gimeno-Orna JA, Faure-Nogueras E, Sancho-Serrano MA: Usefulness of total cholesterol/HDL-cholesterol ratio in the management of diabetic dyslipidemia. *Diabet Med* 22:26–31, 2004.

Giorgino F, Laviola L, Cavallo Perin P, Solnica B, Fuller J, Chaturvedi N: Factors associated with progression to macroalbuminuria in microalbuminuric type 1 diabetic patients: the EURODIAB Prospective Complications Study. *Diabetologia* 47:1020–1028, 2004.

Giri S, Shaw LJ, Murthy DR, Travin MI, Miller DD, Hachamovitch R, Borges-Neto S, Berman DS, Waters DD, Heller GV: Impact of diabetes on the risk stratification using stress single-photon emission computed tomography myocardial perfusion imaging in patients with symptoms suggestive of coronary artery disease. *Circulation* 105:32–40, 2002.

Girling JC, de Swiet M: Thyroxine dosing during pregnancy in women with primary hypothyroidism. *Br J Obstet Gynecol* 99:368–370, 1992.

Giunti S, Bruno G, Veglio M, Gruden G, Webb DJ, Livingstone S, Chaturvedi N, Fuller JH, Perin PC; the EURODIAB IDDM Complications Study Group: Electrocardiographic left ventricular hypertrophy in type 1 diabetes. Prevalence and relation to coronary heart disease and cardiovascular risk factors: the EURODIAB IDDM Complications Study. *Diabetes Care* 28: 2255–2257, 2005.

Glastras SJ, Craig ME, Verge CF, Chan AK, Cusumano JM, Donaghue KC: The role of autoimmunity at diagnosis of type 1 diabetes in the development of thyroid and celiac disease and microvascular complications. *Diabetes Care* 28:2170–2175, 2005.

Glinoer D, De Nayer P, Bourdoux P, Lemone M, Robyn C, Van Steirteghem A, Kinthaert J, Lejeune B: Regulation of maternal thyroid during pregnancy. *J Clin Endocrinol Metab* 71:276–287, 1990.

Glinoer D, Soto MF, Bourdoux P, Lejeune B, Delange F, Lemone M, Kinthaert J, Robijn C, Grun JP, De Nayer P: Pregnancy in patients with mild thyroid abnormalities: maternal and neonatal repercussions. *J Clin Endocrinol Metab* 73:421–427, 1991.

Glinoer D, DeNayer P, Robyn C, Lejeune B, Kinthaert J, Meuris S: Serum levels of intact human chorionic gonadotropin (hCG) and its free alpha and beta subunits, in relation to maternal thyroid stimulation during normal pregnancy. *J Endocrinol Invest* 16:881–888, 1993.

Glinoer D, Riahi M, Grun JP, Kinthaert J: Risk of subclinical hypothyroidism in pregnant women with asymptomatic autoimmune thyroid disorders. *J Clin Endocrinol Metab* 79:197–204, 1994.

Glinoer D: Thyroid hyperfunction during pregnancy. *Thyroid* 8:859–864, 1998.

Glinoer D: What happens to the normal thyroid during pregnancy? *Thyroid* 9: 631–635, 1999.

Glinoer D, Delange F: The potential repercussions of maternal, fetal, and neonatal hypothyroxinemia on the progeny. *Thyroid* 10:871–887, 2000a.

Glinoer D: Thyroid autoimmuniy, thyroid dysfunction, and the risk of miscarriage. Editorial. *Am J Reprod Immunol* 43:202–203, 2000b.

Glinoer D: Pregnancy and iodine. *Thyroid* 11:471–481, 2001.

Glinoer D: Miscarriage in women with positive anti-TPO antibodies: is thyroxine the answer? Editorial. *J Clin Endocrinol Metab* 91:2500–2502, 2006.

Goetze JP, Rehfeld JF, Videbaek R, Friis-Hansen L, Kastrup J: B-type natriuretic peptide and its precursor in cardiac venous blood from failing hearts. *Eur J Heart Fail* 7:69–74, 2005.

Goldberg, IJ: Diabetic dyslipidemia: causes and consequences. *J Clin Endocrinol Metab* 86: 965–971, 2001.

Goldberg RB, Jacobson TA: Effects of niacin on glucose control in patients with dyslipidemia. *Mayo Clin Proc* 83:470–478, 2008.

Goldstein R, Levy E, Shafrir E: Increased maternal-fetal transport of fat in diabetes assessed by polyunsaturated fatty acid content in fetal lipids. *Biol Neonate* 47:343–349, 1985.

Goldstein LB, Adams R, Alberts MJ, Appel LJ, Brass LM, Bushnell CD, Culebras A, DeGraba TJ, Gorelick PB, Guyton JR, Hart RG, Howard G, Kelly-Hayes M, Nixon JV, Sacco RL: Primary prevention of ischemic stroke: a guideline from the American Heart Association/American Stroke Association Stroke Council: cosponsored by the Atherosclerotic Peripheral Vascular Disease Interdisciplinary Working Group; Cardiovascular Nursing Council; Clinical Cardiology Council; Nutrition, Physical Activity, and Metabolism Council; and the Quality of Care and Outcomes Research Interdisciplinary Working Group: the American Academy of Neurology affirms the value of this guideline. *Circulation* 113:e873–e923, 2006 <DOI: 10.1161/01. STR.0000223048.70103.F1>.

Golembiewska E, Ciechanowski K, Safranow K, Kedzierska K, Kabat-Koperska J: Renal handling of uric acid in patients with type 1 diabetes in relation to glycemic control. *Arch Med Res* 36:32–35, 2005.

Golik A, Weissgarten J, Cotariu D, Cohen N, Zaidenstein R, Ramot Y, Averbukh Z, Modai D: Renal uric acid handling in non-insulin-dependent patients with elevated glomerular filtration rates. *Clin Sci (Lond)* 85:713–716, 1993.

Gonsales-Valerio E, Lopes Ramos JG, Martins-Costa SH, Muller AL: Variation in the urinary protein/creatinine ratio at four different periods of the day in hypertensive pregnant women. *Hypertens Preg* 24:213–221, 2005.

Gonzalez GC, Capel I, Rodriguez-Espinoza J, Mauricio D, de Leiva A, Perez A: Thyroid autoimmunity at onset of type 1 diabetes as a predictor of thyroid dysfunction. *Diabetes Care* 30:1611–1612, 2007.

Gonzalez-Clemente JM, Pinies JA, Calle-Pacual A, Saavedra A, Sanchez C, Bellido D, Martin-Folgueras T, Moraga I, Recasens A, Girbes J, Sanchez-Zamarano MA, Mauricio D; the PADiD Study Group: Cardiovascualr risk factor management is poorer in diabetic patients with undiagnosed peripheral arterial disease than in those with known coronary heart disease or cerebrovascular disease. Results of a nationwide study in tertiary diabetes centers. *Diabet Med* Mar 13 2008 (Epub ahead of print).

Gonzalez-Gonzalez NL, Ramirez O, Mozas J, Melchor J, Armas H, Garcia-Hernandez JA, Caballero A, Hernandez M, Diaz-Gomez MN, Jimenez A, Parache J, Bartha JL: Factors influencing pregnancy outcome in women with type 2 versus type 1 diabetes mellitus. *Acta Obstet Gynecol Scand* 87:43–49, 2008.

Goodwin TM, Montoro M, Mestman JH, Pekary AE, Hershman JM: The role of chorionic gonadotropin in transient hyperthyroidism of hyperemesis gravidarum. *J Clin Endocrinol Metab* 75:1333–1337, 1992.

Goodwin G, Volkening LK, Laffel LMB: Younger age at onset of type 1 diabetes in concordant sibling pairs is associated with increased risk for autoimmune thyroid disease. *Diabetes Care* 29:1397–1398, 2006.

Goraya TY, Leibson CL, Palumbo PJ, Weston SA, Killian JM, Pfeifer EA, Jacobsen SJ, Frye RL, Roger VL: Coronary atherosclerosis in diabetes mellitus. A population-based autopsy study. *J Am Coll Cardiol* 40:946–953, 2002.

Gordin D, Hiilesmaa V, Fagerudd J, Ronnback M, Forsblom C, Kaaja R, Teramo K, Groop P-H; FinnDiane Study Group: Preeclampsia but not pregnancy-induced hypertension is a risk factor for diabetic nephropathy in type 1 diabetic women. *Diabetologia* 50:516–522, 2007.

Gordon MC, Landon MB, Boyle J, Stewart KS, Gabbe SG: Coronary artery disease in insulin-dependent diabetes mellitus of pregnancy (class H): a review of the literature. *Obstet Gynecol Surv* 51:437–444, 1996a.

Gordon M, Landon MB, Samuels P, Hissrich S, Gabbe SG: Perinatal outcome and long-term follow-up associated with modern management of diabetic nephropathy. *Obstet Gynecol* 87:401–409, 1996b.

Gosmanov NR, Szoke E, Israelian Z, Smith T, Cryer PE, Gerich JE, Meyer C: Role of the decrement in intraislet insulin for the glucagon response to hypoglycemia in humans. *Diabetes Care* 28:1124–1131, 2005.

Gotoh M, Li C, Yatoh M, Iguchi A, Hirooka Y: Serum uric acid concentrations in type 2 diabetes: its significant relationship to serum 1,5-anhydroglucitol concentrations. *Endocr Regul* 39:119–125, 2005.

Gowda RM, Khan IA, Mehta NJ, Vasavada BC, Sacchi TJ: Cardiac arrhythmias in pregnancy: clinical and therapeutic considerations. *Int J Cardiol* 88:129–133, 2003.

Grab Grab D, Paulus WE, Erdmann M, Terinde R, Oberhoffer R, Lang D, Muche R, Kreienberg R: Effects of low-dose aspirin on uterine and fetal blood flow during pregnancy: results of a randomized, placebo-controlled, double-blind trial. *Ultrasound Obstet Gynecol* 15:19–27, 2000.

Grady EF, Sechi LA, Griffen CA, Schambelan M, Kalinyak JE: Expression of AT2 receptors in the developing rat fetus. *J Clin Invest* 88:921–933, 1991.

Granberg V, Ejskjaer N, Peakman M, Sundkvist G: Autoantibodies to autonomic nerves associated with cardiac and peripheral autonomic neuropathy. *Diabetes Care* 28:1959–1964, 2005.

Grandi AM, Piantanida E, Franzetti I, Bernasconi M, Maresca A, Marnini P, Guasti L, Venco A: Effect of glycemic control on left ventricular diastolic function in type 1 diabetes mellitus. *Am J Cardiol* 97:71–76, 2006.

Graner M, Varpula M, Kahri J, Salonen RM, Nyyssonen K, Nieminen MS, Taskinen MR, Syvanne M: Association of carotid intima-media thickness with angiographic severity and extent of coronary artery disease. *Am J Cardiol* 97:624–629, 2006.

Gray RS, Borsey DQ, Seth J, Herd R, Brown NS, Clarke BF: Prevalence of subclinical thyroid failure in insulin-dependent diabetes. *J Clin Endocrinol Metab* 50:1034–1037, 1980.

Gray RS, Borsey DQ, Irvine WJ, Seth J, Clarke BF: Natural history of thyroid function in diabetics with impaired thyroid reserve: a four-year controlled study. *Clin Endocrinol* 19:445–451, 1983.

Gray RO, Butler PC, Beers TR, Kryshak EJ, Rizza RA: Comparison of the ability of bread versus bread plus meat to treat and prevent subsequent hypoglycemia in patients with insulin-dependent diabetes mellitus. *J Clin Endocrinol Metab* 81:1508–1511, 1996.

Greco P, Vimercati A, Giorgino F, Loverro G, Selvaggi L: Reversal of fetal hydrops and fetal tachyarrhythmia associated with maternal diabetic coma. *Eur J Obstet Gynecol Reprod Biol* 93:33–35, 2000.

Green SM, Rothrock SG, Ho JD, Gallant RD, Borger R, Thomas TL, Zimmerman GJ: Failure of adjunctive bicarbonate to improve outcome in severe pediatric diabetic ketoacidosis. *Ann Emerg Med* 31:41–48, 1998.

Greene MF, Hare JW, Krache M, Phillippe M, Barss VA, Saltzman DH, Nadel A, Younger MD, Heffner L, Scherl JE: Prematurity among insulin-requiring diabetic gravid women. *Am J Obstet Gynecol* 161:106–111, 1989.

Greenland P, Smith SC, Grundy SM: Improving coronary heart disease risk assessment in asymptomatic people. Role of traditional risk factors and noninvasive cardiovascular tests. *Circulation* 104:1863–1867, 2001.

Grenfell A, Brudenell JM, Doddridge MC, Watkins PJ: Pregnancy in diabetic women who have proteinuria. *Quar J Med* 228:379–386, 1986a.

Grenfell A, Bewick M, Brudenell JM, Carr JV, Parsons V, Snowden S, Watkins PJ: Diabetic pregnancy following renal transplantation. *Diabet Med* 3:177–179, 1986b.

Grewal J, McKelvie R, Lonn E, Tait P, Carlsson J, Gianni M, Jarnert C, Persson H: BNP and NT-proBNP predict echocardiographic severity of diastolic dysfunction. *Eur J Heart Fail* 10:252–259, 2008.

Griffin KA, Picken MM, Bakris GL, Bidani AK: Class differences in the effects of calcium channel blockers in the rat remnant kidney model. *Kidney Int* 55: 1849–1860, 1999.

Griffin KA, Picken M, Bakris GL, Bidani AK: Comparative effects of selective T- and L-type calcium channel blockers in the remnant kidney model. *Hypertension* 37:1268–1272, 2001.

Griffin KA, Hacioglu R, bu-Amarah I, Loutzenhiser R, Williamson GA, Bidani AK: Effects of calcium channel blockers on "dynamic" and "steady-state" renal autoregulation. *Am J Physiol* 286:F1136–F1143, 2004.

Grill V, Gutniak M, Bjorkman O, Lindqvist G, Reichard P, Widen L: Cerebral blood flow and substrate utilization in insulin-treated diabetic subjects. *Am J Physiol* 258:E813–E820, 1990.

Grinstein G, Muzumdar R, Aponte L, Vuguin P, Saenger P, Di Martino-Nardi J: Presentation and 5-year follow-up of type 2 diabetes mellitus in African-American and Caribbean-Hispanic adolescents. *Horm Res* 60:121–126, 2003.

Groop PH, Elliott T, Ekstrand A, Franssila-Kallunki A, Friedman R, Viberti GC, Taskinen MR: Multiple lipoprotein abnormalities in type 1 diabetic patients with renal disease. *Diabetes* 45:974–979, 1996.

Groop P-H, Thomas MC: Brain natriuretic peptide: microalbuminuria for cardiac disease and diabetes? Commentary. *Diabetologia* 48:3–5, 2005.

Gross JL, de Azevedo MJ, Silveiro SP, Canani LH, Caramori ML, Zelmanovitz T: Diabetic nephropathy: diagnosis, prevention, and treatment. *Diabetes Care* 28:176–188, 2005.

Grubb AO: Cystatin C—properties and use as a diagnostic marker. *Adv Clin Chem* 35:63–99, 2000.

Grun JP, Meuris S, De Nayer P, Glinoer D: The thyrotropic role of human chorionic gonadotropin (hCG) in the early stages of twin (versus single) pregnancies. *Clin Endocrinol* 46:719–725, 1997.

Grundy SM, Benjamin IJ, Burke GL, Chait A, Eckel RH, Howard BV, Mitch W, Smith SC, Sowers JR: Diabetes and cardiovascular disease. A statement for healthcare professionals from the American Heart Association. *Circulation* 100:1134–1146, 1999.

Grundy SM, Garber A, Goldberg R, Havas S, Holman R, Lamendola C, Howard WJ, Savage P, Sowers J, Vega GL: AHA conference proceedings. Prevention Conference VI. Diabetes and cardiovascular disease. Writing Group IV: Lifestyle and medical management of risk factors. *Circulation* 105:e153–e158, 2002a.

Grundy SM, Howard B, Smith S Jr, Eckel R, Redberg R, Bonow RO: Prevention Conference VI: Diabetes and Cardiovascular Disease: executive summary: a conference proceeding for healthcare professionals from a special writing group of the American Heart Association. *Circulation* 105:2231–2239, 2002b.

Grundy SM: Low-density lipoprotein, non-high-density lipoprotein, and apolipoprotein B as targets of lipid-lowering therapy. Editorial. *Circulation* 106:2526–2529, 2002c.

Grundy SM, Vega GL, McGovern ME, Tulloch BR, Kendall DM, Fitz-Patrick D, Ganda OP, Rosenson RS, Buse JB, Robertson DD, Sheehan JP; Diabetes Multicenter Research Group: Efficacy, safety, and tolerability of once-daily niacin for the treatment of dyslipidemia associated with type 2 diabetes: results of the assessment of diabetes control and evaluation of the efficacy of niaspan trial. *Arch Intern Med* 162:1568–1576, 2002d.

Grundy SM, Cleeman JI, Merz NB, Brewer HB Jr, Clark LT, Hunninghake DB, Pasternak RC, Smith SC Jr, Stone NJ; for the Coordinating Committee of the National Cholesterol Education Program: Implications of recent clinical trials for the National Cholesterol Education Program Adult Treatment Panel III Guidelines. *Circulation* 110:227–239, 2004.

Grunewald C, Garoff L, Lunell N-O, Nisell H, Nylund L, Sarby B, Thornstrom S: Oral isradipine and feto-maternal hemodynamics in hypertensive pregnancy. *Clin Exper Hyper Preg* B11:195–205, 1992.

GSIG—Gruppo di Studio Ipertensione in Gravidanza: Nifedipine versus expectant management in mild to moderate hypertension in pregnancy. *Br J Obstet Gynecol* 105:718–722, 1998.

Gudbjornsdottir S, Cederholm J, Nilsson PM, Eliasson B; the Steering Committee of the Swedish National Diabetes Register: The National Diabetes Register in Sweden. An implementation of the St. Vincent Declaration for Quality Improvement in Diabetes Care. *Diabetes Care* 26:1270–1276, 2003.

Gueyffier F, Boutitie F, Boissel J-P, Pocock S, Coope J, Cutler J, Ekbom T, Fagard R, Friedman L, Perry M, Prineas R, Schron E: Effect of antihypertensive drug treatment on cardiovascular outcomes in women and men: a meta-analysis of individual patient data from randomized controlled trials. The INDANA Investigators. *Ann Intern Med* 126:761–767, 1997.

Guglielmi MD, Pierdomenico SD, Salvatore L, Romano F, Tascione E, Pupillo M, Porreca E, Imbastaro T, Cuccurullo F, Mezzetti A: Impaired left ventricular diastolic function and vascular postischemic vasodilation associated with microalbuminuria in IDDM patients. *Diabetes Care* 18:353–360, 1995.

Guillaume J, Schussler GC, Goldman J: Components of the total serum thyroid hormone concentrations during pregnancy: high free thyroxine and blunted thyrotropin (TSH) response to TSH-releasing hormone in the first trimester. *J Clin Endocrinol Metab* 60:678–684, 1985.

Gum PA, Kottke-Marchant K, Poggio ED, Gurm H, Welsh PA, Brooks L, Sapp SK, Topol EJ: Profile and prevalence of aspirin resistance in patients with cardiovascular disease. *Am J Cardiol* 88:230–235, 2001.

Gum PA, Kottke-Marchant K, Welsh PA, White J, Topol EJ: A prospective, blinded determination of the natural history of aspirin resistance among stable patients with cardiovascular disease. *J Am Coll Cardiol* 41:961–965, 2003.

Gunczler P, Lanes R, Lopez E, Essa S, Villaroel O, Revel-Chion R: Cardiac mass and function, carotid artery intima-media thickness and lipoprotein(a) levels in children and adolescents with type 1 diabetes mellitus of short duration. *J Pediatr Endocrinol Metab* 15:181–186, 2002.

Gunczler P, Lanes R, Soros A, Verdu L, Ramon Y, Guevara B, Beer N: Coronary artery calcification, serum lipids, lipoproteins, and peripheral inflammatory markers in adolescents and young adults with type 1 diabetes. *J Pediatr* 149: 320–323, 2006.

Gunenc O, Cicek N, Gorkemli H, Celik C, Acar A, Akyurek C: The effect of methyldopa treatment on uterine, umbilical and fetal middle cerebral artery blood flows in preeclamptic patients. *Arch Gynecol Obstet* 266:141–144, 2002.

Gungor N, Thompson T, Sutton-Tyrell K, Janosky J, Arslanian S: Early signs of cardiovascular disease in youth and obesity and type 2 diabetes. *Diabetes Care* 28:1219–1221, 2005.

Gunton JE, McElduff A, Sulway M, Stiel J, Kelso I, Boyce S, Fulcher G, Robinson B, Clifton-Bligh P, Wilmshurst E: Outcome of pregnancies complicated by pre-gestational diabetes mellitus. *Aust N Z J Obstet Gynecol* 40:38–43, 2000.

Gupta U, Cook JC, Tassinari MS, Hurtt ME: Comparison of developmental toxicology of aspirin (acetylsalicylic acid) in rats using selected dosing paradigms. *Birth Defects Res B Dev Reprod Toxicol* 68:27–37, 2003.

Guy DA, Sandoval D, Richardson MA, Tate D, Flakoll PJ, Davis SN: Differing physiological effects of epinephrine in type 1 diabetes and nondiabetic humans. *Am J Physiol Endocrinol Metab* 288:E178–E186, 2005a.

Guy DA, Sandoval D, Richardson MA, Tate D, Davis SN: Effects of glycemic control on target organ responses to epinephrine in type 1 diabetes. *Am J Physiol Endocrinol Metab* 289:E258–E265, 2005b.

Guyton JR, Blazing MA, Hagar J, Kashyap ML, Knopp RH, McKenney JM, Nash DT, Nash SD: Extended-release niacin vs gemfibrozil for the treatment of low levels of high-density lipoprotein cholesterol. Niaspan-Gemfibrozil Study Group. *Arch Intern Med* 160:1177–1184, 2000.

Gylling H, Tuominen JA, Koivisto VA, Miettinen TA: Cholesterol metabolism in type 1 diabetes. *Diabetes* 53:2217–2222, 2004.

Haase M, Morgera S, Bamberg C, Halle H, Martini S, Dragun D, Neumayer HH, Budde K: Successful pregnancies in dialysis patients including those suffering from cystinosis and familial Mediterranean fever. *J Nephrol* 19: 677–681, 2006.

Haddow JE, Palomaki GE, Allan WC, Williams JR, Knight GJ, Gagnon J, O'Heir CE, Mitchell ML, Hermos RJ, Waisbren SE, Faix JD, Klein RZ: Maternal thyroid deficiency during pregnancy and subsequent neuropsychological development of the child. *N Engl J Med* 341:549–555, 1999.

Haelterman E, Breart G, Paris-Llado J, Dramaix M, Tchobroutsky C: Effect of uncomplicated chronic hypertension on the risk of small-for-gestational age birth. *Am J Epidemiol* 15:689–695, 1997.

Haffner SM, Lehto S, Ronnemaa T, Pyorala K, Laakso M: Mortality from coronary heart disease in subjects with type 2 diabetes and in nondiabetic subjects with and without prior myocardial infarction. *N Engl J Med* 339:229–234, 1998a.

Haffner SM: The importance of hyperglycemia in the nonfasting state to the development of cardiovascular disease. *Endocr Rev* 19:583–592, 1998b.

Haffner SM: Management of dyslipidemia in adults with diabetes. Technical review. *Diabetes Care* 21:160–178, 1998c.

Hagay ZJ: Diabetic ketoacidosis in pregnancy: etiology, pathophysiology, and management. *Clin Obstet Gynecol* 37:39–49, 1994a.

Hagay ZJ, Weissman A, Lurie S, Insler V: Reversal of fetal distress following intensive treatment of maternal diabetic ketoacidosis. *Am J Perinatol* 11:430–432, 1994b.

Hagay ZJ, Schacter M, Pollack A, Levy R: Development of proliferative retinopathy in a new type 2 diabetic patient following rapid metabolic control. *Eur J Obstet Gynecol Reprod Biol* 57:211–213, 1994c.

Hagay Z, Weissman A: Management of diabetic pregnancy complicated by coronary artery disease and neuropathy. *Obstet Gynecol Clin North Am* 23:205–220, 1996.

Haire-Joshu D, Glasgow RE, Tibbs TL: Smoking and diabetes. *Diabetes Care* 22:1887–1898, 1999.

Hajjar I, Kotchen TA: Trends in prevalence, awareness, treatment, and control of hypertension in the United States, 1988–2000. *JAMA* 290:199–206, 2003.

Hale PJ, Crase J, Nattrass M: Metabolic effects of bicarbonate in the treatment of diabetic ketoacidosis. *Br Med J* 289:1035–1038, 1984.

Hall DR, Odendaal HJ, Steyn DW, Smith M: Nifedipine or prazosin as a second agent to control early severe hypertension in pregnancy: a randomized controlled trial. *BJOG* 107:759–765, 2000.

Hallan S, Asberg A, Lindberg M, Johnsen H: Validation of the Modification of Diet in Renal Disease formula for estimating GFR with special emphasis on calibration of the serum creatinine assay. *Am J Kidney Dis* 44:84–93, 2004.

Halligan A, O'Brien E, O'Malley K, Mee F, Atkins N, Conroy R, Walshe JJ, Darling M: Twenty-four hour ABPM in a primigravid population. *J Hypertens* 11: 869–873, 1993.

Hanefeld M, Fischer S, Julius U, Schulze J, Schwanebeck, Schmechel H, Ziegelasch HJ, Lindner J; the DIS Group: Risk factors for myocardial infarction and death in newly detected NIDDM: the Diabetes Intervention Study, 11–year follow-up. *Diabetologia* 39:1577–1583, 1996.

Hanff LM, Vulto AG, Bartels PA, Roofthooft DW, Bijvank BN, Steegers EA, Visser W: Intravenous use of the calcium-channel blocker nicardipine as second-line treatment in severe, early-onset pre-eclamptic patients. *J Hypertens* 23:2319–2326, 2005.

Hanson U, Persson B: Outcome of pregnancies complicated by type 1 insulin-dependent diabetes in Sweden: acute pregnancy complications, neonatal mortality and morbidity. *Am J Perinatol* 10:330–333,1993.

Hanson U, Persson B: Epidemiology of pregnancy-induced hypertension and preeclampsia in type 1 (insulin-dependent) diabetic pregnancies in Sweden. *Acta Obstet Gynecol Scand* 77:620–624, 1998.

Hanssens M, Keirse MJ, Vankelecom F, Van Assche FA: Fetal and neonatal effects of treatment with angiotensin-converting enzyme inhibitors in pregnancy. *Obstet Gynecol* 78:128–135, 1991.

Hansson L, Zanchetti A, Carruthers SG, Dahlof B, Elmfeldt D, Julius S, Menard J, Rahn KH, Wedel H, Westerling S; the HOT Study Group: Effects of intensive blood-pressure lowering and low-dose aspirin in patients with hypertension: principal results of the Hypertension Optimal Treatment (HOT) randomized trial. *Lancet* 351:1755–1762, 1998.

Hansson GK: Inflammation, atherosclerosis, and coronary artery disease. *N Engl J Med* 352:1685–1695, 2005.

Harborne LR, Alexander CE, Thomson AJ, O'Reilly DS, Greer IA: Outcomes of pregnancy complicated by thyroid disease. *Aust N Z J Obstet Gynecol* 45: 239–242, 2005.

Hardin NJ: The myocardial and vascular pathology of diabetic cardiomyopathy. *Coron Artery Dis* 7:99–108, 1996.

Hardman AE, Aldred HE: Walking during the postprandial period decreases alimentary lipemia. *J Cardiovasc Risk* 2:71–78, 1995.

Hare JW, White P: Pregnancy in diabetes complicated by vascular disease. *Diabetes* 26:953–955, 1977.

Hare JW, Kitzmiller JL: Diabetes and Graves' disease complicating pregnancy. *Obstet Gynecol* 51:655–658, 1978.

Hare JW: Diabetic neuropathy and coronary heart disease. In: Reece EA, Coustan DR, eds. *Diabetes Mellitus in Pregnancy: Principles and Practice.* New York: Churchill-Livingstone; 1988:517–518.

Hare JW: Complicated diabetes complicating pregnancy. *Baillieres Clin Obstet Gynecol* 5:349–367, 1991.

Hare JW: Diabetic complications of diabetic pregnancies. *Semin Perinatol* 18: 451–458, 1994.

Harjutsalo V, Katoh S, Sarti C, Tajima N, Tuomilehto J: Population-based assessment of familial clustering of diabetic nephropathy in type 1 diabetes. *Diabetes* 53:2449–2454, 2004.

Harper A, Murnaghan GA: Maternal and fetal hemodynamics in hypertensive pregnancies during maternal treatment with intravenous hydralazine or labetalol. *Br J Obstet Gynecol* 98:453–459, 1991.

Harrison MJ, Weisblatt E: A sex difference in the effect of aspirin on "spontaneous" platelet aggregation in whole blood. *Thromb Haemost* 50:773–774, 1983.

Harshfield GA, Alpert BS, Pulliam DA, Somes GW, Wilson DK: Ambulatory blood pressure recordings in children and adolescents. *Pediatrics* 94:180–184, 1994.

Hart PD, Bakris GL: Should beta-blockers be used to control hypertension in people with chronic kidney disease? *Semin Nephrol* 27:555–564, 2007.

Hartikainen-Sorri A-L, Heikkinen JE, Koivisto M: Pharmacokinetics of clonidine during pregnancy and nursing. *Obstet Gynecol* 69:598–600, 1987.

Harvey SJ, Miner JH: Breaking down the barrier: evidence against a role for heparan sulfate in glomerular permselectivity. *J Am Soc Nephrol* 18:672–674, 2007.

Hassouna A, Loubani M, Matata BM, Fowler A, Standen NB, Galinanes M: Mitochondrial dysfunction as the cause of the failure to precondition the diabetic human myocardium. *Cardiovasc Res* 69:450–458, 2006.

Hathout EH, Thomas W, El-Shaawy M, Nahab F, Mace JW: Diabetic autoimmune markers in children and adolescents with type 2 diabetes. *Pediatrics* 107(6): e102–e105, 2001.

Hauth JC, Ewell MG, Levine RJ, Esterlitz JR, Sibai B, Curet LB, Catalano PM, Morris CD; for the Calcium for Preeclampsia Prevention Study Group: Pregnancy outcomes in healthy nulliparas who developed hypertension. *Obstet Gynecol* 95:24–28, 2000.

Havel RJ, Kane JP: Introduction: structure and metabolism of plasma lipoproteins. In: Scriver CR, Beaudet AL, Sly WS, and ValleD, eds., Childs B, Kinzler KW, Vogelstein B, associate eds. *Molecular and Metabolic Bases of Inherited Disease.* 8th ed. Vol. 2. New York: McGraw-Hill; 2001:2705–2716.

Havel RJ, Hamilton RL: Hepatic catabolism of remnant lipoproteins: where the action is. Editorial. *Arterioscler Thromb Vasc Biol* 24:213–215, 2004.

Hayaishi-Okano R, Yamasaki Y, Katakami N, Ohtoshi K, Gorogawa S-I, Kuroda A, Matsuhisa M, Kosugi K, Nishikawa N, Kajimoto Y, Hori M: Elevated C-reactive protein associates with early-stage carotid atherosclerosis in young subjects with type 1 diabetes. *Diabetes Care* 25:1432–1438, 2002.

Hayashi K, Nagahama T, Oka K, Epstein M, Saruta T: Disparate effects of calcium antagonists on renal microcirculation. *Hypertens Res* 19:31–36, 1996.

Hayashi K, Ozawa Y, Fujiwara K, Wakino S, Kumagai H, Saruta T: Role of actions of calcium antagonists on efferent arterioles—with special references to glomerular hypertension. *Am J Nephrol* 23:229–244, 2003.

Hayden MR, Tyagi SC: Uric acid: a new look at an old risk marker for cardiovascular disease, metabolic syndrome, and type 2 diabetes mellitus: the urate redox shuttle. *Nutr Metab* 1:10, 2004.

Hays L, Reid C, Doran M, Geary K: Use of methadone for the treatment of diabetic neuropathy. *Diabetes Care* 28:485–487, 2005.

HDSG—Hypertension in Diabetes Study Group: Hypertension in Diabetes Study (HDS): I. Prevalence of hypertension in newly presenting type 2 diabetic patients and the association with risk factors for cardiovascular and diabetic complications. *J Hypertens* 11:309–317, 1993.

He K, Song Y, Daviglus ML, Liu K, Van Horn L, Dyer AR, Greenland P: Accumulated evidence on fish consumption and coronary heart disease mortality. A meta-analysis of cohort studies. *Circulation* 109:2705–2711, 2004.

He FJ, Markandu ND, MacGregor GA: Modest salt reduction lowers blood pressure in both isolated systolic hypertension and combined hypertension. *Hypertension* 46:66–70, 2005.

Heard AR, Dekker GA, Chan A, Jacobs DJ, Vreeburg SA, Priest KR: Hypertension during pregnancy in South Australia, Part 1: pregnancy outcomes. *Aust N Z J Obstet Gynecol* 44:404–409, 2004.

Hebert MF, Carr DB, Anderson GD, Blough D, Green GE, Brateng DA, Kantor E, Benedetti TJ, Easterling TR: Pharmacokinetics and pharmacodynamics of atenolol during pregnancy and postpartum. *J Clin Pharmacol* 45:25–33, 2005.

Heikkinen T, Ekblad U, Laine K: Transplacental transfer of amitriptyline and nortriptyline in isolated perfused human placenta. *Psychopharmacology* 153: 450–454, 2001.

Held C, Hjemdahl P, Eriksson SV, Bjorkander I, Forslund L, Rehnqvist N: Prognostic implications of intima-media thickness and plaques in the carotid and femoral arteries in patients with stable angina pectoris. *Eur Heart J* 22:11–14, 2001.

Helewa ME, Burrows RF, Smith J, Williams K, Brain P, Rabkin SW: Report of the Canadian Hypertension Society Consensus Conference: 1. Definitions, evaluation and classification of hypertensive disorders in pregnancy. *Can Med Assoc J* 157:715–725, 1997.

Heller GV: Evaluation of the patient with diabetes mellitus and suspected coronary artery disease. *Am J Med* 118:9S-14S, 2005.

Hellmuth E, Damm P, Molsted-Pedersen L, Bendtson I: Prevalence of nocturnal hypoglycemia in first trimester of pregnancy in patients with insulin treated diabetes mellitus. *Acta Obstet Gynecol Scand* 79:958–962, 2000.

Hellstedt T, Kaaja R, Teramo K, Immonen I: The effect of pregnancy on mild diabetic retinopathy. *Graefes Arch Clin Exp Ophthalmol* 235:437–441, 1997.

Hemachandra A, Ellis D, Lloyd CE, Orchard TJ: The influence of pregnancy on IDDM complications. *Diabetes Care* 18:950–954, 1995.

Hemingway H, McCallum A, Shipley M, Manderbacka K, Martikainen P, Keskimaki I: Incidence and prognostic implications of stable angina pectoris among women and men. *JAMA* 295:1404–1411, 2006.

Hemingway H, Langenberg C, Damant J, Frost C, Pyorala K, Barrett-Connor E: Prevalence of angina in women versus men. A systematic review and meta-analysis of international variations across 31 countries. *Circulation* 117: 1526–1536, 2008.

Henderson JN, Allen KV, Deary IJ, Frier BM: Hypoglycemia in insulin-treated type 2 diabetes: frequency, symptoms and impaired awareness. *Diabet Med* 20: 1016–1021, 2003.

Henricsson M, Nilsson A, Janzon L, Groop L: The effect of glycemic control and the introduction of insulin therapy on retinopathy in non-insulin-dependent diabetes mellitus. *Diabet Med* 14:123–131, 1997.

Henry RM, Kamp O, Kostense PJ, Spijkerman AM, Dekker JM, van Elijck R, Nijpels G, Heine RJ, Bouter LM, Stehouwer CD: Left ventricular mass increases with deteriorating glucose tolerance, especially in women: independence of increased arterial stiffness or decreased flow-mediated dilation: the Hoorn study. *Diabetes Care* 27:522–529, 2004.

Hepburn DA, Beary IJ, Frier BM, Patrick AW, Quinn JD, Fisher BM: Symptoms of acute insulin-induced hypoglycemia in humans with and without IDDM. Factor-analysis based approach. *Diabetes Care* 14:949–957, 1991.

Hepburn DA, Deary IJ, Frier BM: Classification of symptoms of hypoglycemia in insulin-treated diabetic patients using factor-analysis: relationship to hypoglycemia unawareness. *Diabet Med* 9:70–75, 1992.

Herder C, Schneitler S, Rathmann W, Haastert B, Schneitler H, Winkler H, Bredahl R, Hahnloser E, Martin S: Low-grade inflammation, obesity, and insulin resistance in adolescents. *J Clin Endocrinol Metab* 92:4569–4574, 2007.

Herlitz J, Malmberg K: How to improve the cardiac prognosis for diabetes. *Diabetes Care* 22 (Suppl 2):B89–B96, 1999.

Herman B, Goldbourt U: Uric acid and diabetes: observations in a population study. *Lancet* 2:240–243, 1982.

Herman WH, Shahinfar S, Carides GW, Dasbach EJ, Gerth WC, Alexander CM, Cook JR, Keane WF, Brenner BM: Losartan reduces the costs associated with diabetic end-stage renal disease: the RENAAL study economic evaluation. *Diabetes Care* 26:683–687, 2003.

Hermida RC, Ayala DE: Sampling requirements for ambulatory blood pressure monitoring in the diagnosis of hypertension in pregnancy. *Hypertension* 42:619–624, 2003a.

Hermida RC, Ayala DE, Mojon A, Fernandez JR, Alonso I, Aguilar MF, Ucieda R, Iglesias M: Differences in circadian blood pressure variability during gestation between healthy and complicated pregnancies. *Am J Hypertens* 16:200–208, 2003b.

Hermida RC, Ayala DE, Iglesias M: Differences in circadian pattern of ambulatory pulse pressure between healthy and complicated pregnancies. *Hypertension* 44:316–321, 2004.

Hermida RC, Ayala DE: Reference thresholds for 24-h, diurnal, and nocturnal ambulatory blood pressure mean values in pregnancy. *Blood Press Monit* 10: 33–41, 2005.

Herrera E, Lasuncion MA, Gomez-Coronado D, Aranda P, Lopez-Luna P, Maier I: Role of lipoprotein lipase activity on lipoprotein metabolism and the fate of circulating triglycerides in pregnancy. *Am J Obstet Gynecol* 158:1575–1583, 1988.

Herrera E: Metabolic adaptations in pregnancy and their implications for the availability of substrates to the fetus. *Eur J Clin Nutr* 54 (Suppl 1):S47–S51, 2000.

Herrera E, Ortega H, Alvino G, Giovanni N, Amusquivar E, Cetin I: Relationship between plasma fatty acid profile and antioxidant vitamins during normal pregnancy. *Eur J Clin Nutr* 58:1231–1238, 2004.

Hiatt WR, Hoag S, Hamman RF: Effect of diagnostic criteria on the prevalence of peripheral arterial disease: the San Luis Valley Diabetes Study. *Circulation* 91:1472–1479, 1995.

Hiatt WR: Medical treatment of peripheral arterial disease and claudication. *N Engl J Med* 344:1608–1621, 2001.

Higby K, Suiter CR, Phelps JY, Siler-Khodr T, Langer O: Normal values of urinary albumin and total protein excretion during pregnancy. *Am J Obstet Gynecol* 171:984–989, 1994.

Higby K, Suiter CR, Siler-Khodr T: A comparison between two screening methods for detection of microproteinuria. *Am J Obstet Gynecol* 173:1111–1114, 1995.

Hiilesmaa V, Suhonen L, Teramo K: Glycemic control is associated with preeclampsia but not with pregnancy-induced hypertension in women with type 1 diabetes mellitus. *Diabetologia* 43:1534–1539, 2000.

Hillier TA, Pedula KL: Complications in young adults with early-onset type 2 diabetes: losing the relative protection of youth. *Diabetes Care* 26:2999–3005, 2003.

Hinchcliffe SA, Lynch MR, Sargent PH, Howard CV, Van Velzen D: The effect of intrauterine growth retardation on the development of renal nephrons. *Br J Obstet Gynecol* 99:296–301, 1992.

Hink HU, Santianam N, Dikalov S, McCann L, Nguyen AD, Parthasarathy S, Harrison DG, Fukai T: Peroxidase properties of extracellular superoxide dismutase: role of uric acid in modulating in vivo activity. *Arterioscler Thromb Vasc Biol* 22:1402–1408, 2002.

Hirsch JT, Criqui MH, Treat-Jacobson D, Regensteiner JG, Olin JW, Krook SH, Hunninghake DB, Comerota AJ, Walsh ME, McDermott MM, Hiatt WR: Peripheral arterial disease detection, awareness, and treatment in primary care. *JAMA* 286:1317–1324, 2001.

Hjertberg R, Faxelius G, Belfrage P: Comparison of outcome of labetalol or hydralazine therapy during hypertension in pregnancy in very low birth weight infants. *Acta Obstet Gynecol Scand* 72:611–615, 1993.

Hodis HN, Mack WJ, LaBree L, Selzer RH, Liu CR, Liu CH, Azen SP: The role of carotid arterial intima-media thickness in predicting clinical coronary events. *Ann Intern Med* 128:262–269, 1998.

Hoffman BB: Adrenoceptor-activating and other sympathomimetic drugs. Adrenoceptor antagonist drugs. In: Katzung BG, ed. *Basic and Clinical Pharmacology.* 9th ed. New York: Lange Medical Books/McGraw-Hill; 2004:122–159.

Hogstedt S, Lindberg B, Peng DR, Regardh C-G, Rane A: Pregnancy-induced increase in metoprolol metabolism. *Clin Pharmacol Ther* 37:688–692, 1985.

Hokanson JE, Austin MA: Plasma triglyceride level is a risk factor for cardiovascular disease independent of high-density lipoprotein level: a meta-analysis of population-based prospective studies. *J Cardiovasc Risk* 3:213–219, 1996.

Holbrook RH, Voss EM, Gibson RN: Ovine fetal cardiorespiratory response to nicardipine. *Am J Obstet Gynecol* 161:718–721, 1989.

Holden KP, Jovanovic L, Druzin ML, Peterson CM: Increased fetal activity with low maternal blood glucose levels in pregnancies by diabetes. *Am J Perinatol* 1: 161–164, 1984.

Holder M, Holl RW, Barth J, Hecker W, Heinze E, Leichter HE, Teller W: Influence of long-term glycemic control on the development of cardiac autonomic neuropathy in pediatric patients with type 1 diabetes. *Diabetes Care* 20: 1042–1043, 1997.

Holl RW, Bohm B, Loos U, Grabert M, Heinze E, Homoki J: Thyroid autoimmunity in children and adolescents with type 1 diabetes mellitus. Effect of age, gender and HLA type. *Horm Res* 52:113–118, 1999a.

Holl RW, Pavlovic M, Heinze E, Thon A: Circadian blood pressure during the early course of type 1 diabetes. Analysis of 1,011 ambulatory blood pressure recordings in 354 adolescents and young adults. *Diabetes Care* 22:1151–1157, 1999b.

Holl RW, Grabert M, Thon A, Heinze E: Urinary excretion of albumin in adolescents with type 1 diabetes. Persistent versus intermittent microalbuminuria and relationship to duration of diabetes, sex, and metabolic control. *Diabetes Care* 22:1555–1560, 1999c.

Holley JL, Bernardini J, Quadri KHM, Greenberg A, Laifer SA: Pregnancy outcomes in a prospective matched control study of pregnancy and renal disease. *Clin Nephrol* 45:77–82, 1996.

Holley JL, Reddy SS: Pregnancy in dialysis patients: a review of outcomes, complications, and management. *Semin Dial* 16:384–388, 2003.

Hollingsworth DR, Grundy SM: Pregnancy-associated hypertriglyceridemia in normal and diabetic women. Differences in insulin-dependent, non-insulin-dependent, and gestational diabetes. *Diabetes* 31:1092–1097, 1982.

Hollingsworth DR, Moore TR: Postprandial walking exercise in pregnant insulin-dependent (type 1) diabetic women: reduction of plasma lipid levels but absence of a significant effect on glycemic control. *Am J Obstet Gynecol* 157:1359–1363, 1987.

Hollowell JG, Staehling NW, Flanders WD, Hannon WH, Gunter EW, Spencer CA, Braverman LE: Serum TSH, T4, and thyroid antibodies in the United States population (1988 to 1994): National Health and Nutrition Examination Survey (NHANES III). *J Clin Endocrinol Metab* 87:489–499, 2002.

Holman RR, Coleman RL, Shine BSF, Stevens RJ: Non-HDL cholesterol is less informative than the total-to-HDL cholesterol ratio in predicting cardiovascular risk in type 2 diabetes. *Diabetes Care* 28:1796–1797, 2005.

Holness MJ, Greenwood GK, Smith ND, Sugden MC: Hyperthyroidism impairs pancreatic beta cell adaptations to late pregnancy and maternal liporegulation in the rat. *Diabetologia* 48:2305–2312, 2005.

Holstein A, Plaschke A, Egberts E-H: Clinical characterization of severe hypoglycemia: a prospective population-based study. *Exp Clin Endocrinol Diabetes* 111:364–369, 2003.

Holzgreve H, Nakov R, Beck K, Janka HU: Antihypertensive therapy with verapamil SR plus trandolapril versus atenolol plus chlorthalidone on glycemic control. *Am J Hypertens* 16:381–386, 2003.

Hoogendoorn EH, Hermus AR, de Vegt F, Ross HA, Verbeek ALM, Kiemeny LALM, Swinkels DW, Sweep FCGJ, den Heijer M: Thyroid function and prevalence of anti-thyroperoxidase antibodies in a population with borderline sufficient iodine intake: influences of age and sex. *Clin Chem* 52:104–111, 2006.

HOPE—The Heart Outcomes Prevention Evaluation (HOPE)-2 Investigators: Homocysteine lowering with folic acid and B vitamins in vascular disease. *N Engl J Med* 354:1567–1577, 2006.

Horvat M, Maclean H, Goldberg L, Crock GW: Diabetic retinopathy in pregnancy: a 12 year prospective survey. *Br J Ophthalmol* 64:398–403, 1980.

Horvath JS, Phippard A, Korda A, Henderson-Smart DJ, Child A, Tiller DJ: Clonidine hydrochloride—a safe and effective antihypertensive agent in pregnancy. *Obstet Gynecol* 66:634–638, 1985.

Hother-Nielsen O, Faber O, Sorensen NS, Beck-Nielsen H: Classification of newly diagnosed diabetic patients as insulin-requiring or non-insulin-requiring based on clinical and biochemical variables. *Diabetes Care* 11:531–537, 1988.

Hou SH, Orlowski J, Pahl M, Ambrose S, Hussey M, Wong D: Pregnancy in women with end stage renal disease: treatment of anemia and preterm labor. *Am J Kidney Dis* 21:16–22, 1993.

Hou S: Frequency and outcome of pregnancy in women on dialysis. *Am J Kidney Dis* 23:60–63, 1994.

Hou S, Firanek C: Management of the pregnant dialysis patient. *Adv Ren Replace Ther* 5:24–30, 1998.

Hou S: Pregnancy in chronic renal insufficiency and end-stage renal disease. *Am J Kidney Dis* 33:235–252, 1999.

Hou S: Pregnancy in women on dialysis. In: Nissenson AR, Fine RN, eds. *Dialysis Therapy.* 3rd ed. Philadelphia: Hanley & Belfus; 2002:519–522.

Hou S: Pregnancy in renal transplant recipients. *Adv Ren Replace Ther* 10:40–47, 2003.

Houlihan CA, Tsalamandris C, Akdeniz A, Jerums G: Albumin-to-creatinine ratio: a screening test with limitations. *Am J Kidney Dis* 39:1183–1189, 2002.

Houlihan DD, Dennedy MC, Ravkumar N, Morrison JJ: Antihypertensive therapy and the feto-placental circulation: effects on umbilical artery resistance. *J Perinat Med* 32:315–319, 2004.

Hovind P, Rossing P, Tarnow L, Toft H, Parving J, Parving H-H: Remission of nephrotic-range albuminuria in type 1 diabetic patients. *Diabetes Care* 24: 1972–1977, 2001.

Hovind P, Tarnow L, Rossing K, Rossing P, Eising S, Larsen N, Binder C, Parving HH: Decreasing incidence of severe diabetic microangiopathy in type 1 diabetes. *Diabetes Care* 26:1258–1264, 2003.

Hovind P, Tarnow L, Rossing P, Carstensen B, Parving HH: Improved survival in patients obtaining remission of nephritic range albuminuria in diabetic nephropathy. *Kidney Int* 66:1180–1186, 2004a.

Hovind P, Tarnow L, Rossing P, Jensen BR, Graae M, Torp I, Binder C, Parving HH: Predictors for the development of microalbuminuria and macroalbuminuria in patients with type 1 diabetes: inception cohort study. *BMJ* 328:1105, 2004b.

How HY, Sibai B, Lindheimer M, Caritis S, Hauth J, Klebanoff M, MacPherson C, Van Dorsten P, Miodovnik M, Landon M, Paul R, Meis P, Thurnau G, Dombrowski M, Roberts J: Is early-pregnancy proteinuria associated with an increased rate of preeclampsia in women with pregestational diabetes mellitus? *Am J Obstet Gynecol* 190:775–778, 2004.

Howard BV, Robbins DC, Sievers ML, Lee ET, Rhoades D, Devereux RB, Cowan LD, Gray RS, Welty TK, Go OT, Howard WJ: LDL cholesterol as a strong predictor of coronary heart disease in diabetic individuals with insulin resistance and low LDL: the Strong Heart Study. *Arterioscler Thromb Vasc Biol* 20:830–835, 2000.

Howard BV, Rodriguez BL, Bennett PH, Harris MI, Hamman R, Kuller LH, Pearson TA, Wylie-Rosett J: Diabetes and cardiovascular disease. Writing Group I: epidemiology. American Heart Association Prevention Conference VI. *Circulation* 105:e132–e137, May 7, 2002.

Howard BV, Best LG, Galloway JM, Howard WJ, Jones K, Lee ET, Ratner RE, Resnick HE, Devereux RB: Coronary heart disease risk equivalence in diabetes depends on concomitant risk factors. *Diabetes Care* 29:391–397, 2006.

Howard BV, Roman MJ, Devereux RB, Fleg JL, Galloway JM, Henderson JA, Howard WJ, Lee ET, Mete M, Poolaw B, Ratbner RE, Russell M, Silverman A, Stylianou M, Umans JG, Wang W, Weir MR, Weissman NJ, Wilson C, Yeh F, Zhu J: Effect of lower targets for blood pressure and LDL cholesterol on atherosclerosis in diabetes: the SANDS randomized trial. *JAMA* 299:1678–1689, 2008.

Hsia SH, Connelly PW, Hegele RA: Successful outcome in severe pregnancy-associated hyperlipemia: a case report and literature review. *Am J Med Sci* 309:213–221, 1995.

Hu FB, Stampfer MJ, Solomon CG, Liu S, Willett WC, Speizer FE, Nathan DM, Manson JE: The impact of diabetes mellitus on mortality from all causes and coronary heart disease in women: 20 years of follow-up. *Arch Int Med* 161: 1717–1723, 2001.

Hu FB, Bronner L, Willett WC, Stampfer MJ, Rexrode KM, Albert CM, Hunter D, Manson JE: Fish and omega-3 fatty acid intake and risk of coronary heart disease in women. *JAMA* 287:1815–1821, 2002.

Hu FB, Cho E, Rexrode KM, Albert CM, Manson JE: Fish and long-chain omega-3 fatty acid intake and risk of coronary heart disease and total mortality in diabetic women. *Circulation* 107:1852–1857, 2003.

Hu F, Morrissey P, Yao J, Xu Z: Development of AT(1) and AT(2) receptors in the ovine fetal brain. *Brain Res Dev Brain Res* 150:51–61, 2004.

Hubel CA, McLaughlin MK, Evans RW, Hauth BA, Sims CJ, Roberts JM: Fasting serum triglycerides, free fatty acids, and malondialdehyde are increased in preeclampsia, are positively correlated, and decrease within 48 hours post partum. *Am J Obstet Gynecol* 174: 975–982, 1996.

Hubel CA, Shakir Y, Gallaher MJ, McLaughlin MK, Roberts JM: Low-density lipoprotein particle size decreases during normal pregnancy in association with triglyceride increases. *J Soc Gynecol Investig* 5:244–250, 1998.

Hughes AB: Fetal heart rate changes during diabetic ketosis. *Acta Obstet Gynecol Scand* 66:71–73, 1987.

Hulton SA, Thomson PD, Cooper PA, Rothberg AD: Angiotensin-converting enzyme inhibitors in pregnancy may result in neonatal renal failure. *S Afr Med J* 78:673–676, 1990.

Hung JH, Yen MY, Pan YP, Hsu LP: The effect of methyldopa on retinal artery circulation in preeclamptic gravidae. *Ultrasound Obstet Gynecol* 15:513–519, 2000.

Hunter S, Robson SC: Adaptation of the maternal heart in pregnancy. *Br Heart J* 68:540–543, 1992.

Hurst RT, Lee RW: Increased incidence of coronary atherosclerosis in type 2 diabetes mellitus: mechanisms and management. *Ann Intern Med* 139:824–834, 2003.

Ibrahim H, Mondress M, Tello A, Fan Y, Koopmeiners J, Thomas W: An alternative formula to the Cockcroft-Gault and the Modification of Diet in Renal Diseases formulas in predicting GFR in individuals with type 1 diabetes. *J Am Soc Nephrol* 16:1051–1060, 2005.

Idris I, Srinivasan R, Simm A, Page RC: Maternal hypothyroidism in early and late gestation: effects on neonatal and obstetric outcome. *Clin Endocrinol (Oxf)* 63:560–565, 2005.

Idzior-Walus B, Mattock MB, Solnica B, Stevens L, Fuller JH: Factors associated with plasma lipids and lipoproteins in type 1 diabetes mellitus: the EURODIAB IDDM Complications Study. *Diabet Med* 18:786–796, 2001.

Iglesias A, Montelongo A, Herrera E, Lasuncion MA: Changes in cholesteryl ester transfer protein activity during normal gestation and postpartum. *Clin Biochem* 27:63–68, 1994.

Iijima T, Tada H, Hidaka Y, Mitsuda N, Murata Y, Amino N: Effects of autoantibodies on the course of pregnancy and fetal growth. *Obstet Gynecol* 90:364–369, 1997.

Incerti J, Zelmanovitz T, Camargo JL, Gross JL, de Azevedo MJ: Evaluation of tests for microalbuminuria screening in patients with diabetes. *Nephrol Dial Transplant* 20:2402–2407, 2005.

Ingelfinger JR, Woods LL: Perinatal programming, renal development, and adult renal function. *Am J Hypertens* 15:46S–49S, 2002.

Ingelsson E, Schaefer EJ, Contois JH, McNamara JR, Sullivan L, Keyes MJ, Pencina MJ, Schoonmaker C, Wilson PWF, D'Agostino RB, Vasan RS: Clinical utility of different lipid measures for prediction of coronary heart disease in men and women. *JAMA* 298:776–785, 2007.

Inzucchi SE: Noninvasive assessment of the diabetic patient for coronary artery disease. Editorial. *Diabetes Care* 24:1519–1521, 2001.

Ioachimescu AG, Brennan DM, Hoar BM, Kashyap SR, Hoogwerf BJ: Serum uric acid, mortality and glucose control in patients with type 2 diabetes mellitus: a PreCIS database study. *Diabet Med* 24:1369–1374, 2007.

IOM—Institute of Medicine, Food and Nutrition Board: *Dietary Reference Intakes: Energy, Carbohydrates, Fiber, Fat, Fatty Acids, Cholesterol, Protein, and Amino Acids.* Washington, DC: National Academies Press; 2002. Available at: http://www.nap.edu/catalog.php?record_id=10490. Accessed March 12, 2008.

IOM—Institute of Medicine, Food and Nutrition Board: *Dietary Reference Intakes for Water, Potassium, Sodium, Chloride, and Sulfate.* Washington, DC: National Academies Press; 2004. Available at: http://www.nap.edu/catalog.php?record_id=10925. Accessed March 12, 2008.

Irfan S, Arain TM, Shaukat A, Shahid A: Effect of pregnancy on diabetic nephropathy and retinopathy. *J Coll Physicians Surg Pak* 14:75–78, 2004.

Iribarren C, Karter AJ, Go AS, Ferrara A, Liu JY, Sidney S, Selby JV: Glycemic control and heart failure among adult patients with diabetes. *Circulation* 103:2668–2673, 2001.

Isezuo SA, Ekele BA: Eclampsia and abnormal Qtc. *West Afr J Med* 23:123–127, 2004.

Israelian Z, Gosmanov NR, Szoke E, Schorr M, Bokhari S, Cryer PE, Gerich JE, Meyer C: Increasing the decrement in insulin secretion improves glucagon responses to hypoglycemia in advanced type 2 diabetes. *Diabetes Care* 28:2691–2696, 2005.

Israelian Z, Szoke E, Woerle J, Bokhari S, Schorr M, Schwenke DC, Cryer PE, Gerich JE, Meyer C: Multiple defects in counterregulation of hypoglycemia in modestly advanced type 2 diabetes mellitus. *Metabolism* 55:593–598, 2006.

Iwasaki R, Ohkuchi A, Furuta I, Ojima T, Matsubara S, Sato, Minakami H: Relationship between blood pressure level in early pregnancy and subsequent changes in blood pressure during pregnancy. *Acta Obstet Gynecol Scand* 81:918–925, 2002.

Iwase M, Sonoki K, Sasaki N, Ohdo S, Higuchi S, Hattori H, Iida M: Lysophosphatidylcholine contents in plasma LDL in patients with type 2 diabetes mellitus: relation with lipoprotein-associated phopholipase A2 and effects of simvastatin treatment. *Atherosclerosis* 196:931–936, 2008.

Jabs WJ, Theissing E, Nitschke M, Bechtel JF, Duchrow M, Mohamed S, Jahrbeck B, Sievers HH, Steinhoff J, Bartels C: Local generation of C-reactive protein in diseased coronary artery venous bypass grafts and normal vascular tissue. *Circulation* 108:1428–1431, 2003a.

Jabs WJ, Logering BA, Gerke P, Kreft B, Wolber EM, Klinger MH, Fricke L, Steinhoff J: The kidney as a second site of human C-reactive protein formation in vivo. *Eur J Immunol* 33:152–161, 2003b.

Jacob S, Henriksen EJ: Metabolic properties of vasodilating beta blockers: management considerations for hypertensive diabetic patients and patients with the metabolic syndrome. *J Clin Hypertens* 6:690–696, 2004.

Jacobs MJ, Kleisli T, Pio JR, Malik S, L'Italien GJ, Chen RS, Wong ND: Prevalence and control of dyslipidemia among persons with diabetes in the United States. *Diabetes Res Clin Pract* 70:263–269, 2005a.

Jacobs AK, Eckel RH: Evaluating and managing cardiovascular disease in women. Understanding a woman's heart. *Circulation* 111:383–384, 2005b.

Jacoby RM, Nesto RW: Acute myocardial infarction in the diabetic patient: pathophysiology, clinical course and prognosis. *J Am Coll Cardiol* 20:736–744, 1992.

Jaeger C, Hatziagelaki E, Petzoldt R, Bretzel RG: Comparative analysis of organ-specific autoantibodies and celiac disease-associated antibodies in type 1 diabetic patients, their first-degree relatives, and healthy control subjects. *Diabetes Care* 24:27–32, 2001.

Jaffer FA, O'Donnel CJ, Larson MG, Chan SK, Kissinger KV, Kupka MJ, Salton C, Botnar RM, Levy D, Manning WJ: Age and sex distribution of subclinical aortic atherosclerosis: a magnetic resonance imaging examination of the Framingham Heart Study. *Arterioscl Thromb Vasc Biol* 22:849–854, 2002.

Jain L: Effect of pregnancy-induced and chronic hypertension on pregnancy outcome. *J Perinatol* 17:425–427, 1997.

James AH, Bushnell CD, Jamison MG, Myers ER: Incidence and risk factors for stroke in pregnancy and the puerperium. *Obstet Gynecol* 106:509–516, 2005.

James AH, Jamison MG, Biswas MS, Brancazio LR, Swamy GK, Myers ER: Acute myocardial infarction in pregnancy. A United States population-based study. *Circulation* 113:1564–1571, 2006.

James AH, Brancazio LR, Price T: Aspirin and reproductive outcomes. *Obstet Gynecol Surv* 63:49–57, 2008.

Janand-Delenne B, Savin B, Habib G, Bory M, Vaguen P, Lassmann-Vague V: Silent myocardial ischemia in patients with diabetes. Who to screen. *Diabetes Care* 22:1396–1400, 1999.

Jandeleit-Dahm KA, Lassila M, Allen TJ: Advanced glycation end products in diabetes-associated atherosclerosis and renal disease: interventional studies. *Ann N Y Acad Sci* 1043:759–766, 2005.

Jannet D, Carbonne B, Sebban E, Milliez J: Nicardipine versus metoprolol in the treatment of hypertension during pregnancy: a randomized comparative trial. *Obstet Gynecol* 84:354–359, 1994.

Jarrett RJ: Type 2 (non-insulin-dependent) diabetes mellitus and coronary heart disease: chicken, egg, or neither? *Diabetologia* 26:99–102, 1984.

Jarvisalo MJ, Putto-Laurila A, Jartti L, Lehtimaki T, Solakivi T, Ronnemaa T, Raitakari OT: Carotid artery intima-media thickness in children with diabetes mellitus. *Diabetes* 51:493–498, 2002.

Javorka M, Javorkova J, Tonhajzerova I, Javorka K: Parasympathetic versus sympathetic control of the cardiovascular system in young patients with type 1 diabetes mellitus. *Clin Physiol Funct Imaging* 25:270–274, 2005.

Jenkins AJ, Steele J, Janus E, Best J: Increased plasma apolipoprotein(a) levels in IDDM patients with microalbuminuria. *Diabetes* 40:787–790, 1991.

Jenkins AJ, Lyons TJ, Zheng D, Otvos JD, Lackland DT, McGee D, Garvey WT, Klein RL; the DCCT/EDIC Research Group: Serum lipoproteins in the Diabetes Control and Complications Trial/Epidemiology of Diabetes Intervention and Complications cohort. Associations with gender and glycemia. *Diabetes Care* 26:810–818, 2003a.

Jenkins AJ, Lyons TJ, Zheng D, Otvos JD, Lackland DT, McGee D, Garvey WT, Klein RL; the DCCT/EDIC Research Group: Lipoproteins in the DCCT/EDIC cohort: associations with diabetic nephropathy. *Kidney Int* 64:817–828, 2003b.

Jensen T, Borch-Johnsen K, Kofoed-Enevoldsen A, Deckert T: Coronary heart disease in young type 1 (insulin-dependent) diabetic patients with and without diabetic nephropathy: incidence and risk factors. *Diabetologia* 30:144–148, 1987.

Jensen MD: Gender differences in regional fatty acid metabolism before and after meal ingestion. *J Clin Invest* 96:2297–2303, 1995.

Jensen JS, Feldt-Rasmussen B, Strandgaard S, Schroll M, Borch-Johnsen K: Arterial hypertension, microalbuminuria, and risk of ischemic heart disease. *Hypertension* 35:898–903, 2000.

Jensen DM, Damm P, Molsted-Pedersen L, Ovesen P, Westergaard JG, Moeller M, Beck-Nielsen H: Outcomes in type 1 diabetic pregnancies. A nationwide, population-based study. *Diabetes Care* 27:2819–2833, 2004.

Jensen JS, Feldt-Rasmussen B, Borch-Johnsen K, Jensen KS, Nordestgaard BG: Increased transvascular lipoprotein transport in diabetes: association with albuminuria and systolic hypertension. *J Clin Endocrinol Metab* 90:4441–4445, 2005.

Jensen-Urstad KJ, Reichard PG, Rosfors JS, Lindblad JE, Jensen-Urstad MT: Early atherosclerosis is retarded by improved long-term blood glucose control in patients with IDDM. *Diabetes* 45:1253–1258, 1996.

Jerums G, Allen TJ, Tsalamandris C, Akdeniz A, Sinha A, Gilbert R, Cooper ME: Relationship of progressively increasing albuminuria to apoprotein(a) and blood pressure in type 2 (non-insulin-dependent) and type 1 (insulin-dependent) diabetic patients. *Diabetologia* 36:1037–1044, 1993.

Jochmann N, Stangl K, Garbe E, Baumann G, Stangl V: Female-specific aspects in the pharmacotherapy of chronic cardiovascular diseases. *Eur Heart J* 26:1585–1595, 2005.

Johansen OE, Birkeland KI, Orvik E, Flesland O, Wergeland R, Ueland T, Smith C, Endresesn K, Aukrust P, Gillestad L: Inflammation and coronary angiography in asymptomatic type 2 diabetic subjects. *Scand J Clin Lab Invest* 67:306–316, 2007.

Johnson RJ, Kang D-H, Feig D, Kivlighn S, Kanellis J, Watanabe S, Tuttle KR, Rodriguez-Iturbe B, Herrera-Acosta J, Mazzali M: Is there a pathogenetic role for uric acid in hypertension and cardiovascular and renal disease? *Hypertension* 41:1183–1190, 2003.

Johnson RJ, Rideout BA: Uric acid and diet—insights into the epidemic of cardiovascular disease. *N Engl J Med* 350:1071–1073, 2004.

Johnson BD, Shaw LJ, Pepine CJ, Reis SE, Kelsey SF, Sopko G, Rogrs WJ, Mankad S, Sharaf BL, Bittner V, Bairey Merz CN: Persistent chest pain predicts cardiovascular events in women without obstructive coronary artery disease: results from the NIH-NHLBI-sponsored Women's Ischemia Syndrome Evaluation (WISE) study. *Eur Heart J* 27:1408–1415, 2006.

Johnston GP: Pregnancy and diabetic retinopathy. *Am J Ophthalmol* 90:519–524, 1980.

Jones HMR, Cummings AJ: A study of the transfer of alpha-methyldopa in the human fetus and newborn infant. *Br J Clin Pharmacol* 6:432–434, 1978.

Jones DC, Hayslett JP: Outcome of pregnancy in women with moderate or severe renal insufficiency. *N Engl J Med* 335:226–232, 1996.

Jones KL: Role of obesity in complicating and confusing the diagnosis and treatment of diabetes in children. *Pediatrics* 121:361–368, 2008.

Jonsdottir LS, Arngrimsson R, Geirsson RT, Sigvaldason H, Sigfusson N: Death rates from ischemic heart disease in women with a history of hypertension in pregnancy. *Acta Obstet Gynecol Scand* 74:772–776, 1995.

Joseph F, Younis N, Sowery J, Soran H, Stanaway S, Bowen-Hones D: Blood pressure control in diabetes: are we achieving the guideline targets? *Pract Diab Int* 20:276–282, 2003.

Jouppila P, Kirkinen P, Koivula A, Ylikorkala O: Labetalol does not alter the placental and fetal blood flow or maternal prostanoids in preeclampsia. *Br J Obstet Gynecol* 93:543–547, 1986.

Jovanovic R, Jovanovic L: Obstetric management when normoglycemia is maintained in diabetic pregnant women with vascular compromise. *Am J Obstet Gynecol* 149:617–623, 1984.

Jovanovic L: Diabetic retinopathy. In: Reece EA, Coustan DR, Gabbe SG, eds. *Diabetes in Women. Adolescence, Pregnancy, and Menopause.* 3rd ed. Philadelphia: Lippincott William & Wilkins; 2004:371–382.

Jovanovic-Peterson L, Peterson CM: De novo clinical hypothyroidism in pregnancies complicated by type 1 diabetes, subclinical hypothyroidism and proteinuria: a new syndrome. *Am J Obstet Gynecol* 159:442–446, 1988.

Junik R, Kozinski M, Debska-Kozinska K: Thyroid ultrasound in diabetic patients without overt thyroid disease. *Acta Radiol* 47:687–691, 2006.

Justesen TI, Petersen JLA, Ekbom P, Damm P, Mathiesen ER: Can measurement of the albumin/creatine ratio in random urine samples replace 24-hour urine collection in screening for micro- and macroalbuminuria in pregnant women with type 1 diabetes mellitus? *Diabetes Care* 29:924–925, 2006.

Juttilainen A, Kortelainen S, Lehto S, Ronnemaa T, Pyorala K, Laakso M: Gender difference in the impact of type 2 diabetes on coronary heart disease risk. *Diabetes Care* 27:2898–2904, 2004.

Juutilainen A, Lehto S, Ronnemaa T, Pyorala K, Laakso M: Type 2 diabetes as a "coronary heart disease equivalent." An 18-year prospective population-based study in Finnish subjects. *Diabetes Care* 28:2901–2907, 2005.

Juutilainen A, Lehto S, Ronnemaa T, Pyorala K, Laakso M: Similarity of the impact of type 1 and type 2 diabetes on cardiovascular mortality in middle-aged subjects. *Diabetes Care* 31:714–719, 2008.

Kaaja R, Sjoberg L, Hellsted T, Immonen I, Sane T, Teramo K: Long-term effects of pregnancy on diabetic complications. *Diabet Med* 13:165–169, 1996.

Kaaja R, Loukovaara S: Progression of retinopathy in type 1 diabetic women during pregnancy. *Curr Diab Rev* 3:85–93, 2007.

Kablak-Ziembicka A, Przewlocki T, Tracz W, Pieniazek P, Musialek P, Sokolowski A: Gender differences in carotid intima-media thickness in patients with suspected coronary artery disease. *Am J Cardiol* 96:1217–1222, 2005.

Kahhale S, Zugaib M, Carrara W, Paula FJ, Sabbaga E, Neme B: Comparative study of chronic hypertensive pregnant women treated and nontreated with pindolol (Portuguese). *Ginecologia e Obstetrica Brasileiras* 8:85–89, 1985.

Kahn JK, Zola B, Juni JE, Vinik AI: Decreased exercise heart rate and blood pressure response in diabetic subjects with cardiac autonomic neuropathy. *Diabetes Care* 9:389–394, 1986.

Kainz A, Harabicz I, Cowlrick IS, Gadqil SD, Hagiwara D: Review of the course and outcome of 100 pregnancies in 84 women treated with tacrolimus. *Transplantation* 70:1718–1721, 2000.

Kairaitis LK, Nankivell BJ, Lawrence S, Nicholl MC, O'Connell PJ, Kable K, Chapman JR, Allen RD: Successful obstetric outcome after simultaneous pancreas and kidney transplantation. *Med J Aust* 170: 368–370, 1999.

Kale A, Kale E, Yalinkaya A, Akdeniz N, Canoruc N: The comparison of amino-terminal probrain natriuretic peptide levels in preeclampsia and normotensive pregnancy. *J Perinat Med* 33:121–124, 2005.

Kalergis M, Schiffrin A, Gougeon R, Jones PJH, Yale J-F: Impact of bedtime snack composition on prevention of nocturnal hypoglycemia in adults with type 1 diabetes undergoing intensive insulin management using lispro insulin before meals. A randomized, placebo-controlled, crossover trial. *Diabetes Care* 26:9–15, 2003.

Kalluri R: Proteinuria with and without renal glomerular podocyte effacement. *J Am Soc Nephrol* 17:2383–2389, 2006.

Kamalesh M, Feigenbaum H, Sawada S: Challenge of identifying patients with diabetes mellitus who are at low risk for coronary events by use of cardiac stress imaging. *Am Heart J* 147:561–563, 2004.

Kamalkannan D, Baskar V, Barton DM, Abdu TAM: Diabetic ketoacidosis in pregnancy. *Postgrad Med J* 79:454–457, 2003.

Kaminsky S, Sibley CP, Maresh M, Thomas CR, D'Souza SW: The effects of diabetes on placental lipase activity in the rat and human. *Pediatr Res* 30:541–543, 1991.

Kamoi K, Miyakoshi M, Soda S, Kaneko S, Nakagawa O: Usefulness of home blood pressure measurement in the morning in type 2 diabetic patients. *Diabetes Care* 25:2218–2223, 2002.

Kanaya AM, Grady D, Barrett-Connor E: Explaining the sex difference in coronary heart disease mortality among patients with type 2 diabetes mellitus: a meta-analysis. *Arch Intern Med* 162:1737–1745, 2002.

Kanellis J, Kang DH: Uric acid as a mediator of endothelial dysfunction, inflammation, and vascular disease. *Semin Nephrol* 25:39–42, 2005.

Kang DH, Finch J, Nakagawa T, Karumanchi SA, Kanellis J, Granger J, Johnson RJ: Uric acid, endothelial dysfunction and preeclampsia: searching for a pathogenetic link. *J Hypertens* 22:229–235, 2004.

Kannel WB, Eaker ED: Psychosocial and other features of coronary heart disease: insights from the Framingham Study. *Am Heart J* 112:1066–1073, 1986.

Kannel WB: Left ventricular hypertrophy as a risk factor: the Framingham experience. *J Hypertens Suppl* 9:S3–S8, 1991.

Kaplan MM: Monitoring thyroxine treatment during pregnancy. *Thyroid* 2:147–152, 1992.

Karnik AA, Fields AV, Shannon RP: Diabetic cardiomyopathy. *Curr Hypertens Rep* 9:467–473, 2007.

Kaspers S, Kordonouri O, Schober E, Grabert M, Hauffa BP, Holl RW; German Working Group for Pediatric Diabetology: Anthropometry, metabolic control, and thyroid autoimmunity in type 1 diabetes with celiac disease: a multicenter survey. *J Pediatr* 145:790–795, 2004.

Katz K, Karliner JS, Resnik R: Effects of a natural volume overload state (pregnancy) on left ventricular performance in normal human subjects. *Circulation* 58: 434–441, 1978.

Katz AM, Zile MR: New molecular mechanism in diastolic heart failure. Editorial. *Circulation* 113:1922–1925, 2006.

Kawasumi M, Tanaka Y, Uchino H, Shimizu T, Tamura Y, Sato F, Mita T, Watada H, Sakai K, Hirose T, Kawamori R: Strict glycemic control ameliorates the increase of carotid IMT in patients with type 2 diabetes. *Endocr J* 53:45–50, 2006.

Kaymaz AA, Telci A, Albeniz I, Belce A, Altug T: Comparison of the metabolic and antioxidant effects of diltiazem and vitamin E on streptozotocin-diabetic rats. *J Vet Med A Physiol Pathol Clin Med* 51:265–267, 2004.

Kazancioglu R, Sahin S, Has R, Turnmen A, Ergin-Karadayi H, Ibrahimoglu L, Bozfakioglu S: The outcome of pregnancy among patients receiving hemodialysis treatment. *Clin Nephrol* 59:379–382, 2003.

Keane WF, Brenner BM, de Zeeuw D, Grunfeld JP, McGill J, Mitch WE, Ribeiro AB, Shahinfar S, Simpson RL, Snapinn SM, Toto R; RENAAL Study Investigators: The risk of developing end-stage renal disease in patients with type 2 diabetes and nephropathy: the RENAAL study. *Kidney Int* 63:1499–1507, 2003a.

Keane WF, Lyle PA; Reduction of Endpoints in NIDDM with the Angiotensin II Receptor Antagonist Losartan Study Group: Recent advances in management of type 2 diabetes and nephropathy: lessons from the RENAAL study. *Am J Kidney Dis* 41 (Suppl 1):S22–S25, 2003b.

Keaney JF Jr, Loscalzo J: Diabetes, oxidative stress, and platelet activation. Editorial. *Circulation* 99:189–191, 1999.

Kempler P, Tesfaye S, Chaturvedi N, Stevens LK, Webb DJ, Eaton S, Kerenyi Z, Tamas G, Ward JD, Fuller JH: Blood pressure response to standing in the diagnosis of autonomic neuropathy: the EURODIAB IDDM Complications Study. *Arch Physiol Biochem* 109:215–222, 2001.

Kempler P, Tesfaye S, Chaturvedi N, Stevens LK, Webb DJ, Eaton S, Kerenyi Z, Tamas G, Ward JD, Fuller JH; EURODIAB IDDM Complications Study Group: Autonomic neuropathy is associated with increased cardiovascular risk factors: the EURODIAB IDDM Complications Study. *Diabet Med* 19:900–909, 2002.

Kershnar AK, Daniels SR, Imperatore G, Palla SL, Pettiti DB, Pettitt DJ, Marcovina S, Dolan LM, Hamman RF, Liese AD, Pihoker C, Rodriguez BL: Lipid abnormalities are prevalent in youth with type 1 and type 2 diabetes: the Search for Diabetes in Youth Study. *J Pediatr* 149:314–319, 2006.

Kestenbaum B, Seliger SL, Easterling TR, Gillen DL, Critxhlow CW, Stehman-Breen CO, Schwartz SM: Cardiovascular and thromboembolic events following hypertensive pregnancy. *Am J Kid Dis* 42:982–989, 2003.

Khaliq A, Foreman D, Ahmed A, Weich H, Gregor Z, McLeod D, Boulton M: Increased expression of placenta growth factor in proliferative diabetic retinopathy. *Lab Invest* 78:109–116, 1998.

Khan NA, McAlister FA, Rabkin SW, Padwal R, Feldman RD, Campbell NR, Leiter LA, Lewanczuk RZ, Schiffrin EL, Hill MD, Arnold M, Moe G, Campbell TS, Herbert C, Milot A, Stone JA, Burgess E, Hemmelgarn B, Jones C, Larochelle P, Ogilvie RI, Houlden R, Herman RJ, Hamet P, Fodor G, Carruthers G, Culleton B, Dechamplain J, Pylypchuk G, Logan AG, Gledhill N, Petrella R, Tobe S, Ytouyz RM; Canadian Hypertension Education Program: The 2006 Canadian Hypertension Education Program recommendations for the management of hypertension: Part II—Therapy. *Can J Cardiol* 15:583–593, 2006.

Khandewal M, Kumanova M, Gaughan JP, Reece EA: Role of diltiazem in pregnant women with chronic renal disease. *J Matern Fetal Neonatal Med* 12:408–412, 2002.

Kharlip J, Naglieri R, Mitchell BD, Ryan KA, Donner TW: Screening for silent coronary heart disease in type 2 diabetes. Clinical application of American Diabetes Association guidelines. *Diabetes Care* 29:692–694, 2006.

Khoury JC, Miodovnik M, Lemasters G, Sibai B: Pregnancy outcome and progression of diabetic nephropathy. What's next? *J Matern Fetal Neonatal Med* 11:238–244, 2002.

Khoury J, Henriksen T, Christophersen B, Tonstad S: Effect of a cholesterol-lowering diet on maternal, cord, and neonatal lipids, and pregnancy outcome: a randomized clinical trial. *Am J Obstet Gynecol* 193:1292–1301, 2005.

Kieler H, Zettergren T, Svensson H, Dickman PW, Larsson A: Assessing urinary albumin excretion in preeclamptic women: which sample to use? *BJOG* 110: 12–17, 2003.

Kilby MD, Neary RH, Mackness MI, Durrington PN: Fetal and maternal lipoprotein metabolism in human pregnancy complicated by type I diabetes mellitus. *J Clin Endocrinol Metab* 83: 1736–1741, 1998.

Kilvert JA, Nicholson HO, Wright AD: Ketoacidosis in diabetic pregnancy. *Diabetic Med* 10:278–281, 1993.

Kim WY, Astrup AS, Stuber M, Tarnow L, Falk E, Botnar RM, Simonsen C, Pietraszek L, Hansen PR, Manning WJ, Andersen NT, Parving HH: Subclinical coronary and aortic atherosclerosis detected by magnetic resonance imaging in type 1 diabetes with and without diabetic nephropathy. *Circulation* 115:228–235, 2007.

Kimball TR, Daniels SR, Khoury SR, Magnotti RA, Turner AM, Dolan LM: Cardiovascular status in young patients with insulin-dependent diabetes mellitus. *Circulation* 90:357–361, 1994.

Kimble LP, McGuire DB, Dunbar SB, Fazio S, De A, Weintraub WS, Strickland OS: Gender differences in pain characteristics of chronic stable angina and perceived physical limitation in patients with coronary artery disease. *Pain* 101:45–53, 2003.

Kimmerle R, Heinemann L, Delecki A, Berger M: Severe hypoglycemia incidence and predisposing factors in 85 pregnancies of type 1 diabetic women. *Diabetes Care* 15:1034–1037, 1992.

Kimmerle R, Zass R-P, Cupisti S, Somville T, Bender R, Pawlowski B, Berger M: Pregnancies in women with diabetic nephropathy: long-term outcome for mother and child. *Diabetologia* 38:227–235, 1995.

Kimura M, Amino N, Tamaki H, Mitsuda N, Miyai K, Tanizawa O: Physiologic thyroid activiation in normal early pregnancy is induced by circulating hCG. *Obstet Gynecol* 75:775, 1990.

King GL, Goodman AD, Buzney S, Moses A, Kahn CR: Receptors and growth-promoting effects of insulin and insulin-like growth factors on cells from bovine retinal capillaries and aorta. *J Clin Invest* 75:1028–1036, 1985.

King DE, Mainous AG III, Buchanan TA, Pearson WS: C-reactive protein and glycemic control in adults with diabetes. *Diabetes Care* 26:1535–1539, 2003.

Kioko EM, Shaw KM, Clarke AD, Warren DJ: Successful pregnancy in a diabetic patient treated with continuous ambulatory peritoneal dialysis. *Diabetes Care* 6:298–300, 1983.

Kishore P, Gabriely I, Cui M-H, Di Vito J, Gajavelli S, Hwang J-H, Shamoon H: Role of hepatic glycogen breakdown in defective counterregulation of hypoglycemia in intensively treated type 1 diabetes. *Diabetes* 55:659–666, 2006.

Kislinger T, Fu C, Huber B, Qu W, Taguchi A, Yan SD, Hofmann M, Yan SF, Pischetsrider M, Stern D, Schmidt AM: Nϵ (carboxymethyl)lysine modifications of proteins are ligands for RAGE that activate cell signaling pathways and modulate gene expression. *J Biol Chem* 274:31740–31749, 1999.

Kitabchi AE, Umpierrez GE, Murphy MB, Barrett EJ, Kreisberg RA, Malone JI, Wall BM: Management of hyperglycemic crises in patients with diabetes mellitus. Technical review. *Diabetes Care* 24:131–153, 2001.

Kitabchi AE: Ketosis-prone diabetes: a new subgroup of patients with atypical type 1 and type 2 diabetes? Editorial. *J Clin Endocrinol Metab* 88:5087–5089, 2003.

Kitabchi AE, Umpierrez GE, Murphy MB, Kreisberg RA: Hyperglycemic crises in adult patients with diabetes. A consensus statement from the American Diabetes Association. *Diabetes Care* 29:2739–2748, 2006.

Kitajima MS, Oka I, Yasuhi M, Fukuda Y, Rii Y, Ishimaru T: Maternal serum triglyceride at 24–32 weeks' gestation and newborn weight in nondiabetic women with positive diabetic screens. *Obstet Gynecol* 97: 776–780, 2001.

Kitamura A, Hoshino T, Kon T, Ogawa R: Patients with diabetic neuropathy are at risk of a greater intraoperative reduction in core temperature. *Anesthesiology* 92:1311–1318, 2000.

Kitzmiller JL, Brown ER, Phillippe M, Stark AR, Acker D, Kaldany A, Singh S, Hare J: Diabetic nephropathy and perinatal outcome. *Am J Obstet Gynecol* 141: 741–751, 1981.

Kitzmiller JL: Diabetic ketoacidosis and pregnancy. *Contemp Obstet Gynecol* 20: 141–147, 1982.

Kitzmiller, JL, Gavin LA, Gin GD, Jovanovic-Peterson L, Main EK, Zigrang WD: Preconception care of diabetes. Glycemic control prevents congenital anomalies. *JAMA* 265:731–736, 1991.

Kitzmiller JL, Main E, Ward B, Theiss T, Peterson DL: Insulin lispro and the development of proliferative diabetic retinopathy during pregnancy. *Diabetes Care* 22:874–876, 1999.

Kitzmiller JL: Diabetic nephropathy in pregnancy. In: Mogensen CE, ed. *The Kidney and Hypertension in Diabetes Mellitus.* 6th ed. London: Taylor & Francis; 2004a:647–686.

Kitzmiller JL: Clinical diabetic nephropathy before and during pregnancy. In: Reece EA, Coustan DR, Gabbe SG, eds. *Diabetes in Women. Adolescence, Pregnancy, and Menopause.* 3rd ed. Philadelphia: Lippincott Williams & Wilkins; 2004b:383–423.

Klein BEK, Klein R, Meuer SM, Moss SE, Dalton DD: Does the severity of diabetic retinopathy predict perinatal outcome? *J Diabetes Complications* 2:179–184, 1988.

Klein BEK, Moss SE, Klein R: Effect of pregnancy on progression of diabetic retinopathy. *Diabetes Care* 13:34, 1990.

Klein RZ, Haddow JE, Faix JD, Brown RS, Hermos RJ, Pulkkinen A, Mitchell ML: Prevalence of thyroid deficiency in pregnant women. *Clin Endocrinol (Oxf)* 35:41–46, 1991.

Klein RL, Hunter SJ, Jenkins AJ, Zheng D, Semler AJ, Clore J, Garvey WT; the DCCT/EDIC Study Group: Fibrinogen is a marker for nephropathy and peripheral vascular disease in type 1 diabetes. Studies of plasma fibrinogen and fibrinogen gene polymorphism in the DCCT/EDIC cohort. *Diabetes Care* 26:1439–1448, 2003.

Klein BEK, Klein R, McBride PE, Cruikshanks KJ, Palta M, Knudtson MD, Moss SE, Reinke JO: Cardiovascular disease, mortality, and retinal microvascular characteristics in type 1 diabetes. Wisconsin Epidemiologic Study of Diabetic Retinopathy. *Arch Intern Med* 164:1917–1924, 2004.

Klein RL, McHenry MB, Lok KH, Hunter SJ, Le NA, Jenkins AJ, Zheng D, Semler A, Page G, Brown WV, Lyons TJ, Garvey WT; the DCCT/EDIC Research

Group: Apolipoprotein C-III protein concentrations and gene polymorphisms in type 1 diabetes: associations with microvascular disease complications in the DCCT/EDIC cohort. *J Diabetes Complications* 19:18–25, 2005.

Klinzing P, Markert UR, Liesaus K, Peiker G: Case report: successful pregnancy and delivery after myocardial infarction and essential thrombocythemia treated with clopidrogel. *Clin Exp Obstet Gynecol* 28:215–216, 2001.

Knerr I, Dost A, Lepler R, Raile K, Schober E, Rascher W, Holl RW; the Diabetes Data Acquisition System for Prospective Surveillance (DPV) Scientific Initiative Germany and Austria: Tracking and prediction of arterial blood pressure from childhood to young adulthood in 868 patients with type 1 diabetes. A multicenter longitudinal survey in Germany and Austria. *Diabetes Care* 31: 726–727, 2008.

Knight EL, Verhave JC, Spiegelman D, Hillege HL, deZeeuw D, Curhan GC, deJong P: Factors influencing serum cystatin C levels other than renal function and the impact on renal function measurement. *Kidney Int* 65:1416–1421, 2004.

Knopp RH, Warth MR, Carrol CJ: Lipid metabolism in pregnancy. I. Changes in lipoprotein triglyceride and cholesterol in normal pregnancy and the effects of diabetes mellitus. *J Reprod Med* 10:95–101, 1973.

Knopp R H, Chapman M, Bergelin R, Wahl PW, Warth MR, Irvine S: Relationships of lipoprotein lipids to mild fasting hyperglycemia and diabetes in pregnancy. *Diabetes Care* 3: 416–420, 1980.

Knopp RH, Montes A, Childs M, Mafuchi LJR: Metabolic adjustments in normal and diabetic pregnancy. *Clin Obstet Gynecol* 24:21–49, 1981.

Knopp RH, Bergelin RO, Wahl PW, Walden CE, Chapman M, Irvine S: Population-based lipoprotein lipid reference values for pregnant women compared to nonpregnant women classified by sex hormone usage. *Am J Obstet Gynecol* 143: 626–637, 1982.

Knopp RH, Warth MR, Charles D, Childs M, Li JR, Mabuchi H, Van Allen MI: Lipoprotein metabolism in pregnancy, fat transport to the fetus, and the effects of diabetes. *Biol Neonate* 50:297–317, 1986.

Knopp RH, Bonet B, Lasuncion MA, Montelongo A, Herrera E: Lipoprotein metabolism in pregnancy. In: Herrera E, Knopp RH, eds. *Perinatal Biochemistry.* Boca Raton, FL: CRC Press; 1992a:19–51.

Knopp RH, Magee MS, Walden CE, Bonet B, Benedetti TJ: Prediction of infant birth weight by GDM screening tests. Importance of plasma triglyceride. *Diabetes Care* 15:1605–1613, 1992b.

Knopp RH, Van Allen MI, McNeely M, Walden CE, Plovie B, Shiota K, Brown Z: Effect of insulin-dependent diabetes on plasma lipoproteins in diabetic pregnancy. *J Reprod Med* 38: 703–710, 1993.

Knopp RH: Hormone-mediated changes in nutrient metabolism in pregnancy: a physiological basis for normal fetal development. *Ann N Y Acad Sci* 817: 251–271, 1997.

Knopp R, Bonet B, Zhu X-D: Lipid metabolism in pregnancy. In: Cowett R, ed. *Principles of Perinatal-Neonatal Metabolism.* New York: Springer-Verlag; 1998:221–258.

Knopp RH: Drug treatment of lipid disorders. *N Engl J Med* 341:498–511, 1999.

Knopp R, Aikawa K: Estrogen, female gender and heart disease. In: Topol E, ed. *The Textbook of Cardiovascular Medicine.* Philadelphia: Lippincott Williams & Wilkins; 2002:171–188.

Knopp RH, Retzlaff B, Fish B, Walden C, Wallick S, Anderson M, Aikawa K, Kahn SE: Effects of insulin resistance and obesity on lipoproteins and sensitivity to egg feeding. *Arterioscler Thromb Vasc Biol* 23:1437–1443, 2003a.

Knopp RH, Retzlaff B, Aikawa K, Kahn SE: Management of patients with diabetic hyperlipidemia. *Am J Cardiol* 91:24E-28E, 2003b.

Knopp RH, Paramsothy P, Retzlaff BM, Fish B, Walden C, Dowdy A, Tsunehara C, Aikawa K, Cheung MC: Sex differences in lipoprotein metabolism and dietary response: basis in hormonal differences and implications for cardiovascular disease. *Curr Cardiol Rep* 8:452–459, 2006a.

Knopp RH, d'Emden M, Smilde JG, Pocock SJ: Efficacy and safety of atorvastatin in the prevention of cardiovascular end points in subjects with type 2 diabetes: the Atorvastatin Study for Prevention of Coronary Heart Disease Endpoints in non-insulin-dependent diabetes mellitus (ASPEN). *Diabetes Care* 29:1478–1485, 2006b.

Knopp RH, Paramsothy P: Oxidized LDL and abdominal obesity: a key to understanding the metabolic syndrome. Editorial. *Am J Clin Nutr* 83:1–2, 2006c.

Knuttgen D, Weidemann D, Doehn M: Diabetic autonomic neuropathy: abnormal cardiovascular reactions under general anesthesia. *Klin Wochenschr* 68:1168–1172, 1990.

Kobayashi M, Yamazaki K, Hirao K, Oishi M, Kanatsuka A, Yamauchi M, Takagi H, Kawai K; Japan Diabetes Clinical Data Management Study Group: The status of diabetes control and antidiabetic drug therapy in Japan—a cross-sectional survey of 17,000 patients with diabetes mellitus (JDDM 1). *Diabetes Res Clin Pract* 73:198–204, 2006.

Koch M, Gradaus F-C, Lescjke M, Grabensee B: Relevance of conventional cardiovascular risk factors for the prediction of coronary artery disease in diabetic patients on renal replacement therapy. *Nephrol Dial Transplant* 12:1187–1191, 1997.

Kohner EM: Diabetic retinopathy in pregnancy. In: Dornhorst A, Hadden DR, eds. *Diabetes and Pregnancy: An International Approach to Diagnosis and Management.* London: John Wiley & Sons Ltd.; 1996:155–165.

Koistinen MJ: Prevalence of asymptomatic myocardial ischemia in diabetic subjects. *BMJ* 301:92–95, 1990.

Koivikko ML, Salmela PI, Airaksinen KEJ, Tapanainen JS, Ruokonen A, Makikallio TH, Huikuri HV: Effects of sustained insulin-induced hypoglycemia on cardiovascular autonomic regulation in type 1 diabetes. *Diabetes* 54:744–750, 2005.

Koivisto VA, Stevens LK, Mattock M, Ebeling P, Muggeo M, Stephenson J, Idzior-Walus B; the EURODIAB IDDM Complications Study Group: Cardiovascular disease and its risk factors in IDDM in Europe. *Diabetes Care* 19:689–697, 1996.

Koka V, Wang W, Huang XR, Kim-Mitsuyama S, Truong LD, Lan HY: Advanced glycation end products activate a chymase-dependent angiotensin II-generating pathway in diabetic complications. *Circulation* 113:1353–1360, 2006.

Koklu E, Akcakus M, Kurtoglu S, Kokiu S, Yikilmaz A, Coskun A, Gunes T: Aortic intima-media thickness and lipid profile in macrosomic newborns. *Eur J Pediatr* 166:333–338, 2007.

Kollerits B, Auinger M, Reisig V, Kastenbauer T, Lingenhel A, Irsigler K, Prager R, Kronenberg F: Lipoprotein(a) as a predictor of cardiovascular disease in a prospectively followed cohort of patients with type 1 diabetes. *Diabetes Care* 29:1661–1663, 2006.

Kondo T, Vicent D, Suzuma K, Yanagisawa M, King GL, Holzenberger M, Kahn CR: Knockout of insulin and IGF-1 receptors on vascular endothelial cells protects against neovascularization. *J Clin Invest* 111:1835–1842, 2003.

Kong APS, So WY, Szeto CC, Chan NN, Luk A, Ma RCW, Ozaki R, Ng VWS, Ho CS, Lam CWK, Chow CC, Cockram CS, Chan JCN, Tong PCY: Assessment of glomerular filtration rate in addition to albuminuria is important in managing type II diabetes. *Kidney Int* 69:383–387, 2006.

Konstantin-Hansen KF, Hesseldahl H, Pederson SM: Microalbuminuria as a predictor of pre-eclampsia. *Acta Obstet Gynecol Scand* 71:343–346, 1992.

Kontush A, Chapman MJ: Why is HDL functionally deficient in type 2 diabetes? *Curr Diab Rep* 8:51–59, 2008.

Kooistra L, Crawford S, van Baar AL, Brouwers EP, Pop VJ: Neonatal effects of maternal hypothyroxinemia during early pregnancy. *Pediatrics* 117:161–167, 2006.

Kordonouri O, Klinghammer A, Lang EB, Gruters-Kieslich A, Grabert M, Holl RW; on behalf of the DPV-Initiative of the German Working Group for Pediatric Diabetology: Thyroid autoimmunity in children and adolescents with type 1 diabetes. A multi-center survey. *Diabetes Care* 25:1346–1350, 2002a.

Kordonouri O, Deiss D, Danne T, Dorow A, Bassir C, Gruters-Kieslich A: Predictivity of thyroid autoantibodies for the development of thyroid disorders in children and adolescents with type 1 diabetes. *Diabet Med* 19:518–521, 2002b.

Kordonouri O, Hartmann R, Deiss D, Wilms M, Gruters-Kieslich: Natural course of autoimmune thyroiditis in type 1 diabetes: association with gender, age, diabetes duration, and puberty. *Arch Dis Child* 90:411–414, 2005.

Korosoglou G, Humpert PM, Halbgewachs E, Bekeredjian R, Filusch A, Buss SJ, Morcos M, Bierhaus A, Katus HA, Nawroth PP, Kuecherer H: Evidence of left ventricular contractile asynchrony by echocardiographic phase imaging in patients with type 2 diabetes mellitus and without clinically evident heart disease. *Am J Cardiol* 98:1525–1530, 2006.

Korytskowski MT, Mokan M, Veneman TF, Mitrakou A, Cryer PE, Gerich JE: Reduced β-adrenergic sensitivity in patients with type 1 diabetes and hypoglycemia unawareness. *Diabetes Care* 21:1939–1943, 1998.

Kosmala W, Kucharski W, Przewlocka-Kosmala M, Mazurek W: Comparison of left ventricular function by tissue doppler imaging in patients with diabetes mellitus without systemic hypertension versus diabetes mellitus with systemic hypertension. *Am J Cardiol* 94:395–399, 2004.

Kozer E, Nikfar S, Costei A, Boskovic R, Nulman I, Koren G: Aspirin consumption during the first trimester of pregnancy and congenital anomalies: a meta-analysis. *Am J Obstet Gynecol* 187:1623–1630, 2002.

Kragelund C, Gustafsson I, Omland T, Gronning B, Kober L, Faber J, Strande S, Stefensen R, Hildebrandt P: Prognostic value of NH2-terminal pro B-type natriuretic peptide in patients with diabetes and stable coronary heart disease. *Diabetes Care* 29:1411–1413, 2006.

Krahenmann F, Hucha A, Atar D: Troponin measurement in the diagnosis of myocardial injury during pregnancy and delivery: two cases. *Am J Obstet Gynecol* 183:1308–1310, 2000.

Krakoff J, Lindsay RS, Looker HC, Nelson RG, Hanson RL, Knowler WC: Incidence of retinopathy and nephropathy in youth-onset compared with adult-onset type 2 diabetes. *Diabetes Care* 26:76–81, 2003.

Kramer HJ, Nguyen QD, Curhan G, Hsu CY: Renal insufficiency in the absence of albuminuria and retinopathy among adults with type 2 diabetes mellitus. *JAMA* 289:3273–3277, 2003.

Kramer H, Molitch ME: Screening for kidney disease in adults with diabetes. *Diabetes Care* 28:1813–1816, 2005.

Krantz DS, Olson MB, Francis JL, Phankao C, Bairey Merz CN, Sopko G, Vido DA, Shaw LJ, Sheps DS, Pepine CJ, Matthews KA: Anger, hostility, and cardiac symptoms in women with suspected coronary artery disease: the Women's Ischemia Syndrome Evaluation (WISE) study. *J Women's Health (Larchmt)* 15:1214–1223, 2006.

Krauss RM, Eckel RH, Howard B, Appel LJ, Daniels SR, Deckelbaum RJ, Erdman JW, Kris-Etherton P, Goldberg IJ, Kotchen TA, Lichtenstein AH, Mitch WE, Mullis R, Robinson K, Wylie-Rosett J, St Jeor S, Suttie J, Tribble DL, Bazzarre TL: AHA Dietary Guidelines. Revision 2000: a statement for healthcare professionals from the Nutrition Committee of the American Heart Association. *Circulation* 102:2284–2299, 2000.

Krauss RM: Lipids and lipoproteins in patients with type 2 diabetes. *Diabetes Care* 27:1496–1504, 2004.

Kreisberg RA, Oberman A: Medical management of hyperlipidemia/dyslipidemia. *J Clin Endocrinol Metab* 88:2445–2461, 2003.

Kristensen K, Lindstrom V, Schmidt C, Blirup-Jensen S, Grubb A, Wide-Swensson D, Strevens H: Temporal changes of the plasma levels of cystatin C, beta-trace protein, beta2-microglobulin, urate and creatinine during pregnancy indicate continuous alterations in the renal filtration process. *Scand J Lab Clin Invest* 67:612–618, 2007a.

Kristensen K, Wide-Swensson D, Schmidt C, Blirup-Jensen S, Lindstrom V, Strevens H, Grubb A: Cystatin C, beta2-microglobulin and beta-trace protein in preeclampsia. *Acta Obstet Gynecol Scand* 86:921–926, 2007b.

Kristensen K, Larsson I, Hansson SR: Increased cystatin C expression in the preeclamptic placenta. *Mol Hum Reprod* 13:189–195, 2007c.

KROC Collaborative Study Group: Blood glucose control and evolution of diabetic retinopathy and albuminuria. *N Engl J Med* 311:365–368, 1984.

Krolewski AS, Kosinski EJ, Warram JH, Leland OS, Busick EJ, Asmal AC, Rand LI, Christlieb AR, Bradley RF: Magnitude and determinants of coronary artery disease in juvenile-onset, insulin-dependent diabetes mellitus. *Am J Cardiol* 59:750–755, 1987.

Krolewski AS, Canessa M, Warram JH, Laffel LMB, Christlieb AR, Knowler WC, Rand LI: Predisposition to hypertension and susceptibility to renal disease in insulin-dependent diabetes mellitus. *N Engl J Med* 318:140–145, 1988.

Krolewski AS, Barzilav J, Warram JH, Martin BC, Pfeifer M, Rand LI: Risk of early-onset proliferative retinopathy in IDDM is closely related to cardiovascular autonomic neuropathy. *Diabetes* 41:430–437, 1992.

Krolewski M, Eggers PW, Warram JH: Magnitude of end-stage renal disease in IDDM: a 35 year follow-up study. *Kidney Int* 50:2041–2046, 1996.

Krutzen E, Olofsson P, Baeck S-E, Nilsson-Ehle P: Glomerular filtration rate in pregnancy: a study in normal subjects and in patients with hypertension, preeclampsia and diabetes. *Scand J Lab Invest* 52:387–392, 1992.

Kubota N, Terauchi Y, Yamauchi T, Kubota T, Moroi M, Matsui J, Eto K, Yamashita T, Kamon J, Satoh H, Yano W, Froguel P, Nagai R, Kimura S, Kadowaki T, Noda T: Disruption of adiponectin causes insulin resistance and neointimal formation. *J Biol Chem* 277:25863–25866, 2002.

Kudat H, Akkaya V, Sozen AB, Salman S, Demirel S, Ozcan M, Atilgan D, Yilmaz MT, Guven O: Heart rate variability in diabetes patients. *J Int Med Res* 34: 291–296, 2006.

Kuga T, Sadoshima J, Tomoike H, Kanaide H, Akaike N, Nakamura M: Actions of $Ca2^+$ antagonists on two types of $Ca2^+$ channels in rat aorta smooth muscle cells in primary culture. *Circ Res* 67:469–480, 1990.

Kugiyama K, Ota Y, Takazoe K, Moriyama Y, Kawano H, Miyao Y, Sakamoto T, Soejima H, Ogawa H, Doi H, Sugiyama S, Yasue H: Circulating levels of secretory type II phospholipase A_2 predict coronary events in patients with coronary artery disease. *Circulation* 100:1280–1284, 1999.

Kuhn DC, Crawford MA, Stuart MJ, Botti JJ, Demers LM: Alterations in transfer and lipid distribution of arachidonic acid in placentas of diabetic pregnancies. *Diabetes* 39:914–918, 1990.

Kuller JA, D'Andrea NM, McMahon MJ: Renal biopsy and pregnancy. *Am J Obstet Gynecol* 184:1093–1096, 2001.

Kullo IJ, BaileyKR, Kardia SL, Mosley TH Jr, Boerwinkle E, Turner ST: Ethnic differences in peripheral arterial disease in the NHLBI Genetic Epidemiology Network of Arteriopathy (GENOA) study. *Vasc Med* 8:237–242, 2003.

Kuo VS, Koumantakis G, Gallery EDM: Proteinuria and its assessment in normal and hypertensive pregnancy. *Am J Obstet Gynecol* 167:723–728, 1992.

Kurtz TW. False claims of blood pressure-independent protection by blockade of the renin angiotensin aldosterone system? *Hypertension* 41:193–196, 2003.

Kushlan MC, Gollan JL, Ma WL, Ockner RK: Sex differences in hepatic uptake of long chain fatty acids in single-pass perfused rat liver. *J Lipid Res* 22:431–436, 1981.

Kutteh WH, Yetman DL, Carr AC, Beck LA, Scott RT Jr: Increased prevalence of antithyroid antibodies identified in women with recurrent pregnancy loss but not in women undergoing assisted reproduction. *Fertil Steril* 71:843–848, 1999.

Kuzkaya N, Weissmann N, Harrison DG, Dikalov S: Interactions of peroxynitrite with uric acid in the presence of ascorbate and thiols: implications for uncoupling endothelial nitric oxide synthase. *Biochem Pharmacol* 70:343–354, 2005.

Kwan BCH, Kronenberg F, Beddhu S, Cheung AK: Lipoprotein metabolism and lipid management in chronic kidney disease. *J Am Soc Nephrol* 18:1246–1261, 2007.

Kyle GC: Diabetes and pregnancy. *Ann Intern Med* 59 (Suppl 3):1–82, 1963.

Kyle PM, Fielder JN, Pullar B, Horwood LJ, Moore MP: Comparison of methods to identify significant proteinuria in pregnancy in the outpatient setting. *BJOG* 115:523–527, 2008.

Laatikainen L, Teramo K, Hieta-Heikurainen H, Koivisto V, Pelkonen R: A controlled study of the influence of continuous insulin infusion treatment on diabetic retinopathy during pregnancy. *Acta Med Scand* 221:367–376, 1987.

Laclide-Drouin H, Masutti JP, Hatier R, Dauca M, Grignon G: Effect of clofibrate on the peroxisomes of the intestine of the rat during fetal development. *Ital J Anat Embryol* 100 (Suppl 1):411–417, 1995.

LaCroix AZ, Haynes SG, Savage DD, Havlik RJ: Rose questionnaire angina among United States black, white, and Mexican-American women and men. Prevalence and correlates from the Second National and Hispanic Health and Nutrition Examination Surveys. *Am J Epidemiol* 129:669–686, 1989.

Ladner HE, Danielsen B, Gilbert WM: Acute myocardial infarction in pregnancy and the puerperium: a population-based study. *Obstet Gynecol* 105:480–484, 2005.

Laffel LM, McGill JB, Gans DJ; North American Microalbuminuria Study Group: The beneficial effect of angiotensin-converting enzyme inhibition with captopril on diabetic nephropathy in normotensive IDDM patients with microalbuminuria. *Am J Med* 99:497–504, 1995.

Laffel L: Ketone bodies: a review of physiology, pathophysiology and application of monitoring to diabetes. *Diabetes Metab Res Rev* 15:412–426, 1999.

LaFranchi SH, Haddow JE, Hollowell JG: Is thyroid inadequacy during gestation a risk factor for adverse pregnancy and developmental outcomes? *Thyroid* 15:60–71, 2005.

Lahdenpera M, Groop PH, Tilly-Kiesi M, Kuusi T, Elliott TG, Viberti GC, Taskinen MR: LDL subclasses in IDDM patients: relation to diabetic nephropathy. *Diabetologia* 37:681–688, 1994.

Lain KY, Markovic N, Ness RB, Roberts JM: Effect of smoking on uric acid and other metabolic markers throughout normal pregnancy. *J Clin Endocrinol Metab* 90:5743–5746, 2005.

Laing SP, Swerdlow AJ, Slater DS, Botha JL, Burden AC, Waugh NR, Smith AW, Hill RD, Bingley PJ, Patterson CC, Qiao Z, Keen H: The British Diabetic Association Cohort Study. II. Cause-specific mortality in patients with insulin-treated diabetes mellitus. *Diabet Med* 16:466–471, 1999.

Laing SP, Swerdlow AJ, Slater SD, Burden AC, Morris A, Waugh NR, Gatling W, Bingley PJ, Patterson CC: Mortality from heart disease in a cohort of 23,000 patients with insulin-treated diabetes. *Diabetologia* 46:760–765, 2003a.

Laing SP, Swerdlow AJ, Carpenter LM, Slater SD, Burden AC, Botha JL, Morris AD, Waugh NR, Gatling W, Gale EAM, Patterson CC, Qiao Z, Keen H: Mortality from cerebrovascular disease in a cohort of 23,000 patients with insulin-treated diabetes. *Stroke* 34:418–421, 2003b.

Laird-Meeter K, van de Ley G, Bom TH, Wladimoroff JW, Roelandt J: Cardiocirculatory adjustments during pregnancy: an echocardiographic study. *Clin Cardiol* 2:328–332, 1979.

Lajer M, Tarnow L, Jorsal A, Teerlink T, Parving H-H, Rossing P: Plasma concentration of asymmetric dimethylarginine (ADMA) predicts cardiovascular morbidity and mortality in type 1 diabetic patients with diabetic nephropathy. *Diabetes Care* 31:747–752, 2008.

Lam C, Lim KH, Kang DH, Karumanchi SA: Uric acid and preeclampsia. *Semin Nephrol* 25:56–60, 2005.

Lambot M-A, Vermeylen D, Noel J-C: Angiotensin-II-receptor inhibitors in pregnancy. *Lancet* 357:1619–1620, 2001.

Lamparter S, Sun Y, Weber KT: Angiotensin II receptor blockade during gestation attenuates collagen formation in the developing rat heart. *Cardiovasc Res* 43:165–172, 1999.

Landin-Olsson M, Karlsson FA, Lernmark A, Sundkvist G; the Diabetes Incidence Study in Sweden Group: Islet cell and thyrogastric antibodies in 633 consecutive 15-to-34-yr-old patients in the Diabetes Incidence Study in Sweden. *Diabetes* 41:1022–1027, 1992.

Landon MB: Diabetic nephropathy and pregnancy. *Clin Obstet Gynecol* 50:998–1006, 2007.

Lanfredini M, Florina P, Grazia M, Veronelli M, Mello A, Astori E, Dall'Aglio P, Craveri A: Fasting and post-methionine load homocysteine values are correlated with microalbuminuria and could contribute to worsening vascular damage in non-insulin-dependent diabetes mellitus patients. *Metabolism* 47:915–921, 1998.

Lang GD, Lowe GDO, Walker JJ, Forbes CD, Prentice CRM, Calder AA: Blood rheology in preeclampsia and intrauterine growth retardation: effects of blood pressure reduction with labetalol. *Br J Obstet Gynecol* 91:438–443, 1984.

Langan SJ, Deary IJ, Hepburn DA, Frier BM: Cumulative cognitive impairment following recurrent severe hypoglycemia in adult patients with insulin-treated diabetes mellitus. *Diabetologia* 34:337–344, 1991.

Lange LA, Bowden DW, Langefeld CD, Wagenknecht LE, Carr JJ, Rich SS, Riley WA, Freedman BI: Heritability of carotid artery intima-medial thickness in type 2 diabetes. *Stroke* 33:1876–1881, 2002.

Lanska DJ, Kryscio RJ: Stroke and intracranial venous thrombosis during pregnancy and puerperium. *Neurology* 51:1622–1628, 1998.

Lanska DJ, Kryscio RJ: Risk factors for peripartum and postpartum stroke and intracranial venous thrombosis. *Stroke* 31:1274–1282, 2000.

Lansky AJ, Hochman JS, Ward PA, Mintz GS, Fabunmi R, Berger PB, New G, Grines CL, Pietras CG, Kern MJ, Leon MB, Mehran R, White C, Mieres JH, Moses JW, Stone GW, Jacobs AK: Percutaneous coronary intervention and adjunctive pharmacotherapy in women: a statement for healthcare professionals from the American Heart Association. *Circulation* 111:940–953, 2005.

Lapolla A, Cardone C, Negrin P, Midena E, Marini S, Gardellin C, Bruttomesso D, Fedele D: Pregnancy does not induce or worsen retinal and peripheral nerve dysfunction in insulin-dependent diabetic women. *J Diabetes Complications* 12:74–80, 1998.

Lapolla A, Dalfra MG, Masin M, Bruttomesso D, Piva I, Crepaldi C, Tortul C, Dalla Barba B, Fedele D: Analysis of outcome of pregnancy in type 1 diabetes treated with insulin pump or conventional insulin therapy. *Acta Diabetol* 40:143–149, 2003.

Larinkari J, Laatikainen L, Ranta T, Morenen P, Pesonen K, Laatikainen T: Metabolic control and serum hormone levels in relation to retinopathy in diabetic pregnancy. *Diabetologia* 22:327–332, 1982.

Larsen J, Brekke M, Sandvik L, Arnesen H, Hanssen KF, Dahl-Jorgensen K: Silent coronary atheromatosis in type 1 diabetic patients and its relation to long-term glycemic control. *Diabetes* 51:2637–2641, 2002.

Larsen JR, Sjoholm H, Hanssen KF, Sandvik L, Berg TJ, Dahl-Jorgensen K: Optimal blood glucose control during 18 years preserves peripheral nerve function in patients with 30 years' duration of type 1 diabetes. *Diabetes Care* 26:2400–2404, 2003.

Larsen JR, Sjoholm H, Berg TJ, Sandvik L, Brekke M, Hanssen KF, Dahl-Jorgensen K: Eighteen years of fair glycemic control preserves cardiac autonomic function in type 1 diabetes. *Diabetes Care* 27:963–966, 2004.

Larsen JR, Brekke M, Bergensen L, Sandvik L, Arnesen H, Hanssen KF, Dahl-Jorgensen K: Mean HbA1C over 18 years predicts carotid intima-media thickness in women with type 1 diabetes. *Diabetologia* 48:776–779, 2005a.

Larsen M, Colmorn LB, Bonnelycke M, Kaaja R, Immonen I, Sander B, Loukovaara S: Retinal artery and vein diameters during pregnancy in diabetic women. *Invest Ophthalmol Vis Sci* 46:709–713, 2005b.

Larsson CA, Gullberg B, Merlo J, Rastam L, Lindblad U: Female advantage in AMI mortality is reversed in patients with type 2 diabetes in the Skaraborg Project. *Diabetes Care* 28:2246–2248, 2005.

Laudenbach V, Mantz J, Lagercrantz H, Desmonts J-M, Evrard P, Gressens P: Effects of α2-adrenoceptor agonists on perinatal excitotoxic brain injury. Comparison of clonidine and dexmedetomidine. *Anesthesiology* 96:134–141, 2002.

Lauenborg J, Mathiesen E, Ovesen P, Westergaard JG, Ekbom P, Moelsted-Pedersen L, Damm P: Audit on stillbirths in women with pregestational type 1 diabetes. *Diabetes Care* 26:1385–1389, 2003.

Laurberg P, Nygaard B, Glinoer D, Grussendorf M, Orgiazzi J: Guidelines for TSH-receptor antibody measurements in pregnancy: results of an evidence-based symposium organized by the European Thyroid Association. *Eur J Endocrinol* 139:584–586, 1998.

Lauritzen T, Larsen HW, Frost-Larsen K, Deckert T; the Sten Study Group: Effect of one year of normal blood glucose levels on retinopathy in insulin-dependent diabetes. *Lancet* 1:200–204, 1983.

Lauszus FF, Klebe JG, Rasmussen GW, KlebeTM, Dorup J, Christensen T: Renal growth during pregnancy in insulin-dependent diabetic women. A prospective study of renal volume and clinical variables. *Acta Diabetol* 32:225–229, 1995.

Lauszus FF, Gron PL, Klebe JG: Pregnancies complicated by diabetic proliferative retinopathy. *Acta Obstet Gynecol Scand* 77:814–818, 1998.

Lauszus F, Klebe JG, Bek T: Diabetic retinopathy in pregnancy during tight metabolic control. *Acta Obstet Gynecol Scand* 79:367–370, 2000.

Lauszus FF, Rasmussen OW, Lousen T, Klebe TM, Klebe JG: Ambulatory blood pressure as predictor of preeclampsia in diabetic pregnancies with respect to urinary albumin excretion rate and glycemic regulation. *Acta Obstet Gynecol Scand* 80:1096–1103, 2001.

Lauszus FF, Klebe JG, Bek T, Flyvbjerg A: Increased serum IGF-I during pregnancy is associated with progression of diabetic retinopathy. *Diabetes* 52:852–856, 2003.

Lauszus FF, Rosgaard A, Lousen T, Rasmussen OW, Klee TM, Klebe JG: Precision, consistency, and reproducibility of blood pressure in diabetic and non-diabetic pregnancy: the appraisal of repeated measurements. *Acta Obstet Gynecol Scand* 86:1063–1070, 2007.

Lavado-Autric R, Auso E, Garcia-Velasco JV, del Carmen Arufe M, del Rey FE, Berbel P, Morreale de Escobar G: Early maternal hypothyroxinemia alters histogenesis and cerebral cortex cytoarchitecture of the progeny. *J Clin Invest* 111:1073–1082, 2003.

Lavine SJ, Gellman SD: Treatment of heart failure in patients with diabetes mellitus. *Drugs* 62:285–307, 2002.

Lavoratti G, Seracini D, Fiorini P, Cocchi C, Materassi M, Donzelli G, Pela I: Neonatal anuria by ACE inhibitors during pregnancy. *Nephron* 76:235–236, 1997.

Law MR, Frost CD, Wald NJ: By how much does dietary salt reduction lower blood pressure? III: analysis of data from trials of salt reduction. *BMJ* 302:819–824, 1991.

Lawson ML, Gerstein HC, Tsui E, Zinman B: Effect of intensive therapy on early macrovascular disease in young individuals with type 1 diabetes. A systematic review and meta-analysis. *Diabetes Care* 22 (Suppl 2):B35–B39, 1999.

Leather HM, Baker P, Humphreys DM, Chadd MA: A controlled trial of hypotensive agents in hypertension in pregnancy. *Lancet* 2:488–490, 1968.

Lebeau SO, Mandel SJ: Thyroid disorders during pregnancy. *Endocrinol Metab Clin North Am* 35:117–136, 2006.

Lechmanova M, Parizek A, Halaska M, Slavicek J, Kittnar O: Changes in the electrical heart field and hemodynamic parameters in the 34th to 40th weeks of pregnancy and after delivery. *Arch Gynecol Obstet* 266:145–151, 2002a.

Lechmanova M, Kittnar O, Micek M, Slavicek J, Dohnalova A, Havranek S, Kolarik J, Parizek A: QT dispersion and T-loop morphology in late pregnancy and after delivery. *Physiol Res* 51:121–129, 2002b.

Lee CJ, Hsieh TT, Chiu TH, Chen KC, Lo LM, Hung TH: Risk factors for preeclampsia in an Asian population. *Int J Gynecol Obstet* 70:327–333, 2000.

Lee SP, Harris ND, Robinson RT, Davies C, Ireland R, Macdonald IA, Heller SR: Effects of atenolol on QTc interval lengthening during hypoglycemia in type 1 diabetes. *Diabetologia* 48:1269–1272, 2005.

Lee JE, Kim YG, Choi YH, Huh W, Kim DJ, Oh HY: Serum uric acid is associated with microalbuminuria in prehypertension. *Hypertension* 47:962–967, 2006.

Leese GP, Wang J, Broomhall J, Kelly P, Marsden A, Morrison W, Frier BM, Morris AD; DARTS/MEMO Collaboration: Frequency of severe hypoglycemia requiring emergency treatment in type 1 and type 2 diabetes: a population-based study of health service resource use. *Diabetes Care* 26:1176–1180, 2003.

Legato MJ, Gelzer A, Goland R, Ebner SA, Rajan S, Villagra V, Kosowski M; Writing Group for the Partnership for Gender-Specific Medicine: Gender-specific care of the patient with diabetes: review and recommendations. *Gend Med* 3:131–158, 2006.

Leguizamon GF, Reece EA: Diabetic neuropathy and coronary heart disease. In: Reece EA, Coustan DR, Gabbe SG, eds. *Diabetes in Women. Adolescence, Pregnancy, and Menopause.* Philadelphia: Lippincott Williams & Wilkins; 2004:425–432.

Leguizamon GF, Zeff NP, Fernandez A: Hypertension and the pregnancy complicated by diabetes. Narrative review. *Curr Diabetes Rep* 6:297–304, 2006.

Lehto S, Ronnemaa T, Haffner SM, Kallio V, Laakso M: Dyslipidemia and hyperglycemia predict coronary heart disease events in middle-age patients with NIDDM. *Diabetes* 46:1354–1359, 1997.

Lehto S, Niskanen L, Ponnemaa T, Laakso M: Serum uric acid is a strong predictor of stroke in patients with non-insulin-dependent diabetes mellitus. *Stroke* 29:635–639, 1998.

Lehto S, Ronnemaa T, Pyorala K, Laakso M: Poor glycemic control predicts coronary heart disease events in patients with type 1 diabetes without nephropathy. *Arterioscler Thromb Vasc Biol* 19:1014–1019, 1999.

Leitao CB, Canani LH, Polson PB, Molon MP, Pinotti AF, Gross JL: Urinary albumin excretion rate is associated with increased ambulatory blood pressure in normoalbuminuric type 2 diabetic patients. *Diabetes Care* 28:1724–1729, 2005.

Lejeuene B, Grun JP, deNayer P, Servais G, Glinoer D: Antithyroid antibodies underlying thyroid abnormalities and miscarriage or pregnancy induced hypertension. *Reprod Sci* 100:669–672, 1993.

Lemann J, Bidani AK, Bain RP, Lewis EJ, Rohde RD: Use of the serum creatinine to estimate glomerular filtration rate in health and early diabetic nephropathy. *Am J Kidney Dis* 16:236–243, 1990.

Lemley KV, Blouch K, Abdullah I, Boothroyd DB, Bennett PH, Myers BD, Nelson RG: Glomerular permselectivity at the onset of nephropathy in type 2 diabetes mellitus. *J Am Soc Nephrol* 11:2095–2105, 2000.

Leonhardt A, Bernert S, Watzer B, Schmitz-Ziegler G, Seyberth HW: Low-dose aspirin in pregnancy: maternal and neonatal aspirin concentrations and neonatal prostanoid formation. *Pediatrics* 111:e77–e81, 2003.

Leopold JA, Loscalzo J: Oxidative enzymopathies and vascular disease. *Arterioscler Thromb Vasc Biol* 25:1332–1340, 2005.

Lepore G, Maglio ML, Nosari I, Dodesini AR, Trevisan R: Cost-effectiveness of two screening programs for microalbuminuria in type 2 diabetes. *Diabetes Care* 25:2103–2104, 2002.

Leslie RD, Williams R, Pozzilli P: Type 1 diabetes and latent autoimmune diabetes in adults: one end of the rainbow. *J Clin Endocrinol Metab* 91:1654–1659, 2006.

Leung AS, Millar LK, Koonings PP, Montoro M, Mestman J: Perinatal outcome in hypothyroid pregnancies. *Obstet Gynecol* 81:349–353, 1993.

Levey AS, Berg RL, Gassman J, Hall PM, Walker WG; Modification of Diet in Renal Disease Study Group: Creatinine filtration, secretion and excretion during progressive renal disease. *Kidney Int* 36: (Suppl 27):S73–S80, 1989.

Levey AS, Bosch JP, Lewis JB, Greene T, Rogers N, Roth D; for the Modification of Diet in Renal Disease Study Group: A more accurate method to estimate glomerular filtration rate from serum creatinine: a new prediction equation. *Ann Intern Med* 130:461–470, 1999.

Levey AS, Coresh J, Balk E, Kausz AT, Levin A, Steffes MW, Hogg RJ, Perrone RD, Lau J, Eknoyan G: National Kidney Foundation practice guidelines for chronic kidney disease: evaluation, classification and stratification. *Ann Intern Med* 139:137–147, 2003.

Levey AS, Eckhardt K-U, Tsukamoto Y, Levin A, Coresh J, Rossert J, de Zeeuw D, Hostetter TH, Lamiere N, Eknoyan G: Definition and classification of chronic kidney disease: a position statement from Kidney Disease: Improving Global Outcomes (KDIGO). *Kidney Int* 67:2089–2100, 2005.

Levey AS, Coresh J, Greene T, Marsh J, Stevens LA, Kusek JW, Van Lente F; Chronic Kidney Disease Epidemiology Collaboration: Expressing the Modification of Diet in Renal Disease Study Equation for estimating glomerular filtration rate with standardized serum creatinine values. *Clin Chem* 53:766–772, 2007.

Levin RI: The puzzle of aspirin and sex. Editorial. *N Engl J Med* 352:1366–1368, 2005.

Levitas IM, Kristal JJ: Stress exercise testing of the young diabetic for the detection of unknown coronary artery disease. *Isr J Med Sci* 8:845–847, 1972.

Levy CJ, Kinsley BT, Bajaj M, Simonsen DC: Effect of glycemic control on glucose counterregulation during hypoglycemia in NIDDM. *Diabetes Care* 21:1330–1338, 1998.

Lewis EJ, Hunsicker LG, Bain RP, Rohde RD; the Collaborative Study Group: The effect of angiotensin-converting–enzyme inhibition on diabetic nephropathy. *N Engl J Med* 329:1456–1462, 1993.

Lewis EJ, Hunsicker LG, Clarke WR, Berl T, Pohl MA, Lewis JB, Ritz E, Atkins RC, Rohde R, Raz I: Renoprotective effect of the angiotensin-receptor antagonist irbesartan in patients with nephropathy due to type 2 diabetes. *N Engl J Med* 345:851–869, 2001.

Lewis J, Greene T, Appel L, Contreras G, Douglas J, Lash J, Toto R, Van Lente F, Wang X, Wright JT Jr; for the AASK Study Group: A comparison of iothalamate-GFR and serum creatinine-based outcomes: acceleration in the rate of GFR decline in the African American Study of Kidney Disease and Hypertension. *J Am Soc Nephrol* 15:3175–3183, 2004.

Leys D, Bandu L, Henon H, Lucas C, Mounier-Vehier F, Rondepierre P, Godefroy O: Clinical outcome in 287 consecutive young adults (15 to 45 years) with ischemic stroke. *Neurology* 59:26–33, 2002.

Libby P, Nathan DM, Abraham K, Brunzell JD, Fradkin JE, Haffner SM, Hsueh W, Rewers M, Roberts T, Savage PJ, Skarlatos S, Wassef M, Rabadan-Diehl C: Report of the National Heart, Lung, and Blood Institute—National Institute of

Diabetes and Digestive and Kidney Diseases Working Group on cardiovascular complications of type 1 diabetes mellitus. *Circulation* 111:3489–3493, 2005a.

Libby P, Theroux P: Pathophysiology of coronary artery disease. *Circulation* 111:3481–3488, 2005b.

Lichtenstein AH, Appel LJ, Brands M, Carnethon M, Daniels S, Franch HA, Franklin B, Kris-Etherton P, Harris WS, Howard B, Karanja N, Lefevre M, Rudel L, Sacks F, Van Horn L, Winston M, Wylie-Rosett J: Diet and lifestyle recommendations revision 2006. A scientific statement from the American Heart Association Nutrition Committee. *Circulation* 114:82–96, 2006.

Liem A, Reynierse-Buitenwerf GH, Zwindermann AH, Jukema JW, van Veldhuisen DJ: Secondary prevention with folic acid: effects on clinical outcomes. *J Am Coll Cardiol* 41:2105–2113, 2003.

Lieske JC, de la Vega LSP, Gettman MT, Slezak JM, Bergstralh EJ, Melton LJ III, Leibson CL: Diabetes mellitus and the risk of urinary tract stones: a population-based case-control study. *Am J Kidney Dis* 48:897–904, 2006.

Liguori A, D'Armiento FP, Palagiano A, Palinski W, Napoli C: Maternal C-reactive protein and developmental programming of atherosclerosis. *Am J Obstet Gynecol* 198:281.e1–281.e5, 2008.

Lim KH, Friedman SA, Ecker JL, Kao L, Kilpatrick SJ: The clinical utility of serum uric acid measurements in hypertensive diseases of pregnancy. *Am J Obstet Gynecol* 178:1067–1071, 1998.

Lindeberg S, Sandstrom B, Lundborg P, Regardh C-G: Disposition of the adrenergic blocker metoprolol in the late-pregnant woman, the amniotic fluid, the cord blood and the neonate. *Acta Obstet Gynecol Scand* 118:61–64, 1984.

Lindegaard MLS, Damm P, Mathiesen ER, Nielsen LB: Placental triglyceride accumulation in maternal type 1 diabetes is associated with increased lipase gene expression. *J Lipid Res* 47:2581–2588, 2006.

Lindheimer MD, Katz AI: Pregnancy in the renal transplant patient. *Am J Kidney Dis* 19:173, 1992.

Lindow SW, Davies N, Davey DA, Smith JA: The effect of sublingual nifedipine on uteroplacental blood flow in hypertensive pregnancy. *Br J Obstet Gyncol* 95:1276–1281, 1988.

Lindow SW, Davey DA: The variability of urinary protein and creatinine excretion in patients with gestational proteinuric hypertension. *Br J Obstet Gynecol* 99:869–872, 1992.

Linnemann B, Janka HU: Prolonged QTc interval and elevated heart rate identify the type 2 diabetic patient at high risk for cardiovascular death. The Bremen Diabetes Study. *Exp Clin Endocrinol Diabetes* 111:215–222, 2003.

Lip GYH, Beevers M, Churchill D, Shaffer LM, Beevers DG: Effect of atenolol on birth weight. *Am J Cardiol* 79:1437–1438, 1997a.

Lip GY, Churchill D, Beevers M, Auckett A, Beevers DG: Angiotensin-converting-enzyme inhibitors in early pregnancy. *Lancet* 350:1446–1447, 1997b.

Liu H, Momotani N, Noh JY, Ishikawa N, Takebe K, Ito K: Maternal hypothyroidism during early pregnancy and intellectual development of progeny. *Arch Intern Med* 154:785–787, 1994.

Liu JE, Robbins DC, Palmieri V, Bella JN, Roman MJ, Fabsitz R, Howard BV, WeltyTK, Lee ET, Devereux RB: Association of albuminuria with systolic and diastolic left ventricular dysfunction in type 2 diabetes. The Strong Heart Study. *J Am Coll Cardiol* 41:2022–2028, 2003.

Liu J, Sempos C, Donahue RP, Dorn J, Trevisan M, Grundy SM: Joint distribution of non-HDL and LDL cholesterol and coronary heart disease risk prediction among individuals with and without diabetes. *Diabetes Care* 28:1916–1921, 2005.

Liu J, Sempos CT, Donahue RP, Dorn J, Trevisan M, Grundy SM: Non-high-density lipoprotein and very-low-density lipoprotein cholesterol and their risk predictive values in coronary heart disease. *Am J Cardiol* 98:1363–1368, 2006.

Llorente-Cortes V, Otero-Vinas M, Sanchez S, Rodriguez C, Badimon L: Low-density lipoprotein upregulates low-density lipoprotein receptor-related protein expression in vascular smooth muscle cells. *Circulation* 106:3104–3110, 2002.

Llorente-Cortes V, Badimon L: LDL receptor-related protein and the vascular wall. Implications for atherothrombosis. *Arterioscler Thromb Vasc Biol* 25:497–504, 2005.

Lloyd CE, Kuller LH, Ellis D, Becker DJ, Wing RR, Orchard TJ: Coronary heart disease in IDDM. Gender differences in risk factors but not risk. *Arterioscler Thromb Vasc Biol* 16:720–726, 1996.

Lloyd-Jones DM, Sutton-Tyrell K, Patel AS, Matthews KA, Pasternak RC, Everson-Rose SA, Scuteri A, Chae CU: Ethnic variation in hypertension among premenopausal and perimenopausal women. Study of Women's Health Across the Nation. *Hypertension* 46:689–695, 2005.

Lo SSS, Leslie RDG, St John Sutton M: Effects of type 1 diabetes mellitus on cardiac function: a study of monozygotic twins. *Br Heart J* 73:450–455, 1995.

LoBue C, Goodlin R: Treatment of fetal distress during diabetic ketoacidosis. *J Reprod Med* 20:101–104, 1978.

Lonn E, Mathew J, Pogue J, Johnstone D, Danisa K, Bosch J, Baird M, Dagenais G, Sleight P, Yusuf S; Heart Outcomes Prevention Evaluation Study Investigators: Relationship of electrocardiographic left ventricular hypertrophy to mortality and cardiovascular morbidity in high-risk patients. *Eur J Cardiovasc Prev Rehabil* 10:420–428, 2003.

Looker HC, Krakoff J, Funahashi T, Matsuzawa Y, Tanaka S, Nelson RG, Knowler WC, Lindsay RS, Hanson RL: Adiponectin concentrations are influenced by renal function and diabetes duration in Pima Indians with type 2 diabetes. *J Clin Endocrinol Metab* 89:4010–4017, 2004.

Lopez-Espinoza I, Dhar H, Humphreys S, Redman CWG: Urinary albumin excretion during pregnancy. *Brit J Obstet Gynecol* 93:176–181, 1986.

Lopez-Virella MF, Klein RL, Virella G: Modification of lipoproteins in diabetes. *Diabetes Metab Rev* 12:69–90, 1996.

Lopez-Virella MF, McHenry MB, Lipsitz S, Yim E, Wilson PF, Lackland DT, Lyons T, Jenkins AJ, Virella G; the DCCT/EDIC Research Group: Immune complexes containing modified lipoproteins are related to the progression of internal carotid intima-media thickness in patients with type 1 diabetes. *Atherosclerosis* 190:359–369, 2007.

Lorenz MW, von Kegler S, Steinmetz H, Markus HS, Sitzer M: Carotid intima-media thickening indicates a higher vascular risk across a wide range: prospective data from the Carotid Athersclerosis Progression Study (CAPS). *Stroke* 37:87–92, 2006.

Lorenzi M, Gerhardinger C: Early cellular and molecular changes induced by diabetes in the retina. *Diabetologia* 44:791–804, 2001.

Loscalzo J: Homocysteine trials—clear outcomes for complex reasons. *N Engl J Med* 354:1629–1632, 2006.

Loukovaara S, Kaaja R, Immonen I: Macular capillary blood flow velocity by blue-field entoptoscopy in diabetic and healthy women during pregnancy and the postpartum period. *Graefes Arch Clin Exp Ophthalmol* 240:977–982, 2002.

Loukavaara S, Harju M, Kaaja R, Immonen I: Retinal capillary blood flow in diabetic and nondiabetic women during pregnancy and postpartum period. *Invest Ophthalmol Vis Sci* 44:1486–1491, 2003a.

Loukovaara S, Harju M, Kaaja RJ, Immonen IJ: Topographic changes in the central macula coupled with contrast sensitivity loss in diabetic pregnancy. *Graefes Arch Clin Exp Ophthalmol* 241:607–614, 2003b.

Loukovaara S, Immonen I, Koistinen R, Rudge J, Teramo KA, Laatikainen L, Hiilesmaa V, Kaaja RJ: Angiopoietic factors and retinopathy in pregnancies complicated with type 1 diabetes. *Diabet Med* 21:697–704, 2004.

Loukovaara S, Immonen I, Koistinen R, Hiilesmaa V, Kaaja R: Inflammatory markers and retinopathy in pregnancies complicated with type 1 diabetes. *Eye* 19:422–430, 2005a.

Loukovaara S, Immonen IJ, Yandie TG, Nicholls G, Hillesmaa VK, Kaaja RJ: Vasoactive mediators and retinopathy during type 1 diabetic pregnancy. *Acta Ophthalmol Scand* 83:57–62, 2005b.

Loukovaara S, Immonen IJ, Koistinen R, Rutanen EM, Hiilesmaa V, Loukovaara M, Kaaja RJ: The insulin-like growth factor system and type 1 diabetic retinopathy during pregnancy. *J Diabetes Complications* 19:297–304, 2005c.

Lovestam-Adrian M, Agardh C-D, Aberg A, Agardh E: Pre-eclampsia is a potent risk factor for deterioration of retinopathy during pregnancy in type 1 diabetic patients. *Diabet Med* 14:1059–1065, 1997.

Low PA, Benrud-Larson LM, Sletten DM, Opfer-Gehrking TL, Weigand SD, O'Brien PC, Suarez GA, Dyck PJ: Autonomic symptoms and diabetic neuropathy. A population-based study. *Diabetes Care* 27:2942–2947, 2004.

Lowy C: Endocrine emergencies in pregnancy. *Clin Endocrinol Metab* 9:569–581, 1980.

LRCP—Lipid Research Clinics Program. Lipid Metabolism Branch, Division of Heart and Vascular Diseases, National Heart, Lung, and Blood Institute. *The Lipid Research Clinics Population Studies Data Book.* Bethesda, MD: Department of Health and Human Services, Public Health Service, National Institutes of Health; 1980.

Lu W, Resnick HE, Jablonski KA, Jones KL, Jain AK, Howard WJ, Robbins DC, Howard BV: Non-HDL cholesterol as a predictor of cardiovascular disease in type 2 diabetes: the Strong Heart Study. *Diabetes Care* 26:16–23, 2004.

Lubbe WF, Hodge JV: Combined α- and β-adrenoceptor antagonism with prazosin and oxprenolol in control of severe hypertension in pregnancy. *N Z Med J* 94:169–172, 1981.

Luescher TF, Cosentino F: The classification of calcium antagonists and their selection in the treatment of hypertension. A reappraisal. *Drugs* 55:509–517, 1998.

Luescher TF, Creager MA, Beckman, Cosentino F: Diabetes and vascular disease. Pathophysiology, clinical consequences, and medical therapy: part II. *Circulation* 108:1655–1661, 2003.

Lunell NO, Hjemdahl P, Fredholm BB, Nisell H, Persson B, Wager J: Circulatory and metabolic effects of a combined alpha- and beta-adrenoceptor blocker (labetalol) in hypertension of pregnancy. *Br J Clin Pharmacol* 12:345–348, 1981.

Lunell N-O, Nylund L, Lewander R, Sarby B: Acute effect of an antihypertensive drug, labetalol, on uteroplacental blood flow. *Br J Obstet Gynecol* 89:640–644, 1982.

Lurbe A, Redon J, Pascual JM, Tacons J, Alvarez V, Batlle DC: Altered blood pressure during sleep in normotensive subjects with type 1 diabetes. *Hypertension* 21:227–235, 1993.

Lurbe E, Redon J, Kesani A, Pascual JM, Tacons J, Alvarez V, Batlle D: Increase in nocturnal blood pressure and progression to microalbuminuria in type 1 diabetes. *N Engl J Med* 347:797–805, 2002.

Lydakis C, Beevers DG, Beevers M, Lip GYH: Obstetric and neonatal outcome following chronic hypertension in pregnancy among different ethnic groups. *QJM* 91:837–844, 1998.

Lydakis C, Lip GYH, Beevers M, Beevers DG: Atenolol and fetal growth in pregnancies complicated by hypertension. *Am J Hypertens* 12:541–547, 1999.

Lykkesfeldt G, Bock JE, Pedersen FD, Meinertz H, Faergeman O: Excessive hypertriglyceridemia and pancreatitis in pregnancy. Association with deficiency of lipoprotein lipase. *Acta Obstet Gynecol Scand* 60:79–82, 1981.

Lyons TJ, Jenkins AJ, Zheng D, Klein RL, Otvos JD, Yu Y, Lackland DT, McGee D, McHenry MB, Lopes-Virella M, Garvey WT; DCCT/EDIC Research Group: Nuclear magnetic resonance-determined lipoprotein subclass profile in the DCCT/EDIC cohort: associations with carotid intima-media thickness. *Diabet Med* 23:955–966, 2006.

Lysko PG, Webb CL, Gu JL, Ohlstein EH, Ruffolo RR Jr, Yue TL: A comparison of carvedilol and metoprolol antioxidant activities in vitro. *J Cardiovasc Pharmacol* 36:277–281, 2000.

Ma PT, Yamamoto T, Goldstein JL, Brown MS: Increased mRNA for low-density lipoprotein receptor in livers of rabbits treated with 17 alpha-ethinyl estradiol. *Proc Natl Acad Sci U S A* 83:792–796, 1986.

Maahs DM, Ogden LG, Kinney GL, Wadwa P, Snell-Bergeon JK, Dabelea D, Hokanson JE, Ehrlich J, Eckel RH, Rewers M: Low plasma adiponectin levels predict progression of coronary artery calcification. *Circulation* 111:747–753, 2005a.

Maahs DM, Kinney GL, Wadwa P, Snell-Bergeon J, Dabelea D, Hokanson J, Ehrlich J, Garg S, Eckel RH, Rewers MJ: Hypertension prevalence, awareness, treatment, and control in an adult type 1 diabetes population and a comparable general population, *Diabetes Care* 28:301–306, 2005b.

Maahs DM, Snively BM, Bell RA, Dolan-L, Hirsch I, Imperatore G, Linder B, Marcovina SM, Mayer-Davis EJ, Pettitt DJ, Rodriguez BL, Dabelea D: Higher prevalence of elevated albumin excretion in youth with type 2 than type 1 diabetes: the SEARCH for Diabetes in Youth Study. *Diabetes Care* 30:2593–2598, 2007.

Maara G, Cotroneo P, Pitocco D, Manto A, Di Leo MAS, Ruotolo V, Caputo S, Giradina B, Ghirlanda B, Santini SA: Early increase of oxidative stress and reduced antioxidant defenses in patients with uncomplicated type 1 diabetes. A case for gender difference. *Diabetes Care* 25:370–375, 2002.

Mabie WC, Gonzalez AR, Sibai BM, Amon E: A comparative trial of labetalol and hydralazine in the acute management of severe hypertension complicating pregnancy. *Obstet Gynecol* 70:328–333, 1987.

Mabie WC, DiSessa TG, Crocker LG, Sibai BM, Arheart KL: A longitudinal study of cardiac output in normal human pregnancy. *Am J Obstet Gynecol* 170:849–856, 1994.

Mabley JG, Soriano FG: Role of nitrosative stress and poly(ADP-ribose) polymerase activation in diabetic vascular dysfunction. *Curr Vasc Pharmacol* 3:247–252, 2005.

Macarthur A, Cook L, Pollard JK, Brant R: Peripartum myocardial ischemia: a review of Canadian deliveries from 1970 to 1998. *Am J Obstet Gynecol* 194:1027–1033, 2006.

Macdonald J, Marcora S, Jibani M, Roberts G, Kumwenda M, Glover R, Barron J, Lemmey A: GFR estimation using cystatin C is not independent of body composition. *Am J Kidney Dis* 48:712–719, 2006.

MacGregor AS, Price JF, Hau CM, Lee AJ, Carson MN, Fowkes FGR: Role of systolic blood pressure and plasma triglycerides in diabetic peripheral arterial disease. The Edinburgh Artery Study. *Diabetes Care* 22:453–458, 1999.

MacIsaac RJ, Tsalamandris C, Thomas MC, Premaratne E, Panagiotopoulos S, Smith TJ, Poon A, Jenkins MA, Ratnaike SI, Power DA, Jerums G: Estimating glomerular filtration rate in diabetes: a comparison of cystatin C- and creatinine-based methods. *Diabetologia* 49:1686–1689, 2006.

MacIsaac RJ, Tsalamandris C, Thomas MC, Premaratne E, Panagiotopoulos S, Smith TG, Poon A, Jenkins MA, Ratnaike SI, Power DA, Jerums G: The accuracy of cystatin C and commonly used creatinine-based methods for detecting moderate and mild chronic kidney disease in diabetes. *Diabet Med* 24:443–448, 2007.

Mackie ADR, Doddridge MC, Gamsu HR, Brudenell JM, Nicolaides KH, Drury PL: Outcome of pregnancy in patients with insulin-dependent diabetes mellitus and nephropathy with moderate renal impairment. *Diabet Med* 13:90–96, 1996.

Mackinnon AD, Jerrard-Dunne P, Sitzer M, Buehler A, von Kegler S, Markus HS: Rates and determinants of site-specific progression of carotid artery intima-media thickness: the carotid atherosclerosis progression study. *Stroke* 35:2150–2154, 2004.

MacPhee CH, Moores KE, Boyd HF, Dhanak D, Ife RJ, Leach CA, Leake DS, Milliner KJ, Patterson RA, Suckling KE, Tew DG, Hickey DM: Lipoprotein-associated phospholipase A2, platelet-activating factor acetylhydrolase, generates two bioactive products during the oxidation of low-density lipoprotein: use of a novel inhibitor. *Biochem J* 338:479–487, 1999.

MacRury SM, Pinion S, Quin JD, O'Reilly DS, Lunan CB, Lowe GD, MacCuish AC: Blood rheology and albumin excretion in diabetic pregnancy. *Diabet Med* 12:51–55, 1995.

Madsen EM, Lindegaard LS, Andersen CB, Damm P, Nielsen LB: Human placenta secretes apolipoprotein B-100–containing lipoproteins. *J Biol Chem* 279:55271–55276, 2004.

Maeda K, Tsutamoto T, Wada A, Hisanaga T, Kinoshita M: Plasma brain natriuretic peptide as a biochemical marker of high left ventricular end-diastolic pressure in patients with symptomatic left ventricular dysfunction. *Am Heart J* 135:825–832, 1998.

Maehira F, Miyagi I, Eguchi Y: Sex- and age-related variations in the in vitro heparin-releasable lipoprotein lipase from mononuclear leukocytes in blood. *Biochim Biophys Acta* 1042:344–351, 1990.

Magee LA, Schick B, Donnenfeld AE, Sage SR, Conover B, Cook L, McElhatton PR, Schmidt MA, Koren G: The safety of calcium channel blockers in human pregnancy: a prospective, multicenter cohort study. *Am J Obstet Gynecol* 174:823–828, 1996.

Magee LA, von Dadelszen P, Bohun CM, Rey E, El-Zibdeh M, Stalker S, Ross S, Hewson S, Logan AG, Ohlsson A, Naeem T, Thornton JG, Abdalla M, Walkinshaw S, Brown M, Davis G, Hannah ME: Serious perinatal complications of non-proteinuric hypertension: an international, multicenter, retrospective cohort study. *J Obstet Gynecol Can* 25:372–382, 2003a.

Magee LA, Cham C, Waterman EJ, Ohlsson A, von Dadelszen P: Hydralazine for treatment of severe hypertension in pregnancy: meta-analysis. *BMJ* 327:955–960, 2003b.

Magee LA, Duley L: Oral beta-blockers for mild-to-moderate hypertension during pregnancy (Cochrane Review). In: *The Cochrane Library.* Issue 2. Chichester, UK: John Wiley & Sons, Ltd.; 2004.

Magnusson M, Melander O, Israelsson B, Grubb A, Groop L, Jovinge S: Elevated levels of Nt-proBNP in patients with type 2 diabetes without overt cardiovascular disease. *Diabetes Care* 27:1929–1935, 2004a.

Magnusson AL, Waterman IJ, Wennergren M, Jansson T, Powell TL: Triglyceride hydrolase activities and expression of fatty acid binding proteins in the human placenta in pregnancies complicated by intrauterine growth restriction and diabetes. *J Clin Endocrinol Metab* 89:4607–4614, 2004b.

Main EK, Main DM, Gabbe SG: Factors predicting perinatal outcome in pregnancies complicated by diabetic nephropathy (class F). *Diabetes* 33 (Suppl 1):201A, 1984.

Maisel AS, Krishnaswamy P, Nowak RM, McCord J, Hollander JE, Duc P, Omland T, Storrow AB, Abraham WT, Wu AHB, Clopton P, Steg PG, Westheim A, Knudsen CW, Perez A, Kazanegra R, Herrmann HC, McCullough PA: The Breathing Not Properly Multinational Study Investigators: Rapid measurement of B-type natriuretic peptide in the emergency diagnosis of heart failure. *N Engl J Med* 347:161–167, 2002.

Makimattila S, Schlenzka A, Mantysaari M, Bergholm R, Summanen P, Saar P, Erkkila H, Yki-Jarvinen H: Predictors of abnormal cardiovascular autonomic function measured by frequency domain analysis of heart rate variability and conventional tests in patients with type 1 diabetes. *Diabetes Care* 23:1686–1693, 2000.

Malamitsi-Puchner A, Brianan DD, Kontara L, Boutsikou M, Baka S, Hassiakos D, Marmarinos A, Gourgiotis D: Serum cystatin C in pregnancies with normal and restricted fetal growth. *Reprod Sci* 14:37–42, 2007.

Maldonado M, Hampe CS, Gaur LK, D'Amico S, Iyer D, Hammerle LP, Bolgiano D, Rodriguez L, Rajan A, Lernmark A, Balasubramanyam A: Ketosis-prone diabetes: dissection of a heterogenous syndrome using an immunogenetic and beta-cell functional classification, prospective analysis, and clinical outcomes. *J Clin Endocrinol Metab* 88:5090–5098, 2003.

Maldonado MR, Otiniano ME, Lee R, Rodriguez L, Balasubramanyam A: Characteristics of ketosis-prone diabetes in a multiethnic indigent community. *Ethn Dis* 14:243–249, 2004.

Maldonado M, Otiniano ME, Cheema F, Rodriguez L, Balasubramanyam A: Factors associated with insulin discontinuation in subjects with ketosis-prone diabetes with preserved beta-cell function. *Diabet Med* 22:1744–1750, 2005.

Malik S, Lopez V, Chen R, Wu W, Wong ND: Undertreatment of cardiovascular risk factors among persons with diabetes in the United States. *Diabetes Res Clin Pract* 77:126–133, 2007.

Man EB, Brown JF, Serunian SA: Maternal hypothyroxinemia: psycho-neurological deficits in progeny. *Ann Clin Lab Sci* 21:227–239, 1991.

Man in 'T-Veld AJ, Schalekamp MADH: How intrinsic sympathomimetic activity modulates the hemodynamic responses to β-adrenoceptor antagonists. A clue to the nature of their antihypertensive mechanism. *Br J Pharmacol* 13:245S-257S, 1982.

Manalich R, Reyes L, Herrera M, Melendi C, Fundora I: Relationship between weight at birth and the number and size of renal glomeruli in humans: a histomorphometric study. *Kidney Int* 58:771–773, 2000.

Mancia G, Parati G: Office compared with ambulatory blood pressure in assessing response to antihypertensive treatment: a meta-analysis. *J Hypertens* 22:435–445, 2004.

Mandel SJ, Larsen PR, Seely EW, Brent GA: Increased need for thyroxine during pregnancy in women with primary hypothyroidism. *N Engl J Med* 323:91–96, 1990.

Mandel SJ, Spencer CA, Hollowell JG: Are detection and treatment of thyroid insufficiency in pregnancy feasible? *Thyroid* 15:44–53, 2005.

Manji N, Boelaert K, Sheppard MC, Holder RL, Gough SC, Franklyn JA: Lack of association between serum TSH or free T4 and body mass index in euthyroid subjects. *Clin Endocrinol (Oxfd)* 64:125–128, 2006.

Manske CL, Wilson RF, Wang Y, Thomas W: Prevalence of, and risk factors for, angiographically determined coronary artery disease in type I-diabetic patients with nephropathy. *Arch Intern Med* 152:2450–2455, 1992a.

Manske CL, Wang Y, Rector T, Wilson RF, White CW: Coronary revascularization in insulin-dependent diabetic patients with chronic renal failure. *Lancet* 340:998–1002, 1992b.

Manske CL, Thomas W, Wang Y, Wilson RF: Screening diabetic transplant candidates for coronary artery disease: identification of a low risk subgroup. *Kidney Int* 44:617–621, 1993.

Manson JE, Stampfer MJ, Colditz GA, Willett WC, Rosner B, Speizer FE, Hennekens CH: A prospective study of aspirin use and primary prevention of cardiovascular disease in women. *JAMA* 266:521–527, 1991.

Many A, Hubel CA, Roberts JM: Hyperuricemia and xanthine oxidase in preeclampsia, revisited. *Am J Obstet Gynecol* 174:288–291, 1996.

Marcovecchio M, Mohn A, Chiarelli F: Type 2 diabetes mellitus in children and adolescents. *J Endocrinol Invest* 28:853–863, 2005.

Maritim AC, Sanders RA, Watkins JB 3rd: Diabetes, oxidative stress, and antioxidants: a review. *J Biochem Mol Toxicol* 17:24–38, 2003.

Mark DB, Felker GM: B-type natriuretic peptide—a biomarker for all seasons? Editorial. *N Engl J Med* 350:718–720, 2004.

Markus HS, Labrum R, Bevan S, Reindl M, Egger G, Wiederman CJ, Xu Q, Kiechl S, Willeit J: Genetic and acquired inflammatory conditions are synergistically associated with early carotid atherosclerosis. *Stroke* 37(9): 2253–2259, 2006.

Marques JL, George E, Peacey SR, Harris ND, Macdonald IA, Cochrane T, Heller SR: Altered ventricular polarization during hypoglycemia in patients with diabetes. *Diabet Med* 14:648–654, 1997.

Marso SP, Hiatt WR: Peripheral arterial disease in patients with diabetes. *J Am Coll Cardiol* 47:921–929, 2006.

Martin RA, Jones KL, Mendoza A, Barr M Jr, Benirschke K: Effect of ACE inhibition on the fetal kidney: decreased renal blood flow. *Teratology* 46:317–321, 1992.

Martin U, Davies C, Hayavi S, Hartland A, Dunne F: Is normal pregnancy atherogenic? *Clin Sci (Lond)* 96:421–425, 1999.

Martin A, O'Sullivan AJ, Brown M: Body composition and energy metabolism in normotensive and hypertensive pregnancy. *Br J Obstet Gynecol* 108:1263–1271, 2001.

Martin JN Jr, Thigpen BD, Moore RC, Rose CH, Cushman J, May W: Stroke and severe preeclampsia and eclampsia: a paradigm shift focusing on systolic blood pressure. *Obstet Gynecol* 105:246–254, 2005.

Martin CL, Albers J, Herman WH, Cleary P, Waberski B, Greene DA, Stevens MJ, Feldman EL: Neuropathy among the Diabetes Control and Complications Trial cohort 8 years after trial completion. *Diabetes Care* 29:340–344, 2006.

Martinovic J, Benachi A, Laurent N, Daika-Dahmane F, Gubler MC: Fetal toxic effects and angiotensin-II receptor antagonists. *Lancet* 358:241–242, 2001.

Masaoka S, Lev-Ran A, Hill LR, Vakil G, Hon EH: Heart rate variability in diabetes: relationship to age and duration of the disease. *Diabetes Care* 8:64–68, 1985.

Masding MG, Jones JR, Bartley E, Sandeman DD: Assessment of blood pressure in patients with type 2 diabetes: comparison between home blood pressure monitoring, clinic blood pressure measurement and 24-h ambulatory blood pressure monitoring. *Diabet Med* 18:431–437, 2001.

Masding MG, Stears AJ, Burdge GC, Wootton SA, Sandeman DD: Premenopausal advantages in postprandial lipid metabolism are lost in women with type 2 diabetes. *Diabetes Care* 26:3243–3249, 2003.

Maser RD, Steenkiste AR, Dorman JS, Nielsen VK, Bass EB, Manjoo Q, Drash AL, Becker DJ, Kuller LH, Greene DA, Orchard TJ: Epidemiological correlates of diabetic neuropathy. Report from the Pittsburgh Epidemiology of Diabetic Complications Study. *Diabetes* 38:1456–1461, 1989.

Maser RE, Mitchell BD, Vinik AI, Freeman R: The association between cardiovascular autonomic neuropathy and mortality in individuals with diabetes. A meta-analysis. *Diabetes Care* 26:1895–1901, 2003.

Maser RE, Lenhard MJ: Cardiovascular autonomic neuropathy due to diabetes mellitus: clinical manifestations, consequences, and treatment. *J Clin Endocrinol Metab* 90:5896–5903, 2005.

Mason GF, Petersen KF, Rothman DL, Shulman GI: Increased brain monocarboxylate acid transport and utilization in type 1 diabetes. *Diabetes* 55:929–934, 2004.

Masse J, Forest JC, Moutquin JM, Marcoux S, Brideau NA, Bleanger M: A prospective study of several potential biologic markers for early prediction of the development of preeclampsia. *Am J Obstet Gynecol* 169:501–508, 1993.

Mastaitis JW, Wurmbach E, Cheng H, Sealfon SC, Mobbs CV: Acute induction of gene expression in brain and liver by insulin-induced hypoglycemia. *Diabetes* 54:952–958, 2005.

Mastorikou M, Mackness M, Mackness B: Defective metabolism of oxidized phospholipids by HDL from people with type 2 diabetes. *Diabetes* 55:3099–3103, 2006.

Matalon S, Sheiner E, Levy A, Mazor M, Wiznitzer A: Relationship of treated maternal hypothyroidism and perinatal outcome. *J Reprod Med* 51:59–63, 2006.

Matejkova-Behanova M, Zamrazil V, Vondra K, Vrbikova J, Kucera P, Hill M, Andel M: Autoimmune thyroiditis in non-obese subjects with initial diagnosis of type 2 diabetes mellitus. *J Endocrinol Invest* 25:779–784, 2002.

Matsuda Y, Ikenoue T, Matsuda K, Sameshima H, Ibara S, Hokanishi H, Sakamoto H: The effect of nicardipine on maternal and fetal hemodynamics and uterine blood flow in chronically instrumented pregnant goats. *Asia Oceania J Obstet Gynaecol* 19:191–198, 1993.

Mattock MB, Cronin N, Cavallo-Perin P, Idzior-Walus B, Penno G, Bandinelli S, Standl E, Kofinis A, Fuller JH; EURODIAB IDDM Complications Study: Plasma lipids and urinary albumin excretion rate in type 1 diabetes mellitus. *Diabet Med* 18:59–67, 2001.

Mauvais-Jarvis F, Sobngwi E, Porcher R, Riveline JP, Kevorkian JP, Vaisse C, Charpentier G, Guillausseau PJ, Vexiau P, Gautier JF: Ketosis-prone type 2 diabetes in patients of sub-Saharan African origin: clinical pathophysiology and natural history of β-cell dysfunction and insulin resistance. *Diabetes* 53:645–653, 2004.

Maxwell SR, Thomason H, Sandler D, LeGuen C, Baxter MA, Thorpe GH, Jones AF, Barnett AH: Antioxidant status in patients with uncomplicated insulin-dependent and non-insulin-dependent diabetes mellitus. *Eur J Clin Invest* 27:484–490, 1997.

May O, Arildsen H, Damsgaard EM, Mickley H: Prevalence and prediction of silent ischemia in diabetes mellitus: a populaton-based study. *Cardiovasc Res* 34:241–247, 1997.

May HT, Horne BD, Anderson JL, Wolfert RL, Muhlestein JB, Renlund DG, Clarke JL, Kolek MJ, Bair TL, Pearson RR, Sudhir K, Carlquist JF: Lipoprotein-associated phospholipase A₂ independently predicts the angiographic diagnosis of coronary artery disease and coronary death. *Am Heart J* 152:997–1003, 2006.

Mazurkiewicz JC, Watts GF, Warburton FG, Slavin BM, Lowy C, Koukkou E: Serum lipids, lipoproteins and apolipoproteins in pregnant non-diabetic patients. *J Clin Pathol* 47:728–731, 1994.

McAllister AS, Atkinson AB, Johnston GD, McCance DR: Endothelial function in offspring of type 1 diabetic patients with and without diabetic nephropathy. *Diabet Med* 16:298–303, 1999.

McAnulty JH, Metcalfe J, Ueland K: Heart disease and pregnancy. In: Fuster V, Alexander RW, O'Rourke RA, eds. *Hurst's The Heart.* 11th ed. New York: McGraw-Hill; 2004:2211–2288.

McAuley JW, Anderson GD: Treatment of epilepsy in women of reproductive age. Pharmacokinetic considerations. *Clin Pharmacokinet* 41:559–579, 2002.

McCance DR, Traub AI, Harley JMG, Hadden DR, Kennedy L: Urinary albumin excretion in diabetic pregnancy. *Diabetologia* 32:236–239, 1989.

McCance DR, Hanson RL, Pettitt DJ, Jacobsson LTH, Bennett PH, Bishop DT: Diabetic nephropathy: a risk factor for diabetes mellitus in offspring. *Diabetologia* 38:221–226, 1995.

McCanlies E, O'Leary LA, Foley TP, Kramer MK, Burke JP, Libman A, Swan JS, Steenkiste AR, McCarthy BJ, Trucco M, Dorman JS: Hashimoto's thyroiditis and insulin-dependent diabetes mellitus: differences among individuals with and without abnormal thyroid function. *J Clin Endocrinol Metab* 83:1548–1551, 1998.

McCowan LM, Buist RG, North RA, Gamble G: Perinatal morbidity in chronic hypertension. *Br J Obstet Gynecol* 103:123–129, 1996.

McCrimmon RJ, Fan X, Ding Y, Zhu W, Jacob RJ, Sherwin RS: Potential role for AMP-activated protein kinase in hypoglycemia sensing in the ventromedial hypothalamus. *Diabetes* 53:1953–1958, 2004.

McDermott MM, Criqui MH, Liu K, Guralnik JM, Greenland P, Martin GJ, Pearce W: Lower ankle/brachial index, as calculated by averaging the dorsalis pedis and posterior tibial arterial pressures, and association with leg functioning in peripheral arterial disease. *J Vasc Surg* 32:1164–1171, 2000.

McDermott MM, Greenland P, Liu K, Guralnik JM, Criqui MH, Dolan NC, Chan C, Celic L, Pearce WH, Schneider JR, Sharma L, Clark E, Gibson D, Martin GJ: Leg symptoms in peripheral arterial disease. Associated clinical characteristics and functional impairment. *JAMA* 286:1599–1606, 2001.

McDermott MM, Liu K, Criqui MH, Ruth K, Goff D, Saad MF, Wu C, Homma S, Sharrett AR: Ankle-brachial index and subclinical cardiac and carotid disease. The Multi-Ethnic Study of Atherosclerosis. *Am J Epidemiol* 162:33–41, 2005.

McElvy SS, Miodovnik M, Rosenn B, Khoury JC, Siddiqi T, Dignan PSJ, Tsang RC: A focused preconceptional and early pregnancy program in women with type 1 diabetes reduces perinatal mortality and malformation rates to general population levels. *J Maternal-Fetal Med* 9:14–20, 2000.

McElvy SS, Demarini S, Miodovnik M, Khoury JC, Rosenn B, Tsang RC: Fetal weight and progression of diabetic retinopathy. *Obstet Gynecol* 97:587–592, 2001.

McFarlane SI, Jacober SJ, Winer N, Kaur J, Castro JP, Wui MA, Gliwa A, Von Gizycki H, Sowers JR: Control of cardiovascular risk factors in patients with diabetes and hypertension at urban academic medical centers. *Diabetes Care* 25:718–723, 2002.

McFarlane SI, Salifu MO, Makaryus J, Sowers JR: Anemia and cardiovascular disease in diabetic nephropathy. *Curr Diab Rep* 6:213–218, 2006.

McGee AR, Boyko EJ: Physical examination and chronic lower-extremity ischemia. A critical review. *Arch Intern Med* 158:1357–1364, 1998.

McGregor E, Stewart G, Junor BJ, Rodger RS: Successful use of recombinant human erythropoietin in pregnancy. *Nephrol Dial Transplant* 6:292–293, 1991.

McGregor VP, Banerer S, Cryer PE: Elevated endogenous cortisol reduces autonomic neuroendocrine and symptom responses to subsequent hypoglycemia. *Am J Physiol* 282:E770–E777, 2002.

McGrory CH, Groshek MA, Sollinger HW, Moritz MJ, Armenti VT: Pregnancy outcomes in female pancreas-kidney transplants. *Transplant Proc* 31:652–653, 1999.

McKay DB, Josephson MA, Armenti VT, August P, Coscia LA, Davis CL, Davison JM, Easterling T, Friedman JE, Hou S, Karlix J, Lake KD, Lindheimer M, Matas AJ, Moritz MJ, Riely CA, Ross LF, Scott JR, Wagoner LE, Wrenshall L, Adams PL, Bumgardner GL, Fine RN, Goral S, Krams SM, Martinez OM, Tolkoff-Rubin N, Pavlakis M, Scantlebury V; Women's Health Committee of the American Society of Transplantation: Reproduction and transplantation: report on the AST Consensus Conference on Reproductive Issues and Transplantation. *Am J Transplant* 5:1592–1599, 2005.

McKenney J: New perspectives on the use of niacin in the treatment of lipid disorders. *Arch Intern Med* 164:697–705, 2004.

McKinnon B, Li H, Richard K, Mortimer R: Synthesis of thyroid binding proteins transthyretin and albumin by human trophoblast. *J Clin Endocrinol Metab* 90:6714–6720, 2006.

McMurray RG, Katz VL, Berry MJ, Cefalo RC: The effect of pregnancy on metabolic responses during rest, immersion, and aerobic exercise in the water. *Am J Obstet Gynecol* 158:481–486, 1988.

McMurry MP, Connor WE, Goplerud CP: The effects of dietary cholesterol upon the hypercholesterolemia of pregnancy. *Metabolism* 30:869–879, 1981.

McQuaid KR, Laine L: Systematic review and meta-analysis of adverse events of low-dose aspirin and clopidogrel in randomized controlled trials. *Am J Med* 119: 624–638, 2006.

Meier C, Staub J-J, Roth C-B, Guglielmetti M, Kunz M, Miserez AR, Drewe J, Huber P, Herzog R, Muller B: TSH-controlled L-thyroxine therapy reduces cholesterol levels and clinical symptoms in subclinical hypothyroidism: a double-blind, placebo-controlled trial (Basel Thyroid Study). *J Clin Endocrinol Metab* 86:4860–4866, 2001.

Meier JJ, Deifuss S, Klamann A, Launhardt V, Schmiegel WH, Nauck MA: Plasma glucose at hospital admission and previous metabolic control determine myocardial infarct size and survival in patients with and without type 2 diabetes. The Langendreer Myocardial Infarction and Blood Gluose in Diabetic Patients Assessment (LAMBDA). *Diabetes Care* 28:2551–2553, 2005.

Meijer J-W G, Smit AJ, Lefrandt JD, van der Hoeven JH, Hoogenberg K, Links TP: Back to basics in diagnosing diabetic polyneuropathy with the tuning fork! *Diabetes Care* 28:2201–2205, 2005.

Melander A, Niklasson B, Ingemarsson I, Liedholm H, Schersten B, Sjoberg N-O: Transplacental passage of atenolol in man. *Eur J Clin Pharmacol* 14:93–94, 1978.

Mendelson MA, Lang RM: Pregnancy and cardiovascular disease. *In*: Barron WM, Lindheimer MD, eds. *Medical Disorders During Pregnancy*. 3rd ed. St Louis: Mosby; 2000; pp:147–192.

Menuet R, Lavie CJ, Milani RV: Importance and management of dyslipidemia in the metabolic syndrome. *Am J Med Sci* 330:295–302, 2005.

Mercuro G, Vitale C, Cerquetani E, Zoncu S, Fini M, Rosano GMC: Effect of hyperuricemia upon endothelial function in patients at increased cardiovascular risk. *Am J Cardiol* 94:932–935, 2004.

Merimee TJ, Fineberg SE: Homeostasis during fasting. II. Hormone substrate differences between men and women. *J Clin Endocrinol Metab* 37:698–702, 1973.

Merzouk H, Madani S, Korso N, Bouchenak M, Prost J, Belleville J: Maternal and fetal serum lipid and lipoprotein concentrations and compositions in type 1 diabetic pregnancy: relationship with maternal glycemic control. *J Lab Clin Med* 136:441–448, 2000a.

Merzouk H, Bouchenak M, Loukidi B, Madani S, Prost J, Belleville J: Fetal macrosomia related to maternal poorly controlled type 1 diabetes strongly impairs serum lipoprotein concentrations and composition. *J Clin Pathol* 53:917–923, 2000b.

Merzouk H, Khan NA: Implications of lipids in macrosomia of diabetic pregnancy: can n-3 polyunsaturated fatty acids exert beneficial effects? *Clin Sci* 105:519–529, 2003.

Mesa A, Jessurun C, Hernandez A, Adam K, Brown D, Vaughn WK, Wilansky S: Left ventricular diastolic function in normal human pregnancy. *Circulation* 99:511–517, 1999.

Messer PM, Hauffa BP, Olbricht T, Benker G, Kotulla P, Reinwein D: Antithyroid drug treatment of Graves' disease in pregnancy: long-term effects on somatic growth, intellectual development and thyroid function of the offspring. *Acta Endocrinol* 123:311–316, 1990.

Mestman JH: Hyperthyroidism in pregnancy. *Endocrinol Metab Clin North Am* 27:127–149, 1998.

Meyer NL, Mercer BM, Friedman SA, Sibai BM: Urinary dipstick protein: a poor predictor of absent or severe proteinuria. *Am J Obstet Gynecol* 170:137–141, 1994.

Mieres JH, Shaw LJ, Arai A, Budoff MJ, Flamm SD, Hundley G, Marwick TH, Mosca L, Patel AR, Quinones MA, Redberg RF, Taubert KA, Taylor AJ, Thomas GS, Wenger NK; AHA Cardiac Imaging Committee, Council on Clinical Cardiology; Cardiovascular Imaging and Intervention Committee, Council on Cardiovascular Radiology and Intervention: The role of noninvasive testing in the clinical evaluation of women with suspected coronary artery disease. *Circulation* 111:682–696, 2005.

Miettinen TA, Gylling H, Tuominen J, Simonen P, Koivisto V: Low synthesis and high absorption of cholesterol characterize type 1 diabetes. *Diabetes Care* 27: 53–58, 2004.

Mildenberger RR, Bar-Shlomo B, Druck MN, Jablonsky G, Morch JE, Hilton JD, Kenshole AB, Forbath N, McLaughlin PR: Clinically unrecognized ventricular dysfunction in young diabetic patients. *J Am Coll Cardiol* 4:234–238, 1984.

Millar LK, Wing DA, Leung AS, Koonings PP, Montoro MN, Mestman JH: Low birth weight and preeclampsia in pregnancies complicated by hyperthyroidism. *Obstet Gynecol* 84:946–949, 1994.

Miller EH: Metabolic management of diabetes in pregnancy. *Semin Perinatol* 18: 414–431, 1994.

Miller TE, Estrella E, Myerburg RJ, de Viera JG, Moreno N, Rusconi P, Ahearn ME, Baumbach L, Kurlansky P, Wilff G, Bishopric NH: Recurrent third-trimester fetal loss and maternal mosaicism for long-QT syndrome. *Circulation* 109:3029–3034, 2004.

Miller WG, Myers GL, Ashwood ER, Killeen AA, Wang E, Thienpont LM, Siekmann L: Creatinine measurement. State of the art in accuracy and interlaboratory harmonization. *Arch Pathol Lab Med* 129:297–304, 2005.

Miller TD, Redberg RF, Wackers FJT: Screening asymptomatic diabetic patients for coronary artery disease. *J Am Coll Cardiol* 48:761–764, 2006.

Mills JL, Knopp RH, Simpson JL, Jovanovic-Peterson L, Metzger BE, Holmes LB, Aarons JH, Brown Z, Reed GF, Bieber FR: Lack of relation of increased malformation rates in infants of diabetic mothers to glycemic control during organogenesis. *N Engl J Med* 318:671–676, 1988.

Min Y, Lowy C, Ghebremeskel K, Thomas B, Offley-Shore B, Crawford MC: Unfavorable effect of type 1 and type 2 diabetes on maternal and fetal essential fatty acid status: a potential marker of fetal insulin resistance. *Am J Clin Nutr* 82:1162–1168, 2005.

Mineo C, Deguchi H, Griffin JH, Shaul PW: Endothelial and antithrombotic actions of HDL. *Circ Res* 98:1352–1364, 2006.

Mintz GS, Painter JA, Pichard AD, Kent KM, Satler LF, Popma JJ, Chuang YC, Bucher TA, Sokolowicz LE, Leon MB: Atherosclerosis in angiographically "normal" coronary artery reference segments: an intravascular ultrasound study with clinical correlations. *J Am Coll Cardiol* 25:1479–1485, 1995.

Miodovnik M, Lavin JP, Harrington DJ, Leung LS, Seeds AE, Clark KE: Effect of maternal ketoacidemia on the pregnant ewe and the fetus. *Am J Obstet Gynecol* 144:585–593, 1982a.

Miodovnik M, Lavin JP, Harrington DJ, Leung L, Seeds AE, Clark KE: Cardiovascular and biochemical effects of infusion of beta hydroxybutyrate into the fetal lamb. *Am J Obstet Gynecol* 144:594–600, 1982b.

Miodovnik M, Rosenn BM, Khoury JC, Grigsby JL, Siddiqi TA: Does pregnancy increase the risk for development and progression of diabetic retinopathy? *Am J Obstet Gynecol* 174:1180–1191, 1996.

Miranova MA, Klein RL, Virella GT, Lopez-Virella MF: Anti-modified LDL antibodies, LDL-containing human complexes, and susceptibility of LDL to in vitro oxidation in patients with type 2 diabetes. *Diabetes* 49:1033–1041, 2000.

MiSAD—Milan Study on Atherosclerosis and Diabetes (MiSAD) Group: Prevalence of unrecognized silent myocardial ischemia and its association with atherosclerotic risk factors in non-insulin-dependent diabetes mellitus. *Am J Cardiol* 79:134–139, 1997.

Misiani R, Marchesi D, Tiraboschi L, Pagni R, Goglio A, Amuso G, Muratore D, Bertuletti P, Massazza M: Urinary albumin excretion in normal pregnancy and pregnancy-induced hypertension. *Nephron* 59:416–422, 1991.

Misra UK, Gawdi G, Gonzalez-Gronow M, Pizzo SV: Coordinate regulation of the α_2-macroglobulin signaling receptor and the low-density lipoprotein receptor-related protein/α_2-macroglobulin receptor by insulin. *J Biol Chem* 274:25785–25791, 1999.

Missant C, Teunkens A, Vandermeersch E, Van de Velde M: Intrathecal clonidine prolongs labor analgesia but worsens fetal outcome: a pilot study. *Can J Anesth* 51:696–701, 2004.

Mitamura Y, Tashimo A, Nakamura Y, Ohtsuka K, Mizue Y, Nishihira J: Vitreous levels of placenta growth factor and vascular endothelial growth factor in patients with proliferative diabetic retinopathy. *Diabetes Care* 25:2352, 2002.

Mitrakou A, Ryan C, Veneman T, Mokan M, Jenssen T, Kiss I, Durrant J, Cryer P, Gerich J: Hierarchy of glycemic thresholds for counterregulatory hormone secretion, symptoms, and cerebral dysfunction. *Am J Physiol* 260:E67–E74, 1991.

Mittendorfer B, Patterson BW, Klein S: Effect of sex and obesity on basal VLDL-triacylglycerol kinetics. *Am J Clin Nutr* 77:573–579, 2003.

Moar VA, Jeffries MA, Mutch IMM, Ounsted MK, Redman CWG: Neonatal head circumference and the treatment of maternal hypertension. *Br J Obstet Gynecol* 85:933–937, 1978.

Mogensen CE, Christensen CK: Predicting diabetic nephropathy in insulin-dependent patients. *N Engl J Med* 311:89–93, 1984.

Mogensen CE, Schmitz O: The diabetic kidney: from hyperfiltration and microalbuminuria to endstage renal failure. *Med Clin North Am* 72:1465–1492, 1988.

Mogensen CE, Vestbo E, Poulson PL, Christiansen C, Damsgaard EM, Eiskjer H, Froland A, Hansen KW, Nielsen S, Pedersen MM: Microalbuminuria and potential confounders. A review and some observations on variability of urinary albumin excretion. Commentary. *Diabetes Care* 18:572–581, 1995a.

Mogensen CE, Keane WF, Bennett PH, Jerums G, Parving HH, Passa P, Steffes MW, Striker GE, Viberti GC: Prevention of diabetic renal disease with special reference to microalbuminuria. *Lancet* 346:1080–1084, 1995b.

Mohler ER 3rd, Treat-Jacobson D, Reilly MP, Cunningham KE, Miani M, Criqui MH, Hiatt WR, Hirsch AT: Utility and barriers to performance of the ankle-brachial index in primary care practice. *Vasc Med* 9:253–260, 2004.

Mohn A, Di Michele S, Di Luzio R, Tumini S, Chiarelli F: The effect of subclinical hypothyroidism on metabolic control in children and adolescents with type 1 diabetes mellitus. *Diabet Med* 19:70–73, 2002.

Mohsin F, Craig ME, Cusumano J, Chan AKF, Hing S, Lee JW, Silink M, Howard NJ, Donaghue KC: Discordant trends in microvascular complications in adolescents with type 1 diabetes from 1990 to 2002. *Diabetes Care* 28: 1974–1980, 2005.

Molden E, Asberg A, Christensen H: CYP2D6 is involved in *O*-methylation of diltiazem. An in vitro study with transfected human liver cells. *Eur J Clin Pharmacol* 56:575–579, 2000.

Molden E, Johansen PW, Boe GH, Bergan S, Christensen H, Rugstad HE, Rootwelt H, Reubsaet L, Lehne G: Pharmacokinetics of diltiazem and its metabolites in relation to *CYP2D6* genotype. *Clin Pharmacol Ther* 72:333–342, 2002.

Moloney JBM, Drury IM: The effect of pregnancy on the natural course of diabetic retinopathy. *Am J Ophthalmol* 93:745, 1982.

Momotani N, Noh J, Oyanagi H, Ishikawa N, Ito K: Antithyroid drug therapy for Graves' disease during pregnancy. Optimal regimen for fetal thyroid status. *N Engl J Med* 315:24–28, 1986.

Momotani N, Noh JY, Ishikawa N, Ito K: Effects of propylthiouracil and methimazole on fetal thyroid status in mothers with Graves' hyperthyroidism. *J Clin Endocrinol Metab* 82:3633–3636, 1997.

Momotani N, Yamashita R, Makino F, Noh JY, Ishikawa N, Ito K: Thyroid function in wholly breast-feeding infants whose mothers take high doses of propylthiouracil. *Clin Endocrinol (Oxf)* 53:177–181, 2000.

Mone SM, Sanders SP, Colan SD: Control mechanisms for physiological hypertrophy of pregnancy. *Circulation* 94:667–672, 1996.

Montan S, Liedholm H, Lingman G, Marsal K, Sjoberg N-O, Solum T: Fetal and uteroplacental hemodynamics during short-term atenolol treatment of hypertension in pregnancy. *Br J Obstet Gynecol* 94:312–317, 1987.

Montan S, Ingemarsson I, Marsal K, Sjoberg N-O: Randomized controlled trial of atenolol and pindolol in human pregnancy: effects on fetal hemodynamics. *BMJ* 304:946–949, 1992.

Montan S, Anandakumar C, Arulkumaran S, Ingemarsson I, Ratnam SS: Effects of methyldopa on uteroplacental and fetal hemodynamics in pregnancy-induced hypertension. *Am J Obstet Gynecol* 168:152–156, 1993.

Montan S: Drugs used in hypertensive diseases in pregnancy. *Curr Opin Obstet Gynecol* 16:111–115, 2004.

Montelongo A, Lasuncion MA, Pallardo LF, Herrera E: Longitudinal study of plasma lipoproteins and hormones during pregnancy in normal and diabetic women. *Diabetes* 41:1651–1659, 1992.

Montes A, Walden CE, Knopp RH, Cheung M, Chapman MB, Albers JJ: Physiologic and supraphysiologic increases in lipoprotein lipids and apoproteins in late pregnancy and postpartum. Possible markers for the diagnosis of "prelipemia." *Arteriosclerosis* 4: 407–417, 1984.

Montoro MM, Collea JV, Frasier SD, Mestman JH: Successful outcome of pregnancy with hypothyroidism. *Ann Intern Med* 94:31–34, 1981.

Montoro MN, Myers VP, Mestman JH, Yunhua X, Anderson BG, Golde SH: Outcome of pregnancy in diabetic ketoacidosis. *Am J Perinatol* 10:17–20, 1993.

Montoro MN: Management of hypothyroidism during pregnancy. *Clin Obstet Gynecol* 40:65–80, 1997.

Montoro MM: Diabetic ketoacidosis in pregnancy. In: Reece EA, Coustan DR, Gabbe SG, eds. *Diabetes in Women. Adolescence, Pregnancy, and Menopause.* 3rd ed. Philadelphia: Lippincott Williams & Wilkins; 2004:344–350.

Montouris G: Gabapentin exposure in human pregnancy: results from the Gabapentin Pregnancy Registry. *Epilepsy Behav* 4:310–317, 2003.

Monzani F, Caraccio N, Kozakowa M, Dardano A, Vittone F, Virdis A, Taddei S, Palombo C, Ferrannini E: Effect of levothyroxine replacement on lipid profile and intima-media thickness in subclinical hypothyroidism: *J Clin Endocrinol Metab* 89:2099–2106, 2004.

Moodley J, Gangaram R, Khanyile R, Ojwang PJ: Serum cystatin C for assessment of glomerular filtration rate in hypertensive disorders of pregnancy. *Hypertens Preg* 23:309–317, 2004.

Moreno PR, Murcia AM, Palacios I, Leon MN, Bernardi VH, Fuster V, Fallon JT: Coronary composition and macrophage infiltration in atherectomy specimens from patients with diabetes mellitus. *Circulation* 102:2180–2184, 2002.

Moretti NM, Fairlie FM, Aki S, Khouri AD, Sibai BM: The effect of nifedipine therapy on fetal and placental Doppler waveforms in preeclampsia remote from term. *Am J Obstet Gynecol* 163:1844–1848, 1990.

Moriarity JT, Folsom AR, Iribarren C, Nieto FJ, Rosamond WD: Serum uric acid and risk of coronary heart disease: Atherosclerosis Risk in Communities (ARIC) Study. *Ann Epidemiol* 10:136–143, 2000.

Morigi M, Angioletti S, Imberti B, Donadelli R, Micheletti G, Figliuzzi M, Remuzzi A, Zoja C, Remuzzi G: Leukocyte-endothelial interaction is augmented by high glucose concentrations and hyperglycemia in a NF-kB-dependent fashion. *J Clin Invest* 101:1905–1915, 1998.

Morreale de Escobar G, Allan WC, Haddow JE, Palomaki GE, Williams JR, Mitchell ML, Hermos RJ, Faix JD, Klein RZ: Maternal thyroid deficiency and pregnancy complications: implications for population screening. *J Med Screen* 7:127–130, 2000a.

Morreale de Escobar G, Obregon MJ, Escobar del Rey F: Is neuropsychological development related to maternal hypothyroidism or to maternal hypothyroxinemia? *J Clin Endocrinol Metab* 85:3975–3987, 2000b.

Morreale de Escobar G, Obregon MJ, Escobar del Rey F: Role of thyroid hormone during early brain development. *Eur J Endocrinol* 151:1–14, 2004.

Morris LR, Murphy MB, Kitabchi AE: Bicarbonate therapy in severe diabetic ketoacidosis. *Ann Intern Med* 105:836–840, 1986.

Mortensen HB, Hougaard P, Ibsen KK, Parving HH: Relationship between blood pressure and urinary albumin excretion rate in young Danish type 1 diabetic patients: comparison to nondiabetic children. Danish Group of Diabetes in Childhood. *Diabet Med* 11:155–161, 1994.

Mortensen HB: Microalbuminuria in young patients with type 1 diabetes. In: Mogensen CE, ed. *The Kidney and Hypertension in Diabetes Mellitus.* 6th ed. London: Taylor & Francis; 2004:457–477.

Mortimer RH, Cannell GR, Addison RS, Johnson LP, Roberts MS, Bernus I: Methimazole and propylthiouracil equally cross the perfused human term placental lobule. *J Clin Endocrinol Metab* 82:3099–3102, 1997.

Mosca L (chair); American Heart Association Expert Panel/Writing Group: Appel LJ, Benjamin EJ, Berra K, Chandra-Strobos N, Fabunmi RP, Grady D, Haan CK, Hayes SN, Judelson DR, Keenan NL, McBride P, Oparil S, Ouyang P, Oz MC, Mendeksohn ME, Pasternak RC, Pinn VW, Robertson RM, Schenk-Gustafsson K, Sila CA, Smith SC, Sopko G, Taylor AL, Walsh BW, Wenger NK, Williams CL: Evidence-based guidelines for cardiovascular disease prevention in women. AHA guidelines. *Circulation* 109:672–693, 2004a.

Mosca L; for the Expert Panel/Writing Group: Summary of the American Heart Association's evidence-based guidelines for cardiovascular disease prevention in women. *Aterioscler Thromb Vasc Biol* 24:394–396, 2004b.

Mosca L, Linfante AH, Benjamin EJ, Berra K, Hayes SN, Walsh B, Fabunmi RP, Kwan J, Mills T, Simpson SL: Physician awareness and adherance to cardiovascular disease prevention guidelines in the United States. *Circulation* 111:499–510, 2005.

Moss SE, Klein R, Kessler SD, Fichie KA: Comparison between ophthalmoscopy and fundus photography in determining severity of diabetic retinopathy. *Ophthalmology* 92:62–67, 1985.

Moss AJ, Zareba W, Hall WJ, Schwartz PJ, Crampton RS, Benhorin J, Vincent GM, Locati EH, Priori SG, Napolitano C, Medina A, Zhang L, Robinson JL, Timothy K, Towbin JA, Andrews ML: Effectiveness and limitations of beta-blocker therapy in congenital long QT syndrome. *Circulation* 101:616–623, 2000.

Mouradian M, Abourizk N: Diabetes mellitus and thyroid disease. *Diabetes Care* 6:512–520, 1983.

Moutquin J-M, Garner PR, Burrows RF, Rey E, Helewa ME, Lange IR, Rabkin SW: Report of the Canadian Hypertension Society Consensus Conference: 2. Nonpharmacologic management and prevention of hypertensive disorders in pregnancy. *CMAJ* 157:907–919, 1997.

Movahed MR: Diabetes as a risk factor for cardiac conduction defects: a review. *Diabetes Obes Metab* 9:276–281, 2007.

Mozaffarian D, Prineas RJ, Stein PK, Siscovick DS: Dietary fish and *n*-3 fatty acid intake and cardiac electrocardiographic parameters in humans. *J Am Coll Cardiol* 48:478–484, 2006.

Mueller C, Scholer A, Laule-Kilian K, Martina B, Schindler C, Buser P, Pfisterer M, Perruchoud AP: Use of B-type natriuretic peptide in the evaluation and management of acute dyspnea. *N Engl J Med* 350:647–654, 2004.

Mueller C, Laule-Kilian K, Christ A, Perruchoud AP: The use of B-type natriuretic peptide in the management of patients with diabetes and acute dyspnea. *Diabetologia* 49:629–636, 2006.

Mulnier HE, Seaman HE, Raleigh VS, Soedamah-Muthu SS, Colhoun HM, Lawrenson RA, De Vries CS: Risk of stroke in people with type 2 diabetes in the U.K.: a study using the General Practice Research Data Base. *Diabetologia* 49:2859–2865, 2006.

Murakami T, Michelagnoli S, Longhi R, Gianfranceschi G, Pazzucconi F, Calabresi L, Sirtori CR, Franceschini G: Triglycerides are major determinants of cholesterol esterification/transfer and HDL remodeling in human plasma. *Arterioscler Thromb Vasc Biol* 15:1819–1828, 1995.

Murphy NP, Ford-Adams ME, Ong KK, Harris ND, Keane SM, Davies C, Ireland RH, MacDonald IA, Knight EJ, Edge JA, Heller SR, Dunger DB: Prolonged cardiac repolarization during spontaneous nocturnal hypoglycemia in children and adolescents with type 1 diabetes. *Diabetologia* 47:1940–1947, 2004.

Murray DP, O'Brien T, Mulrooney R, O'Sullivan DJ: Autonomic dysfunction and silent myocardial ischaemia on exercise testing in diabetes mellitus. *Diabet Med* 7:580–584, 1990.

Murthy K, Stevens LA, Stark PC, Levey AS: Variation in the serum creatinine assay calibration: a practical application to glomerular filtration rate estimation. *Kidney Int* 68:1884–1887, 2005.

Muscelli E, Natali A, Bianchi S, Bigazzi R, Galvan AQ, Sironi AM, Frascerra S, Ciocaro D, Ferrannini E: Effect of insulin on renal sodium and uric acid handling in essential hypertension. *Am J Hypertens* 9:746–752, 1996.

Mussap M, Dalla Vestra M, Fioretto P, Saller A, Varagnolo M, Nosadini R, Plebani M: Cystatin C is a more sensitive marker than serum creatinine for the estimation of GFR in type 2 diabetic subjects. *Kidney Int* 61:1453–1461, 2002.

Mutch LMM, Moar VA, Ounsted MK, Redman CWG: Hypertension during pregnancy, with and without specific hypotensive treatment: 1. Perinatal factors and neonatal morbidity. *Early Hum Dev* 1:47–57, 1977a.

Mutch LMM, Moar VA, Ounsted MK, Redman CWG: Hypertension in pregnancy with and without specific hypotensive treatment: 2. The growth and development of the infant in the first year of life. *Early Hum Dev* 1:59–67, 1977b.

Myers MG, Tobe SW, McKay DW, Bolli P, Hemmelgarn BR, McAlister FA; the Canadian Hypertension Education Program: New algorithm for the diagnosis of hypertension. Canadian Hypertension Education Program Recommendations (2005). *Am J Hypertens* 18:1369–1374, 2005.

Myers GL, Miller WG, Coresh J, Fleming J, Greenberg N, Greene T, Hostetter T, Levey AS, Panteghini M, Welch M, Eckfeldt JH; the National Kidney Disease Education Program Laboratory Working Group: Recommendations for improving serum creatinine measurement: a report from the Laboratory Working Group of the National Kidney Disease Education Program. *Clin Chem* 52:5–18, 2006.

Nabhan F, Emanuele MA, Emanule N: Latent autoimmune diabetes of adulthood. Unique features that distinguish it from type 1 and 2. *Postgrad Med* 117:7–12, 2005.

Nader S, Mastrobattista J: Recurrent hyperthyroidism in consecutive pregnancies characterized by hyperemesis. *Thyroid* 6:465, 1996.

Nader S: Thyroid disease and other endocrine disorders in pregnancy. *Obstet Gynecol Clin North Am* 31:257–285, 2004.

Naghavi M, Falk E, Hecht HS, Jamieson MJ, Kaul S, Berman D, Fayad Z, Budoff MJ, Rumberger J, Naqvi TZ, Shaw LJ, Faergeman O, Cohn J, Bahr R, Koenig W, Demirovic J, Arking D, Herrera VLM, Badimon J, Goldstein JA, Rudy YA, Airaksinen J, Schwartz RS, Riley WA, Mendes RA, Douglas P, Shah PK; the SHAPE Task Force: From vulnerable plaque to vulnerable patient—Part III: Executive Summary of the Screening for Heart Attack Prevention and Education (SHAPE) Task Force Report. *Am J Cardiol* 98 (Suppl):2H-15H, 2006.

Naito J, Koretsune Y, Sakamoto N, Shutta R, Yoshida J, Yasuoka Y, Yoshida S, Chin W, Kusuoka H, Inoue M: Transmural heterogeneity of myocardial integrated backscatter in diabetic patients without overt cardiac disease. *Diabetes Res Clin Pract* 52:11–20, 2001.

Naka Y, Bucciarelli LG, Wendt T, Lee LK, Rong LL, Ramasamy R, Yan SF, Schmidt AM: RAGE axis. Animal models and novel insights into the vascular complications of diabetes. *Arterioscler Thromb Vasc Biol* 24:1342–1349, 2004.

Nakagawa T, Kang DH, Feig D, Sanchez-Lozada LG, Srinivas TR, Sautin Y, Ejaz AA, Segal M, Johnson RJ: Unearthing uric acid: an ancient factor with recently found significance in renal and cardiovascular disease. *Kidney Int* 69:1722–1725, 2006.

Nakamura K, Yamagishi SI, Adachi H, Kurita-Nakamura Y, Matsui T, Yochida T, Sato A, Imaizumi T: Elevation of soluble form of receptor for advanced glycation end products (sRAGE) in diabetic subjects with coronary artery disease. *Diabetes Metab Res Rev* 23:368–371, 2006.

Nandkeoliar MK, Dharmalingam M, Marcus SR: Diabetes mellitus in Asian children and adolescents. *J Pediatr Endocrinol Metab* 20:1109–1114, 2007.

Napoli C, D'Armiento FD, Mancini FP, Postiglione A, Witztum JL, Palumbo G, Palinski W: Fatty streak formation occurs in human fetal aortas and is greatly enhanced by maternal hypercholesterolemia. Intimal accumulation of low density lipoprotein and its oxidation precede monocyte recruitment into early atherosclerotic lesions. *J Clin Invest* 100:2680–2690, 1997.

Napoli C, Glass CK, Witztum JL, Deutsch R, D'Armiento FP, Palinski W: Influence of maternal hypercholesterolemia during pregnancy on progression of early atherosclerotic lesions in childhood: Fate of Early Lesions in Children (FELIC) study. *Lancet* 354:1234–1241, 1999.

Napoli A, Sabbatini A, Di Biase N, Marceca M, Colatrella A, Falluca F: Twenty-four-hour blood pressure monitoring in normoalbuminuric normotensive type 1 diabetic women during pregnancy. *J Diabetes Complications* 17:292–296, 2003.

Nasir K, Redberg RF, Budoff MJ, Hui E, Post WS, Blumenthal RS: Utility of stress testing and coronary calcification measurement for detection of coronary artery disease in women. *Arch Intern Med* 164:1610–1620, 2004.

Natarajan S, Liao Y, Cao G, Lipsitz SR, McGee DL: Sex differences in risk for coronary heart disease mortality associated with diabetes and established coronary heart disease. *Arch Intern Med* 163:1735–1740, 2003.

Nathan DM, Lachin J, Cleary P, Orchard T, Brillon DJ, Backlund JY, O'Leary DH, Genuth S; Diabetes Control and Complications Trial; Epidemiology of Diabetes Interventions and Complications Research Group: Intensive diabetes therapy and carotid intima-media thickness in type 1 diabetes mellitus. *N Engl J Med* 348:2294–2303, 2003.

Nayar B, Singhal A, Aggarwal R, Malhotra N: Losartan-induced fetal toxicity. *Indian J Pediatr* 70:138–142, 2003.

NBP—National High Blood Pressure Education Program Working Group; Gifford RW, August PA, Cunningham G, Green LA, Lindheimer MD, McNellis D, Roberts JM, Sibai BM, Taler SJ: Report on high blood pressure in pregnancy. National Heart, Lung, and Blood Institute. *Am J Obstet Gynecol* 183:S1–S22, 2000.

NBP—National High Blood Pressure Education Program Working Group on High Blood Pressure in Children and Adolescents: The Fourth Report on the diagnosis, evaluation, and treatment of high blood pressure in children and adolescents. Sponsored by the National Heart, Lung, and Blood Institute and endorsed by the American Academy of Pediatrics. *Pediatrics* 114 (Suppl 2): 555–576, 2004.

NCEP—National Cholesterol Education Program, Expert Panel on Detection, Evaluation, and Treatment of High Blood Cholesterol in Adults: Executive summary of the Third Report of the National Cholesterol Education Program (NCEP) Expert Panel on Detection, Evaluation, and Treatment of High Blood Cholesterol in Adults (Adult Treatment Panel III). *JAMA* 285:2486–2497, 2001.

NCEP—National Cholesterol Education Program (NCEP), Expert Panel on Detection, Evaluation, and Treatment of High Blood Cholesterol in Adults (Adult Treatment Panel III): Third report of the National Cholesterol Education Program (NCEP) Expert Panel on Detection, Evaluation, and Treatment of High Blood Cholesterol in Adults (Adult Treatment Panel III). Final report. *Circulation* 106:3143–3421, 2002.

Neale D, Burrow G: Thyroid disease in pregnancy. *Obstet Gynecol Clin North Am* 31:893–905, 2004.

Negro R, Formoso G, Mangieri T, Pezzarossa A, Dazzi D, Hassan H: Levothyroxine treatment in euthyroid pregnant women with autoimmune thyroid disease: effects on obstetrical complications. *J Clin Endocrinol Metab* 91:2587–2591, 2006.

Neithardt AB, Dooley SL, Borensztajn J: Prediction of 24-hour protein excretion in pregnancy with a single voided urine protein-to-creatine ratio. *Am J Obstet Gynecol* 186:883–886, 2002.

Ness RB, Markovic N, Bass D, Harger G, Roberts JM: Family history of hypertension, heart disease, and stroke among women who develop hypertension in pregnancy. *Obstet Gynecol* 102:1366–1371, 2003.

Nesto RW, Phillips RT, Kett KG, Hill T, Perper E, Young E, Leland OS: Relationship of angina to ischemia in diabetics and nondiabetics: assessment by exercise thallium scintigraphy. *Ann Intern Med* 108:170–175, 1988.

Nesto RW: Screening for asymptomatic coronary artery disease in diabetes. *Diabetes Care* 22:1393–1395, 1999.

Nesto RW: Beyond low-density lipoprotein: addressing the atherogenic lipid triad in type 2 diabetes mellitus and the metabolic syndrome. *Am J Cardiovasc Drugs* 5:379–387, 2005.

Newman EJ, Rahman FS, Lees KR, Weir CJ, Walters MR: Elevated serum urate concentration independently predicts poor outcome following stroke in patients with diabetes. *Diabetes Metab Res Rev* 22:79–82, 2006.

Newton CA, Raskin P: Diabetic ketoacidosis in type 1 and type 2 diabetes mellitus. Clinical and biochemical differences. *Arch Intern Med* 164: 1925–1931, 2004.

Niakan E, Harati Y, Rolak LA, Comstock JP, Rokey R: Silent myocardial infarction and diabetic cardiovascular autonomic neuropathy. *Arch Intern Med* 146: 2229–2230, 1986.

Nichols GA, Hillier TA, Erbey JR, Brown JB: Congestive heart failure in type 2 diabetes: prevalence, incidence, and risk factors. *Diabetes Care* 24:1614–1619, 2001.

Nichols GA, Gullion CM, Koro CE, Ephross SA, Brown JB: The incidence of congestive heart failure in type 2 diabetes. An update. *Diabetes Care* 27: 1879–1884, 2004.

Nicholson A, White IR, Macfarlane P, Brunner E, Marmot M: Rose questionnaire angina in younger men and women: gender differences in the relationship to cardiovascular risk factors and other reported symptoms. *J Clin Epidemiol* 52:337–346, 1999.

Nielsen S, Guo Z-K, Albu JB, Klein S, O'Brien PC, Jensen MD: Energy expenditure, sex, and endogenous fuel availability in humans. *J Clin Invest* 111:981–988, 2003.

Nielsen LR, Muller C, Damm P, Mathiesen ER: Reduced prevalence of early preterm delivery in women with type 1 diabetes and microalbuminuria—possible effect of early antihypertensive treatment during pregnancy. *Diabet Med* 23:426–431, 2006.

Nielsen LR, Pedersen-Bjergaard U, Thorsteinsson B, Johansen M, Damm P, Mathiesen ER: Hypoglycemia in pregnant women with type 1 diabetes. Predictors and role of metabolic control. *Diabetes Care* 31:9–14, 2008.

Nies BM, Dreiss RJ: Hyperlipidemic pancreatitis in pregnancy: a case report and review of the literature. *Am J Perinatol* 7:166–169, 1990.

Nieto FJ, Iribarren C, Gross MD, Comstock GW, Cutler RG: Uric acid and serum antioxidant capacity: a reaction to atherosclerosis? *Atherosclerosis* 148:131–139, 2000.

Nieuwdorp M, van Haeften TW, Gouverneur MCLG, Mooij HL, van Lieshout MHP, Levi M, Meijers JCM, Holleman F, Hoekstra JBL, Vink H, Kastelein JJP, Stroes ESG: Loss of endothelial glycocalyx during acute hyperglycemia coincides with endothelial dysfunction and coagulation activation in vivo. *Diabetes* 55:480–486, 2006.

Nieves DJ, Cnop M, Retzlaff B, Walden CE, Brunzell JD, Knopp RH, Kahn SE: The atherogenic lipoprotein profile associated with obesity and insulin resistance is largely attributed to intra-abdominal fat. *Diabetes* 52:172–179, 2003.

Nilsson PM, Gudbjornsdottir S, Eliasson B, Cederholm J; the Screening Committee of the National Diabetes Register in Sweden: Hypertension in diabetes: trends in clinical control in repeated national surveys from Sweden 1996–99. *J Hum Hypertens* 17:37–44, 2003.

Nisell H, Trygg M, Back R: Urine albumin/creatinine ratio for the assessment of albuminuria in pregnancy hypertension. *Acta Obstet Gynecol Scand* 85:1327–1330, 2006.

Nishibata K, Nagashima M, Tsuji A, Hasegawa S, Nagai N, Goto M, Hayashi H: Comparison of casual blood pressure and twenty-four-hour ambulatory blood pressures in high school students. *J Pediatr* 127:34–39, 1995.

Nishimura RA, Abel MD, Hatle LK, Tajik AJ: Assessment of diastolic function of the heart: background and current applications of Doppler echocardiography. II: clinical studies. *Mayo Clin Proc* 64:181–204, 1989.

Nishimura R, Dorman JS, Bosnyak Z, Tajima N, Becker DJ, Orchard TJ; Diabetes Epidemiology Research International Mortality Study Group: Incidence of ESRD and survival after renal replacement therapy in patients with type 1 diabetes: a report from the Allegheny Count Registry. *Am J Kidney Dis* 42:117–124, 2003.

Niskanen L, Laaksonen DE, Lindstrom J, Eriksson JG, Keinanen-Kiukaanniemi S, Ilanne-Parikka P, Aunola S, Hamalainen H, Tuomilehto J, Uusitupa M; the Finnish Diabetes Prevention Study Group: Serum uric acid as a harbinger of metabolic outcome in subjects with impaired glucose tolerance. *Diabetes Care* 29:709–711, 2006.

Nissen SE, Gurley JC, Grines CL, Booth DC, McClure R, Berk M, Fischer C, DeMaria AN: Intravascular ultrasound assessment of lumen size and wall morphology in normal subjects and patients with coronary artery disease. *Circulation* 84:1087–1099, 1991.

NKF—National Kidney Foundation: Kidney Disease Outcome Quality Initiative (K/DOQI) clinical practice guidelines for chronic kidney disease: evaluation, classification, and stratification. *Am J Kidney Dis* 39 (Suppl 1):S1–S266, 2002.

Nordmann A, Frach B, Walker T, Martina B, Battegay E: Reliability of patients measuring blood pressure at home: prospective observational study. *BMJ* 319:1172, 1999.

Nordstrom L, Spetz E, Wallstrom K, Walinder O: Metabolic control and pregnancy outcome among women with insulin-dependent diabetes mellitus. A twelve-year follow-up in the county of Jamtland, Sweden. *Acta Obstet Gynecol Scand* 77:284–289, 1998.

Nordwall M, Bojestig M, Arnqvist HJ, Ludvigsson J: Declining incidence of severe retinopathy and persisting decrease of nephropathy in an unselected population of type 1 diabetes: the Linkoping Diabetes Complications Study. *Diabetologia* 47:1266–1272, 2004.

Norgaard K, Feldt-Rasmussen B, Borch-Johnsen K, Saelan H, Deckert T: Prevalence of hypertension in type 1 (insulin-dependent) diabetes mellitus. *Diabetologia* 33:407–410, 1990.

Norgard B, Puho E, Czeizel AE, Skriver MV, Sorensen HT: Aspirin use during early pregnancy and the risk of congenital abnormalities: a population-based case-control study. *Am J Obstet Gynecol* 192:922–923, 2005.

Norwood VF, Craig MR, Mansel HJ, Gomez RA: Differential expression of angiotensin II receptors during early renal morphogenesis. *Am J Physiol* 272: R662–R668, 1997.

Noto H, Chitkara P, Raskin P: The role of lipoprotein-associated phospholipase A(2) in the metabolic syndrome and diabetes. *J Diabetes Complications* 20:343–348, 2006.

Novelli GP, Valensise H, Vasapollo B, Larciprete G, Altomare F, Di Pierro G, Casalino B, Galante A, Arduini D: Left ventricular concentric geometry as a risk factor in gestational hypertension. *Hypertension* 41:469–475, 2003.

Nyengaard JR, Ido Y, Kilo C, Williamson JR: Interactions between hyperglycemia and hypoxia. Implications for diabetic retinopathy. *Diabetes* 53:2931–2938, 2004.

Nylund L, Lunell N-O, Lewander R, Sarby B, Thornstrom S: Labetalol for the treatment of hypertension in pregnancy. Pharmacokinetics and effects on the uteroplacental blood flow. *Acta Obstet Gynecol Scand* 118:71–73, 1984.

O'Brien IA, McFadden JP, Corrall RJ: The influence of autonomic neuropathy on mortality in insulin-dependent diabetes. *Q J Med* 79:495–502, 1991.

O'Brien KD, Reichenbach DD, Marcovina SM, Kuusisto J, Alpers CE, Otto CM: Apolipoproteins B, (a), and E accumulate in the morphologically early lesion of 'degenerative' valvular aortic stenosis. *Arterioscler Thromb Vasc Biol* 16:523–532, 1996.

O'Brien E, Asmar R, Beilin L, Imai Y, Mancia G, Mengden T, Myers M, Padfield P, Palatini P, Parati G, Pickering T, Redon J, Staessen J, Stergiou G, Verdecchia P; on behalf of the European Society of Hypertension Working Group on Blood Pressure Monitoring: European Society of Hypertension recommendations for conventional, ambulatory and home blood pressure measurement. *J Hypertens* 21:821–848, 2003.

O'Donoghue M, Kenney P, Oestreicher E, Anwaruddin S, Baggish AL, Krauser DG, Chen A, Tung R, Cameron R, Januzzi JL Jr: Usefulness of aminoterminal pro-brain natriuretic peptide testing for the diagnostic and prognostic evaluation of dyspneic patients with diabetes mellitus seen in the emergency department (from the PRIDE study). *Am J Cardiol* 100:1336–1340, 2007.

O'Leary PC, Feddema PH, Michelangeli VP, Leedman PJ, Chew GT, Knuiman M, Kaye J, Walsh JP: Investigations of thyroid hormones and antibodies based on a community health survey: the Busselton thyroid study. *Clin Endocrinol (Oxfd)* 64:97–104, 2006.

Oakley C, Child A, Jung B, Prebitero P, Tornos P, Klein W, Garcia MAA, Blomstrom-Lundqvist C, de Backer G, Dargie H, Deckers J, Flather M, Hradec J, Mazzotta G, Oto A, Parkhomenko A, Silber S, Torbicki A, Trappe H-J, Dean V, Poumeyrol-Jumeau D; Task Force on the Management of Cardiovascular Diseases During Pregnancy of the European Society of Cardiology: Expert consensus document on management of cardiovascular diseases during pregnancy. *Eur Heart J* 24:761–781, 2003.

Obata T, Kinemuchi H, Aomine M: Protective effect of diltiazem, a L-type calcium channel antagonist, on bisphenol A-enhanced hydroxyl radical generation by 1-methyl-4-phenylpyridinium ion in rat striatum. *Neurosci Lett* 16:211–213, 2002.

Oberbauer R, Nenov V, Weidekamm C, Haas M, Szekeres T, Mayer G: Reduction in mean glomerular pore size coincides with the development of large shunt pores in patients with diabetic nephropathy. *Exp Nephrol* 9:49–53, 2001.

Ochsenbein-Kolble N, Roos M, Gasser T, Huch R, Zimmermann R: Cross sectional study of automated blood pressure measurements throughout pregnancy. *Br J Obstet Gynecol* 111:319–325, 2004.

Odegard RA, Vatten IJ, Nilsen ST, Salvesen KA, Austgulen R: Risk factors and clinical manifestations of preeclampsia. *Br J Obstet Gynecol* 107:1410–1416, 2000.

Odermarsky M, Nilsson A, Lernmark A, Sjoblad S, Liuba P: Atherogenic vascular and lipid phenotypes in young patients with type 1 diabetes are associated with diabetes high-risk HLA genotype. *Am J Physiol* 293:H3175–H3179, 2007.

Oei H-H, van der Meer IM, Hofman A, Koudstaal PJ, Stijnen T, Breteler MMB, Witteman JCM: Lipoprotein-associated phospholipase A$_2$ activity is associated with risk of coronary heart disease and ischemic stroke. The Rotterdam Study. *Circulation* 111:570–575, 2005.

Ogburn PL, Kitzmiller JL, Hare JW, Phillippe M, Gabbe SG, Miodovnik M, Tagatz GE, Nagel TC, Williams PP, Goetz FC, Barbosa JJ, Sutherland DE: Pregnancy following renal transplantation in class T diabetes mellitus. *JAMA* 255:911–915, 1986.

Ohkubo T, Imai Y, Tsuji I, Nagai K, Kato J, Kikuchi N, Nishiyama A, Aihara A, Sekino M, Kikuya M, Ito S, Satoh H: Home blood pressure measurement has a stronger predictive power for mortality than does screening blood pressure measurement: a population-based observation in Ohasama, Japan. *J Hypertens* 16:971–975, 1998.

Ohrt V: The influence of pregnancy on diabetic retinopathy with special regard to the reversible changes shown in 100 pregnancies. *Acta Ophthalmol* 62:603–616, 1984.

Okamoto Y, Arita Y, Nishida M, Muraguchi M, Ouchi N, Takahashi M, Igura T, Inui Y, Kihara S, Nakamura T, Yamashita S, Funahashi T, Matsuzawa Y: An adipocyte-derived plasma protein, adiponectin, adheres to injured vascular walls. *Horm Metab Res* 32:47–50, 2000.

Okin PM, Wright JT, Nieminen MS, Jern S, Taylor AL, Philips R, Papademetriou V, Clark LT, Ofili EO, Randall OS, Oikarinen L, Viitasalo M, Toivonen L, Julius S, Dahlof B, Devereux RB: Ethnic differences in electrocardiographic criteria for left ventricular hypertrophy: the LIFE study. Losartan Intervention For Endpoint. *Am J Hypertens* 15:663–671, 2002.

Okin PM, Devereux RB, Gerdts E, Snapinn SM, Harris KE, Jern S, Kjeldsen SE, Julius S, Edelman JM, Lindholm LH, Dahlof B; for the LIFE Study Investigators: Impact of diabetes mellitus on regression of electrocardiographic left ventricular hypertrophy and the prediction of outcome during antihypertensive therapy. *Circulation* 113:1588–1596, 2006.

Okuda Y, Adrogue HJ, Field JB, Nohara H, Yamashita K: Counterproductive effects of sodium bicarbohydrate in diabetic ketoacidosis. *J Clin Endocrinol Metab* 81:314–320, 1996.

Okundaye I, Abrinko P, Hou S: Registry of pregnancy in dialysis patients. *Am J Kidney Dis* 31:766–773, 1998.

Olofsson P, Krutzen E, Nilsson-Ehle P: Iohexol clearance for assessment of glomerular filtration rate in diabetic pregnancy. *Eur J Obstet Gynecol Reprod Biol* 64:63–67, 1996.

Olsen BS, Sjolie A-K, Hougaard P, Johannesen J, Borch-Johnsen K, Marinelli K, Thorsteinsson B, Pramming S, Mortensen HB; the Danish Study Group of Diabetes in Childhood: A 6-year nationwide cohort study of glycemic control in young people with type 1 diabetes. Risk markers for the development of retinopathy, nephropathy, and neuropathy. *J Diabetes Complications* 14:295–300, 2000.

Olson JC, Edmundowicz D, Becker DJ, Kuller LH, Orchard TJ: Coronary calcium in adults with type 1 diabetes. A stronger correlate of clinical coronary artery disease in men than women. *Diabetes* 49:1571–1578, 2000.

Olson JC, Erbey JR, Forrest KY, Williams K, Becker DJ, Orchard TJ: Glycemia (or, in women, estimated glucose disposal rate) predict lower extremity arterial disease events in type 1 diabetes. *Metabolism* 51:248–254, 2002.

Omori Y, Minei S, Testuo T, Nemoto K, Shimuzu M, Sanaka M: Current status of pregnancy in diabetic women. A comparison of pregnancy in IDDM and NIDDM mothers. *Diabetes Res Clin Pract* 24 (Suppl):S273–S278, 1994.

Ong KL, Cheung BMY, Man YB, Lau CP, Lam KSL: Prevalence, awareness, treatment, and control of hypertension among United States adults 1999–2004. *Hypertension* 49:69–75, 2007.

Orchard TJ, Strandness DE Jr: Assessment of peripheral vascular disease in diabetes. Report and recommendations of an international workshop sponsored by the American Diabetes Association and the American Heart Association. September 18–20, 1992. New Orleans, Louisiana. *Circulation* 88:819–828, 1993.

Orchard TJ, Stevens LK, Forrest KYZ, Fuller JH: Cardiovascular disease in insulin dependent diabetes mellitus: similar rates but different risk factors in the U.S. compared with Europe. *Int J Epidemiol* 27:976–983, 1998.

Orchard TJ, Virella G, Forrest KYZ, Evans RW, Becker DJ, Lopes-Virella MF: Antibodies to oxidized LDL predict coronary artery disease in type 1 diabetes: a nested case-control study from the Pittsburgh Epidemiology of Diabetes Complications Study. *Diabetes* 48:1454–1458, 1999.

Orchard TJ, Forrest KY-Z, Kuller LH, Becker DJ: Lipid and blood pressure treatment goals for type 1 diabetes. 10-year incidence data from the Pittsburgh Epidemiology of Diabetes Complications Study. *Diabetes Care* 24:1053–1059, 2001.

Orchard TJ, Olson JC, Erbey, Williams K, Forrest KY-Z, Kinder LS, Ellis D, Becker DJ: Insulin resistance-related factors, but not glycemia, predict coronary artery disease in type 1 diabetes: 10-year follow-up data from the Pittsburgh Epidemiology of Diabetes Complications Study. *Diabetes Care* 26:1374–1379, 2003.

Orchard TJ, Costacou T, Kretowski A, Nesto RW: Type 1 diabetes and coronary artery disease. Review. *Diabetes Care* 29:2528–2538, 2006.

Ortega-Gonzalez C, Liao-Lo A, Ramirez-Peredo J, Carino-Biol N, Lira J, Parra A: Thyroid peroxidase antibodies in Mexican-born healthy pregnant women, in women with type 2 or gestational diabetes mellitus and in their offspring. *Endocr Pract* 6:244–248, 2000.

Osicka TM, Houlihan CA, Chan JG, Jerums G, Comper WD: Albuminuria in patients with type 1 diabetes is directly linked to changes in the lysosome-mediated degradation of albumin during renal passage. *Diabetes* 49:1579–1584, 2000.

Otto CM: *Textbook of Clinical Echocardiography.* 3rd ed. St Louis, MO: W.B. Saunders Co.; 2004.

Ouchi N, Kihara S, Arita Y, Maeda K, Kuriyama H, Okamoto Y, Hotta K, Nishida M, Takahashi M, Nakamura T, Yamashita S, Funahashi T, Matsuzawa Y: Novel modulator for endothelial adhesion molecules. Adipocyte-derived plasma protein adiponectin. *Circulation* 100:2473–2476, 1999.

Ouedraogo R, Wu X, Xu S-Q, Fuchsel L, Motoshima H, Mahadev K, Hough K, Scalia R, Goldstein BJ: Adiponectin suppression of high-glucose-induced reactive oxygen species in vascular endothelial cells. Evidence of involvement of a cAMP signaling pathway. *Diabetes* 55:1840–1846, 2006.

Ovalle F, Fanelli CG, Paramore DS, Craft S, Cryer PE: Brief twice weekly episodes of hypoglycemia reduce detection of clinical hypoglycemia in type 1 diabetes mellitus. *Diabetes* 47:1472–1479, 1998.

Pacher P, Obrosova IG, Mabley JG, Szabo C: Role of nitrosative stress and peroxynitrite in the pathogenesis of diabetic complications. Emerging new therapeutical strategies. *Curr Med Chem* 12:267–275, 2005.

Pacher P, Szabo C: Role of peroxynitrite in the pathogenesis of cardiovascular complications of diabetes. *Curr Opin Pharmacol* 6:136–141, 2006.

Paech MJ, Banks SL, Gurrin LC, Yeo ST, Pavy TJG: A randomized, double-blinded trial of subarachnoid bupivacaine and fentanyl, with or without clonidine, for combined spinal/epidural analgesia during labor. *Anesth Analg* 95:1396–1401, 2002.

Page EW, Christianson R: The impact of mean arterial pressure in the middle trimester upon the outcome of pregnancy. *Am J Obstet Gynecol* 125:740–746, 1976a.

Page EW, Christianson R: Influence of blood pressure changes with and without proteinuria upon outcome of pregnancy. *Am J Obstet Gynecol* 126:821–833, 1976b.

Pajunen P, Taskinen M-R, Nieminen MS, Syvanne M: Angiographic severity and extent of coronary artery disease in patients with type 1 diabetes mellitus. *Am J Cardiol* 86:1080–1085, 2000.

Paladini D, Lamberti A, Teodoro A, Arienzo M, Tartaglione A, Martinelli P: Tissue Doppler imaging of the fetal heart. *Ultrasound Obstet Gynecol* 16:530–535, 2000.

Palatini P, Penzo M, Racioppa A, Zugno E, Guzzardi G, Anaclerio M, Pessina AC: Clinical relevance of nighttime blood pressure and of daytime blood pressure variability. *Arch Intern Med* 152:1855–1860, 1992.

Palmer JP, Hampe CS, Chiu H, Goel A, Brooks-Worrell BM: Is latent autoimmune diabetes in adults distinct from type 1 diabetes or just type 1 diabetes at an older age? *Diabetes* 54 (Suppl 2):S62–S67, 2005.

Palmieri V, Capaldo B, Russo C, Iaccarino M, Di Minno G, Riccardi G, Celentano A: Left ventricular chamber and myocardial systolic function reserve in patients with type 1 diabetes mellitus: insight from traditional and Doppler tissue imaging echocardiography. *J Am Soc Echocardiogr* 19:848–856, 2006.

Pambianco G, Costacou T, Ellis D, Becker DJ, Klein R, Orchard TJ: The 30-year natural history of type 1 diabetes complications: the Pittsburgh Epidemiology of Diabetes Complications Study experience. *Diabetes* 55:1463–1469, 2006.

Parisi VM, Salinas J, Stockmar EJ: Fetal vascular responses to maternal nicardipine administration in the hypertensive ewe. *Am J Obstet Gynecol* 161:1035–1039, 1989a.

Parisi VM, Salinas J, Stockmar EJ: Placental vascular responses to maternal nicardipine administration in the hypertensive ewe. *Am J Obstet Gynecol* 161:1039–1043, 1989b.

Park JJ, Swan PD: Effect of obesity and regional adiposity on the QTc interval in women. *Int J Obes Relat Metab Disord* 21:1104–1110, 1997.

Parker CR Jr, Hauth JC, Goldenberg RL, Cooper RL, Dubard MB: Umbilical cord serum levels of thromboxane B2 in term infants of women who participated in a placebo-controlled trial of low-dose aspirin. *J Matern-Fetal Med* 9:209–215, 2000.

Parving HH, Lehnert H, Brochner-Mortensen J, Gomis R, Andersen S, Arner P: The effect of irbesartan on the development of diabetic nephropathy in patients with type 2 diabetes. *N Engl J Med* 345:870–878, 2001a.

Parving H-H: Diabetic nephropathy: prevention and treatment. *Kidney Int* 60: 2041–2055, 2001b.

Pasternak RC, Criqui MH, Benjamin EJ, Fowkes FGR, Isselbacher EM, McCullough PA, Wolf PA, Zheng Z-J: Atherosclerotic vascular disease conference. Writing Group I: Epidemiology. American Heart Association Conference Proceedings. *Circulation* 109:2605–2612, 2004.

Pavkov ME, Bennett PH, Knowler WC, Krakoff J, Sievers ML, Nelson RG: Effect of youth-onset type 2 diabetes mellitus on incidence of end-stage renal disease and mortality in young and middle-aged Pima Indians. *JAMA* 296:421–426, 2006.

Pearce EN: Diagnosis and management of thyrotoxicosis. Clinical review. *BMJ* 332:1369–1373, 2006.

Pearson GD, Veille J-C, Rahimtoola S, Hsia J, Oakley CM, Hosenpud JD, Ansari A, Baughman KL: Peripartum cardiomyopathy. National Heart, Lung, and Blood Institute and Office of Rare Diseases (National Institutes of Health) Workshop recommendations and review. *JAMA* 283:1183–1188, 2000.

Pecis M, Azevedo MJ, Moraes RS, Ferlin EL, Gross JL: Autonomic dysfunction and urinary albumin excretion rate are associated with an abnormal blood pressure pattern in normotensive normoalbuminuric type 1 diabetic patients. *Diabetes Care* 23:989–993, 2000.

Pedersen EB, Rasmussen AB, Johannesen P, Kristensen S, Lauritsen JG, Mogensen CE, Soelling K, Wohlert M: Urinary excretion of albumin, beta-2-microglobulin and light chains in pre-eclampsia, essential hypertension in pregnancy and normotensive pregnant and non-pregnant control subjects. *Scand J Clin Lab Invest* 41:777–784, 1981.

Pejic RN, Lee DT: Hypertriglyceridemia. *J Am Board Fam Med* 19:310–316, 2006.

Pekelharing HL, Aalders NL, Visser GH, van Doormaal JJ, Bouma BN, Kleinveld HA, van Rijn HJ: Method-dependent increase in lipoprotein(a) in insulin-dependent diabetes during pregnancy. *Metabolism* 44:1606–1611, 1995.

Penny JA, Halligan A, Shennan AH, Lambert PC, Jones D, de Swiet M, Taylor DJ: Automated, ambulatory, or conventional blood pressure measurement in pregnancy: which is the better predictor of severe hypertension? *Am J Obstet Gynecol* 178:521–526, 1998.

Pepine CJ, Abrams J, Marks RG, Morris JJ, Scheidt SS, Handberg E; the TIDES Investigators: Characteristics of a contemporary population with angina pectoris. *Am J Cardiol* 74:226–231, 1994.

Pepine CJ, Kerensky RA, Lambert CR, Smith KM, von Mering GO, Sopko G, Bairey Merz CN: Some thoughts on the vasculopathy of women with ischemic heart disease. *J Am Coll Cardiol* 47 (Suppl 3):S30–S35, 2006.

Perez A, Carreras G, Caixas A, Castellvi A, Caballero A, Bonet R, Ordonez-Llanos J, de Leiva A: Plasma lipoprotein(a) levels are not influenced by glycemic control in type 1 diabetes. *Diabetes Care* 21:1517–1520, 1998.

Perez A, Wagner AM, Carreras G, Gimenez G, Sanchez-Quesada JL, Rigla M, Gomez-Gerique JA, Pou JM, de Leiva A: Prevalence and phenotype distribution of dyslipidemia in type 1 diabetes mellitus. Effect of glycemic control. *Arch Intern Med* 160:2756–2762, 2000.

Perez-Aytes A, Ledo A, Boso V, Saenz P, Roma E, Poveda JL, Vento M: In utero exposure to mycophenolate mofetil: a characteristic phenotype? *Am J Med Genet* A 146:1–7, 2008.

Perez-Maraver M, Carrera MJ, Micalo T, Sahun M, Vinzia C, Soler J, Montanya E: Renoprotective effect of diltiazem in hypertensive type 2 diabetic patients with persistent microalbuminuria despite ACE inhibitor treatment. *Diabetes Res Clin Pract* 70:13–19, 2005.

Pergola PE, Kancharia A, Riley DJ: Kidney transplantation during the first trimester of pregnancy: immunosuppression with mycophenolate mofetil, tacrolimus, and prednisone. *Transplantation* 71:994–997, 2001.

Perkins BA, Olaleye D, Zinman B, Bril V: Simple screening tests for peripheral neuropathy in the diabetes clinic. *Diabetes Care* 24:250–256, 2001.

Perkins BA, Ficociello LH, Silva KH, Finkelstein DM, Warram JH, Krolewski AS: Regression of microalbuminuria in type 1 diabetes. *N Engl J Med* 348: 2285–2293, 2003.

Perkins BA, Nelson RG, Ostrander BEP, Blouch KL, Krolewski AS, Myers BD, Warram JH: Detection of renal function decline in patients with diabetes and normal or elevated GFR by serial measurements of serum cystatin C concentration: results of a 4–year follow-up study. *J Am Soc Nephrol* 16: 1404–1421, 2005a.

Perkins BA, Krowlewski AS: Early nephropathy in type 1 diabetes: a new perspective on who will and who will not progress. *Curr Diab Rep* 5:455–463, 2005b.

Perkins BA, Bril V: Early vascular risk factor modification in type 1 diabetes. Editorial. *N Engl J Med* 352:408–409, 2005c.

Perkins BA, Ficociello LH, Ostrander BE, Silva KH, Weinberg J, Warram JH, Krolewski AS: Microalbuminuria and the risk for early progressive renal function decline in type 1 diabetes. *J Am Soc Nephrol* 18:1353–1361, 2007.

Perrin NE, Torbjornsdotter TB, Jaremko GA, Berg UB: Follow-up of kidney biopsies in normoalbuminuric patients with type 1 diabetes. *Pediatr Nephrol* 19: 1004–1013, 2004.

Perrone RD, Madias NE, Levey AS: Serum creatinine as an index of renal function: new insights into old concepts. *Clin Chem* 38:1933–1953, 1992.

Perros P, McCrimmon RJ, Shaw G, Frier BM: Frequency of thyroid dysfunction in diabetic patients: value of annual screening. *Diabet Med* 12:622–627, 1995.

Perros P, Singh RK, Ludlam CA, Frier BM: Prevalence of pernicious anemia in patients with type 1 diabetes mellitus and autoimmune thyroid disease. *Diabet Med* 17:749–751, 2000.

Perseghin G, Lattuada G, Danna M, Serini LP, Maffi P, De Cobelli F, Battezzati A, Secchi A, Del Machio A, Luzi L: Insulin resistance, intramyocellular lipid content, and plasma adiponectin in patients with type 1 diabetes. *Am J Physiol* 285:E1174–E1181, 2003.

Peterson CM, Jovanovic-Peterson L, Mills JL, Conley MR, Knopp RH, Reed GF, Aarons JH, Holmes LB, Brown Z, Van Allen M, Schmeltz R, Metzger BE; the National Institute of Child Health and Human Development—The Diabetes in Early Pregnancy Study: The Diabetes in Early Pregnancy Study: Changes in cholesterol, triglycerides, body weight, and blood pressure. *Am J Obstet Gynecol* 166:513–518, 1992.

Pettitt DJ, Saad MF, Bennett PH, Nelson RG, Knowler WC: Familial predisposition to renal disease in two generations of Pima Indians with type 2 (non-insulin-dependent) diabetes mellitus. *Diabetologia* 33:438–443, 1990.

Phelps RL, Sakol P, Metzger BE, Jampol LM, Freinkel N: Changes in diabetic retinopathy during pregnancy: correlations with regulation of hyperglycemia. *Arch Ophthalmol* 104:1806–1810, 1986.

Philpott S, Boynton PM, Feder G, Hemingway H: Gender differences in description of angina symptoms and health problems immediately prior to angiography: the ACRE study. *Soc Sci Med* 52:1565–1575, 2001.

Phippard AF, Fischer WE, Horvath JS, Child AG, Korda AR, Henderson-Smart D, Duggin GG, Tiller DJ: Early blood pressure control improves pregnancy outcome in primigravid women with mild hypertension. *Med J Aust* 154: 378–382, 1991.

Picano E: Diabetic cardiomyopathy: the importance of being earliest. Editorial. *J Am Coll Cardiol* 42:454–457, 2003a.

Picano E: Stress echocardiography: a historical perspective. *Am J Med* 114:126–130, 2003b.

Piccini JP, Klein L, Gheorghiade M, Bonow RO: New insights into diastolic heart failure: role of diabetes mellitus. A symposium. *Am J Med* 116:64S–75S, 2004.

Pichard L, Gillet G, Fabre I, Dalet-Beluche I, Bonfils C, Thenot J-P, Maurel P: Identification of the rabbit and human cytochromes P-450IIIA as the major enzymes involved in the *N*-demethylation of diltiazem. *Drug Metab Dispos* 18:711–719, 1990.

Pickering TG, Davidson K, Gerin W, Schwartz JE: Masked hypertension. *Hypertension* 40:795–796, 2002.

Pickering TG, Hall JE, Appel LJ, Falkner BE, Graves J, Hill MN, Jones DW, Kurtz T, Sheps SG, Rocella EJ: Recommendations for blood pressure measurement in humans and experimental animals. Part 1: Blood pressure measurement in humans. A statement for professionals from the Subcommittee of Professional and Public Education of the American Heart Association Council on High Blood Pressure Research. *Hypertension* 45:142–161, 2005.

Pickering TG, Shimbo D, Haas D: Ambulatory blood-pressure monitoring. *N Engl J Med* 354:2368–2374, 2006.

Pickles CJ, Symonds EM, Broughton Pipkin F: The fetal outcome of early intervention therapy in pregnancy-induced hypertension. A multicenter randomized double blind controlled trial of labetalol versus placebo. *Br J Obstet Gynecol* 96:38–43, 1989.

Pickles CJ, Broughton Pipkin F, Symonds EM: A randomized placebo controlled trial of labetalol in the treatment of mild to moderate pregnancy induced hypertension. *Br J Obstet Gynecol* 99:964–968, 1992.

Piconi L, Quagliaro L, Da Ros R, Assaloni R, Giugliano D, Esposito K, Szabo C, Ceriello A: Intermittent high glucose enhances ICAM-1, VCAM-1, E-selectin and interleukin-6 expression in human umbilical endothelial cells in culture: the role of poly(ADP-ribose) polymerase. *J Thromb Haemost* 2:1453–1459, 2004.

Pieper GM, Jordan M, Dondlinger LA, Adams MB, Roza AM: Peroxidative stress in diabetic blood vessels: reversed by pancreatic islet transplantation. *Diabetes* 44:884–889, 1995.

Pietrement C, Malot L, Santerne B, Roussel B, Motte J, Morville P: Neonatal acute renal failure secondary to maternal exposure to telmisartan, angiotensin II receptor antagonist. *J Perinatol* 23:254–255, 2003.

Piha SJ, Halonen JP: Effect of disease duration on cardiac autonomic reflexes in young patients with insulin-dependent diabetes mellitus. *Diabetes Res Clin Pract* 18:61–67, 1992.

Pinhas-Hamiel O, Dolan LM, Daniels SR, Standiford D, Khoury PR, Zeitler P: Increased incidence of non-insulin-dependent diabetes mellitus among adolescents. *J Pediatr* 128:608–615, 1996.

Pinhas-Hamiel O, Zeitler P: Type 2 diabetes in adolescents—no longer rare. *Pediatr Rev* 19:434–435, 1998.

Pinhas-Hamiel O, Zeitler P: The global spread of type 2 diabetes mellitus in children and adolescents. *J Pediatr* 146:693–700, 2005.

Pinhas-Hamiel O, Zeitler P: Acute and chronic complications of type 2 diabetes mellitus in children and adolescents. *Lancet* 369:1823–1831, 2007.

Pirhonen JP, Erkkola RU, Ekblad UU: Uterine and fetal flow velocity waveforms in hypertensive pregnancy: the effect of a single dose of nifedipine. *Obstet Gynecol* 76:37–41, 1990a.

Pirhonen JP, Erkkola RU, Ekblad UU, Nyman L: Single dose of nifedipine in normotensive pregnancy: nifedipine concentrations, hemodynamic responses, and uterine and fetal flow velocity waveforms. *Obstet Gynecol* 76:807–811, 1990b.

Pirhonen JP, Erkkola RU, Makinen JI, Ekblad UU: Single dose of labetalol in hypertensive pregnancy: effects on maternal hemodynamics and uterine and fetal flow velocity waveforms. *J Perinat Med* 19:167–171, 1991.

Pitocco D, Di Stasio E, Romitelli F, Zaccardi F, Tavazzi B, Manto A, Caputo S, Musella T, Zuppi C, Santini SA, Ghirlanda G: Hypouricemia linked to an overproduction of nitric oxide is an early marker of oxidative stress in female subjects with type 1 diabetes. *Diabetes Metab Res Rev* Feb 6 2008 (Epub ahead of print).

Pitt BD, Waters D, Brown WV, van Boven AJ, Schwartz L, Title LM, Eisenberg D, Shurzinske L, McCormick LS: Aggressive lipid-lowering therapy compared with angioplasty in stable coronary artery disease. Atorvastatin versus Revascularization Treatment Investigators. *N Engl J Med* 341:70–77, 1999.

Plouin P-F, Breart G, Maillard F, Papiernik E, Relier J-P; the Labetalol Methyldopa Study Group: Comparison of antihypertensive efficacy and perinatal safety of labetalol and methyldopa in the treatment of hypertension in pregnancy: a randomized controlled trial. *Br J Obstet Gynecol* 95:868–876, 1988.

Podjarny E, Haskiah A, Pomeranz A, Bernheim J, Green J, Rathaus M, Bernheim J: Effect of diltiazem and methyldopa on gestation-related renal complications in rats with adriamycin nephrosis. Relationship to glomerular prostanoid synthesis. *Nephrol Dial Transplant* 10:1598–1602, 1995.

Podjarny E, Benchetrit S, Katz B, Green J, Bernheim J: Effect of methyldopa on renal function in rats with L-NAME-induced hypertension in pregnancy. *Nephron* 88:354–359, 2001.

Poggio ED, Nef P, Wang X, Greene T, Van Lente F, Dennis VW, Hall PM: Performance of the Cockcroft-Gault and Modification of Diet in Renal Disease equations in estimating GFR in ill hospitalized patients. *Am J Kidney Dis* 46:242–252, 2005.

Pombar X, Strassner HT, Fenner PC: Pregnancy in a woman with class H diabetes mellitus and previous coronary artery bypass graft: a case report and review of the literature. *Obstet Gynecol* 85:825–829, 1995.

Poornima IG, Parikh P, Shannon RP: Diabetic cardiomyopathy: the search for a unifying hypothesis. *Circ Res* 98:596–605, 2006.

Pop VJ, de Vries E, van Baar AL, Waelkens JJ, de Rooy HA, Horsten M, Donkers MM, Komproe IH, van Son MM, Vader HL: Maternal thyroid peroxidase antibodies during pregnancy: a marker of impaired child development? *J Clin Endocrinol Metab* 80:3561–3566, 1995.

Pop VJ, Kuijpens JL, van Baar AL, Verkerk G, van Son MM, de Vijlder JJ, Vulsma T, Wiersinga WM, Drexhage HA, Vader HL: Low maternal free thyroxine concentrations during early pregnancy are associated with impaired psychomotor development in infancy. *Clin Endocrinol* 50:149–155, 1999.

Pop VJ, Brouwers EP, Vader HL, Vulsma T, van Baar AL, de Vijlder JJ: Maternal hypothyroxinemia during early pregnancy and subsequent child development: a 3-year follow-up study. *Clin Endocrinol* 59:282–288, 2003.

Pop VJ, Vulsma T: Maternal hypothyroxinemia during (early) gestation. Commentary. *Lancet* 365:1604–1606, 2005.

Poppas A, Shroff SG, Korcaz CE, Hibbard JU, Berger DS, Lindheimer MD, Lang RM: Serial assessment of the cardiovascular system in normal pregnancy. Role of arterial compliance and pulsatile arterial load. *Circulation* 95:2407–2415, 1997.

Poppe K, Glinoer D: Thyroid autoimmunity and hypothyroidism before and during pregnancy. *Hum Reprod Update* 9:149–161, 2003.

Porta M, Allione A: Current approaches and perspectives in the medical treatment of diabetic retinopathy. *Pharmacol Therapeut* 103:167–177, 2004.

Poulaki V, Qin W, Joussen AM, Hurlbut P, Wiegand SJ, Rudge J, Yancopoulos GD, Adamis AP: Acute intensive insulin therapy exacerbates diabetic blood-retinal barrier breakdown via hypoxia-inducible factor-1α and VEGF. *J Clin Invest* 109:805–815, 2002.

Poulaki V, Joussen AM, Mitsiades CS, Iliaki EF, Adamis AP: Insulin-like growth factor-I plays a pathogenetic role in diabetic retinopathy. *Am J Pathol* 165:457–469, 2004.

Powers RW, Bodnar LM, Ness RB, Cooper KM, Gallaher MJ, Frank MP, Daftary AR, Roberts JM: Uric acid concentrations in early pregnancy among preeclamptic women with gestational hyperuricemia at delivery. *Am J Obstet Gynecol* 194:160, 2006.

PPP—Primary Prevention Project Collaborative Group: Low-dose aspirin and vitamin E in people at cardiovascular risk: a randomized trial in general practice. *Lancet* 357:89–95, 2001.

Pratt DE, Kaberlein G, Dudkiewicz A, Karande V, Gleicher N: The association of antithyroid antibodies in euthyroid nonpregnant women with recurrent first trimester abortions in the next pregnancy. *Fertil Steril* 60:1001–1005, 1993.

Premawardhana LD, Parkes AB, Ammari F, John R, Darke C, Adams H, Lazarus JH: Postpartum thyroiditis and long-term thyroid status: prognostic influence of thyroid peroxidase antibodies and ultrasound echogenicity. *J Clin Endocrinol Metab* 85:71–75, 2000.

Prevost RR, Akl SA, Whybrew WD, Sibai BM: Oral nifedipine pharmacokinetics in pregnancy-induced hypertension. *Pharmacotherapy* 12:174–177, 1992.

Prevost G, Phan TM, Mounier-Vehier C, Fontaine P: Control of cardiovascular risk factors in patients with type 2 diabetes and hypertension in a French national study (Phenomen). *Diabetes Metab* 31:479–485, 2005.

Price JH, Hadden DR, Archer DB, Harley JM: Diabetic retinopathy in pregnancy. *Br J Obstet Gynecol* 91:11–17, 1984.

Pryde PG, Sedman AB, Nugent CE: Angiotensin-converting enzyme inhibitor fetopathy. *J Am Soc Nephrol* 3:1575–1582, 1993.

Psallas M, Tentolouris N, Papadogiannis D, Doulgerakis D, Kokkinos A, Cokkinos DV, Katsilambros N: QT dispersion: comparison between participants with type 1 and 2 diabetes and association with microalbuminuria in diabetes. *J Diabetes Complications* 20:88–97, 2006.

PSC—Prospective Studies Collaboration: Age-specific relevance of usual blood pressure to vascular mortality: a meta-analysis of individual data for one million adults in 61 prospective studies. *Lancet* 360:1903–1913, 2002.

Purdy LP, Hantsch CE, Molitsch ME, Metzger BE, Phelps RL, Dooley SL, Kou SH: Effect of pregnancy on renal function in patients with moderate-to-severe diabetic renal insufficiency. *Diabetes Care* 19:1067–1074, 1996.

Purnell JQ, Marcovina SM, Hokanson JE, Kennedy H, Cleary PA, Steffes MW, Brunzell JD: Levels of lipoprotein(a), apolipoprotein B, and lipoprotein cholesterol distribution in IDDM. Results from follow-up in the Diabetes Control and Complications Trial. *Diabetes* 44:1218–1226, 1995.

Purnell JQ, Hokanson JE, Marcovina SM, Steffes MW, Cleary PA, Brunzell JD: Effects of excessive weight gain with intensive therapy of type 1 diabetes on lipid levels and blood pressure: results from the Diabetes Control and Complications Trial. *JAMA* 280:140–146, 1998.

Purnell JQ, Dev RK, Steffes MW, Cleary PA, Palmer JP, Hirsch IB, Hokanson JE, Brunzell JD: Relationship of family history of type 2 diabetes, hypoglycemia, and autoantibodies to weight gain and lipids with intensive and conventional therapy in the Diabetes Control and Complications Trial. *Diabetes* 52: 2623–2629, 2003.

Puzey MS, Ackovic KL, Lindow SW, Gonin R: The effect on nifedipine on fetal umbilical artery Doppler waveforms in pregnancies complicated by hypertension. *S Afr Med J* 79:192–194, 1991.

Pyorala K, Lehto S, De Bacquer D, De Sutter J, Sans S, Keil U, Wood D, De Backer G: Risk factor management in diabetic and non-diabetic patients with coronary heart disease: findings from the EUROASPIRE I and II surveys. *Diabetologia* 47:1257–1265, 2004.

Quadri KHM, Bernardini J, Greenberg A, Laifer S, Syed A, Holley JL: Assessment of renal function during pregnancy using a random urine protein to creatinine ratio and Cockcroft-Gault formula. *Am J Kidney Dis* 24:416–420, 1994.

Quinn M, Angelico MC, Warram JH, Krolewski AS: Familial factors determine the development of diabetic nephropathy in patients with IDDM. *Diabetologia* 39:940–945, 1996.

Quyyumi AA: Women and ischemic heart disease: pathophysiologic implications from the Women's Ischemia Syndrome Evaluation (WISE) study and future research steps. *J Am Coll Cardiol* 47: (Suppl 3):S66–S71, 2006.

Radaideh AR, Nusier MK, Amari FL, Bateiha AE, El-Khateeb MS, Naser AS, Ajlouni KM: Thyroid dysfunction in patients with type 2 diabetes mellitus in Jordan. *Saudi Med J* 25:1046–1050, 2004.

Rader DJ: Inflammatory markers of coronary risk. Editorial. *N Engl J Med* 343:1179–1182, 2000.

Rader DJ: Molecular regulation of HDL metabolism and function: implications for novel therapies. *J Clin Invest* 116:3090–3100, 2006.

Raev DC: Which left ventricular function is impaired earlier in the evolution of diabetic cardiomyopathy? An echocardiographic study of young type 1 diabetic patients. *Diabetes Care* 17:633–639, 1994.

Raggi P, Bellasi A, Ratti C: Ischemia imaging and plaque imaging in diabetes: complementary tools to improve cardiovascular risk management. *Diabetes Care* 28:2787–2794, 2005.

Ragonese P, Ferrazza A, Paolini A, Reale F: Left ventricular diastolic filling in type 1 diabetes mellitus: a pulsed Doppler echocardiographic study. *Eur J Med* 1:69–74, 1992.

Rahman W, Rahman FZ, Yassin S, Al-Suleiman SA, Rahman J: Progression of retinopathy during pregnancy in type 1 diabetes mellitus. *Clin Experiment Ophthalmol* 35:231–236, 2007.

Raja SN, Hatthornthwaite JA: Combination therapy for neuropathic pain—which drugs, which combination, which patients? Editorial. *N Engl J Med* 352: 1373–1375, 2005.

Rajagopalan N, Miller TD, Hodge DO, Frye RL, Gibbons RJ: Identifying high-risk asymptomatic diabetic patients who are candidates for screening stress single-photon emission computed tomography imaging. *J Am Coll Cardiol* 45:43–49, 2005.

Rajan SK, Gokhale SM: Cardiovascular function in patients with insulin-dependent diabetes mellitus: a study using noninvasive methods. *Ann N Y Acad Sci* 958:425–430, 2002.

Raju B, McGregor VP, Cryer PE: Cortisol elevations comparable to those that occur during hypoglycemia do not cause hypoglycemia-associated autonomic failure. *Diabetes* 52:2083–2089, 2003.

Raju B, Cryer PE: Loss of the decrement in intraislet insulin plausibly explains loss of the glucagon response to hypoglycemia in insulin deficient diabetes. *Diabetes* 54:757–764, 2005.

Raju B, Arbelaez AM, Breckenridge SM, Cryer PE: Nocturnal hypoglycemia in type 1 diabetes: an assessment of preventive bedtime treatments. *J Clin Endocrinol Metab* 91:2087–2092, 2006.

Ramanathan V, Goral S, Tanriover B, Feurer ID, Kazancioglu R, Shaffer D, Helderman JH: Screening asymptomatic diabetic patients for coronary artery disease prior to renal transplantation. *Transplantation* 79:1453–1458, 2005.

Ramos JG, Martins-Costa SH, Mathias MM, Guerin YL, Barros EG: Urinary protein/creatinine ratio in hypertensive pregnant women. *Hypertens Preg* 18: 209–218, 1999.

Rana BS, Lim PO, Naas AA, Ogston SA, Newton RW, Jung RT, Morris AD, Struthers AD: QT interval abnormalities are often present at diagnosis in diabetes and are better predictors of cardiac death than ankle brachial pressure index and autonomic function tests. *Heart* 91:44–50, 2005.

Rana BS, Davies JI, Band MM, Pringle SD, Morris A, Struthers AD: B-type natriuretic peptide can detect silent myocardial ischemia in asymptomatic type 2 diabetes. *Heart* 92:916–920, 2006.

Rao GN, Corson MA, Berk BC: Uric acid stimulates vascular smooth muscle proliferation by increasing platelet derived growth factor A-chain expression. *J Biol Chem* 266:8604–8608, 1991.

Rasanen J, Jouppila P: Uterine and fetal hemodynamics and fetal cardiac function after atenolol and pindolol infusion. A randomized study. *Eur J Obstet Gynecol Reprod Biol* 62:195–201, 1995.

Rashba EJ, Zareba W, Moss AJ, Hall WJ, Robinson J, Locati EH, Schwartz PJ, Andrews M: Influence of pregnancy on the risk for cardiac events in patients with hereditary long QT syndrome. LQTS investigators. *Circulation* 97: 451–456, 1998.

Rathmann W, Ziegler D, Jahnke M, Haastert B, Gries FA: Mortality in diabetic patients with cardiovascular autonomic neuropathy. *Diabet Med* 10:820–824, 1993a.

Rathmann W, Hauner H, Dannehl K, Gries FA: Association of elevated serum uric acid with coronary heart disease in diabetes mellitus. *Diabetes Metab* 19: 159–166, 1993b.

Ray JG, Burrows RF, Burrows EA, Vermeulen MJ: MOS HIP: McMaster outcome study of hypertension in pregnancy. *Early Hum Dev* 64:129–143, 2001a.

Ray JG, Vermeulen MJ, Burrows EA, Burrows RF: Use of antihypertensive medications in pregnancy and the risk of adverse pregnancy outcomes: McMaster Outcome Study of Hypertension in Pregnancy 2 (MOS HIP 2). *BMC Pregnancy and Childbirth* 1:6, 2001b. Available at: www.biomedcentral.com/1471–2393/1/6. Accessed Apr 17, 2008.

Rayburn W, Piehl E, Jacober S, Schork A, Ploughman L: Severe hypoglycemia during pregnancy: its frequency and predisposing factors in diabetic women. *Int J Gynecol Obstet* 24:263–268, 1986.

Rayburn W, Piehl E, Sanfield J, Compton A: Reversing severe hypoglycemia during pregnancy with glucagon therapy. *Am J Perinatol* 4:259–261, 1987.

Razvi S, Ingoe L, Keeka G, Oates C, McMillan C, Weaver JU: The beneficial effect of L-thyroxine on cardiovascular risk factors, endothelial function, and quality of life in subclinical hypothyroidism: randomized, crossover trial. *J Clin Endocrinol Metab* 92:1715–1723, 2007.

Redberg RF, Greenland P, Fuster V, Pyorala K, Blair SN, Folsom AR, Newman AB, O'Leary DH, Orchard TJ, Psaty B, Schwartz JS, Starke R, Wilson PWF: AHA Conference Proceedings. Prevention Conference VI. Diabetes and Cardiovascular Disease. Writing Group III: Risk assessment in persons with diabetes. *Circulation* 105:e144–e152, 2002. Available at: http://circ.ahajournals.org/cgi/reprint/105/18/e144?maxtoshow=&HITS=10&hits=10&RESULTFORMAT=&fulltext-Risk+assessment+in+persons ı with ı diabetes&searchid-1&FIRSTINDEX=0&resourcetype=HWCIT. Accessed Apr 9, 2008.

Reddy SS, Holley JL: Management of the pregnant chronic dialysis patient. *Adv Chronic Kidney Dis* 14:146–155, 2007.

Redman CWG, Beilin LJ, Bonnar J, Ounsted MK: Fetal outcome in trial of antihypertensive treatment in pregnancy. *Lancet* 2:753–756, 1976.

Redman CWG, Beilin LG, Bonnar J: Treatment of hypertension in pregnancy with methyldopa: blood pressure control and side effects. *Br J Obstet Gynecol* 84: 419–426, 1977.

Reece EA, Coustan DR, Hayslett JP, Holford T, Coulehan J, O'Connor TZ, Hobbins JC: Diabetic nephropathy: pregnancy performance and fetomaternal outcome. *Am J Obstet Gynecol* 159:56–66, 1988.

Reece EA, Winn HN, Hayslett JP, Coulehan J, Wan M, Hobbins JC: Does pregnancy alter the rate of progression of diabetic nephropathy? *Am J Perinatol* 7:193–197, 1990.

Reece EA, Lockwood CJ, Tuck S, Coulehan J, Homko C, Wisnitzer A, Puklin J: Retinal and pregnancy outcomes in the presence of diabetic proliferative retinopathy. *J Reprod Med* 39:799–804, 1994.

Reece EA, Hagay Z, Roberts AB, DeGennaro N, Homko CJ, Connolly-Diamond, M, Sherwin R, Tamborlane WV, Diamond MP: Fetal Doppler and behavioral responses during hypoglycemia induced with the insulin clamp technique in pregnant diabetic women. *Am J Obstet Gynecol* 172:151–155, 1995.

Reece EA, Homko CJ, Hagay Z: Diabetic retinopathy in pregnancy. *Obstet Gynecol Clin North Am* 23:161–171, 1996.

Reece EA, Leguizamon G, Homko C: Pregnancy performance and outcomes associated with diabetic nephropathy. *Am J Perinatol* 15:413–421, 1998a.

Reece EA, Leguizamon G, Homko C: Stringent controls in diabetic nephropathy associated with optimization of pregnancy outcomes. *J Matern-Fetal Med* 7: 213–216, 1998b.

Reece EA, Homko C, Miodovnik M, Langer O: A consensus report of the Diabetes in Pregnancy Study Group of North America Conference 2002. *J Matern Fetal Neonatal Med* 12:362–364, 2002.

Reichard P, Pihl M, Rosenqvist U, Sule J: Complications in IDDM are caused by elevated blood glucose level: the Stockholm Diabetes Intervention Study (SDIS) at 10-year follow-up. *Diabetologia* 39:1483–1488, 1996.

Reichard P, Jensen-Urstad K, Ericsson M, Jensen-Urstad M, Lindblad LE: Autonomic neuropathy—a complication less pronounced in patients with type 1 diabetes mellitus who have lower blood glucose levels. *Diabet Med* 17:860–866, 2000.

Rein AJ, O'Donnell C, Geva T, Nir A, Perles Z, Hashimoto I, Li XK, Sahn DJ: Use of tissue velocity imaging in the diagnosis of fetal cardiac arrythmias. *Circulation* 106:1827–1833, 2002.

Reinehr T, Schober E, Wiegand S, Thon A, Holl R; DPV-Wiss Study Group: Beta-cell autoantibodies in children with type 2 diabetes mellitus: subgroup or misclassification? *Arch Dis Child* 91:473–477, 2006.

Reiter CEN, Gardner TW: Retinal insulin and insulin signaling: implications for diabetic retinopathy. *Prog Retin Eye Res* 22:545–562, 2003.

Remuzzi G: Nephropathic nature of proteinuria. *Curr Opin Nephrol Hypertens* 8: 655–663, 1999.

Remuzzi G, Benigni A, Remuzzi A: Mechanisms of progression and regression of renal lesions of chronic nephropathies and diabetes. Scientific review. *J Clin Invest* 116:288–296, 2006.

Remuzzi G, Cravedi P, Costantini M, Lesti M, Ganeva M, Gherardi G, Ene-Iordache B, Gotti E, Donati D, Salvadori M, Sandrini S, Segoloni G, Federico S, Rigotti P, Sparacino V, Ruggenenti P; the MYSS Follow-Up Study Group: Mycophenolate mofetil versus azathioprine for prevention of chronic allograft dysfunction in renal transplantation: the MYSS Follow-Up randomized controlled trial. *J Am Soc Nephrol* 18:1880–1888, 2007.

Resnik JL, Hong C, Resnik R, Kazanegra R, Beede J, Bhalla V, Maisel A: Evaluation of B-type natriuretic peptide (BNP) levels in normal and preeclamptic women. *Am J Obstet Gynecol* 193:450–454, 2005.

Retnakaran R, Hanley AJ, Raif N, Connelly PW, Sermer M, Zinman B: C-reactive protein and gestational diabetes: the central role of maternal obesity. *J Clin Endocrinol Metab* 88:3507–3512, 2003.

Retnakaran R, Cull CA, Thorne KI, Adler AI, Holman RR; the UKPDS Study Group: Risk factors for renal dysfunction in type 2 diabetes. U.K. Prospective Diabetes Study 74. *Diabetes* 55:1832–1839, 2006.

Rewers M, Shetterly SM, Baxter J, Marshall JA, Hamman RF: Prevalence of coronary heart disease in subjects with normal and impaired glucose tolerance and non-insulin-dependent diabetes mellitus in a biethnic Colorado population. The San Luis Valley Diabetes Study. *Am J Epidemiol* 135: 1321–1327, 1992.

Rey E: Effects of methyldopa on umbilical and placental artery blood flow velocity waveforms. *Obstet Gynecol* 80:783–787, 1992.

Rey E, Couturier A: The prognosis of pregnancy in women with chronic hypertension. *Am J Obstet Gynecol* 171:410–416, 1994.

Rey E, LeLorier J, Burgess E, Lange I, Leduc L: Report of the Canadian Hypertension Society Consensus Conference: 3. Pharmacologic treatment of hypertensive disorders in pregnancy. *Can Med Assoc J* 157:1245–1254, 1997.

Rey E, Pilon F, Boudreault J: Home blood pressure levels in pregnant women with chronic hypertension. *Hypertens Pregnancy* 26:403–414, 2007.

Rhodes RW, Ogburn PL: Treatment of severe diabetic ketoacidosis in the early third trimester in a patient with fetal distress. *J Reprod Med* 299:621–624, 1984.

Richards M, Nicholls MG, Espiner EA, Lainchbury JG, Troughton RW, Elliott J, Frampton CM, Crozier IG, Yandle TG, Doughty R, MacMahon S, Sharpe N; the Christchurch Cardioendocrine Research Group and the Australia-New Zealand Heart Failure Group: Comparison of B-type natriuretic peptides for assessment of cardiac function and prognosis in stable ischemic heart disease. *J Am Coll Cardiol* 47:52–60, 2006.

Ridker PM, Hennekens CH, Tofler GH, Lipinska I, Buring JE: Anti-platelet effects of 100 mg alternate day oral aspirin: a randomized, double-blind, placebo-controlled trial of regular and enteric coated formulations in men and women. *J Cardiovasc Risk* 3:209–212, 1996.

Ridker PM, Hennekens CH, Buring JE, Fifai N: C-reactive protein and other markers of inflammation in the prediction of cardiovascular disease in women. *N Engl J Med* 342:836–843, 2000.

Ridker PM, Cook NR, Lee I-M, Gordon D, Gaziano JM, Manson JE, Hennekens CH, Buring JE: A randomized trial of low-dose aspirin in the primary prevention of cardiovascular disease in women. *N Engl J Med* 352:1293–1304, 2005.

Rigalleau V, Lasseur C, Perlemoine C, Barthe N, Raffaitin C, Liu C, Chauveau P, Baillet-Blanco L, Beauvieux M-C, Combe C, Gin H: Estimation of glomerular filtration rate in diabetic subjects. Cockcroft formula or Modification of Diet in renal disease study equation? *Diabetes Care* 28:838–843, 2005.

Riihimaa PH, Knip M, Hirvela H, Tapanainen P: Metabolic characteristics and urine albumin excretion rate in relation to pubertal maturation in type 1 diabetes. *Diabetes Metab Res Rev* 16:269–275, 2000.

Riihimaa PH, Suominen K, Knip M, Tapanainen P, Tolonen U: Cardiovascular autonomic reactivity is decreased in adolescents with type 1 diabetes. *Diabet Med* 19:932–938, 2002.

Riley WJ, Toskes PP, Maclaren NK, Silverstein JH: Predictive value of gastric parietal cell autoantibodies as a marker for gastric and hematologic abnormalities associated with insulin-dependent diabetes. *Diabetes* 31:1051–1055, 1982.

Risberg A, Larsson A, Olsson K, Lyrenas S, Sjoquist M: Relationship between urinary albumin and albumin/creatinine ratio during normal pregnancy and preeclampsia. *Scand J Clin Lab Invest* 64:17–24, 2004.

Ritz E, Orth SR: Nephropathy in patients with type 2 diabetes mellitus. *N Engl J Med* 341:1127–1133, 1999.

Ritz E: Albuminuria and vascular damage—the vicious twins. Essay. *N Engl J Med* 348:2349–2352, 2003.

Robert M, Sepandj F, Liston RM, Dooley KC: Random protein-creatinine ratio for the quantitation of proteinuria in pregnancy. *Obstet Gynecol* 90:893–895, 1997.

Roberts M, Lindheimer MD, Davison JM: Altered glomerular permselectivity to neutral dextrans and heteroporous membrane modeling in human pregnancy. *Am J Physiol* 270:F338–F343, 1996.

Roberts LJ II, Morrow JD: The generation and actions of isoprostanes. *Biochim Biophys Acta* 1345:121–135, 1997.

Roberts JM, Bodnar LM, Lain KY, Hubel CA, Markovic N, Ness RB, Powers RW: Uric acid is as important as proteinuria in identifying fetal risk in women with gestational hypertension. *Hypertension* 46:1263–1269, 2005.

Robinson RT, Harris ND, Ireland RH, Lee S, Newman C, Heller SR: Mechanisms of abnormal cardiac repolarization during insulin-induced hypoglycemia. *Diabetes* 52:1469–1474, 2003.

Robinson RT, Harris ND, Ireland RH, Macdonald IA, Heller SR: Changes in cardiac repolarization during clinical episodes of nocturnal hypoglycemia in adults with type 1 diabetes. *Diabetologia* 47:312–315, 2004.

Robson SC, Hunter S, Boys RJ, Dunlop W: Serial study of factors influencing changes in cardiac output during human pregnancy. *Am J Physiol* 256:H1060–H1065, 1989.

Rochon C, Tauveron I, Dejax C, Benoits P, Capitan P, Fabricio A, Berry C, Champedon C, Thieblot P, Grizard J: Response of glucose disposal to hyperinsulinemia in human hypothyroidism and hyperthyroidism. *Clin Sci* 104:7–15, 2003.

Rodby RA, Rohde RD, Sharon Z, Pohl MA, Bain RP, Lewis EJ: The urine protein to creatinine ratio as a predictor of 24-hour urine protein excretion in type 1 diabetic patients with nephropathy. *Am J Kidney Dis* 26:904–909, 1995.

Rodgers BD, Rodgers DE: Clinical variables associated with diabetic ketoacidosis during pregnancy. *J Reprod Med* 36:797–800, 1991.

Rodriguez BL, Fujimoto WY, Mayer-Davis EJ, Imperatore G, Williams DE, Bell RA, Wadwa RP, Palla SL, Liu LL, Kershinar A, Daniels SR, Linder B; the SEARCH for Diabetes in Youth Study Group: Prevalence of cardiovascular disease risk factors in U.S. children and adolescents with diabetes. *Diabetes Care* 29:1891–1896, 2006.

Rodriguez-Thompson D, Lieberman ES: Use of a random urinary protein-to-creatinine ratio for the diagnosis of significant proteinuria during pregnancy. *Am J Obstet Gynecol* 185:808–811, 2001.

Roelants F, Lavand'homme PM, Mercier-Fuzier V: Epidural administration of neostigmine and clonidine to induce labor analgesia. *Anesthesiology* 102:1205–1210, 2005.

Rogers RC, Sibai BM, Whybrew WD: Labetolol pharmacokinetics in pregnancy-induced hypertension. *Am J Obstet Gynecol* 162:362–366, 1990.

Rogus JJ, Warram JH, Krolewski AS: Genetic studies of late diabetic complications. The overlooked importance of diabetes duration before complication onset. *Diabetes* 51:1655–1662, 2002.

Rohrer L, Hersberger M, von Eckardstein A: High density lipoproteins in the intersection of diabetes mellitus, inflammation and cardiovascular disease. *Curr Opin Lipidol* 15:269–278, 2004.

Romao JE Jr, Luders C, Kahhale S, Pascoal IJ, Abensur H, Sabbaga E, Zugaib M, Marcondes M: Pregnancy in women on chronic dialysis. A single-center experience with 17 cases. *Nephron* 78:416–422, 1998.

Ros HS, Lichtenstein P, Bellocco R, Peterson G, Cnattingius S: Pulmonary embolism and stroke in relation to pregnancy: how can high-risk women be identified? *Am J Obstet Gynecol* 186:198–203, 2002.

Rosa FW, Bosco LA, Graham CF, Milstien JB, Dreis M, Creamer J: Neonatal anuria with maternal angiotensin-converting enzyme inhibition. *Obstet Gynecol* 74:371–374, 1989.

Rosano GM, Vitale C, Fragasso G: Metabolic therapy for patients with diabetes mellitus and coronary artery disease. *Am J Cardiol* 98:14J-18J, 2006.

Rose GA: The diagnosis of ischemic heart pain and intermittent claudication in field surveys. *Bull World Health Organization* 27:645–658, 1962.

Rosenbloom AL, Joe JR, Young RS, Winter WE: Emerging epidemic of type 2 diabetes in youth. *Diabetes Care* 22:345–354, 1999.

Rosenn B, Miodovnik M, Kranias G, Khoury J, Combs CA, Mimouni F, Siddiqi TA, Lipman MJ: Progression of diabetic retinopathy in pregnancy: association with hypertension in pregnancy. *Am J Obstet Gynecol* 166:1214–1218, 1992.

Rosenn BM, Miodovnik M, Holcberg G, Khoury JC, Siddiqi TA: Hypoglycemia: the price of intensive insulin therapy for pregnant women with insulin-dependent diabetes mellitus. *Obstet Gynecol* 85:417–422, 1995a.

Rosenn B, Siddiqi TA, Miodovnik M: Normalization of blood glucose in insulin-dependent diabetic pregnancies and the risks of hypoglycemia: a therapeutic dilemma *Obstet Gynecol Surv* 50:56–61, 1995b.

Rosenn BM, Miodovnik M, Khoury JC, Siddiqi TA. Counterregulatory hormonal responses to hypoglycemia during pregnancy. *Obstet Gynecol* 87:568–574, 1996.

Rosenn BM, Miodovnik M: Medical complications of diabetes mellitus in pregnancy. *Clin Obstet Gynecol* 43:17–31, 2000.

Rosenthal T, Oparil S: The effect of antihypertensive drugs on the fetus. *J Hum Hypertens* 16:293–298, 2002.

Ross R: Atherosclerosis: an inflammatory disease. *N Engl J Med* 340:115–126, 1999.

Rossing P, Breum L, Major-Pedersen A, Sato A, Winding H, Pietersen A, Kastrup J, Parving HH: Prolonged QTc interval predicts mortality in patients with type 1 diabetes mellitus. *Diabet Med* 18:199–205, 2001.

Rossing P, Hougaard P, Parving HH: Risk factors for development of incipient and overt diabetic nephropathy in type 1 diabetic patients: a 10-year prospective observational study. *Diabetes Care* 25:859–864, 2002a.

Rossing K, Jacobsen P, Hommel E, Mathiesen E, Svenningsen A, Rossing P, Parving H-H: Pregnancy and progression of diabetic nephropathy. *Diabetologia* 45:36–41, 2002b.

Rossing K, Christensen PK, Hovind P, Parving HH: Remission of nephritic-range albuminuria reduces risk of end-stage renal disease and improves survival in type 2 diabetic patients. *Diabetologia* 48:2241–2247, 2005.

Rossing P, Rossing K, Gaede P, Pedersen O, Parving H-H: Monitoring kidney function in type 2 diabetic patients with incipient and overt diabetic nephropathy. *Diabetes Care* 29:1024–1030, 2006.

Ross-McGill H, Hewison J, Hirst J, Dowswell T, Holt A, Brunskill P, Thornton JG: Antenatal home blood pressure monitoring: a pilot randomized controlled trial. *BJOG* 107:217–221, 2000.

Rotchell YE, Cruickshank JK, Gay MP, Griffiths J, Stewart A, Farrell B, Ayers S, Hennis A, Grant A, Duley L, Collins R: Barbados Low Dose Aspirin Study in Pregnancy (BLASP): a randomized trial for the prevention of preeclampsia and its complications. *Br J Obstet Gynecol* 105:286–292, 1998.

Rothenbacher D, Koenig W, Brenner H: Comparison of N-terminal pro-B-natriuretic peptide, C-reactive protein, and creatinine clearance for prognosis in patients with known coronary heart disease. *Arch Intern Med* 166:2455–2460, 2006.

Ruberte J, Ayuso E, Navarro M, Carretero A, Nacher V, Haurigot V, George M, Llombart C, Casellas A, Costa C, Bosch A, Bosch F: Increased ocular levels of IGF-1 in transgenic mice lead to diabetes-like eye disease. *J Clin Invest* 113:1149–1157, 2004.

Rubin PC, Butters L, Kelman AW, Fitzsimons C, Reid JL: Labetalol disposition and concentration-effect relationships during pregnancy. *Br J Clin Pharmacol* 15:465–470, 1983a.

Rubin PC, Butters L, Reid JL: Clinical pharmacological studies with prazosin during pregnancy complicated by hypertension. *Br J Clin Pharmacol* 16:543–547, 1983b.

Rudberg S, Ullman E, Dahlquist G: Relationship between early metabolic control and the development of microalbuminuria; a longitudinal study in children with type 1 (insulin-dependent) diabetes mellitus. *Diabetologia* 36:1309–1314, 1993.

Rudberg S, Stattin EL, Dahlquist G: Familial and perinatal risk factors for micro- and macroalbuminuria in young IDDM patients. *Diabetes* 47:1121–1126, 1998.

Rule AD, Larson TS, Bergstralh EJ, Slezak JM, Jacobsen SJ, Cosio FG: Using serum creatinine to estimate glomerular filtration rate: accuracy in good health and in chronic kidney disease. *Ann Intern Med* 141:929–937, 2004.

Rule AD, Bergstralh EJ, Slezak JM, Bergert J, Larson TS: Glomerular filtration rate estimated by cystatin C among different clinical presentations. *Kidney Int* 69:399–405, 2006.

Russell RR III, Chyun D, Song S, Sherwin RS, Tamborlane WV, Lee FA, Pfeifer MA, Rife F, Wackers FJT, Young LH: Cardiac responses to insulin-induced hypoglycemia in nondiabetic and intensively treated type 1 diabetic patients. *Am J Physiol* 281:E1029–E1036, 2001.

Russo LM, Bakris GL, Comper WD: Renal handling of albumin: a critical review of basic concepts and perspective. *Am J Kidney Dis* 39:899–919, 2002.

Rutledge T, Reis SE, Olson MB, Owens J, Kelsey SF, Pepine CJ, Mankad S, Rogers WJ, Merz CN, Sopko G, Cornell CE, Sharaf B, Matthews KA, Vaccarino V: Depression symptom severity and reported treatment history in the prediction of cardiac risk in women with suspected myocardial ischemia: the NHLBI-sponsored WISE study. *Arch Gen Psychiatry* 63:874–880, 2006.

Rutter MK, McComb JM, Brady S, Marshall SM: Silent myocardial ischemia and microalbuminuria in asymptomatic subjects with non-insulin-dependent diabetes mellitus. *Am J Cardiol* 83:27–31, 1999.

Rutter MK, Wahid ST, McComb JM, Marshall SM: Significance of silent ischemia and microalbuminuria in predicting coronary events in asymptomatic patients with type 2 diabetes. *J Am Coll Cardiol* 40:56–61, 2002.

Rutter MK, Nesto RW: The changing costs and benefits of screening for asymptomatic coronary heart disease in patients with diabetes. *Nat Clin Pract Endocrinol Metab* 3:26–35, 2007.

Ryan CM, Williams TM, Finegold DN, Orchard TJ: Cognitive dysfunction in adults with type 1 (insulin-dependent) diabetes mellitus of long duration: effects of recurrent hypoglycemia and other chronic complications. *Diabetologia* 36:329–334, 1993.

Saadine JB, Engelgau MM, Beckles GL, Gregg EW, Thompson TJ, Narayan KM: A diabetes report card for the United States: quality of care in the 1990s. *Ann Intern Med* 136:565–574, 2002.

Sacco M, Pellegrini F, Roncaglioni MC, Avanzini F, Tognoni G; on behalf of the PPP Collaborative Group: Primary prevention of cardiovascular events with low-dose aspirin and vitamin E in type 2 diabetic patients. Results of the Primary Prevention Project (PPP) trial. *Diabetes Care* 26:3264–3272, 2003.

Sacks DA, Chen W, Greenspoon JS, Wolde-Tsadik G: Should the same glucose values be targeted for type 1 as for type 2 diabetics in pregnancy? *Am J Obstet Gynecol* 177:1113–1119, 1997.

Sacks DB, Bruns DE, Goldstein DE, Maclaren NK, McDonald JM, Parrot M: Guidelines and recommendations for laboratory analysis in the diagnosis and management of diabetes mellitus. *Clin Chem* 48:436–472, 2002.

Sacks GP, Seyani L, Lavery S, Trew G: Maternal C-reactive protein levels are raised at 4 weeks gestation. *Hum Reprod* 19:1025–1030, 2004.

Sadaniantz A, Kocheril AG, Emaus SP, Garber CE, Parisi AF: Cardiovascular changes in pregnancy evaluated by two-dimensional and Doppler echocardiography. *Am J Soc Echocard* 5:253–258, 1992.

Safar ME, Smulyan H: The blood pressure measurement—revisited. Editorial. *Am Heart J* 152:417–419, 2006.

Safley DM, Marso SP: Diabetes and percutaneous coronary intervention in the setting of acute coronary syndrome. *Diabetes Vasc Dis Res* 2:128–135, 2005.

Sagnella GA: Measurement and significance of circulating natriuretic peptides in cardiovascular disease. *Clin Sci* 95:519–529, 1998.

Saji H, Yamanaka M, Hagiwara A, Ijiri F: Losartan and fetal toxic effects. *Lancet* 357:363, 2001.

Sakamoto H, Misumi K, Matsuda Y, Ikenoue T: Effects of antihypertensive drugs on maternal and fetal hemodynamics and uterine blood flow in pregnant goats—comparison of nicardipine and labetalol. *J Vet Med Sci* 58:515–519, 1996.

Salam AM: Acute myocardial infarction in the first trimester of pregnancy. *Asian Cardiovasc Thorac Ann* 13:175–177, 2005.

Salles GF, Deccache W, Cardoso CR: Usefulness of QT-interval parameters for cardiovascular risk stratification in type 2 diabetic patients with arterial hypertension. *J Hum Hypertens* 19:241–249, 2005.

Salmela KT, Kyllonen LEJ, Holmberg C, Groenhagen-Riska C: Impaired renal function after pregnancy in renal transplant recipients. *Transplantation* 56:1372–1375, 1993.

Salonen R, Salonen JT: Progression of carotid atherosclerosis and its determinants: a population-based ultrasonography study. *Atherosclerosis* 81:33–40, 1990.

Sam F, Kerstetter DL, Pimental DR, Mulukutia S, Tabaee A, Bristow MR, Colucci WS, Sawyer DB: Increased reactive oxygen species production and functional alterations in antioxidant enzymes in human failing myocardium. *J Card Fail* 11:473–480, 2005.

Samadi A, Mayberry RM: Maternal hypertension and spontaneous preterm births among black women. *Obstet Gynecol* 91:899–904, 1998.

Sampson MJ, Chambers JB, Sprigings DC, Drury PL: Abnormal diastolic function in patients with type 1 diabetes and early nephropathy. *Br Heart J* 64:266–271, 1990.

Sampson MJ, Drury PL: Accurate estimation of glomerular filtration rate in diabetic nephropathy from age, body weight, and serum creatinine. *Diabetes Care* 15:609–612, 1992.

Sanchez-Lozada LG, Tapia E, Avila-Casado C, Soto V, Franco M, Santamaria J, Nakagawa T, Rodriguez-Iturbe B, Johnson RJ, Herrera-Acosta J: Mild hyperuricemia induces glomerular hypertension in normal rats. *Am J Physiol* 283: F1105–F1110, 2002.

Sanchez-Lozada LG, Nakagawa T, Kang D-H, Feig DI, Franco M, Johnson RJ, Herrera-Acosta J: Hormonal and cytokine effects of uric acid. *Curr Opin Nephrol Hypertens* 15:30–33, 2006.

Sander GE, Giles TD: Diabetes mellitus and heart failure. *Am Heart Hosp J* 1:273–280, 2003.

Sandoval DA, Ertl AC, Richardson A, Tate DB, Davis SN: Estrogen blunts neuroendocrine and metabolic responses to hypoglycemia. *Diabetes* 52:1749–1755, 2003.

Sangiorgi G, Rumberger JA, Severson A, Edwards WD, Gregoire J, Fitzpatrick LA, Schwartz RS: Arterial calcification and not lumen stenosis is highly correlated with atherosclerotic plaque burden in humans: a histologic study of 723 coronary artery segments using nondecalcifying methodology. *J Am Coll Cardiol* 31:126–133, 1998.

Sansom M, Vermeijden JR, Smout AJPM, Roelofs J, van Dam PS, Martens EP, Eelkman-Rooda SJ, van Berge-Henegouwen GP: Prevalence of delayed gastric emptying in diabetic patients and relationship to dyspeptic symptoms. A prospective study in unselected diabetic patients. *Diabetes Care* 26:3116–3122, 2003.

Saotome T, Minoura S, Terashi K, Sato T, Echizen H, Ishizaki T: Labetalol in hypertension during the third trimester of pregnancy: its antihypertensive effect and pharmacokinetic-dynamic analysis. *J Clin Pharmacol* 33:979–988, 1993.

Sarnak MJ, Levey AS, Schoolwerth AC, Coresh J, Culleton B, Hamm LL, McCullough PA, Kasiske BL, Kelepouris E, Klag MJ, Parfrey P, Pfeffer M, Raij L, Spinosa DJ, Wilson PW; American Heart Association Councils on Kidney in Cardiovascualr Disease, High Blood Pressure Research, Clinical Cardiology, and Epidemiology and Prevention: Kidney disease as a risk factor for development of cardiovascular disease: a statement from the American Heart Association. *Circulation* 108:2154–2169, 2003.

Sartipy P, Camejo G, Svensson L, Hurt-Camejo E: Phospholipase A_2 modification of low density lipoproteins forms small high density particles with increased affinity for proteoglycans and glycosaminoglycans. *J Biol Chem* 274:25913–25920, 1999.

Sarwar N, Danesh J, Eiriksdottir G, Sigurdsson G, Wareham N, Bingham S, Boekholdt SM, Khaw K-T, Gudnason V: Triglycerides and the risk of coronary heart disease. 10,158 incident cases among 262,525 participants in 29 western prospective studies. *Circulation* 115:450–458, 2007.

Sastry S, Riding G, Morris J, Taberner D, Cherry N, Heagerty A, McCollum C: Young adult myocardial infarction and ischemic stroke. *J Am Coll Cardiol* 48:686–691, 2006.

Sato A, Tarnow L, Parving HH: Prevalence of left ventricular hypertrophy in type I diabetic patients with diabetic nephropathy. *Diabetologia* 42:76–80, 1999.

Sato A, Tarnow L, Nielsen FS, Knudsen E, Parving HH: Left ventricular hypertrophy in normoalbuminuric type 2 diabetic patients not taking antihypertensive treatment. *QJM* 98:879–884, 2005.

Sator MO, Joura EA, Gruber DM, Obruca A, Zeisler H, Egarter C, Muber JC: Non-invasive detection of alterations of the carotid artery in pregnant women with high frequency ultrasound. *Ultrasound Obstet Gynecol* 13:260–262, 1999.

Sattar N, Greer IA, Louden J, Lindsay G, McConnell M, Shepherd J, Packard CJ: Lipoprotein subfraction changes in normal pregnancy: threshold effect of plasma triglyceride on appearance of small, dense low density lipoprotein. *J Clin Endocrinol Metab* 82:2483–2491, 1997.

Saudan PJ, Brown MA, Farrell T, Shaw L: Improved methods of assessing proteinuria in hypertensive pregnancy. *Br J Obstet Gynecol* 104:1159–1164, 1997.

Saudan P, Brown MA, Buddle ML, Jones M: Does gestational hypertension become pre-eclampsia? *Br J Obstet Gynecol* 105:1177–1184, 1998.

Savvidou MD, Gerrts L, Nicolaides KH: Impaired vascular reactivity in pregnant women with insulin-dependent diabetes. *Am J Obstet Gynecol* 186:84–88, 2002.

Saydah SH, Fradkin J, Cowie CC: Poor control of risk factors for vascular disease among adults with previously diagnosed diabetes. *JAMA* 291:2495–2499, 2004.

Scanu AM: Lp(a) lipoprotein—coping with heterogeneity. *N Engl J Med* 349:2089–2090, 2003.

Scardo JA, Vermillion ST, Newman RB, Chauhan SP, Hogg BB: A randomized, double-blind, hemodynamic evaluation of nifedipine and labetalol in preeclamptic hypertensive emergencies. *Am J Obstet Gynecol* 181:862–866, 1999.

Schaefer C: Angiotensin II-receptor-antagonists: further evidence of fetotoxicity but not teratogenicity. *Birth Defects Res (Part A) Clin Mol Teratol* 67:591–594, 2003.

Schannwell CM, Schmitz L, Schoebel FC, Zimmerman T, Marx R, Plehn G, Leschke M, Strauer BE: Left ventricular diastolic function in pregnancy in patients with arterial hypertension. A prospective study with M-mode echocardiography and Doppler echocardiography. *Z Kardiol* 90:427–436, 2001.

Schannwell CM, Schneppenheim M, Perings S, Plehn G, Strauer BE: Left ventricular diastolic dysfunction as an early manifestation of diabetic cardiomyopathy. *Cardiology* 98:33–39, 2002a.

Schannwell CM, Zimmermann T, Schneppenheim M, Plehn G, Marx R, Strauer BE: Left ventricular hypertrophy and diastolic dysfunction in healthy pregnant women. *Cardiology* 97:73–78, 2002b.

Schannwell CM, Schneppenheim M, Perings SM, Zimmerman T, Plehn G, Strauer BE: Alterations of left ventricular function in women with insulin-dependent diabetes mellitus during pregnancy. *Diabetologia* 46:267–275, 2003.

Schartl M, Bocksch W: How to assess coronary artery remodeling by intravascular ultrasound. *Am Heart J* 152:414–416, 2006.

Schaumberg DA, Glynn RJ, Jenkins AJ, Lyons TJ, Rifai N, Manson JE, Ridker PM, Nathan DM: Effect of intensive glycemic control on levels of markers of inflammation in type 1 diabetes mellitus in the Diabetes Control and Complications Trial. *Circulation* 111:2446–2453, 2005.

Scheetz MJ, King GL: Molecular understanding of hyperglycemia's adverse effects for diabetic complications. *JAMA* 288:2579–2588, 2002.

Scheidt-Nave C, Barrett-Connor E, Wingard DL: Resting electrocardiographic abnormalities suggestive of asymptomatic heart disease associated with non-insulin-dependent diabetes mellitus in a defined population. *Circulation* 81:899–906, 1990.

Schiel R, Muller UA, Beltschikow W, Stein G: Trends in the management of arterial hypertension in patients with type 1 and insulin-treated type 2 diabetes mellitus over a period of 10 years (1989/1990–1994/1995). Results of the JEVIN trial. *J Diabetes Complicationsl* 20:273–279, 2006.

Schmid KE, Davidson WS, Myatt L, Woolett LA: The transport of cholesterol across a placental cell monolayer: implications for net transport of sterol from the maternal to the fetal circulation. *J Lipid Res* 44:1909–1918, 2003.

Schmidt IM, Chellakooty M, Boisen KA, Damgaard IN, Kai CM, Olgaard K, Main KM: Impaired kidney growth in low-birth-weight children: distinct effects of maturity and weight for gestational age. *Kidney Int* 68:731–740, 2005.

Schneider MB, Umpierrez GE, Ramsey RD, Mabie WC, Bennett KA: Pregnancy complicated by diabetic ketoacidosis. Maternal and fetal outcomes. *Diabetes Care* 26:958–959, 2003.

Schnyder G, Roffi M, Flammer Y, Pin R, Hess OM: Effect of homocysteine-lowering therapy with folic acid, vitamin B12, and vitamin B6 on clinical outcome after percutaneous coronary intervention: the Swiss Heart Study: a randomized controlled trial. *JAMA* 288:973–979, 2002.

Schocket LS, Grunwald JE, Tsang AF, DuPont J: The effects of pregnancy on retinal hemodynamics in diabetic versus nondiabetic mothers. *Am J Ophthalmol* 128:477–484, 1999.

Schott M, Feldkemp J, Bathan C, Fritzen R, Scherbaum WA, Seissler J: Detecting TSH-receptor antibodies with the recombinant TBII assay: technical and clinical evaluation. *Horm Metab Res* 32:429–435, 2000.

Schouten EG, Dekker JM, Meppelimk P, Kolk FJ, Vanderbroucke JP, Pool J: QT interval prolongation predicts cardiovascular mortality in an apparently healthy population. *Circulation* 84:1516–1523, 1991.

Schram MT, Chaturvedi N, Schalkwijk CG, Fuller JH, Stehouwer CDA: Markers of inflammation are cross-sectionally associated with microvascular complications and cardiovascular disease in type 1 diabetes: the Eurodiab Prospective Complications Study. *Diabetologia* 48:370–378, 2005.

Schroder W, Heyl W, Hill-Grasshoff B, Rath W: Clinical value of detecting microalbuminuria as a risk factor for pregnancy-induced hypertension in insulin-treated diabetic pregnancies. *Eur J Obstet Gynecol Reprod Biol* 91:155–158, 2000.

Schubert FP, Abernathy MP: Alternate evaluations of proteinuria in the gravid hypertensive patient. *J Reprod Med* 51:709–714, 2006.

Schulze MB, Shai I, Manson JE, Li T, Rifai TL, Jiang R, Hu FB: Joint role of non-HDL cholesterol and glycohemoglobin in predicting future coronary heart disease events among women with type 2 diabetes. *Diabetologia* 47:2129–2136, 2004.

Schwab KO, Menche U, Schmeisl G, Lohse MJ: Hypoglycemia-dependent β2–adrenoceptor downregulation: a contributing factor to hypoglycemia unawareness in patients with type 1 diabetes? *Horm Res* 62:137–141, 2004.

Schwab KO, Doerfer J, Hecker W, Grulich-Henn J, Wiemann D, Kordonouri O, Beyer P, Holl RW; the DPV Initiative of the German Working Group for Pediatric Diabetology: Spectrum and prevalence of atherogenic risk factors in 27,358 children, adolescents, and young adults with type 1 diabetes. Cross-sectional data from the German diabetes documentation and quality management system (DPV). *Diabetes Care* 29:218–225, 2006.

Schwab KO, Doerfer J, Krebs A, Krebs K, Schorb E, Hallermann K, Superti-Furga A, Zieger B, Marz W, Schmidt-Trucksass A, Winkler K: Early atherosclerosis in childhood type 1 diabetes: role of raised systolic blood pressure in the absence of dyslipidemia. *Eur J Pediatr* 166:541–548, 2007.

Schwartz PJ, Stramba-Badiale M, Segantini A, Austoni P, Bosi G, Giorgetti R, Grancini F, Marni ED, Perticone F, Rosti D, Salice P: Prolongation of the QT interval and the sudden infant death syndrome. *N Engl J Med* 338:1709–1714, 1998.

Schwartz PJ: Stillbirths, sudden infant deaths, and long-QT syndrome. Puzzle or mosaic, the pieces of the jigsaw are being fitted together. *Circulation* 109: 2930–2932, 2004.

Schwedler SB, Filep JG, Galle J, Wanner C, Potempa LA: C-reactive protein: a family of proteins to regulate cardiovascular function. *Am J Kidney Dis* 47:212–222, 2005.

Scognamiglio R, Avogaro A, Casara D, Crepaldi C, Marin M, Palisi M, Mingardi R, Erle G, Fasoli G, Volta SD: Myocardial dysfunction and adrenergic innervation in patients with insulin-dependent diabetes mellitus. *J Am Coll Cardiol* 31: 404–412, 1998.

Scognamiglio R, Negut C, de Kreuzenberg SV, Palisi M, Tiengo A, Avogaro A: Abnormal myocardial perfusion and contractile recruitment during exercise in type 1 diabetic patients. *Clin Cardiol* 28:93–99, 2005a.

Scognamiglio R, Negut C, De Kreutzenberg SV, Tiengo A, Avogaro A: Postprandial myocardial perfusion in healthy subjects and in type 2 diabetic patients. *Circulation* 112:179–184, 2005b.

Scognamiglio R, Negut C, Ramondo A, Tiengo A, Avogaro A: Detection of coronary artery disease in asymptomatic patients with type 2 diabetes mellitus. *J Am Coll Cardiol* 47:65–71, 2006.

Scott AR, Tattersall RB, McPherson M: Improvement of postural hypotension and severe diabetic autonomic neuropathy during pregnancy. Letter and comments. *Diabetes Care* 11:369–370, 1988.

Scott A, Toomath R, Bouchier D, Bruse R, Crook N, Carroll D, Cutfield R, Dixon P, Doran J, Dunn P, Hotu C, Khant M, Lonsdale M, Lunt H, Wiltshire E, Wu D: First national audit of the outcomes of care in young people with diabetes in New Zealand: high prevalence of nephropathy in Maori and Pacific Islanders. *N Z Med J* 119:U2015, 2006.

Sebastian C, Scherlag M, Kugelmass A, Schechter E: Primary stent implantation for acute myocardial infarction during pregnancy: use of abciximab, ticlopidine, and aspirin. *Catheter Cardiovasc Diagn* 45:275–279, 1998.

Seely EW: Hypertension in pregnancy: a potential window into long-term cardiovascular risk in women. *J Clin Endocrinol Metab* 84:1858–1861, 1999.

Seely EW, Solomon CG: Insulin resistance and its potential role in pregnancy-induced hypertension. *J Clin Endocrinol Metab* 88:2393–2398, 2003.

Segel SA, Fanelli CG, Dence CS, Markham J, Videen TO, Paramore DS, Powers WJ, Cryer PE: Blood-to-brain glucose transport, cerebral glucose metabolism and cerebral blood flow are not increased following hypoglycemia. *Diabetes* 50: 1911–1917, 2001.

Segel SA, Paramore DS, Cryer PE: Hypoglycemia-associated autonomic failure in advanced type 2 diabetes. *Diabetes* 51:724–733, 2002.

Sejil S, Janand-Delenne B, Avierinos JF, Habib G, Labastie N, Raccah D, Vague P, Lassmann-Vague V: Six-year follow-up of a cohort of 203 patients with diabetes after screening for silent myocardial ischemia. *Diabet Med* 23:1186–1191, 2006.

Seki H, Takeda S, Kinoshita K: Long-term treatment with nicardipine for severe pre-eclampsia. *Int J Gynaecol Obstet* 76:135–141, 2002.

Selvarajah D, Wilkinson ID, Emery CJ, Harris ND, Shaw PJ, Witte DR, Griffiths PD, Tesfaye S: Early involvement of the spinal cord in diabetic peripheral neuropathy. *Diabetes Care* 29:2664–2669, 2006.

Selvin E, Erlinger TP: Prevalence of and risk factors for peripheral arterial disease in the United States: results from the National Health and Nutrition Examination Survey, 1999–2000. *Circulation* 110:738–743, 2004a.

Selvin E, Marinopoulos S, Berkenblit G, Rami T, Brancati FL, Powe NR, Golden SH: Meta-analysis: glycosylated hemoglobin and cardiovascular disease in diabetes mellitus. *Ann Intern Med* 141:421–431, 2004b.

Selvin E, Coresh J, Golden SH, Brancati FL, Folsom AR, Steffes MW: Glycemic control and coronary heart disease risk in persons with and without diabetes. The Atherosclerosis Risk in Communities Study. *Arch Intern Med* 165:1910–1916, 2005.

Sen S, Ozmert G, Turan H, Caliskan E, Onbasili A, Kaya D: The effects of spinal anesthesia on QT interval in preeclamptic patients. *Anesth Analg* 103: 1250–1255, 2006.

Senior PA, Welsh RC, McDonald CG, Paty BW, Shapiro AMJ, Ryan EA: Coronary artery disease is common in nonuremic, asymptomatic type 1 diabetic islet transplant candidates. *Diabetes Care* 28:866–872, 2005.

Seow KM, Tang MH, Chuang J, Wang YY, Chen DC: The correlation between renal function and systolic or diastolic blood pressure in severe preeclamptic women. *Hypertens Preg* 24:247–257, 2005.

Serup L: Influence of pregnancy on diabetic retinopathy. *Acta Endocrinol Copenhagen* 277 (Suppl):122–124, 1986.

Shade GH, Ross G, Bever FN, Uddin Z, Devireddy L, Gardin JM: Troponin I in the diagnosis of acute myocardial infarction in pregnancy, labor, and post partum. *Am J Obstet Gynecol* 187:1719–1720, 2002.

Shah BR, Hux JE, Austin PC: Diabetes is not treated as a coronary artery disease risk equivalent. *Diabetes Care* 30:381–383, 2007.

Shankar A, Klein R, Klein BEK, Nieto FJ, Moss SE: Relationship between low-normal blood pressure and kidney disease in type 1 diabetes. *Hypertension* 49: 48–54, 2007.

Shaw LJ, Bairey Merz CN, Pepine CJ, Reis SE, Bittner V, Kelsey SF, Olson M, Johnson BD, Mankad S, Sharaf BL, Rogers WJ, Wessel TR, Arant CB, Pohost GM, Lerman A, Quyyumi AA, Sopko G; the WISE Investigators: Insights from the NHLBI-sponsored Women's Ischemia Syndrome Evaluation (WISE) study: Part I: gender differences in traditional and novel risk factors, symptom evaluation, and gender-optimized diagnostic strategies. *J Am Coll Cardiol* 47: S4–S20, 2006a.

Shaw LJ, Bairey Merz N, Pepine CJ, Reis SE, Bittner V, Kip KE, Kelsey SF, Olson M, Johnson D, Mankad S, Sharaf BL, Rogers WJ, Pohost GM, Sopko G; the Women's Ischemia Syndrome Evaluation (WISE) Investigators: The economic burden of angina in women with suspected ischemic heart disease. Results from the National Institutes of Health—National Heart, Lung, and Blood Institute-sponsored Women's Ischemia Syndrome Evaluation. *Circulation* 114:894–904, 2006b.

Sheffield JS, Cunningham FG: Thyrotoxicosis and heart failure that complicate pregnancy. *Am J Obstet Gynecol* 190:211–217, 2004.

Sheth BP: Does pregnancy accelerate the rate of progression of diabetic retinopathy? *Curr Diab Rep* 2:327–330, 2002.

Shichiri M, Kishikawa H, Ohkubo Y, Wake N: Long-term results of the Kumomoto Study on optimal diabetes control in type 2 diabetic patients. *Diabetes Care* 25 (Suppl 2): B21–B29, 2000.

Shirodaria C, Antoniades C, Lee J, Jackson CE, Robson MD, Francis JM, Moat SJ, Ratnatunga C, Pillai R, Refsum H, Neubauer S, Channon KM: Global improvement of vascular function and redox state with low-dose folic acid. Implications for folate therapy in patients with coronary artery disease. *Circulation* 115:2262–2270, 2007.

Shivalkar B, Dhondt D, Goovaerts I, Van Gaal L, Bartunek J, Van Crombrugge P, Vrints C: Flow mediated dilatation and cardiac function in type 1 diabetes mellitus. *Am J Cardiol* 97:77–82, 2006.

Shotan A, Ostrzega E, Mehra A, Johnson JV, Elkayam U: Incidence of arrhythmias in normal pregnancy and relation to palpitations, dizziness and syncope. *Am J Cardiol* 79:1061–1064, 1997.

Sibai BM, Grossman RA, Grossman HG: Effects of diuretics on plasma volume in pregnancies with long-term hypertension. *Am J Obstet Gynecol* 150:831–835, 1984.

Sibai BM, Mabie WC, Shamsa F, Villar MA, Anderson GD: A comparison of no medication versus methyldopa or labetolol in chronic hypertension during pregnancy. *Am J Obstet Gynecol* 162:960–966, 1990.

Sibai BM, Barton JR, Aki S, Sarinoglu C, Mercer BM: A randomized prospective comparison of nifedipine and bed rest versus bed rest alone in the management of preeclampsia remote from term. *Am J Obstet Gynecol* 167:879–884, 1992.

Sibai BM, Linheimer M, Hauth J, Caritis S, VanDorsten P, Klebanoff M, MacPherson C, Landon M, Miodovnik M, Paul R, Meis P, Dombrowski M; for the NICHHD Network of Maternal-Fetal Medicine Units: Risk factors for preeclampsia, abruptio placentae, and adverse neonatal outcomes among women with chronic hypertension. *N Engl J Med* 339:667–671, 1998.

Sibai BM, Caritis SN, Hauth JC, MacPherson C, VanDorsten JP, Klebanoff M, Landon M, Paul RH, Meis PJ, Miodovnik M, Dombrowski MP, Thurnau GR, Moawad AH, Roberts J; for the National Institute of Child Health and Human Development Maternal-Fetal Medicine Units Network: Preterm delivery in women with pregestational diabetes mellitus or chronic hypertension relative to women with uncomplicated pregnancies. *Am J Obstet Gynecol* 183:1520–1524, 2000a.

Sibai BM, Caritas S, Hauth J, Lindheimer M, VanDorsten JP, MacPherson C, Klebanoff M, Landon M, Miodovnik M, Paul R, Meis P, Dombrowski M, Thurnau G, Roberts J, McNellis D; for the National Institute of Child Health and Human Development Network of Maternal-Fetal Medicine Units: Risks of preeclampsia and adverse neonatal outcomes among women with pregestational diabetes mellitus. *Am J Obstet Gynecol* 182:364–369, 2000b.

Sibai BM: Risk factors, pregnancy complications, and prevention of hypertensive disorders in women with pregravid diabetes mellitus. *J Matern-Fetal Med* 9: 62–65, 2000c.

Sibal L, Law HN, Gebbie J, Dashora UK, Agarwal SC, Home P: Predicting the development of macrovascular disease in people with type 1 diabetes: A 9-year follow-up study. *Ann N Y Acad Sci* 1084:191–207, 2006.

Sibley SD, Hokanson JE, Steffes MW, Purnell JQ, Marcovina SM, Cleary PA, Brunzell JD: Increased small dense LDL and intermediate-density lipoprotein with albuminuria in type 1 diabetes. *Diabetes Care* 22:1165–1170, 1999.

Siegel RD, Cupples A, Schaefer EJ, Wilson PWF: Lipoproteins, apolipoproteins, and low-density lipoprotein size among diabetics in the Framingham Offspring Study. *Metabolism* 45:1267–1272, 1996.

Sifontis NM, Coscia LA, Constatinescu S, Lavelanet AF, Moritz MJ, Armenti VT: Pregnancy outcomes in solid organ transplant recipients with exposure to mycophenolate mofetil or sirolimus. *Transplantation* 82:1698–1702, 2006.

Silaste M-L, Rantala M, Alfthan G, Aro A, Witzum JL, Kesaniemi YA, Horkko S: Changes in dietary fat intake alter plasma levels of oxidized low-density lipoprotein and lipoprotein(a). *Arterioscler Thromb Vasc Biol* 24:498–503, 2004.

Silliman K, Tall AR, Kretchmer N, Forte TM: Unusual high-density lipoprotein subclass distribution during late pregnancy. *Metabolism* 42:1592–1599, 1993.

Silliman K, Shore V, Forte TM: Hypertriglyceridemia during late pregnancy is associated with the formation of small dense low-density lipoproteins and the presence of large buoyant high-density lipoproteins. *Metabolism* 43:1035–1041, 1994.

Silver MA, Maisel A, Yancy CW, McCullough PA, Burnett JC Jr, Francis GS, Mehra MR, Peacock WF 4th, Fonarow G, Gibler WB, Morrow DA, Hollander J; BNP Consensus Panel: BNP consensus panel 2004: a clinical approach for the diagnostic, prognostic, screening, treatment monitoring, and therapeutic roles for natriuretic peptides in cardiovascular diseases. *Congest Heart Fail* 10 (Suppl 3): 1–30, 2004.

Silverstein J, Klingensmith G, Copeland K, Plotnick L, Kaufman F, Laffel L, Deeb L, Grey M, Anderson B, Holzmeister LA, Clark N: Care of children and adolescents with type 1 diabetes. A statement of the American Diabetes Association. *Diabetes Care* 28:186–210, 2005.

Silverstone A, Trudinger BJ, Lewis PJ, Bulpitt CJ: Maternal hypertension and intra-uterine fetal death in mid-pregnancy. *Br J Obstet Gynecol* 87:457–461, 1980.

Simons LA, Simons J: Diabetes and coronary heart disease. Editorial. *N Engl J Med* 339:1714–1715, 1998.

Simpson AE, Brammar WJ, Pratten MK, Cockcroft N, Elcombe CR: Placental transfer of the hypolipidemic drug, clofibrate, induces CYP4A expression in 18.5–day fetal rats. *Drug Metab Dispos* 24:547–554, 1996.

Sims AAH: Serial studies of renal function in pregnancy complicated by diabetes mellitus. *Diabetes* 10:190–197, 1961.

Sinclair SH, Nesler C, Foxman B, Nichols CW, Gabbe S: Macular edema and pregnancy in insulin-dependent diabetes. *Am J Ophthalmol* 97:154–167, 1984.

Singh A, Satchell SC, Neal CR, McKenzie EA, Tooke JE, Mathieson PW: Glomerular endothelial glycocalyx constitutes a barrier to protein permeability. *J Am Soc Nephrol* 18:2885–2893, 2007.

Sipahi I, Tuzcu EM, Schoenhagen P, Wolski KE, Nicholls SJ, Balog C, Crowe TD, Nissen SE: Effects of normal, pre-hypertensive, and hypertensive blood pressure levels on progression of coronary atherosclerosis. *J Am Coll Cardiol* 48:833–838, 2006.

Skalen K, Gustafsson M, Rydberg EK, Hulten LM, Wiklund O, Innerarity TL, Boren J: Subendothelial retention of atherogenic lipoproteins in early atherosclerosis. *Nature* 417:750–754, 2002.

Skannal DG, Miodovnik M, Dungy-Poythress LJ, First R: Successful pregnancy after combined renal-pancreas transplantation: a case report and literature review. *Am J Perinatol* 13:383–387, 1996.

Skrivarhaug T, Bangstad HJ, Stene LC, Sandvik L, Hanssen KF, Joner G: Long-term mortality in a nationwide cohort of childhood-onset type 1 diabetic patients in Norway. *Diabetologia* 49:298–305, 2006.

Skuza KA, Sills IN, Stene M, Rapaport R: Prediction of neonatal hyperthyroidism in infants born to mothers with Graves' disease. *J Pediatr* 128:264–267, 1996.

Smallridge RC, Ladenson PW: Hypothyroidism in pregnancy: consequences to neonatal health. *J Clin Endocrinol Metab* 86:2349–2353, 2001.

Smallridge RC, Glinoer D, Hollowell JG, Brent G: Thyroid function inside and outside of pregnancy: what do we know and what don't we know? *Thyroid* 15:54–59, 2005.

Smith AC, Toto R, Bakris GL: Differential effects of calcium channel blockers on size selectivity of proteinuria in diabetic glomerulopathy. *Kidney Int* 54:889–896, 1998.

Smith LEH, Perruzzi C, Soker S, Kinose F, Xu X, Robinson G, Driver S, Bischoff J, Zhang B, Schaeffer JM, Senger DR: Regulation of vascular endothelial growth factor-dependent retinal neovascularization by insulin-like growth factor-1 receptor. *Nature Med* 5:1390–1395, 1999.

Smith SC, Milani RV, Arnett DK, Crouse JR III, McDermott MM, Ridker PM, Rosenson RS, Taubert KA, Wilson PWF: Atherosclerotic vascular disease conference. Writing Group II: risk factors. American Heart Association Conference Proceedings. *Circulation* 109:2613–2616, 2004.

Smith SC, Allen J, Blair SN, Bonow RO, Brass LM, Fonarow GC, Grundy SM, Hiratzka L, Jones D, Krumholz HM, Mosca L, Pasternak RC, Pearson T, Pfeffer MA, Taubert KA: AHA/ACC guidelines for secondary prevention for patients with coronary and other atherosclerotic vascular disease: 2006 update. Endorsed by the National Heart, Lung, and Blood Institute. *Circulation* 113:2363–2372, 2006.

Smith MC, Moran P, Ward MK, Davison JM: Assessment of glomerular filtration rate during pregnancy using the MDRD formula. *BJOG* 115:109–112, 2008.

Smithson MJ: Screening for thyroid dysfunction in a community population of diabetic patients. *Diabet Med* 15:148–150, 1998.

Snell-Bergeon JK, Hokanson JE, Jensen L, MacKenzie T, Kinney G, Dabelea D, Eckel RH, Ehrlich J, Garg S, Rewers M: Progression of coronary artery calcification in type 1 diabetes. The importance of glycemic control. *Diabetes Care* 26:2923–2928, 2003.

Sniderman AD, Scantlebury T, Cianflone K: Hypertriglyceridemic hyperapoB: the unappreciated atherogenic dyslipoproteinemia in type 2 diabetes mellitus. *Ann Intern Med* 135:447–459, 2001.

Sniderman AD, Lamarche B, Tilley J, Seccombe D, Frohlich J: Hypertriglyceridemic hyperapoB in type 2 diabetes. *Diabetes Care* 25:579–582, 2002.

Sniderman AD, Furberg CD, Keech A, Roeters van Lennep J, Frohlich J, Jungner I, Walldius G: Apolipoprotein versus lipids as indices of coronary risk and as targets for statin treatment. Viewpoint. *Lancet* 361:777–780, 2003.

Sniderman AD, Jungner I, Holme I, Aastveit A, Walldius G: Errors that result from using the TC/HDL-C ratio rather than the apoB/apoA-I ratio to identify the lipoprotein-related risk of vascular disease. *J Intern Med* 259:455–461, 2006.

Snow V, Aronson MD, Hornbake ER, Mottur-Pilson C, Weiss KB; for the Clinical Efficacy Assessment Subcommittee of the American College of Physicians: Lipid control in the management of type 2 diabetes mellitus: a clinical practice guideline from the American College of Physicians. *Ann Intern Med* 140: 644–649, 2004.

Sobal G, Menzel EJ, Sinzinger H: Calcium antagonists as inhibitors of in vitro low density lipoprotein oxidation and glycation. *Biochem Pharmacol* 61:373–379, 2001.

Soedamah-Muthu SS, Colhoun HM, Abrahamian H, Chan NN, Mangill R, Reboldi GP, Fuller JH; EURODIAB Prospective Complications Study Group: Trends in hypertension management in type 1 diabetes across Europe, 1989/1990–1997/1999. *Diabetologia* 45:1362–1371, 2002.

Soedamah-Muthu SS, Chang YF, Otvos J, Evans RW, Orchard TJ; Pittsburgh Epidemiology of Diabetes Complications Study Group: Lipoprotein subclass measurements by nuclear magnetic resonance spectroscopy improve the prediction of coronary artery disease in type 1 diabetes. A prospective report from the Pittsburgh Epidemiology of Diabetes Complications Study. *Diabetologia* 46:674–682, 2003.

Soedamah-Muthu SS, Chaturvedi N, Toeller M, Ferriss B, Reboldi P, Michel G, Manes C, Fuller JH; the EURODIAB Prospective Complications Study Group: Risk factors for coronary heart disease in type 1 diabetic patients in Europe. The EURODIAB Prospective Complications Study. *Diabetes Care* 27:530–537, 2004.

Soedamah-Muthu SS, Fuller JH, Mulnier HE, Raleigh VS, Lawrenson RA. Colhoun HM: All-cause mortality rates in patients with type 1 diabetes mellitus compared with a non-diabetic population for the U.K. general practice research data base, 1992—1999. *Diabetologia* 49:660–666, 2006a.

Soedamah-Muthu SS, Fuller JH, Mulnier HE, Raleigh VS, Lawrenson RA, Colhoun HM: High risk of cardiovascular disease in patients with type 1 diabetes in the U.K. A cohort study using the General Practice Research Database. *Diabetes Care* 29:798–804, 2006b.

Soffers HE, Kester AD, Kaiser V, Rinkens PE, Kitzlaar PJ, Knottnerus JA: The diagnostic value of the measurement of the ankle-brachial systolic pressure index in primary health care. *J Clin Epidemiol* 49:1401–1405, 1996.

Song YQ, Stanmfer MJ, Liu SM: Meta-analysis: apolipoprotein E genotypes and risk for coronary artery disease. *Ann Intern Med* 141:137–147, 2004.

Song K-H, Ko SH, Kim H-W, Ahn Y-B, Lee J-M, Son H-S, Yoon K-H, Cha B-Y, Lee K-W, Son H-Y: Prospective study of lipoprotein(a) as a risk factor for deteriorating renal function in type 2 diabetic patients with overt proteinuria. *Diabetes Care* 28:1718–1723, 2005.

Song G, Bazer FW, Spencer TE: Differential expression of cathepsons and cystatin C in ovine uteroplacental tissues. *Placenta* 28:1091–1098, 2007.

Sorajja P, Chareonthaitawee P, Rajagopalan N, Miller TD, Frye RL, Hodge DO, Gibbons RJ: Improved survival in asymptomatic diabetic patients with high-risk SPECT imaging treated with coronary artery bypass grafting. *Circulation* 112: I311–I316, 2005.

Sorensen HT, Steffensen FH, Olesen C, Nielsen GL, Pedersen L, Olsen J: Pregnancy outcome in women exposed to calcium channel blockers. *Reprod Toxicol* 12:383–384, 1998.

Sorensen HT, Czeizel AE, Rockenbauer M, Steffensen FH, Olsen J: The risk of limb deficiencies and other congenital abnormalities in children exposed in utero to calcium channel blockers. *Acta Obstet Gynecol Scand* 80:397–401, 2001.

Sorensen TK, Williams MA, Lee I-M, Dashow EE, Thompson ML, Luthy DA: Recreational physical activity during pregnancy and risk of preeclampsia. *Hypertension* 41:1273–1280, 2003.

Soria A, Bocos C, Herrera E: Opposite response to fenofibrate treatment in pregnant and virgin rats. *J Lipid Res* 43:74–81, 2002.

Soria A, Gonzalez Mdel C, Vidal H, Herrera E, Bocos C: Triglyceridemia and peroxisome proliferator-activated receptor-alpha expression are not connected in fenofibrate-treated pregnant rats. *Mol Cell Biochem* 273:97–107, 2005.

Soubrane G, Coscas G: Influence of pregnancy on the evolution of diabetic retinopathy. *Int Ophthalmol Clin* 38:187–194, 1998.

Souma ML, Cabaniss CD, Nataraj A, Khan Z: The Valsalva maneuver: a test of autonomic nervous system function in pregnancy. *Am J Obstet Gynecol* 145: 274–278, 1983.

Sovik O, Thordarson H: Dead-in-bed syndrome in young diabetic patients. *Diabetes Care* 22 (Suppl 2):B40–B42, 1999.

Sowers JR, Epstein M, Frohlich ED: Diabetes, hypertension, and cardiovascular disease. *Hypertension* 37:1053–1059, 2001.

Spallone V, Bernardi L, Ricordi L, Solda P, Maiello MR, Calciati A, Gambardella S, Pratino P, Menzinger G: Relationship between the circadian rhythms of blood pressure and sympathovagal balance in diabetic autonomic neuropathy. *Diabetes* 42:1745–1752, 1993.

Spallone V, Gambardelia S, Maiello MR, Barini A, Frontoni S, Menzinger G: Relationship between autonomic neuropathy, 24-hour blood pressure profile, and nephropathy in normotensive IDDM patients. *Diabetes Care* 17:578–584, 1994.

Spallone V, Maiello MR, Cicconetti E, Menzinger G: Autonomic neuropathy and cardiovascular risk factors in insulin-dependent and non-insulin-dependent diabetes. *Diabetes Res Clin Pract* 34:169–179, 1997a.

Spallone V, Menzinger G: Diagnosis of cardiovascular autonomic neuropathy in diabetes. *Diabetes* 46 (Suppl 2):S67–S76, 1997b.

Spencer CA, Hollwell JG, Kazarosyan M, Bravereman LE: National Health and Nutrition Examination Survey III thyroid-stimulating hormone (TSH)-thyroperoxidase antibody relationships demonstrate that TSH upper reference limits may be skewed by occult thyroid dysfunction. *J Clin Endocrinol Metab* 92:4236–4240, 2007.

Sprafka JM, Bender AP, Jagger HG: Prevalence of hypertension and associated risk factors among diabetic individuals. The Three-City Study. *Diabetes Care* 11:17–22, 1988.

Spranger M, Aspey BS, Harrison MJG: Sex differences in antithrombotic effect of aspirin. *Stroke* 20:34–37, 1989.

Spyer G, Hattersley AT, MacDonald IA, Amiel S, MacLeod KM: Hypoglycemic counterregulation at normal glucose concentrations in patients with well controlled type 2 diabetes. *Lancet* 356:1970–1974, 2000.

St Clair L, Ballantyne CM: Biological surrogates for enhancing cardiovascular risk prediction in type 2 diabetes mellitus. *Am J Cardiol* 99:80B-88B, 2007.

St Goar FG, Pinto FJ, Alderman EL, Fitzgerald PJ, Stinson EB, Billingham ME, Popp RL: Detection of coronary atherosclerosis in young adult hearts using intravascular ultrasound. *Circulation* 86:756–763, 1992.

Staessen JA, Den Hond E, Celis H, Fagard R, Keary L, Vandehoven G, O'Brien ET; for the Treatment of Hypertension Based on Home or Office Blood Pressure (THOP) Trial Investigators: Antihypertensive treatment based on blood pressure measurement at home or in the physician's office. A randomized controlled trial. *JAMA* 291:955–964, 2004.

Stagnaro-Green A, Roman SH, Cobin RH, El-Harazy E, Alvarez-Marfany M, Davies TF: Detection of at-risk pregnancy by means of highly sensitive assays for thyroid autoantibodies. *JAMA* 264:1422–1425, 1990.

Stamilio DM, Sehdev HM, Morgan MA, Propert K, Macones GA: Can antenatal clinical and biochemical markers predict the development of severe preeclampsia? *Am J Obstet Gynecol* 182:589–594, 2000.

Stangenberg M, Persson B, Stange L, Carlstrom K: Insulin-induced hypoglycemia in pregnant diabetics. Maternal and fetal cardiovascular reactions. *Acta Obstet Gynecol Scand* 62:249–252, 1983.

Stanley CW, Gottlieb R, Zager R, Eisenberg J, Richmond R, Moritz MJ, Armenti VT: Developmental well-being in offspring of women receiving cyclosporine post-renal transplant. *Transplant Proc* 31:241–242, 1999.

Starkman HS, Cable G, Halaq V, Hecht H, Donnelly CM: Delineation of prevalence and risk factors for early coronary artery disease by electron beam computed tomography in young adults with type 1 diabetes. *Diabetes Care* 26:433–436, 2003.

Steel JM: Autonomic neuropathy in pregnancy. *Diabetes Care* 12:170–171, 1989.

Steel JM, Johnstone FD, Hepburn DA, Smith AF: Can prepregnancy care of diabetic women reduce the risk of abnormal babies? *BMJ* 301:1070–73, 1990.

Steer P: Factors influencing relative weights of placenta and newborn infant. Maternal hemoglobin and blood pressure should have been regarded as continuous variables. Letter. *Br Med J* 315:1542, 1997.

Steer PJ, Little MP, Kold-Jensen T, Chapple J, Elliott P: Maternal blood pressure in pregnancy, birth weight, and perinatal mortality in first births: prospective study. *BMJ* 329:1312–1314, 2004.

Steffenson FH, Nielsen GL, Sorensen HT, Olesen C, Olsen J: Pregnancy outcome with ACE-inhibitor use in early pregnancy. *Lancet* 351:596, 1998.

Stehouwer CDA, Fischer HRA, Hackeng WHL, den Ottolander GJH: Identifying patients with incipient diabetic nephropathy. Should 24–hour collections be used? *Arch Intern Med* 150:373–375, 1990.

Stehouwer CD, Gall MA, Hougaard P, Jakobs C, Parving H-H: Plasma homocysteine concentration predicts mortality in non-insulin-dependent diabetic patients with and without albuminuria. *Kidney Int* 55:308–314, 1999.

Stehouwer CDA, Gall M-A, Twisk JWR, Knudsen E, Emeis JJ, Parving H-H: Increased urinary albumin excretion, endothelial dysfunction, and chronic low grade inflammation in type 2 diabetes. Progressive, interrelated, and independently associated with risk of death. *Diabetes* 51:1157–1165, 2002.

Stein PK, Hagley MT, Cole PL, Domitrovich PP, Kleiger RE, Rottman JN: Changes in 24–hour heart rate variability during normal pregnancy. *Am J Obstet Gynecol* 180:978–985, 1999.

Steinhauff S, Pehlivanli S, Bakovic-Alt R, Meiser BM, Becker BF, von Scheidt W, Weis M: Beneficial effects of quinaprilat on coronary vasomotor function, endothelial oxidative stress, and endothelin activation after human heart transplantation. *Transplantation* 27:1859–1865, 2004.

Steinke JM, Sinaiko AR, Kramer MS, Suissa S, Chavers BM, Mauer M; for the International Diabetic Nephropathy Study Group: The early natural history of nephropathy in type 1 diabetes. III. Predictors of 5-year urinary albumin excretion rate patterns in initially normoalbuminuric patients. *Diabetes* 54:2164–2171, 2005.

Stenstrom G, Gottsater A, Bakhtadze E, Berger B, Sundkvist G: Latent autoimmune diabetes in adults: definition, prevalence, beta-cell function, and treatment. *Diabetes* 54 (Suppl 2):S68–S72, 2005.

Stephenson JM, Kenny S, Stevens LK, Fuller JH, Lee E; the WHO Multinational Study Group: Proteinuria and mortality in diabetes: the WHO Multinational Study of Vascular Disease in Diabetes. *Diabet Med* 12:149–155, 1995.

Stergiou G, Mengden T, Padfield PL, Parati G, O'Brien E; on behalf of the Working Group on Blood Pressure Monitoring of the European Society of Hypertension: Self monitoring of blood pressure at home is an important adjunct to clinic measurements. Editorial. *BMJ* 329:870–871, 2004.

Stergiou GS, Salgami EV, Tzamouranis DG, Roussias LG: Masked hypertension assessed by ambulatory blood pressure versus home blood pressure monitoring: is it the same phenomenon? *Am J Hypertens* 18:772–778, 2005.

Stern MP: Diabetes and cardiovascular disease: the "common soil" hypothesis. *Diabetes* 44:369–374, 1995.

Stettler C, Allemann S, Juni P, Cull CA, Holman RR, Egger M, Krahenbuhl S, Diem P: Glycemic control and macrovascular disease in types 1 and 2 diabetes mellitus: meta-analysis of randomized trials. *Am Heart J* 152:27–38, 2006.

Stettler C, Bearth A, Allemann S, Zwahlen M, Zanchin L, Deplazes M, Christ ER, Teuscher A, Diem P: QT_c interval and resting heart rate as long-term predictors of mortality in type 1 and type 2 diabetes mellitus: a 23-year follow-up. *Diabetologia* 50:186–194, 2007.

Stevens MJ: Oxidative-nitrosative stress as a contributing factor to cardiovascular disease in subjects with diabetes. *Curr Vasc Pharmacol* 3:253–266, 2005.

Stevens LA, Coresh J, Greene T, Levey AS: Assessing kidney function—measured and estimated glomerular filtration rate. *N Engl J Med* 354:2473–2483, 2006.

Stevens LA, Manzi J, Levey AS, Chen J, Deysher AE, Greene T, Poggio ED, Schmid CH, Steffes MW, Zhang YL, Van Lente F, Coresh J: Impact of creatinine calibration on performance of GFR estimating equations in a pooled individual patient database. *Am J Kidney Dis* 50:21–35, 2007a.

Stevens LA, Coresh J, Feldman HI, Greene T, Lash JP, Nelson RG, Rahman M, Deysher AE, Zhang YL, Schmid CH, Levey AS: Evaluation of the Modification of Diet in Renal Disease study equation in a large diverse population. *J Am Soc Nephrol* 18:2749–2757, 2007b.

Stevens LA, Coresh J, Schmid CH, Feldman HI, Froissart M, Kusek J, Rossert J, Van Lente F, Bruce RD 3rd, Zhang YL, Greene T, Levey AS: Estimating GFR using serum cystatin C alone and in combination with serum creatinine: a pooled analysis of 3,418 individuals with CKD. *Am J Kidney Dis* 51:395–406, 2008.

Stone JL, Lockwood CJ, Berkowitz GS, Alvarez M, Lapinski R, Berkowitz RL: Risk factors for severe preeclampsia. *Obstet Gynecol* 83:357–361, 1994.

Stone ML, Craig ME, Chan AK, Lee JW, Verge CF, Donaghue KC: Natural history and risk factors for microalbuminuria in adolescents with type 1 diabetes. A longitudinal study. *Diabetes Care* 29:2072–2077, 2006.

Strain WD, Chaturvedi N, Bulpitt CJ, Rajkumar C, Shore AC: Albumin excretion rate and cardiovascular risk. Could the association be explained by early microvacular dysfunction? *Diabetes* 54:1816–1822, 2005.

Stratton IM, Adler AI, Neil HAW, Matthews DR, Manley SE, Cull CA, Hadden D, Turner RC, Holman RR; UK Prospective Diabetes Study Group: Epidemiological association of glycemia with macrovascular and microvascular complications of type 2 diabetes. (UKPDS 35). *BMJ* 321:405–412, 2000a.

Stratton IM, Adler AI, Neil HA, Matthews DR, Manley SE, Cull CA, Hadden D, Turner RC, Holman RR: Association of glycemia with macrovascular and microvascular complications of type 2 diabetes (UKPDS 35). *BMJ* 321: 405–412, 2000b.

Strevens H, Wide-Swensson D, Torffvit O, Grubb A: Serum cystatin C for assessment of glomerular filtration rate of pregnant and nonpregnant women. Indications of altered filtration process in pregnancy. *Scand J Lab Invest* 62: 141–148, 2002.

Strevens H, Wide-Swensson D, Grubb A, Hensen A, Horn T, Ingemarsson I, Larsen S, Nyengaard JR, Torffvit O, Willner J, Olsen S: Serum cystatin C reflects glomerular endotheliosis in normal, hypertensive and preeclamptic pregnancies. *BJOG* 110:825–830, 2003.

Struthers AD, Donnan PT, Lindsay P, McNaughton D, Broomhall J, MacDonald TM: Effect of allopurinol on mortality and hospitalizations in congestive heart failure: a retrospective cohort study. *Heart* 87:229–234, 2002.

Sturgiss SN, Davison JM: Perinatal outcome in renal allograft recipients: prognostic significance of hypertension and renal function before and during pregnancy. *Obstet Gynecol* 78:573–577, 1991.

Sturgiss SN, Davison JM: Effect of pregnancy on long-term function of renal allografts. *Am J Kidney Dis* 19:167–172, 1992.

Subtil D, Goeusse P, Ouech F, Lequien P, Biausque S, Breart G, Uzan S, Marquis P, Parmentier D, Churlet A; Essai Regional Aspirine Mere-Enfant (ERASME) Collaborative Group: Aspirin (100 mg) used for prevention of pre-eclampsia in nulliparous women. *BJOG* 110:475–484, 2003.

Sudano I, Spieker LE, Hermann F, Flammer A, Corti R, Noll G, Luscher TF: Protection of endothelial function: targets for nutritional and pharmacological interventions. *J Cardiovasc Pharmacol* 47 (Suppl 2):S136–S150, S172–S176, 2006.

Sullebarger JT, Fontanet HL, Matar FA, Singh SS: Percutaneous coronary intervention for myocardial infarction during pregnancy: a new trend? *J Invasive Cardiol* 15:725–728, 2003.

Sultan A, Piot C, Mariano-Goulart D, Rasamisoa M, Renard E, Avignon A: Risk factors for silent myocardial ischemia in high-risk type 1 diabetic patients. *Diabetes Care* 27:1745–1747, 2004.

Sumnik Z, Drevinek P, Snajderova M, Kolouskova S, Sedlakova P, Pechova M, Vavrinec J, Cinek O: HLA-DQ polymorphisms modify the risk of thyroid autoimmunity in children with type 1 diabetes mellitus. *J Pediatr Endocrinol Metab* 16:851–858, 2003.

Sundkvist LB: Autonomic neuropathy predicts deterioration in glomerular filtration rate in patients with IDDM. *Diabetes Care* 16:773–779, 1993.

Sundquist K, Li X: Type 1 diabetes as a risk factor for stroke in men and women aged 15–49: a nation-wide study from Sweden. *Diabet Med* 23:1261–1267, 2006.

Surks MI, Ortiz E, Daniels GH, Sawin CT, Col NF, Cobin RH, Franklyn JA, Hershman JM, Burman KD, Denke MA, Gorman C, Cooper RS, Weissman NJ: Subclinical thyroid disease. Scientific review and guidelines for diagnosis and management. *JAMA* 291:228–238, 2004.

Surks MI, Goswami G, Daniels GH: The thyrotropin reference range should remain unchanged. Commentary. *J Clin Endocrinol Metab* 90:5489–5496, 2005.

Surks MI, Hollowell JG: Age-specific distribution of serum thyrotropin and antithyroid antibodies in the U.S. population: implications for the prevalence of subclinical hypothyroidism. *J Clin Endocrinol Metab* 92:4575–4582, 2007.

Suys BE, Huybrechts SJ, De Wolf D, Op De Beeck L, Matthys D, Van Overmeire B, Du Caju MV, Rooman RP: QTc interval prolongation and QTc dispersion in children and adolescents with type 1 diabetes. *J Pediatr* 141:59–63, 2002.

Suys BE, Katier N, Rooman RPA, Matthys D, De Beeck LO, Du Caju MVL, De Wolf D: Female children and adolescents with type 1 diabetes have more pronounced early echocardiographic signs of diabetic cardiomyopathy. *Diabetes Care* 27:1947–1953, 2004.

Suys B, Heuten S, De Wolf D, Verherstraeten M, de Beck LO, Matthys D, Vrints C, Rooman R: Glycemia and corrected QT interval prolongation in young type 1 diabetic patients. What is the relation? *Diabetes Care* 29:427–429, 2006.

Svensson M, Sundkvist G, Arnqvist HJ, Bjork E, Blohme G, Bolinder J, Henricsson M, Nystrom L, Torffvit O, Waernbaum I, Ostman J, Eriksson JW: Signs of nephropathy may occur early in young adults with diabetes despite modern diabetes management. Results from the nationwide population-based Diabetes Incidence Study in Sweden (DISS). *Diabetes Care* 26:2903–2909, 2003.

Svensson M, Nystrom L, Schon S, Dahlquist G; the Swedish Childhood Diabetes Study and the Swedish Registry for Active Treatment of Uremia: Age at onset of childhood-onset type 1 diabetes and the development of end-stage renal disease. A nationwide population-based study. *Diabetes Care* 29:538–542, 2006.

Svetkey LP: Management of prehypertension. *Hypertension* 45:1056–1061, 2005.

Tabacova S, Little R, Tsong Y, Vega A, Kimmel CA: Adverse pregnancy outcomes associated with maternal enalapril antihypertensive treatment. *Pharmacoepidemiol Drug Saf* 12:633–646, 2003.

Taegtmeyer H, McNulty P, Young ME: Adaptation and maladaptation of the heart in diabetes: Part I. General concepts. *Circulation* 105:1727–1733, 2002.

Takahashi Y, Kawabata I, Shinohara A, Tamaya T: Transient fetal blood flow redistribution induced by maternal diabetic ketoacidosis diagnosed by Doppler ultrasonography. *Prenat Diagn* 20:524–525, 2000.

Takebayashi K, Aso Y, Matsumoto R, Wakabayashi S, Inukai T: Association between the corrected QT intervals and combined intimal-medial thickness of the carotid artery in patients with type 2 diabetes. *Metabolism* 53:1152–1157, 2004.

Taku K, Umegaki K, Sato Y, Taki Y, Endoh K, Watanabe S: Soy isoflavones lower serum total and LDL cholesterol in humans: a meta-analysis of 11 randomized controlled trials. *Am J Clin Nutr* 85:1148–1156, 2007.

Tall AR, Jiang X-C, Luo Y, Silver D: Lipid transfer proteins, HDL metabolism, and atherogenesis. *Arterioscler Thromb Vasc Biol* 20:1185–1188, 2000.

Tall AR: Protease variants, LDL, and coronary heart disease. Editorial. *N Engl J Med* 354:1310–1312, 2006.

Tamaki H, Amino N, Takeoka K, Mitsuda N, Miyai K, Tanazawa O: Thyroxine requirement during pregnancy for replacement therapy of hypothyroidism. *Obstet Gynecol* 76:230–233, 1990.

Tan GD, Lewis AV, James TJ, Altmann P, Taylor RP, Levy JC: Clinical usefulness of cystatin C for the estimation of glomerular filtration rate in type 1 diabetes: reproducibility and accuracy compared with standard measures and iohexol clearance. *Diabetes Care* 25:2004–2009, 2002.

Tan TO, Cheng YW, Caughey AB: Are women who are treated for hypothyroidism at risk for pregnancy complications? *Am J Obstet Gynecol* 194:e1–e3, 2006.

Tanaka H, Hvllienmark L, Thulesius O, Brismar T, Ludvigsson J, Ericson MO, Lindblad LE, Tamai H: Autonomic function in children with type 1 diabetes mellitus. *Diabet Med* 15:402–411, 1998.

Tanaka M, Jaamaa G, Kaiser M, Hills E, Soim A, Zhu M, Shcherbatykh IY, Samelson R, Bell E, Zdeb M, McNutt L-A: Racial disparity in hypertensive disorders of pregnancy in New York State: a 10-year longitudinal population-based study. *Am J Public Health* 97:163–170, 2007.

Tang WHW: Biomarker screening for cardiac dysfunction: the more the merrier? Editorial. *Am Heart J* 152:1–3, 2006.

Tannock L, O'Brien KD, Knopp R, Retzlaff BM, Fish B, Wener MH, Kahn SE, Chait A: Cholesterol feeding increases CRP and SAA in lean insulin-sensitive individuals, but not insulin-resistant individuals. *Circulation* 108 (Suppl IV): IV784, 2003.

Tarn AC, Drury PL: Blood pressure in children, adolescents and young adults with type 1 (insulin-dependent) diabetes. *Diabetologia* 29:275–281, 1986.

Tarnow L, Hildebrandt P, Hansen BV, Borch-Johnsen K, Parving H-H: Plasma NT-pro-brain natriuretic peptide as an independent predictor of mortality in diabetic nephropathy. *Diabetologia* 48:149–155, 2005.

Tarnow L, Gall MA, Hansen BV, Hovind P, Parving HH: Plasma N-terminal pro-B-type natriuretic peptide and mortality in type 2 diabetes. *Diabetologia* 49: 2256–2262, 2006.

Taskinen M-R: Diabetic dyslipidemia: from basic research to clinical practice. Claude Bernard Lecture. *Diabetologia* 46:733–749, 2003.

Taskiran M, Rasmussen V, Rasmussen B, Fritz-Hansen T, Larsson HB, Jensen GB, Hilsted J: Left ventricular dysfunction in normotensive type 1 diabetes patients: the impact of autonomic neuropathy. *Diabet Med* 21:524–530, 2004.

Tattersall RB, Gill GV: Unexplained deaths of type 1 diabetic patients. *Diabet Med* 8:49–58, 1991.

Tavel ME: Stress testing in cardiac evaluation: current concepts with emphasis on the ECG. *Chest* 119:907–925, 2001.

Tawakol A, Forgione MA, Stuehlinger M, Alpert NM, Cooke JP, Loscalzo J, Fischman AJ, Creager MA, Gewirtz H: Homocysteine impairs coronary vasodilator function in humans. *J Am Coll Cardiol* 40:1051–1058, 2002.

Taylor AA, Davison JM: Albumin excretion in normal pregnancy. *Am J Obstet Gynecol* 177:1559–1560, 1997.

Taylor EN, Stampfer MJ, Cuhhan GC: Diabetes mellitus and the risk of nephrolithiasis. *Kidney Int* 68:1230–1235, 2005.

Temple RC, Aldridge VA, Sampson MJ, Greenwood RH, Heyburn PJ, Glenn A: Impact of pregnancy on the progression of diabetic retinopathy in type 1 diabetes. *Diabet Med* 18:573–577, 2001.

Teno S, Uto Y, Nagashima H, Endoh Y, Iwamoto Y, Omori Y, Takizawa T: Association of postprandial hypertriglyceridemia and carotid intima-media thickness in patients with type 2 diabetes. *Diabetes Care* 23:1401–1406, 2000.

terBraak EWMT, Evers I, Erkelens DW, Visser GHA: Maternal hypoglycemia during pregnancy in type 1 diabetes: maternal and fetal consequences. *Diabetes Metab Res Rev* 18:96–105, 2002.

TerMaaten JC, Voorburg A, Heine RJ, Ter Wee PM, Donker AJ, Gans RO: Renal handling of urate and sodium during acute physiological hyperinsulinemia in healthy subjects. *Clin Sci Lond* 92:51–58, 1997.

Tesfaye S, Chaturvedi N, Eaton SEM, Ward JD, Manes C, Ionescu-Tirgoviste C, Witte DR, Fuller JH; for the EURODIAB Prospective Complications Study Group: Vascular risk factors and diabetic neuropathy. *N Engl J Med* 352:341–350, 2005.

Tester DJ, Ackerman MJ: Sudden infant death syndrome: how significant are the cardiac channelopathies? *Cardiovasc Res* 67:388–396, 2005.

Thadhani R, Stampfer MJ, Hunter DJ, Manson JE, Solomon CG, Curhan GC: High body mass index and hypercholesterolemia: risk of hypertensive disorders of pregnancy. *Obstet Gynecol* 94:543–550, 1999.

Thangaratinam S, Ismail KM, Sharp S, Coomarasamy A, Khan KS; Tests in Prediction of Preeclampsia Severity review group: Accuracy of serum uric acid in predicting complications of preeclampsia: a systematic review. *BJOG* 113:369–378, 2006.

Theochari MA, Vyssoulis GP, Toutouzas PK, Bartsocas CS: Arterial blood pressure changes in children and adolescents with insulin-dependent diabetes mellitus. *J Pediatr* 129:667–670, 1996.

Thomas PK: Classification, differential diagnosis, and staging of diabetic peripheral neuropathy. *Diabetes* 46 (Suppl 2):S54–S57, 1997.

Thomas W, Shen Y, Molitch ME, Steffes MW: Rise in albuminuria and blood pressure in patients who progressed to diabetic nephropathy in the Diabetes Control and Complications Trial. *J Am Soc Nephrol* 12:333–340, 2001.

Thomas MC, MacIsaac RJ, Tsalamandris C, Molyneaux L, Goubina I, Fulcher G, Yue D, Jerums G: Anemia in patients with type 1 diabetes. *J Clin Endocrinol Metab* 89:4359–4363, 2004.

Thomson SC, Vallon V, Blantz RC: Kidney function in early diabetes: the tubular hypothesis of glomerular function. Invited review. *Am J Physiol* 286:F8–F15, 2004.

Thorpe-Beeston JG, Nicolaides KH, Felton CV, Butler J, McGregor AM: Maturation of the secretion of thyroid hormone and thyroid-stimulating hormone in the fetus. *N Engl J Med* 324:532–536, 1991.

Tibaldi JM, Lorber DL, Nerenberg A: Diabetic ketoacidosis and insulin resistance with subcutaneous terbutaline infusion: a case report. *Am J Obstet Gynecol* 163:509–510, 1990.

Tjoa ML, van Vugt JM, Go AT, Blankenstein MA, Oudejans CB, van Wijk IJ: Elevated C-reactive protein levels during first trimester of pregnancy are indicative of preeclampsia and intra-uterine growth restriction. *J Reprod Immunol* 59:29–37, 2003.

Toba H, Nakagawa Y, Miki S, Shimuzu T, Yoshimura A, Inoue R, Asayama J, Kobara M, Nakata T: Calcium channel blockades exhibit anti-inflammatory and antioxidative effects by augmentation of endothelial nitric oxide synthase and the inhibition of angiotensin converting enzyme in the N^G-nitro-L-arginine methyl ester-induced hypertensive rat aorta: vasoprotective effects beyond the blood pressure-lowering effects of amlodipine and manidipine. *Hypertens Res* 28: 689–700, 2005.

Toba H, Shimizu T, Miki S, Inoue R, Yoshimura A, Tsukamoto R, Sawai N, Kobara M, Nakata T: Calcium [corrected] channel blockers reduce angiotensin II-induced superoxide generation and inhibit lectin-like oxidized low-density lipoprotein receptor-1 expression in endothelial cells. *Hypertens Res* 29:105–116, 2006.

Toescu V, Nuttall SL, Martin U, Nightingale P, Kendall MJ, Brydon P: Changes in plasma lipids and markers of oxidative stress in normal pregnancy and pregnancies complicated by diabetes. *Clin Sci* 106:93–98, 2004.

Tomaselli L, Trischitta V, Vinci C, Frittitta L, Squatrito S, Vigneri R: Evaluation of albumin excretion rate in overnight versus 24–h urine. *Diabetes Care* 12: 585–587, 1989.

Toole JF, Malinow MR, Chambless LE, Spence JD, Pettigrew LC, Howard VJ, Sides EG, Wang CH, Stampfer M: Lowering homocysteine in patients with ischemic stroke to prevent recurrent stroke, myocardial infarction, and death: the Vitamin Intervention for Stroke Prevention (VISP) randomized controlled trial. *JAMA* 291:565–575, 2004.

Torbjornsdotter TB, Jaremko GA, Berg UB: Ambulatory blood pressure and heart rate in relation to kidney structure and metabolic control in adolescents with type 1 diabetes. *Diabetologia* 44:865–873, 2001.

Torbjornsdotter TB, Jaremko GA, Berg UB: Nondipping and its relation to glomerulopathy and hyperfiltration in adolescents with type 1 diabetes. *Diabetes Care* 27:510–516, 2004.

Towler DA, Havlin CD, Craft S, Cryer PE: Mechanisms of the awareness of hypoglycemia: perception of neurogenic (predominantly cholinergic) rather than neuroglycopenic symptoms. *Diabetes* 42:1791–1798, 1993.

Trovik TS, Jaeger R, Jorde R, Sager G: Reduced sensitivity to β-adrenoceptor stimulation and blockade in insulin-dependent diabetic patients with hypoglycemia unawareness. *Br J Clin Pharmacol* 38:427–432, 1994.

Trovik TS, Vaartun A, Jorde R, Sager G: Dysfunction in the β2–adrenergic signal pathway in patients with insulin-dependent diabetes mellitus (IDDM) and unawareness of hypoglycemia. *Eur J Clin Pharmacol* 48:327–332, 1995.

Tryggvason G, Indridason OS, Thorsson AV, Hreidarsson AB, Palsson R: Unchanged incidence of diabetic nephropathy in type 1 diabetes: a nation-wide study in Iceland. *Diabet Med* 22:182–187, 2005.

Tsalamandris C, Allen TJ, Gilbert RE, Sinha A, Panagiotopolous S, Cooper ME, Jerums G: Progressive decline in renal function in diabetic patients with and without albuminuria. *Diabetes* 43:649–655, 1994.

Tseng C-H: Lipid abnormalities associated with urinary albumin excretion rate in Taiwanese type 2 diabetic patients. *Kidney Int* 67:1547–1553, 2005.

Tsimakis S, Brilakis ES, Miller ER, McConnell JP, Lennon RJ, Kornman KS, Witzum JL, Berger PB: Oxidized phospholipids, Lp(a) lipoprotein, and coronary artery disease. *N Engl J Med* 353:46–57, 2005.

Tsujino T, Kawasaki D, Masuyama T: Left ventricular diastolic dysfunction in diabetic patients: pathophysiology and therapeutic implications. *Am J Cardiovasc Drugs* 6:219–230, 2006.

Tu A-Y, Cgeung MC, Zhu X, Knopp RH, Albers JJ: Low-density lipoprotein inhibits secretion of phospholipids transfer protein in human trophoblastic BeWo cells. *Exp Biol Med* 229:1046–1052, 2004.

Turgan N, Habif, S, Kabaroglu CG, Mutaf I, Ozmen D, Bayindir O, Uysal A: Effects of the calcium channel blocker amlodipine on serum and aortic cholesterol, lipid peroxidation, antioxidant status and aortic histology in cholesterol-fed rabbits. *J Biomed Sci* 10:65–72, 2003.

Turner RC, Millns H, Neil HA, Stratton IM, Manley SE, Matthews DR, Holman RR; the United Kingdom Prospective Diabetes Study Group: Risk factors for coronary disease in non-insulin dependent diabetes mellitus: United Kingdom prospective diabetes study (UKPDS: 23). *BMJ* 316:823–828, 1998.

UKHSG—UK Hypoglycemia Study Group: Risk of hypoglycemia in types 1 and 2 diabetes: effects of treatment modalities and their duration. *Diabetologia* 50:1140–1147, 2007.

UKPDS—UK Prospective Diabetes Study Group: Intensive blood glucose control with sulfonylureas or insulin compared with conventional treatment and risk of complications in patients with type 2 diabetes. (UKPDS 33). *Lancet* 352: 837–853, 1998a.

UKPDS—U.K. Prospective Diabetes Study Group: Tight blood pressure control and risk of macrovascular and microvascular complications in type 2 diabetes (UKPDS 38). *BMJ* 317:703–713, 1998b.

UKPDS—U.K. Prospective Diabetes Study Group: Efficacy of atenolol and captopril in reducing risk of macrovascular and microvascular complications in type 2 diabetes (UKPDS 39). *BMJ* 317:713–720, 1998c.

Umpierrez GE, Casals MMC, Gebhart SSP, Mixon PS, Clark WS, Phillips LS: Diabetic ketoacidosis in obese African-Americans. *Diabetes* 44:790–795, 1995.

Umpierrez GE, Woo W, Hagopian WA, Isaacs SD, Palmer JP, Gaur LK, Nepom GT, Clark WS, Mixon PS, Kitabchi AE: Immunogenetic analysis suggests different pathogenesis for obese and lean African-Americans with diabetic ketoacidosis. *Diabetes Care* 22:1517–1523, 1999.

Umpierrez GE, Latif KA, Murphy MB, Lambeth HC, Stentz F, Bush A, Kitabchi AE: Thyroid dysfunction in patients with type 1 diabetes. A longitudinal study. *Diabetes Care* 26:1181–1185, 2003.

Umpierrez GE, Smiley D, Kitabchi AE: Narrative review: ketosis-prone type 2 diabetes mellitus. *Ann Intern Med* 144:350–357, 2006a.

Umpierrez GE: Ketosis-prone type 2 diabetes. Time to revise the classification of diabetes. Editorial. *Diabetes Care* 29:2755–2757, 2006b.

Utermann G: The mysteries of lipoprotein(a). *Science* 246:904–910, 1989.

Vaarasmaki M, Hartikainen A-L, Anttila M, Pirttiaho H: Out-patient management does not impair outcome of pregnancy in women with type 1 diabetes. *Diabetes Res Clin Pract* 47:111–117, 2000.

Vaarasmaki M, Antilla M, Pirttiaho H, Hartikainen A-L: Are recurrent pregnancies a risk in Type 1 diabetes? *Acta Obstet Gynecol Scand* 81:1110–1115, 2002.

Vaidya B, Anthony S, Bilous M, Shields B, Drury J, Hutchison S, Bilous R: Detection of thyroid dysfunction in early pregnancy: universal screening or targeted high-risk case finding? *J Clin Endocrinol Metab* 92:203–207, 2007.

Vakkilainen J, Steiner G, Ansquer JC, Aubin F, Rattier S, Foucher C, Hamsten A, Taskinen MR; DAIS Group: Relationships between low-density lipoprotein particle size, plasma lipoproteins, and progression of coronary artery disease: the Diabetes Atherosclerosis Intervention Study (DAIS). *Circulation* 107:1733–1737, 2003.

Valabhji J, McColl AJ, Richmond W, Schachter M, Rubens MB, Elkeles RS: Total antioxidant status and coronary artery calcification in type 1 diabetes. *Diabetes Care* 24:1608–1613, 2001.

Valabhji J, Watson M, Cox J, Poulter C, Elwig C, Elkeles RS: Type 2 diabetes presenting as diabetic ketoacidosis in adolescence. *Diabet Med* 20:416–417, 2003.

Valensi P, Attali JR, Gagant S: Reproducibility of parameters for assessment of diabetic neuropathy. The French Group for Research and Study of Diabetic Neuropathy. *Diabet Med* 10:933–939, 1993.

Valensi P, Huard JP, Giroux C, Attali JR: Factors involved in cardiac autonomic neuropathy in diabetic patients. *J Diabetes Complications* 11:180–187, 1997.

Valensi P, Sachs R-N, Harfouche B, Lormeau B, Paries J, Cosson E, Paycha F, Leutenegger M, Attali JR: Predictive value of cardiac autonomic neuropathy in diabetic patients with or without silent myocardial ischemia. *Diabetes Care* 24:339–343, 2001.

Valensi P, Paries J, Attali JR; French Group for Research and Study of Diabetic Neuropathy: Cardiac autonomic neuropathy in diabetic patients: influence of diabetes duration, obesity, and microangiopathic complications—the French multicenter study. *Metabolism* 52:815–820, 2003.

Valensi P, Paries J, Brulport-Cerisier V, Torremocha F, Sachs RN, Vanzetto G, Cosson E, Lormeau B, Attali JR, Marechaud R, Estour B, Halimi S: Predictive value of silent myocardial ischemia for cardiac events in diabetic patients: influence of age in a French multicenter study. *Diabetes Care* 28:2722–2727, 2005.

Valensise H, Vasapollo B, Novelli GP, Pasqualetti P, Galante A, Arduini D: Maternal total vascular resistance and concentric geometry: a key to identify uncomplicated gestational hypertension. *BJOG* 113:1044–1052, 2006.

Valle R, Bagolin E, Canali C, Giovinazzo P, Barro S, Aspromonte N, Carbonieri E, Milani L: The BNP assay does not identify mild left ventricular diastolic dysfunction in asymptomatic diabetic patients. *Eur J Echocardiogr* 7:40–44, 2006.

Valsania P, Zarich SW, Kowalchuk GJ, Kosinski E, Warram JH, Krolewski AS: Severity of coronary artery disease in young patients with insulin-dependent diabetes mellitus. *Am Heart J* 122:695–700, 1991.

van Wijngaarden P, Coster DJ, Williams KA: Inhibitors of ocular neovascularization. Promises and potential problems. Commentary. *JAMA* 293:1509–1513, 2005.

Vanderheyden M, Bartunek A, Claeys G, Manoharan G, Beckers JF, Ide L: Head to head comparison of N-terminal pro-B-type natriuretic peptide and B-type natriuretic peptide in patients with/without left ventricular systolic dysfunction. *Clin Biochem* 39:640–645, 2006.

Vanderpump MPJ, Tunbridge WMG, French JM, Appleton D, Bates D, Clark F, Grimley Evans J, Hasan DM, Rodgers H, Tunbridge F, Young ET: The incidence of thyroid disorders in the community: a twenty-year follow-up of the Whickham Survey. *Clin Endocrinol* 43:55–68, 1995.

vanHeerebeek L, Borbely A, Niessen HWM, Bronzwaer JGF, van der Velden J, Stienen GJM, Linke WA, Laarman GJ, Paulus WJ: Myocardial structure and function differ in systolic and diastolic heart failure. *Circulation* 113:1966–1973, 2006.

vanHeerebeek L, Hamdani N, Handoko L, Falcao-Pires I, Musters RJ, Kupreishvili K, Ijsselmuiden AJJ, Schalkwijk CG, Bronzwaer JGF, Diamant M, Bobbely A, van der Velden J, Stienen GJM, Laarman GJ, Niessen HWM, Paulaus WJ: Diastolic stiffness of the failing diabetic heart. Importance of fibrosis, advanced glycation end products, and myocyte resting tension. *Circulation* 117:43–51, 2008.

VanLierde B, Buysschaert M, de Hertogh R, Loumaye R, Thomas K: Intravenous administration of ritodrine to pregnant insulin-dependent diabetics. Metabolic impact. *J Gynecol Obstet Biol Reprod* 11:869–875, 1982.

VanLoon AJ, Derksen JT, Bos AF, Rouwe CW: In utero diagnosis and treatment of fetal goitrous hypothyroidism, caused by maternal use of propylthiouracil. *Prenat Diagn* 15:599–604, 1995.

vanStuijvenberg ME, Schabart I, Labadarios D, Nel JT: The nutritional status and treatment of patients with hyperemesis gravidarum. *Am J Obstet Gynecol* 172:1585–1591, 1995.

Vanzetto G, Boizel R, Halimi S, Ormezzano O, Belle L, Fagret D, Machecourt J: Effects of a myocardial ischemia-guided therapeutic program on survival and incidence of coronary events in asymptomatic patients with diabetes: the ARCADIA study. *Diabetes Metab* 33:459–465, 2007.

Vaquero E, Lazzarin N, De Carolis C, Valensise H, Moretti C, Romanini C: Mild thyroid abnormalities and recurrent spontaneous abortion: diagnostic and therapeutic approach. *Am J Reprod Immunol* 43:204–208, 2000.

Vasan R: Biomarkers of cardiovascular disease. Molecular basis and practical considerations. *Circulation* 113:2335–2362, 2006.

Vassalotti JA, Stevens LA, Levey AS: Testing for chronic kidney disease: a position statement from the National Kidney Foundation. *Am J Kidney Dis* 50:169–180, 2007.

Veglio M, Borra M, Stevens LK, Fuller JH, Cavallo Perin P: The relationship between QTc interval prolongation and diabetic complications: the EURODIAB IDDM Complication Study Group. *Diabetologia* 42:68–75, 1999.

Veglio M, Sivieri R, Chinaglia A, Scagliono L, Cavallo-Perin P: QT interval prolongation and mortality in type 1 diabetic patients. A 5–year cohort prospective study. *Diabetes Care* 23:1381–1383, 2000.

Veglio M, Giunti S, Stevens LK, Fuller JH, Perin PC; the EURODIAB IDDM Complications Study Group: Prevalence of Q-T interval dispersion in type 1 diabetes and its relation with cardiac ischemia. *Diabetes Care* 25:702–707, 2002.

Veneman T, Mitraqkou A, Mokan M, Cryer P, Gerich J: Induction of hypoglycemia unawareness by asymptomatic nocturnal hypoglycemia. *Diabetes* 42:1233–1237, 1993.

Verdecchia P, O'Brien E, Pickering T, Staessen JA, Parati G, Myers M, Palatini P; European Society of Hypertension Working Group on Blood Pressure Monitoring: When can the practicing physician suspect white coat hypertension? Statement from the Working Group on Blood Pressure Monitoring of the European Society of Hypertension. *Am J Hypertens* 16:87–91, 2003.

Verdecchia P, Angeli F: How can we use the results of ambulatory blood pressure monitoring in clinical practice? Editorial commentary. *Hypertension* 46:25–26, 2005.

Vered Z, Poler SM, Gibson P, Wlody D, Perez JE: Noninvasive detection of the morphologic and hemodynamic changes during normal pregnancy. *Clin Cardiol* 14:327–334, 1991.

Verhave JC, Fesler P, Ribstein J, du Callier G, Mimran A: Estimation of renal function in subjects with normal serum creatinine levels: influence of age and body mass index. *Am J Kidney Dis* 46:233–241, 2005.

Verier-Mine O, Chaturvedi N, Webb D, Fuller JH: Is pregnancy a risk factor for microvascular complications? The EURODIAB Prospective Complications Study. *Diabet Med* 22:1503–1509, 2005.

Vermillion ST, Scardo JA, Newman RB, Chauhan SP: A randomized, double-blind trial of oral nifedipine and intravenous labetalol in hypertensive emergencies of pregnancy. *Am J Obst Gynecol* 181:858–861, 1999.

Viberti GC, Hill RD, Jarrett RJ, Argyropoulos A, Mahmud U, Keen H: Microalbuminuria as a predictor of clinical nephropathy in insulin-dependent diabetes mellitus. *Lancet* 1:1430–1432, 1982.

Vidaeff AC, Carroll MA, Ramin SM: Acute hypertensive emergencies in pregnancy. Systematic review. *Crit Care Med* 33 (Suppl):S307–S312, 2005.

Vigil-DeGrazia P, Lasso M, Ruiz E, Vega-Malek JC, de Mena FT, Lopez JC; the HYLA Treatment Study Group: Severe hypertension in pregnancy: hydralazine or labetalol. A randomized clinical trial. *Eur J Obstet Gynecol Reprod Biol* 128:157–162, 2006.

Vinereanu D, Nicolaides E, Tweddel AC, Fraser AG: "Pure" diastolic dysfunction is associated with long-axis systolic dysfunction. Implications for the diagnosis and classification of heart failure. *Eur J Heart Fail* 7:820–828, 2005.

Vinge E, Lindegard B, Nilsson-Ehle P, Grubb A: Relationships among serum cystatin C, serum creatinine, lean tissue mass and glomerular filtration rate in healthy adults. *Scand J Lab Clin Invest* 59:587–592, 1999.

Vinik AI, Maser RE, Mitchell BD, Freeman R: Diabetic autonomic neuropathy. Technical review. *Diabetes Care* 26:1553–1579, 2003.

Vinik AI, Erbas T: Cardiovascular autonomic neuropathy: diagnosis and management. *Curr Diab Rep* 6:424–430, 2006.

Virella G, Thorpe SR, Alderson NL, Stephan EM, Atchley D, Wagner F, Lopes-Virella MF; DCCT/EDIC Research Group: Autoimmune response to advanced glycosylation end-products of human low density lipoprotein. *J Lipid Res* 443:487–493, 2003.

Visser M, Bouter LM, McQuillan GM, Wener MH, Harris TB: Elevated C-reactive protein levels in overweight and obese adults. *JAMA* 282:2131–2135, 1999.

Vlassara H, Brownlee M, Manogue KR, Dinarello CA, Pasagian A: Cachectin/TNF and IL-1 induced by glucose-modified proteins: role in normal tissue remodeling. *Science* 240:1546–1548, 1988.

Von Bibra H, Thrainsdottir IS, Hansen A, Dounis V, Malmberg K, Ryden L: Tissue doppler imaging for the detection and quantification of myocardial dysfunction in patients with type 2 diabetes mellitus. *Diabetes Vasc Dis Res* 2:24–30, 2005.

von Dadelszen P, Ornstein MP, Bull SB, Logan AG, Koren G, Magee LA. Fall in mean arterial pressure and fetal growth restriction in pregnancy hypertension: a meta-analysis. *Lancet* 355:87–92, 2000.

von Dadelszen P, Magee LA: Fall in mean arterial pressure and fetal growth restriction in pregnancy hypertension: an updated metaregression analysis. *J Obstet Gynecol Can* 24:941–945, 2002.

Vondra K, Vrbikova J, Sterzl I, Bilek R, Vondrova M, Zamrazil V: Thyroid antibodies and their clinical relevance in young adults with type 1 diabetes during the first 12 years after diabetes onset. *J Endocrinol Invest* 27:728–732, 2004.

Vondra K, Vrbikova J, Dvorakova K: Thyroid gland diseases in adult patients with diabetes mellitus. *Minerva Endocrinol* 30:217–236, 2005.

Vreeburg SA, Jacobs DJ, Dekker GA, Heard AR, Priest KR, Chan A: Hypertension during pregnancy in South Australia, Part 2: risk factors for adverse maternal and/or perinatal outcome—results of multivariable analysis. *Aust N Z J Obstet Gynecol* 44:410–418, 2004.

Vulsma T, Gons MH, De Vijlder JM: Maternal-fetal transfer of thyroxine in congenital hypothyroidism due to a total organification defect or thyroid agenesis. *N Engl J Med* 321:13–16, 1989.

Wackers FJ, Young LH, Inzucchi SE, Chyun DA, Davey JA, Barrett EJ, Taillefer R, Wittlin SD, Heller GV, Filipchuk N, Engel S, Ratner RE, Iskandrian AE; Detection of Ischemia in Asymptomatic Diabetes Investigators: Detection of silent myocardial ischemia in asymptomatic diabetic subjects: the DIAD study. *Diabetes Care* 27:1954–1961, 2004.

Wackers FJ, Chyun DA, Young LH, Heller GV, Iskandrian AE, Davey JA, Barrett EJ, Taillefer R, Wittlin SD, Filipchuk N, Ratner RE, Inzucchi SE: Resolution of asymptomatic myocardial ischemia in patients with type 2 diabetes mellitus in the DIAD study. *Diabetes Care* 30:2892–2898, 2007.

Wadwa RP, Kinney GL, Maahs DM, Snell-Bergeon J, Hokanson JE, Garg SK, Eckel RH, Rewers M: Awareness and treatment of dyslipidemia in young adults with type 1 diabetes. *Diabetes Care* 28:1051–1056, 2005.

Wadwa RP, Kinney GL, Ogden L, Snell-Bergeon JK, Maahs DM, Cornell E, Tray RP, Rewers M: Soluble interleukin-2 receptor as a marker for progression of coronary artery calcification in type 1 diabetes. *Int J Biochem Cell Biol* 38:996–1003, 2006.

Waeber G, Waeber B, Nussberger J, Brunner HR: Ambulatory blood pressure monitoring in adolescent untreated hypertensive patients. *Clin Exp Hypertens* A8:611–614, 2006.

Wagenknecht LE, Bowden DW, Carr JJ, Langefeld CD, Freedman BI, Rich SS: Familial aggregation of coronary artery calcium in families with type 2 diabetes. *Diabetes* 50:861–866, 2001.

Wagner AM, Perez A, Calvo F, Bonet R, Castellvi A, Ordonez J: Apolipoprotein(B) identifies dyslipidemic phenotypes associated with cardiovascular risk in normocholesterolemic type 2 diabetic patients. *Diabetes Care* 22:812–817, 1999.

Wagner AM, Perez A, Zapico E, Ordonez-Llanos J: Non-HDL cholesterol and apolipoprotein B in the dyslipidemic classification of type 2 diabetic patients. *Diabetes Care* 26:2048–2051, 2003.

Wagner AM, Perez A, Sanchez-Quesada JL, Ordonez-Llanos J: Triglyceride-to-HDL cholesterol ratio in the dyslipidemic classification of type 2 diabetes. *Diabetes Care* 28:1798–1800, 2005.

Walden CE, Knopp RH, Wahl PW, Beach KW, Strandness E Jr: Sex differences in the effect of diabetes mellitus on lipoprotein triglyceride and cholesterol concentrations. *N Engl J Med* 311:953–959, 1984.

Walker JJ, Greer I, Calder AA: Treatment of acute pregnancy-related hypertension: labetalol and hydralazine compared. *Postgrad Med J* 59 (Suppl 3):168–170, 1983.

Walker S, Permezel M, Brennecke S, Tuttle L, Ugoni A, Higgins J: The effect of hospitalization on ambulatory blood pressure in pregnancy. *Aust N Z J Obstet Gynecol* 42:490–493, 2002.

Walker JA, Illions EH, Huddleston JF, Smallridge RC: Racial comparisons of thyroid function and autoimmunity during pregnancy and the postpartum period. *Obstet Gynecol* 106:1365–1371, 2005.

Wallace C, Newhouse SJ, Braund P, Zhang F, Tobin M, Falchi M, Ahmadi K, Dobson RJ, Marcano AC, Hajat C, Burton P, Deloukas P, Brown M, Connell JM, Dominiczak A, Lathrop GM, Webster J, Farrall M, Spector T, Samani NJ, Caulfield MJ, Munroe PB: Genome-wide association study identifies genes for biomarkers of cardiovascular disease: serum urate and dyslipidemia. *Am J Hum Genet* 82:139–149, 2008.

Walldius G, Jungner I, Holme I, Aastveit AH, Kolar W, Steiner E: High apolipoprotein B, low apolipoprotein A-I, and improvement in the prediction of fatal myocardial infarction (AMORIS study): a prospective study. *Lancet* 358:2026–2033, 2001.

Walldius G, Aastveit AH, Jungner I: Stroke mortality and the apoB/apoA-I ratio: results of the AMORIS prospective study. *J Intern Med* 259:259–266, 2006a.

Walldius G, Jungner I: The apoB/apoA-I ratio: a strong, new risk factor for cardiovascular disease and a target for lipid-lowering therapy—a review of the evidence. *J Intern Med* 259:493–519, 2006b.

Walls J: Relationship between proteinuria and progressive renal disease. *Am J Kidney Dis* 37 (Suppl 2):S13–S16, 2001.

Walsh MG, Zgibor J, Borch-Johnsen K, Orchard TJ; the DiaComp Investigators: A multinational comparison of complications assessment in type 1 diabetes. The DiaMond Substudy of Complications (DiaComp) level 2. *Diabetes Care* 27:1610–1617, 2004.

Walsh MG, Zgibor J, Borch-Johnsen K, Orchard TJ: A multinational assessment of complications in type 1 diabetes: the DiaMond substudy of complications (DiaComp) Level 1. *Diabetes Vasc Dis Res* 3:84–92, 2006.

Wang TJ, Larson MG, Levy D, Benjamin EJ, Leip EP, Omland T, Wolf PA, Vasan R: Plasma natriuretic peptide levels and the risk of cardiovascular events and death. *N Engl J Med* 350:655–663, 2004.

Wang JC, Criqui MH, Denenberg JO, McDermott MM, Golomb BA, Fronek A: Exertional leg pain in patients with and without peripheral arterial disease. *Circulation* 112:3501–3508, 2005a.

Wang Q, Zhu X, Xu Q, Ding X, Chen YE, Song Q: Effect of C-reactive protein on gene expression in vascular endothelial cells. *Am J Physiol* 288:H1539–H1545, 2005b.

Wang TJ, Gona P, Larson MG, Tofler GH, Levy D, Newton-Cheh C, Jacques PF, Rifai N, Selhub J, Robins SJ, Benjamin EJ, D'Agostino RB, Vasan RS: Multiple biomarkers for the prediction of first major cardiovascular events and death. *N Engl J Med* 355:2631–2639, 2006a.

Wang JG, Staessen JA, Li Y, Van Bortel LM, Nawrot T, Fagard R, Messerli FH, Safar M: Carotid intima-media thickness and antihypertensive treatment: a meta-analysis of randomized controlled trials. *Stroke* 37:1933–1940, 2006b.

Wang YR: Lack of effect of guideline changes on hypertension control for patients with diabetes in the U.S., 1995–2005. *Diabetes Care* 30:49–52, 2007.

Waring WS, Webb DJ, Maxwell SR: Systemic uric acid administration increases serum antioxidant capacity in healthy volunteers. *J Cardiovasc Pharmacol* 38:365–371, 2001.

Warram JH, Gearin G, Laffel L, Krolewski AS: Effect of duration of type 1 diabetes on the prevalence of stages of diabetic nephropathy defined by urinary albumin/creatinine ratio. *J Am Soc Nephrol* 7:930–937, 1996.

Warram J, Krolewski A: Use of the albumin/creatinine ratio in patient care and clinical studies. In: Mogensen CE, ed. *The Kidney and Hypertension in Diabetes Mellitus.* 4th ed. Boston: Kluwer; 1998:85–96.

Warth MR, Arky RA, Knopp RH: Lipid metabolism in pregnancy. III. Altered lipid composition in intermediate, very low, low, and high-density lipoprotein fractions. *J Clin Endocrinol Metab* 41:649–655, 1975.

Warth MR, Knopp RH: Lipid metabolism in pregnancy. V. Interactions of diabetes, body weight, age and high carbohydrate diet. *Diabetes* 26:1056–1062, 1977.

Wartofsky L, Dickey RA: The evidence for a narrower thyrotropin reference range is compelling. Commentary. *J Clin Endocrinol Metab* 90:5483–5488, 2005.

Watala C, Golanski J, Pluta J, Boncler M, Rozalski M, Luzak B, Kropiwnicka A, Drzewoski J: Reduced sensitivity of platelets from type 2 diabetic patients to acetylsalicylic acid (aspirin)—its relation to metabolic control. *Thromb Res* 113:101–113, 2004.

Watanabe D, Suzuma K, Matsui S, Kurimoto M, Kiryu J, Kita M, Suzuma I, Ohashi H, Ojima T, Murakami T, Kobayashi T, Masuda S, Nagao M, Yoshimura N, Takagi H: Erythropoietin as a retinal angiogenic factor in proliferative diabetic retinopathy. *N Engl J Med* 353:782–797, 2005.

Watschinger B, Brunner C, Wagner A, Schnack C, Prager R, Weissel M, Burghuber OC: Left ventricular diastolic impairment in type 1 diabetic patients with microalbuminuria. *Nephron* 63:145–151, 1993.

Waugh J, Perry IJ, Halligan AWF, de Swiet M, Lambert PC, Penny JA, Taylor DJ, Jones DR, Shennan A: Birth weight and 24-hour ambulatory blood pressure in nonproteinuric hypertensive pregnancy. *Am J Obstet Gynecol* 183:633–637, 2000.

Waugh J, Habiba MA, Bosio P, Shennan A, Halligan AWF: Patient initiated home blood pressure recordings are accurate in hypertensive pregnant women. *Hypertens Preg* 22:93–97, 2003a.

Waugh J, Bell SC, Kilby MD, Lambert PC, Blackwell CN, Shennans A, Halligan A: Urinary microalbumin/creatinine ratios: reference range in uncomplicated pregnancy. *Clin Sci* 104:103–107, 2003b.

Waugh JJS, Bell SC, Kilby MD, Blackwell CN, Seed P, Shennan AH, Halligan AWF: Optimal bedside urinalysis for the detection of proteinuria in hypertensive pregnancy: a study of diagnostic accuracy. *BJOG* 112:412–417, 2005a.

Waugh J, Bell SC, Kilby MD, Lambert P, Shennan A, Halligan A: Urine protein estimation in hypertensive pregnancy: which thresholds and laboratory assay best predict clinical outcome? *Hypertens Pregnancy* 24:291–302, 2005b.

Weerasekera DS, Piris H: The significance of serum uric acid, creatinine and urinary microprotein levels in predicting preeclampsia. *J Obstet Gynecol* 23:17–19, 2003.

Weimert NA, Tanke WF, Sims JJ: Allopurinol as a cardioprotective during coronary artery bypass graft surgery. *Ann Pharmacother* 37:1708–1711, 2003.

Weinberger MH: Salt restriction in the treatment of isolated systolic and combined hypertension. Is that enough? Editorial commentary. *Hypertension* 46:31–32, 2005.

Weinbrenner T, Schroder H, Escurriol V, Fito M, Elosua R, Vila J, Marrugat J, Covas MI: Circulating oxidized LDL is associated with increased waist circumference independent of body mass index in men and women. *Am J Clin Nutr* 83:30–35, 2006.

Weiner DA, Ryan TJ, Parsons L, Fisher LD, Chaitman BR, Sheffield T, Tristani FE: Significance of silent myocardial ischemia during exercise testing in patients with diabetes mellitus: a report from the Coronary Artery Surgery Study (CASS) Registry. *Am J Cardiol* 68:729–734, 1991.

Weinrauch LA, Burger A, Gleason RE, Lee AT, D'Elia JA: Left ventricular mass reduction in type 1 diabetic patients with nephropathy. *J Clin Hypertens (Greenwich)* 7:159–164, 2005.

Weir MR: Diltiazem: ten years of clinical experience in the treatment of hypertension. *J Clin Pharmacol* 35:220–232, 1995.

Weiss RE, Brown RL: Doctor...could it be my thyroid? Editorial. *Arch Intern Med* 168:568–569, 2008.

Weissman A, Lowenstein L, Peleg A, Thaler I, Zimmer EZ: Power spectral analysis of heart rate variability during the 100-g oral glucose tolerance test in pregnant women. *Diabetes Care* 29:571–574, 2006.

Weitz C, Khouzami V, Maxwell K, Johnson JWC: Treatment of hypertension in pregnancy with methyldopa: a randomized double blind study. *Int J Gynecol Obstet* 25:35–40, 1987.

Weitz JI, Byrne J, Clagett GP, Farkouh ME, Porter JM, Sackett DL, Strandness DE Jr, Taylor LM: Diagnosis and treatment of chronic arterial insufficiency of the lower extremities: a critical review. American Heart Association medical/scientific statement. *Circulation* 94:3026–3049, 1996.

Weksler BB, Pett SB, Alonso D, Richter RC, Stelzer P, Subramanian V, Tack-Goldman K, Gay WA Jr: Differential inhibition by aspirin of vascular and platelet prostaglandin synthesis in atherosclerotic patients. *N Engl J Med* 308:800–805, 1983.

Wender-Ozegowska E, Kozlik J, Bicsysko R, Ozgowski S: Changes of oxidative stress parameters in diabetic pregnancy. *Free Radic Res* 38:795–803, 2004.

Wender-Ozegowska E, Michalowska-Wender G, Zawiejska A, Pietryga M, Brazert J, Wender M: Concentration of chemokines in peripheral blood in first trimester of diabetic pregnancy. *Acta Obstet Gynecol Scand* 87:14–19, 2008.

Wenger N, Hurst J, Strozier V: Electrocardiographic changes in pregnancy. *Am J Cardiol* 13:774–778, 1964.

Werler MM, Sheehan JE, Mitchell AA: Maternal medication use and risks of gastroschisis and small intestinal atresia. *Am J Epidemiol* 155:26–31, 2002.

Weston PJ, Glancy JM, McNally PG, Thurston H, de Bono DP: Can abnormalities of ventricular repolarization identify insulin-dependent diabetic patients at risk of sudden cardiac death? *Heart* 78:56–60, 1997.

Weston PJ, Gill GV: Is undetected autonomic dysfunction responsible for sudden death in type 1 diabetes mellitus? The "dead in bed" syndrome revisited. *Diabet Med* 16:626–631, 1999.

Westphal SA: The occurrence of diabetic ketoacidosis in non-insulin-dependent diabetes and newly diagnosed diabetic adults. *Am J Med* 101:19–24, 1996.

Whaley-Connell A, Sowers JR: Hypertension mangement in type 2 diabetes mellitus: recommendations of the Joint National Committee VII. *Endocrinol Metab Clin North Am* 34:63–75, 2005.

Whaley-Connell AT, Sowers JR, McFarlane SI, Norris KC, Chen SC, Qiu Y, Wang C, Stevens LA, Vassalotti JA, Collins AJ; Kidney Early Evaluation Program Investigators: Diabetes mellitus in CKD: Kidney Early Evaluation Program (KEEP) and National Health and Nurition and Examination Survey (NHANES) 1999–2004. *Am J Kidney Dis* 51:S21–S29, 2008.

Whelton PK, Barzilay J, Cushman WC, Davis BR, Iiamathi E, Kostis JB, Leenen FH, Louis GT, Margolis KL, Mathis DE, Moloo J, Nwachuku C, Panebianco D, Parish DC, Pressel S, Simmons DL, Thadani U; ALLHAT Collaborative Research Group: Clinical outcomes in antihypertensive treatment of type 2 diabetes, impaired fasting glucose concentration, and normoglycemia: Antihypertensive and Lipid-Lowering Treatment to Prevent Heart Attack Trial (ALLHAT). *Arch Intern Med* 165:1401–1409, 2005.

Whitelaw A: Maternal methyldopa treatment and neonatal blood pressure. *Br Med J* 283:471, 1981.

Whitely L, Padmanabhan S, Hole D, Isles C: Should diabetes be considered a coronary heart disease risk equivalent? Results from 25 years of follow-up in the Renfrew and Paisley Survey. *Diabetes Care* 28:1588–1593, 2005.

Whiteman VE, Homko CJ, Reece EA: Management of hypoglycemia and diabetic ketoacidosis in pregnancy. *Obstet Gynecol Clin North Am* 23:87–107, 1996.

Whitsel EA, Boyko EJ, Rautaharju PM, Raghunathan TE, Lin D, Pearce RM, Weinmann SA, Siscovick DS: Electrocardiographic QT interval prolongation and risk of primary cardiac arrest in diabetic patients. *Diabetes Care* 28:2045–2047, 2005.

Wide-Swensson D, Ingemarsson I, Anderson K-E, Anandakumar C, Arulkumaran S, Ratnam SS: Isradipine reduces blood pressure, but not placental blood flow in pregnancy induced hypertension. *Clin Exper Hypertens Preg* B10:49–60, 1991.

Wide-Swensson DH, Ingemarsson I, Lunell N-O, Forman A, Skajaa K, Lindberg B, Lindeberg S, Marsal K, Andersson K-E: Calcium channel blockade (isradipine) in treatment of hypertension in pregnancy: a randomized placebo-controlled study. *Am J Obstet Gynecol* 173:872–878, 1995.

Wiegmann TB, Chonko AM, Barnerd MJ, MacDougall ML, Folscroft J, Stephenson J, Kyner JL, Moore WV: Comparison of albumin excretion rate obtained with different times of collection. *Diabetes Care* 13:864–871, 1990.

Wikstrom A-K, Wikstrom J, Larsson A, Olovsson M: Random albumin/creatinine ratio for quantification of proteinuria in manifest preeclampsia. *BJOG* 113: 930–934, 2006.

Wilcosky T, Harris R, Weisfeld L: The prevalence and correlates of Rose questionnaire angina among women and men in the Lipid Research Clinics Program Prevalence study population. *Am J Epidemiol* 125:400–409, 1987.

Wild SH, Byrne CD: ABC of obesity. Risk factors for diabetes and coronary heart disease. *BMJ* 333:1009–1011, 2006.

Wildman RP, Muntner P, Chen J, Sutton-Tyrell K, He J: Relation of inflammation to peripheral arterial disease in the national health and nutrition examination survey, 1999–2002. *Am J Cardiol* 96:1579–1583, 2005.

Wilkinson CP, Ferris FL 3rd, Klein RE, Lee PP, Agardh CD, Davis M, Dills D, Kampik A, Paraajaegaram R, Verdaguer JT; the Global Diabetic Retinopathy Project Group: Proposed international clinical diabetic retinopathy and diabetic macular disease severity scales. *Ophthalmology* 110:1677–1682, 2003.

Willems D, Dorchy H, Dufrasne D: Serum lipoprotein(a) in type 1 diabetic children and adolescents: relationships with HbA1C and subclinical complications. *Eur J Pediatr* 155:175–178, 1996.

Williams SB, Goldfine AB, Timimi FK, Ting HH, Roddy MA, Simonson DC, Creager MA: Acute hyperglycemia attenuates endothelium-dependent vasodilation in humans *in vivo*. *Circulation* 97:1695–1701, 1998.

Williams KP, Galerneau F: The role of serum uric acid as a prognostic indicator of the severity of maternal and fetal complications in hypertensive pregnancies. *J Obstet Gynecol Can* 24:628–632, 2002.

Williams RI, Masani ND, Buchalter MB, Fraser AG: Abnormal myocardial strain rate in noncompaction of the left ventricle. *J Am Soc Echocardiogr* 16:293–296, 2003.

Williams B: Evolution of hypertensive disease: a revolution in guidelines. *Lancet* 368:6–8, 2006.

Wilmer WA, Hebert LA, Lewis EJ, Rohde RD, Whittier F, Cattran D, Levey AS, Lewis JB, Spitalewitz S, Blumenthal S, Bain RP: Remission of nephritic syndrome in type 1 diabetes: long-term followup of patients in the Captopril Study. *Am J Kidney Dis* 34:308–314, 1999.

Wilson HK, Keuer SP, Lea AS, Boyd AE 3rd, Eknoyan G: Phosphate therapy in diabetic ketoacidosis. *Arch Intern Med* 142:517–520, 1982.

Wilson PW, D'Agostino RB, Levy D, Belanger AM, Silberhatz H, Kannel WB: Prediction of coronary heart disease using risk factor categories. *Circulation* 97:1837–1847, 1998.

Wilson GA, Coscia LA, McGrory CH, Dunn SR, Radomski JS, Maritz MJ, Armenti VT: National Transplantation Pregnancy Registry: postpregnancy graft loss among female pancreas-kidney transplants. *Transplant Proc* 33:1667–1669, 2001.

Wilson BJ, Watson MS, Prescott GJ, Sunderland S, Campbell DM, Hannaford P, Smith WCS: Hypertensive diseases of pregnancy and risk of hypertension and stroke in later life: results from cohort study. *BMJ* 326:845–849, 2003.

Wilson AM, Boyle AJ, Fox P: Management of ischemic heart disease in women of childbearing age. *Intern Med J* 34:694–697, 2004.

Wilson AM, Swan JD, Ding H, Zhang Y, Whitbourn RJ, Gurry J, Yii M, Wilson AC, Hill M, Triggle C, Best JD, Jenkins AJ: Widespread vascular production of C-reactive protein (CRP) and a relationship between serum CRP, plaque CRP and intimal hypertrophy. *Atherosclerosis* 191:175–181, 2007.

Wilton LV, Shakir S: A postmarketing surveillance study of gabapentin as add-on therapy for 3,100 patients in England. *Epilepsia* 43:983–992, 2002.

Wing DA, Millar LK, Koonings PP, Montoro MN, Mestman JH: A comparison of propylthiuracil versus methimazole in the treatment of hyperthyroidism in pregnancy. *Am J Obstet Gynecol* 170:90–95, 1994.

Winkler K, Wetzka B, Hoffman MM, Friedrich I, Kinner M, Baumstark MW, Wieland H, Marz W, Zahradnik HP: Low density lipoprotein subfractions during pregnancy: accumulation of buoyant LDL with advancing gestation. *J Clin Endocrinol Metab* 85:4543–4550, 2000.

Winocour PH, Taylor RJ: Early alterations of renal function in insulin-dependent diabetic pregnancies and their importance in predicting pre-eclamptic toxemia. *Diabetes Res* 10:159–164, 1989.

Witczak BJ, Hartmann A, Jenssen T, Foss A, Endresen K: Routine coronary angiography in diabetic nephropathy patients before transplantation. *Am J Transplant* 6:2403–2408, 2006.

Witte DR, Tesfaye S, Chaturvedi N, Eaton SE, Kempler P, Fuller JH; EURODIAB Prospective Complications Study Group: Risk factors for cardiac autonomic neuropathy in type 1 diabetes. *Diabetologia* 48:164–171, 2005.

Wofford JL, Kahl FR, Howard GR, McKinney WM, Toole JF, Crouse JR: Relation of extent of extracranial carotid artery atherosclerosis as measured by B-mode ultrasound to the extent of coronary atherosclerosis. *Arterioscler Thromb* 11:1786–1794, 1991.

Wolf M, Sandler L, Hsu K, Vossen-Smirnakis K, Ecker JL, Thadhani R: First trimester C-reactive protein and subsequent gestational diabetes. *Diabetes Care* 26:819–824, 2003.

Wolf G, Chen S, Ziyadeh FN: From the periphery of the glomerular capillary wall toward the center of disease. Podocyte injury comes of age in diabetic nephropathy. *Diabetes* 54:1626–1634, 2005.

Wolfberg AJ, Lee-Paritz A, Peller AJ, Lieberman ES: Obstetric and neonatal outcomes associated with maternal hypothyroid disease. *J Matern Fetal Neonatal Med* 17:35–38, 2005.

Wolff SP, Dean RT: Glucose autoxidation and protein modification: their potential role of autoxidative glycosylation in diabetes. *Biochem J* 245:243–250, 1987.

Wolff K, Carlstrom K, Fyhrquist F, Hemsen A, Lunell N-O, Nisell H: Plasma endothelin in normal and diabetic pregnancy. *Diabetes Care* 20:653–656, 1997.

Wolfsdorf J, Glaser N, Sperling MA: Diabetic ketoacidosis in infants, children, and adolescents. A consensus statement from the American Diabetes Association. *Diabetes Care* 29:1150–1159, 2006.

Wolk R, Cobbe SM, Hicks MN, Kane KA: Functional, structural and dynamic bases of electrical heterogeneity in healthy and diseased cardiac muscle: implications for arrhythmogenesis and antiarrhythmic drug therapy. *Pharmacol Therapeutics* 84:207–231, 1999.

Wolkow PP, Niewczas MA, Perkins B, Ficociello LH, Lipinski B, Warram JH, Krolewski AS: Association of urinary inflammatory markers and renal decline in microalbuminuric type 1 diabetes. *J Am Soc Nephrol* 19:789–797, 2008.

Woolett LA: Maternal cholesterol in fetal development: transport of cholesterol from the maternal to the fetal circulation. *Am J Clin Nutr* 82:1155–1161, 2005.

Wooton PT, Stephens JW, Hurel SJ, Durand H, Cooper J, Ninio E, Humphries SE, Talmud PJ: Lp-PLA2 activity and PLA2G7 A379V genotype in patients with diabetes mellitus. *Atherosclerosis* 189:149–156, 2006.

Wredling R, Levander S, Adamson U, Lins PE: Permanent neurophysiological impairment after recurrent episodes of severe hypoglycemia in man. *Diabetologia* 33:152–157, 1990.

Wright A, Steele P, Bennett JR, Watts G, Polak A: The urinary excretion of albumin in normal pregnancy. *Brit J Obstet Gynecol* 94:408–412, 1987.

Wright AD, Cull CA, Macleod KM, Holman RR; the UKPDS Group: Hypoglycemia in type 2 diabetic patients randomized to and maintained on monotherapy with diet, sulfonylurea, metformin, or insulin for 6 years from diagnosis: UKPDS73. *J Diabetes Complications* 20:395–401, 2006.

Wu AH, Omland T, Duc P, McCord J, Nowak RM, Hollander JE, Herrmann HC, Steg PG, Wold KC, Storrow AB, Abraham WT, Perez A, Kamin R, Clopton P, Maisel AS, McCullough PA: The effect of diabetes on B-type natriuretic peptide concentrations in patients with acute dyspnea: an analysis from the Breathing Not Properly Multinational Study. *Diabetes Care* 27:2398–2404, 2004.

Wylie BR, Kong J, Kozak SE, Marshall CJ, Tong SO, Thompson DM: Normal perinatal mortality in type 1 diabetes mellitus in a series of 300 consecutive pregnancy outcomes. *Am J Perinatol* 19:169–176, 2002.

Wyne KL, Woolett LA: Transport of maternal LDL and HDL to the fetal membranes and placenta of the Golden Syrian hamster is mediated by receptor-dependent and receptor-independent processes. *J Lipid Res* 39:518–530, 1998.

Xiong X, Mayes D, Demianczuk N, Olson DM, Davidge ST, Newburn-Cook C, Saunders LD: Impact of pregnancy-induced hypertension on fetal growth. *Am J Obstet Gynecol* 180:207–213, 1999.

Yamaguchi H, Yoshida J, Yamamoto K, Sakata Y, Mano T, Akehi N, Hori M, Lim YJ, Mishima M, Masuyama T: Elevation of plasma brain natriuretic peptide is a hallmark of diastolic heart failure independent of ventricular hypertrophy. *J Am Coll Cardiol* 43:55–60, 2004.

Yamasaki Y, Kawamori R, Matsushima H, Nishizawa H, Kodama M, Kajimoto Y, Morishima T, Kamada T: Atherosclerosis in carotid artery of young type 1 diabetes patients monitored by ultrasound high-resolution B-mode imaging. *Diabetes* 43:634–639, 1994.

Yamazaki K, Sato K, Shizume K, Kanaji Y, Ito Y, Obara T, Nakagawa T, Koizumi T, Nishimura R: Potent thyrotropic activity of human chorionic gonadotropin variants in terms of ^{125}I incorporation and de novo synthesized thyroid hormone release in human thyroid follicles. *J Clin Endocrinol Metab* 80:473–479, 1995.

Yan SD, Schmidt AM, Anderson GM, Zhang J, Brett J, Zou YS, Pinsky D, Stern D: Enhanced cellular oxidant stress by the interaction of advanced glycation end products with their receptors/binding proteins. *J Biol Chem* 269:9889–9897, 1994.

Yan SF, Ramasamy R, Naka Y, Schmidt AM: Glycation, inflammation, and RAGE: a scaffold for the macrovascular complications of diabetes and beyond. *Circ Res* 93:1159–1169, 2003.

Yang CCH, Chao T-C, Kuo TBJ, Yin C-S, Chien HI: Preeclamptic pregnancy is associated with increased sympathetic and decreased parasympathetic control of HR. *Am J Physiol* 278:H1269–H1273, 2000.

Yang SP, Ho LJ, Cheng SM, Hsu YL, Tsao TP, Chang DM, Lai JH: Cervedilol differentially regulates cytokine production from activated human peripheral blood mononuclear cells. *Cardiovasc Drugs Ther* 18:183–188, 2004.

Yang Q, Guo CY, Cupples LA, Levy D, Wilson PW, Fox CS: Genome-wide search for genes affecting serum uric acid levels: the Framingham Heart Study. *Metabolism* 54:1435–1441, 2005.

Yankowitz J, Piraino B, Laifer A, Frassetto L, Gavin L, Kitzmiller JL, Crombleholme W: Use of erythropoietin in pregnancies complicated by severe anemia of renal failure. *Obstet Gynecol* 80:485–488, 1992.

Yavuz T, Akcay A, Omeroglu RE, Bundak R, Sukur M: Ultrasonic evaluation of early atherosclerosis in children and adolescents with type 1 diabetes mellitus. *J Pediatr Endocrinol Metab* 15:1131–1136, 2002.

Yip SK, Leung TN, Fung HY: Exposure to angiotensin-converting enzyme inhibitors during first trimester: is it safe to fetus? *Acta Obstet Gynecol Scand* 77:570–571, 1998.

Yip G, Wang M, Zhang Y, Fung JW, Ho PY, Sanderson JE: Left ventricular long axis function in diastolic heart failure is reduced in both diastole and systole: time for a redefinition? *Heart* 87:121–125, 2002.

Yla-Herttuala S, Palinski W, Rosenfeld ME, Parthasarathy S, Carew TE, Butlar S, Witztum JL, Steinberg D: Evidence for the presence of oxidatively modified low density lipoprotein in atherosclerotic lesions of rabbit and man. *J Clin Invest* 84:1086–1095, 1989.

Yokoyama H, Okudaira M, Otani T, Watanabe C, Takaike H, Miura J, Yamada H, Mutou K, Satou A, Uchigata Y, Iwamoto Y: High incidence of diabetic nephropathy in early-onset Japanese NIDDM patients. Risk analysis. *Diabetes Care* 21:1080–1085, 1998.

Yoshi T, Iwai M, Li Z, Chen R, Ide A, Fukunaga S, Oshita A, Mogi M, Higaki J, Horiuchi M: Regression of atherosclerosis by amlodipine via anti-inflammatory and anti-oxidative stress actions. *Hypertens Res* 29:457–466, 2006.

Yoshimura M, Hershman JM: Thyrotropic action of human chorionic gonadotropin. *Thyroid* 5:425–434, 1995.

Young RA, Buchanan RJ, Kinch RAH: Use of the protein/creatinine ratio of a single voided urine specimen in the evaluation of suspected pregnancy-induced hypertension. *J Fam Pract* 42:385–389, 1996.

Young ME, McNulty P, Taegtmeyer H: Adaptation and maladaptation of the heart in diabetes: Part II. Potential mechanisms. *Circulation* 105:1861–1870, 2002.

Young LH: Diastolic function and type 1 diabetes. Editorial. *Diabetes Care* 27: 2081–2083, 2004.

Yu E, Guo H, Wu T: Factors associated with discontinuing insulin therapy after diabetic ketoacidosis in adult diabetic patients. *Diabet Med* 18:895–899, 2001.

Yu CM, Lin H, Ho PC, Yang H: Assessment of left and right ventricular systolic and diastolic synchronicity in normal subjects by tissue Doppler echocardiography and the effects of age and heart rate. *Echocardiography* 20:19–27, 2003a.

Yu CK, Papageorghiou AT, Parra M, Palma Dias R, Nicolaides KH; Fetal Medicine Foundation Second Trimester Screening Group: Randomized controlled trial using low-dose aspirin in the prevention of pre-eclampsia in women with abnormal uterine artery Doppler at 23 weeks gestation. *Ultrasound Obstet Gynecol* 22:233–239, 2003b.

Yuan Z, Shioji K, Kihara Y, Takenaka H, Onozawa Y, Kishimoto C: Cardioprotective effects of carvedilol on acute autoimmune myocarditis: anti-inflammatory effects associated with antioxidant property. *Am J Physiol Heart Circ Physiol* 286: H83–H90, 2004.

Zaidi M, Robert AR, Fesler R: Computer assisted study of ECG indices of the dispersion of ventricular depolarization. *J Electrocardiol* 29:199–211, 1996.

Zammitt NN, Frier BM: Hypoglycemia in type 2 diabetes. Pathophysiology, frequency, and effects of different treatment modalities. *Diabetes Care* 28: 2948–2961, 2005.

Zandbergen AAM, Sijbrands EJ, Lamberts SW, Bootsma AH: Normotensive women with type 2 diabetes and microalbuminuria are at high risk for macrovascular disease. *Diabetes Care* 29:1851–1855, 2006.

Zandbergen AAM, Vogt L, de Zeeuw D, Lamberts SWJ, Ouwendijk RJTH, Baggen MGA, Bootsma AH: Change in albuminuria is predictive of cardiovascular outcome in normotensive patients with type 2 diabetes and microalbuminuria. *Diabetes Care* 30:3119–3121, 2007.

Zarich SW, Arbuckle BE, Cohen LR, Roberts M, Nesto RW: Diastolic abnormalities in young asymptomatic diabetic patients assessed by pulsed Doppler echocardiography. *J Am Coll Cardiol* 12:114–120, 1988.

Zarich SW, Nesto RW: Diabetic cardiomyopathy. *Am Heart J* 118:1000–1012, 1989.

Zarich S, Waxman S, Freeman RT, Mittleman M, Hegarty P, Nesto RW: Effects of autonomic nervous system dysfunction on the circadian pattern of myocardial ischemia in diabetes mellitus. *J Am Coll Cardiol* 24:956–962, 1994.

Zeina AR, Odeh M, Rosenschein U, Zaid G, Barmeir E: Coronary artery disease among asymptomatic diabetic and nondiabetic patients undergoing coronary computed tomography angiography. *Coron Artery Dis* 19:37–41, 2008.

Zerbini G, Bonfanti R, Meschi F, Bognetti E, Paesano PL, Gianolli L, Querques M, Maestroni A, Calori G, Del Maschio A, Fazio F, Luzi L, Chiumello G: Persistent renal hypertrophy and faster decline of glomerular filtration rate precede the development of microalbuminuria in type 1 diabetes. *Diabetes* 55:2620–2625, 2006.

Zetterstrom K, Lindeberg SN, Haglund B, Hanson U: Maternal complications in women with chronic hypertension: a population-based cohort study. *Acta Obstet Gynecol Scand* 84:419–424, 2005.

Zetterstrom K, Lindeberg SN, Haglund B, Hanson U: Chronic hypertension as a risk factor for offspring to be born small for gestational age. *Acta Obstet Gynecol Scand* 85:1046–1050, 2006.

Zgibor JC, Orchard TJ: Has control of hyperlipidemia and hypertension in patients with type 1 diabetes improved over time? *Diabetes* 50:A255, 2001.

Zgibor JC, Wilson RR, Orchard TJ: Has control of hypercholesterolemia and hypertension in type 1 diabetes improved over time? *Diabetes Care* 28:521–526, 2005.

Zgibor JC, Piatt GA, Ruppert K, Orchard TJ, Roberts MS: Deficiencies of cardio-vascular risk prediction models for type 1 diabetes. *Diabetes Care* 29: 1860–1865, 2006.

Zhang J, Klebanoff MA: Low blood pressure during pregnancy and poor perinatal outcomes: an obstetric paradox. *Am J Epidemiol* 153:642–646, 2001.

Ziegler D, Laux G, Dannehl K, Spuler M, Muhlen H, Mayer P, Gries FA: Assessment of cardiovascular autonomic function: age-related normal ranges and reproducibility of spectral analysis, vector analysis, and standard tests of heart rate variation and blood pressure responses. *Diabet Med* 9:166–175, 1992a.

Ziegler D, Dannehl K, Muhlen H, Spuler M, Gries FA: Prevalence of cardiovascular autonomic dysfunction assessed by spectral analysis, vector analysis, and standard tests of heart rate variation and blood pressure responses at various stages of diabetic neuropathy. *Diabet Med* 9:806–814, 1992b.

Ziegler D, Gries FA, Muhlen M, Rathmann W, Spuler M, Lessmana F: Prevalence and clinical correlates of cardiovascular autonomic and peripheral diabetic neuropathy in patients attending diabetes centers. The DIACAN Multicenter Study Group. *Diabetes Metab* 19:143–151, 1993.

Ziegler D: Cardiovascular autonomic neuropathy: clinical manifestations and measurement. *Diabetes Rev* 7:300–315, 1999.

Zile MR, Brutsaert DL: New concepts in diastolic dysfunction and diastolic heart failure: Part I. Diagnosis, prognosis, and measurements of diastolic function. *Circulation* 105:1387–1393, 2002.

Zile MR: Heart failure with preserved ejection fraction: is this diastolic heart failure? *J Am Coll Cardiol* 41:1519–1522, 2003.

Zile MR, Baicu CF, Gaasch WH: Diastolic heart failure. Abnormalities in active relaxation and passive stiffness of the left ventricle. *N Engl J Med* 350: 1953–1959, 2004.

Zimmerman D: Fetal and neonatal hyperthyroidism. *Thyroid* 9:727–733, 1999.

Zoeller RT: Transplacental thyroxine and fetal brain development. *J Clin Invest* 111:954–957, 2003.

Zuspan FP, Rayburn WF: Blood pressure self-monitoring during pregnancy: practical considerations. *Am J Obstet Gynecol* 164:2–6, 1991.

PART (3)

Obstetrical Management of Women with Preexisting Diabetes Mellitus

PRENATAL AND ANTEPARTUM FETAL ASSESSMENT

—— *Original contribution by Deborah L. Conway MD and Patrick M. Catalano MD*

Applications of techniques to monitor fetal condition and growth across gestation have accompanied improvements in glycemic control that are associated with reduced perinatal mortality and morbidity in pregnancies complicated by PDM. Major fetal conditions (influenced by maternal hyperglycemia and vascular disease) that are subject to assessment include congenital anomalies, cardiovascular function, restriction of growth or excess size and fat deposition, fetal hypoxia or acidosis, and fetal lung maturation. When no fetal anomalies are present and metabolic control is excellent, rates of fetal death in diabetic women can be comparable with a nondiabetic population. However, major congenital malformations, suboptimal glycemic control, poor patient adherence, and presence of vascular disease or comorbid conditions increase the risk for fetal loss. Therefore, strategies for avoiding these losses should employ tests that can detect fetal compromise early, but with sufficient specificity to minimize unnecessary intervention. The roster of sequential laboratory evaluations suggested for women with PDM throughout pregnancy is presented in Table III.1.

Ultrasonography and Markers Used to Assess Fetal Growth, Structure, and Genotype

First-Trimester Ultrasonography and Biomarkers

Women with type 1 and type 2 diabetes have increased rates of spontaneous abortion when periconceptional metabolic control has been poor (early studies reviewed in Kitzmiller 96, Temple 02, Jovanovic 05, Temple 06). In the first trimester of pregnancy, monitoring fetal well-being consists primarily of ensuring that a pregnancy is progressing and will continue. Transvaginal and transabdominal ultrasonography provides evidence that an early fetus is alive and furnishes important gestational age information that may be critical in clinical decision-making later in pregnancy. Crown–rump length (CRL) is a more accurate indicator of gestational age than the mean gestational

TABLE III.1 Techniques and Purpose of Fetal Assessment Used in Pregnant Women with PDM According to Gestational Age

Testing Modality	Timing	Comments
Ultrasound, transvaginal or transabdominal Crown–rump length Fetal cardiac activity NT thickness at 12–13 weeks; couple with free β-hCG, PAPP-A	First trimester	Important to confirm living fetus, establish gestational age, and estimate due date as early as possible; elevated NT measurement is associated with fetal Down syndrome, and specific congenital anomalies (cardiac defects, diaphragmatic hernia, skeletal and neurological abnormalities) more common in women with PDM.
Maternal serum marker screening	First trimester (with or without ultrasonic NT measurement) Second trimester (triple[1] or quad[2] marker test, or MSAFP alone)	PDM is associated with an increased risk of open neural tube defects (detected by second-trimester triple or quad marker test, or MSAFP alone).
Ultrasound, transabdominal Fetal biometric measurements Fetal anatomy	Second trimester	Important to establish gestational age when this has not been done earlier in pregnancy; detailed fetal anatomical examination and fetal echocardiography should be considered in all women with PDM, but particularly in those at highest risk for congenital anomalies.[3]
Ultrasound, transabdominal Fetal growth rate Amniotic fluid volume	Third trimester	Following fetal growth by ultrasound examinations at regular intervals may be warranted when a pregnancy is at risk for fetal growth restriction (hypertension or vascular complications) or excessive fetal growth (poor glycemic control), or in lower-risk women when a fundal height–dates discrepancy is noted.
Nonstress test	Third trimester	Abnormal NST and BPP tests suggest possible decreased fetal oxygenation status, but are affected by other factors. Optimal testing regimen.
Biophysical profile	Third trimester	And ideal time to initiate testing are not known. However, women with hypertensive disorders, vascular disease, or evidence of fetal growth restriction should begin testing earlier, with a frequency of every 3–7 days.
Doppler velocimetry of umbilical artery (middle cerebral artery, ductus venosus, umbilical vein)	Third trimester	The utility of this testing has not been established in the absence of hypertensive disease, vasculopathy, or fetal growth restriction. It may be useful adjunctive testing in these settings.

Testing Modality	Timing	Comments
Amniotic fluid markers of fetal lung maturity	Before delivery in indicated cases	Positive tests suggest a low risk of RDS in the newborn infant

[1]*Maternal serum alpha-fetoprotein (MSAFP), unconjugated estriol, chorionic gonadotropin.*
[2]*All components of the triple marker test, plus inhibin.*
[3]*Elevated first-trimester hemoglobin A1C value, abnormal multiple marker results; abnormality suspected on basic ultrasound study or personal history of a prior birth affected by congenital anomalies.*

β-hCG, β-*human chorionic gonadotropin; BPP, biophysical profile; MSAFP, maternal serum alpha-fetoprotein; NST, nonstress test; NT, nuchal transparency; PAPP-A, pregnancy-associated plasma protein-A; PDM, preexisting diabetes mellitus; RDS, respiratory distress syndrome.*

sac diameter. Cardiac motion usually is observed when the embryo length is ≥5 mm (ACOG 04a). Because the occurrence of pregnancy often necessitates changes in treatment modality for these women (such as changing from oral agents to insulin), it is prudent to promptly confirm the viability of the pregnancy. On the other hand, efforts to optimize glucose levels should proceed for the benefit of the woman whether or not fetal viability can be confirmed with US.

There has been controversy whether "early fetal growth delay" occurs in type 1 diabetes. In an early cross-sectional study in Denmark, fetuses of diabetic women at 5–13 weeks gestation averaged 5.5 days smaller than control fetuses, and a subset of fetuses ≥9 days smaller than expected had a 20% frequency of fetal anomalies (Pedersen 79,81). The difficulty in determining the onset of pregnancy may be relevant to these findings. A subsequent study in the same laboratory changed the "small group" to discrepancies of ≥6 days from the regular LMP or rise in BBT (27% of viable singleton diabetic pregnancies) and found that group to be associated with elevated A1C levels (Pedersen 84) and impaired psychomotor development at age 4 (Petersen 88). Two other reports supported the association of early embryonic "growth delay" with poor glycemic control at conception (Tchobroustsky 85, Mulder 91a); however, none of these European studies were controlled for smoking or drinking alcohol in early and perhaps unrecognized pregnancy. Studies in Edinburgh (Steel 84,95) and San Diego (Cousins 88) did not confirm differences in early embryonic growth in carefully dated diabetic and control pregnancies.

In the prospective National Institute of Child Health and Human Development (NICHHD) Diabetes and Early Pregnancy Study, mean CRL at 8 weeks did not differ in 269 diabetic women and 289 control women; however, at 12 weeks, mean measurements were 58.5 ± 8.8 mm vs. 60.6 ± 8.7 mm; p = 0.04) (Brown 92). Early fetal growth delay, which is defined as sonographic gestational age ≥6 days less than menstrual gestational age, was present in 9.9% of nondiabetic subjects at 10–15 weeks compared with 32 of 256 (12.5%) normal fetuses of diabetic subjects and 4 of 13 (30.8%) malformed fetuses of diabetic subjects (p = 0.06; normal vs. malformed) (Brown 92). Early fetal growth delay did not predict eventual BW. A1C levels did not differ in subjects with or without growth delay. Women who both smoked tobacco and drank alcohol had increased growth delay. Investigators concluded that "in clinical practice, inaccuracies in menstrual dating and sonographic measurements will probably obscure and confound the interpretation of subtle delays in fetal growth" (Brown 92). A retrospective survey of 38 pregnancies with PDM and 81 controls who had first-trimester

US examinations found that 28.9% of the former had a difference ≥6 days between postmenstrual age and "delayed" US age compared with 18.5% in controls (p = 0.02). Congenital anomalies were common in the diabetic group (18.4%), but no association was found between anomalies and "growth delay" (Reece 97). We may conclude that pregnancies are difficult to "date" by the last menstrual period in diabetic women and that early US is indicated for this purpose, which helps establish the timing of later evaluations and procedures.

In nondiabetic and diabetic gestations, increasing evidence suggests that early US scanning reduces the gestational age estimate in 23–41% of women, causing 40-week post-onset-of-menses due dates to often be readjusted (Yang 02, Bennett 04, Morin 05). Many investigators believe that early sonography is the best method to date pregnancy due to the frequency of delayed ovulation in women with regular menstrual cycles (Goldenberg 89, Rowlands 93, Gardosi 98, Nguyen 99, Khalish 04, Dietz 07).

The growth and structure of the yolk sac may be affected by poorly controlled diabetes, at least experimentally (Reece 04). Even though the yolk sac contains no yolk in humans, it is the embryonic source of blood cells, blood vessels, primitive germ cells, and epithelia of the gastrointestinal and respiratory tracts. Four to six weeks postconception, the provisceral yolk sac is inactive and the extruded remnant is attached to the embryo (Moore 98). In clinical use, routine US evaluation of the yolk sac remnant in women with PDM was not helpful due to wide variability (Reece 88). Yet in a recent study using a three-dimensional US approach, yolk sac volume was greater in women with PDM than in controls at 5–9 weeks gestation; it also decreased faster after an equal peak volume at 10 weeks until it was no longer visable after 12 weeks in both groups (Cosmi 05). Yolk sac diameter was significantly larger for gestational age in 60 women with type 1 diabetes (especially in those with elevated A1C) than in 60 healthy pregnancy controls (Ivanisevic 06). The clinical and diagnostic implications of these results are unclear.

An emerging technology uses first-trimester (12–13 weeks) sonographic measurements of nuchal translucency (NT) thickness as a risk predictor for congenital heart and other defects (Souka 98, Ghi 01, McAuliffe 04, Atzei 05, Bahado-Singh 05, Makrydimas 05, Maymon 05, Johnson 07, Weiner 07), which are then best identified at 18–22 weeks (McAuliffe 05a,b, Saltveldt 06, Westin 06). In a preliminary study of 74 pregnant women with type 1 diabetes, no association was found between fetal NT thickness and A1C or level of glycemic control (Bartha 03). The mean or median Δ NT (difference of the measured fetal NT from the normal median NT at the measured CRL) was not significantly different in 206 pregnancies with type 1 diabetes compared with 16,366 controls (Spencer 03b,c,05).

NT thickness is also used to screen for chromosomal abnormalities during the late first trimester in concert with maternal serum-free β-hCG and pregnancy-associated plasma protein-A (PAAP-A), both of trophoblast origin (Krantz 00, Spencer 03a, Wapner 03, Dugoff 04, Krantz 04, Nicolaides 04, Avgidou 05, Kagan 06, Perni 06, Holmgren 08). Fetal aneuploidy is not increased by maternal diabetes per se. The ACOG and others have suggested clinical management guidelines for the prenatal diagnosis of aneuploidies (Reddy 06, ACOG 07, Breathnach 07). PAAP-A is of special interest because it is identified as a protease for IGF binding protein-4 (Lawrence 99). It is speculated that low PAAP-A levels are associated with higher levels of IGF binding protein, thus leading to lower levels of free IGF. IGF is important in placentation (Irwin 99), which could help explain the association of very low first-trimester PAAP-A levels with intrauterine growth restriction (IUGR) later in pregnancy (Smith 02, Dugoff 04, Krantz 04, Smith 06). It remains unresolved whether maternal weight-adjusted free β-hCG or PAAP-A levels are different in women with diabetes compared with controls (Aso 04) and whether adjustments are needed to calculate the risks of chromosomal defects or IUGR in women with PDM (Castracane 85, Braunstein 89, Pedersen 98, Ong 00, Spencer 05).

Second-Trimester Fetal Assessment

Second-trimester fetal assessment focuses on screening for risk of fetal chromosome abnormalities (which are not increased with diabetes) as well as detection of major fetal malformations, the rates of which are greater (4–15%) with increasing first-trimester A1C levels and absence of intensified preconception care of diabetes (Inkster 06, Temple 06, Jonasson 07). The increased risk of malformation exists in both type 1 and type 2 diabetes populations, and there are high rates in ethnic minorities. The crude RR was 2.5–7.7 for major malformations compared with the background population or tight-glycemic-control group in recent studies (early studies reviewed in Cousins 91 and Kitzmiller 96; Omori 94, Reece 98, Cundy 00, Dunne 00, McElvy 00, Schaefer-Graf 00, Suhonen 00, Vaarasmaki 00, Hadden 01, Farrell 02, Platt 02, Sheffield 02, Temple 02, Penney 03, Vangen 03, Evers 04, Jensen 04, Ray 04a, Clausen 05, McElduff 05a, Verheijen 05, Guerin 07). The association with diabetes in a large population-based registry from 1980 to 1996 was strongest for renal agenesis (adjusted prevalence odds ratio [POR] 14.8), obstructive congenital abnormalities of the genital tract (POR 4.3), cardiovascular congenital abnormalities (POR 3.4), and multiple congenital abnormalities (POR 4.3) (Nielsen 05). Testing for abnormalities takes two forms: maternal serum marker screening (α-fetoprotein [AFP], free β-hCG, inhibin A, unconjugated estriol) and anotomical survey by US.

All diabetic pregnant women without abnormalities identified by NT studies at 12–13 weeks should be offered multiple serum marker screening at 15–20 weeks gestation, with appropriate referral to a perinatologist/perinatal genetic counselor for any abnormal result. Early data indicated that AFP concentrations decreased with poor glycemic control in women with PDM and with maternal weight >200 lb (Wald 79, Milunsky 82, Baumgarten 88, Greene 88, Martin 90, Henriques 93, Evans 02a), causing laboratories to use correction factors to standardize multiples of the median for diabetic pregnancies. Some investigators have recently proposed that with improved glycemic control, adjustment of AFP values for PDM is no longer justified (Evans 02b). Midtrimester measurements of β-hCG and unconjugated estriol do not need to be adjusted for PDM (Evans 96, Peled 03). Moderately elevated maternal serum AFP values in diabetic and other pregnancies with normal amniotic fluid AFP levels (and no NTDs) have been associated with increased risk for various obstetrical complications (Greene 91, Yaron 99).

Women with PDM should be offered a detailed US examination at 18–22 weeks gestation, with measurements of biparietal diameter (BPD), HC, abdominal circumference (AC), and femoral diaphysis length (FL) for dating confirmation and growth information (ACOG 04a). Timing of the US study is often adjusted according to maternal body habitus. The midtrimester study should include a systematic evaluation of fetal anatomy, such as the Essential Elements of the Fetal Anatomic Ultrasound Survey promulgated by the American College of Radiology (ACR 03, ACOG 04a). Detailed study is important for signs of NTDs and cardiac anomalies, including a four-chamber view of the fetal heart and outflow tracts (ACOG 04a). Comprehensive fetal ultrasonography may be more efficient at identifying NTDs than maternal AFP screening (Greene 91, Albert 96, Norem 05). The sensitivity of fetal sonography at 18–22 weeks gestation in early studies was 59–80% for detection of noncardiac defects in fetuses of diabetic mothers, with maternal obesity a limiting factor (Gomez 88, Pijlman 89, Greene 91, Albert 96). The standard four-chamber cardiac view missed 44–67% of cardiac anomalies in diabetic (Greene 91, Albert 96) and nondiabetic pregnancies (Wigton 93, Crane 94).

Although fetal echocardiography—performed by a qualified perinatologist, cardiologist, radiologist, or US technician at 18–22 weeks gestation—may be appropriate for all women with PDM (Copel 87, Pijlman 89, Shields 93, Veille 93, Meyer-Wittkopf 96, Smith 97), it is certainly recommended for those at increased risk for fetal anomalies. Such pregnancies would include those with elevated A1C levels in the first trimester, increased NT thickness, abnormal serum multiple marker results, and abnormal findings on standard US, as well as a history of cardiac defects in prior offspring. The majority of neonatally confirmed cardiac defects in IDMs that are not identified by the standard four-chamber US view involve lesions of the cardiac septum and outflow tracts (Copel 87, Pijlman 89, Albert 96, Meyer 96, Smith 97, Ferencz 90). Color Doppler ultrasonography is helpful in detecting septal defects and in visualizing the central opening of a single atrioventricular valve (Gabrielli 04). The yield of abnormal fetal echocardiograms in a diabetic population ranges from 2% to 7% depending on the degree of risk in the sample (Smythe 92, Cooper 95, Gladman 97, Friedberg 04). The sensitivity of fetal echocardiography with multiple images to detect cardiac lesions in IDMs ranges from 82% to 98% and is limited by maternal obesity (Smythe 92, Cooper 95, Albert 96, Gladman 97, Smith 97, Tometzki 99, Friedberg 04). The sensitivity range is similar to that obtained in prescreened and unselected populations (Davis 90, Stumpflen 96, Berghella 01, Meyer-Wittkopf 01, Perolo 01, Carvalho 02, Randall 05). In a large series with good follow-up, the cardiac lesions with the highest frequencies of inaccurate fetal diagnosis were coarctation of the aorta (30.1%), mitral atresia (30.0%), tricuspid atresia (11.6%), complete transposition (20.0%), and common arterial trunk (28.6%) (Allan 94). Three-dimensional approaches may improve diagnostic capability (Chan 04, Benacerraf 05, Goncalves 05).

Late first- and second-trimester imaging of bilateral flow velocity waveforms in maternal uterine arteries (Nylund 82) by continuous, pulsed, or color Doppler studies have been evaluated as an imperfect predictor of preterm preeclampsia and IUGR (Trudinger 85a, Bower 93, Harrington 97, Albaiges 00, Chien 00, Martin 01, Chappell 02, Aardema 04, Dugoff 05, Toal 08). Signs of early diastolic notch, increased pulsatility or resistance index, or elevated systolic/diastolic (S/D) ratio reflect abnormal uteroplacental vascular resistance (Ochi 98), often associated with decreased trophoblast invasion and lack of physiological remodeling of spiral arterioles (Lin 95, Prefumo 04, Belkacemi 05). Primarily used in research studies, this technique has not been widely applied in diabetic pregnant women (Bracero 89a, Kofinas 91, Salvesen 92, Haddad 93, Salvesen 93a, Zimmerman 94). Abnormal uteroplacental vascular impedance was associated with pregestational diabetic vasculopathy in most studies (Kofinas 91, Haddad 93, Pietryga 05). In one small study of women with type 1 diabetes, significant increases in placental site arcuate artery Doppler S/D ratios were associated with decidual arteriolar fibrinoid necrosis, foam cell deposition (atherosis), and thrombosis (Barth 96).

Third-Trimester Fetal Ultrasonography

There are several purposes for fetal US examinations beyond the second trimester ($\geq$26 weeks gestation). The first is to assess estimated fetal weight (EFW) to detect IUGR (Bernstein 00, Doctor 01, Chauhan 06) with or without head sparing so that tests of fetal well-being can be applied. The 10th percentile of growth for gestational age predicts increased risk of neonatal death in all U.S. pregnancies, which varies by gestational age at birth: neonatal mortality rate ratio of 3.1 at 26 weeks, 1.4 at 30 weeks, 2.6 at 34 weeks, and 1.2 at 38 weeks (Boulet 06). The OR for IUGR was 6.0 (95%

CI 1.5–23.3) for IDMs with microvascular disease compared with other IDMs (Howarth 07). The second purpose is to detect excessive fetal size and fatness as a marker of glycemic control (early studies in PDM reviewed by Ben-Haroush 04; Combs 00, Holcomb 00, Wong 01, Best 02, Jaffe 02, Greco 03, Coomarasamy 05, Langer 05, Sacks 07). Except for FL, fetal biometric measurements at 24–29 weeks gestation and beyond reflect glycemic control as well as fetal size determined by gestational age and maternal weight gain (Ogata 80, Landon 89a, Keller 90, Reece 90, Greene 95, Koukkou 97, Wong 02, Ben-Haroush 07).

Another purpose for third-trimester US is estimation of AF volume, which may be abnormally increased or decreased in women with diabetes (Cousins 87, Reece 98, Girz 92, Rosenn 93, Dashe 00, Carpenter 04, Underwood 05). In poorly controlled diabetes, a linear relationship was found between amniotic fluid index (AFI) and BW percentiles (Vink 06).

- The AFI is a summation of AF depth-of-pocket measurements in four quadrants of the intrauterine space.
- AFI ≥20 cm is defined as polyhydramnios.
- AFI <5 cm or largest vertical pocket ≤2 cm defines oligohydramnios (Manning 90, Magann 03).

A fourth purpose for fetal US examinations is to detect fetal cardiac hypertrophy and possible impaired cardiac function (Gardiner 06, Wong 07). Signs of this condition include increased right ventricular wall thickness and interventricular septal thickness, decreased ventricular compliance and filling, and impaired fractional shortening of the ventricles, all of which can be associated with fetal death (Leslie 82, Sardesai 01) or heart failure after delivery (Rasanen 87, Rizzo 91a, Weber 91, Rizzo 92, Vielle 92, Gandhi 95, Rizzo 95a, Tsyvian 98, Weiner 99, Wong 03a, Prefumo 05).

Follow-up US examinations can be performed at regular intervals in women at high risk of poor fetal growth, such as those with coexisting hypertension or vascular disease. They can also be performed as indications arise in lower-risk diabetic women, such as fundal height–dates discrepancies. Although there is limited accuracy from late third-trimester fetal US measurements (Sacks 00) in predicting the macrosomic (>4,000–4,500 gm) fetus of the diabetic mother (sensitivity 68–80%; specificity 78–96%; NPV 81–87%; 71–82% of EFWs within 10% of actual BW) (Tamura 85, Alsulyman 97, Combs 00, Best 02, Ben-Haroush 03, Farrell 04), there is consensus that such measurements are more accurate than predictions based on gestational age or physical examination of the maternal abdomen in obese women. Algorithms including clinical risk factors for macrosomia, high AFI, and US EFW >75th percentile or >4,000 gm may increase the predictive value for severe macrosomia (Hackmon 07, Pates 08).

Measures of fetal fat correlate with accelerated growth velocity in large fetuses of diabetic mothers (Bernstein 92, Kehl 96, Bernstein 98). Retrospective studies in women with PDM sought to relate a measure of fetal adiposity (AC >60th–75th percentile) to a measure of fetal hyperinsulinemia (elevated AF insulin concentration) (Kainer 97), yet in the most recent study, the majority of cases with AC >75th percentile had normal AF insulin (Schaefer-Graf 03). Controversy surrounds whether focus on the fetal AC (AC >35–38 cm) (Jazayeri 99, Gilby 00, Bethune 03, Loetworawanit 06), especially in relation to HC, improves the prediction of difficult vaginal birth in diabetic women (Landon 89a, Johnstone 96, Wong 01, Farrell 04, Maticot-Baptista 07). Other techniques that attempt to predict risk of shoulder dystocia at delivery have not achieved wide clinical usage (Elliott 82, Kitzmiller 87, Mintz 89, Cohen 96,99). A retrospective US study within 14 days of delivery showed that a positive difference between fetal abdominal diameter and BPD (AD – BPD ≥2.6 cm) yielded a risk rate for shoulder dystocia of 38.5% in diabetic women (Miller 07). Prospective controlled studies of these techniques are needed to demonstrate their costs and benefits, but such studies are difficult to perform given the requirements of informed consent.

Antepartum Assessment for Fetal Hypoxia

The pathophysiology of fetal death in diabetic women is incompletely understood, but fetal hyperglycemia, hyperinsulinemia, hypoxia, and acidosis certainly play a role (Robillard 78, Seeds 79, Carson 80, Miodovnik 82, Philipps 82a, Milley 84, Philipps 84, Mimouni 86a, Clark 88, Mimouni 88a, Hay 89, Bradley 92, Salvesen 92,93a,b,c, Mohsin 06, Dudley 07). The risk of stillbirth with type 1 diabetes is well known, but association with type 2 diabetes is at least as great, with obesity a probable factor (Nohr 05, deValk 06, Guenter 06, Macintosh 06, Cundy 07, Lapolla 07). Maternal hypertension and diabetic vasculopathy are contributory (Gonzalez-Gonzalez 08), and fetal venous thrombosis has been noted with very poor glycemic control (Oppenheimer 65, Foley 81). Some cases of fetal demise are associated with acute fetal cardiac hypertrophy (Leslie 82, Sardesai 01). Chronic fetal hypoxia is marked by increased fetal erythropoietin (Widness 81, Philipps 82b, Shannon 86, Teramo 87, Stonestreet 89, Widness 90, Salvesen 93d, Mamopoulos 94, Salvesen 95, Jazayeri 98, Teramo 04) that is produced by trophoblast and various fetal tissues (Conrad 96, Dame 98, Fairchild 99, Davis 03) and not transferred across the human placenta (Schneider 95).

The placenta may show histological abnormalities compatible with impaired placental function in diabetic pregnancies (Emmrich 76, Jones 76, Kitzmiller 81, Asmussen 82a,b, Teasdale 83, Bjork 84, Semmler 85, Teasdale 85, Mayhew 93,94, Barth 96, Mayhew 02, Evers 03, Mayhew 03, Desoye 04, Galettis 04, Mayhew 04). Some experimental evidence suggests that hyperglycemia affects fetoplacental vasoactive prostaglandin release (Jeremy 83, Crandell 85, Rakoczi 88, Roth 90, Saldeen 96). Placental oxidative stress found in hyperglycemic diabetes can cause vascular dysfunction in the placenta (Lyall 98, Leitch 99, Kossenjans 00, Myatt 00, Coughlan 04). In the fetoplacental circulation, K_{ATP} and K_V channels contribute to baseline vascular tone and hypoxia-induced vasoconstriction (Hampl 02); in diabetes, vascular K_{ATP} channel function is impaired (Bisseling 05). Increased baseline vascular tone of the fetal–placental vascular bed in diabetes is apparently not related to NO-mediated effects (Lyall 98, di Iulio 99, Bisseling 03) or increased vascular response to thromboxane (Wilkes 94). Studies of diabetes-induced differences in placental expression of other angiopoietic/vasoactive factors (Janota 03, Leach 04), including fibroblast and placental growth factors (Burleigh 04, Ong 04, Loukovaara 05) and placental erythropoietin (Resch 03, Jain 06), are preliminary.

Surveillance for signs of placental insufficiency and fetal hypoxia usually begins in the third trimester by using a variety of testing modalities (Table III.1) (Fuentes 96, Landon 96, Harman 97, Bocking 03, Siddiqi 03, Kontopoulos 04, Malcus 04, Graves 07). Antepartum fetal asssment has been a valuable approach to safely prolonging the pregnancies of women with PDM (Gabbe 03). Biophysical signs of fetal hypoxemia include acute loss of: (a) breathing movements, (b) tone and purposeful movements, and (c) fetal heart rate (FHR) reactivity and variability, with or without decelerations of the FHR, as well as effects of chronic hypoxia on reduction of AF volume (Manning 95). Some evidence states that "fetal breathing movements disappear early in the course of progressive hypoxemia, whereas fetal movements disappear with more advanced disease" (Manning 95). To appropriately interpret the clinical results obtained, it is helpful to understand how the diabetic state affects these fetal biophysical parameters. Differences exist in fetal sleep/wake cycles between diabetic and nondiabetic pregnancies (Dierker 82). Specifically, it appears that term fetuses and neonates of women with PDM have delayed development of the relatively longer sleep/wake cycles that are typically found in normal term fetuses and newborns. Other studies show an early delay in gestational development of normal fetal movement patterns (except fetal breathing movements), especially with poor periconceptional glycemic control (Visser 85, Mulder 91b,c). In the third trimester, there may be fewer fetal movements and FHR accelerations, but more fetal breathing movements in fetuses of mothers with diabetes compared with controls depending on the level of glycemic control (Kariniemi 83, Mulder 90, Devoe 94, Mulder 95, Weiner 96, Allen 99, Tincello 01, Robertson 03, Rosenn 04).

Data are conflicting regarding the influence of maternal blood glucose on fetal biophysical parameters. In the postprandial state, both fetal breathing movements and total fetal activity were found to be increased in diabetic women compared with nondiabetic controls (Natale 78, Patrick 80, Roberts 80, de Vries 87). Studies of induced maternal hyperglycemia in normal pregnancies have shown increased (Miller 78, Aladjem 79, Gelman 80, Graca 81, Bocking 84, Eller 92, Gillis 92), decreased (Edelberg 87, Allen 99, Zimmer 00), or no change in fetal activity or FHR reactivity (Lewis 78, Natale 83, Divon 85, Druzin 86, Bocking 89). Maternal glucose infusion tends to increase fetal breathing activity (Natale 78, Bocking 82, Divon 85). Induced maternal hypoglycemia to ~40 mg/dL (2.2 mM) associated with a rise in maternal catecholamines has led to an increase in the frequency and amplitude of FHR accelerations (Bjorklund 96), increased fetal activity (Holden 84), or no change in fetal parameters (Reece 95).

Early outpatient antepartum fetal surveillance programs for diabetic women reported in the 1980s (Coustan 80, Schneider 80, Teramo 83, Golde 84, Miller 85, Olofsson 86a, Dicker 88, Johnson 88) replaced strategies of daily fetal monitoring (estriol, FHR) of patients who were hospitalized at 34–37 weeks gestation (Gabbe 77a, Kitzmiller 78, Leveno 79, Whittle 79, Jorge 81) due to the previously noted increased risk (4–7%) of fetal demise near term (Delaney 70, Karlsson 72, Essex 73, Pedersen 74, Drury 77, Jervell 79, Connell 85). Thus, the goal of weekly or semi-weekly ambulatory monitoring in the third trimester was to prevent stillbirth by prompt delivery of babies showing indirect evidence of possible fetal hypoxemia and to avoid preterm delivery in patients with normal assessment. This strategy was highly successful at centers of excellence, and antepartum fetal surveillance became the standard of care, although reduced perinatal mortality occurred concurrently with application of improved techniques of glycemic control (see the section titled "Introduction"). In the absence of RCTs of either fetal surveillance or glycemic control, it is impossible to state which strategy contributed the most to improved outcomes. Other difficulties in assessing the predictive power of fetal surveillance techniques are that multiple methods were often used in the same patients and that imprecise end points ("fetal distress" in labor, condition at birth, neonatal complications or death) were influenced by many clinical variables in addition to possible antepartum fetal hypoxia.

Forms of third-trimester fetal surveillance (Malcus 04) include (a) the nonstress test (NST) (continuous external FHR monitoring for 20–60 min in which healthy FHR reactivity is marked by long-term accelerations and short-term "beat-to-beat" variability) (Devoe 02), (b) contraction stress testing (CST) (external FHR monitoring during stimulation of uterine contractions in which uteroplacental insufficiency and fetal hypoxia is suggested by decelerations of the FHR persisting beyond the end of the contraction), (c) estimation of reduced AF volune (Magann 02), (d) the biophysical profile (BPP), and (e) Doppler velocimetry of the umbilical artery (Westergaard 01, Albuquerque 04). The BPP is obtained by real-time US and external FHR monitoring (or biophysical score, in which a "score" [0-10] of fetal condition is based on the sum of fetal trunk movements, tone of fetal limbs, rapid fetal chest wall motion ("breathing"), pocket of AF >2 cm, and reactivity of FHR, with 2 points given for each parameter) (Manning 95, Manning 02).

The performance of NSTs confirmed by BPP or CST (Coustan 80, Teramo 83, Golde 84, Miller 85, Olofsson 86a, Ostlund 91, Landon 92, Kjos 95), primary BPP (Dicker 88, Johnson 88), or primary CST (Schneider 80, Lagrew 93) in identifying the presence or absence of fetal compromise has been investigated in pregnancies complicated by PDM (Ammala 83, Bourgeois 90, Bracero 96, Tincello 98, Brown 99, Wylie 02), with most observational studies showing low sensitivity, specificity, and PPVs but high predictive values of a negative test (>95%). The frequency of pregnancies with nonreassuring tests leading to delivery of the baby ranged from 3.0% to 22.5%, with a median value of 10.2%. Excluding one study of 42 patients without good glycemic control and four stillbirths (Miller 85), there were four stillbirths in 1,501 pregnancies (0.27%) of women with PDM and only one false negative antepartum test, but >40% had false positive tests (Schneider 80, Golde 81, Ammala 83, Teramo 83, Olofsson 86a, Dicker 88, Johnson 88, Ostlund 91, Landon 92, Lagrew 93, Kjos 95, Wylie 02). The low stillbirth rates at centers of excellence are generally not matched by the continuing excessive rates of 1.8–4.5% in recent population-based surveys or regional series of pregnant women with either type 1 or type 2 diabetes (Hanson 93, Cnattingius 94, Cundy 00, Dunne 00, Vaarasmaki 00, Hadden 01, Platt 02, Lauenborg 03, Penney 03, Vangen 03, Wood 03, Evers 04, Jensen 04, dos santos Silva 05, McElduff 05a, Verheijen 05, deValk 06, Macintosh 06, Cundy 07, Bell 08, Gonzalez-Gonzalez 08).

The ability to draw conclusions from studies of fetal surveillance is compromised for many reasons. Several studies include insulin-treated gestational diabetic women under the designation of "insulin dependent." Because comorbid vascular complications are less common in GDM than in PDM, inclusion of women with GDM may diminish the apparent usefulness of antenatal testing in detecting fetal compromise in women with type 1 and type 2 diabetes. In addition, the overall quality of metabolic control and intensity of glucose monitoring vary widely between reports, making it difficult to meaningfully assess the impact of metabolic control on fetal biophysical parameters. Further, the algorithm for choice of surveillance modality differs from one study to another, with few head-to-head comparisons of the performance of various modalities. Finally, and perhaps most importantly, we lack solid evidence that any antenatal fetal surveillance modality or testing algorithm reduces perinatal mortality because there are no RCTs comparing a monitored group to an unmonitored group, and sample sizes are too small to provide meaningful data on this relatively rare outcome. Given these limitations, an "optimal" testing strategy cannot be determined at this time (Reece 02).

The NST is the mainstay of antenatal fetal surveillance in most clinical settings and is usually performed at 3–7-day intervals. In women with diabetes, a reactive NST predicts an absence of fetal compromise in >95% of cases within 2 days of the test; conversely, an abnormal result has a significantly lower predictive value for adverse perinatal events, such as fetal intolerance of labor and low Apgar scores (Olofsson 86a).

For women living at a distance from perinatal centers, telemetry has been applied for ambulatory and home FHR monitoring (Hod 03). Among women with PDM, various authors report the rate of "nonreactive" NST results to be ~10% for a single test (Golde 84, Miller 85, Landon 92). However, this rate can be safely reduced by either repeating the NST or by obtaining reassurance of fetal well-being by means of another modality, such as the CST or BPP. By adding these follow-up tests, the rate of abnormal results is quite low, while the perinatal mortality rate in nonanomalous fetuses also remains low (Golde 84, Ostlund 91, Salveson 93, Bracero 96). Thus, there appears to be no increased risk of poor outcome if other evidence of fetal well-being can be obtained after an initially nonreactive NST. Similar rates of abnormal results have been described for the BPP as first-line testing in women with PDM (Dicker 88, Johnson 88).

In a unique study of fetal pH in umbilical venous (UV) blood obtained by cordocentesis before delivery at 27–39 weeks in 31 women with PDM (6 with nephropathy), low-range UV pH and pO2 were strongly related to acute but not chronic maternal and UV glucose concentrations (Salvesen 93b). Computerized assessment of FHR variability and BPP were performed prior to cordocentesis. Mild fetoplacental acidemia (UV pH <7.350; <5th percentile for normal pregnancy) was noted in 12 cases (38.7%); of those, eight had FHR variability <5th percentile for normal pregnancy, and four had a nonreassuring BPP score of 4–6. Of 11 cases with low FHR variability, eight had UV pH <7.35; of four cases with nonreassuring BPP, all had pH <7.35. Four of the cases with "low" fetal pH were delivered preterm in women with nephropathy. Only two cases of UV pH <7.30 were found at cordocentesis; both had UV glucose >180 mg/dL (>10 mM) and reassuring BBP scores of 8, but with low FHR variability. Of 11 cases with low FHR variability, six had UV glucose >126 mg/dL (>7.0 mM) compared with only 1 of 20 cases with normal FHR variability (Salvesen 93b).

The utility of third-trimester Doppler velocimetry studies of the umbilical artery in managing the pregnancy complicated by diabetes is controversial (Trudinger 85b, Bracero 86, Landon 89b, Salvesen 92,93a, Bracero 96, Maulik 02, Rosenn 04, Tan 05). Waveform measurements are based on the relationship between the S/D flow and are variously expressed as S/D, pulsitility index, or resistance index (Rosenn 04). Increased umbilical artery resistance is associated with a reduced number of small fetoplacental arteries in nondiabetic pregnancies (especially in those with FGR) (Giles 85, McCowan 87, Bracero 89b, Fok 90), but this finding is inconsistent in women with PDM (Bracero 93, Sysmanowski 94). A minority of cases of increased S/D ratio are associated with fetal hypoxia and acidemia assessed by cordocentesis (Weiner 90, Salvesen 92,93a,b) or examination at delivery (Figueras 05). However, the Cochrane Systematic Review of 11 RCTs on the measurement of Doppler umbilical artery waveforms versus other surveillance techniques in high-risk pregnancies showed a trend toward reduction in perinatal deaths (OR 0.71; 95% CI 0.50–1.01) with fewer hospital admissions and fewer inductions of labor. In this analysis, the method was especially useful in pregnancies with hypertension or presumed impaired fetal growth (Neilson 02). Another meta-analysis demonstrated the value of umbilical artery Doppler surveillance in pregnancies associated with FGR or hypertensive disease of pregnancy (Westergaard 01). In an RCT in women with various high-risk factors (including 11% diabetes; only 7% suspected FGR), umbilical artery Doppler was associated with fewer cesarean deliveries for fetal distress than the NST, but had no effect on condition at birth (Williams 03). In a large growth restriction intervention trial conducted in European countries, immediate versus delayed delivery (1.5–10.8 days) did not improve birth outcome of 182 fetuses with reduced, 205 with absent, or 33 with reversed end-diastolic flow on umbilical artery waveform analysis (GRIT 03).

Other investigators focus on Doppler assessment of the fetal middle cerebral artery (Vyas 91, Vergani 05) or fetal venous blood flows (Hoffstaetter 02, Baschat 04a,b, Schwarze 05) to identify cardiac decompensation and improve the prediction of pre-term fetuses who are at such high intrauterine risk that they should be considered for early delivery. Umbilical or middle cerebral arterial studies provide information on downstream distribution of CO (Baschat 04a), but further evaluation of fetal cardiac function is useful (Hecher 95a, Rizzo 95b, Severi 00). Declining forward cardiac function marks cardiovascular deterioration in growth-restricted fetuses (Baschat 04a) and is often accompanied by acidemia (Hecher 95b, Rizzo 96). Although fetal venous Doppler parameters may best predict fetal acidemia and neonatal complications, use of this technology still begs the question of the optimal timing of delivery to reduce neonatal and developmental morbidity in growth-restricted preterm babies.

Doppler velocimetry examination in fetuses of women with PDM revealed no significant differences in umbilical artery pulsatility index at 26 and 36 weeks compared with controls in an early study, but fetal aortic velocities and flows were greater in the diabetic gestations (Olofsson 87). The latter finding was not confirmed in studies of well-controlled diabetic women (Salvesen 93a, Grunewald 96). Another study demonstrated an increase in umbilical artery peak systolic velocities in diabetic pregnant women compared with controls matched for gestational age, but the pulsatility index did not differ. The authors suggested that there was an increase in fetal systemic arteriolar placental afterload (Ursem 99). An increase in FGR, fetal distress in labor, stillbirth, and neonatal metabolic derangements has been found if the umbilical artery S/D ratio is elevated >3.0 in the bulk of observational studies in PDM (Bracero 86,89, Landon 89b, Dicker 90, Ishimatsu 91, Johnstone 92, Salvesen 92, Zimmerman 92, Salvesen 93d, Reece 94, Grunewald 96, Fadda 01, Wong 03b, Tan 05). In a prospective blinded study in 39 women with type 1 diabetes, the sensitivity and PPV of elevated umbilical artery S/D for condition at birth was low, but the timing of the single examination was often many weeks before delivery (Ben-Ami 95).

Impaired glycemic control was associated with higher resistance in the umbilical artery in only 3 (Bracero 86, Fadda 01, Bracero 02) of 12 studies (Landon 89b, Dicker 90, Degani 91, Ishimatsu 91, Johnstone 92, Zimmerman 92, Salvesen 93d, Reece 94, Grunewald 96). Significantly elevated S/D ratios were often found in diabetic women with vasculopathy or hypertension compared with those without (Landon 89b, Dicker 90, Salvesen 93, Reece 94, Landon 96, Wong 03b). However, inaccurate measurement of umbilical artery blood flow can lead to false positive findings and unnecessary intervention, and normal S/D ratios have been recorded in other cases of confirmed fetal compromise (Siddiqi 03). Therefore, if used, this mode of fetal surveillance should be confined to women with vasculopathy, hypertension, or growth-restricted fetuses and should be performed by ultrasonographers familiar with appropriate techniques to obtain accurate measurements. Doppler studies of fetal middle cerebral artery flow are not as well documented in pregnancies complicated by PDM (Salvesen 93a, Ishimatsu 95).

The optimal gestational week to begin fetal testing is not known. One group of investigators evaluated the results of antenatal fetal testing in 614 insulin-treated diabetic women (71% GDM or recent type 2 diabetes) for three outcomes: fetal death, occurrence of an abnormal CST, or intervention because of abnormal test results (Lagrew 93). The surveillance algorithm consisted of weekly CSTs with an interval mid-week NST. An abnormal CST occurred in 7.4% of patients, with the earliest at

28 weeks. Delivery because of abnormal test results confirmed by BPP occurred in 11.6% of these women, with the earliest at 27 weeks in a patient with superimposed preeclampsia. Three stillbirths occurred, two of which were undergoing antenatal fetal testing. In terms of the time frame at initiation of testing, 49% of all women who had a positive CST were at <34 weeks gestation; 21% of those delivered due to abnormal tests. Comparing women with and without abnormal test results and/or intervention for abnormal test results, it appears that FGR poses an increased risk for both of these outcomes, particularly at <34 weeks gestation. The majority of the women who had a growth-restricted infant also had hypertension. In fact, among diabetic women without evidence of hypertension or FGR, no intervention was required because of abnormal fetal testing at <35 weeks gestation (Lagrew 93).

These data suggest that the patient's clinical condition and comorbid conditions should be taken into account when determining when to initiate fetal surveillance. For example, women at highest risk for early fetal compromise include those in poor glycemic control, those with vascular disease or uncontrolled hypertension, and those with evidence for FGR. In such cases, testing should begin at 26–28 weeks gestation. For all other women with type 1 and type 2 diabetes, initiation of fetal testing might be delayed until approximately 34–36 weeks gestation. It should be noted, however, that the necessity of fetal surveillance in these lower-risk women has not been tested in an RCT. Similarly, no testing modality has been shown to be superior to any other in the setting of diabetes, although few head-to-head comparisons of testing algorithms have been reported.

In the third trimester, the simplest form of primary fetal surveillance for fetal hypoxia is to instruct all pregnant women to perform fetal movement counts daily and report persistently diminished fetal movement (<4/h or <10 in 2 h) to their care provider immediately (Neldham 80, Rayburn 82, Sadovsky 83, Moore 89). In women with diabetes, additional secondary means of surveillance as discussed in this section are recommended to provide reassurance that the fetus is not compromised (Marden 97, Velasquez 02).

Assessment of Fetal Lung Maturity

Pulmonary surfactant is composed of glycerophospholipids and surfactant-associated proteins that reduce surface tension at the alveolar–air interface and prevent end-expiratory atelectasis after delivery (Dobbs 89, Weaver 91). Fetal hyperglycemia and hyperinsulinemia are associated with impaired action or production of components of pulmonary surfactant (disaturated dipalmitoylphosphatidylcholine [DSPC], phosphatidylglycerol [PG], surfactant apoproteins) in human fetal lung tissue (Smith 75, Bourbon 85a, Snyder 87, Dekowski 92) and most animal models (Neufeld 79, Demottaz 80, Sosenko 80, Tyden 80, Eriksson 83, Mulay 83, Sosenko 83, Tsai 83, Warburton 83a,b, Engle 84, Patel 84, Bourbon 85b,86, Guttentag 92), including Rhesus monkeys (Epstein 76). In the early years of monitoring pregnancies complicated by PDM, excess rates (12.9–20.6%) of pulmonary surfactant deficiency and respiratory distress syndrome (RDS) were found in IDMs delivered at ≥35 weeks gestation (Usher 71, Karlsson 72, Robert 76, Drury 77, Jervell 79) and not exclusively in those delivered by CS (White 85).

The AF lecithin–sphingomyelin ratio (L/S) measured by thin-layer chromatography (TLC) was developed as a test to predict RDS because lecithin contains DSPC as its major surface-active fraction. DSPC concentration in AF increases steadily after

32–34 weeks, but sphingomyelin does not (Kulovich 79, James 84a); therefore, the ratio is used to control for intersubject variation in the volume of AF (Gluck 71,73, Buhi 75, Morrison 77). Assessment of fetal lung maturity by amniocentesis and measurement of L/S became the standard of care before elective delivery of diabetic women at <39 weeks gestation, and the frequency of RDS at ≥35 weeks declined to 2.7–5.0% (Gabbe 77, Kitzmiller 78, Coustan 80). In the absence of RCTs, it is difficult to determine how much of this improvement was due to tightened glycemic control (Curet 79, Dudley 85, Landon 87), a reduction in fetal hypoxia and acidosis (Cruz 76), or use of the new technology.

False normal results of L/S were noted to be more common in pregnancies complicated by diabetes; 19 of 23 studies showed that L/S ratios of 2.0–2.9 that were expected to be "mature" did not always predict the absence of RDS in IDMs (Gabert 73, Lemons 73, Whitfield 73, Dunn 74, Mukherjee 74, Gabbe 77b, Tchobroutsky 78, Andrews 79, Skjaeraasen 79, Tabsh 82, James 84b, Dudley 85, Landon 87, Karcher 05). The false normal prediction rate ranged from 8.3% to 28.5% in nine reports in which authors provided the denominator (Duhring 75, Cruz 76, Dahlenburg 77, Kitzmiller 78, Mueller-Heubach 78, Curet 79, Hallman 79, Amenta 83, Lavin 83). These excessive rates could be related to difficulties with the L/S technique, diabetes-related increases in phosphatidylinositol (Moore 02) or phosphatidylserine appearing at the lecithin spot in single-dimension TLC (James 84ab), decreased sphingomyelin in diabetes (Gebhardt 79,82), increased rate of cesarean delivery at <39 weeks gestation in diabetic women, or causes of respiratory distress other than surfactant deficiency in the infants. In any case, a "supramature" L/S of 3.5 was demanded before elective delivery in many programs, and investigators also explored other measures of fetal lung maturity (Dilena 97).

Fetal type II pneumocytes synthesize and secrete surfactant-associated glycoproteins (apolipoproteins), and the major component known as SP-A (or 35 kd protein) has an important role in surfactant function (Nogee 88, Weaver 91). Insulin can inhibit SP-A synthesis and mRNA expression in human fetal lung explants, and authors speculate that this could contribute to RDS in diabetic pregnanies with "mature" L/S and fetal hyperinsulinemia (Snyder 87, Dekowski 92). In a clinical study of diabetic women, AF SP-A measured by enzyme-linked immunoassay >2 µg/mL predicted the absence of RDS. SP-A was <2 µg/mL in five AF samples with an L/S ratio of 2.0–3.4; three infants developed RDS. In 10 other samples, SP-A was <2 µg/mL and the L/S ratio was <2.0, exhibiting six cases of RDS (Katyal 84). Decreased AF SP-A in diabetic women with "mature" L/S ratios was confirmed in a separate study (Snyder 88). In a third study of women delivered within 24 h of amniocentesis at ≥35 weeks gestation, RDS was described in 8 of 37 control infants with SP-A <4 µg/mL versus five of an unknown denominator of infants of women with PDM. Mean SP-A levels did not differ in 30 controls and in infants of women with PDM matched by gestational age (McMahon 87). Surfactant protein can be falsely elevated with severe preeclampsia (Hallman 89). To our knowledge, there has been no further evaluation of SP-A in pregnancies complicated by PDM, and no one has examined the relationship between SP-A and fetal insulin production.

DSPC is the major contributor to surface activity in the pulmonary alveolus (Torday 79, Dobbs 89). The AF concentration of DSPC is decreased in inadequately controlled diabetic women (James 84a, Tsai 87), but the assay is time consuming and expensive (Tanasijevic 96). In well-controlled diabetes, the progressive increase in AF DSPC after 32–34 weeks gestation did not differ between diabetic and control women (Farrell 84, Delgado 00).

The presence or absence of the stable PG measured in AF by TLC was tested many times as a predictor of RDS in IDMs (Cunningham 78, Kulovich 79, Skjaeraasen 79, Tsai 79, Whittle 82, Farrell 84, Ferroni 84, James 84b, Amon 86, Curet 89, Heimberger 99). In an early study of 23 cases in which the L/S ratio was between 2.0 and 3.0, PG was positive in only five (no RDS) and was absent in 18 samples (4 RDS) (Hallman 79). In other studies, only 16.7% of AF samples from diabetic women contained PG when the L/S ratio was >2.0 (Cunningham 82), and PG was absent in 24% of AF samples from women with PDM at term in spite of good glycemic control (Ojomo 90). Investigators confirmed the delayed appearance of PG in the AF of women with PDM (James 84a, Tsai 84, Ylinen 87, Piper 93, Moore 02), which is perhaps related to elevated fetal plasma myoinositol levels with pneumocyte production of phosphatidylinositol predominating over PG (Hallman 79, Bourbon 85a,86). Therefore, positive PG marks fetal maturity in PDM, but with a high false negative rate (Piper 95). Positive PG most closely correlated to an L/S ratio ≥3.0 or lamellar body counts ≥50,000 in clear AF specimens obtained from 76 diabetic women (20 MNT-treated GDM) (Ghidini 02). Controversy surrounds whether PG itself contributes to surfactant activity in the neonatal lung (Hallman 76, Beppu 83, Hallman 85).

To avoid difficult chromatographic assays, simpler tests were developed to estimate fetal lung maturity. The foam stability or "shake" test received some early attention (Mukherjee 74, Amenta 83, Amon 86, Piazze 99), but had problems with interpretation of results and false negativity. AF levels of cholesterol palmitate (substrate for DSPC) (Ludmir 87) did not correlate with fetal lung maturity in pregnancies complicated by diabetes (Ludmir 88). AF optical density at 650 nm was considered a marker of fetal maturity in diabetic women (most of whom had GDM) in one laboratory (Kjos 90).

Fluorescent polarization (determined by the freedom of rotation of a fat-soluble fluorescent dye probe introduced into AF samples uncontaminated with blood or meconium) is inversely proportional to the L/S ratio because the surface tension of surfactant components and the intrinsic microviscosity of the total lipid aggregates are interrelated (Petersen 83, Ivie 87). The degree of fluorescence polarization was originally measured with a specialized microviscosimeter (Blumenfeld 78, Golde 79), but this technique was infrequently used in women with PDM (Barkai 82, Neufeld 85, Simon 87). An alternate method of measuring fluorescence polarization using a different fluorescent probe and the Abbott TDx analyzer predicted RDS satisfactorily in infants of 77 diabetic mothers in preliminary studies (Tait 87, Towey 93). The current method calibrates fluorescence polarization, and surfactant concentration is converted to the surfactant/albumin value, which correlates best with gestational age, L/S values, and neonatal outcome (Russell 89). By using the automated TDx-FLM analyzer to measure the surfactant/albumin ratio (>70 mg/gm indicated unlikely RDS), this assay provided consistent results (Steinfeld 92, Herbert 93, Hagen 93), including results in pregnancies complicated by diabetes (Livingston 95, Tanasijevic 96, Del Valle 97, Delgado 00, McElrath 04, Bildirrici 05, Karcher 05). The second-generation assay is TDx-FLM$_{II}$, with a cutoff of 55 mg/gm at ≥35 weeks in samples collected by amniocentesis or vaginal pool (Kesselman 03, McElrath 04, Winn-McMillan 05). Predictive accuracy is improved if test results are presented as a probability of RDS according to gestational age (Pinette 02, McElrath 04, Bildiricci 05, Karcher 05, Parvin 05).

Fetal type II pneumocytes secrete lamellar bodies that carry the phospholipids of surfactant into the tracheal and amniotic fluid (Ghidini 05). Lamellar body counts can be measured quickly in the platelet channel of an automated hematologic cell counter

(Ashwood 90, Dalence 95, Lewis 99). In a recent study, lamellar body count and TDx-FLM_{II} had equal accuracy, either positive or negative (Karcher 05). AF samples from 104 diabetic pregnant women were included in a multicenter comparison of methods to assess fetal lung maturity, and the authors concluded that lamellar body counts performed as well as L/S and PG analysis in the diabetic subgroup (Neerhof 01a). In a small study of 31 women with PDM, use of a lamellar body count >37,000/μL resulted in 81% sensitivity, 100% specificity, and a PPV of 100% in predicting an L/S ratio >2.0 and presence of PG. Because no cases of RDS were found in the infants, a much larger series is required to establish the level of false positivity (DeRoche 02). Lamellar body counts >50,000/μL had 92% sensitivity and a zero false-positive rate in predicting positive PG in the AF of a mixed group of 75 women with GDM or PDM (Ghidini 02). A protocol for standardization of preparation and measurement of fluid samples may increase the consistency of results with this method across institutions (Neerhof 01b).

Predictive values (Richardson 85) of the L/S, PG, and TDx-FLM assays for absence or presence of RDS in pooled studies of women with PDM are presented in Table III.2. Because most data are not actually dichotomous, likelihood ratos may be preferred even though they are not widely applied in obstetrics (Grimes 05). The question remains whether amniocentesis and fetal lung maturity testing is necessary before an elective delivery of any diabetic woman at <38–39 weeks gestation (Piper 02). With "modern management" of PDM in pregnancy, several authors found no delay in fetal lung maturity with diabetes compared with controls (Dudley 85, Fadel 86, Mimouni 87a, Curet 89, Kjos 90, Piper 98, Piazze 99, Kjos 02). Due to the low rate of RDS in women with PDM delivered vaginally at term after "good glycemic control" in the third trimester, RCTs are impractical to prove whether amniocentesis is necessary for

TABLE III.2 Predictive Values of Common Tests for Fetal Lung Maturity

Lecithin/Sphingomyelin Ratio	RDS Present	RDS Absent
<2.0	46 PNV 22.5%; sensitivity 0.52	158 (77.5% false negative)
≥2.0 (positive predicts no RDS)	42 (5.6% false positive)	738 PPV 94.6%; specificity 0.82
Phosphatidylglycerol		
Absent	13 PNV 9.3%; sensitivity 1.00	127 (90.7% false negative)
Present (positive predicts no RDS)	0 (none false positive)	212 PPV 100%; specificity 0.625
Fluorescence polarization TDx-FLM		
<70 g/gm surfactant/albumin	9 PNV 15.3%; sensitivity 0.75	50 (84.7% false negative)
≥70 g/gm (positive predicts no RDS)	3 (0.7% false positive)	419 PPV 99.3%; specificity 0.89

Pooled analyses of retrospective studies of pregnancies complicated by preexisting diabetes, delivered at ≥34 weeks gestation. References cited in text. For L/S, data pooled from Whitfield 73, Dunn 74, Duhring 75, Dahlenburg 77, Gabbe 77, Mueller-Heubach 78, Curet 79, Tabsh 82, Amenta 83, Lavin 83, Tsai 84, Dudley 85. For phosphatidylglycerol test, data pooled from Cunningham 78, Hallman 79, Cunningham 82, Whittle 82, James 84b, Amon 86, Curet 89, Ojomo 90. For TDx-FLM test, data pooled from Livingston 95, Tanasijevic 96, Del Valle 97.

PNV, predictive negative value; PPV, predictive positive value; RDS, respiratory distress syndrome with mild cases of transient tachypnea excluded.

such patients attempting a vaginal delivery at ≥37 weeks and to establish glycemic control targets for prevention of RDS. The ACOG clinical management guideline currently advises amniocentesis to determine fetal lung maturity for delivery at <39 weeks gestation "in poorly controlled patients," without definition of poor glycemic control (ACOG 05a).

It remains controversial whether elective cesarean delivery of diabetic women (primary or repeat) "in good control" is safe at 38 weeks gestation without amniocentesis in the well-dated pregnancy or whether it is best delayed to 39 weeks gestation (Keszler 92, Hook 97, Wax 02). The incidence of significant respiratory morbidity in infants of nondiabetic pregnancies delivered at 38 weeks, 0–6 days' gestation by elective CS without labor was 4.2–6.2% compared with 1.5–1.8% at 39 weeks (Morrison 95, Stutchfield 05, Hansen 08), and we expect no less morbidity in IDMs. The consensus panel recommends waiting until 39 weeks. There is no evidence on which to base a recommendation to perform amniocentesis before elective induction of labor at 38 weeks gestation in patients with "good glycemic control" as defined in Part I of this document. Induction of labor is occasionally considered to be "indicated" at 37–38 weeks gestation in a diabetic patient without good glycemic control without regard to assessment of fetal lung maturity.

Recommendations

- Pregnancies complicated by PDM should be dated by US measurements early in prenatal care. (E)
- First-trimester NT thickness may be offered to diabetic women at 11–13 weeks gestation as a screening test for congenital heart defects and other pregnancy complications; NT can be coupled with serum PAAP-A and free β-hCG measurements as a screen for chromosomal defects. (E)
- Maternal serum marker screening for chromosomal and open NTDs should be offered to all diabetic women <35 years of age between 15–20 weeks gestation, with appropriate referral if abnormal results are obtained. Women ≥35 years of age can undergo serum marker screening or be referred directly for genetic counseling/prenatal diagnostic testing. (E)
- All women with PDM should undergo assessment of fetal anatomy by detailed US in the second trimester. Whenever feasible, this test should be performed by a provider skilled in detection of fetal anomalies. Fetal echocardiography can be considered for those at high risk of cardiac defects. (E)
- US measurements of fetal body size in the third trimester can be used to assess the effectiveness of glycemic control, especially if estimates of fetal adiposity by measurement of AC >75th percentile for gestational age and increased AFI are incorporated. (E)
- All diabetic women should be instructed to perform fetal movement counts daily in the third trimester and to report decreased or absent fetal movement immediately. (E)
- Ongoing assessment of fetal well-being using the NST or BPP should be performed in the third trimester for women with diabetes. Such testing should begin at ~28 weeks gestation in highest-risk pregnancies and by 34–36 weeks gestation in other cases. (E)

- Assessment of fetal lung maturity should be considered before elective vaginal delivery of diabetic women at <39 weeks gestation, particularly in those who have not met glycemic targets (Part I) and before elective CS at <39 weeks gestation. When either form of delivery is indicated for maternal or fetal well-being at ≥34 weeks gestation, clinicians may need to proceed without assessment of fetal lung maturity. (E)
- Prior to delivery at <34 weeks gestation, consideration should be given to the benefits and risks of maternal corticosteroid treatment to enhance fetal lung maturation. (A)

MANAGEMENT OF PREGNANCY COMPLICATIONS

—— *Original contribution by Patrick M. Catalano MD and Deborah L. Conway MD*

Preterm Labor and Delivery

An increased risk of preterm delivery (<37 weeks gestation) is evident in women with PDM, with RRs of 2.3–7.0 compared with control populations (Cousins 87, Greene 89, Hanson 93, Rosenn 93, Aucott 94, Reece 98, Vaarasmaki 00, Evers 04, Jensen 04, Lepercq 04, Guenter 06). The increased risk of preterm birth with chronic diabetes adjusted for relevant factors is found in all ethnic groups in the U.S., and this study includes a majority of women with type 2 diabetes (Rosenberg 05). Published rates in observational studies vary from 16.6–18.9% in Japanese (Zhu 97) and Finnish (Vaarasmaki 00) populations to 26.0% in a 46-center survey in France (GDFSG 91), 37.9% in a large North American multicenter prospective cohort (Sibai 00a,b), 41.7% in a population survey in Denmark (Jensen 04), and 43.4% at a referral center in Toronto (Ray 01). Prior to application of methods of intensified glycemic control, iatrogenic preterm delivery of diabetic women to prevent stillbirth was a major factor.

Indications for preterm delivery in four studies conducted in1984–2002 and providing sufficient detail are presented in Table III.3. Spontaneous preterm deliveries constituted 37.3%, 53.9%, and 39.0% of all preterm deliveries, respectively, in the three studies providing data in all categories (Greene 89, Rosenn 93, Lepercq 04). Preeclampsia is a leading cause of the indicated preterm deliveries (Zhu 97). In those studies that stratified preterm deliveries by gestational age, premature rupture of the membranes and premature labor were leading factors at 35–36 weeks gestation, while occurrence of preeclampsia was distributed from 28 to 36 weeks. Polyhydramnios is inconsistently associated with preterm delivery in these studies. Diabetes-related risk factors for preterm delivery in women with PDM include poor glucose control (Roversi 82, Rosenn 93, Reece 98, Lepercq 04, Lauszus 06), underlying microvascular disease and hypertension with FGR (particularly DN with proteinuria), and superimposed preeclampsia (Mimouni 88b, Greene 89, Sibai 00a, Cundy 02, Evers 04). The highest reported risks of preterm delivery were 54% and 60% in Danish (Ekbom 01) and North American (Combs 93) cohorts with DN, with the primary reason for these preterm deliveries being the onset of preeclampsia.

The risk of spontaneous preterm labor is increased in women with PDM, especially those with inadequate glycemic control (Roversi 82, Mimouni 88c, Kovilam 02). In two major U.S. referral centers, the rate of spontaneous preterm labor with intact membranes leading to treatment was 23–31% of diabetic women, a two- to threefold

TABLE III.3 Indications for Preterm Delivery at <37 Weeks Gestation

Author (year)	Greene 1989	Rosenn 1993*	Lepercq 2004	Lauszus 2006**
Patients (N)	420	254	168	71
Preterm delivery (%)	110 (26.2)	76 (29.9)	41 (24.4)	16 (22.5)
Preeclampsia	36	12	14	—
Fetal distress	15	12	4	3
Other indicated delivery	18	5	7	4
PTL	14	41	3	1
PPROM	27	6	13	8

Authors provided details of pregnancies complicated by preexisting diabetes mellitus.

*Excluded major malformations.

**Excluded micro- and macroalbuminuria.

PPROM, preterm premature rupture of the membranes; PTL, spontaneous premature labor. Fetal distress suspected based on nonreassuring fetal assessments, including failure of fetal growth.

increase compared with nondiabetic control populations. About 70% of the treated diabetic patients were delivered preterm (Mimouni 88b, Greene 89, Rosenn 93). On the other hand, preterm labor was recorded in 9.2% of 423 women with PDM participating in the California statewide program (Cousins 91). Preterm delivery remains a major contributor to neonatal mortality, morbidity, and costs (Goldenberg 02, McIntire 08). Reasons for the association of hyperglycemia with premature labor are unclear, but authors speculate about links to inflammation or oxidative stress. UTI was associated with preterm labor in two observational studies of diabetic women (Rosenn 93, Reece 98). Premature labor is diagnosed by finding a cervix dilated at the internal os in the presence of uterine contactions. Current obstetrical techniques used to predict the risk of preterm delivery in women with premature contractions or history of spontaneous preterm birth include measurement of cervical length by US and assay of fetal fibronectin in vaginal pool specimens (Goldenberg 96, Iams 03, Owen 04, Yost 04). Women with a cervix longer than 3 cm or absence of fibronectin are at low risk of preterm delivery, and no evidence exists that these parameters are modified by diabetes.

Commonly used tocolytic agents in the treatment of preterm labor include magnesium sulfate, prostaglandin synthesis inhibitors, and CCBs (nifedipine) (Oei 99, Tsatsaris 01, King 03, Lyell 07). In Europe, an oxytocin receptor blocker (atosiban) is licensed for the treatment of preterm labor (Moutquin 00, Romero 00, Valenzuela 00, Coomaraswamy 03, Lamont 03, Beattie 04). Although none of these agents have successfully prevented preterm births at <37 weeks gestation in properly controlled trials (Goldenberg 02), their use may prolong gestation to a clinically significant extent. While each of these agents has specific contraindications based on underlying medical conditions, general use in women with diabetes is not contraindicated. However, because magnesium sulfate is currently a very widely used tocolytic agent in the U.S., care must be taken in treating premature labor in women with DN because magnesium concentrations are dependent on renal clearance. β-Adrenergic agonists used in the treatment of preterm labor, such as ritodrine or terbutaline, will adversely affect maternal glucose metabolism (Gundogdu 79, Lenz 79, Wager 81), even to the point of KTA

(Thomas 77, Desir 78). Therefore, this class of medications is currently used much less often in women with diabetes and requires intensified glucose monitoring and intravenous insulin administration (Barnett 80, Miodovnik 85).

The only prophylaxis attempting to prevent preterm delivery that has demonstrated improved neonatal outcome in prospective double-blind randomized trials in women at risk of primary or recurrent preterm birth with singleton gestations is the use of 17 α-hydroxyprogesterone (250 mg i.m. weekly from 20 to 36 weeks) (Johnson 75, Yemeni 85, Meis 03,05, Gonzalez-Quintaro 07, Rebarber 07a) or 100 mg natural progesterone daily by vaginal suppository from 24 to 34 weeks (daFonseca 03). Such treatment is deemed cost-effective (Petrini 05, Odibo 06) and is supported by clinical guidelines (ACOG 03). Four-year follow-up studies of 193 children exposed to 17 α-hydroxyprogesterone in utero during the second and third trimesters revealed no physical or neurodevelopmental sequelae (Northern 07). Even though the use of progesterone may adversely affect maternal glucose control, there are as yet no studies to assess the affect of intramuscular or vaginal progesterone (used to prevent preterm birth) (Dodd 05, Mackenzie 06) on glucose metabolism in women with PDM. Use of 17 α-hydroxyprogesterone caproate increased the rate of GDM in 557 treated women compared with a control group (Rebarber 07b).

Administration of antenatal glucocorticoids is indicated to enhance lung maturity for all fetuses at acute risk of preterm delivery at 24–33 weeks gestation to reduce the risk of RDS, intraventricular hemorrhage, and death (NIH 95,01, ACOG 02a, Crane 03, Neilson 07). Some clinical evidence suggests that two doses of betamethasone given intramuscularly 24 h apart is preferable to four doses of dexamethasone given intramuscularly 12 h apart due to lessened mortality and long-term morbidity in the offspring of treated mothers (Jobe 04, Spinillo 04, Lee 06). However, an RCT showed no significant differences in outcomes except for lessened neonatal intraventricular hemorrhage after maternal dexamethasone (Elimian 07). Additional studies are needed to establish the lowest effective dose of either corticosteroid (Jobe 04) as well as whether the benefit of repeated courses of treatment in patients at continuing high risk of preterm delivery outweighs the possibility of long-term complications in the infants (Aghajafari 01, ACOG 02a, Crane 03, Crowther 03, Guinn 04, Crowther 06). Long-term follow-up studies of offspring of mothers given single courses of betamethasone or dexamethasone compared with placebo show no drug-related impairment of childhood development (MacArthur 82, CGAST 84) or adult cognitive function (Dessens 00, Dalziel 05).

Although no evidence exists concerning the effectiveness of antenatal corticosteroids in diabetic or preeclamptic pregnancies, "this lack of confirmation, however, should not preclude their use in these clinical situations because the risks appear minimal" (Wapner 04). Of course, corticosteroids cause hyperglycemia in diabetic patients, and recent evidence points to the role of subclinical infection or inflammation as potential factors in the etiology of preterm labor, which may also adversely affect glucose control. Therefore, the aggressive use of insulin—whether via subcutaneous or intravenous administration—and frequent glucose monitoring needs to be instituted after antenatal glucocorticoid therapy and continued for a number of days to adequately control blood glucose (Barondiot 07). A published algorithm for increasing the daily subcutaneous insulin dose by 27%, 45%, 40%, 31%, and 11% for the 5 days following betamethasone treatment has been shown to prevent severe hyperglycemia, KTA, and severe hypoglycemia (Mathiesen 02). Another protocol was based on supplementary i.v. insulin according to need (range 32–88 units/day) (Kaushal 03).

Urinary Tract Infection

Data are sparse on UTI during pregnancy in women with PDM (Abdelgadir 03), despite the possible linkage to premature birth and worsening glycemic control. Pyelonephritis was included as a prognostically bad sign for increase in the risk of perinatal death in an influential early Danish study of type 1 diabetes in pregnancy (Pedersen 65,74). A systematic review of articles published from 1965 to 1985 revealed an incidence of pyelonephritis of 3.4% in 620 women with PDM (Cousins 87), which was similar to the rate of 3.5% noted in a single-center study in 1990 of 288 pregnant women with PDM (Reece 98). In the latter study, pyelonephritis was not more common in women with diabetic microvascular disease. Pyelonephritis was recorded in 2.1% of 423 women with PDM in the California statewide program in 1986–1988 (Cousins 91). Symptomatic UTIs confirmed by culture were found in 12% of pregnant women with type 1 diabetes in Cincinnati, with a crude RR of 2.0 compared with nondiabetic controls (Stamler 90). In a French 46-center survey conducted in 1986–1988, UTI defined as a combination of pyelonephritis or asymptomatic bacteriuria was noted in 25% of 232 pregnant women with type 1 diabetes and 24% of 78 women with type 2 diabetes (GDFSG 91).

Asymptomatic bacteriuria was somewhat increased (7%) in pregnant diabetic women compared with controls in early studies in Boston (Pometta 67) and Copenhagen (18%) (Vejlsgaard 73a). The rate was highest in women with diabetic microangiopathy (Vejlsgaard 73b). Bacteriuria was associated with increased risk of preterm delivery (Vejlsgaard 73c). The prevalence of significant bacteriuria was 43% in a study of 120 pregnant women with diabetes compared with 15% in 60 controls in Poland; the incidence was less in the third trimester in patients with improved glucose control. Staphylococcus and *Escherichia coli* culture occurred more frequently (Bieganska 02). To our knowledge, no prospective studies have been conducted on the benefits and costs of treatment of asymptomatic bacteriuria in pregnant women with diabetes. It is therefore difficult to make an evidence-based recommendation on the routine use of urine cultures or other screening tests in diabetic pregnancies.

Preeclampsia

Hypertensive disorders are frequent in women with PDM (Feig 06, Becker 07). Classification and diagnosis of the hypertensive disorders of pregnancy as well as management of chronic and gestational hypertension in pregnancy are considered in Part II in the section titled "Blood Pressure Control." Preeclampsia (new or sudden worsening of hypertension and proteinuria, perhaps with other signs of target organ damage) is associated with increased maternal morbidity, possible fetal hypoxia, and neonatal morbidity associated with prematurity (Table III.4). The prevalence of preeclampsia ranges from 12.5% to 29.2 % in women with type 1 diabetes (Diamond 85, Siddiqi 91, Zhu 97, Hanson 98, Hiilesmaa 00, Sibai 00b, Ekbom 01, Ray 01, Vaarasmaki 02, Wylie 02, Evers 04) and from 12.0% to 30.9 % in women with type 2 diabetes (Omori 94, Sacks 97, Zhu 97, Cundy 02). These rates represented a three- to sevenfold increase in studies that compared PDM to pregnancies in nondiabetic women (Garner 90, Ros 98, Lee 00, Vangen 03, Jensen 04, Duckitt 05, Rosenberg 05, Feig 06, Catov 07).

The increased association of preeclampsia with chronic diabetes, adjusted for relevant factors, is found in all ethnic groups in the U.S. except for non-Hispanic Asians, and there is probable interplay between diabetes and excess maternal weight in their

TABLE III.4 Pregnancy Outcome Associated with Preeclampsia in Observational Studies Providing Details of Pregnancies Complicated by Preexisting Diabetes

Author (year)	Frequency of Preeclampsia	Preterm Delivery	Infant Small for Gestational Age	NICU Admittance	Perinatal Death
Diamond, 1985	41/199 (20.6%)	NA	2.4%	37.5% respiratory distress; 20% hypoglycemia; 27.5% hyperbilirubinemia	1 stillborn
Sibai, 2000b	92/462 (19.9%)	56.5% <37 weeks	5.4%	65.2%	1 stillborn
Cundy, 2002	39/200 (19.5%)	23.1% <36 weeks	5.1%	69%	None

NICU, neonatal intensive care unit; NA, not available.

contribution to development of preeclampsia (Ray 01, Bo 03, Rosenberg 05). Prevalence is highest in initial pregnancies (Vaarasmaki 02) and in those with elevated A1C levels (Hanson 98, Ekbom 00, Hiilesmaa 00, Combs 93, Rosenn 93, Hsu 96,98, Temple 06), chronic hypertension (Combs 93, Sibai 00, Vaarasmaki 02), or micro/macroalbuminuria (Winocour 89, Sibai 00b, Ekbom 01, Lauszus 01, Cundy 02). An RCT of improved postprandial glucose control in women with type 1 diabetes demonstrated a significantly reduced incidence of preeclampsia (Manderson 03). Preeclampsia in women with type 1 diabetes predicted a higher rate of incipient/overt DN and CHD 11 years after pregnancy (Gordin 07). Analysis of data on preeclampsia and diabetes is complicated by the number of diabetic women that enter pregnancy with obesity, baseline hypertension, and/or early-to-advanced DN.

Reasons for the increased rate of preeclampsia in women with PDM are unknown, but they are probably multifactorial and involve response of the maternal kidneys and systemic vasculature to placental factors. Diabetes-associated reasons that have been proposed include failure of trophoblast-induced modification of uterine spiral arteries and development of atherosis (Kitzmiller 81, Semmler 85), preexisting diabetic microangiopathy (Hanson 88, Reece 98), enhancement of oxidative stress by hyperglycemia (Walsh 98, Kossenjans 00, Ekbom 01), and imbalance in the fetoplacental NO pathway (Bisseling 05). Emerging research focuses on the pathogenesis of preeclampsia, which may provide more insight into the linkage between diabetes and this serious placental–renal–vascular disorder (Solomon 04, Gupta 05, Lam 05, Roberts 05, Thadhani 05, Mignini 06) and thereby suggest the means of its prevention.

To date, prophylactic measures, such as the use of aspirin, have not reduced the frequency of preeclampsia in women with PDM (Caritis 98), although there is controversy surrounding whether aspirin would be helpful in pregnant women with diabetic microangiopathy (Duley 03,06). Conventional meta-analysis showed a modest benefit of aspirin to reduce preeclampsia in the general obstetrical population, although the largest individual RCTs did not (Duley 04). A meta-analysis of individual patient data in RCTs of aspirin showed "hypertensive disorder of pregnancy events" (including gestational hypertension, as well as preeclampsia and eclampsia) in 60 of 439 (13.7%) women with PDM randomized to an antiplatelet drug versus 82 of 466 (17.6%) women with PDM in control groups. The RR calculation was 0.76 (95% CI 0.56–1.04) associated with drug use compared with 0.91 (95% CI 0.84–0.99) for drug use in

11,641 women without PDM (interaction p value = 0.26) (Askie 07). Editorialists commented that aspirin might produce an anti-inflammatory effect, as well as inhibition of platelet aggregation and dilation of blood vessels, and whether treating 50 high-risk women to prevent one case of preeclampsia is worthwhile will depend on individual patient–doctor counseling (Roberts 07).

Controversy also surrounds whether calcium supplementation during pregnancy reduces the frequency of preeclampsia or its severity (Atallah 02, Hofmeyr 05, Villar 06a), and this hypothesis is not well tested in diabetic women. The most recent systematic review of trials showed an RR of 0.22 (95% CI 0.12–0.42) for preeclampsia with calcium supplementation in women at high risk for preeclampsia (5 trials, 587 women) and an RR of 0.36 (95% CI 0.18–0.70) in women with low baseline calcium intake (7 trials, 10,154 women). No significant reduction in preeclampsia was found if there was adequate dietary calcium intake (RR 0.62; 95% CI 0.32–01.20; 4 trials, 5,022 women) (Hofmeyr 07). RCTs of antioxidants to prevent preeclampsia have failed in the general population (see the section titled "Medical Nutrition Therapy" in Part I), and RCTs in women with diabetes are currently in progress. To date, no clinically effective biochemical or biophysical screening tests for preeclampsia in nondiabetic women have been conducted (Conde-Agudelo 04), but these putative tests are not well tested in diabetic women.

Management of preeclampsia in women with diabetes should not differ compared with women with normal glucose tolerance. However, renal status in women with DN requires strict attention to fluid, electrolyte, and magnesium sulfate therapy. Because delivery is the only definitive treatment for women who develop preeclampsia, criteria for delivery are based on maternal and fetal severity as well as gestational age. Treatment of diabetic women with the onset of preeclampsia who are remote from term requires specific attention to the use of antenatal glucocorticoids to enhance lung maturation, which is discussed earlier in the section titled "Preterm Labor and Delivery." Intravenous synthetic corticosteroids have been used to treat women with severe preeclampsia complicated by hemolysis, thrombocytopenia, and elevated liver enzymes (Magann 94, Martin 03), but most RCTs focused on postpartum treatment (van Runnard Heimel 04). Antenatal use of this protocol in diabetic women would require an intensively monitored intravenous insulin regimen to prevent severe hyperglycemia. Acute treatment of severe systolic (>155–160) or diastolic (>110) hypertension in preeclampsia is important to prevent maternal vascular complications (Cunningham 00,05, Martin 05, Duley 06). Hydralazine, nicardipine, nifedipine, and labetalol have been used effectively in these emergency situations (Vermillion 99, Aali 02, Duley 02, Elatrous 02, Magee 03).

Standard obstetrical treatment for the prevention and treatment of convulsions in women with preeclampsia is intravenous magnesium sulfate (Scardo 95, Sibai 05a, Duley 06). Although it is not the standard therapy for seizures in general medical practice, prospective randomized clinical trials have found magnesium sulfate superior to placebo or other anticonvulsive medications, such as phenytoin or diazepam, for seizure prophylaxis in women with severe preeclampsia (ECG 95, Lucas 95, Coetzee 98, MTG 02, Belfort 03); trials were conducted in the setting of use of various antihypertensive agents to control severe hypertension (Sibai 05b). The use of magnesium sulfate in women with mild preeclampsia and diabetes is controversial because there are currently no prospective trials with sufficient power to definitively determine the utility of magnesium sulfate in this clinical situation (Sibai 05b). Controversy has surrounded the safety of concomitant use of nifedipine and magnesium sulfate in preeclampsia (Waisman 88, Snyder 89, Impey 93, Ben Ami 94), but a recent controlled analysis of 162 cases found no increase in neuromuscular weakness or hypotension (Magee 05).

Recommendations

- Screen diabetic women with premature uterine contractions or previous preterm delivery with measurement of cervical length by US or assay of fetal fibronectin in vaginal pool samples to establish risk of preterm birth. (A)

- 17 α-Hydroxyprogesterone significantly decreases the risk of preterm delivery in women with prior preterm delivery, but is not successful as a tocolytic agent for established preterm labor. As yet, no data exist regarding any potential adverse affects of weekly progesterone injections on maternal glucose metabolism in women with PDM. (A)

- Tocolytic agents used to treat preterm labor and prolong gestation include magnesium sulfate, prostaglandin synthesis inhibitors, and CCBs. β-Adrenergic agonists, such as terbutaline, should be used as a last choice to treat premature labor in women with diabetes because they cause substantial hyperglycemia. (E)

- Antenatal glucocorticoids should be used to enhance fetal lung maturation between 24 and 34 weeks gestation if there is a significant clinical risk of preterm delivery. However, antenatal steroids adversely affect maternal glucose control, and intensive insulin therapy and frequent glucose monitoring is required to prevent hyperglycemia. (A)

- Agents such as aspirin or calcium have not been shown to prevent preeclampsia in women with PDM. Studies of antioxidant therapy in diabetic women are ongoing, and therefore no recommendation can be made. Antioxidant vitamins in nondiabetic pregnant women have not reduced preeclampsia. (A; E for diabetic pregnancy)

- Management of preeclampsia in diabetic women includes careful fetal assessment, use of betamethasone to enhance fetal lung maturity before delivery between 24 and 34 weeks gestation coupled with intensive insulin therapy, use of intravenous magnesium sulfate to prevent convulsions, and short-term antihypertensive therapy to keep systolic pressure <155–160 and diastolic pressure <110 (not to be confused with systolic BP targets of 110–129 and diastolic BP targets of 65–79 for chronic hypertension in diabetes). (A; E for diabetic pregnancy)

MANAGEMENT OF DELIVERY

—— *Original contribution by Deborah L. Conway MD and Patrick M. Catalano MD*

Planning Delivery

The issue of the timing of delivery in women with PDM is controversial due to the lack of adequate prospective studies (Conway 02, Sacks 02). Few studies are RCTs evaluating the risk and benefit of timing or mode of delivery. Furthermore, many studies include both pregestational and gestational diabetic women, and risks may be diluted by inclusion of the latter group. Apprehension of clinical factors has influenced the timing of delivery in women with PDM: (a) inadequately controlled diabetes (type 1 or type 2) and the increased risk of stillbirth balanced with a possible delay in fetal lung maturation and (b) fear of traumatic vaginal delivery and shoulder dystocia balanced with possible increased mother/infant complications with CS. In persisting maternal hyperglycemia due to the risk of fetal hypoxia, many authors recommend induction of labor at 37 weeks gestation after confirming fetal lung maturity (Rasmussen 92, Hod 98, Sacks 03, Visser 03, Coustan 04). An emerging consensus suggests that well-monitored diabetic women achieving excellent glycemic control as defined in Part I, without obstetrical complications, can await spontaneous labor up to 39–40 weeks gestation (Murphy 84, McAuliffe 99, Kjos 02, Sacks 02, Gabbe 03, Coustan 04, Kjos 04).

There is an increased risk of shoulder dystocia (4.7–11.4%) in vaginal deliveries reported in observational studies of women with PDM, which may include more difficult cases of diabetes that are referred to centers of excellence (Bahar 96, Sacks 97, Blackwell 00a, Ray 01, Wylie 02, Feig 06). The frequency of shoulder dystocia was 4.6%, 6.4%, and 14.0% of vaginal deliveries in recent population surveys of women with PDM in Norway, Canada, and the Netherlands, respectively (Vangen 03, Visser 03, Feig 06). Adjusted ORs were 2.4–6.0 for shoulder dystocia associated with maternal diabetes (Acker 85, Langer 91, Robinson 03, Vangen 03, Feig 06). Because shoulder dystocia is defined as "a delivery that requires additional obstetrical maneuvers following failure of gentle downward traction on the fetal head to effect delivery of the shoulders" (ACOG 02b), it is recognized that data collection is subjective and that varying degrees of severity are included.

Risk of shoulder dystocia increases with increasing BW in both diabetic and nondiabetic populations, varying from 8% to 23% across the 4,000–4,500-gm range in the largest study of diabetic women (including GDM) (Nesbitt 98) (Table III.5). In

TABLE III.5 Shoulder Dystocia in Vaginal Births of Infants of Women with Diabetes* and Nondiabetic Controls, Stratified by Birth Weight

	Acker 1985		Langer 1991		Nesbitt 1998			
	DM	Controls	DM	Controls	DM NSVD	DM Assist	ND NSVD	ND Assist
Number	144	14,577	1,589	74,390	NA	NA	NA	NA
BW ≥4,000 gm	25.0%	8.8%	20.6%	7.6%	NA	NA	NA	NA
Total shoulder dystocia (%)	15 (10.4)	294 (2.0)	50 (3.2)	406 (0.5)	NA	NA	NA	NA
3,500–3,749 gm	4/43 (9.3)	94/4,249	NA	NA	(3.0)	(4.0)	(1.8)	(2.0)
3,750–3,999	"	" (2.2)	3/254 (1.2)	71/7,050 (1.0)	(5.8)	(8.5)	(2.8)	(4.0)
4,000–4,249	6/26 (23.1)	107/1,074	4/132 (3.0)	86/3,317 (2.6)	(8.4)	(12.2)	(5.2)	(8.6)
4,250–4,499	"	" (10.0)	6/87 (6.9)	73/1,472 (5.0)	(12.3)	(16.7)	(9.1)	(12.9)
4,500–4,750	5/10 (50.0)	47/208	12/55 (21.8)	43/571 (7.5)	(19.9)	(27.3)	(14.3)	(23.0)
4,750–4,999	"	" (22.6)	10/28 (35.7)	26/202 (12.9)	(23.5)	(34.8)	(21.1)	(29.0)
≥5,000	"	"	10/26 (38.5)	10/112 (8.9)	NA	NA	NA	NA

Acker and Langer data are from single centers of referral; Nesbitt data are from California births in 1992, with 175,886 vaginal births of infants weighing >3,500 gm.

For BW ≥4,000 gm, the denominator is term-size vaginal births in the study.

*Includes women with gestational diabetes.

DM, diabetes mellitus; ND, nondiabetic; NSVD, normal spontaneous vaginal delivery; Assist, vaginal delivery assisted by use of forceps or vacuum extractor; NA, not available; ", numbers pooled with subset above.

two other studies, fetal macrosomia with BW ≥4,000 gm predicted 73.3% and 84.0% of the cases of shoulder dystocia (Acker 85, Langer 91). However, in a nationwide survey of type 1 diabetic pregnancies in the Netherlands with 179 vaginal deliveries in 1999–2000, 40% of the cases of shoulder dystocia occurred with a BW of 3,000–3,999 gm. Frequency of shoulder dystocia was 3.8% at 3,000–3,500 gm, 14.3% at 3,500–4,000 gm, 30.0% at 4,000–4,500 gm, and 66.7% at ≥4,500 gm (Visse 03). Due to increased truncal adiposity in IDMs compared with equivalent weight controls (Modanlou 82, Brans 83, Bernstein 92, Ballard 93, Catalano 95, Kehl 96, McFarland 98, Cohen 99) and perhaps also due to increased obesity in diabetic women, the risk of shoulder dystocia may be greater than in nondiabetic populations even at BWs of 3,000–3,999 gm (Acker 85, Langer 91, Nesbitt 98, Visser 03). For infants with BW >4,000 gm, shoulder circumference was found to be larger in IDMs compared with nondiabetic mothers (McFarland 98). This finding confirmed an earlier study that determined the difference between mean shoulder circumference minus HC to be 7.4 cm vs. 3.2 cm for infants at a BW >4,000 gm (p < 0.001) and 3.6 cm in IDMs at a BW of 2,501–4,000 gm compared with 1.7 cm in infants of nondiabetic mothers in the same BW range (p < 0.001) (Modanlou 82).

Any type of infant birth trauma was found in 20–44% of cases of shoulder dystocia in diabetic women, including fracture of the clavicle or humerus, facial palsy, and brachial plexus palsy (Acker 85, Langer 91, Nesbit 98, Wylie 02, Visser 03, Mehta 06). In one large study of 50 IDMs delivered with shoulder dystocia, the frequency of perinatal mortality was 28% and birth trauma 36%; 38% had a 5-min Apgar score <7 compared with 2.2%, 3.5%, and 5.8%, respectively, in 1,539 IDMs delivered without shoulder dystocia (Langer 91). In this study, as in most analyses of shoulder dystocia, diabetes included both PDM and GDM. Risk of brachial plexus injury (anterior shoulder) is not as common, but the few serious, permanent cases can be devastating to development of the child (Levine 84, Pollock 00, Wolf 00, Gherman 03, Mehta 06). Frequency of obstetrical brachial plexus injury has been 0.5–6.2% of vaginal deliveries of women with PDM (Acker 85, Mimouni 92, Ecker 97, Nesbitt 98, Wylie 02, Visser 03, Mehta 06) versus 0.05%, 0.15%, 0.19%, and 0.21% in population surveys of births of nondiabetic women, respectively (McFarland 86, Gregory 98, Gilbert 99, Mollberg 05). In a 10-year population survey of all births in Sweden, the adjusted OR for brachial plexus palsy associated with diabetes in pregnancy was 2.4, even when controlling for infant BW (Mollberg 05). Studies of diabetic women show that 4.0–13.3% of shoulder dystocia cases result in brachial plexus injury, with the risk increasing with operative delivery and greater BW (Acker 85, Mimouni 92, Ecker 97, Nesbitt 98, Wylie 02, Visser 03, Mehta 06). A retrospective multicenter study of 624 deliveries with shoulder dystocia found that the rate of brachial plexus injury per case of impacted shoulders varied from 3% to 10% at different centers (Chauban 07). Much larger surveys of births in background populations demonstrate that only 43.6–74.1% of cases of brachial palsy are associated with recorded shoulder dystocia (Jennett 92, Graham 97, Gregory 98, Gilbert 99). Malpresentation is a factor in many other cases, even if delivered by CS.

Evidence regarding the imperfect methods of antepartum assessment for macrosomia and the risk of shoulder dystocia is noted in the section titled "Third-Trimester Fetal Ultrasonography." Debate is ongoing as to whether abnormal patterns of labor predict a higher risk of shoulder dystocia in diabetic women (Benedetti 78, Acker 85, Langer 91, McFarland 95). In the California population study, shoulder dystocia rates were higher in diabetic women requiring operative delivery versus spontaneous delivery at any BW >3,500 gm (Nesbitt 98). Noting the difficulty in predicting shoulder dystocia, the ACOG does not recommend primary cesarean delivery in diabetic women unless EFW is >4,500 gm (ACOG 02b). In published opinions by diabetes and pregnancy authorities, this EFW threshold has varied from 4,000 to 4,500 gm; thus, no consensus has been reached (Gabbe 77a, Kitzmiller 78, Spellacy 85, Cousins 87, Langer 91, Hod 98, Gabbe 03, Oats 03, Visser 03, Coustan 04). Some evidence suggests that maternal weight and height might enter into the prediction of risk of birth injury as well as fetal macrosomia (Gudmunnsson 05, Mazouni 06).

No RCTs have been conducted comparing primary CS with attempted vaginal delivery in women with PDM and EFW of 4,000–4,500 gm. Peripartum maternal morbidity may be comparable between vaginal delivery of a macrosomic infant and cesarean delivery without labor for suspected fetal macrosomia, but prior cesarean delivery does increase the chance of adverse events in subsequent pregnancies (Conway 02). One group of investigators calculated that "if all diabetic subjects whose infants weigh ≥4,250 gm were delivered by cesarean section, the overall cesarean section rate would increase by only 0.26% and would result in the elimination of 76% of the cases of shoulder dystocia" (Langer 91). Others used a computer model to estimate the cost-effectiveness of "elective"cesarean delivery of diabetic women at different EFW thresholds (Rouse 96). Baseline parameters that were entered into the model for diabetic women included 17.1% BW at 4,000–4,499 gm and, at this range of BW, CS rate of 18%, shoulder dystocia rate of 13.9%, and an 18% frequency of brachial plexus injury with shoulder dystocia, with 6.7% of those being permanent injuries. The authors estimated that, in one million diabetic women using a 4,000-gm threshold for primary cesarean delivery, there would be 158,004 additional CSs, 22,365 fewer shoulder dystocias, and 323 fewer permanent brachial plexus injuries at an additional cost of $283 million ($283.00 per patient; $876,161 per permanent injury avoided). Costs included the cost of occupational therapy visits for rehabilitation of brachial plexus injury for 1 year, but not NICU costs associated with vaginal birth trauma, physician visits, surgical therapy, lifetime costs, or costs of litigation, all of which presumably would reduce the cost per permanent injury avoided (Rouse 96).

Another approach in reducing shoulder dystocia and birth injury of IDMs has been to induce labor before macrosomia becomes too severe (Levy 02). In Dublin, Ireland, observational studies of pregnancies in diabetic women (majority being multiparous) show low CS and birth trauma rates with a policy of noninterference; however, they reported fetal deaths at term (37–41 weeks gestation) (Drury 83, Rasmussen 92). The single RCT in "compliant" insulin-treated patients in Los Angeles (93.5% GDM) with EFW <3,800 gm compared active induction of labor at 38 weeks gestation (n = 100) with expectant management up to 42 weeks (n = 100) unless fetal distress, preeclampsia, or maternal hyperglycemia supervened. Mean gestational age at delivery was 39 weeks in the active induction group and 40 weeks in the expectant group. Spontaneous labor before induction or CS without labor was 30% vs. 51%, induction of labor 70% vs. 49%, CS 25% vs. 31%, BW ≥4,000 gm 15% vs. 27% (p = 0.05), and mild shoulder dystocia 0% vs. 3%, respectively; no birth trauma occurred in either group. The difficulty of conducting this type of study is indicated by the fact that 744 insulin-treated women were unable or unwilling to participate during the 3.5 years of this RCT (Kjos 93). Although this study was underpowered to detect differences in perinatal outcome, expectant management was not superior to active induction of labor. A consensus group interpreted this study as demonstrating no increase in cesarean delivery in the induced group and significant reduction in macrosomic babies (Reece 02).

In Israel, a prospective observational study of induction of labor at 38–39 weeks gestation if EFW was <4,500 gm yielded shoulder dystocia in 1 of 74 vaginal deliveries of insulin-treated women with GDM (infant 4,250 gm at 39 weeks gestation, birth asphyxia, neonatal death) and a CS rate of 22.9%. Authors compared results with a previous protocol in which 164 patients were allowed to progress to spontaneous labor up to 41 weeks gestation unless EFW was >4,500 gm or obstetrical complications occurred. Seven cases of shoulder dystocia in 137 vaginal deliveries occurred in this group as well as a CS rate of 18.9%; BW was >4,200 gm in five of these shoulder dystocia cases. There was a brachial plexus injury in two infants: spontaneous delivery, 3,600 gm at 39 weeks; spontaneous delivery, 4,250 gm at 41 weeks (Lurie 96). In a much larger prospective observational study of 1,078 diabetic women in San Antonio (91% GDM), expectant management was used if US EFW between 37 and 38 weeks gestation was appropriate for gestational age. CS was performed with EFW ≥4,250 gm (4.9%), and labor was induced if EFW showed LGA (8.6%). The overall incidence of shoulder dystocia was 1.5% (7.4% in 68 infants ≥4,000 gm delivered vaginally), and the CS rate was 25.1%. The authors contrasted these figures with a 2.8% overall incidence of shoulder dystocia (18.8% in 85 infants ≥4,000 gm delivered vaginally) and a 21.7% CS rate in a previous 3-year period in which US-based intervention was not used in 1,227 patients (Conway 98).

Thus, we lack high-level evidence upon which to base a recommendation for or against induction of labor or primary cesarean delivery of women with PDM and EFW <4,500 gm. The Cochrane review titled "Elective Delivery in Diabetic Pregnant Women" also concluded that limited data from the single RCT do not allow one to draw conclusions about risks of maternal or neonatal morbidity with either approach and that "women's views on elective delivery and prolonged surveillance should be assessed in future trials." Reviewers did note that results of the single RCT "suggested that there might be little advantage in delaying delivery beyond 38–39 weeks in insulin-treated diabetic pregnant women" (Boulvain 01).

The ACOG clinical practice guideline provides no support for routine induction of labor at <40 weeks gestation, citing difficulties with accurate determination of the size of the large fetus (ACOG 05a). "Early delivery may be indicated in some patients with vasculopathy, nephropathy, poor glucose control, or a prior stillbirth. In contrast, patients with well-controlled diabetes may be allowed to progress to their expected date of delivery as long as antenatal testing remains reassuring. To prevent traumatic birth injury, cesarean delivery may be considered if the estimated fetal weight is greater than 4500 gm in women with diabetes" (ACOG 05a). A consensus report of the Diabetes in Pregnancy Study Group of North America proposes that: "At 38 weeks gestation, an evaluation of the diabetic woman's obstetrical history, diabetic control, and fetal size should be undertaken. Induction should be strongly considered for women who are poorly controlled, poorly compliant or where there is evidence of excessive fetal growth...Consideration may be given to delivery by cesarean section for estimated fetal weight of 4,250–4,500 gm or more, based on clinical evaluation, obstetric history and following discussion with the patient" (Reece 02). The Australasian Diabetes in Pregnancy Society consensus guidelines for the management of type 1 and type 2 diabetes in relation to pregnancy state: "The need for induction of labor or assisted delivery should be based on obstetric and fetal indications. Where the estimated birthweight is >4,250–4,500 gm, the risk of shoulder dystocia warrants consideration of elective cesarean section" (McElduff 05b). However, in this guideline, suspected macrosomia becomes an indicated cesarean delivery.

Pending future studies, given the lack of high-level evidence and the imprecise guidelines, the diabetic patient and her obstetrician have a decision to make as term pregnancy approaches (Hankins 06). Based on the RCT and observational cohort studies, we can only recommend that the decision to induce labor or perform cesarean delivery may be individualized when the EFW is between 4,000 and 4,500 gm (Conway 02, Sacks 03, Coustan 04). Primary CS is recommended in most cases when EFW is >4,499 gm. This clinical conundrum arising at the end of diabetic pregnancies can be minimized by excellent glycemic control throughout gestation, which is associated with reduced rates of fetal macrosomia, preeclampsia, and nonreassuring fetal testing.

The decision to attempt a vaginal birth after one previous CS in a diabetic woman should be based on usual obstetrical criteria (ACOG 04b). The decision will no doubt be influenced by all of the diabetes-related factors plus the policy of the medico–legal liability carrier. In one small study, the successful vaginal birth after cesarean rate was 14 of 32 (43.7%) in women with PDM and insulin-treated GDM, and no unusual complications were witnessed (Blackwell 00a). In a larger analysis of 1,092 diabetic women (mostly GDM) in Los Angeles with prior cesarean delivery, 59.4% attempted a trial of labor and 56.9% of those succeeded at vaginal delivery. Factors predicting success included prior vaginal delivery, lack of hypertension or obesity, and spontaneous labor (Kjos 04). Data on complications were not reported.

Managing Labor and Vaginal Delivery

Ripening the cervix with dinoprostone or misoprostol and induction of labor with controlled infusion of oxytocin do not have specific untoward effects in diabetic women without a uterine scar (Kjos 93, Lurie 96, Conway 98, Goldberg 01, Incerpi 01, Rozenberg 04, Yogev 04.

Characteristics of Labor in Diabetic Women

Data are surprisingly sparse on the characteristics of labor in diabetic women. We do not know whether the likelihood of failed induction or prolonged labor is greater in diabetic than nondiabetic women when controlling for gestational age and maternal/fetal weight. In a population survey of 1,532 deliveries of women with PDM in Ontario, Canada, in 2001, labor was induced in 33%, and 8.4% had "obstructed labor" (various ICD-9 codes) (Feig 06). Failure of induction to enter the active phase of labor was recorded in 7% of diabetic patients in Los Angeles (Kjos 93) compared with 26.5% in a smaller study in Detroit (Blackwell 00a). Active management of labor with early amniotomy and oxytocin augmentation reduces time in the first stage of labor, but does not reduce CS rates in nulliparous women (Sadler 00). It is presumed but not proven that the results apply to diabetic patients (McAuliffe 99, Sacks 03) because RCTs have not been conducted in this group. Arrest of labor in the active phase is variously defined as no or slow (<1cm/h) dilatation of the cervix beyond 2–4 h (Rouse 99, Sacks 03). Arrest disorders were described in 9.0%, 19.4%, and 23.9% of diabetic women in labor in three reports (Acker 85, Kjos 93, McFarland 95) compared with 6–8% in nondiabetic women with BWs of 3,000–4,499 gm (Table III.6) (Acker 86). In one study, a prolonged second stage >2 h was noted in 8.7% of diabetic women (McFarland 95). For comparison, the distribution of labor patterns among different

TABLE III.6 Patterns of Labor in Nondiabetic Women Delivering Vaginally with Infants of Different Birth Weights and Diabetic Women with Infants >4,000 gm

Labor Pattern	3,000–3,499 gm [SD %]	3,500–3,999 gm [SD %]	4,000–4,499 gm [SD %]	≥4,500 gm [SD %]	DM ≥4,000 gm [SD %]
Normal, n (%)	4,408 (70.5) [0.6]	2,875 (67.7) [1.8]	716 (66.7) [10.5]	133 (63.9) [17.3]	25 (69.4) [24.0]
Prolonged latent phase	644 (10.3) [0.6]	461 (10.8) [2.6]	84 (7.8) [6.0]	17 (8.2) [35.3]	1 (2.8) [0.0]
Protraction disorder	581 (9.3) [0.7]	466 (11.0) [4.3]	213 (19.8) [10.8]	31 (14.9) [22.6]	3 (8.3) [66.7]
Precipitate labor	567 (9.1) [0.7]	411 (9.7) [1.9]	41 (3.8) [0.0]	23 (11.1) [26.1]	4 (11.1) [75.0]
Arrest disorders	373 (6.0) [1.3]	317 (7.5) [5.0]	84 (7.8) [10.7]	20 (9.6) [55.0]	4 (11.1) [25.0]
Shoulder dystocia	40 (0.6)	94 (2.2)	107 (10.0)	47 (22.6)	11 (30.6)
Total gravidas	6,252	4,249	1,074	208	36

Protraction or arrest disorders occurred in the first or second stages of labor, defined according to Friedman 78. At the time of the study, nonrepeat cesarean sections were performed in 13% of all gravidas. DM includes preexisting and gestational diabetes. Data from Acker 85 and 86.

SD, shoulder dystocia.

infant BW groups in 11,783 nondiabetic women delivering in Boston in 1975–1982 are provided in Table III.6 (Friedman 78, Acker 85,86).

Controlled data are conflicting regarding whether epidural analgesia prolongs labor or predisposes to CS. Increased use of oxytocin augmentation and more operative vaginal deliveries are inconsistently associated with neuraxial blockade (Sacks 03, Sharma 03, Kotaska 06, Nageotte 06). RCTs have not been performed in diabetic women, but there are few reasons to withhold epidural or other analgesia from diabetic patients in the active phase of labor. Epidural analgesia attenuates the increase in plasma catecholamines during painful labor in nondiabetic women (Shnider 83). Pain decreases insulin sensitivity (Greisen 01), so epidural analgesia may smooth glucose and BP control during labor (Tsen 03). Although poorly studied, there is no evidence that the pharmacokinetics and pharmacodynamics of anesthetic agents are modified by diabetes in pregnancy (Wissler 04). No published data exist on possible interactions between diabetic complications and labor anesthesia during pregnancy (Wissler 04). Based on nonpregnancy experience, patients with autonomic cardiovascular dysfunction may have greater potential for hypotension during regional anesthesia (McAnulty 00). Noninvasive preanesthetic testing for autonomic neuropathy may be wise, and these patients may benefit from more vigorous intravenous hydration and more frequent BP measurement before and during anesthesia (Wissler 04). Ephedrine administration during initiation of epidural analgesia for labor results in better maintenance of maternal mean arterial pressure and fewer nonreassuring FHR changes that appear 15–25 min after induction of analgesia (Kreiser 04). Placental transfer of ephedrine does not affect neonatal outcome (Hughes 85). Intrathecal opioids used for labor analgesia can produce fetal bradycardia (Mardirosoff 02). Regarding maternal hypertension, evidence suggests that labor epidural anesthesia is safe for pregnant women with severe hypertensive disease and does not increase frequencies of cesarean delivery, pulmonary edema, or renal failure (Hogg 99).

Observational series show rates of operative vaginal delivery to be 10.2–22.0% in diabetic women, which are higher compared with nondiabetic women, even in nondiabetic women delivering macrosomic infants (Drury 83, Acker 85, McFarland 95, Vangen 03). Whether deliveries are assisted by use of forceps or vacuum extractor seems to be based on local preference. Fetal macrosomia and instrumental vaginal delivery are strong risk predictors for anal sphincter injury in large obstetrical datasets (Hudelist 05, Sheiner 05, Andrews 06, deLeeuw 08). Mediolateral episiotomy at a proper angle protects the anal sphincter during forceps or vacuum extraction deliveries (deLeeuw 08). Risks for severe perineal trauma associated with diabetes are subsumed under macrosomia. The rate of second- to fourth-degree vaginal tears was 18.4% of all vaginal births in one series of 196 women with PDM (Ray 01).

An association exists between operative vaginal delivery and increased risk of shoulder dystocia in most studies of diabetic women (Benedetti 78, Langer 91, McFarland 95, Bofill 97, Nesbitt 98, Levy 06, Sheiner 06, Athukorala 07), which points to the need for careful clinical decision-making and patient consultation during labor (Hankins 06). Most midpelvic deliveries should be discouraged in diabetic women (Acker 85). Due to risks of shoulder dystocia in diabetic women with an EFW >3,500 gm, labor should be managed with proper anticipation and preparation for this possibility (O'Leary 90), including the securement of appropriate facilities, anesthesia, and well-trained personnel "mobilized to aid the clinician and to deal with this acute obstetrical emergency in a skillful and expeditious fashion" (Acker 85). The ACOG Practice Bulletin states that no evidence suggests that any one obstetrical delivery maneuver (McFarland 96, Gherman 98) is "superior to another in releasing an impacted shoulder or reducing the chance of injury," but that hyperflexion and abduction of the hips (Gonik 83, Gherman 00) coupled with suprapubic (not fundal) pressure is a reasonable initial approach (ACOG 02b). "Despite the introduction of ancillary obstetric maneuvers, such as McRoberts maneuver and a generalized trend towards the avoidance of fundal pressure, it has been shown that the rate of shoulder dystocia-associated brachial plexus palsy has not decreased" (Gherman 06). Indeed, the rate has increased over 15 years as the rate of shoulder dystocia has gradually risen (MacKenzie 07), possibly associated with increasing maternal obesity and diabetes.

Metabolic Management of Labor and Delivery

Maternal hyperglycemia during labor is associated with increased risk of fetal hypoxia indicators (threshold blood glucose >150 mg/dL; >8.3 mM) (Mimouni 88a) as well as neonatal hyperinsulinemia and reactive hypoglycemia (Hall 77, Sosenko 79, Kuhl 82, Knip 83, Stenninger 97, Fraser 99, Stenninger 08) (threshold blood glucose >90–110 mg/dL; >5–6 mM) (Light 72, Oakley 72, Yeast 78, Andersen 85, Miodovnik 87, Agrawal 00). In the largest published experience with 233 insulin-treated pregnant patients, the lowest risk of neonatal hypoglycemia occurred when intrapartum maternal glucose was maintained at <100 mg/dL (<5.6 mM), and intrapartum hyperglycemia had more effect on neonatal hypoglycemia than did antepartum glucose levels (Curet 97). Persistent (Koivisto 72, Stenninger 98) and even transient neonatal hypoglycemia (Fluge 75, Dalgic 02) may be associated with long-term effects on neurodevelopmental outcome (Haworth 76). The presence of initial hypoglycemia is an important risk factor for perinatal brain injury in infants that are depressed at birth with fetal acidemia (Salhab 04). In a previous experimental study, insulin-induced hypoglycemia had a greater impact on perinatal hypoxic–ischemic damage than fasting-induced hypoglycemia (Yager 92). "Meticulous attention to avoiding maternal hypoglycemia during labor can prevent neonatal hypoglycemia" (Hawkins 07).

In an early metabolic study of labor in six women with type 1 diabetes using a complex glucose-controlled insulin infusion system, average dextrose infusion rates were 0, 0, 2.9, 3.0, 6.4, and 6.5 gm/h to maintain normoglycemia (83–94 mg/dL; 4.6–5.2 mM). Initial insulin infusion rates of 0, 9, 2, 17, 17, and 10 units/h were required to attain normoglycemia, respectively, and subsequent rates of 0.2, 0.7, 1.6, 6.7, 3.9, and 1.9 units/h were needed to maintain normoglycemia. The authors noted the necessity of immediately reducing the insulin infusion at delivery to avoid a precipitous fall in maternal glucose level (Nattrass 78). Subsequent investigators using a similar commercial glucose-controlled insulin infusion system (Biostator) in 12 women with type 1 diabetes (who were maintained euglycemic in the antepartum period) found that an average glucose infusion rate of 2.5 mg/kg/min was required to maintain maternal glucose at 70–90 mg/dL (3.9–5.0 mM), even when the insulin requirement declined to zero in the first stage of labor, regardless of oxytocin infusion or use of epidural anesthesia. The authors speculated that the drop in insulin requirement in insulin-dependent women was due to the exercise of labor (Jovanovic 83). Other investigators agreed that some diabetic women, even in type 1 diabetes, will not require insulin to remain normoglycemic with modern management of the first stage of labor; however, insulin requirement usually increases in the second stage (Golde 82, Jovanovic 83) and perhaps with maternal stress in the first stage of labor (Kitzmiller 02).

With the possibility of labor being prolonged beyond 6–8 h in fasting diabetic women and the presumed risks of ketogenesis, it is wise to provide nutritional support in the form of controlled infusions of intravenous dextrose in electrolyte solutions (Jovanovic 04). The latter help to maintain uteroplacental blood flow and prevent maternal hypotension with regional block anesthesia. Glucose infusion rates of 90–120 mg/min (5.6–8.2 gm/h; 1.2 mg/kg/min; ∼100–150 cc/h of 5% dextrose solutions) are successful at preventing maternal hypoglycemia or ketonemia, and intravenous insulin infusion of 0.005–0.05 units/kg/h will usually prevent maternal hyperglycemia if blood glucose is sampled hourly during active labor (Golde 82, Mimouni 87, Miodovnik 87).

One small RCT did not use dextrose infusions in the labor of 15 previously insulin-treated women (13 GDM, 2 type 2 diabetes) if maternal fingerstick blood glucose measured hourly was at 101–140 mg/dL (5.6–7.8 mM) and withheld Regular insulin infusion until maternal blood glucose was >141 mg/dL (Rosenberg 06). This was compared with a graded insulin infusion started at maternal blood glucose levels >81 mg/dL (>4.5 mM) along with 5% dextrose in normal saline at 125 mL/h in 20 women (15 GDM, 5 type 2 diabetes). Mean maternal blood glucose was 103.9 ± 8.7 mg/dL, and three women were treated with insulin infusion. There were intrapartum episodes of blood glucose >141 mg/dL (>7.8 mM) in five women (33%) in the "rotating fluids" arm compared with mean maternal blood glucose values of 103.2 ± 17.9 mg/dL in the insulin infusion arm in five women (25%) with episodes of intrapartum blood glucose >141 mg/dL. The authors did not comment on signs of fetal well-being in labor, but no newborn infants in either group were recorded with 1- or 5-min Apgar scores <7. Neonatal hypoglycemia (heelstick plasma glucose <35 mg/dL; [<1.9 mM] in first 24 h of life) was noted in 4 of 21 (19%) neonates in the maternal insulin-infusion group (43% of 21 admitted to NICU for unclear reasons) and 1 of 15 (6.7%) neonates in the maternal "rotating fluids" group (13.3% of 15 admitted to NICU; NS due to small numbers).

The authors noted that their study is not applicable to management of insulin-deficient women (Rosenberg 06), and additional research is needed to determine the optimal intrapartum metabolic management of women with type 2 diabetes.

Review of the aggregate experience with glucose and insulin requirements during labor and delivery suggests that maintaining normoglycemia during labor and delivery is necessary to minimize neonatal hypoglycemia (Jovanovic 04). Many authors reported simplified protocols for intrapartum insulin management in observational studies, but no head-to-head comparisons have been made (West 77, Linzey 78, Yeast 78, Jovanovic 80, Caplan 82, Haigh 82, Bowen 84, Miodovnik 87, Feldberg 88, Lean 90, Njenga 92). Two well-tested examples are provided in Table III.7 (Jovanovic 80, Kitzmiller 02,

TABLE III.7 Two Protocols for Insulin Management of Labor and Delivery.

	A.	B.
Intravenous fluids	Intravenous infusion of normal saline is begun. Once active labor begins or glucose levels decrease to <70 mg/dL, infusion is changed to 5% dextrose and delivered at a rate of 100–150 cc/h to achieve a glucose level of ~100 mg/dL (5.6 mM).	BG >130 mg/dL, LR at 125 mL/h BG <130 mg/dL, begin D5LR at 125 mL/h
Initiating insulin	Regular (short-acting) insulin is administered by intravenous infusion at a rate of 1.25 units/h if glucose levels are >100 mg/dL.	Mix 25 units Regular insulin in 250 mL normal saline (1 U: 10 mL) Algorithm (see below)

Protocol B Algorithm		
Maternal Plasma Glucose in mg/dL (mM)	Insulin (units/h)	Individualized Dose
<70 (<3.9)	0.0	
71–90 (3.9–5.0)	0.5	
91–110 (5.1–6.1)	1.0	
111–130 (6.2–7.2)	2.0	
131–150 (7.3–8.3)	3.0	
151–170 (8.4–9.4)	4.0	
171–190 (9.5–10.6)	5.0	
>190 (>10.6)	Check ketones	

The usual dose of intermediate-acting insulin is given at bedtime, but the usual morning dose is withheld. In both protocols, glucose levels are checked hourly using a bedside meter allowing for adjustment in the insulin or glucose infusion rate. Protocols differ in the blood glucose thresholds at which to infuse dextrose-containing solutions and Regular short-acting insulin. Many nursing clinicians believe it is simpler to always infuse 5% dextrose, as with perioperative management of diabetic patients (Hirsch 91, Gavin 92, ACE 04). Data discussed in the text suggest a maternal glucose target <100 mg/dL (<5.6 mM) to minimize neonatal hypoglycemia. Protocol A is taken from ACOG 05a based on data from Jovanovic 80 and Coustan 04.
Protocol B is taken from Kitzmiller 02 and assumes that many patients with type 1 diabetes will have a small insulin requirement to remain normoglycemic.

LR, lactated Ringer's solution; D5LR, 5% dextrose lactated Ringer's solution.

Coustan 04, ACOG 05a). Perfusion of the insulin-containing tubing and catheter system before insertion will prevent dose deficiency due to insulin adsorption to the plastic (Peterson 76). Principles of intravenous therapy for labor or cesarean delivery are similar to those used in the perioperative management of diabetes except that no insulin is often needed for many hours postpartum (Hirsch 91, Gavin 92, ACE 04). Intravenous insulin protocols are also useful to prevent hyperglycemia in fasting diabetic patients during times of antepartum stress, such as administration of corticosteroids. However, subcutaneous boluses of short-acting insulin will be necessary in the patient who is eating.

Intrapartum Fetal Monitoring

Due to the increased risks of fetal hypoxia and acidosis in labor associated with maternal hyperglycemia, diabetic vasculopathy, and preeclampsia (Teramo 83, Mimouni 86a, Olofsson 86b, Cousins 87, Mimouni 88a, Bradley 92, Salvesen 93a,95), intrapartum FHR monitoring has been widely used in women with PDM. Although the effect of intrapartum electronic fetal monitoring (EFM) on prevention of perinatal brain injury is arguable for children of normoglycemic women (Thacker 01, Graham 06), there seems little doubt that proper interpretation of EFM in the setting of diabetes reduces the frequency of intrapartum stillbirth and fetal acidosis at birth, which in turn reduces the frequency of respiratory distress in the infant. Intermittent and continuous FHR monitoring may be comparable in low-risk patients (Vintzileos 95a,b), but the ACOG recommends continuous external Doppler or internal (scalp electrode) monitoring in the high-risk situation of diabetes (ACOG 05b).

The ACOG and the NIH published similar guidelines for the interpretation of electronic FHR monitoring (FIGO 87, NIH 97, ACOG 05b, Amer-Wahlin 07). The clinician must understand the implications of changes over time in baseline rate, variability, presence of accelerations, and periodic or episodic decelerations and must interpret FHR patterns during labor according to gestational age, medications, prior fetal assessment, and obstetrical and medical conditions (ACOG 05b). The term "fetal distress" (generally referring to an ill fetus) should be replaced by "nonreassuring fetal status," followed by a further description of the findings: repetitive variable decelerations, fetal tachycardia (>160 bpm) or bradycardia (<110 bpm), late decelerations, or low BPP (ACOG 05c). Some evidence suggests higher basal FHR and significantly lower accelerations and short-term variability in maternal diabetes compared with controls (Weiner 96, Tincello 98,01, Ruozi-Berretta 04).

The goal of EFM interpretation is to "predict fetal asphyxial exposure before decompensation and neonatal morbidity" (Low 99). Conversely, it is recognized that EFM has poor inter- and intraobserver reliability as well as a high false positive rate and that false interpretations can increase the rate of cesarean and operative deliveries (Sykes 83, ACOG 05b). With careful interpretation, predictive FHR patterns over a narrow 1-h window (including minimal baseline variability and late or prolonged decelerations) "can be a useful screening test for fetal asphyxia. However, supplementary tests are required to confirm the diagnosis and to identify the large number of false-positive patterns to avoid unnecessary interventions" (Low 99). Direct fetal blood sampling by cordocentesis is considered invasive and impractical during labor; the method is used primarily in research studies (Bradley 92, Salvesen 93b).

If there is decreased or absent FHR variability without spontaneous accelerations >10–15 bpm, a variety of techniques (especially scalp stimulation with a digit or Allis clamp or vibroacoustic stimulation) can be used to stimulate fetal response (Skupski 02).

When there is an acceleration following stimulation, fetal acidosis is unlikely and labor can continue (ACOG 05b). Hyperstimulation (≥ 6 contractions in 10 min) or hypertonus (single contraction lasting ≥ 2 min) can be treated with β-adrenergic agents (ACOG 05b), which will increase blood glucose. When a nonreassuring FHR tracing persists, fetal scalp sampling for pH (Berg 87, Huch 94) or fetal pulse oximetry can be used to determine whether to allow labor to continue (Kuhnert 98, Seelbach-Gobel 99). We are not aware of subgroup analyses of diabetic women in published trials of fetal pulse oximetry, in which 3 of 4 RCTs showed benefit in reduction of CSs for nonreassuring FHR patterns (Garite 00, Kuhnert 04, Bloom 06, East 06a,b).

Repolarization of myocardial cells in preparation for the next cardiac contraction (marked by the ST segment and T wave on the fetal ECG) is affected by a negative energy balance associated with fetal hypoxia (Rosen 75,76, Hokegard 81, Rosen 84, Westgate 01). A rise in the ST segment shows a fetus responding to hypoxia, and a negative ST wave shows a fetus that is unable to respond or has not had time to react (Luzzietti 03). In Europe, 2 of 3 RCTs showed that coupling of cardiotocography with ST-segment and T-wave analysis (STAN) by scalp electrode ECG increased the sensitivity of EFM, lowered the rate of CSs for nonreassuring fetal patterns, and reduced the number of babies born with metabolic acidosis (Westgate 93, Luzietti 99, Amer-Wahlin 01, Sundstrom 01, Neilson 06, Ojala 06). This technique requires a dedicated medical device that produces poor fetal ECG signal quality 11% of the time (Dervaitis 04). Increasing STAN usage in large Dutch and Swedish communities provided consistent improvements in fetal outcome without increasing operative interventions for nonreassuring FHR patterns (Kwee 04, Noren 06). Evaluation of the availability of ST-segment information for FHR tracing analysis in California showed significantly greater observer agreement on required interventions and their timing compared with standard visual analysis of FHR patterns (Ross 04). An ongoing European Union–sponsored fetal ECG project seeks to extend evaluation and training in STAN technology to many perinatal centers in Europe (Luzietti 03). Infrequent problems reported with expanded use of STAN (Doria 07, Westerhuis 07) led to European consensus conferences to develop clinical guidelines (Amer-Wahlin 07).

Maternal diabetes has been an indication for STAN usage in Europe. A retrospective case–control study of participants in two multicenter trials of STAN assessed ST-segment changes in 104 cases with PDM or GDM. ST depression was present on the fetal ECG in 22% of fetuses of mothers with diabetes compared with 12% of 207 controls (OR 2.6, 95% CI 1.4–4.7, adjustment for BW and nulliparity). ST-segment elevation was present in 47.1% of diabetic patients and 41% of controls (OR 1.4, 95% CI 0.9–2.3; p = 0.18). The authors speculated that the increased rate of ST depression probably did not indicate fetal hypoxia, "but an altered ability of the myocardium to respond to the stress of labor" (Yli 08).

Cesarean Delivery

Characteristics of Cesarean Delivery in Diabetic Women

Pregnancies in women with PDM prior to 1985 had high rates of CS: 44.0% primary and 13.4% repeat in diabetic women without known microvascular disease and 56.7% primary (p < 0.005) and 19.6% repeat for diabetic women with microvascular disease (Cousins 87). Recent observational studies of women with PDM continue to bear this out (total CS rates 30.0–60.2%) (Hanson 93, Elmallah 97, Sacks 97, Zhu 97, Nordstrom 98, Reece 98, McElvy 00, Wylie 02, Ehrenberg 04,

Kjos 04). High rates are also reported (34.9–62.0%; median 51%) in recent population-based surveys of diabetic women in North America and Europe, with RRs of 2.6–6.5 compared with control populations, even when adjusted for maternal factors and BW (CDC 93, Hawthorne 97, Remsberg 99, Levy 02, Vangen 03, Jensen 04, Feig 06, Guenter 06). In the 191 well-controlled pregnancies in the multicenter DCCT, 61 women were delivered by CS without labor and 46 had cesarean delivery after a trial of labor for a total CS rate of 56.0%, even though the rate of BW >4,500 gm was only 10.5% (DCCT 96).

Common coded indications for cesarean delivery without labor in diabetic women, listed in decreasing order of frequency, include prior CS, suspected macrosomia, pre-eclampsia, nonreassuring fetal status, malpresentation, and various obstetrical diagnoses (Miodovnik 87, Kjos 93, Remsberg 99, Blackwell 00a,b, Kjos 04). Common coded indications for CS after labor in diabetic women, also listed in order of decreasing frequency, include arrest disorders, failed induction of labor, and nonreassuring fetal status (Drury 83, Kjos 93, Blackwell 00a,b, Kjos 04). Independent risk factors for the high rates of CS identified in multivariate analysis include prior cesarean deliveries, maternal BMI, fetal macrosomia, and preeclampsia (Remsberg 99, Ehrenberg 04, Kjos 04). Controversy surrounds the determination of how much a policy that encourages induction of labor will increase the cesarean rate in diabetic women (Conway 98, Levy 02, Kjos 04). However, it is widely recognized and supported by controlled analyses that physician decision-making is a major influence on rates of CS in women with PDM (Naylor 96, Buchanan 98, Conway 02, Sacks 02). Indeed, the rising tide of patient self-selected cesarean delivery in many hospitals (NIH 06) will degrade the evaluation of cesarean delivery frequency as an indicator of management of diabetic pregnancies.

Informed consent for truly elective cesarean deliveries (Hankins 06) should consider data on the cesarean-related increase in serious maternal morbidity (Villar 06b, Liu 07), especially with an increasing number of repeat cesarean deliveries in the same woman (Silver 06). Clinicians should also consider the possible increased frequency of wound complications and septic pelvic thrombophlebitis in diabetic women with abdominal deliveries (Diamond 86, Stamler 90, Riley 96, Takoudes 04). The use of prophylactic antibiotics is established practice for prevention of postoperative morbidity after cesarean deliveries in high-risk patients (labor, ruptured membranes, prolonged surgery, excessive bleeding) (Duff 86,87, ACOG 03). The only observational (and retrospective) study that did not show increased wound infections in diabetic patients was conducted in a setting using prophylactic antibiotics in diabetic and control women (Riley 96); thus, most clinicians consider diabetic women to be at high risk for postoperative morbidity after elective CS. Three meta-analyses of 12 RCTs in low-risk patients undergoing elective cesarean delivery also concluded that antibiotic prophylaxis was effective in reducing the incidence of postoperative fever, endometritis, and wound infections (Chelmow 01, Smaill 02, Hopkins 03).

Pregnancy-Related Venous Thromboembolism

Although the risk of VTE increases four- to sixfold in pregnancy and especially in the puerperium (Andersen 98, ACOG 01, Heit 05, Blanco-Molina 07) after operative delivery (Treffers 83, Gherman 99, Simpson 01), no controlled data are known to us on the risk reduction of postoperative thromboembolism in obese diabetic women delivered by CS. Pulmonary embolism is the leading cause of maternal mortality in developed countries (Franks 90, Berg 03). Cesarean delivery carries a fivefold higher risk of thrombosis compared with vaginal delivery in nondiabetic women (Macklon 96, Lindqvist 99, Quinones 05). Data from a multicenter study of 30,132 cesarean deliveries without labor in 1999–2002 (23% with maternal medical disease) showed frequencies of deep venous thrombosis (DVT) and pulmonary embolus of 0.27% and 0.21%, respectively, after the first cesarean delivery compared with 0.14% and 0.08%, respectively, after the third cesarean delivery (Silver 06). Another epidemiological survey of >1,000 cesarean deliveries yielded a prevalence of postoperative pulmonary embolus of 0.47% (Jacobsen 04).

Diabetes (PDM and GDM) was an independent risk factor for VTE in the antepartum period in a case–control study taken from a register of 613,232 pregnancies in Norway (Jacobsen 08). A query of the U.S. Nationwide Inpatient Sample for 2000–2001 provided data on the risk of pregnancy-related VTE associated with diabetes (James 06a). The frequency of DVT was 0.07% and pulmonary embolism was 0.015% among more than eight million pregnancy admissions with deliveries, but the frequency of DVT was 7.31% and pulmonary embolism was 2.39% among 73,834 postpartum readmissions. Total rate for DVT was 1.36 per 1,000 deliveries and 0.36 per 1,000 deliveries for pulmonary embolism. The rate of pregnancy-related thromboembolic events by race included 2.64 per 1,000 deliveries for black women, 1.75 for white women, 1.25 for Hispanic women, and 1.07 for Asian women. The OR for increased risk of pregnancy-related VTE associated with diabetes (including GDM) was 2.0 (95% CI 1.4–2.7) compared with significant ORs (univariate analysis) of 51.8 for thrombophilia, 7.1 for heart disease, 4.4 for obesity, 2.1 for cesarean deliveries, 1.8 for hypertension, and 1.7 for smoking (James 06a).

An analysis of the circumstances surrounding US-confirmed DVT in pregnant or postpartum patients was conducted as part of a large U.S. multicenter registry of 2,892 consecutive women with DVT (James 05). Sites of DVT during pregnancy or postpartum are elaborated in Table III.8. None of these women experienced concomitant pulmonary embolism. The most common presenting symptoms were swelling (88% in pregnancy, 79% in postpartum women), extremity discomfort (79% in pregnancy, 95% postpartum), difficulty walking (21% in pregnancy, 32% postpartum), and erythema (26% in both groups) (James 05). Other data concur that DVT is most likely to arise in the left leg in

TABLE III.8 Sites of Pregnancy-Related Deep Vein Thrombosis in 53 Consecutive Patients

Site	34 Pregnant Women	19 Postpartum Women
Left leg	26 (76%)	9 (47%)
Proximal without calf involvement	18 (53%)	2 (11%)
Proximal with calf involvement	7 (21%)	6 (32%)
Calf only	1 (3%)	1 (5%)
Right leg	4 (12%)	7 (37%)
Proximal without calf involvement	3 (9%)	2 (11%)
Proximal with calf involvement	0	3 (16%)
Calf only	1 (3%)	2 (11%)
Left upper extremity	0	3 (16%)
Right upper extremity	2 (6%)	0
Pelvis	4 (12%)	2 (11%)

DVT confirmed by ultrasound in the first trimester in 28.3%, at 14–28 weeks gestation in 17.0%, in the third trimester in 18.9%, and 1–6 weeks postpartum in 35.8%.
Modified from James 05. Used with permission.

association with pregnancy and that more than one-half of the events occur in the first and second trimester (Gherman 99, Ray 99). Prescribed bed rest during pregnancy increases the risk of thromboembolic events (Kovacevich 00). In a meta-analysis of 14 studies using objective testing to diagnose DVT in pregnancy or the puerperium, the estimated relative distribution of 100 DVT events would be 0.23 per day during pregnancy and 0.82 per day in the postpartum period (Ray 99).

Thrombophilia tests were more likely to be positive in women with venous VTE in the first trimester of pregnancy, using data from a European registry of consecutive patients with objectively confirmed, symptomatic acute VTE (848 women aged <47 years, of whom 72 were pregnant and 64 postpartum) (Blanco-Molina 07). A study of 15 women after cesarean delivery who were at moderate to high risk for venous thrombosis but without US evidence of DVT revealed that 46% were positive for definite thrombosis in the iliac or common femoral veins using magnetic resonance venography (Rodger 06). The clinical meaning of this recent finding is unknown, as is the relevance to diabetic pregnant women who have such a high rate of cesarean delivery.

Another form of serious postoperative venous thrombosis marked by severe headache is cerebral venous thrombosis or thrombosis of intracranial cerebral venous sinuses. In multivariate logistic analysis based on a U.S. sample (administrative data) of 1,408,015 deliveries in 1993–1994, risk increased threefold with cesarean delivery (95% CI 2.3–4.2) to a prevalence of 33 per 100,00 deliveries. Risk increased 1.9-fold with hypertension (95% CI 1.2–3.0) and 14-fold with excessive vomiting (95% CI 3.2–65), but not with PDM (Lanska 00). However, this issue deserves further study because cerebral venous thrombosis is reported with the dehydration of DKA (DeKeyser 04). Historical data on the increased frequency of severe transient "pregnancy headache" in poorly controlled type 1 diabetes have been alleged to be associated with intracranial venous thrombosis (White 71).

A joint committee on clinical efficacy of the American College of Physicians and the American Academy of Family Physicians recently reviewed the diagnosis (Segal 07a) and management of VTE (Segal 07b) and provided clinical practice guidelines (Qaseem 07, Snow 07). The target patient population for the clinical practice guideline on diagnosis of VTE is all adults who have a probability of developing DVT or pulmonary embolism, including pregnant individuals. The joint committee made four recommendations on diagnosis (Qaseem 07):

Use a validated clinical prediction rule to estimate pretest probability of VTE (Wells 97, Chagnon 02, Moores 04) and to use as a basis for interpretation of subsequent tests. The Wells rule performs less well in patients with comorbidities (Qaseem 07). The risk prediction score performed well in an analysis of 116 consecutive pregnancies with a historical risk of VTE, allowing avoidance of antenatal thromboprophylaxis in patients with low scores (Dargaud 05). On the other hand, many clinicians believe pregnancy itself is a risk predictor for the likelihood of thrombosis, especially in diabetic women after cesarean delivery.

Obtain a high-sensitivity D-dimer assay (reflects increased thrombin activity and fibrinolysis) in selected patients with a low pretest probability of VTE (Kearon 06). D-dimer levels increase along with fibrinogen in the second half of physiological pregnancy up to 685 µg/L (Francalanci 95, Eichinger 05, Kline 05). D-dimer levels increase further during labor and decrease quickly during the first 3 days after delivery, but do not decline to "normal" levels until 4 weeks postpartum (Boehlen 05).

Use compression US to diagnose symptomatic thrombosis in the proximal vein of the lower limb (less sensitive with DVT limited to the calf). Negative compression ultrasonography of the lower limb veins in 107 pregnant or postpartum women was a good predictor of low risk of subsequent thromboembolic events over 3 months (LeGal 06). Contrast venography is still considered the definitive test to rule out diagnosis of DVT in postpartum women (Qaseem 07).

Patients with intermediate or high pretest probability of pulmonary embolism require diagnostic imaging studies: perfusion lung scan with a low dose to the fetus or pulmonary angiography postpartum (Stone 05, Qaseem 07). Helical computed tomography has never been validated in pregnant women (Righini 05). The inadequacy of data on the reliability of VTE diagnostic tests during or after pregnancy was recently reviewed (Nijkeuter 06, Krivak 07).

After review of 11 observational studies of pregnant and puerperal women (Segal 07b), the joint committee concluded that there is not adequate evidence for definitive recommendations for types of anticoagulation management of VTE in pregnant women (Snow 07). "Clinicians should avoid vitamin K antagonists in pregnant women because these drugs cross the placenta and are associated with embryopathy between 6 and 12 weeks gestation, as well as fetal bleeding (including intracranial hemorrhage) at delivery. Neither low molecular weight heparin (LMWH) nor unfractionated heparin crosses the placenta, and neither is associated with embryopathy or fetal bleeding" (Snow 07). For management of VTE in general, the joint committee recommended that LMWH rather than unfractionated heparin should be used whenever possible for initial inpatient treatment of DVT (less mortality and major bleeding) and that either unfractionated heparin or LMWH is appropriate for initial treatment of pulmonary embolism (additional trials needed, but LMWH is quickly and consistently therapeutic). Compression stockings should be used routinely to prevent postthrombotic syndrome (limb pain, edema) beginning within 1 month of diagnosis of proximal DVT and continuing for 1 year after diagnosis. Anticoagulation should be maintained for 3 to 6 months for VTE secondary to transient risk factors and for >12 months for recurrent VTE. The risk–benefit ratio is not known for durations >4 years (Snow 07).

Regarding prevention of VTE, studies in nondiabetic women suggest that use of compression leg stimulators provide benefit (Agu 99, Amaragiri 00, Gray 06) and cost-effectiveness as long as the incidence of postcesarean DVT is at least 0.68% (Casele 06). A Cochrane Review of four trials of antenatal thromboprophylaxis and four studies of postnatal prophylaxis after CS concluded that "there is insufficient evidence on which to base recommendations for thromboprophylaxis during pregnancy and the early postnatal period. Large scale randomized trials of currently-used interventions should be conducted" (Gates 02,04). A decision analysis based on available observational and trial data estimated that use of pneumatic pressure stockings compared with routine postoperative care would reduce VTE events from 1,350 to 675 in a theoretical cohort of one million women having cesarean deliveries (Quinones 05). Universal heparin prophylaxis would produce a similar reduction of VTE events, but would cause 2,000–15,000 cases of heparin-induced thrombocytopenia (Fausett 01), 1,000–7,522 cases of subsequent thrombosis after discontinuation of heparin, and 1,004 cases of major bleeding. These complications would be significantly reduced by using a protocol of universal screening for inherited thrombophilia (5% baseline prevalence) and heparin prophylaxis in screen-positive patients only, which would leave 950 VTE events in the theoretical population (Quinones 05).

Anesthesia for Cesarean Delivery

Preoperative assessment of diabetic women should take into account the possible problems associated with obesity and heart disease, along with the other complications of diabetes (Tsen 03, Ray 04b, Amour 08, Smith 08, Soens 08). Consideration of the need for anticoagulant therapy may influence the choice of anesthesia for CS in diabetic patients with cardiac disease (Spencer 94, Kaufman 03, Tsen 03).

Regional block (spinal, epidural) anesthesia has been widely and successfully used for CS in diabetic women (Wissler 04, Bloom 05). Prevention and treatment of hypotension is a major concern, especially in those with DAN (Tsen 03). Hypotension during lumbar epidural block for CS is associated with decreased placental intervillous blood flow measured by xenon washout (Huovinen 79). Early studies showed an association of umbilical cord and neonatal acidosis with spinal and epidural anesthesia for CS in women with PDM, probably related to use of dextrose-containing fluids for volume expansion and to episodes of maternal hypotension (Datta 77,81). High-volume infusion of dextrose solutions before delivery is also associated with neonatal acidosis in nondiabetic pregnancies (Oakley 72, Robillard 78, Kenepp 80, Mendiola 82). When dextrose-free solutions were used for volume expansion in diabetic women and hypotension was prevented by prompt treatment with ephedrine (Datta 82a), there was no difference in acid–base values in infants of diabetic versus control mothers having spinal (Datta 82b) or epidural (Ramanathan 91) anesthesia for CS. Either epidural or spinal anesthesia has equivalent efficacy and safety for CS in women with severe preeclampsia without coagulopathy (Wallace 95, Visalyaputra 05).

When general inhalation anesthesia is chosen for CS, intubation is indicated due to the increased risk of gastric regurgitation and pulmonary aspiration in pregnancy (Hawkins 97, Wissler 04). This risk is exacerbated if there is diabetic gastroparesis. One authority recommends the preanesthetic administration of metoclopromide (10 mg i.v.) to minimize risk of aspiration in women with PDM (Wissler 04). Direct laryngoscopy and intubation may be more difficult in diabetic patients with "stiff joint" syndrome (aka, diabetic scleredema) due to limited movement of the atlantocipital joint (Hogan 88, Wissler 04). Careful preanesthetic patient evaluation is necessary.

Perioperative glycemic control is important to decrease risks of fetal hypoxia and acidosis (Miodovnik 87), neonatal hypoglycemia (Ramanathan 91), and postoperative wound infections (Riley 96). Epidural anesthesia was more successful than general anesthesia in blocking the hyperglycemic effect of abdominal surgery in nonpregnant patients by decreasing glucose production (Lattermann 02), but such an investigation has not been performed for CS. The maternal insulin requirement usually drops precipitously after delivery; therefore, intravenous insulin therapy is the most flexible method of perioperative treatment (Miodovnik 87, Wissler 04).

Recommendations

- Assuming excellent glucose control, adherence to treatment, and lack of maternal or fetal compromise, women with PDM may await spontaneous labor up to 39–40 weeks gestation without evaluation of fetal lung maturity. (E)
- To reduce the risk of stillbirth or birth asphyxia with persisting poor glycemic control, consider induction of labor or CS at 37–38 weeks gestation after evaluation of fetal lung maturity. (E)

- If there is a medical, surgical, or obstetrical reason for early delivery that outweighs the risk of RDS in the infant, evaluation for fetal lung maturity is not required. (E)
- Consideration should be given to cesarean delivery at 39 weeks gestation based on the patient's clinical history and physical evaluation if EFW is >4,499 gm. (B)
- Because BW at term is strongly dependent on gestational age, if the EFW is 4,000–4,499 gm at 37–38 weeks gestation, the decision on induction of labor at 37–38 weeks after evaluation of fetal lung maturity *or* CS at 39 weeks may be individualized. (E)
- Planning vaginal birth after one previous CS in women with PDM should take into account the aforementioned recommendations as well as criteria from the ACOG. (C)
- With vaginal delivery of women with PDM, the obstetrical team should be prepared for management of shoulder dystocia. The delivering physician should use caution with operative delivery if the EFW is >3,500 gm, and midpelvic operative deliveries should be avoided. (B)
- Continuous EFM is recommended for diabetic women in labor, with interpretation according to ACOG criteria. If the FHR pattern is nonreassuring, supplementary tests should be considered prior to proceeding to operative vaginal or cesarean delivery. (B)
- Strict intrapartum or perioperative glycemic control is recommended with controlled intravenous glucose and insulin infusions to reduce risks of fetal hypoxia/acidosis and neonatal hypoglycemia as well as maternal hypoglycemia. (B)
- There is usually no reason to withhold requested epidural analgesia from diabetic women in labor. Epidural, spinal, or general inhalation anesthesia with intubation can be used for CS with attention to the prevention or treatment of maternal hypotension and hyperglycemia. Preanesthetic evaluation is advisable for DAN, gastroparesis, and possible difficult intubation. (C)
- The obstetrical team and parents-to-be should communicate with the pediatric caregiver well prior to delivery to enhance smooth transition of care for the baby. Delivery should be planned for a facility with neonatal care options appropriate for the anticipated complexity of management. (E)

INFANTS AND CHILDREN OF DIABETIC MOTHERS

—— *Original contribution by Edward S. Ogata MD*

Background

Despite advances in normalizing glucose balance in mothers with PDM, IDMs (Cordero 93, Weintrob 96, Schwartz 00, Nold 04) remain at risk for developing RDS (Mimouni 87a, Aucott 94), transient tachypnea of the newborn (TTN) (Gross 83, Kjos 90), hypertrophic cardiomyopathy and possible heart failure (Breitweser 80, Reller 88, Seppanen 97, Vela-Huerta 00, Kozak-Barany 04, Demiroren 05, Kozak-Barany 07, Ullmo 07), hypoglycemia (Andersen 85, Stenninger 97, Gunton 00, Watson 03), hypocalcemia, hypomagnesemia (Tsang 72,75,76, Mimouni 86b,87b), and perhaps decreased bone mineral content (Mimouni 88d, Lapillonne 97), hyperbilirubinemia

(Taylor 63, Stevenson 76, Aucott 94), polycythemic hyperviscosity syndrome (Mimouni 86c), poor feeding (Bromker 06), tissue iron deficiency (Amarnaff 89, Georgieff 90, Petry 92, Siddappa 04, Verner 07), compromised arachidonic acid/DHA and prostacyclin generation status (Stuart 85, Ghebremeskel 04), signs of delayed brain maturation and disturbed neurobehavioral organization (Schulte 69a,b,c, Yogman 82, Visser 85, Mulder 87, Rizzo 90, deRegnier 00), and congenital malformations (Schaefer-Graf 00, Suhonen 00, Farrell 02, Sheffield 02, Wang 02), with an emphasis on congenital heart disease (Loffredo 01, Abu-Sulaiman 04). The frequencies of common neonatal morbidities are presented in Table III.9 (Cousins 91, GDFSG 91, Hanson 93, Hunter 93, Wylie 02).

In the DCCT multicenter trial of intensified diabetes control that was applied to all subjects becoming pregnant, neonatal complications of 191 liveborn infants of women with type 1 diabetes included 18.8% respiratory distress (all types), 38.2% hypoglycemia, 4.2% hypocalcemia, 4.7% major malformations, and 1.05% neonatal mortality (DCCT 96). In all of the studies, the various morbidities may cluster in the same infant (Breitweser 80, Landon 87, Amarnoff 89, Persson 93) and are at least as common in infants of mothers with type 2 as in type 1 diabetes (Omori 94, Sacks 97, Watson 03, Clausen 05, Verheijen 05). The high rate of cesarean deliveries contributes to respiratory disease in IDMs (Kjos 90, Keszler 92, Morrison 95, Wax 02). While preterm delivery and difficult birth contribute to excess neonatal morbidity as well (Gross 83, Aucutt 94, Zhu 97, Nesbitt 98, Leperq 04), term infants of poorly controlled diabetic mothers can also have problems (Miodovnik 87). As a result, preparation for delivery and the possibility of specialized neonatal care is critical.

Observational studies of women with PDM suggest that tight glycemic control before and during pregnancy will minimize morbidity in infants of mothers with PDM (see the section titled "Glycemic Control and Perinatal Outcome" in Part I). Admittedly, RCTs of intensified glycemic control are mostly lacking (Demarini 94, Manderson 03) due to the reluctance of investigators to randomly assign pregnant women with PDM to a poorly controlled group. The importance of glycemic control during pregnancy is supported by a landmark RCT in women with GDM in which treatment with MNT and insulin reduced serious perinatal morbidity compared with routine care (Crowther 05).

It is widely recognized that hyperglycemia at the beginning of pregnancy is a teratogen, but that excellent glycemic control is associated with rates of congenital malformation that differ little from controls (Kitzmiller 96, Nielsen 06).

Maternal hyperglycemia after the first trimester leads to increased fetal insulin production (measured as insulin in AF or as C-peptide in umbilical cord or neonatal blood) (Baird 62, Salvesen 93c, Krew 94, Lindsay 03,04, Westgate 06), which predicts (1) excessive size and fatness at birth and in later life, (2) cardiomegaly at birth, and (3) neonatal hypoglycemia (Hall 77, Sosenko 79, Hall 80, Freyschuss 82, Kuhl 82, Sosenko 82, Knip 83, Metzger 90, Silverman 93, Curet 97, Stenninger 97, Weiss 98, Fraser 99). Initial neonatal hypoglycemia is also associated with low glucagon secretion (Bloom 72, Luyckx 72, Williams 79, Knip 93) but normal catecholamine response (Hertel 85) in IDMs. Catecholamines are thought to counteract the inhibitory effect of insulin on lipolysis so that the plasma concentration of NEFAs and glycerol increases after birth in IDMs (Hertel 86), although to a lower level in hyperinsulinemic, hypoglycemic infants (Andersen 82). Hypoglycemic, hyperinsulinemic IDMs were also noted to have lower levels of certain amino acids at 2 h of age than normoglycemic infants (Hertel 82). Good glycemic control in the mothers resulted in appropriate

TABLE III.9 Neonatal Morbidity in Recent Series of Infants of Mothers with Preexisting Diabetes

	Cousins 1991	GDFSG 1991	Hanson 1993	Hunter 1993	Wylie 2002
Site	California statewide, n (%)	French multicenter, n (%)	Swedish population, n (%)	Hamilton, Ontario, n (%)	Vancouver, British Columbia, n (%)
Liveborn infants	370	273	481	230	271
Delivery <37 weeks	101 (27.3)	71 (26.0)	121 (24.6)	56 (24.3)	124 (45.8)
Macrosomia	115 (31.0) [>90th percentile] 80 (21.6) [>4,000 gm]	73 (26.9) [>90th percentile]	96 (20.0) [>90th percentile]	75 (32.6) [>90th percentile]	98 (36) [>90th percentile] 11 (4.1) [>4,500 gm]
LBW	21 (5.70) [<10th percentile]	4 (1.5) [<10th percentile]	5 (1.0) [<10th percentile]	NA	NA
Hypoglycemia	92 (24.9) [<30 mg/dL]	88 (32.2) [<54 mg/dL]	39 (8.1) [<30 mg/dL + symptoms]	86 (37) [glucose infusion]	60 (22) [<40 mg/dL]
RDS	22 (5.9)	7 (2.6)	8 (1.7)	10 (4.4) [ventilated]	NA
Mild respiratory distress (TTN)	16 (4.3)	29 (10.6)	16 (3.3)	34 (14.8)	NA
Hyperbilirubinemia	90 (24.3) [>15 mg/dL, 38 weeks] [>10 mg/dL, 34–37 weeks]	35 (12.8) [>15.2 mg/dL]	80 (16.6) [>17.5 mg/dL]	44 (19.1) [>14.6 mg/dL]	41 (15) [phototherapy]
Polycythemia	13 (3.5) [Hct >65 %]	9 (3.3) [Hct >70%]	11 (2.3) [Hct >70]	32 (15.7) [>hgb gm/dL]	Zero*
Hypocalcemia	6 (1.6) [<8.0 mg/dL]	15 (5.5) [<6.8 mg/dL]	NA	21 (17.8) [<8.0 mg/dL]	Zero*
Major malformations	23/374 (6.1) [includes fetal deaths]	12 (4.4)	16 (4.8)	11 (4.8)	18 (6.6) [includes terminations]
Neonatal/infant death	5 (1.35) [malformations NS]	7 (2.6) [5 malformations]	5 (1.0) [malformations NS]	4 (1.7) [4 malformations]	3 (1.1) [1 malformation]

Note the variance in frequencies and [definitions]. Total r.eonatal death rate 21 of 1,446 (1.45%).
*Not routinely tested.

GDFSG, Gestation and Diabetes in France Study Group; Hct, hematocrit; LBW, low birth weight; malf, malformations; NA, not applicable; RDS, respiratory distress syndrome; TTN, transient tachypnea of the newborn.; NS, not stated

counterregulatory responses in the neonatal period (Artal 88). IDMs are able to respond to exogenous glucagon with a rise in plasma glucose (Wu 75).

Links between maternal hyperglycemia and other forms of neonatal morbidity are not as well understood. Improved glycemic control in the lone RCT in women with PDM reduced hypocalcemia in their infants (Demarini 94). Hypocalcemia in infants of mothers with PDM (Mimouni 86b,90) has been related to decreased maternal (Martinez 91) and neonatal (Salle 81) 25(OH)D levels, decreased maternal magnesium levels via increased urinary loss (Mimouni 89), increased placental calcium uptake (Strid 03), and decreased fetal osteocalcin and parathyroid hormone levels (Cruikshank 83, Martinez 94, Verhaeghe 95). Feed intolerance in the infant may be related to increased levels of amylin peptide, an inhibitor of gastric motility that is co-secreted with insulin (Kairamkonda 05). Maternal hyperglycemia (and chronic fetal hypoxia) have been linked to increased fetal erythropoiesis and decreased iron indexes at birth (Widness 81, Georgieff 90, Widness 90, Teramo 04, Verner 07). Maternal A1C levels correlate with increased pro-BNP found in IDMs, but its relationship with neonatal cardiac function is unstudied (Halse 05, Girsen 08). Healthy newborns of mothers with type 1 diabetes have reduced plasma levels of arachidonic acid and DHA that are important in neurovisual and vascular development (Ghebremeskel 04, Min 05). There is evidence for increased markers of oxidative stress, inflammation, and endothelial activation in seemingly healthy IDMs, perhaps related to maternal–fetal hyperglycemia or hyper-fatty acidemia (Loukovaara 05b, Rajdl 05, Nelson 07a, Fadini 08). All of these in utero processes associated with diabetes should be studied for possible links to subsequent disease in the offspring.

Macrosomic IDMs have increased LPL activity (Rovamo 86) and LDL-hypercholesterolemia (Akisu 99, Merzouk 99, Akcakus 07). Analysis of two systematic studies of cord lipids in IDMs shows the influence of route of delivery and degrees of fetal insulinemia, adiposity, and leptin concentration on levels of FFA, TGs, cholesterol, and apo- and lipoproteins (Kilby 98, Nelson 07b). The effect of maternal diabetes on fetal and long-term dyslipidemia needs additional study (Manderson 02). Interestingly, female IDMs in the largest study had higher insulin, cholesterol, HDL-C, and LDL-C levels than males (Nelson 07b). Female infants of nondiabetic mothers also have higher cord insulin and proinsulin levels than males (despite lower weight) (Shields 07), and the authors and others speculated that girls have greater insulin resistance than boys or greater β-cell responsiveness (Wilkin 06, Yajnik 07).

Population-based surveys continue to show excessive early (first month) and late (1–12 months) mortality in IDMs (0.9–5.9% of liveborn infants, median 1.2%; crude RR 1.7–9.5, median 2.8) (Connell 85, Hanson 93, Cnattingius 94, Casson 97, Gunton 00, Platt 02, Penney 03, Evers 04, Jensen 04, Santos-Silva 05). Common causes of infant mortality include congenital malformations, disorders of immaturity, hypoxic–ischemic encephalopathy, and sepsis. Congenital malformations remain the leading contributor to mortality and long-term morbidity in IDMs (Connel 85, Hunter 93, Cnattingius 94, Hadden 01, Evers 04, Verheijen 05), pointing to the continuing need for improvement of preconception care of diabetic women (Kitzmiller 96).

Communication

Ideally, the physician (pediatrician, family practitioner, or neonatologist if necessary) who will be responsible for child care should be identified during the pregnancy to assure smooth transition of care for the infant at delivery. This allows the practioner to become familiar with the family and with any issues during pregnancy that could possibly affect the offspring. Such communication is particularly important if specific concerns are identified in the fetus, such as congenital malformations, which will require coordinated specialized neonatal care.

Neonatal Care

Preparation for Resuscitation

The obstetrician must ensure that personnel skilled in neonatal resuscitation are immediately available at delivery. For apparently uncomplicated delivery, a physician or nurse skilled in neonatal resuscitation should be in attendance. For any delivery with potential complications (difficult delivery due to macrosomia, nonreassuring fetal status), it is preferable that a resuscitation team be in attendance. Ideally, a neonatal intensive care nursery should be immediately available.

Neonatal Care

A complete physical examination should be accomplished in a timely manner after delivery; this is not only important to screen for routine neonatal problems, but also to screen for polycythemia/hyperviscosity, respiratory distress, congenital malformations (Nold 04), and other disorders that are problematic in IDMs (Schwartz 00). Neonatal anthropometric measures can be used to estimate fat mass (Whitelaw 77, Brans 83, Catalano 95). IDMs were noted to have more sluggish motor processes and reflex functioning than control infants on day 1 of life, with improved scores on day 2. IDMs may require increased efforts to facilitate sensitive maternal responding during their first days of life (Pressler 99).

All IDMs should be screened for hypoglycemia during at least the first 24 h after birth. In normal infants, the nadir of 45–60 mg/dL (2.5–3.3 mM) occurs at 30–60 min of life, reaching a plateau steady state of 72–90 mg/dL (4–5 mM) by 2–4 h (Kalhan 00a, Cowett 04). Insulin levels drop and alternative substrates are mobilized (glycerol, FFAs, β-hydroxybutyrate) (Chen 65, Bloom 72, Persson 73, Kalhan 77, King 82, Kuhl 82, Knip 83, Hertel 86, Ogata 86, Patel 92, Kalhan 00b). In IDMs, glucose kinetics was normal if maternal glycemic control was excellent (Cowett 83, Baarsma 93). Low plasma glucose values <36 mg/dL (<2 mM) require close monitoring as well as intervention if they are persistent (Cornblath 00) to prevent convulsions and/or impaired neurodevelopment. Target therapeutic values should be 72–90 mg/dL (4–5 mM) (Kalhan 00b).

Assess for hyperbilirubinemia (>13 mg/dL) if the infant is jaundiced, and consider the need for phototherapy (Nold 04). Calcium should be measured at 6, 24, and 48 h, with serum magnesium obtained if calcium is low (<2 mM) (Nold 04). Infants with symptomatic hypocalcemia (<7 mg/dL) and hypomagnesemia (<1.5 mg/dL) (jitteriness, sweating, tachypnea, irritability, seizures) should be treated, accompanied by continuous ECG monitoring (Nold 04). Hypomagnesemia may contribute to the convulsive problems of hypocalcemia (Donati-Genet 04), but prophylactic treatment of hypomagnesemia did not reduce the incidence of hypocalcemia in IDMs (Mehta 98). Preexisting maternal diabetes was independently associated with a fourfold increase in the rate of neonatal seizures in term infants in a case–control study utilizing the Colorado Birth Certificate Registry. Contributing factors were thought to be hypoglycemia, hypocalcemia, or maternal diabetic vasculopathy with reduced fetal oxygenation (Hall 06).

The possibility of these neonatal problems occurring after 48 h of life is minimal. All efforts should be made to ensure that the mother is capable of caring for her infant before discharge. If the neonatal period is uneventful, follow-up of the infant can be conducted on a routine schedule.

Follow-Up of Children of Diabetic Mothers

Early follow-up studies of children of diabetic mothers found an increased proportion with lower intelligence scores and neurodevelopmental abnormalities, especially in those with poor glycemic control at onset of pregnancy (Pedersen 84, Petersen 88,89), in those born to mothers with acetonuria while hospitalized late in pregnancy, and in those born SGA or with congenital malformations (Churchill 69, Yssing 74, Bibergeil 75, Yssing 75, Haworth 76, Stehbens 77, Cummins 80). These data were collected at a time when poor glycemic control was the rule. For children born in Sweden in 1984–1990, maternal insulin-dependent diabetes doubled the risk (OR 2.09; 95% CI 1.41–3.09) for cerebral palsy by 4 years of age (Thorngren-Jerneck 06). Cognitive scores in a small sample of young adult male offspring of women with type 1 diabetes who were delivered in 1976–1984 showed an inverse relation to maternal A1C (Nielsen 07).

Further studies confirmed that IDMs with higher fasting β-hydroxybutyrate levels in the second and third trimesters had lower intelligence and psychomotor development scores independent of perinatal complications (Rizzo 91b,94,95c). The authors interpreted these results as a reflection of poorer general metabolic regulation (including lipid dysregulation) in the mothers of children with psychomotor disturbances, which supports the case for intensified glycemic control during pregnancy. Fortunately, maternal hypoglycemic events were not related to poor infant outcome (Rizzo 91b). Continued follow-up of this cohort of children of diabetic mothers to ages 7–11 revealed that maternal antepartum levels of fasting blood glucose, A1C, and β-hydroxybutyrate had negative correlations with measures of childhood intelligence (Rizzo 97a) but not with measures of childhood behavioral adjustment (Rizzo 97b). In other studies, elevated glycosylated hemoglobin as a measure of gestational glycemic control correlated with smaller infant brain size at 3 years (which predicted language development) (Sells 94) as well as with impaired eye–hand coordination and gross and fine motor development in school-age children of diabetic mothers (Ornoy 98, Ratzon 00, Ornoy 01, Kowalczyk 02, Ornoy 05). In these and other reports (Hadden 84, Persson 84, Yamashita 96), offspring of mothers with careful metabolic regulation throughout pregnancy had normal intelligence and psychomotor testing.

Although persistent or recurrent neonatal hypoglycemia in premature infants can contribute to adverse neurodevelopmental outcomes (Lucas 88, Boluyt 06), not all studies of diabetic pregnancies demonstrated this association in children who had experienced transient or persistent neonatal hypoglycemia after mostly near-term or term deliveries (Francois 74, Tuncer 74, Haworth 76, Cummins 80, Persson 84). Other studies of IDMs, while controlling for perinatal problems including hypoglycemia, found subtle deficits in neonatal auditory recognition memory as well as psychomotor development and recognition memory at 1 year. The findings were associated with lower cord ferritin levels, independent of maternal iron status but influenced by maternal glycemic control (Georgieff 90, Nelson 00, Siddapa 04, DeBoer 05, deRegnier 07). Investigators speculate that risk factors could include chronic fetal hypoxia, reactive neonatal hypoglycemia, and especially tissue iron deficiency (Nelson 00, Tamura 02, Burden 07).

Considerable interest surrounds the intrauterine "programming" of fetal metabolic and endocrine functions as adaptive responses to inadequate or excessive supply of nutrients or hormones that devolve into major health risks in youth and adulthood (Hales 91, Barker 93, Mughal 05, Kaijser 08, Palinski 08, Skilton 08). A subtle example is lower urinary excretion of calcium and magnesium (but not sodium) in children of diabetic mothers, perhaps due to persistent upregulation of renal reabsorption of calcium and magnesium (Mughal 05). Another effect is increased cardiovascular risk factors (dyslipidemia, endothelial adhesion factors) in children of mothers with type 1 diabetes (Manderson 02). More prominent "programming" effects in older children of diabetic mothers focus on subsequent (1) obesity (Hagbard 59, Breidahl 66, Farquhar 69, Verdy 74, Shah 75, Weitz 76, Pettitt 83,87,88, Metzger 90, Silverman 91, Plagemann 97a, Silverman 98, Touger 05, Hillier 07), (2) impaired glucose tolerance (Amendt 76, Pettitt 93, McCance 94, Silverman 95, Pribylova 96, Plagemann 97b, Dabelea 00, Weiss 00, Hunter 04, Clausen 08), (3) impaired acute insulin secretion (Gautier 01, Klupa 02, Stride 02), and (4) increased BP (Pribylova 96, Nilsson 99, Cho 00, Bunt 05). Thus, optimal metabolic regulation of diabetic pregnant women may contribute to the improved health of succeeding generations, with substantially greater impact than the widely parent-feared "genetic" inheritance of type 1 or type 2 diabetes (White 60, Dabelea 01, Tuomi 03). In a large retrospective observational study of offspring of women with type 1 diabetes during pregnancy, the 20-year cumulative risk of type 1 diabetes was $2.1 \pm 0.5\%$ (Warram 84,88). The long-term risk of type 2 diabetes in offspring of women who had type 2 diabetes in pregnancy is much greater (Pettitt 88, Lindsay 00, Sobngwi 03, Tougher 05, McLean 06, Singh 06).

Recommendations

- Predelivery pediatric consultation and planning of newborn care is important due to persisting excess neonatal morbidity and mortality in IDMs. (E)
- Prepare for possible infant resuscitation at delivery with (1) a skilled physician or nurse for an apparently uncomplicated delivery, or (2) a resucitation team for a delivery with possible complications such as prematurity, congenital malformations, nonreassuring fetal assessment, or fetal macrosomia. (B)
- Enhance successful breast-feeding and early transfer of protective colostrum by placing the newborn at the breast soon after delivery. Encourage mother/baby skin contact as a heat source for the infant. Keep the baby with the mother as much as possible during the first few days of life. (A)
- Prepare parents for the need of (1) examination of the infant for conditions requiring treatment and (2) screening laboratory tests for hypoglycemia and perhaps hyperviscosity, hyperbilirubinemia, or hypocalcemia. (E)
- Ensure that the mother is capable of caring for her infant before discharge. (E)
- Encourage a 2-week visit with the pediatric physician or nurse practitioner. (E)
- Facilitate long-term follow-up of all infants to detect late-onset problems and assist with quality assessment of the diabetes and pregnancy treatment program. (E)

MATERNAL MORTALITY

—— *Original contribution by John L. Kitzmiller MD, MS*

The maternal mortality ratio (MMR) (expressed as deaths per 100,000 live births over a given period) is a major measure of obstetrical care quality, access to care, and health of a population of reproductive-aged women (Atrash 95, Graham 02, Welsch 04, Wildman 04). An ACOG–CDC study group proposed definitions of maternal mortality that focus on pregnancy-related death during gestation or within 1 year of

TABLE III.10 Definitions of Aspects of Maternal Mortality

- *Pregnancy-associated death:* Death of a woman from any cause while she was pregnant or within 1 year of termination of pregnancy, regardless of duration and site of pregnancy.
- *Pregnancy-related death:* Death of a woman while pregnant or within 1 year of termination of pregnancy, regardless of duration and site of pregnancy, from any cause related to or aggravated by her pregnancy or its management.
- *Direct death:* Death resulting from obstetrical complications of the pregnant state (pregnancy, labor, puerperium), from interventions, omissions, incorrect treatment, or from a chain of events resulting from any of the above.
- *Indirect death:* Death resulting from previously existing disease or disease that developed during pregnancy and that was not due to direct obstetrical causes, but which was aggravated by the physiological effects of pregnancy.
- *Early death:* Death that occurred during pregnancy or within 42 days of its end.
- *Late death:* Death that occurred between 43 and 365 days after the end of pregnancy.
- *Pregnancy outcome:* Result of conception and ensuing pregnancy, including undelivered, ectopic pregnancy, induced abortion, stillbirth, or live birth.

Data taken from the Maternal Mortality Study Group of the American College of Obstetricians and Gynecologists and the U.S. Centers for Disease Control and Prevention (Atrash 92, Deneux-Tharaux 05).

termination of pregnancy (Atrash 92). Pregnancy-related deaths are classified as direct or indirect and early or late (Table III.10). The new system is an advance on ICD-10 codes that have included cases occurring only through 42 days after delivery. Approximately 10% of maternal deaths occur >42 days postpartum, including 14% of deaths caused by infection, 9% by complications of anesthesia, 9% by cerebrovascular accident, 16% by other medical conditions, and 46% by cardiomyopathy (Berg 03).

Four recent analyses (Finland, France, Massachusetts, North Carolina) revealed that 52–65% of all pregnancy-associated deaths were not pregnancy related (Deneux-Tharaux 05). Of those that are pregnancy related, the major direct obstetrical causes of death in the U.S. in 1991–1997 were hemorrhage (18.2% of all pregnancy-related deaths), hypertensive disorders of pregnancy (19.9%), infection (13.2%), AF embolism (8.6%), cardiomyopathy (7.7%), and anesthesia complications (1.6%). Major indirect causes of death were thrombotic embolism (10.2%), cerebrovascular accidents not related to preeclampsia (4.7%), and other medical conditions (mainly CVD, diabetes, and hemoglobinopathies) (18.2%) (Berg 03). Similar proportional causality figures were published in an analysis of 290 maternal deaths in 1992–1997 in 11 countries in Europe (Wildman 04).

Current studies show that indirect deaths are underreported (Turner 02, Deneux-Tharaux 05). The recent timing of maternal deaths in Europe was 15.6% antepartum, 11.4% with interruption of pregnancy (including ectopic pregnancy), 31.5% intrapartum (including the first 24 h after delivery), 36.6% postpartum, and 4.8% late (Wildman 04). The U.S. total pregnancy-related maternal mortality ratio (PRMMR) for 1991–1997 was 11.5 (Berg 03), which was slightly higher than ratios recorded in Western Europe during a similar time period (Wildman 04). The PRMMR for black women in the U.S. was 29.6 compared with 7.9 for white women and 11.1 for women of other races (Berg 03). For women having their first cesarean delivery without labor in a multicenter prospective study in the U.S. in 1999–2002, the total MMR was 194/100,000

(Silver 06). Cesarean delivery was associated with increased MMR in Latin America after adjustment for risk factors (Villar 06b) but not in Canada (Liu 07). A population-based case–control study in France showed cesarean delivery was associated with a significantly increased risk of maternal death from complications of anesthesia, puerperal infection, and VTE (Deneux-Tharaux 06).

As deaths from hemorrhage, embolism, and anesthesia have declined since 1979–1986 in the U.S., proportionate mortality from infection, cardiomyopathy, and other causes has increased (Atrash 90, Berg 96,03, Whitehead 03). Pregnancy-related mortality in the U.S. increases with maternal age regardless of parity, time of entry into prenatal care, and level of education (Callaghan 03). Among white women, the RRs for death from hemorrhage, infection, embolisms, hypertensive disorders of pregnancy, cardiomyopathy, cerebrovascular accidents, or other medical conditions ranged from 1.8 to 2.7 of those aged 35–39 years (compared with 25–29-year-old women) and from 2.5 to 7.9 for those ≥40 years of age. Among black women, the RRs for death from these conditions ranged from 2.0 to 4.1 for those aged 35–39 years and from 4.3 to 7.6 for those ≥40 years of age (Callaghan 03). Deaths from CVD are particularly linked to advanced maternal age. White women aged 35–39 years and ≥40 years were 3.9 and 8.2 times more likely to die of CVD, respectively, than their younger counterparts. The RR was 10.6 for black women ≥40 years of age compared with 25–29-year-old black women (Callaghan 03).

Recent large population surveys in the U.S. and Canada using hospital administrative data (ICD-9 codes) found in-hospital case fatality rates to be 7.3%, 5.6%, and 1.8%, respectively, for MIs associated with pregnancy or the puerperium (Ladner 05, James 06b, Macarthur 06). In these analyses, crude RRs of MMRs associated with MI compared with all maternal deaths vary from 4.0 to 142 (James 05, Macarthur 06). Independent ORs for diabetes as a risk factor for MI associated with pregnancy were 4.3, 3.6, and 60.4, respectively (James 05, Ladner 05, Macarthur 06). However, clinical factors related to individual deaths associated with diabetes were not detectable in these surveys. Investigators noted that the accuracy of identifying outcomes in these national/regional databases was dependent on disease recognition by physicians and accurate coding by hospital data abstractors. Therefore, large prospective patient-specific studies using case–control methodology will be necessary to determine the role of risk factors, such as diabetes, in gestational cardiovascular mortality.

Due to lack of a denominator of a large number of livebirths born to women with PDM, it is difficult to define the PRMMR for diabetic women. At the University Central Hospital in Helsinki in 1975–1997, five maternal deaths occurred among 972 pregnant women with type 1 diabetes (MMR ~514) (Leinonen 01). One death occurred after spontaneous abortion due to KTA, one at 10 weeks due to dead-in-bed syndrome, one at 14 weeks due to hypoglycemia, one postpartum due to spinal anesthesia, and one postpartum due to brain stem infarction; two patients had DN (Leinonen 01). In a 1-year (1999–2000) Netherlands survey of 323 type 1 diabetes pregnancies, two maternal mortalities occurred (MMR ~619): one due to hypoglycemia and cardiac arrest at 17 weeks and one during delivery due to AF embolism (Evers 04). However, it is unlikely that these series capture all aborting pregnancies or even all births to women with PDM. Of 3,463 deliveries of diabetic women (ICD-9 code 250.0) in Canada in 1991–2001, there were two in-hospital maternal deaths (MMR ~55) (Wen 05). Other recent population-based surveys of diabetic pregnant women in Denmark (Jensen 04), Norway (Vangen 03), Ontario (Feig 06), and Scotland (Penney 03) provide a total denominator of 11,705 pregnancies, but the reports do not mention maternal mortality. A review of the effect of pregnancy on the diabetic mother in 1956–1961 noted 40 maternal deaths among 6,957 cases of PDM (MMR ~575) reported by four authors, which stated that the deaths were due to "diabetic coma, toxemia, and obstetrical, anesthetic, and maternal vascular accidents" (Kyle 63). In a survey of 793 maternal deaths in Los Angeles County in 1957–1974 representing a total PRMMR of 36, mortalities occurred in 24 diabetic pregnant patients (3.0% of total deaths) (Gabbe 76). Causes of death were infection (6), hemorrhage (5), KTA (4), hypoglycemia (3), anesthetic complications (3), preeclampsia (2), and leukemia (1).

Recommendations

- Prospective studies using large databases are needed to determine the actual PRMMR for diabetic patients and whether the ratio is actually ~50 times greater than that of nondiabetic women.
- Studies of proportional causality and case-by-case analysis of preventability are important "to inform specific prevention strategies" (Deneux-Tharaux 05).

Part 3 Reference

Aali BS, Nejad SS: Nifediine or hydralazine as a first-line agent to control hypertension in severe preeclampsia. *Acta Obstet Gynecol Scand* 81:25–30, 2002.

Aardema MW, Saro MCS, Lander M, de Wolf BTHM, Oosterhof H, Aanoudse JG: Second trimester Doppler ultrasound screening of the uterine arteries differentiates between subsequent normal and poor outcomes of hypertensive pregnancy: two different pathophysiological entities? *Clin Sci* 106:377–382, 2004.

Abdelgadir M, Elbagir M, Eltom A, Eltom M, Berne C: Factors affecting perinatal morbidity and mortality in pregnancies complicated by diabetes mellitus in Sudan. *Diabetes Res Clin Pract* 60:41–47, 2003.

Abu-Sulaiman RM, Subaih B: Congenital heart disease in infants of diabetic mothers: echocardiographic study. *Pediatr Cardiol* 25:137–140, 2004.

ACE—American College of Endocrinology Task Force on Inpatient Diabetes Metabolic Control: American College of Endocrinology position statement on inpatient diabetes and metabolic control. *Endocr Pract* 10 (Suppl 2):4–9, 2004.

Acker DB, Sachs BP, Friedman EA: Risk factors for shoulder dystocia. *Obstet Gynecol* 66:762–768, 1985.

Acker DB, Sachs BP, Friedman EA: Risk factors for shoulder dystocia in the average-weight infant. *Obstet Gynecol* 67:614–618, 1986.

ACOG—American College of Obstetricians and Gynecologists: Thromboembolism in pregnancy. ACOG Practice Bulletin #21. *Int J Obstet Gynecol* 75:203–212, 2001.

ACOG—American College of Obstetricians and Gynecologists: Committee on Obstetric Practice: Antenatal corticosteroid therapy for fetal maturation. ACOG Committee Opinion. *Obstet Gynecol* 99:871–873, 2002a.

ACOG—American College of Obstetricians and Gynecologists: Shoulder dystocia. Clinical management guidelines for obstetrician-gynecologists. ACOG Practice Bulletin #40. *Obstet Gynecol* 100:1045–1049, 2002b.

ACOG—American College of Obstetricians and Gynecologists: Use of progesterone to prevent preterm birth. Practice committee opinion. *Obstet Gynecol* 102: 1115–1116, 2003a.

ACOG—American College of Obstetricians and Gynecologists: Prophylactic antibiotics in labor and delivery. ACOG Practice Bulletin #47. Clinical Management Guidelines for Obstetrician-Gynecologists. *Obstet Gynecol* 102:875–882, 2003b.

ACOG—American College of Obstetricians and Gynecologists: Ultrasonography in pregnancy. ACOG Practice Bulletin #58. *Obstet Gynecol* 1449–1458, 2004a.

ACOG—American College of Obstetricians and Gynecologists: Vaginal birth after previous cesarean delivery. Clinical management guidelines for obstetrician-gynecologists. ACOG Practice Bulletin #54. *Obstet Gynecol* 104:203–211, 2004b.

ACOG—American College of Obstetricians and Gynecologists: Pregestational diabetes mellitus. Clinical management guidelines for obstetrician-gynecologists. ACOG Practice Bulletin #60. *Obstet Gynecol* 105:675–685, 2005a.

ACOG—American College of Obstetricians and Gynecologists: Intrapartum fetal heart rate monitoring. Clinical management guidelines for obstetrician-gynecologists. ACOG Practice Bulletin #70. *Obstet Gynecol* 106:1453–1461, 2005b.

ACOG—American College of Obstetricians and Gynecologists, Committee on Obstetric Practice: Inappropriate use of the terms fetal distress and birth asphyxia. Committee Opinion #326. *Obstet Gynecol* 106:1469–1470, 2005c.

ACOG—American College of Obstetricians and Gynecologists: Invasive prenatal testing for aneuploidy. Practice Bulletin #88. *Obstet Gynecol* 110:1459–1467, 2007.

ACR—American College of Radiology: ACR practice guideline for the performance of antepartum obstetrical ultrasound. In: *ACR Practice Guidelines and Technical Standards.* Philadelphia: ACR, 2003:625–631.

Aghajafari F, Murphy K, Willan A, Ohlsson A, Amankwah K, Matthews S, Hannah M: Multiple courses of antenatal corticosteroids: a systematic review and meta-analysis. *Am J Obst Gynecol* 185:1073–1080, 2001.

Agrawal RK, Lui K, Gupta JM: Neonatal hypoglycemia in infants of diabetic mothers. *J Pediatr Child Health* 36:354–356, 2000.

Akcakus M, Kokiu E, Baykan A, Yikilmaz A, Coskun A, Gunes T, Kortoglu S, Narin N: Macrosomic newborns of diabetic mothers are associated with increased aortic intima-media thickness and lipid concentrations. *Horm Res* 67:277–283, 2007.

Agu O, Hamilton G, Baker D: Graduated compression stockings in the prevention of venous thromboembolism. *Br J Surg* 86:992–1004, 1999.

Akisu M, Darcan S, Oral R, Kultursay N: Serum lipid and lipoprotein composition of infants of diabetic mothers. *Indian J Pediatr* 66:381–386, 1999.

Aladjem S, Feria A, Rest J, Gull K, O'Connor M: Effect of maternal glucose load on fetal activity. *Am J Obstet Gynecol* 134:276–280, 1979.

Albaiges G, Misselfelder-Lobos H, Lees C, Parra M, Nicolaides KH: One-stage screening for pregnancy complications by color Doppler assessment of the uterine arteries at 23 weeks gestation. *Obstet Gynecol* 96:559–564, 2000.

Albert TJ, Landon MB, Wheller JJ, Samuels P, Cheng RF, Gabbe S: Prenatal detection of fetal anomalies in pregnancies complicated by insulin-dependent diabetes mellitus. *Am J Obstet Gynecol* 174:1424–1428, 1996.

Albuquerque CA, Smith KR, Johnson C, Chao R, Harding R: Influence of maternal tobacco smoking during pregnancy on uterine, umbilical and fetal cerebral artery blood flows. *Early Hum Dev* 80:31–42, 2004.

Allan LD, Sharland GK, Milburn A, Lockhart SM, Groves AMM, Anderson RH, Cook AC, Fagg NLK: Prospective diagnosis of 1,006 consecutive cases of congenital heart disease in the fetus. *J Am Coll Cardiol* 23:1452–1458, 1994.

Allen CL, Kisilevsky BS: Fetal behavior in diabetic and nondiabetic pregnant women: an exploratory study. *Dev Psychobiol* 35:69–80, 1999.

Alsulyman OM, Ouzounian JG, Kjos SL: The accuracy of intrapartum ultrasonographic fetal weight estimation in diabetic pregnancies. *Am J Obstet Gynecol* 177:503–506, 1997.

Amaragiri SV, Lees TA: Elastic compression stockings for prevention of deep vein thrombosis. *Cochrane Database Syst Rev* 2000;(3):CD001484.

Amarnaff UM, Ophoven JJ, Mills MM, Murphy EL, Georieff MK: The relationship between decreased iron stores, serum iron and neonatal hypoglycemia in large-for-date newborn infants. *Acta Paediatr Scand* 78:538–543, 1989.

Amendt P, Michaelis D, Hildman W: Clinical and metabolic studies in children of diabetic mothers. *Endokrinologie* 67:351–361, 1976.

Amenta JS, Silverman JA: Amniotic fluid lecithin, phosphatidylglycerol, L/S ratio, and foam stability test in predicting respiratory distress in the newborn. *J Clin Pathol* 79:52–64, 1983.

Amer-Wahlin I, Hellsten C, Noren H, Hagberg H, Herbst A, Kjellmer I, Lilja H, Lindoff C, Mansson M, Martensson L, Olofsson P, Sundstrom A, Marsal K: Cardiotocography versus cardiotocography plus ST analysis of the fetal ECG: a Swedish randomized controlled trial. *Lancet* 358:534–538, 2001.

Amer-Wahlin I, Ingemarsson I, Marsal K, Herbst A: Fetal heart rate patterns and ECG ST segment changes preceding metabolic acidemia at birth. *BJOG* 112:160–165, 2005.

Amer-Wahlin I, Arulkumaran S, Hagberg H, Marsal K, Visser GHA: Fetal electrocardiogram: ST waveform analysis in intrapartum surveillance. *BJOG* 114:1191–1193, 2007.

Ammala P, Kariniemi V: Short-term variability of fetal heart rate during insulin-dependent diabetic pregnancies. *J Perinat Med* 11:97–102, 1983.

Amon E, Lipshitz J, Sibai BM, Abdella TN, Whybrew MS, El-Nazer A: Quantitative analysis of amniotic fluid phospholipids in diabetic pregnant women. *Obstet Gynecol* 68:373–378, 1986.

Amour J, Kersten JR: Diabetic cardiomyopathy and anesthesia: bench to bedside. *Anesthesiology* 108:524–530, 2008.

Andersen GE, Hertel J, Kuhl C, Molsted-Pedersen L: Metabolic events in infants of diabetic mothers during first 24 hours after birth. II. Changes in plasma lipids. *Acta Paediatr Scand* 71:27–32, 1982.

Andersen O, Hertel J, Schmolker L, Kuhl C: Influence of the maternal plasma glucose concentration at delivery on the risk of hypoglycemia in infants of insulin-dependent diabetic mothers. *Acta Paediatr Scand* 74:268–273, 1985.

Andersen BS, Steffensen FH, Sorenson HT, Nielsen GL, Olsen J: The cumulative incidence of venous thromboembolism during pregnancy and puerperium—an 11 year Danish population-based study of 63,000 pregnancies. *Acta Obstet Gynecol Scand* 77:170–173, 1998.

Andrews AG, Brown JB, Jeffery PE, Horacek I: Amniotic fluid palmitic acid/stearic acid, lecithin/sphingomyelin ratios, and palmitic acid concentrations in the assessment of fetal lung maturity in diabetic pregnancies. *Br J Obstet Gynecol* 86:959–964, 1979.

Andrews V, Sultan AH, Thakar R, Jones PW: Risk factors for obstetric anal sphincter injury: a prospective study. *Birth* 33:117–122, 2006.

Artal R, Doug N, Wu P, Sperling MA: Circulating catecholamines and glucagon in infants of strictly controlled diabetic mothers. *Biol Neonate* 53:121–125, 1988.

Ashwood ER, Oldroyd RG, Palmer SE: Measuring the number of lamellar body particles in amniotic fluid. *Obstet Gynecol* 75:289–292, 1990.

Askie LM, Duley L, Hendrson-Smart DJ, Stewart LA; the PARIS Collaborative Group: Antiplatelet agents for prevention of preeclampsia: a meta-analysis of individual patient data. *Lancet* 369:1791–1797, 2007.

Asmussen I: Ultrastructure of the villi and fetal capillaries of the placentas delivered by nonsmoking diabetic women (White group D). *Acta Path Microbiol Immunol Scand* 90 (section A):95–101, 1982a.

Asmussen I: Vascular morphology in diabetic placentas. *Contrib Gynecol Obstet* 9: 76–85, 1982b.

Aso Y, Okumura K-I, Wakabayashi S, Takebayashi K, Taki S, Inukai T: Elevated pregnancy-associated plasma protein-A in sera from type 2 diabetic patients with hypercholesterolemia: associations with carotid atherosclerosis and toe-brachial index. *J Clin Endocrinol Metab* 89:5713–5717, 2004.

AST—Antenatal Steroid Therapy Collaborative Group: Effects of antenatal dexamethasone administration in the infant: long-term follow-up. *J Pediatr* 104:259–267, 1984.

Atallah AN, Hofmeyr GJ, Duley L: Calcium supplementation during pregnancy for preventing hypertensive disorders and related problems. *Cochrane Database Syst Rev* 2002;(1):CD001059.

Athukorala C, Crowther CA, Willson K; Australian Carbohydrate Intolerance Study in Pregnant Women (ACHOIS) Trial Group: Women with gestational diabetes mellitus in the ACHOIS trial: risk factors for shoulder dystocia. *Aust N Z J Obstet Gynecol* 47:37–41, 2007.

Atrash HK, Koonin LM, Lawson HW, Franks AL, Smith JC: Maternal mortality in the United States, 1979–1986. *Obstet Gynecol* 76:1055–1060, 1990.

Atrash HK, Rowley D, Hogue CJ: Maternal and perinatal mortality. *Curr Opin Obstet Gynecol* 4:61–71, 1992.

Atrash HK, Alexander S, Berg CJ: Maternal mortality in developed countries: not just a concern of the past. *Obstet Gynecol* 86:700–705, 1995.

Atzei A, Gajewska K, Huggon IC, Allan L, Nicolaides KH: Relationship between nuchal translucency thickness and prevalence of major cardiac defects in fetuses with normal karyotype. *Ultrasound Obstet Gynecol* 26:154–157, 2005.

Aucott SW, Williams TG, Hertz RH, Kalhan SC: Rigorous management of insulin-dependent diabetes mellitus during pregnancy. *Acta Diabetol* 31:126–129, 1994.

Avgidou K, Papageorghiou A, Bindra R, Spencer K, Nicolaides KH: Prospective first-trimester screening for trisomy 21 in 30,564 pregnancies. *Am J Obstet Gynecol* 192:1761–1767, 2005.

Baarsma R, Reijngoud D-J, van Asselt WA, Doormal JJ, Berger R, Okken A: Postnatal glucose kinetics in newborns of tightly controlled insulin-dependent diabetic mothers. *Pediatr Res* 34:443–447, 1993.

Bahado-Singh RO, Wapner R, Thom E, Zachary J, Platt L, Mahoney MJ, Johnson A, Silver RK, Pergament E, Filkins K, Hogge WA, Wilson RD, Jackson LG, for the First Trimester Maternal Serum Biochemistry and Fetal Nuchal Translucency Screening (BUN) Study Group: Elevated first-trimester nuchal translucency increases the risk of congenital heart defects. *Am J Obstet Gynecol* 192: 1357–1361, 2005.

Bahar AM: Risk factors and fetal outcome in cases of shoulder dystocia compared with normal deliveries of a similar birthweight. *Br J Obstet Gynecol* 103:868–872, 1996.

Baird JD, Farquhar JW: Insulin-secreting capacity in newborn infants of normal and diabetic women. *Lancet* 1:71–72, 1962.

Ballard JL, Rosenn B, Khoury JC, Miodovnik M: Diabetic fetal macrosomia: significance of disproportionate growth. *J Pediatr* 122:155–159, 1993.

Barkai G, Mashiach S, Lanzer D, Kayam Z, Brish M, Goldman B: Determination of fetal lung maturity from amniotic fluid microviscosity in high-risk pregnancy. *Obstet Gyecol* 59:615–623, 1982.

Barker DJP, Gluckman PD, Godfrey KM, Harding JE, Owen JA, Robinson JS: Fetal nutrition and cardiovascular disease in adult life. *Lancet* 341:938–941, 1993.

Barnett AH, Stubbs SM, Mander AM: Management of premature labor in diabetic pregnancy. *Diabetologia* 18:365–368, 1980.

Barondiot C, Morel O, Vieux R, Sery GA, Floriot M, Hascoet JM: Antenatal betamethasone during pregnancy with severe diabetes: is better worse than good? *Arch Pediatr* 14:989–992, 2007.

Barth WH Jr, Genest DR, Riley LE, Frigeletto FD Jr, Benacerraf BR, Greene MF: Uterine arcuate artery Doppler and decidual microvascular pathology in pregnancies complicated by type 1 diabetes mellitus. *Ultrasound Obstet Gynecol* 8:98–103, 1996.

Bartha JL, Wood J, Kyle PM, Soothill PW: The effect of metabolic control on fetal nuchal translucency in women with insulin-dependent diabetes: a preliminary study. *Ultrasound Obstet Gynecol* 21:451–454, 2003.

Baschat AA, Guclu S, Kush ML, Gembruch U, Weiner CP, Harman CR: Venous Doppler in the prediction of acid-base status of growth-restricted fetuses with elevated placental blood flow resistance. *Am J Obstet Gynecol* 191:277–284, 2004a.

Baschat A: Pathophysiology of fetal growth restriction: implications for diagnosis and surveillance. *Obstet Gynecol Surv* 59:617–627, 2004b.

Baumgarten A, Robinson J: Prospective study of an inverse relationship between maternal glycosylated hemoglobin and serum alpha-fetoprotein concentrations in pregnant women with diabetes. *Am J Obstet Gynecol* 159:77–81, 1988.

Beattie RB, Helmer H, Khan KS, Lamont RF, McNamara H, Svare J, Tsatsaris V, Van Geijn HP (Steering Group of the International Preterm Labor Council): Emerging issues over the choice of nifedipine, beta-agonists and atosiban for tocolysis in spontaneous preterm labor—a proposed systematic review by the International Preterm Labour Council. *J Obstet Gynecol* 24:213–215, 2004.

Becker T, Vermeulen MJ, Wyatt PR, Meier C, Ray JG: Prepregnancy diabetes and risk of placental vascular disease. *Diabetes Care* 30:2496–2498, 2007.

Belfort MA, Anthony J, Saade GR, Allen JC Jr, for the Nimodipine Study Group: A comparison of magnesium sulfate and nimodipine for the prevention of preeclampsia. *N Engl J Med* 348:304–311, 2003.

Belkacemi L, Lash GE, Macdonald-Goodfellow SK, Caldwell JD, Graham CH: Inhibition of human trophoblast invasiveness by high glucose concentrations. *J Clin Endocrinol Metab* 90:4846–4851, 2005.

Bell R, Bailey K, Cresswell T, Hawthorne G, Critchley J, lewis-Barned N; Norhtern Diabetic Pregnancy Survey Steering Group: Trends in prevalence and outcomes of pregnancy in women with preexisting type 1 and type II diabetes. *BJOG* 115:445–452, 2008.

Ben-Ami M, Giladi Y, Shalev E: The combination of magnesium sulfate and nifedipine: a cause of neuromuscular blockade. *Br J Obstet Gynecol* 101:262–263, 1994.

Ben-Ami M, Battino S, Geslevich Y, Shalev E: A random single Doppler study of the umbilical artery in the evaluation of pregnancies complicated by diabetes. *Am J Perinatol* 12:437–438, 1995.

Benacerraf BR, Benson CB, Abuhamad AZ, Copel JA, Abramowicz JS, DeVoe GR, Doubilet PM, Lee W, LevToaff AS, Merz E, Nelson TR, O'Neill MJ, Parsons AK, Platt LD, Pretorius DH, Timor-Tritsch IE: Three- and 4-dimensional ultrasound in obstetrics and gynecology. Proceedings of the American Institute of Ultrasound in Medicine Consensus Conference. *J Ultrasound Med* 24:15987–1597, 2005.

Benedetti TJ, Gabbe SG: Shoulder dystocia: a complication of fetal macrosomia and prolonged second stage of labor with midpelvic delivery. *Obstet Gynecol* 53: 526–529, 1978.

Ben-Haroush A, Yogev Y, Mashiach R, Hod M, Meisner I: Accuracy of sonographic estimation of fetal weight before induction of labor in diabetic pregnancies and pregnancies with suspected fetal macrosomia. *J Perinat Med* 31:225–230, 2003.

Ben-Haroush A, Yogev Y, Hod M: Fetal weight estimation in diabetic pregnancies and suspected fetal macrosomia. *J Perinat Med* 32:113–121, 2004.

Ben-Haroush A, Chen R, Hadar E, Hod M, Yogev Y: Accuracy of a single fetal weight estimation at 29–34 weeks in diabetic pregnancies: can it predict large-for-gestational-age infants at term? *Am J Obstet Gynecol* 197:497.e1–497.e6, 2007.

Bennett KA, Crane JMG, O'Shea P, Lacelle J, Hutchens D, Copel JA: First trimester ultrasound screening is effective in reducing postterm labor induction rates: a randomized controlled trial. *Am J Obstet Gynecol* 190:1077–1081, 2004.

Beppu OS, Clements JA, Goerke J: Phosphatidyl glycerol-deficient lung surfactant has normal properties. *J Appl Physiol* 55:496–502, 1983.

Berg CJ, Atrash HK, Koonin LM, Tucker M: Pregnancy-related mortality in the United States, 1987–1990. *Obstet Gynecol* 88:161–167, 1996.

Berg CJ, Chang J, Callaghan WM, Whitehead SJ: Pregnancy-related mortality in the United States, 1991–1997. *Obstet Gynecol* 101:289–296, 2003.

Berg van den P, Schmidt S, Gesche J, Saling E: Fetal distress and the condition of the newborn using cardiotocography and fetal blood analysis during labor. *Br J Obstet Gynecol* 94:72–75, 1987.

Berghella V, Pagotto L, Kaufman M, Huhta JC, Wapner RJ: Accuracy of prenatal diagnosis of congenital heart defects. *Fetal Diagn Ther* 16:407–412, 2001.

Bernstein IM, Catalano PM: Influence of fetal fat on the ultrasound estimation of fetal weight in diabetic mothers. *Obstet Gynecol* 79:561–563, 1992.

Bernstein IM, Catalano PM: Fetal body composition and ultrasonographic estimates of fetal weight. Letter. *Am J Obstet Gynecol* 179:558, 1998.

Bernstein IM, Horbar JD, Badger GJ, Ohlsson A, Golan A: Morbidity and mortality among very-low-birth weight neonates with intrauterine growth restrction: the Vermont Oxford network. *Am J Obstet Gynecol* 182:198–206, 2000.

Best G, Pressman EK: Ultrasonographic prediction of birth weight in diabetic pregnancies. *Obstet Gynecol* 99:740–744, 2002.

Bethune M, Bell R: Evaluation of the measurement of the fetal fat layer, interventricular septum and the abdominal circumference percentile in the prediction of macrosomia in pregnancies affected by gestational diabetes. *Ultrasound Obstet Gynecol* 22:586–590, 2003.

Bibergeil H, Godel E, Amendt P: Diabetes and pregnancy: early and late prognosis of children of diabetic mothers. In: Camerini-Davalos RA, Cole HS, eds. *Early Diabetes in Early Life*. New York: Academic Press, 1975:427–434.

Bieganska E, Wender-Ozegowska E, Pietryga M, Meissner W, Mitkowska-Wozniak H, Meller S, Biczysko R: Urinary tract infections of diabetic pregnancy. *Ginekol Pol* 73:817–822, 2002.

Bildiricci I, Moga CN, Gronowski AM, Sadovsky Y: The mean weekly increment of amniotic fluid TDx-FLM II ratio is constant during the latter part of pregnancy. *Am J Obstet Gynecol* 193:1685–1690, 2005.

Bisseling TM, Wouterse AC, Steegers EA, Elving L, Russel FG, Smits P: Nitric oxide mediated vascular tone in the fetal placental circulation of patients with type 1 diabetes mellitus. *Placenta* 24:974–978, 2003.

Bisseling TM, Versteegen MG, van der Wal S, Peereboom-Stegeman JJHC, Borggreven JMPM, Steegers EAP, van der Laak JAWM, Russel FGM, Smits P: Impaired KATP channel function in the fetoplacental circulation of patients with type 1 diabetes mellitus. *Am J Obstet Gynecol* 192:973–979, 2005.

Bjork O, Persson B: Villous structure in different parts of the cotyledon in placentas of insulin-dependent diabetic women. *Acta Obstet Gynecol Scand* 63:37–43, 1984.

Bjorklund AO, Adamson UKC, Almstrom NHH, Enocksson EA, Gennser GM, Lins P-E S, Westgren LMR: Effects of hypoglycemia on fetal heart activity and umbilical artery Doppler velocity waveforms in pregnant women with insulin-dependent diabetes mellitus. *Br J Obstet Gynecol* 103:413–420, 1996.

Blackwell SC, Hassan SS, Wolfe HM, Michaelson J, Berry SM, Sorokin Y: Vaginal birth after cesarean in the diabetic gravida. *J Reprod Med* 45:987–990, 2000a.

Blackwell SC, Hassan SS, Wolfe HM, Michaelson J, Berry SM, Sorokin Y: Why are cesarean delivery rates so high in diabetic pregnancies? *J Perinat Med* 28: 316–320, 2000b.

Blanco-Molina A, Trujillo-Santos J, Criado J, Lopez L, Lecumberri R, Gutierrez R, Monreal M; RIETE Investigators: Venous thromboembolism during pregnancy or postpartum: findings from the RIETE Registry. *Thromb Haemost* 97:186–190, 2007.

Bloom SR, Johnston DI: Failure of glucagon release in infants of diabetic mothers. *Br Med J* 4:453–454, 1972.

Bloom SL, Spong CY, Weimer SJ, Landon MB, Rouse DJ, Varner MW, Moawad AH, Caritis SN, Harper M, Wapner RJ, Sorokin Y, Miodovnik M, O'Sullivan MJ, Sibai B, Langer O, Gabbe SG; National Institute of Child Health and Human Development Maternal-Fetal Medicine Units Network: Complications of anesthesia for cesarean delivery. *Obstet Gynecol* 106: 281–287, 2005.

Bloom SL, Spong CY, Thom E, Varner MW, Rouse DJ, Weininger S, Ramin SM, Caritis SN, Peaceman A, Sorokin Y, Sciscione A, Carpenter M, Mercer B, Thorp J, Malone F, Harper M, Iams J, Anderson G; National Institute of Child Health and Human Development Maternal-Fetal Medicine Units Network: Fetal pulse oximetry and cesarean delivery. *N Engl J Med* 355:2195–2202, 2006.

Blumenfeld TA, Stark RI, James LS, George JD, Dyrenfurth I, Freda VJ, Shinitzky M: Determination of fetal lung maturity by fluorescence polarization of amniotic fluid. *Am J Obstet Gynecol* 130:782–787, 1978.

Bo S, Menato G, Signorile A, Bardelli C, Lezo A, Gallo ML, Gambino R, Cassader M, Massobrio M, Pagano G: Obesity or diabetes: what is worse for the mother and for the baby? *Diabetes Metab* 29:175–178, 2003.

Bocking A, Adamson L, Cousin A, Campbell K, Carmichael L, Natale R, Patrick J: Effects of intravenous glucose injections on human fetal breathing movements and gross body movements at 38 to 40 weeks gestational age. *Am J Obstet Gynecol* 142:606–611, 1982.

Bocking A, Adamson L, Carmichael L, Patrick J, Probert C: Effect of intravenous glucose injection on human maternal and fetal heart rate at term. *Am J Obstet Gynecol* 148:414–420, 1984.

Bocking AD: Observations of biophysical activities in the normal fetus. *Clin Perinatol* 16:583–594, 1989.

Bocking AD: Assessment of fetal heart rate and fetal movements in detecting oxygen deprivation in-utero. *Eur J Obstet Gynecol Reprod Biol* 110:108–112, 2003.

Boehlen F, Epiney M, Boulvain M, Irion O, de Moerloose P: Changes in D-dimer levels during pregnancy and the postpartum period: results of two studies. *Rev Med Suisse* 26:296–298, 2005.

Bofill JA, Rust OA, Devidas M, Roberts WE, Morrison JC, Martin JN Jr: Shoulder dystocia and operative vaginal delivery. *J Matern-Fetal Med* 6: 220–224, 1997.

Boluyt N, van Kempen A, Offringa M: Neurodevelopment after neonatal hypoglycemia: a systematic review and design of an optimal future study. *Pediatrics* 117:2231–2243, 2006.

Boulet SL, Alexander GR, Salihu HM, Kirby RS, Carlo WA: Fetal growth risk curves: defining levels of fetal growth restriction by neonatal death risk. *Am J Obstet Gynecol* 195:1571–1577, 2006.

Boulvain M, Stan C, Irion O: Elective delivery in diabetic pregnant women. *Cochrane Database Syst Rev* 2001;(2):CD0011997.

Bourbon JR, Farrell PM: Fetal lung development in the diabetic pregnancy. *Pediatr Res* 19:253–267, 1985a.

Bourbon JR, Pignol B, Marin L, Rieutort M, Tordet C: Maturation of fetal rat lung in diabetic pregnancies of graded severity. *Diabetes* 34:734–743, 1985b.

Bourbon JR, Doucet E, Rieutort M, Pignol B, Tordet C: Role of myo-inositol in impairment of fetal lung phosphatidylglycerol biosynthesis in the diabetic pregnancy: physiological consequences of a phosphatidylglycerol-deficient surfactant in the newborn rat. *Exp Lung Res* 11:195–207, 1986.

Bourgeois F, Duffer J: Outpatient obstetric management of women with type 1 diabetes. *Am J Obstet Gynecol* 163:1065–1073, 1990.

Bowen DJ, Daykin AP, Nancekievill ML, Norman J: Insulin-dependent diabetic patients during surgery and labor. Use of continuous intravenous insulin-glucose-potassium infusions. *Anesthesiology* 39:407–411, 1984.

Bower S, Bewley S, Campbell S: Improved prediction of preeclampsia by two-stage screening of uterine arteries using the early diastolic notch and color Doppler imaging. *Obstet Gynecol* 82:78–83, 1993.

Bracero L, Schulman H, Fleischer A, Farmakides G, Rochelson B: Umbilical artery velocimetry in diabetes and pregnancy. *Obstet Gynecol* 68:654–658, 1986.

Bracero LA, Jovanovic L, Rochelson B, Bauman W, Farmakides G: Significance of umbilical and uterine artery velocimetry in the well-controlled pregnant diabetic. *J Reprod Med* 34:273–276, 1989a.

Bracero LA, Beneck D, Kirshenbaum N, Peiffer M, Stalter P, Schulman H: Doppler velocimetry and placental disease. *Am J Obstet Gynecol* 161:388–393, 1989b.

Bracero LA, Beneck D, Shulman H: Doppler velocimetry, placental morphology and outcome in insulin-dependent diabetes. *Ultrasound Obstet Gynecol* 3:236–239, 1993.

Bracero LA, Figueroa R, Byrne DW, Han HJ: Comparison of umbilical Doppler velocimetry, nonstress testing, and biophysical profile in pregnancies complicated by diabetes. *J Ultrasound Med* 15:301–308, 1996.

Bracero LA, Haberman S, Byrne DW: Maternal glycemic control and umbilical artery Doppler velocimetry. *J Matern Fetal Neonatal Med* 12:342–348, 2002.

Bradley RJ, Brudenell JM, Nicolaides KH: Fetal acidosis and hyperlactinemia diagnosed by cordocentesis in pregnancies complicated by maternal diabetes mellitus. *Diabet Med* 8:464–468, 1992.

Brans YW, Shannon DL, Hunter MA: Maternal diabetes and neonatal macrosomia. II. Neonatal anthropomorphic measurements. *Early Hum Dev* 8:297–305, 1983.

Braunstein GD, Mills JL, Reed GF, Jovanovic LG, Holmes LB, Aarons J, Simpson JL; the NICHHD-Diabetes in Early Pregnancy Study Group: Comparison of serum placental hormone levels in diabetic and normal pregnancy. *J Clin Endocrinol Metab* 68:3–8, 1989.

Breathnach FM, Malone FD: Screening for aneuploidy in first and second trimesters: is there an optimal paradigm? *Curr Opin Obstet Gynecol* 19:176–182, 2007.

Breidahl HD: The growth and development of children born to mothers with diabetes. *Med J Aust* 1:268–270, 1966.

Breitweser JA, Meyer RA, Sperling MA, Tsang RC, Kaplan S: Cardiac septal hypertrophy in hyperinsulinemic infants. *J Pediatr* 96:535 539, 1980.

Bromiker R, Rachamim A, Hammerman C, Schimmel M, Kaplan M, Medoff-Cooper B: Immature sucking patterns in infants of mothers with diabetes. *J Pediatr* 149: 640 643, 2006.

Brown ZA, Mills JL, Metzger BE, Knopp RH, Simpson JL, Jovanovic-Peterson L, Scheer K, Van Allen MI, Aarons JH, Reed GF; National Institute of Child Health and Human Development Study: Early sonographic evaluation for fetal growth delay and congenital malformations in pregnancies complicated by insulin-requiring diabetes. *Diabetes Care* 15:613–619, 1992.

Brown S, Kyne-Grzebalski D, Mwangi B, Taylor R: Effect of management policy upon 120 type 1 diabetic pregnancies: policy decisions in practice. *Diabet Med* 16:472–476, 1999.

Buchanan TA, Kjos SL, Schaefer U, Peters RK, Xiang A, Byrne J, Berkowitz K, Montoro M: Utility of fetal measurement in the management of gestational diabetes mellitus. *Diabetes Care* 21(Suppl 2):B99–B106, 1998.

Buhi WC, Spellacy WN: Effects of blood or meconium on the determination of the amniotic fluid lecithin/sphingomyelin ratio. *Am J Obstet Gynecol* 121:321–323, 1975.

Bunt JC, Tataranni PA, Salbe AD: Intrauterine exposure to diabetes is a determinant of hemoglobin A1C and systolic blood pressure in Pima Indian children. *J Clin Endocrinol Metab* 90:325–329, 2005.

Burden MJ, Westerlund AJ, Armony-Sivan R, Nelson CA, Jacobson SW, Lozoff ZB, Angelilli ML, Jacobson JL: An event-related-potential study of attention and recognition memory in infants with iron deficiency anemia. *Pediatrics* 120:e336–e345, 2007.

Burleigh DW, Stewart K, Grindle KM, Kay HH, Golos TG: Influence of maternal diabetes on placental fibroblast growth factor-2 expression, proliferation, and apoptosis. *J Soc Gynecol Investig* 11:36–41, 2004.

Callaghan WM, Berg CJ: Pregnancy-related mortality among women aged 35 years and older, United States, 1991–1997. *Obstet Gynecol* 102:1015–1021, 2003.

Caplan RH, Pagliara AS, Beguin EA, Smiley CA, Bina-Frymark M, Goettl KA, Hartigan JM, Tankersley JC, Peck TM: Constant intravenous insulin infusion during labor and delivery in diabetes mellitus. *Diabetes Care* 5:6–10, 1982.

Caritis SN, Sibai B, Hauth J, Lindheimer M, Klebanoff M, Thom E, VanDorsten P, Landon M, Paul R, Miodovnik M, Meis P, Thurnau G; for the NICHHD-MFMU: Low-dose aspirin to prevent preeclampsia in women at high risk. *N Engl J Med* 338:701–705, 1998.

Carpenter MW: Amniotic fluid in non-diabetic and diabetic pregnancies. In: Hod M, Jovanovic L, Di Renzo GC, de Leiva A, Langer O, eds. *Textbook of Diabetes and Pregnancy.* London: Martin Durnitz, 2004:148–157.

Carson BS, Philipps AF, Simmons MA, Battaglia FC, Meschia G: Effects of sustained insulin infusion upon glucose uptake and oxygenation of the bovine fetus. *Pediatr Res* 14:147–152, 1980.

Carvalho JS, Mavrides E, Shinebourne EA, Campbell S, Thilaganathan B: Improving the effectiveness of routine prenatal screening for major congenital heart defects. *Heart* 88:387–391, 2002.

Casele H, Grobman WA: Cost-effectiveness of thromboprophylaxis with intermittent pneumatic compression at cesarean delivery. *Obstet Gynecol* 108:535–540, 2006.

Castracane VD, Jovanovic L, Mills JL: Effect of normoglycemia before conception on early pregnancy hormone profiles. *Diabetes Care* 8:473–476, 1985.

Catalano PM, Thomas AJ, Avallone DA, Amini SB: Anthropometric estimation of neonatal body composition. *Am J Obstet Gynecol* 173:1176–1181, 1995.

Catov JM, Ness RB, Kip KE, Olsen J: Risk of early or severe preeclampsia related to pre-existing conditions. *Int J Epidemiol* Jan 25, 2007.

CDC—Centers for Disease Control and Prevention, Morbidity and Mortality Weekly Report: Pregnancy complications and perinatal outcomes among women with diabetes: North Carolina, 1989–1990. *JAMA* 270:2424–2425, 1993.

Chagnon I, Bounameaux H, Aujesky D, Roy PM, Gourdier AL, Cirnuz J, Perneger T, Perrier A: Comparison of two clinical prediction rules and implicit assessment among patients with suspected pulmonary embolism. *Am J Med* 113:269–275, 2002.

Chan KL, Liu X, Ascah KJ, Beuchesne LM, Burwash IG: Comparison of real-time 3-dimensional echocardiography with conventional 2-dimensional echocardiography in the assessment of structural heart disease. *J Am Soc Echocardiogr* 17:976–980, 2004.

Chappell LC, Seed PT, Briley A, Kelly FJ, Hunt BJ, Charnock Jones DS, Mallet AI, Poston L: A longitudinal study of biochemical variables in women at risk of preeclampsia. *Am J Obstet Gynecol* 187:127–136, 2002.

Chauhan SP, Cole J, Laye MR, Choi K, Sanderson M, Moore RC, Magann EF, King HL, Morrison JC: Shoulder dystocia with and without brachial plexus injury: experience from three centers. *Am J Perinatol* 24:365–371, 2007.

Chelmow D, Ruehli MS, Huang E: Prophylactic use of antibiotics for nonlaboring patients undergoing cesarean delivery with intact membranes: a meta-analysis. *Am J Obstet Gynecol* 184:656–661, 2001.

Chen CH, Adam PAJ, Laskowski DE, McCann ML, Schwartz R: The plasma free fatty acid composition and blood glucose of normal and diabetic pregnant women and of their newborns. *Pediatrics* 36:843–855, 1965.

Chien PFW, Arnott N, Gordon A, Owen P, Khan KS: How useful is uterine artery Doppler flow velocimetry in the prediction of preeclampsia, intrauterine growth retardation and perinatal death? An overview. *BJOG* 107:196–208, 2000.

Cho NH, Silverman BL, Rizzo TA, Metzger BE: Correlations between the intrauterine metabolic environment and blood pressure in adolescent offspring of diabetic mothers. *J Pediatr* 136:587–592, 2000.

Churchill JA, Berendes HW, Nemore J: Neuropsychological deficits in children of diabetic mothers. *Am J Obstet Gynecol* 105:257–268, 1969.

Clark KE, Miodovnik M, Skillman CA, Mimouni F: Review of fetal cardiovascular and metabolic responses to diabetic insults in the pregnant ewe. *Am J Perinatol* 5:312–318, 1988.

Clausen TD, Mathiesen E, Ekbom P, Hellmuth E, Mandrup-Poulsen T, Damm P: Poor pregnancy outcome in women with type 2 diabetes. *Diabetes Care* 28: 323–328, 2005.

Clausen TD, Mathiesen ER, Hansen T, Pedersen O, Jensen DM, Lauenborg J, Damm P: High prevalence of type 2 diabetes and pre-diabetes in adult offspring of women with gestational diabetes mellitus or type 1 diabetes: the role of intrauterine hyperglycemia. *Diabetes Care* 31:340–346, 2008.

Cnattinguis S, Berne C, Nordstrom M: Pregnancy outcome and infant mortality in diabetic women in Sweden. *Diabet Med* 11:696–700, 1994.

Coetzee E, Dommisse J, Anthony J: A randomized controlled trial of intravenous magnesium sulfate versus placebo in the management of women with severe preeclampsia. *Br J Obstet Gynecol* 105:300–303, 1998.

Cohen B, Penning S, Major C, Ansley D, Porto M, Garite T: Sonographic prediction of shoulder dystocia in infants of diabetic mothers. *Obstet Gynecol* 88:10–13, 1996.

Cohen BF, Penning S, Ansley D, Porto M, Garite T: The incidence and severity of shoulder dystocia correlates with a sonographic measurement of asymmetry in patients with diabetes. *Am J Perinatol* 16:197–201, 1999.

Combs CA, Rosenn B, Kitzmiller JL, Khoury JC, Wheeler BC, Miodovnik M: Early-pregnancy proteinuria in diabetes related to preeclampsia. *Obstet Gynecol* 82:802–807, 1993.

Combs CA, Rosenn B, Miodovnik M, Siddiqi TA: Sonographic EFW and macrosomia: is there an optimum formula to predict diabetic fetal macrosomia? *J Matern-Fetal Med* 9:55–61, 2000.

Conde-Agudelo A, Villar J, Lindheimer M: World Health Organization systematic review of screening tests for preeclampsia. *Obstet Gynecol* 104:1367–1391, 2004.

Connell FA, Vadheim C, Emanuel I: Diabetes in pregnancy: a population-based study of incidence, referral for care, and perinatal mortality. *Am J Obstet Gynecol* 151:598–603, 1985.

Conrad KP, Benyo BF, Westyerhausen-Larsen A, Miles TM: Expression of erythropoietin by the human placenta. *FASEB J* 10:760–768, 1996.

Conway DL, Langer O: Elective delivery of infants with macrosomia in diabetic women: reduced shoulder dystocia versus increased cesarean deliveries. *Am J Obstet Gynecol* 178:922–925, 1998.

Conway DL: Delivery of the macrosomic infant: cesarean section versus vaginal delivery. *Sem Perinatol* 26:225–231, 2002.

Coomarasamy A, Knox EM, Gee H, Song F, Khan KS: Effectiveness of nifedipine versus atosiban for tocolysis in preterm labour: a meta-analysis with an indirect comparison of randomized trials. *Br J Obstet Gynecol* 110:1045–1049, 2003.

Coomarasamy A, Connock M, Thornton J, Khan KS: Accuracy of ultrasound biometry in the prediction of macrosomia: a systematic quantitative review. *Br J Obstet Gynecol* 112:1461–1466, 2005.

Cooper MJ, Enderlein MA, Dyson DC, Roge CL, Tarnoff H: Fetal echocardiography: retrospective review of clinical experience and an evaluation of indications. *Obstet Gynecol* 86:577–582, 1995.

Copel JA, Pilu G, Green J, Hobbins JC, Kleinman CS: Fetal echocardiographic screening for congenital heart disease: the importance of the four-chamber heart view. *Am J Obstet Gynecol* 157:648–655, 1987.

Cordero L, Landon M: Infant of the diabetic mother. *Clin Perinatol* 20:635–645, 1993.

Cornblath M, Hawdon JM, Williams AF, Aynsley-Green A, Ward-Platt MP, Schwartz R, Kalhan SC: Controversies regarding definition of neonatal hypoglycemia: suggested operational thresholds. *Pediatrics* 105:1141–1145, 2000.

Cosmi E, Piazze JJ, Ruozi A, Anceschi MM, La Torre R, Andrisani A, Litta P, Nardelli GB, Ambrosini G: Structural-tridimensional study of yolk sac in pregnancies complicated by diabetes. *J Perinat Med* 33:132–136, 2005.

Coughlan MT, Vervaart PP, Permezel M, Georgiou HM, Rice GE: Altered placental oxidative stress status in gestational diabetes mellitus. *Placenta* 25:78–84, 2004.

Cousins L: Pregnancy complications among diabetic women: review 1965–1985. *Obstet Gynecol Surv* 42:140–149, 1987.

Cousins L, Key TC, Schorzman L, Moore TR: Ultrasonographic assessment of early fetal growth in insulin-treated diabetic pregnancies. *Am J Obstet Gynecol* 159:1186–1190, 1988.

Cousins L: The California Diabetes and Pregnancy Program: a statewide collaborative program for the preconception and prenatal care of diabetic women. *Bailliere's Clin Obstet Gynecol* 5:443–459, 1991.

Coustan DR, Berkowitz RL, Hobbins JC: Tight metabolic control of overt diabetes in pregnancy. *Am J Med* 68:845–852, 1980.

Coustan DR: Delivery: timing, mode, and management. In: Reece EA, Coustan DR, Gabbe SG, eds. *Diabetes in Women: Adolescence, Pregnancy, and Menopause.* 3rd ed. Philadelphia: Lippincott Williams & Wilkins, 2004:433–440.

Cowett RM, Susa JB, Giletti B, Oh W, Schwartz R: Glucose kinetics in infants of diabetic mothers. *Am J Obstet Gynecol* 146:781–786, 1983.

Cowett RM, Farrag HM: Selected principles of perinatal-neonatal glucose metabolism. *Semin Neonatol* 9:37–47, 2004.

Crandell SS, Fischer DJ, Morris FH: Effects of ovine maternal hyperglycemia on fetal regional blood flows and metabolism. *Am J Physiol* 249:454–460, 1985.

Crane JP, LeFevre ML, Winborn RC, Evans JK, Ewigman BG, Bain RP, Frigoletto FD, McNellis D; the RADIUS Study Group: A randomized trial of prenatal ultrasonographic screening: impact on the detection, management, and outcome of anomalous fetuses. *Am J Obstet Gynecol* 171:392–399, 1994.

Crane J, Armson A, Brunner M, De La Ronde S, Farine D, Keenan-Lindsay L, Leduc L, Schneider C, Van Aerde J; Executive Committee of the Society of Obstetricians and Gynecologists of Canada: Antenatal corticosteroid therapy for fetal maturation. *J Obstet Gynecol Can* 25:45–52, 2003.

Crowther CA, Harding J: Repeat doses of prenatal corticosteroids for women at risk of preterm birth for preventing neonatal respiratory disease. *Cochrane Database Syst Rev* 2003:CD003935.

Crowther CA, Hiller JE, Moss JR, McPhee AJ, Jeffries WS, Robinson JS; the Australian Carbohydrate Intolerance Study (ACHOIS) in Pregnant Women Trial Group: Effect of treatment of gestational diabetes on pregnancy outcomes. *N Engl J Med* 352:2477–2486, 2005.

Crowther CA, Haslam RR, Hiller JE, Doyle LW, Robinson JS; the Australasian Collaborative Trial of Repeat Doses of Steroids (ACTORDS) Study Group: Neonatal respiratory distress syndrome after repeat exposure to antenatal corticosteroids: a randomized controlled trial. *Lancet* 367:1913–1919, 2006.

Cruikshank DP, Pitkin RM, Varner MW, Williams GA, Hargis GK: Calcium metabolism in diabetic mother, fetus, and newborn infant. *Am J Obstet Gynecol* 145:1010–1016, 1983.

Cruz AC, Buhi WC, Birk SA, Spellacy WN: Respiratory distress syndrome with mature lecithin/sphinglomyelin ratios: *Am J Obstet Gynecol* 126:78–82, 1976.

Cummins M, Norrish M: Follow-up of children of diabetic mothers. *Arch Dis Child* 55:259–264, 1980.

Cundy T, Gamble G, Townend K, Henley PG, MacPherson P, Roberts AB: Perinatal mortality in type 2 diabetes mellitus. *Diabet Med* 17:33–39, 2000.

Cundy T, Slee F, Gamble G, Neale L: Hypertensive disorders of pregnancy in women with type 1 and type 2 diabetes. *Diabet Med* 19:482–489, 2002.

Cundy T, Gamble G, Neale L, Elder R, McPherson P, Henley P, Rowan J: Differing causes of pregnancy loss in type 1 and type 2 diabetes. *Diabetes Care* 30:2603–2607, 2007.

Cunningham MD, Desai NS, Thompson SA, Greene JM: Amniotic fluid phosphatidylglycerol in diabetic pregnancies. *Am J Obstet Gynecol* 131:719–724, 1978.

Cunningham MD, McKean HE, Gillespie DH, Greene JW Jr: Improved prediction of fetal lung maturity in diabetic pregnancies: a comparison of chromatographic methods. *Am J Obstet Gynecol* 142:197–204, 1982.

Cunningham FG, Twickler D: Cerebral edema complicating eclampsia. *Am J Obstet Gynecol* 182:94–100, 2000.

Cunningham FG: Severe preeclampsia and eclampsia: systolic hypertension is also important. *Obstet Gynecol* 105:237–238, 2005.

Curet LB, Olson RW, Schneider JM, Zachman RD: Effect of diabetes mellitus on amniotic fluid lecithin/sphingomyelin ratio and respiratory distress syndrome. *Am J Obstet Gynecol* 135:10–13, 1979.

Curet LB, Tsao FHC, Zachman RD, Olson RW, Henderson PA: Phosphatidylglycerol, lecithin/sphingomyelin ratio and respiratory distress syndrome in diabetic and non-diabetic pregnancies. *Int J Obstet Gynecol* 30:105–108, 1989.

Curet LB, Izquierdo LA, Gilson GJ, Schneider JM, Perelman R, Converse J: Relative effects of antepartum and intrapartum maternal blood glucose levels on the incidence of neonatal hypoglycemia. *J Perinatol* 17:113–115, 1997.

da Fonseca EB, Bittar RE, Carvalho MHB, Zugaib M: Prophylactic administration of progesterone by vaginal suppository to reduce the incidence of spontaneous preterm birth in women at increased risk: a randomized placebo-controlled double-blind study. *Am J Obstet Gynecol* 188:419–424, 2003.

Dabelea D, Hanson RL, Lindsay RS, Pettitt DJ, Imperatore G, Gabir MM, Roumain J, Bennett PH, Knowler WC: Intrauterine exposure to diabetes conveys risks for type 2 diabetes and obesity: a study of discordant sibships. *Diabetes* 49: 2208–2211, 2000.

Dabelea D, Pettitt DJ: Intrauterine diabetic environment confers risks for type 2 diabetes mellitus and obesity in the offspring, in addition to genetic susceptibility. *J Pediatr Endocrinol Metab* 14:1085–1091, 2001.

Dahlenburg GW, Martin FIR, Jeffrey PR, Horacek I: Amniotic fluid lecithin/sphingomyelin ratio in pregnancy complicated by diabetes. *Br J Obstet Gynecol* 84:294–299, 1977.

Dalence CR, Bowie LJ, Dohnal JC, Farrell EE, Neerhof MG: Amniotic fluid lamellar body count: a rapid and reliable fetal maturity test. *Obstet Gynecol* 86:235–239, 1995.

Dalgic N, Ergenekon E, Soysal S, Koc E, Atalay Y, Gucuyener K: Transient neonatal hypoglycemia—long-term effects on neurodevelopmental outcome. *J Pediatr Endocrinol Metab* 15:319–324, 2002.

Dalziel SR, Lim VK, Lambert A, McCarthy D, Parag V, Rodgers A, Harding JE: Antenatal exposure to betamethasone: psychological functioning and health-related quality of life 31 years after incusion in randomized controlled trial. *BMJ* 331:665–668, 2005.

Dame C, Fahnenstich H, Freitag P, Hofman D, Abdul-Nour T, Bartmann P, Fandrey J: Erythropoietin mRNA expression in human fetal and neonatal tissue. *Blood* 92:3218–3225, 1998.

Dargaud Y, Rugeri L, Ninet J, Negrier C, Trzeciak MC: Management of pregnant women with increased risk of venous thrombosis. *Int J Obstet Gynecol* 90: 203–207, 2005.

Dashe J, Nathan L, McIntire DD, Leveno KJ: Correlation between amniotic fluid glucose concentration and amniotic fluid volume in pregnancy complicated by diabetes. *Am J Obstet Gynecol* 182:901–904, 2000.

Datta S, Brown WU: Acid-base status in diabetic mothers and their infants following general or spinal anesthesia for cesarean section. *Anesthesiology* 47:272–276, 1977.

Datta S, Brown WU Jr, Ostheimer GW, Weiss JB, Alper MH: Epidural anesthesia for cesarean section in diabetic parturients: maternal and neonatal acid-base status and bupivacaine concentration. *Anesth Analg* 60:574–578, 1981.

Datta S, Alper MH, Ostheimer GW, Weiss JB: Method of ephedrine administration and nausea and hypotension during spinal anesthesia for cesarean section. *Anesthesiology* 56:68–70, 1982a.

Datta S, Kitzmiller JL, Naulty JS, Ostheimer GW, Weiss JB: Acid-base status of diabetic mothers and their infants following spinal anesthesia for cesarean section. *Anesth Analg* 61:662–665, 1982b.

Davis GK, Farquhar CM, Allan LD, Crawford DC, Chapman MG: Structural cardiac abnormalities in the fetus: reliability of prenatal diagnosis and outcome. *Br J Obstet Gynecol* 97:27–31, 1990.

Davis LE, Widness JA, Brace RA: Renal and placental secretion of erythropoietin during anemia or hypoxia in the ovine fetus. *Am J Obstet Gynecol* 189:1764–1770, 2003.

DCCT—Diabetes Control and Complications Trial Research Group: Pregnancy outcomes in the Diabetes Control and Complications Trial. *Am J Obstet Gynecol* 174:1343–1353, 1996.

de Vries JI, Visser GHA, Mulder EJH, Prechtl HFR: Diurnal and other variations in fetal movement and heart rate patterns at 20–22 weeks. *Early Hum Dev* 15:333–348, 1987.

DeBoer T, Wewerka S, Bauer PJ, Georgieff MK, Nelson CA: Explicit memory performance in infants of diabetic mothers at 1 year of age. *Dev Med Child Neurol* 47:525–531, 2005.

Degani S, Paltielli Y, Gonen R, Sharf M: Fetal internal carotid artery pulsed Doppler flow velocity waveforms and maternal plasma glucose levels. *Obstet Gynecol* 77:379–381, 1991.

DeKeyser K, Paemeleire K, De Clerk M, Peeters D, De Reuck JL: Diabetic ketoacidosis presenting as a cerebral venous sinus thrombosis. *Acta Neurol Belg* 104:117–120, 2004.

Dekowski SA, Snyder JM: Insulin regulation of messenger ribonucleic acid for the surfactant-associated proteins in human fetal lung in vitro. *Endocrinology* 131:669–676, 1992.

Del Valle GO, Adair CD, Ramos EE, Gaudier FL, Sanchez-Ramos L, Morales R: Interpretation of the TDx-FLM fluorescence polarization assay in pregnancies complicated by diabetes mellitus. *Am J Perinatol* 14:241–244, 1997.

Delaney JJ, Ptacek J: Three decades of experience with diabetic pregnancies. *Am J Obstet Gynecol* 106:550–556, 1970.

deLeeuw JW, de Wit C, Kuijken JP, Bruinse HW: Mediolateral episiotomy reduces the risk for anal sphincter injury during operative vaginal delivery. *BJOG* 115:104–108, 2008.

Delgado JC, Greene MF, Winkelman JW, Tanasijevic MJ: Comparison of disaturated phosphatidylcholine and fetal lung maturity surfactant/albumin ratio in diabetic and nondiabetic pregnancies. *Am J Clin Pathol* 113:233–239, 2000.

Demarini S, Mimouni F, Tsang RC, Khoury J, Hertzberg V: Impact of metabolic control of diabetes during pregnancy on neonatal hypoglycemia: a randomized study. *Obstet Gynecol* 83:918–922, 1994.

Demiroren K, Cam L, Oran B, Koc H, Baspinar O, Baysal T, Karaasian S: Echocardiographic measurements in infants of diabetic mothers and macrosomic infants of nondiabetic mothers. *J Perinat Med* 33:232–235, 2005.

Demottaz V, Epstein MF, Frantz ID 3rd: Phospholipid synthesis in lung slices from fetuses of alloxan diabetic rabbits. *Pediatr Res* 14:47–49, 1980.

Deneux-Tharaux C, Berg C, Bouvier-Colle M-H, Gissler M, Harper M, Nannini A, Alexander S, Wildman K, Breart G, Buekens P: Under-reporting of pregnancy-related mortality in the United States and Europe. *Obstet Gynecol* 106:684–692, 2005.

Deneux-Tharoux C, Carmona E, Bouvier-Colle MH, Breart G: Postpartum maternal mortality and cesarean delivery. *Obstet Gynecol* 108:541–548, 2006.

deRegnier R-A, Nelson CA, Thomas K, Wewerka S, Georgieff MK: Neurophysiologic evaluation of auditory recognition memory in healthy newborn infants and infants of diabetic mothers. *J Pediatr* 137:777–784, 2000.

deRegnier RA, Long JD, Georgieff MK, Nelson CA: Using event-related potentials to study perinatal nutrition and brain development in infants of diabetic mothers. *Dev Neuropsychol* 31:379–396, 2007.

DeRoche ME, Ingardia CJ, Guerette PJ, Wu AH, LaSala CA, Mandavilli SR: The use of lamellar body counts to predict fetal lung maturity in pregnancies complicated by diabetes mellitus. *Obstet Gynecol* 187:908–912, 2002.

Dervaitis KL, Poole M, Schmidt G, Penava D, Natale R, Gagnon R: ST segment analysis of the fetal electrocardiogram plus fetal heart rate monitoring in labor and its relationship to umbilical cord arterial blood gases. *Am J Obstet Gynecol* 191:879–884, 2004.

Desir D, Coevorden AV, Kirkpatrick C, Caufriez A: Ritodrine-induced acidosis in pregnancy. *Br Med J* 1:1194, 1978.

Desoye G, Myatt L: The placenta. In: Reece EA, Coustan DR, Gabbe SG, eds. *Diabetes in Women. Adolescence, Pregnancy, and Menopause.* 3rd ed. Philadelphia: Lippincott Williams & Wilkins, 2004:147–157.

Dessens AB, Haas HS, Koppe JG: Twenty-year follow-up of antenatal corticosteroid treatment. *Pediatrics* 105:E77, 2000.

DeValk HW, van Nieuwaal NH, Visser GH: Pregnancy outcome in type 2 diabetes mellitus: a retrospective analysis from the Netherlands. *Rev Diabet Stud* 3:134–142, 2006.

Devoe LD, Youssef AA, Castillo RA, Croom CS: Fetal biophysical activities in third-trimester pregnancies complicated by diabetes mellitus. *Am J Obstet Gynecol* 171:298–305, 1994.

Devoe LD, Jones CR: Nonstress test: evidence-based use in high-risk pregnancy. *Clin Obstet Gynecol* 45:986–992, 2002.

Di Iulio JL, Gude NM, King RG, Li CG, Rand MJ, Brennecke SP: Human placental nitric oxide synthase activity is not altered in diabetes. *Clin Sci* 97:123–128, 1999.

Diamond MP, Shah DM, Hester RA, Vaughn WK, Cotton RB, Boehm FH: Complication of insulin-dependent diabetic pregnancies by preeclampsia and/or chronic hypertension: analysis of outcome. *Am J Perinatol* 2:263–267, 1985.

Diamond MP, Entman SS, Salyer SL, Vaughn WK, Boehm FH: Increased risk of endometritis and wound infection after cesarean section in insulin-dependent diabetic women. *Am J Obstet Gynecol* 155:297–300, 1986.

Dicker D, Feldberg D, Yeshaya A, Peleg D, Karp M, Goldman JA: Fetal surveillance in insulin-dependent diabetic pregnancy: predictive value of the biophysical profile. *Am J Obstet Gynecol* 159:800–804, 1988.

Dicker D, Goldman JA, Yeshaya A, Peleg D: Umbilical artery velocimetry in insulin dependent diabetes mellitus (IDDM) pregnancies. *J Perinat Med* 18:391–395, 1990.

Dierker LJ, Pillay S, Sorokin Y, Rosen M: The change in fetal activity periods in diabetic and nondiabetic pregnancies. *Am J Obstet Gynecol* 143:181–185, 1982.

Dietz PM, England LJ, Callaghan WM, Pearl M, Wier ML, Kharrazi M: A comparison of LMP-based and ultrasound-based estimates of gestational age using linked California livebirth and prenatal screening records. *Pediatr Perinat Epidemiol* 21 (Suppl 2):62–71, 2007.

Dilena BA, Ku F, Doyle I, Whiting MJ: Six alternative methods to the lecithin/ sphingomyelin ratio in amniotic fluid for assessing fetal lung maturity. *Ann Clin Biochem* 34:106–108, 1997.

Divon MY, Zimmer EZ, Yeh SY, Vilenski A, Sarna Z, Paldi E, Platt LD: Effect of maternal intravenous glucose administration on fetal heart rate patterns and fetal breathing. *Am J Perinatol* 2:292–294, 1985.

Dobbs LG: Pulmonary surfactant. *Annu Rev Med* 40:431–446, 1989.

Doctor B, O'Riordan MA, Kirchner HL, Shah D, Hack M: Perinatal correlates and neonatal outcomes of small for gestational age infants born at term gestation. *Am J Obstet Gynecol* 185:652–659, 2001.

Dodd JM, Crowther CA, Cincotta R, Flenady V, Robinson JS: Progesterone supplementation for preventing preterm birth: a systematic review and meta-analysis. *Acta Obstet Gynecol Scand* 84:526–533, 2005.

Donati-Genet PCM, Ramelli GP, Bianchetti MG: A newborn infant of a diabetic mother with refractory hypocalcemic convulsions. *Eur J Pediatr* 163:759–760, 2004.

dos Santos Silva I, Higgins C, Swerdlow AJ, Laing SP, Slater SD, Pearson DWM, Morris AD: Birthweight and other pregnancy outcomes in a cohort of women with pre-gestational insulin-treated diabetes mellitus, Scotland, 1979–95. *Diabet Med* 22:440–447, 2005.

Drury MI, Greene AT, Stronge JM: Pregnancy complicated by clinical diabetes mellitus. *Obstet Gynecol* 49:519–522, 1977.

Drury MI, Stronge JM, Foley ME, MacDonald DW: Pregnancy in the diabetic patient: timing and mode of delivery. *Obstet Gynecol* 62:279–282, 1983.

Druzin ML, Foodim J: Effect of maternal glucose ingestion compared with maternal water ingestion on the nonstress test. *Obstet Gynecol* 67:425–426, 1986.

Duckitt K, Harrington D: Risk factors for preeclampsia at antenatal booking: systematic review of controlled studies. *BMJ* 330:565–572, 2005.

Dudley DKL, Black DM: Reliability of lecithin/sphingomyelin ratios in diabetic pregnancy. *Obstet Gynecol* 66:521–524 1985.

Dudley DJ: Diabetic-associated stillbirth: incidence, pathophysiology, and prevention. *Clin Perinatol* 34:611–626, 2007.

Duff P: Pathophysiology and management of post-cesarean endomyometritis. *Obstet Gynecol* 67:269–276, 1986.

Duff P: Prophylactic antibiotics for cesarean delivery: a simple cost-effective strategy for the prevention of postoperative morbidity. *Am J Obstet Gynecol* 157:794–798, 1987.

Dugoff L, Hobbins JC, Malone F, Porter TF, Luthy D, Comstock CH, Hankins G, Berkowitz RL, Merkatz I, Craigo SD, Timor-Tritsch IE, Carr SR, Wolfe HM, Vidaver J, D'Alton ME; for the FASTER Trial Research Consortium: First-trimester maternal serum PAPP-A and free-beta subunit human chorionic gonadotropin concentrations and nuchal translucency are associated with obstetric complications: a population-based screening study (The FASTER Trial). *Am J Obstet Gynecol* 191:1446–1451, 2004.

Dugoff L, Lynch AM, Cioffi-Ragan D, Hobbins JC, Schultz LK, Malone FD, D'Alton ME; for the FASTER Trial Research Consortium: First trimester uterine artery Doppler abnormalities predict subsequent intrauterine growth restriction. *Am J Obstet Gynecol* 193:1208–1212, 2005.

Duhring JL, Thompson SA: Amniotic fluid phospholipids analysis in normal and complicated pregnancies. *Am J Obstet Gynecol* 121:218–220, 1975.

Duley L, Henderson-Smart DJ: Drugs for treatment of very high blood pressure during pregnancy. *Cochrane Database Syst Rev* 2002;(4):CD 001449.

Duley L, Henderson-Smart DJ, Knight M, King JF: Antiplatelet agents for preventing pre-eclampsia and its complications. *Cochrane Database Syst Rev* 2003;(4):CD004659.

Duley L, Meher S, Abalos E: Management of preeclampsia. *BMJ* 332:463–468, 2006.

Dunn LJ, Bush C, Davis SE III, Bhatnagar AS: Use of laboratory and clinical factors in the management of pregnancies complicated by maternal disease. *Am J Obstet Gynecol* 120:622–632, 1974.

Dunne FP, Brydon PA, Proffitt M, Smith T, Gee H, Holder RL: Fetal and maternal outcomes in Indo-Asian compared to Caucasian women with diabetes in pregnancy. *QJM* 93:813–818, 2000.

East CE, Brennecke SP, King JF, Chan FY, Colditz PB; the FOREMOST Study Group: The effect of intrapartum fetal pulse oximetry, in the presence of a nonreassuring fetal heart rate pattern, on operative delivery rates: a multicenter, randomized, controlled trial (the FOREMOST trial). *Am J Obstet Gynecol* 194:606–616, 2006a.

East CE, Gascoigne MB, Doran CM, Brennecke SP, King JF, Colditz PB: A cost-effectiveness analysis of the intrapartum fetal pulse oximetry multicenter randomized controlled trial (the FOREMOST trial). *BJOG* 113:1080–1087, 2006b.

ECG—Eclampsia Collaborative Group: Which anticonvulsant for women with eclampsia? Evidence from the Collaborative Eclampsia Trial. *Lancet* 345: 1455–1463, 1995.

Ecker JL, Greenberg JA, Norwitz ER, Nadel AS, Repke JT: Birth weight as a predictor of brachial plexus injury. *Obstet Gynecol* 89:643–647, 1997.

Edelberg SC, Dierker L, Kalhan S, Rosen MG: Decreased fetal movements with sustained maternal hyperglycemia using the glucose clamp technique. *Am J Obstet Gynecol* 156:1101–1105, 1987.

Ehrenberg HM, Durnwald CP, Catalano P, Mercer BM: The influence of obesity and diabetes on the risk of cesarean delivery. *Am J Obstet Gynecol* 191:969–974, 2004.

Eichinger S: D-dimer testing in pregnancy. *Semin Vasc Med* 5:375–378, 2005.

Ekbom P, Damm P, Norgaard K, Clausen P, Feldt-Rasmussen U, Feldt-Rasmussen B, Nielsen LH, Molsted-Pedersen L, Mathiesen ER: Urinary albumin excretion and 24-hour blood pressure as predictors of preeclampsia in type 1 diabetes. *Diabetologia* 43:927–931, 2000.

Ekbom P, Damm P, Feldt-Rasmussen B, Feldt-Rasmussen U, Molvig J, Mathiesen ER: Pregnancy outcome in type 1 diabetic women with microalbuminuria. *Diabetes Care* 24:1739–1744, 2001.

Elatrous S, Nouira S, Besbes LO, Marghili S, Boussarssar M, Sakkouhi M, Abroug F: Short-term treatment of severe hypertension of pregnancy: prospective comparison of nicardipine and labetalol. *Intensive Care Med* 28:1281–1286, 2002.

Elimiam A, Garry D, Fiqueroa R, Spitzer A, Wiencek V, Quirk JG: Antenatal betamethasone compared with dexamethasone (betacode trial): a randomized controlled trial. *Obstet Gynecol* 110:26–30, 2007.

Eller DP, Stramm SL, Newman RB: The effect of maternal intravenous administration on fetal activity. *Am J Obstet Gynecol* 167:1071–1074, 1992.

Elliott JP, Garite TJ, Freeman RK, McQown DS, Patel JM: Ultrasonic prediction of fetal macrosomia in diabetic patients. *Obstet Gynecol* 60:159–162, 1982.

Elmallah KO, Narchi H, Kulayat NA, Shaban MS: Gestational and pregestational diabetes: comparison of maternal and fetal characteristics and outcome. *Int J Gynecol Obstet* 58:203–209, 1997.

Emmrich P, Fuchs U, Heinke P, Jutzi E, Godel E: The epithelial and capillary basal laminae of the placenta in maternal diabetes mellitus. *Lab Invest* 35:87–92, 1976.

Engle MJ, Perelman RH, McMahon KE, Langan SM, Farrell PM: Relationship between the severity of experimental diabetes and altered lung phospholipids metabolism. *Proc Soc Exp Biol Med* 176:261–267, 1984.

Epstein MF, Farrell PM, Chez RA: Fetal lung lecithin metabolism in the glucose intolerant rhesus monkey pregnancy. *Pediatrics* 57:722–728, 1976.

Ericksson UJ, Tyden O, Berne C: Development of phosphotidylglycerol biosynthesis in the lungs of diabetic rats. *Diabetologia* 24:202–206, 1983.

Essex NL, Pyke DA, Watkins PJ, Brudenell JM, Gamsu HR: Diabetic pregnancy. *Br Med J* 4:89–93, 1973.

Evans MI, O'Brien JE, Dvorin E, Krivchenia EL, Drugan A, Hume RF Jr, Johnson MP: Similarity of insulin-dependent diabetics' and non-insulin-dependent diabetics' levels of beta-hCG and unconjugated estriol with controls: no need to adjust as with AFP. *J Soc Gynecol Invest* 3:20–22, 1996.

Evans MI, Harrison H, O'Brien JE, Huang X, Chervanak FA, Henry GP, Wapner RJ: Maternal weight correction for alpha-fetoprotein: mathematical truncations revisited. *Genet Test* 6:221–223, 2002a.

Evans MI, Harrison HH, O'Brien JE, Dvorin E, Huang X, Krivchenia EL, Reece EA: Correction for insulin-dependent diabetes in maternal serum alpha-fetoprotein testing has outlived its usefulness. *Am J Obstet Gynecol* 187:1084–1086, 2002b.

Evers IM, Kikkels PGJ, Sikkema JM, Visser GHA: Placental pathology in women with type 1 diabetes and in a control group with normal and large-for-gestational-age infants. *Placenta* 24:819–825, 2003.

Evers IM, de Valk HW, Visser GHA: Risk of complications of pregnancy in women with type 1 diabetes: nationwide prospective study in the Netherlands. *BMJ* 328:915–918, 2004.

Fadda GM, Cherchi PL, D'Antona D, Ambrosini G, Marchesoni D, Capobianco G, Dessole S: Umbilical artery pulsatility index in pregnancies complicated by insulin-dependent diabetes mellitus without hypertension. *Gynecol Obstet Invest* 51:173–177, 2001.

Fadel HE, Saad SA, Nelson GH, Davis HC: Effect of maternal-fetal disorders on lung maturation. I. Diabetes mellitus. *Am J Obstet Gynecol* 155:544–553, 1986.

Fadini GP, Baesso I, Agostini C, Cuccato E, Nardelli GB, Lapolla A, Avogaro A: Maternal insulin therapy increases fetal endothelial progenitor cells during diabetic pregnancy. *Diabetes Care* 31:808–810, 2008.

Fairchild-Benyo D, Conrad KP: Expression of the erythropoietin receptor by trophoblast cells in the human placenta. *Biol Reprod* 60:861–870, 1999.

Farquhar JW: Prognosis for babies born to diabetic mothers in Edinburgh. *Arch Dis Child* 44:36–47, 1969.

Farrell PM, Engle MJ, Curet LB, Perelman RH, Morrison JC: Saturated phospholipids in amniotic fluid of normal and diabetic pregnancies. *Obstet Gynecol* 64:77–85, 1984.

Farrell T, Neale L, Cundy T: Congenital anomalies in the offspring of women with type 1, type 2 and gestational diabetes. *Diabet Med* 19:322–326, 2002.

Farrell T, Fraser R, Chan K: Ultrasonic fetal weight estimation in women with pregnancy complicated by diabetes. *Acta Obstet Gynecol Scand* 83:1065–1066, 2004.

Fausett MB, Vogtlander M, Lee RM, Esplin MS, Branch DW, Rodgers GN, Silver RM: Heparin-induced thrombocytopenia is rare in pregnancy. *Am J Obstet Gynecol* 185:148–152, 2001.

Feig DS, Razzaq A, Sykora K, Hux JE, Anderson GM: Trends in deliveries, prenatal care, and obstetrical complications in women with pregestational diabetes. A population-based study in Ontario, Canada, 1996–2001. *Diabetes Care* 29: 232–235, 2006.

Feldberg D, Samuel N, Peleg D, Karp M, Goldman JA: Intrapartum management of insulin-dependent diabetes mellitus (IDDM) gestants. *Acta Obstet Gynecol Scand* 67:333–338, 1988.

Ferencz C, Rubin JD, McCarter RJ, Clark EB: Maternal diabetes and cardiovascular malformations: predominance of double-outlet right ventricle and truncus arteriosus. *Teratology* 41:319–326, 1990.

Ferroni KM, Gross TL, Sokol RJ, Chik L: What affects fetal pulmonary maturation during diabetic pregnancy? *Am J Obstet Gynecol* 150:270–274, 1984.

Figueras F, Eixarch E, Meler E, Palacio M, Puerto B, Coll O, Figueras J, Cararach V, Vanrell AJ: Umbilical artery Doppler and umbilical cord pH at birth in small-for-gestational-age fetuses: valid estimate of their relationship. *J Perinat Med* 33:219–225, 2005.

Fluge G: Neurological findings at follow-up in neonatal hypoglycemia. *Acta Paediatr Scand* 64:629–634, 1975.

Fok RY, Pavlova Z, Benirschke K, Paul RH, Platt LD: The correlation of arterial lesions with umbilical artery Doppler velocimetry in the placentas of small for dates pregnancies. *Obstet Gynecol* 75:578–583, 1990.

Foley ME, Collins R, Stronge JM, Drury MI, MacDonald O: Blood viscosity in umbilical cord blood from babies of diabetic mothers. *J Obstet Gynecol* 2:93–96, 1981.

Francalanci I, Comeglio P, Liotta AA, Cellai AP, Fedi S, Parretti E, Mello G, Prisco D, Abbate R: D-dimer concentrations during normal pregnancy, as measured by ELISA. *Thromb Res* 78:399–405, 1995.

Francois R, Picaud JJ, Ruitton-Ugliengo A, David L, Cartal MJ, Bauer D: The newborn of the diabetic mothers. *Biol Neonate* 24:1–31, 1974.

Franks AL, Atrash HK, Lawson HW, Colberg KS: Obstetrical pulmonary embolism mortality, United States, 1970–85. *Am J Public Health* 80:720–721, 1990.

Fraser RB, Bruce C: Amniotic fluid insulin levels identify the fetus at risk of neonatal hypoglycemia. *Diabet Med* 16:568–572, 1999.

Freyschuss U, Gentz J, Noack G, Persson B: Circulatory adaptation in newborn infants of strictly controlled diabetic mothers. *Acta Paediatr Scand* 71:209–215, 1982.

Friedberg MK, Silverman NH: Changing indications for fetal echocardiography in a University Center population. *Prenat Diagn* 24:781–786, 2004.

Friedman EA: *Labor: Clinical Evaluation and Management.* 2nd ed. New York: Appleton-Century-Crofts; 1978:61–72.

Fuentes A, Chez RA: Role of fetal surveillance in diabetic pregnancies. *J Matern-Fetal Med* 5:85–88, 1996.

Gabbe SG, Mestman JH, Hibbard LT: Maternal mortality in diabetes mellitus: an 18-year survey. *Obstet Gynecol* 48:549–551, 1976.

Gabbe SG, Mestman JH, Freeman RK, Anderson GV, Lowensohn RI, Nochimson D, Cetrulo C, Quilligan EJ: Management and outcome of pregnancy in diabetes mellitus. Classes B to R. *Am J Obstet Gynecol* 129:723–732, 1977a.

Gabbe SG, Lowensohn RI, Mestman JH, Freeman RK, Goebelsmann U: Lecithin/sphingomyelin ratio in pregnancies complicated by diabetes mellitus. *Am J Obstet Gynecol* 128:757–760, 1977b.

Gabbe SG, Graves CR: Management of diabetes mellitus complicating pregnancy. An Expert's View. *Obstet Gynecol* 102:857–868, 2003.

Gabert HA, Bryson MJ, Stenchever MA: The effect of cesarean section on respiratory distress in the presence of a mature lecithin/sphingomyelin ratio. *Am J Obstet Gynecol* 116:366–368, 1973.

Gabrielli S, Pilu G, Reece EA: Prenatal diagnosis and management of congenital malformations in pregnancies complicated by diabetes. In: Reece EA, Coustan DR, Gabbe SG, eds. *Diabetes in Women. Adolescence, Pregnancy, and Menopause.* 3rd ed. Philadelphia: Lippincott Williams & Wilkins; 2004:300–319.

Galettis A, Campbell S, Morris JM, Jackson CJ, Twigg SM, Gallery EDM: Monocyte adhesion to decidual endothelial cells is increased in pregnancies complicated by type 1 diabetes but not by gestational diabetes. *Diabetes Care* 27:2514–2515, 2004.

Gandhi JA, Zhang XY, Maidman JE: Fetal cardiac hypertrophy and cardiac function in diabetic pregnancies. *Am J Obstet Gynecol* 173:1132–1136, 1995.

Gardiner HM, Pasquini L, Wolfenden J, Kulinskaya E, Li W, Henein M: Increased periconceptional maternal glycated hemoglobin in diabetic mothers reduces fetal long axis cardiac function. *Heart* 92:1125–1130, 2006.

Gardosi J, Geirsson RT: Routine ultrasound is the method of choice for dating pregnancy. *Br J Obstet Gynecol* 105:933–936, 1998.

Garite TJ, Dildy GA, McNamara H, Nageotte MP, Boehm FH, Dellinger EH, Knuppel RA, Porreco RP, Miller HS, Sunderji S, Varner MW, Swedlow DB: A multicenter controlled trial of fetal pulse oximetry in the intrapartum management of nonreassuring fetal heart rate patterns. *Am J Obstet Gynecol* 183:1049–1058, 2000.

Garner PR, D'Alton ME, Dudley DK, Huard P, Hardie M: Preeclampsia in diabetic pregnancies. *Am J Obstet Gynecol* 163:505–508, 1990.

Gates S, Brocklehurst P, Davis LJ: Prophylaxis for venous thromboembolic disaease in pregnancy and the early postpartum period. *Cochrane Database Syst Rev* 2002: CD001689.

Gates S, Brocklehurst P, Ayers S, Bowler U: Thromboprophylaxis and pregnancy: two randomized controlled pilot trials that used low-molecular-weight heparin. *Am J Obstet Gynecol* 191:1296–1303, 2004.

Gautier JF, Wilson C, Weyer C, Mott D, Knowler WC, Cavaghan M, Polonsky KS, Bogardus C, Pratley RE: Low acute insulin secretory responses in adult offspring of people with early onset type 2 diabetes. *Diabetes* 50:1828–1833, 2001.

Gavin LA: Perioperative management of the diabetic patient. *Endocrinol Metab Clin North Am* 21:457–475, 1992.

GDFSG—Gestation and Diabetes in France Study Group: Multicenter survey of diabetic pregnancy in France. *Diabetes Care* 14:994–1000, 1991.

Gebhardt DOE, Beintema A, Reman FC, van Gent CM: The lipoprotein composition of amniotic fluid. *Clin Chim Acta* 94:93–100, 1979.

Gebhardt DOE: Explanation for lack of agreement between lecithin/sphingomyelin ratio of amniotic fluid in diabetic pregnancies and occurrence of respiratory distress. *Am J Obstet Gynecol* 142:1068–1069, 1982.

Gelman SR, Spellacy WN, Wood S, Birk SA, Buhi WC: Fetal movement and ultrasound: effect of maternal intravenous glucose injection. *Am J Obstet Gynecol* 157:459–461, 1980.

Georgieff MK, Landon MB, Mills MM, Hedlund BE, Faassen AE, Schmidt RL, Ophoven JJ, Widness JA: Abnormal iron distribution in infants of diabetic mothers: spectrum and maternal antecedents. *J Pediatr* 117:455–461, 1990.

Ghebremeskel K, Thomas B, Lowy C, Min Y, Crawford MA: Type 1 diabetes compromises plasma arachidonic acid and docosahexanoic acids in newborn babies. *Lipids* 39:335–342, 2004.

Gherman RB, Ouzounian JG, Goodwin TM: Obstetric maneuvers for shoulder dystocia and associated fetal morbidity. *Am J Obstet Gynecol* 178:1126–1130, 1998.

Gherman RB, Goodwin TM, Leung B, Byrne JD, Hethumumi R, Montoro M: Incidence, clinical characteristics, and timing of objectively diagnosed venous thromboembolism during pregnancy. *Obstet Gynecol* 94:730–734, 1999.

Gherman RB, Tramont J, Muffley P, Goodwin TM: Analysis of McRoberts maneuver by X-ray analysis. *Obstet Gynecol* 95:43–47, 2000.

Gherman RB, Ouzounian JG, Satin AJ, Goodwin TM, Phelan JP: A comparison of shoulder dystocia-associated transient and permanent brachial plexus palsies. *Obstet Gynecol* 102:544–548, 2003.

Gherman RB, Chauhan S, Ouzounian JG, Lerner H, Gonik B, Goodwin TM: Shoulder dystocia: the unpreventable obstetric emergency with empiric management guidelines. *Am J Obstet Gynecol* 195:657–672, 2006.

Ghi T, Huggon IC, Zosmer N, Nicolaides KH: Incidence of major structural cardiac defects associated with increased nuchal translucency but normal karyotype. *Ultrasound Obstet Gynecol* 18:610–614, 2001.

Ghidini A, Spong CY, Goodwin K, Pessullo JC: Optimal thresholds of the lecithin/sphingomyelin ratio and lamellar body count for the prediction of the presence of phosphatidyl glycerol in diabetic women. *J Matern Fetal Neonatal Med* 12:95–98, 2002.

Ghidini A, Poggi SH, Spong CY, Goodwin KM, Vink J, Pezzullo JC: Role of lamellar body count for the prediction of neonatal respiratory distress syndrome in non-diabetic pregnant women. *Arch Gynecol Obstet* 271:325–328, 2005.

Gilbert WM, Nesbitt TS, Danielsen B: Associated factors in 1611 cases of brachial plexus injury. *Obstet Gynecol* 93:536–540, 1999.

Gilby JR, Williams MC, Spellacy WN: Fetal abdominal circumference measurements of 35 and 38 cm as predictors of macrosomia. A risk predictor for shoulder dystocia. *J Reprod Med* 45:936–938, 2000.

Giles WB, Trudinger BJ, Baird PJ: Fetal umbilical artery waveforms and placental resistance: pathologic correlation. *Br J Obstet Gynecol* 92:31–38, 1985.

Gillis S, Connors G, Potts P, Hunse C, Richardson B: The effect of glucose on Doppler flow velocity waveforms and heart rate pattern in the human fetus. *Early Hum Dev* 30:1–10, 1992.

Girsen A, Ala-Kopsala M, Makikallio K, Vuolteenaho O, Rasanen J: Increased fetal cardiac natriuretic peptide secretion in type-1 diabetic pregnancies. *Acta Obstet Gynecol Scand* 87:307–312, 2008.

Girz BA, Davon MY, Papajohn M, Merkatz IR: Amniotic fluid volume in diabetic pregnancy. *J Matern Fetal Invest* 1:237–240, 1992.

Gladman G, McCrindle BW, Boutin C, Smallhorn JF: Fetal echocardiographic screening of diabetic pregnancies for congenital heart disease. *Am J Perinatol* 14:59–62, 1997.

Gluck L: Biochemical development of the lung: clinical spects of surfactant development, RDS and the intrauterine assessment of lung maturity. *Clin Obstet Gynecol* 14:710–721, 1971.

Gluck L, Kulovich MV: Lecithin/sphingomyelin ratios in amniotic fluid. I. Normal and abnormal pregnancy. *Am J Obstet Gynecol* 115:539–546, 1973.

Goldberg AB, Greenberg MB, Darney PD: Misoprostol and pregnancy. *N Engl J Med* 344:38–47, 2001.

Golde SH, Vogt JF, Gabbe SG, Cabal LA: Evaluation of the FELMA microviscometer in predicting fetal lung maturity. *Obstet Gynecol* 54:639–642, 1979.

Golde SH, Good-Anderson B, Montoro M, Artal R: Insulin requirements during labor: a reappraisal. *Am J Obstet Gynecol* 144:556–559, 1982.

Golde SH, Montoro M, Good-Anderson B, Broussard P, Jacobs N, Loesser C, Trujillo M, Walla C, Phelan J, Platt LD: The role of nonstress tests, fetal biophysical profile, and contraction stress tests in the outpatient management of insulin-requiring diabetic pregnancies. *Am J Obstet Gynecol* 148:269–273, 1984.

Goldenberg RL, Davis RO, Cutter GR, Hoffman HJ, Brumfield CG, Foster JM: Prematurity, postdates, and growth retardation: the influence of use of ultrasonography on reported gestational age. *Am J Obstet Gynecol* 160:462–470, 1989.

Goldenberg RL, Mercer BM, Meis PJ, Copper RL, Das A, McNellis D; for the NICHD Maternal Fetal Medicine Units Network: The preterm prediction study: fetal fibronectin testing and spontaneous preterm birth. *Obstet Gynecol* 87:643–648, 1996.

Goldenberg RL: The management of preterm labor. *Obstet Gynecol* 100:1020–1037, 2002.

Gomez KJ, Dowdy K, Allen G, Tyson-Thomas M, Cruz AC: Evaluation of ultrasound diagnosis of fetal anomalies in women with pregestational diabetes: University of Florida experience. *Am J Obstet Gynecol* 159:584–586, 1988.

Goncalves LF, Lee W, Espinoza J, Romero R: Three- and 4-dimensional ultrasound in obstetric practice. Does it help? *J Ultrasound Med* 24:1599–1624, 2005.

Gonik B, Stringer CA, Held B: An alternate maneuver for management of shoulder dystocia. *Am J Obstet Gynecol* 145:882–884, 1983.

Gonzalez-Gonzalez NL, Ramirez O, Mozas J, Melchor J, Armas H, Garcia-Hernandez JA, Caballero A, Hernandez M, Diaz-Gomez MN, Jimenez A, Parache J, Bartha JL: Factors influencing pregnancy outcome in women with type 2 versus type 1 diabetes mellitus. *Acta Obstet Gynecol Scand* 87:43–49, 2008.

Gonzalez-Quintero VH, Istwan NB, Rhea DJ, Smarkusky L, Hoffman MC, Stanziano GJ: Gestational age at initiation of 17-hydroxyprogesterone caproate (17P) and recurret delivery. *J Matern-Fetal Neonatal Med* 20:249–252, 2007.

Gordin D, Hiilesmaa V, Fagerudd J, Ronnback M, Forsblom C, Kaaja R, Teramo K, Groop PH; FinnDiane Study Group: Preeclampsia but not pregnancy-induced hypertension is a risk factor for diabetic nephropathy in type 1 diabetic women. *Diabetologia* 50:516–522, 2007.

Graca LM, Meirinho M, Sanches JF, Saraiva J: Modification of fetal activity for an intravenous glucose load to the mothers. *J Perinat Med* 9:286–292, 1981.

Graham EM, Forouzan I, Morgan MA: A retrospective analysis of Erb's palsy cases and their relation to birth weight and trauma at delivery. *J Matern-Fetal Med* 6:1–5, 1997.

Graham WJ: Now or never: the case for measuring maternal mortality. *Lancet* 359:701–704, 2002.

Graham EM, Petersen SM, Christo DK, Fox HE: Intrapartum electronic fetal heart rate monitoring and the prevention of perinatal brain injury. Review. *Obstet Gynecol* 108:656–666, 2006.

Graves CR: Antepartum fetal surveillance and timing of delivery in the pregnancy complicated by diabetes mellitus. *Clin Obstet Gynecol* 50:1007–1013, 2007.

Gray G, Ash AK: A survey of pregnant women on the use of graduated elastic compression stockings on the antenatal ward. *J Obstet Gynecol* 26:424–428, 2006.

Greco P, Vimercati A, Scioscia M, Rossi AC, Giorgino F, Selvaggi L: Timing of fetal growth acceleration in women with insulin-dependent diabetes. *Fetal Diagn Ther* 18:437–441, 2003.

Greene MF, Haddow JE, Palomaki GE, Knight GJ: Maternal serum alpha-fetoprotein levels in diabetic pregnancies. *Lancet* 2:345–346, 1988.

Greene MF, Hare JW, Krache M, Phillippe M, Barss VA, Saltzman DH, Nadel A, Younger MD, Heffner L, Scherl E: Prematurity among insulin-requiring diabetic gravid women. *Am J Obstet Gynecol* 161:106–111, 1989.

Greene MF, Benacerraf BR: Prenatal diagnosis in diabetic gravidas: utility of ultrasound and maternal serum alpha-fetoprotein screening. *Obstet Gynecol* 77:520–524, 1991.

Greene MF, Allred EN, Leviton A: Maternal metabolic control and risk of microcephaly among infants of diabetic mothers. *Diabetes Care* 18:166–169, 1995.

Gregory KD, Henry OA, Ramicone E, Chan LS, Platt LD: Maternal and infant complications in high and normal weight infants by method of delivery. *Obstet Gynecol* 92:507–513, 1998.

Greisen J, Juhl CB, Grofte T, Vilstrup H, Jensen TS, Schmitz O: Acute pain induces insulin resistance in humans. *Anesthesiology* 95:578–584, 2001.

Grimes, DA Schulz KF: Refining clinical diagnosis with likelihood ratios. *Lancet* 365:1500–1505, 2005.

GRIT Study Group: A randomized trial of timed delivery for the compromised preterm fetus: short term outcomes and Bayesian interpretation. *BJOG* 110:27–32, 2003.

Gross TL, Sokol RJ, Kwong MS, Wilson M, Kuhnert PM: Transient tachypnea of the newborn: the relationship to preterm delivery and significant neonatal morbidity. *Am J Obstet Gynecol* 146:236–241, 1983.

Grunewald C, Divon M, Lunell NO: Doppler velocimetry in last trimester pregnancy complicated by insulin-dependent diabetes mellitus. *Acta Obstet Gynecol Scand* 75:804–808, 1996.

Gudmunnsson S, Henningsson A-C, Lindqvist P: Correlation of birth injury with maternal height and birthweight. *BJOG* 112:764–767, 2005.

Guenter HH, Scharf A, Hertel H, Hillemanns P, Wenzlaff P, Maul H: Perinatal morbidity in pregnancies of women with preconceptional and gestational diabetes mellitus in comparison with pregnancies of non-diabetic women. Results of the perinatal registry of Lower Saxony, Germany. *Z Geburtshilfe Neonatol* 210:200–207, 2006.

Guerin A, Nisembaum R, Ray JG: Use of GHb concentration to estimate the risk of congenital anomalies in the offspring of women with prepregnancy diabetes. *Diabetes Care* 30:1920–1925, 2007.

Guinn DA: Repeat courses of antenatal corticosteroids: the controversy continues. *Am J Obstet Gynecol* 190:587–588, 2004.

Gundogdu AS, Brown PM, Juul S, Sachs L, Sonksen PH: Comparison of hormonal and metabolic effects of salbutamol infusion in normal subjects and insulin-requiring diabetics. *Lancet* 29:1317–1321, 1979.

Gupta S, Agarwal A, Sharma RK: The role of placental oxidative stress and lipid peroxidation in preeclampsia. *Obstet Gynecol Surv* 60:807–816, 2005.

Guttentag SH, Phelps DS, Warshaw JB, Floros J: Delayed hydrophobic surfactant protein (SP-B, Sp-C) expression in fetuses of streptozotocin-treated rats. *Am J Respir Cell Mol Biol* 7:190–197, 1992.

Hackmon R, Bornstein E, Ferber A, Horani J, O'Reilly-Green CP, Divon MY: Combined analysis with amniotic fluid index and estimated fetal weight for prediction of severe macrosomia at birth. *Am J Obstet Gynecol* 196:333.e1–333.e4, 2007.

Haddad B, Uzan M, Tchobroutsky C, Uzan S, Papiernik-Berkauer E: Predictive value of uterine artery Doppler waveform during pregnancies complicated by diabetes. *Fetal Diag Ther* 8:119–125, 1993.

Hadden DR, Byrne E, Trotter I, Harley JMG, McClure G, McAuley RR: Physical and psychological health of children of type 1 (insulin-dependent) diabetic mothers. *Diabetologia* 26:250–254, 1984.

Hadden DR, Alexander A, McCance DR, Traub AI; on behalf of the Northern Ireland Diabetes Group and the Ulster Obstetrical Society: Obstetric and diabetic care for pregnancy in diabetic women: 10-year outcome analysis, 1985–1995. *Diabet Med* 18:546–553, 2001.

Hagbard L, Olow I, Reinard T: A follow-up study of 514 children of diabetic mothers. *Acta Paediatr Scand* 48:184–197, 1959.

Hagen E, Link JC, Arias F: A comparison of the accuracy of the TDx-FLM assay, lecithin-sphingomyelin ratio, and phosphatidylglycerol in the prediction of neonatal respiratory distress syndrome. *Obstet Gynecol* 82:1004–1008, 1993.

Haigh SE, Tevaarwerk GJ, Harding PE, Hurst C: A method for maintaining noemoglycemia during labor and delivery in insulin-dependent diabetic women. *Can Med Assoc J* 126:487–490, 1982.

Hales CN, Barker DJ, Clark PM, Cox LJ, Fall C, Osmond C, Winter PD: Fetal and infant growth and impaired glucose tolerance at age 64. *BMJ* 303:1019–1022, 1991.

Hall RT, Rhodes PG, Newman RL: Glucose disappearance in infants of diabetic mothers. II. Relationship to lowest neonatal blood glucose and amniotic fluid insulin. *Early Hum Dev* 1:257–264, 1977.

Hall RT, Rhodes RG, Sheehan MB, Braun WJ: Glucose disappearance rates in infants of diabetic mothers. III. Relationship of spontaneous glucose disappearance to glucose tolerance, neonatal hypoglycemia and lowest blood glucose. *Early Hum Dev* 4:187–194, 1980.

Hall DA, Wadwa RP, Gondenberg NA, Norris JM: Maternal risk factors for term neonatal seizures: population-based study in Colorado, 1989–2003. *J Child Neurol* 21:795–798, 2006.

Hallman M, Gluck L: Phosphatidyl glycerol in lung surfactant: III. Possible modifier of surfactant function. *J Lipid Res* 17:257–262, 1976.

Hallman M, Teramo K: Amniotic fluid phopholipid profile as a predictor of fetal maturity in diabetic pregnancies. *Obstet Gynecol* 54:703–707, 1979.

Hallman M, Enhorning G, Possmayer F: Composition and surface activity of normal and phosphatidylglycerol-deficient lung surfactant. *Pediatr Res* 19:286–292, 1985.

Hallman M, Ariomaa P, Hoppu K, Teramo K, Akino T: Surfactant proteins in the diagnosis of fetal lung maturity. II. The 35 kd protein and phospholipids in complicated pregnancy. *Am J Obstet Gynecol* 161:965–969, 1989.

Halse KG, Lindegaard ML, Goetze JP, Damm P, Mathiesen ER, Nielsen LB: Increased plasma pro-B-type natriuretic peptide in infants of women with type 1 diabetes. *Clin Chem* 51:2296–2302, 2005.

Hampl V, Bibova J, Stranak Z, Wu X, Michelakis E, Hashimoto K, Archer SL: Hypoxic fetoplacental vasoconstriction in humans is mediated by potassium channel inhibition. *Am J Physiol* 283:H2440–H2449, 2002.

Hankins GD, Clark SM, Munn MB: Cesarian section on request at 39 weeks: impact on shoulder dystocia, fetal trauma, neonatal encephalopathy, and intrauterine fetal demise. *Semin Perinatol* 30:276–287, 2006.

Hansen AK, Wisborg K, Uldbjerg N, Henriksen TB: Risk of respiratory morbidity in term infants delivered by elective cesarean section: cohort study. *BMJ* 336:85–87, 2008.

Hanson U, Persson B: Outcome of pregnancies complicated by type 1 insulin-dependent diabetes in Sweden: acute pregnancy complications, neonatal mortality and morbidity. *Am J Perinatol* 10:330–333, 1993.

Hanson U, Persson B: Epidemiology of pregnancy-induced hypertension and preeclampsia in type 1 (insulin-dependent) diabetic pregnancies in Sweden. *Acta Obstet Gynecol Scand* 77:620–624, 1998.

Harman CR, Menticoglou SM: Fetal surveillance in diabetic pregnancy. *Curr Opin Obstet Gynecol* 9:83–90, 1997.

Harrington K, Goldfrad C, Carpenter RG, Campbell S: Transvaginal uterine and umbilical artery Doppler examination of 12–16 weeks and the subsequent development of preeclampsia and intrauterine growth retardation. *Ultrasound Obstet Gynecol* 9:94–100, 1997.

Hawkins JL, Koonin LM, Palmer SK, Gibbs CP: Anesthesia-related deaths during obstetric delivery in the United States, 1979–1990. *Anesthesiology* 86:277–284, 1997.

Hawkins JS, Casey BM: Labor and delivery management for women with diabetes. *Obstet Gynecol Clin North Am* 34:323–334, 2007.

Haworth JC, McRae KN, Dilling LA: Prognosis of infants of diabetic mothers in relation to neonatal hypoglycemia. *Dev Med Child Neurol* 18:471–479, 1976.

Hay W, Digiacomo Meznarich HK, Hirst K, Zerbe G: Effects of glucose and insulin on fetal glucose oxidation and oxygen consumption. *Am J Physiol* 256: E704–E713, 1989.

Hecher K, Campbell S, Doyle P, Harrington K, Nicolaides K: Assessment of fetal compromise by Doppler ultrasound investigation of the fetal circulation: arterial, intracardiac, and venous blood flow velocity studies. *Circulation* 91:129–138, 1995a.

Hecher K, Snijders R, Campbell S, Nicolaides K: Fetal venous, intracardiac, and arterial blood flow measurements in intrauterine growth retardation: relationship with fetal blood gases. *Am J Obstet Gynecol* 173:10–15, 1995b.

Heimberger CM, Ghidini A, Lewis KM, Spong CY: Glycosylated hemoglobin as a predictor of fetal pulmonic maturity in insulin-dependent diabetes at term. *Am J Perinatol* 16:257–260, 1999.

Heit JA, Kobbervig CE, James AH, Petterson TM, Bailey KR, Melton LJ 3rd: Trends in the incidence of venous thromboembolism during pregnancy or postpartum: a 30–year population-based study. *Ann Intern Med* 143:697–706, 2005.

Henriques CU, Damm P, Tabor A, Pedersen JF, Molsted-Pedersen L: Decreased alpha-fetoprotein in amniotic fluid and maternal serum in diabetic pregnancy. *Obstet Gynecol* 82:960–964, 1993.

Herbert WNP, Chapman JF, Schnoor MM: Role of the TDx-FLM assay in fetal lung maturity. *Am J Obstet Gynecol* 168:808–812, 1993.

Hertel J, Andersen GE, Brandt NJ, Christensen E, Kuhl C, Molsted-Pedersen L: Metabolic events in infants of diabetic mothers during first 24 hours after birth. III. Changes in plasma amino acids. *Acta Paediatr Scand* 71:33–37, 1982.

Hertel J, Kuhl C, Christensen NJ, Pedersen SA: Plasma noradrenaline and adrenaline in newborn infants of diabetic mothers: relation to plasma lipids. *Acta Paediatr Scand* 74:521–524, 1985.

Hertel J, Kuhl C: Metabolic adaptations during the neonatal period in infants of diabetic mothers. *Acta Endocrinol Suppl (Copenh)* 277:136–140, 1986.

Hiilesmaa V, Suhonen L, Teramo K: Glycemic control is associated with preeclampsia but not with pregnancy-induced hypertension in women with type 1 diabetes mellitus. *Diabetologia* 43:1534–1539, 2000.

Hillier TA, Pedula KL, Schmidt MM, Mullen JA, Charles M-A, Pettitt DJ: Childhood obesity and metabolic imprinting. The ongoing effects of maternal hyperglycemia. *Diabetes Care* 30:2287–2292, 2007.

Hirsch IB, McGill JB, Cryer PE, White PF: Perioperative management of surgical patients with diabetes mellitus. *Anesthesiology* 74:346–359, 1991.

Hod M, Bar J, Peled Y, Fried S, Katz I, Itzhak M, Ashkenazi S, Schindel B, Ben-Rafael Z: Antepartum management protocol. Timing and mode of delivery in gestational diabetes. *Diabetes Care* 21 (Suppl 2):B113–B117, 1998.

Hod M, Kerner R: Telemedicine for antenatal surveillance of high-risk pregnancies with ambulatory and home fetal heart rate recording: an update. *J Perinat Med* 31:195–200, 2003.

Hofmeyr GJ, Atallah A, Duley L: Calcium supplementation during pregnancy for preventing hypertensive disorders and related problems (Cochrane Review). In: *The Cochrane Library*, Issue 1. Chichester, UK: John Wiley and Sons; 2005.

Hofmeyr GJ, Duley L, Atallah A: Dietary calcium supplementation for prevention of preeclampsia and related problems: a systematic review and commentary. *BJOG* 114:933–943, 2007.

Hofstaetter C, Gudmundsson S, Hansmann M: Venous Doppler velocimetry in the surveillance of severely compromised fetuses. *Ultrasound Obstet Gynecol* 20:233–239, 2002.

Hogan K, Rusy D, Springman SR: Difficult laryngoscopy and diabetes mellitus. *Anesth Analg* 67:1162–1165, 1988.

Hogg B, Hauth JC, Caritis SN, Sibai BM, Lindheimer M, Van Dorsten JP, Klebanoff M, MacPherson C, Landon M, Paul R, Miodovnik M, Meis PJ, Thurnau GR, Dombrowski MP, McNellis D, Roberts JM; for the National Institute of Child Health and Human Development Maternal-Fetal Medicine Units Network: Safety of labor epidural anesthesia for women with severe hypertensive disease. *Am J Obstet Gynecol* 181:1096–1101, 1999.

Hokegard KH, Eriksson BO, Kjellmer I, Magno R, Rosen KG: Myocardial metabolism in relation to electrocardiographic changes and cardiac function during graded hypoxia in the fetal lamb. *Acta Physiol Scand* 113:1–7, 1981.

Holcomb WL, Mostello DJ, Gray DL: Abdominal circumference vs. estimated weight to predict large for gestational age birth weight in diabetic pregnancy. *J Clin Imaging* 24:1–7, 2000.

Holden KP, Jovanovic L, Druzin ML, Peterson CM: Increased fetal activity with low maternal blood glucose levels in pregnancies complicated by diabetes. *Am J Perinatol* 1:161–164, 1984.

Holmgren C, Lacoursiere DY: The use of prenatal ultrasound for the detection of fetal aneuploidy. *Clin Obstet Gynecol* 51:48–61, 2008.

Hook B, Kiwi R, Amini SB, Fanaroff A, Hack M: Neonatal morbidity after elective repeat cesarean section and trial of labor. *Pediatrics* 100:348–353, 1997.

Hopkins L, Smaill F: Antibiotic prophylaxis regimens and drugs for cesarean section (Cochrane Review). In: *The Cochrane Library,* Issue 2. Oxford: Update Software; 2003.

Howarth C, Gazis A, James D: Associations of type 1 diabetes mellitus, maternal vascular disease and complications of pregnancy. *Diabet Med* 24:1229–1234, 2007.

Hsu C-D, Tan HY, Hong SF, Nickless NA, Copel JA: Strategies for reducing the frequency of preeclampsia in pregnancies with insulin-dependent diabetes mellitus. *Am J Perinatol* 13:265–268, 1996.

Hsu C-D, Hong S-F, Nickless NA, Copel JA: Glycosylated hemoglobin in insulin-dependent diabetes mellitus related to preeclampsia. *Am J Perinatol* 15:199–202, 1998.

Huch A, Huch R, Rooth G: Guidelines for blood sampling and measurement of pH and blood gas values in obstetrics. Based upon a workshop held in Zurich March 19, 1993 by an *ad hoc* committee. *Eur J Obstet Gynecol Reprod Biol* 54:165–175, 1994.

Hudelist G, Gelle'n J, Singer C, Ruecklinger E, Czerwenka K, Kandolf O, Keckstein J: Factors predicting severe perineal trauma during childbirth: role of forceps delivery routine combined with mediolateral episiotomy. *Am J Obstet Gynecol* 192:875–881, 2005.

Hughes SC, Ward MG, Levinson G, Shnider SM, Wright RG, Gruenke LD, Craig JC: Placental transfer of ephedrine does not affect neonatal outcome. *Anesthesiology* 63:217–219, 1985.

Hunter DJS, Burrows RF, Mohide PT, Whyte RK: Influence of maternal insulin-dependent diabetes mellitus on neonatal morbidity. *Can Med Assoc J* 149:47–52, 1993.

Hunter WA, Cundy T, Rabone D, Hofman PL, Harris M, Regan F, Robinson E, Cutfield WS: Insulin sensitivity in the offspring of women with type 1 and type 2 diabetes. *Diabetes Care* 27:1148–1152, 2004.

Huovinen K, Lehtovirta P, Forss M: Changes in placental intervillous blood flow measured by the 133xenon method during lumbar epidural block for elective cesarean section. *Acta Anesthesiol Scand* 23:529–533, 1979.

Iams JD: Prediction and early detection of preterm labor. *Obstet Gynecol* 101:402–412, 2003.

Impey L: Severe hypotension and fetal distress following sublingual administration of nifedipine to a patient with severe pregnancy induced hypertension at 33 weeks. *Br J Obstet Gynecol* 100:959–961, 1993.

Incerpi MH, Fassett MJ, Kjos SL, Tran SH, Wing DA: Vaginally administered misoprostol for outpatient cervical ripening in pregnancies complicated by diabetes mellitus. *Am J Obstet Gynecol* 185:916–918, 2001.

Inkster ME, Fahey TP, Donnan PT, Leese GP, Mires GJ, Murphy DJ: Poor glycated hemoglobin control and adverse pregnancy outcomes in type 1 and type 2 diabetes mellitus: systematic review of observational studies. *BMC Pregnancy and Childbirth* 6:30, 2006. doi:10.1186/1471-2393-6-30, www.biomedcentral.com. Accessed Apr 22, 2008.

Irwin JC, Suen LF, Martina NA, Mark SP, Guidice LC: Role of the IGF system in trophoblast invasion and preeclampsia. *Hum Reprod* 14:S90–S96, 1999.

Ishimatsu J, Yoshimura O, Manabe A, Hotta M, Matsunaga T, Matsuzaki T, Tetsuou M, Hamada T: Umbilical artery blood flow velocity waveforms in pregnancy complicated by diabetes mellitus. *Arch Gynecol Obstet* 248:123–127, 1991.

Ishimatsu J, Matsuzaki T, Yakushiji M, Hamada T: Blood flow velocity waveforms of the middle cerebral artery in pregnancies complicated by diabetes mellitus. *Kurume Med J* 42:161–166, 1995.

Ivanisevic M, Djelmis J, Jalsovec D, Blijic D: Ultrasonic morphological characteristics of yolk sac in pregnancy complicated by type 1 diabetes mellitus. *Gynecol Obstet Invest* 61:80–86, 2006.

Ivie WM, Swanson JR: Effect of albumin and lamellar bodies on fluorescence polarization of amniotic fluid. *Clin Chem* 33:1194–1197, 1987.

Jacobsen AF, Drolsum A, Klow NE, Dahl GF, Qvigstad E, Sandset PM: Deep vein thrombosis after elective cesarean section. *Thromb Res* 113:283–288, 2004.

Jacobsen AF, Skjeldestad FE, Sandset PM: Incidence and risk patterns of venous thromboembolism in pregnancy and puerperium—register-based case-control study. *Am J Obstet Gynecol* 198:233.e1–7, 2008.

Jaffe R: Identification of fetal growth abnormalities in diabetes mellitus. *Semin Perinatol* 26:190–195, 2002.

Jain V, Lim M, Longo M, Fisk NM: Inhibitory effect of erythropoietin on contractility of human chorionic plate vessels. *Am J Obstet Gynecol* 194:246–251, 2006.

James DK, Chiswick ML, Harkes A, Williams M, Tindall VR: Maternal diabetes and neonatal respiratory distress. I. Maturation of fetal surfactant. *Br J Obstet Gynecol* 91:316–324, 1984a.

James DK, Chiswick ML, Harkes A, Williams M: Maternal diabetes and prediction of neonatal respiratory distress, II: prediction of fetal lung maturity. *Br J Obstet Gynecol* 91:325–329, 1984b.

James AH, Tapson VF, Goldhaber SZ: Thrombosis during pregnancy and the postpartum period. *Am J Obstet Gynecol* 193:216–219, 2005.

James AH, Jamison MG, Brancazio LR, Myers ER: Venous thromboembolism during pregnancy and the postpartum period: incidence, risk factors, and mortality. *Am J Obstet Gynecol* 194:1311–1315, 2006a.

James AH, Jamison MG, Biswas MS, Brancazio LR, Swamy GK, Myers ER: Acute myocardial infarction in pregnancy. A United States population-based study. *Circulation* 113:1564–1571, 2006b.

Janota J, Pomyje J, Toth D, Sosna O, Zivny J, Kuzel D, Stranak Z, Necas E, Zivny JH: Expression of angiopoietic factors in normal and type-1 diabetes human placenta: a pilot study. *Eur J Obstet Gynecol Reprod Biol* 111:153–156, 2003.

Jazayeri A, O'Brien WF, Tsibris JCM, Spellacy WN: Are maternal diabetes and preeclampsia independent stimulators of fetal erythropoietin production? *Am J Perinatol* 15:577–580, 1998.

Jazayeri A, Heffron JA, Phillips R, Spellacy WN: Macrosomia prediction using ultrasound fetal abdominal circumference of 35 centimeters or more. *Obstet Gynecol* 93:523–526, 1999.

Jennett RJ, Tarby TJ, Kreinick CJ: Brachial plexus palsy: an old problem revisited. *Am J Obstet Gynecol* 166:1673–1677, 1992.

Jensen DM, Damm P, Molsted-Pedersen L, Ovesen P, Westergaard JG, Moeller M, Beck-Nielsen H: Outcomes in type 1 diabetic pregnancies. A nationwide, population-based study. *Diabetes Care* 27:2819–2823, 2004.

Jeremy JY, Mikhalidis DP, Dandona P: Simulating the diabetic environment modifies in vitro prostaglandin synthesis. *Diabetes* 32:217–221, 1983.

Jervell J, Moe N, Skjaeraasen J, Blystad W, Egge K: Diabetes mellitus and pregnancy—management and results at Rikshospitalet, Oslo, 1970–77. *Diabetologia* 16:151–155, 1979.

Jobe AH, Soll RF: Choice and dose of corticosteroids for antenatal treatments. *Am J Obstet Gynecol* 190:878–881, 2004.

Johnson JW, Austin KL, Jones GS, Davis GH, King TM: Efficacy of 17-alpha-hydroxyprogesterone caproate in the prevention of premature labor. *N Engl J Med* 293:675–680, 1975.

Johnson JM, Lange IR, Harman CR, Torchia MG, Manning FA: Biophysical profile scoring in the management of the diabetic pregnancy. *Obstet Gynecol* 72: 841–846, 1988.

Johnson B, Simpson LL: Screening for congenital heart disease: a move toward earlier echocardiography. *Am J Perinatol* 24:449–456, 2007.

Johnstone FD, Steel JM, Haddad NG, Hoskins PR, Greer IA, Chambers S: Doppler umbilical artery flow velocity waveforms in diabetic pregnancy. *Br J Obstet Gynecol* 99:135–140, 1992.

Johnstone FD, Prescott RJ, Steel JM, Mao JH, Chambers S, Muir N: Clinical and ultrasound prediction of macrosomia in diabetic pregnancy. *Br J Obstet Gynecol* 103:747–754, 1996.

Jonasson JM, Brismar K, Sparen P, Lambe M, Nyren O, Ostenson C-G, Ye W: Fertility in women with type 1 diabetes. A population-based cohort study in Sweden. *Diabetes Care* 30:2271–2276, 2007.

Jones CJP, Fox H: An ultrastructural and ultrahistochemical study of the placenta of the diabetic woman. *J Pathol* 119:91–99, 1976.

Jorge CS, Artal R, Paul RH, Goebelsmann U, Gratacos J, Yeh SY, Golde SH, Mestman JH: Antepartum fetal surveillance in diabetic pregnant patients. *Am J Obstet Gynecol* 141:641–645, 1981.

Jovanovic L, Peterson CM: Management of the pregnant, insulin-dependent diabetic woman. *Diabetes Care* 3:63–68, 1980.

Jovanovic L, Peterson CM: Insulin and glucose requirements during the first stage of labor in insulin-dependent diabetic women. *Am J Med* 75:607–612, 1983.

Jovanovic L: Glucose and insulin requirements during labor and delivery: the case for normoglycemia in pregnancies complicated by diabetes. *Endocr Pract* 10 (Suppl 2):40–45, 2004.

Jovanovic L, Knopp RH, Kim H, Cefalu WT, Zhu X-D, Lee YJ, Simpson JL, Mills JL; for the Diabetes in Early Pregnancy Study Group: Elevated pregnancy losses at high and low extremes of maternal glucose in early normal and diabetic pregnancy. Evidence for a protective adaptation in diabetes. *Diabetes Care* 28:1113–1117, 2005.

Kagan KO, Avgidou K, Molina FS, Gajewska K, Nicolaides KH: Relation between increased fetal nuchal translucency thickness and chromosomal defects. *Obstet Gynecol* 107:6–10, 2006.

Kaijser M, Edstedt-Bonamy A-K, Akre O, Cnattingius S, Granath F, Norman M, Ekbom A: Perinatal risk factors for ischemic heart disease. Disentangling the roles of birth weight and preterm birth. *Circulation* 117:405–410, 2008.

Kainer F, Weiss PAM, Huettner U, Haas J: Ultrasound growth parameters in relation to levels of amniotic fluid insulin in women with diabetes type 1. *Early Hum Dev* 49:113–121, 1997.

Kairamkonda V, Deorukhkar A, Coombs R, Fraser R, Mayer T: Amylin peptide levels are raised in infants of diabetic mothers. *Arch Dis Child* 90:1279–1282, 2005.

Kalhan SC, Savin SM, Adam PAJ: Attenuated glucose production rate in newborn infants of insulin-dependent diabetic mothers. *N Engl J Med* 296:375–376, 1977.

Kalhan S, Peter-Wohl S: Hypoglycemia: what is it for the neonate? *Am J Perinatol* 17:11–18, 2000a.

Kalhan S, Parimi P: Gluconeogenesis in the fetus and neonate. *Semin Perinatol* 24:94–106, 2000b.

Karcher R, Sykes E, Batton D, Uddin Z, Ross G, Hockman E, Shade GH Jr: Gestational age-specific predicted risk of neonatal respiratory distress syndrome using lamellar body count and surfactant-to-albumin ratio in amniotic fluid. *Am J Obstet Gynecol* 193:1680–1684, 2005.

Kariniemi V, Forss M, Siegberg R, Ammala P: Reduced short-term variability of fetal heart rate in association with maternal hyperglycemia during pregnancy in insulin-dependent diabetic women. *Am J Obstet Gynecol* 147:793–794, 1983.

Karlsson K, Kjellmer I: The outcome of diabetic pregnancies in relation to the mother's blood sugar level. *Am J Obstet Gynecol* 112:213–220, 1972.

Katyal SL, Amenta JS, Singh G, Silverman JA: Deficient lung surfactant apoproteins in amniotic fluid with mature phospholipids profile from diabetic pregnancies. *Am J Obstet Gynecol* 148:48–53, 1984.

Kaufman I, Bondy R, Benjamin A: Peripartum cardiomyopathy and thromboembolism; anesthetic management and clinical course of an obese, diabetic patient. *Can J Anaesth* 50:161–165, 2003.

Kaushal K, Gibson JH, Railton A, Hounsome B, New JP, Young HJ: A protocol for improved glycemic control following corticosteroid therapy in diabetic pregnancies. *Diabet Med* 20:73–75, 2003.

Kearon C, Ginsberg JS, Douketis J, Turpie AG, Bates SM, Lee AY, Crowther MA, Weitz JI, Brill-Edwards P, Wells P, Anderson DR, Kovacs MJ, Linkins LA, Julian JA, Bonilla LR, Gent M; Canadian Pulmonary Embolism Diagnosis Study (CANPEDS) Group: An evaluation of D-dimer in the diagnosis of pulmonary embolism: a randomized trial. *Ann Intern Med* 144:812–821, 2006.

Kehl RJ, Krew MA, Thomas A, Catalano PM: Fetal growth and body composition in infants of women with diabetes mellitus during pregnancy. *J Matern-Fetal Med* 5:273–280, 1996.

Keller JD, Metxger BE, Dooley SL, Tamura RK, Sabbagha RE, Freinkel N: Infants of diabetic mothers with accelerated fetal growth by ultrasonography: are they all alike? *Am J Obstet Gynecol* 163:893–897, 1990.

Kenepp NB, Shelley WC, Kumar S, Gutsche BB, Gabbe S, Delivoria-Papadopoulos MD: Effects on newborn of hydration with glucose in patients undergoing cesarean section with regional anesthesia. *Lancet* 1:645, 1980.

Kesselman EJ, Figueroa R, Garry D, Maulik D: The usefulness of the TDX/TDxFLx Fetal Lung Maturity II assay in the initial evaluation of fetal lung maturity. *Am J Obstet Gynecol* 188:1220–1222, 2003.

Keszler M, Carbone MT, Cox C, Schumacher RE: Severe respiratory failure after elective repeat cesarean delivery: a potentially preventable condition leading to extracorporeal membrane oxygenation. *Pediatrics* 89:670–672, 1992.

Khalish RB, Thaler HT, Chasen ST, Gupta M, Berman SJ, Rosenwaks Z, Chervenak FA: First- and second-trimester ultrasound assessment of gestational age. *Am J Obstet Gynecol* 191:975–978, 2004.

Kilby MD, Neary RH, Mackness MI, Durrington PN: Fetal and maternal lipoprotein metabolism in human pregnancy complicated by type 1 diabetes mellitus. *J Clin Endocrinol Metab* 83:1736–1741, 1998.

King KC, Tsung K-Y, Kalhan SC: Regulation of glucose production in newborn infants of diabetic mothers. *Pediatr Res* 16:608–612, 1982.

King JF, Flenady VJ, Papatsonis DNM, Dekker G, Carbonne B: Calcium channel blockers for inhibiting preterm labour; a systematic review of the evidence and a protocol for administration of nifedipine. *Aust N Z J Obstet Gynaecol* 43: 192–198, 2003.

Kitzmiller JL, Cloherty JP, Younger MD, Tabatabaii A, Rothchild SB, Sosenko I, Epstein MF, Singh S, Neff RK: Diabetic pregnancy and perinatal morbidity. *Am J Obstet Gynecol* 131:560–580, 1978.

Kitzmiller JL, Watt N, Driscoll SG: Decidual arteriopathy in hypertension and diabetes in pregnancy: immunofluorescent studies. *Am J Obstet Gynecol* 141: 773–779, 1981.

Kitzmiller JL, Mall JC, Gin GD, Hendricks SK, Newman RB, Scheerer L: Measurement of fetal shoulder width with computed tomography in diabetic women. *Obstet Gynecol* 70:941–945, 1987.

Kitzmiller JL, Combs CA, Buchanan TA, Kjos S, Ratner RE: Preconception care of diabetes, congenital malformations, and spontaneous abortions. Technical Review. *Diabetes Care* 19:514–541, 1996.

Kitzmiller JL, Gavin L: Preexisting diabctes and pregnancy. In Lavin N, ed. *Manual of Endocrinology and Metabolism.* 3rd ed. Philadelphia: Lipincott Williams & Wilkins; 2002:660–665.

Kjos SL, Walther FJ, Montoro M, Paul RH, Diaz F, Stabler M: Prevalence and etiology of respiratory distress in infants of diabetic mothers: predictive value of fetal lung maturation tests. *Am J Obstet Gynecol* 163:898–903, 1990.

Kjos SL, Henry OA, Montoro M, Buchanan TA, Mestman JH: Insulin-requiring diabetes in pregnancy: a randomized trial of active induction of labor and expectant management. *Am J Obstet Gynecol* 169:611–615, 1993.

Kjos SL, Leung A, Henry OA, Victor MR, Paul RH, Medearis AL: Antepartum surveillance in diabetic pregnancies: predictors of fetal distress in labor. *Am J Obstet Gynecol* 173:1532–1539, 1995.

Kjos SL, Berkowitz KM, Kung B: Prospective delivery of reliably dated term infants of diabetic mothers without determination of fetal lung maturity: comparison to historical controls. *J Matern Fetal Neonatal Med* 12:433–437, 2002.

Kjos SL, Berkowitz K, Xiang A: Independent predictors of cesarean delivery in women with diabetes. *J Matern-Fetal Med* 15:61–67, 2004.

Kline JA, Williams GW, Hernandez-Nino J: D-dimer concentrations in normal pregnancy: new diagnostic thresholds are needed. *Clin Chem* 51:825–829, 2005.

Klupa T, Warram JH, Antonellis A, Pezzolesi M, Nam M, Malecki MT, Doria A, Rich SS, Krolewski AS: Determinants of the development of diabetes (maturity-onset diabetes of the young-3) in carriers of HNF-1α mutations: evidence for parent-of-origin effect. *Diabetes Care* 25:2292–2301, 2002.

Knip M, Lautala P, Leppaluoto J, Akerblom HK, Kouvalainen K: Relation of enteroinsular hormones at birth to macrosomia and neonatal hypoglycemia in infants of diabetic mothers. *J Pediatr* 103:603–611, 1983.

Knip M, Kaapa P, Koivisto M: Hormonal enteroinsular axis in newborn infants of insulin-treated diabetic mothers. *J Clin Endocrinol Metab* 77:1340–1344, 1993.

Kofinas A, Penry M, Swain M: Uteroplacental Doppler flow velocity waveform analysis correlates poorly with glycemic control in diabetic pregnant women. *Am J Perinatol* 8:273–277, 1991.

Koivisto M, Blanco-Sequerios M, Krause U: Neonatal symptomatic and asymptomatic hypoglycemia: a follow-up study of 151 children. *Dev Med Child Neurol* 5:610–614, 1972.

Kontopolous EV, Vintzileos AM: Condition-specific antepartum fetal testing. *Am J Obstet Gynecol* 191:1546–1551, 2004.

Kossenjans W, Eis A, Sahay R, Brockman D, Myatt L: Role of peroxynitrite in altered fetal-placental vascular reactivity in diabetes or preeclampsia. *Am J Physiol* 278: H1311–H1319, 2000.

Kotaska AJ, Klein MC, Liston RM: Epidural analgesia associated with low-dose oxytocin augmentation increases cesarean births: a critical look at the external validity of randomized trials. *Am J Obstet Gynecol* 194:809–814, 2006.

Koukkou E, Young P, Lowy C: The effect of maternal glycemic control on fetal growth in diabetic pregnancies. *Am J Perinatol* 14:547–552, 1997.

Kovacevich GJ, Gaich SA, Lavin JP, Hopkins MP, Crane SS, Stewart J, Nelson D, Lavin LM: The prevalence of thromboembolic events among women with extended bed rest prescribed as part of the treatment for premature labor or preterm rupture of membranes. *Am J Obstet Gynecol* 182:1089–1092, 2000.

Kovilam O, Khoury J, Miodovnik M, Chames M, Spinnato J, Sibai B: Spontaneous preterm delivery in the type 1 diabetic pregnancy: the role of glycemic control. *J Matern Fetal Neonatal Med* 11:245–248, 2002.

Kowalczyk M, Ircha G, Zawodniak-Szalapska M, Cypryk K, Wilczynski J: Psychomotor development in the children of mothers with type 1 diabetes mellitus or gestational diabetes mellitus. *J Pediatr Endocrinol Metab* 15:277–281, 2002.

Kozak-Barany A, Jokinen E, Kero P, Tuominen J, Ronnemaa T, Valimaki I: Impaired left ventricular diastolic function in newborn infants of mothers with pregestational or gestational diabetes with good glycemic control. *Early Hum Dev* 77:13–22, 2004.

Krantz DA, Hallahan TW, Orlandi F, Buchanan P, Larsen JW, Macri JN: First-trimester Down syndrome screening using dried blood biochemistry and nuchal translucency. *Obstet Gynecol* 96:207–213, 2000.

Krantz D, Goetzl L, Simpson JL, Thom E, Zachary J, Hallahan TW, Silver R, Pergament E, Platt LD, Filkins K, Johnson A, Mahoney M, Hogge WA, Wilson RD, Mohide P, Hershey D, Wapner R; for the First Trimester Maternal Serum Biochemistry and Fetal Nuchal Translucency Screening (BUN) Study Group: Association of extreme first-trimester free human chorionic gonadotropin-beta, pregnancy-associated plasma protein A, and nuchal translucency with intrauterine growth restriction and other adverse pregnancy outcomes. *Am J Obstet Gynecol* 191:1452–1458, 2004.

Kreiser D, Katorza E, Seidman DS, Etchin A, Schiff E: The effect of ephedrine on intrapartum fetal heart rate after epidural analgesia. *Obstet Gynecol* 104: 1277–1281, 2004.

Krew MA, Kehl RJ, Thomas A, Catalano PM: Relation of amniotic fluid C-peptide levels to neonatal body composition. *Obstet Gynecol* 84:96–100, 1994.

Krivak TC, Zorn KK: Venous thromboembolism in obstetrics and gynecology. *Obstet Gynecol* 109:761–777, 2007.

Kuhl C, Andersen GE, Hertel J, Molsted-Pedersen L: Metabolic events in infants of diabetic mothers during the first 24 hours after birth. I. Changes in plasma glucose, insulin and glucagon. *Acta Paediatr Scand* 71:19–25, 1982.

Kuhnert M, Seelbach-Gobel B, Butterwegge M: Predictive agreement between the fetal arterial oxygen saturation and fetal scalp pH: results of the German multicenter study. *Am J Obstet Gynecol* 178:330–335, 1998.

Kuhnert M, Schmidt S: Intrapartum management of nonreassuring fetal heart rate patterns: a randomized controlled trial of fetal pulse oximetry. *Am J Obstet Gynecol* 191:1989–1995, 2004.

Kulovich MV, Gluck L: The lung profile II: complicated pregnancy. *Am J Obstet Gynecol* 135:64–70, 1979.

Kwee A, van der Hoorn-van den Beld CW, Veerman J, Dekkers AH, Visser GH: STAN S21 fetal heart rate monitor for fetal surveillance during labor: an observational study in 637 patients. *J Matern Fetal Neonatal Med* 15:400–407, 2004.

Kyle GC: Diabetes and pregnancy. *Ann Intern Med* 59 (Suppl 3):1–82, 1963.

Ladner H, Danielsen B, Gilbert WM: Acute myocardial infarction in pregnancy and the puerperium: a population-based study. *Obstet Gynecol* 105:480–484, 2005.

Lagrew DC, Pircon RA, Towers CV, Dorchester W, Freeman RK: Antepartum fetal surveillance in patients with diabetes: when to start? *Am J Obstet Gynecol* 168:1820–1826, 1993.

Lam C, Lim K-H, Karumanchi A: Circulating angiogenic factors in the pathogenesis and prediction of preeclampsia. *Hypertension* 46:1077–1085, 2005.

Lamont RF and the International Preterm Labour Council: Evidence-based labour ward guidelines for the diagnosis, management and treatment of preterm labour. *J Obstet Gynecol* 23:469–478, 2003.

Landon MB, Gabbe SG, Piana R, Mennuti MT, Main EK: Neonatal morbidity in pregnancy complicated by diabetes mellitus: predictive value of maternal glycemic profiles. *Am J Obstet Gynecol* 156:1089–1095, 1987.

Landon MB, Mintz MC, Gabbe SG: Sonographic evaluation of fetal abdominal growth: predictor of the large-for-gestational-age infant in pregnancies complicated by diabetes mellitus. *Am J Obstet Gynecol* 160:115–121, 1989a.

Landon MB, Gabbe SG, Bruner JP, Ludmir J: Doppler umbilical artery velocimetry in pregnancy complicated by insulin-dependent diabetes mellitus. *Obstet Gynecol* 73:961–965, 1989b.

Landon MB, Langer O, Gabbe SG, Schick C, Brustman L: Fetal surveillance in pregnancies complicated by insulin-dependent diabetes mellitus. *Am J Obstet Gynecol* 167:617–621, 1992.

Landon MB, Gabbe SG: Fetal surveillance and timing of delivery in pregnancy complicated by diabetes mellitus. *Obstet Gynecol Clin North Am* 23:109–123, 1996.

Langer O, Berkus MD, Huff RW, Samueloff A: Shoulder dystocia: should the fetus weighing >4000 grams be delivered by cesarean section? *Am J Obstet Gynecol* 165:831–837, 1991.

Langer O: Ultrasound biometry evolves in the management of diabetes in pregnancy. *Ultrasound Obstet Gynecol* 26:585–595, 2005.

Lanska DJ, Kryscio RJ: Risk factors for peripartum and postpartum stroke and intracranial venous thrombosis. *Stroke* 31:1274–1282, 2000.

Lapillonne A, Guerin S, Braillon P, Claris O, Delmas PD, Salle BL: Diabetes during pregnancy does not alter whole body bone mineral content in infants. *J Clin Endocrinol Metab* 82:3993–3997, 1997.

Lapolla A, Dalfra MG, Di Cianni G, Bonomo H, Parretti E, Mello G; the Scientific Committee of the GISOGD Group: A multicenter study on pregnancy outcome in women with diabetes. *Nutr Metab Cardiovasc Dis* Apr 10, 2007 (Epub ahead of print).

Lattermann R, Carli F, Wykes L, Schricker T: Epidural blockade modifies perioperative glucose production without affecting protein catabolism. *Anethesiology* 97:374–381, 2002.

Lauenborg J, Mathiesen E, Ovesen P, Westergaard JG, Ekbom P, Molsted-Pedersen L, Damm P: Audit on stillbirths in women with pregestational type 1 diabetes. *Diabetes Care* 26:1385–1389, 2003.

Lauszus FF, Rasmussen OW, Lousen T, Klebe TM, Klebe JG: Ambulatory blood pressure as predictor of preeclampsia in diabetic pregnancies with respect to urinary albumin excretion rate and glycemic regulation. *Acta Obstet Gynecol Scand* 80:1096–1103, 2001.

Lauszus FF, Fuglsang J, Flyvbjerg A, Klebe JG: Preterm delivery in normoalbuminuric, diabetic women without preeclampsia: the role of metabolic control. *Eur J Obstet Gynecol Reprod Biol* 124:144–149, 2006.

Lavin JP Jr, Lovelace DR, Miodovnik M, Knowles HC, Barden TP: Clinical experience with one hundred seven diabetic pregnancies. *Am J Obstet Gynecol* 147:742–752, 1983.

Lawrence JB, Oxvig C, Overgaard MT, Sottrup-Jensen L, Gleich GJ, Hays LG, Yates JR III, Conover CA: The insulin-like growth factor (IGF)-dependent IGF binding protein-4 protease secreted by human fibroblasts is pregnancy-associated plasma protein-A. *Proc Natl Acad Sci USA* 96:3149–3153, 1999.

Leach L, Gray C, Staton S, Babawale MO, Gruchy A, Foster C, Mayhew TM, James DK: Vascular endothelial cadherin and β-cadhenin in human fetoplacental vessels of pregnancies complicated by type 1 diabetes: associations with angiogenesis and perturbed barrier function. *Diabetologia* 47:695–709, 2004.

Lean MEJ, Pearson DWM, Sutherland HW: Insulin management during labor and delivery in mothers with diabetes. *Diabet Med* 7:162–164, 1990.

Lee CJ, Hsieh TT, Chiu TH, Chen KC, Lo LM, Hung TH: Risk factors for preeclampsia in an Asian population. *Int J Obstet Gynecol* 70:327–333, 2000.

Lee BH, Stoll BJ, McDoanld SA, Higgins RD; the National Institute of Child Health and Human Development Neonatal Research Network: Adverse neonatal outcomes associated with antenatal dexamethasone versus antenatal betamethasone. *Pediatrics* 117:1503–1510, 2006.

LeGal G, Prins AM, Righini M, Bohec C, Lacut K, Germain P, Vergos JC, Kaczmarek R, Guias B, Collet M, Bressollette L, Oger E, Mottier D:

Diagnostic value of a negative single complete compression ultrasound of the lower limbs to exclude the diagnosis of deep venous thrombosis in pregnant or postpartum women: a retrospective hospital-based study. *Thromb Res* 118:691–697, 2006.

Leinonen PJ, Hiilesmaa VK, Kaaja RJ, Teramo KA: Maternal mortality in type 1 diabetes. *Diabetes Care* 24:1501–1502, 2001.

Leitch I, Osmond D, Falconer J, Clifton V, Walters W, Read M: Vasoactive effects of 8-epi-prostaglandin-F2alpha in the human placenta in vitro. *J Soc Gynecol Invest* 6:195A, 1999.

Lemons JA, Jaffe RB: Amniotic fluid lecithin/sphingomyelin ratio in the diagnosis of hyaline membrane disease. *Am J Obstet Gynecol* 115:233–237, 1973.

Lenz S, Kuhl C, Wang P, Molsted-Pedersen L, Orskov H, Faber OK: The effect of ritodrine on carbohydrate and lipid metabolism in normal and diabetic pregnant women. *Acta Endocrinol* 92:669–679, 1979.

Lepercq J, Coste J, Theau A, Dubois-Laforgue D, Timsit J: Factors associated with preterm delivery in women with type 1 diabetes. A cohort study. *Diabetes Care* 27:2824–2828, 2004.

Leslie J, Shen SC, Strauss L: Hypertrophic cardiomyopathy in a midtrimester fetus born to a diabetic mother. *J Pediatr* 100:631–632, 1982.

Leveno KJ, Hauth JC, Gilstrap LC, Whalley PJ: Appraisal of rigid blood glucose control during pregnancy in the overtly diabetic woman. *Am J Obstet Gynecol* 135:853–862, 1979.

Levine MG, Holroyde J, Woods JR Jr, Siddiqi TA, Scott M-H, Miodovnik M: Birth trauma: incidence and predisposing factors. *Obstet Gynecol* 63:792–794, 1984.

Levy AL, Gonzalez JL, Rappaport VJ, Curet LB, Rayburn WF: Effect of labor induction on cesarean section rates in diabetic pregnancies. *J Reprod Med* 47:932–932, 2002.

Levy A, Sheiner E, Hammel RD, Hershkovitz R, Hallak M, Katz M, Mazor M: Shoulder dystocia: a comparison of patients with and without diabetes mellitus. *Arch Gynecol Obstet* 273:203–206, 2006.

Lewis PJ, Trudinger BJ, Mabgez J: Effect of maternal glucose ingestion on fetal breathing and body movements in late pregnancy. *Br J Obstet Gynecol* 85:86–89, 1978.

Lewis PS, Lauria MR, Dzieczkowski J, Utter GOO, Dombrowski MP: Amniotic fluid lamellar body count: cost-effective screening for fetal lung maturity. *Obstet Gynecol* 93:387–391, 1999.

Light IJ, Keenan WJ, Sutherland JM: Maternal intravenous glucose administration as a cause of hypoglycemia in the infant of the diabetic mother. *Am J Obstet Gynecol* 113:345–350, 1972.

Lin S, Shimuzu I, Suehara N, Nakayama M, Aono T: Uterine artery Doppler velocimetry in relation to trophoblast migration into the myometrium of the placental bed. *Obstet Gynecol* 85:760–765, 1995.

Lindqvist P, Dahlback B, Marsal K: Thrombotic risk during pregnancy: a population study. *Obstet Gynecol* 94:595–599, 1999.

Lindsay RS, Hanson Rl, Bennett PH, Knowler WC: Secular trends in birth weight, BMI, and diabetes in the offspring of diabetic mothers. *Diabetes Care* 23: 1249–1254, 2000.

Lindsay RS, Walker JD, Halsall I, Hales CN, Calder AA, Hamilton BA, Johnstone FD: Insulin and insulin propeptides at birth in offspring of diabetic mothers. *J Clin Endocrinol Metab* 88:1664–1671, 2003.

Lindsay RS, Ziegler AG, Hamilton BA, Calder AA, Johnstone FD, Walker JD: Type 1 diabetes-related antibodies in the fetal circulation: prevalence and influence on cord insulin and birth weight in offspring of mothers with type 1 diabetes. *J Clin Endocrinol Metab* 89:3436–3439, 2004.

Linzey EM: Controlling diabetes with continuous insulin infusion. *Contemp Obstet Gynecol* 12:43–48, 1978.

Liu S, Liston RM, Joseph KS, Heaman M, Sauve R, Kramer MS; the Maternal Health Study Group of the Canadian Perinatal Surveillance System: Maternal mortality and severe morbidity associated with low-risk planned cesarean delivery versus planned vaginal delivery at term. *CMAJ* 176:455–460, 2007.

Livingston EG, Herbert WNP, Hage ML, Chapman JF, Stubbs TM; for the Diabetes and Fetal Maturity Study Group: Use of the TDx-FLM assay in evaluating fetal lung maturity in an insulin-dependent diabetic population. *Obstet Gynecol* 86:826–829, 1995.

Loetworawanit R, Chittacharoen A, Sututvoravut S: Intrapartum fetal abdominal circumference by ultrasonography for predicting fetal macrosomia. *J Med Assoc Thai* 89 (Suppl 4):S60–S64, 2006.

Loffredo CA, Wilson PD, Ferencz C: Maternal diabetes: an independent risk factor for major cardiovascular malformations with increased mortality of affected infants. *Teratology* 64:98–106, 2001.

Loukovaara M, Leinonen P, Teramo K, Andersson S: Concentration of cord serum placenta growth factor in normal and diabetic pregnancies. *Br J Obstet Gynecol* 112:75–79, 2005a.

Loukovaara MJ, Loukovaara S, Leinonen PJ, Teramo KA, Andersson SH: Endothelium-derived nitric oxide metabolites and soluble intercellular adhesion molecule-1 in diabetic and normal pregnancies. *Eur J Obstet Gynecol Reprod Biol* 118:160–165, 2005b.

Low JA, Victory R, Derrick EJ: Predictive value of electronic fetal monitoring for intrapartum fetal asphyxia with metabolic acidosis. *Obstet Gynecol* 93:285–291, 1999.

Lucas A, Morley R, Cole TJ: Adverse neurodevelopmental outcome of moderate neonatal hypoglycemia. *BMJ* 297:1304–1308, 1988.

Lucas MJ, Leveno KJ, Cunningham FG: A comparison of magnesium sulfate with phenytoin for the prevention of preeclampsia. *N Engl J Med* 333:201–205, 1995.

Ludmir J, Alvarez JG, Mennuti MT, Gabbe SG, Touchstone JC: Cholesterol palmitate as a predictor of fetal lung maturity. *Am J Obstet Gynecol* 157:84–88, 1987.

Ludmir J, Alvarez JG, Landon MB, Gabbe SG, Mennuti MT, Touchstone JC: Amniotic fluid cholesterol palmitate in pregnancies complicated by diabetes mellitus. *Obstet Gynecol* 72:360–362, 1988.

Lurie S, Insler V, Hagay ZJ: Induction of labor at 38 to 39 weeks of gstation reduces the incidence of shoulder dystocia in gestational diabetic patients class A2. *Am J Perinatol* 13:293–296, 1996.

Luyckx AS, Massi-Benedetti F, Falorni A, Lefebvre PJ: Presence of pancreatic glucagon in the portal plasma of human neonates. Differences in the insulin and glucagons responses to glucose between normal infants and infants from diabetic mothers. *Diabetologia* 8:296–300, 1972.

Luzietti R, Erkkola R, Hasbargen U, Mattsson LA, Thoulon JM, Rosen KG: European community multicenter trial. "Fetal ECG analysis during labor": ST plus CTG analysis. *J Perinat Med* 27:431–440, 1999.

Luzietti R, Rosen KG: Monitoring in labor. In: Hod M, Jovanovic L, Di Renzo GC, de Leiva A, Langer O, eds. *Textbook of Diabetes and Pregnancy.* London: Martin Dunitz; 2003:418–429.

Lyall F, Gibson JL, Greer IA, Brockman DE, Eis ALW, Myatt L: Increased nitrotyrosine in the diabetic placenta. Evidence for oxidative stress. *Diabetes Care* 21:1753–1758, 1998.

Lyell DJ, Pullen K, Campbell L, Ching S, Druzin ML, Chitkara U, Burrs D, Caughey AB, El-Sayed YY: Magnesium sulfate compared with nifedipine for acute tocolysis of preterm labor. A randomized controlled trial. *Obstet Gynecol* 110:61–67, 2007.

MacArthur BA, Howie RN, Dezoete JA, Elkins J: School progress and cognitive development of 6-year old children whose mothers were treated antenatally with betamethasone. *Pediatrics* 70:99–105, 1982.

Macarthur A, Cook L, Pollard JK, Brant R: Peripartum myocardial ischemia: a review of Canadian deliveries from 1970 to 1999. *Am J Obstet Gynecol* 194:1027–1033, 2006.

Macintosh MC, Flemin KM, Bailey JA, Doyle P, Modder J, Acolet D, Golightly S, Miller A: Perinatal mortality and congenital anomalies in babies of women with type 1 or type 2 diabetes in England, Wales, and Northern Ireland: population-based study. *BMJ* 333:177 (Epub Jun 16, 2006).

Mackenzie R, Walker M, Armson A, Hannah ME: Progesterone for the prevention of preterm birth among women at increased risk: a systematic review and meta-analysis of randomized controlled trials. *Am J Obstet Gynecol* 194:1234–1242, 2006.

MacKenzie IZ, Shah M, Lean K, Dutton S, Newdick H, Tucker DE: Management of shoulder dystocia. Trends in incidence and maternal and neonatal morbidity. *Obstet Gynecol* 110:1059–1068, 2007.

Macklon NS, Greer IA: Venous thromboembolic disease in obstetrics and gynecology: the Scottish experience. *Scot Med J* 41:83–86, 1996.

Magann EF, Bass D, Chauhan SP, Sullivan DL, Martin RW, Martin JN Jr: Antepartum corticosteroids: disease stabilization in patients with HELLP syndrome. *Am J Obstet Gynecol* 171:1148–1153, 1994.

Magann EF, Chauhan SP, Bofill JA, Martin JN Jr: Comparability of the amniotic fluid index and single deepest pocket measurements in clinical practice. *Aust N Z J Obstet Gynaecol* 43:75–77, 2003.

Magee LA, Cham C, Waterman EJ, Ohlsson A, von Dadelszen P: Hydralazine for treatment of severe hypertension in pregnancy: a meta-analysis. *BMJ* 327:955–960, 2003.

Magee LA, Miremadi S, Li J, Cheng C, Ensom MHH, Carleton B, Cote A-M, von Dadelszen P: Therapy with both magnesium sulfate and nifedipine does not increase the risk of serious magnesium-related maternal side effects in women with preeclampsia. *Am J Obstet Gynecol* 193:153–163, 2005.

Makrydimas G, Sotiridis A, Huggon IC, Simpson J, Sharland G, Carvalho JS, Daubeney PE, Ionnidis JPA: Nuchal translucency and fetal cardiac defects: a pooled analysis of major echocardiography centers. *Am J Obstet Gynecol* 192: 89–95, 2005.

Malcus P: Antenatal fetal surveillance. *Curr Opin Obstet Gynecol* 16:123–128, 2004.

Mamopoulos M, Bili H, Tsantali C, Assimakopoulos E, Mantalenakis S, Farmakides G: Erythropoietin umbilical serum levels during labor in women with preeclampsia, diabetes, and preterm labor. *Am J Perinatol* 11:427–429, 1994.

Manderson JG, Mullan B, Patterson CC, Hadden DR, Traub AI, McCance DR: Cardiovascular and metabolic abnormalities in the offspring of diabetic pregnancy. *Diabetologia* 45:991–996, 2002.

Manderson JG, Patterson CC, Hadden DR, Traub AI, Ennis C, McCance DR: Preprandial versus postprandial blood glucose monitoring in type 1 diabetic pregnancy: a randomized controlled trial. *Am J Obstet Gynecol* 189:507–512, 2003.

Manning FA: The use of sonography in the evaluation of the high-risk pregnancy. *Radiol Clin North Am* 28:205–216, 1990.

Manning FA: Dynamic ultrasound-based fetal assessment: the fetal biophysical profile. *Clin Obstet Gynecol* 38:26–44, 1995.

Manning FA: Fetal biophysical profile: a critical appraisal. *Clin Obstet Gynecol* 45:975–985, 2002.

Marden D, McDuffie RS Jr, Allen R, Abitz D: A randomized controlled trial of a new fetal acoustic stimulation test for fetal well-being. *Am J Obstet Gynecol* 176: 1386–1388, 1997.

Mardirosoff C, Dumont L, Boulvain M, Tramer MR: Fetal brachycardia due to intrathecal opiods for labor analgesia: a systematic review. *BJOG* 109:274–281, 2002.

Martin AO, Dempsey LM, Minogue J, Liu K, Keller J, Tamura R, Freinkel N: Maternal serum alpha-fetoprotein levels in pregnancies complicated by diabetes: implications for screening programs. *Am J Obstet Gynecol* 163: 1209–1216, 1990.

Martin AM, Bindra R, Curcio P, Cicero S, Nicolaudes KH: Screening for preeclampsia and fetal growth restriction by uterine artery Doppler at 11–14 weeks of gestation. *Ultrasound Obstet Gynecol* 18:583–586, 2001.

Martin JN Jr, Thigpen BD, Rose CH, Cushman J, Moore A, May WL: Maternal benefit of high-dose intravenous corticosteroid therapy for HELLP syndrome. *Am J Obstet Gynecol* 189:830–834, 2003.

Martin JN Jr, Thigpen BD, Moore RC, Rose CH, Cushman J, May W: Stroke and severe preeclampsia and eclampsia: a paradigm shift focusing on systolic blood pressure. *Obstet Gynecol* 105:246–254, 2005.

Martinez ME, Catalan P, Balaguer G, Lisbona A, Quero J, Reque A, Pallardo LF: 25(OH)D levels in diabetic pregnancies—relation with neonatal hypoglycemia. *Horm Metab Res* 23:38–41, 1991.

Martinez ME, Catalan P, Lisbona A, Sanchez-Cabezudo MJ, Pallardo F, Jans I, Bouillon R: Serum osteocalcin concentrations in diabetic pregnant women and their newborns. *Horm Metab Res* 26:338–342, 1994.

Mathiesen ER, Christensen AB, Hellmuth E, Hornnes P, Stage E, Damm P: Insulin dose during glucocorticosteroid treatment for fetal lung maturation in diabetic pregnancy: test of an algorithm. *Acta Obstet Gynecol Scand* 81:835–839, 2002.

Maticot-Baptista D, Collin A, Martin A, Maillet R, Riethmuller D: Prevention of shoulder dystocia by an ultrasound selection at the beginning of labor of fetuses with large abdominal circumference. *J Gynecol Obstet Biol Reprod (Paris)* 36:42–49, 2007.

Maulik D, Lysikiewicz A, Sicuranza G: Umbilical artery Doppler sonography for fetal surveillance in pregnancies complicated by pregestational diabetes mellitus. *J Matern Fetal Neonatal Med* 12:417–422, 2002.

Mayhew TM, Sorensen FB, Klebe JG, Jackson MR: Oxygen diffusive conductances in placentae from control and diabetic women. *Diabetologia* 36:955–960, 1993.

Mayhew TM, Sorensen FB, Klebe JG, Jackson MR: Growth and maturation of villi in placentae from well-controlled diabetic women. *Placenta* 15:57–65, 1994.

Mayhew TM: Enhanced fetoplacental angiogenesis in pre-gestational diabetes mellitus: the extra growth is exclusively longitudinal and not accompanied by microvascular remodeling. *Diabetologia* 45:1434–1439, 2002.

Mayhew TM, Sampson C: Maternal diabetes mellitus is associated with altered deposition of fibrin-type fibrinoid at the villous surface in term placentae. *Placenta* 24:524–531, 2003.

Mayhew TM, Charnock-Jones DS, Kaufmann P: Aspects of human fetoplacental vasculogenesis and angiogenesis. III. Changes in complicated pregnancies. *Placenta* 25:127–139, 2004.

Maymon R, Weinraub Z, Herman A: Pregnancy outcome of euploid fetuses with increased nuchal translucency: how bad is the news? *J Perinat Med* 33:191–198, 2005.

Mazouni C, Porcu G, Cohen-Solal E, Heckenroth H, Guidicelli B, Bonnier P, Gamerre M: Maternal and anthropomorphic risk factors for shoulder dystocia. *Acta Obstet Gynecol Scand* 85:567–570, 2006.

McAnulty GR, Robertshaw HJ, Hall GM: Anesthetic management of patients with diabetes mellitus. *Br J Anaesth* 85:80–90, 2000.

McAuliffe FM, Foley M, Firth R, Drury I, Stronge JM: Outcome of diabetic pregnancy with spontaneous labour after 38 weeks. *Irish J Med Sci* 168:160–163, 1999.

McAuliffe FM, Hornberger LK, Winsor S, Chitayat D, Chong K, Johnson J-A: Fetal cardiac defects and increased nuchal translucency thickness: a prospective study. *Am J Obstet Gynecol* 191:1486–1490, 2004.

McAuliffe FM, Trines J, Nield LE, Chitayat D, Jaeggi E, Hornberger LK: Early fetal echocardiography—a reliable prenatal diagnosis tool. *Am J Obstet Gynecol* 193:1253–1259, 2005a.

McAuliffe FM, Fong KW, Toi A, Chitayat D, Keating S, Johnsen J-A: Ultrasound detection of fetal anomalies in conjunction with first-trimester nuchal translucency screening; a feasibility study. *Am J Obstet Gynecol* 193:1260–1265, 2005b.

McCance DR, Pettitt DJ, Hanson RL, Jacobsson LT, Knowler WC, Bennett PH: Birth weight and non-insulin dependent diabetes: thrifty genotype, thrifty phenotype, or surviving small baby genotype? *BMJ* 308:942–945, 1994.

McCowan LM, Mullen BM, Ritchie K: Umbilical artery flow velocity waveforms and the placental vascular bed. *Am J Obstet Gynecol* 157:900–902, 1987.

McElduff A, Ross GP, Lagstrom JA, Champion B, Flack JR, Lau S-M, Moses RG, Seneratne S, McLean M, Cheung NW: Pregestational diabetes and pregnancy. An Australian experience. *Diabetes Care* 28:1260–1261, 2005a.

McElduff A, Cheun NW, Mcintyre HD, Lagstrom JA, Oats JJN, Ross GP, Simmons D, Walters BNJ, Wein P: The Australasian Diabetes in Pregnancy Society consensus guidelines for the management of type 1 and type 2 diabetes in relation to pregnancy. *Med J Aust* 183:373–377, 2005b.

McElrath TF, Colon I, Hecht J, Tanasijevic MJ, Norwitz ER: Neonatal respiratory distress syndrome as a function of gestational age and an assay for surfactant-to-albumin ratio. *Obstet Gynecol* 103:463–468, 2004.

McElvy SS, Miodovnik M, Rosenn B, Khoury JC, Siddiqi T, St John Dignan P, Tsang RC: A focused preconceptional and early pregnancy program in women with type 1 diabetes reduces perinatal mortality and malformation rates to general population levels. *J Matern-Fetal Med* 9:14–20, 2000.

McFarland LV, Raskin M, Daling JR, Benedetti TJ: "Erb's/Duchenne's palsy" a consequence of fetal macrosomia and method of delivery. *Obstet Gynecol* 68:784–788, 1986.

McFarland M, Hod M, Piper JM, Xenakis E M-J, Langer O: Are labor abnormalities more common in shoulder dystocia? *Am J Obetet Gynecol* 173:1211–1214, 1995.

McFarland MB, Langer O, Piper JM, Berkus MD: Perinatal outcome and the type and number of maneuvers in shoulder dystocia. *Int J Gynecol Obstet* 55:219–224, 1996.

McFarland MB, Trylovich CG, Langer O: Anthropometric differences in macrosomic infants of diabetic and nondiabetic mothers. *J Matern-Fetal Med* 7:292–295, 1998.

McIntire DD, Leveno KJ: Neonatal mortality and morbidity rates in late preterm births compared with births at term. *Obstet Gynecol* 111:35–41, 2008.

McLean M, Chipps D, Cheung NW: Mother to child transmission of diabetes mellitus: does gestational diabetes program type 2 diabetes in the next generation? *Diabet Med* 23:1213–1215, 2006.

McMahon MJ, Mimouni F, Miodovnik M, Hull WM, Whitsett JA: Surfactant associated protein (SAP-35) in amniotic fluid from diabetic and nondiabetic pregnancies. *Obstet Gynecol* 70:94–98, 1987.

Mehta KC, Kalkwarf HJ, Mimouni F, Khoury J, Tsang RC: Randomized trial of magnesium administration to prevent hypocalcemia in infants of diabetic mothers. *J Perinatol* 18:352–356, 1998.

Mehta SH, Blackwell SC, Bujold E, Sokol RJ: What factors are associated with neonatal injury following shoulder dystocia? *J Perinatol* 26:85–88, 2006.

Meis PJ, Klebanoff M, Thom E, Dombrowski MP, Sibai B, Moawad A, Spong CY, Hauth JC, Miodovnik M, Varner MW, Leveno KJ, Caritis SN, Iams JD, Wapner RJ, Conway D, O'Sullivan MJ, Carpenter M, Mercer B, Ramin SM, Thorp JM, Peaceman AM; for the National Institute of Child Health and Human Development Maternal-Fetal Medicine Units Network: Prevention of recurrent preterm delivery by 17 alpha-hydroxyprogesterone caproate. *N Engl J Med* 348:2379–2385, 2003.

Meis PJ; for the Society for Maternal-Fetal Medicine: 17 Hydroxyprogesterone for the prevention of preterm delivery. *Obstet Gynecol* 105:1128–1135, 2005.

Mendiola J, Grylack LJ, Scanlon JW: Effects of intrapartum maternal glucose infusion on the normal fetus and newborn. *Anesth Analg* 61:32–35, 1982.

Merzouk H, Madani S, Prosy J, Loukidi B, Meghelli-Bouchenak M, Belleville J: Changes in serum lipid and lipoprotein concentrations and compositions at birth and after 1 month of life in macrosomic infants of insulin-dependent diabetic mothers. *Eur J Pediatr* 158:750–756, 1999.

Metzger BE, Silverman BL, Freinkel N, Dooley SL, Ogata ES, Green OC: Amniotic fluid insulin concentration as a predictor of obesity. *Arch Dis Child* 65:1050–1052, 1990.

Meyer-Wittkopf M, Simpson JM, Sharland GK: Incidence of congenital heart defects in fetuses of diabetic mothers: a retrospective study of 326 cases. *Ultrasound Obstet Gynecol* 8:8–10, 1996.

Meyer-Wittkopf M, Cooper S, Sholler G: Correlation between fetal cardiac diagnosis by obstetric and pediatric cardiologist sonographers and comparison with postnatal findings. *Ultrasound Obstet Gynecol* 17:392–397, 2001.

Mignini LE, Villar J, Khan KS: Mapping the theories of preeclampsia: the need for systematic reviews of mechanisms of the disease. *Am J Obstet Gynecol* 194: 317–321, 2006.

Miller FC, Skiba H, Klapholz H: The effect of maternal blood sugar levels on fetal activity. *Obstet Gynecol* 52:662–665, 1978.

Miller JM, Horger EO: Antepartum fetal heart rate testing in diabetic pregnancy. *J Reprod Med* 30:515–518, 1985.

Miller RS, Devine PC, Johnson EB: Sonographic fetal asymmetry predicts shoulder dystocia. *J Ultrasound Med* 26:1523–1528, 2007.

Milley JR, Rosenberg AA, Philipps AF, Molteni RA, Jones MD, Simmons MA: The effect of insulin on ovine fetal oxygen extraction. *Am J Obstet Gynecol* 149: 673–678, 1984.

Milunsky A, Alpert E, Kitzmiller JL, Younger MD, Neff RK: Prenatal diagnosis of neural tube defects. VIII. The importance of serum alpha-fetoprotein screening in diabetic pregnant women. *Am J Obstet Gynecol* 142:1030–1032, 1982.

Mimouni F, Skillman C, Harrington DJ: Effects of maternal hyperglycemia and ketoacidemia on the pregnant ewe and fetus. *Am J Obstet Gynecol* 154:394–401, 1986a.

Mimouni F, Tsang RC, Hertzberg VS, Miodovnik M: Polycythemia, hypomagnesemia, and hypocalcemia in infants of diabetic mothers. *Am J Dis Child* 140:798–800, 1986b.

Mimouni F, Miodovnik M, Siddiqi TA, Butler JB, Holdroyde J, Tsang RC: Neonatal polycythemia in infants of insulin-dependent diabetic mothers. *Obstet Gynecol* 68:370–372, 1986c.

Mimouni F, Miodovnik ZM, Whitsett JA, Holroude JC, Siddiqi TA, Tsang RC: Respiratory distress syndrome in infants of diabetic mothers in the 1980s: no direct adverse effect of maternal diabetes with modern management. *Obstet Gynecol* 69:191–195, 1987a.

Mimouni F, Miodovnik M, Tsang RC, Holroude J, Dignan PS, Siddiqi TA: Decreased maternal serum magnesium concentration and adverse fetal outcome in insulin-dependent diabetic women. *Obstet Gynecol* 70:85–88, 1987b.

Mimouni F, Miodovnik M, Siddiqi TA, Khoury J, Tsang RC: Perinatal asphyxia in infants of insulin-dependent diabetic mothers. *J Pediatr* 113:345–353, 1988a.

Mimouni F, Miodovnik M, Siddiqi TA, Berk MA, Wittekind C, Tsang RC: High spontaneous premature labor rate in insulin-dependent diabetic pregnant women: an association with poor glycemic control and urogenital infection. *Obstet Gynecol* 72:175–180, 1988b.

Mimouni F, Tsang RC: Pregnancy outcome in insulin-dependent diabetes: temporal relationships with metabolic control during specific pregnancy periods. *Am J Perinatol* 5:334–338, 1988c.

Mimouni F, Steichen JJ, Tsang RC, Hertzberg V, Miodovnik M: Decreased bone mineral content in infants of diabetic mothers. *Am J Perinatol* 5:339–343, 1988d.

Mimouni F, Tsang RC, Hertzberg VS, Neumann V, Ellis K: Parathyroid hormone and calcitriol changes in normal and insulin-dependent diabetic pregnancies. *Obstet Gynecol* 74:49–54, 1989.

Mimouni F, Loughead J, Miodovnik M, Khoury J, Tsang RC: Early neonatal predictors of neonatal hypocalcemia in infants of diabetic mothers: an epidemiologic study. *Am J Perinatol* 7:203–206, 1990.

Mimouni F, Miodovnik M, Rosenn B, Khoury J, Siddiqi TA: Birth trauma in insulin-dependent diabetic pregnancies. *Am J Perinatol* 9:205–208, 1992.

Min Y, Lowy C, Ghebremeskel K, Thomas B, Offley-Shore B, Crawford M: Unfavorable effect of type 1 and type 2 diabetes on maternal and fetal essential fatty acid status: a potential marker of fetal insulin resistance. *Am J Clin Nutr* 82:1162–1168, 2005.

Mintz MC, Landon MB, Gabbe SG, Marinelli DL, Ludmir J, Grumbach K, Arger PH, Coleman BG: Shoulder soft tissue width as a predictor of macrosomia in diabetic pregnancies. *Am J Perinatol* 6:240–243, 1989.

Miodovnik M, Lavin JP, Harrington DJ, Leung L, Seeds AE, Clark KE: Effect of maternal ketoacidemia on the pregnant ewe and the fetus. *Am J Obstet Gynecol* 144:585–593, 1982.

Miodovnik M, Peros N, Holroyde JC, Siddiqi TA: Treatment of premature labor in insulin-dependent diabetic women. *Obstet Gynecol* 65:621–627, 1985.

Miodovnik M, Mimouni F, Tsang RC, Skillman C, Siddiqi TA, Butler JB, Holroyde J: Management of the insulin-dependent diabetic woman during labor and delivery. Influences on neonatal outcome. *Am J Perinatol* 4:106–114, 1987.

Modanlou HD, Komatsu G, Dorchester W, Freeman RK, Bosu SK: Large-for-gestational age neonates: anthropometric reasons for shoulder dystocia. *Obstet Gynecol* 60:417–423, 1982.

Mohsin M, Bauman AE, Jalaludin B: The influence of antenatal and maternal factors on stillbirths and neonatal deaths in New South Wales, Australia. *J Biosoc Sci* 38:643–657, 2006.

Mollberg M, Hagberg H, Bager B, Lilja H, Ladfors L: High birthweight and shoulder dystocia: the strongest risk factors for obstetrical brachial plexus palsy in a Swedish population-based study. *Acta Obstet Gynecol Scand* 84:654–659, 2005.

Moore TR, Piacquadio K: A prospective evaluation of fetal movement screening to reduce the incidence of antepartum fetal death. *Am J Obstet Gynecol* 160: 1075–1080, 1989.

Moore KL, Persaud TVN: Placenta and fetal membranes. In: *Before We Are Born. Essentials of Embryology and Birth Defects* 5th ed. Philadelphia: Saunders; 1998:121–151.

Moore TR: A comparison of amniotic fluid fetal pulmonary phospholipids in normal and diabetic pregnancy. *Am J Obstet Gynecol* 186:641–650, 2002.

Moores LK, Collen JF, Woods KM, Shorr AF: Practical utility of clinical prediction rules for suspected acute pulmonary embolism in a large academic institution. *Thromb Res* 113:1–6, 2004.

Morin I, Morin L, Zhang X, Platt RW, Blondel B, Breart G, Usher R, Kramer MS: Determinants and consequences of discrepancies in menstrual and ultrasonographic gestational age estimates. *BJOG* 112:145–152, 2005.

Morrison JC, Whybrew WD, Bucovaz ET, Wiser WL, Fish SA: The lecithin/sphingomyelin ratio in cases associated with fetomaternal disease. *Am J Obstet Gynecol* 127:363–368, 1977.

Morrison JJ, Renne JM, Milton PJ: Neonatal respiratory morbidity and mode of delivery at term: influence of timing of elective cesarean section. *Br J Obstet Gynecol* 102:101–106, 1995.

Moutquin JM, Sherman D, Cohen H, Mohide PT, Hochner-Celnikier D, Fejgin M, Liston RM, Dansereau J, Mazor M, Shalev E, Boucher M, Glezerman M: Double-blind, randomized controlled trial of atosiban and ritodrine in the treatment of preterm labor: a multicenter effectiveness and safety study. *Am J Obstet Gynecol* 182:1191–1199, 2000.

MTG—Magpie Trial Group: Do women with preeclampsia, and their babies, benefit from magnesium sulfate? The Magpie trial: a randomized, placebo-controlled trial. *Lancet* 359:1877–1890, 2002.

Mueller-Heubach E, Caritis SN, Edelstone DI, Turner JH: Lecithin/sphingomyelin ratio in amniotic fluid and its value for the prediction of neonatal respiratory distress syndrome in pregnant diabetic women. *Am J Obstet Gynecol* 130:28–34, 1978.

Mughal MZ, Eelloo JA, Roberts SA, Sibartie S, Maresh M, Sibley CP, Adams JE: Intrauterine programming of urinary calcium and magnesium excretion in children born to mothers with insulin dependent diabetes mellitus. *Arch Dis Child Fetal Neonatal Ed* 90:F332–F336, 2005.

Mukherjee TK, Rajegowda BK, Glass LL, Auerback J, Evans HE: Amniotic fluid shake test versus lecithin/sphingomyelin ratio in the antenatal prediction of respiratory distress syndrome. *Am J Obstet Gynecol* 119:648–652, 1974.

Mulay S, McNaughton L: Fetal lung development in streptozotocin-induced experimental diabetes: cytidylyl transferase activity, disaturated phosphatidyl choline and glycogen levels. *Life Sci* 33:637–644, 1983.

Mulder EJ, O'Brien MJ, Lems YL, Visser GHA, Prechtl HFR: Body and breathing movements in near-term fetuses and newborn infants of type 1 diabetic women. *Early Hum Dev* 24:131–152, 1990.

Mulder EJ, Visser GH: Growth and motor development in fetuses of women with type-1 diabetes. I. Early growth patterns. *Early Hum Dev* 25:91–106, 1991a.

Mulder EJ, Visser GH: Growth and motor development in fetuses of women with type-1 diabetes. II. Emergence of specific movement patterns. *Early Hum Dev* 25:107–115, 1991b.

Mulder EJ, Visser GH, Morssink LP, de Vries JIP: Growth and motor development in fetuses of women with type-1 diabetes. III. First trimester quantity of fetal movement patterns. *Early Hum Dev* 25:117–133, 1991c.

Mulder EJ, Leiblum DM, Visser GH: Fetal breathing movements in late diabetic pregnancy: relationship to fetal heart rate patterns and Braxton-Hicks contractions. *Early Hum Dev* 43:225–232, 1995.

Murphy J, Peters J, Morris P, Hayes TM, Pearson JF: Conservative management of pregnancy in diabetic women. *Br Med J* 288:1203–1205, 1984.

Myatt L, Kossenjans W, Sahay R, Eis A, Brockman D: Oxidative stress causes vascular dysfunction in the placenta. *J Matern Fetal Neonatal Med* 9:79–82, 2000.

Nageotte M: Timing of conduction analgesia in labor. Editorial. *Am J Obstet Gynecol* 194:598–599, 2006.

Natale R, Patrick J, Richardson B: Effects of human maternal venous plasma glucose concentrations on fetal breathing movements. *Am J Obstet Gynecol* 132:36–41, 1978.

Natale R, Richardson B, Patrick J: The effect of maternal hyperglycemia on gross body movements in human fetuses at 32 to 34 weeks gestation. *Early Hum Dev* 8:13–20, 1983.

Nattrass M, Alberti KGMM, Dennis KJ, Gillibrand PN, Letchworth AT, Buckle ALJ: A glucose-controlled insulin infusion system for diabetic women during labor. *Br Med J* 2:599–601, 1978.

Naylor CD, Sermer M, Chen E, Sykora K; for the Toronto Trihospital Gestational Diabetes Investigators: Cesarean delivery in relation to birth weight and gestational glucose tolerance. Pathophysiology or practice style? *JAMA* 275:1165–1170, 1996.

Neerhof MG, Haney EI, Silver RK, Ashwood ER, Lee I, Piazze JJ: Lamellar body counts compared with traditional phopholipid analysis as an assay evaluating fetal lung maturity. *Obstet Gynecol* 97:305–309, 2001a.

Neerhof MG, Donhal JC, Ashwood ER, Lee I, Anceschi MM: Lamellar body counts: a consensus on protocol. *Obstet Gynecol* 97:318–320, 2001b.

Neilson JP, Alfirevic Z: Doppler ultrasound for fetal assessment in high risk pregnancies. *Cochrane Database Syst Rev* 2002;(2):CD000073.

Neilson JP: Fetal echocardiogram (ECG) for fetal monitoring during labor. *Cochrane Database Syst Rev* Issue 2006;(3):CD000116.

Neilson JP: Cochrane update: antenatal corticosteroids for accelerating fetal lung maturation for women at risk of preterm birth. *Obstet Gynecol* 109:189–190, 2007.

Neldham S: Fetal movements as an indicator of fetal well-being. *Lancet* 1:1222–1224, 1980.

Nelson CA, Wewerka S, Thomas KM, Tribby-Walbridge S, deRegnier R-A, Georgieff M: Neurocognitive sequelae of infants of diabetic mothers. *Behav Neurosci* 114:950–956, 2000.

Nelson SM, Sattar N, Freeman DJ, Walker JD, Lindsay RS: Inflammation and endothelial activation is evident at birth in offspring of mothers with type 1 diabetes. *Diabetes* 56:2697–2704, 2007a.

Nelson SM, Feeman DJ, Sattar N, Johnstone FD, Lindsay RS: IGF-1 and leptin associate with fetal HDL cholesterol at birth: examination in offspring of mothers with type 1 diabetes. *Diabetes* 56:2705–2709, 2007b.

Nesbitt TS, Gilbert WM, Herrchen B: Shoulder dystocia and associated risk factors with macrosomic infants born in California. *Am J Obstet Gynecol* 179:476–480, 1998.

Neufeld ND, Sevanian A, Barrett CT, Kaplan SA: Inhibition of surfactant production by insulin in fetal rabbit lung slices. *Pediatr Res* 13:752–754, 1979.

Neufeld ND, Corbo L, Braunstein GD, Rasor J: Amniotic fluid microviscosity analysis in diabetic pregnancies: comparison with other methods of lung maturity assessment using predictive value analysis. *Mt Sinai J Med* 52:110–115, 1985.

Nguyen TH, Larsen T, Engholm G, Moller H: Evaluation of ultrasound-estimated date of delivery in 17,450 spontaneous singleton births. Do we need to change Naegele's rule? *Ultrasound Obstet Gynecol* 14:23–28, 1999.

Nicolaides KH: Nuchal translucency and other first-trimester sonographic markers of chromosomal abnormalities. *Am J Obstet Gynecol* 191:45–67, 2004.

Nielsen GL, Norgard B, Puho E, Rotmman KJ, Sorensen HT, Czeizel AE: Risk of specific congenital abnormalities in offspring of women with diabetes. *Diabet Med* 22:693–696, 2005.

NIH—National Institutes of Health Consensus Development Panel: Effect of corticosteroids for fetal maturation on perinatal outcomes. *JAMA* 273:413–418, 1995.

NIH—National Institutes of Health, National Institute of Child Health and Human Development Research Planning Workshop: Electronic fetal heart rate monitoring: research guidelines for interpretation. *Am J Obstet Gynecol* 177:1385–1390, 1997.

NIH—National Institutes of Health Consensus Development Panel: Antenatal corticosteroids revisited. National Institutes of Health Consensus Development Conference Statement, August 17–18, 2000. *Obstet Gynecol* 98:144–150, 2001.

NIH—National Institutes of Health, State-of-the-Science Conference Statement: Cesarean delivery on maternal request. *Obstet Gynecol* 107:1386–1397, 2006.

Nijkeuter M, Ginsberg JS, Huisman MV: Diagnosis of deep vein thrombosis and pulmonary embolism in pregnancy: a systematic review. *J Thromb Haemost* 4:496–500, 2006.

Nilsson PM: Increased weight and blood pressure in adolescent offspring of diabetic mothers. *J Hum Hypertens* 13:793–795, 1999.

Njenga E, Lind T, Taylor R: Five year audit of peripartum blood glucose control in type 1 diabetic patients. *Diabet Med* 9:567–570, 1992.

Nogee L, McMahon M, Whitsett JA: Hyaline membrane disease and surfactant protein, SAP-35, in diabetes in pregnancy. *Am J Perinatol* 5:374–377, 1988.

Nohr FA, Bech BH, Davies MJ, Freydenberg M, Henriksen TB, Olsen J: Prepregnancy obesity and fetal death: a study within the Danish national Birth Cohort. *Obstet Gynecol* 106:250–259, 2005.

Nold JL, Georgieff MK: Infants of diabetic mothers. *Pediatr Clin North Am* 51: 619–637, 2004.

Nordstrom L, Spetz E, Wallstrom K, Walinder O: Metabolic control and pregnancy outcome among women with insulin-dependent diabetes mellitus. A twelve-year followup in the county of Jutland, Sweden. *Acta Obstet Gynecol Scand* 77:284–289, 1998.

Norem CT, Schoen EJ, Walton DL, Krieger RC, O'Keefe J, To TT, Ray T: Routine ultrasonography compared with maternal serum alpha-fetoprotein for neural tube defect screening. *Obstet Gynecol* 106:747–752, 2005.

Noren H, Blad S, Carlsson A, Flisberg A, Gustavsson A, Lilja H, Wennergren M, Hagberg H: STAN in clinical practice—the outcome of 2 years of regular use in the city of Gothenburg. *Am J Obstet Gynecol* 195:7–15, 2006.

Northern A, Norman GS, Anderson K, Moseley L, DeVito M, Cotroneo M, Swain M, Bousleiman S, Johnson F, Dorman K, Milluzzi C, Tillinghast J-A, Kerr M, Mallett G, Thom E, Pagliaro S, Anderson GD: The National Institute of Child Health and Human Development (NICHD) Maternal-Fetal Medicine Units (MFMU) Network: follow-up of children exposed in utero to 17 a-hydroxyprogesterone caproate compared with placebo. *Obstet Gynecol* 110:865–872, 2007.

Nylund L, Lunell NO, Lewande R, Persson B, Sarby B, Thornstrom S: Utero-placental blood flow in diabetic pregnancies. *Am J Obstet Gynecol* 144:298–302, 1982.

O'Leary JA, Leonetti HB: Shoulder dystocia: prevention and treatment. *Am J Obstet Gynecol* 162:5–9, 1990.

Oakley NW, Beard RW, Turner RC: Effect of sustained maternal hyperglycemia on the fetus in normal and diabetic pregnancies. *Br Med J* 1:466–469, 1972.

Oats JJN, Langer O: Timing and mode of delivery. In: Hod M, Jovanovic L, Di Renzo GC, de Leiva A, Langer O, eds. *Textbook of Diabetes and Pregnancy.* London: Martin Dunitz; 2003:430–441.

Ochi H, Matsubara K, Kusanagi Y, Taniguchi H, Ito M: Significance of a diastolic notch in the uterine artery flow velocity waveform induced by uterine embolization in the pregnant ewe. *Br J Obstet Gynecol* 105:1181–1121, 1998.

Odibo AO, Stamilio DM, Macones GA, Polsky D: 17a-hydroxyprogesterone caproate for the prevention of preterm delivery. A cost-effectiveness analysis. *Obstet Gynecol* 108:492–499, 2006.

Oei SG, Mol BW, de Kleine MJ, Brolmann HA: Nifedipine versus ritodrine for suppression of preterm labor; a meta-analysis. *Acta Obstet Gynecol Scand* 78: 783–788, 1999.

Ogata ES, Sabbagha RE, Metzger BE, Phelps RL, Depp R, Freinkel N: Serial ultrasonography to assess evolving macrosomia. *JAMA* 243:2405–2408, 1980.

Ogata ES: Carbohydrate metabolism in the fetus and neonate and altered neonatal glucoregulation. *Pediatr Clin North Amer* 33:25–45, 1986.

Ojala K, Vaarasmaki M, Makikallio K, Valkama M, Tekay A: A comparison of intrapartum automated fetal electrocardiography and conventional cardiotography—a randomized controlled study. *BJOG* 113:419–423, 2006.

Ojomo EO, Coustan DR: Absence of evidence of pulmonary maturity at amniocentesis in term infants of diabetic mothers. *Am J Obstet Gynecol* 163: 954–957, 1990.

Olofsson P, Sjoberg N-O, Solum T: Fetal surveillance in diabetic pregnancy. I. Predictive value of the non-stress test. *Acta Obstet Gynecol Scand* 65:241–246, 1986a.

Olofsson P, Ingemarsson I, Solum T: Fetal distress during labor in diabetic pregnancy. *Br J Obstet Gynecol* 93:1067–1071, 1986b.

Olofsson P, Lingman G, Marsal K, Sjoberg N-O. Fetal blood flow in diabetic pregnancy. *J Perinat Med* 15:545–553, 1987.

Omori Y, Minei S, Testuo T, Nemoto K, Shimuzu M, Sanaka M: Current status of pregnancy in diabetic women. A comparison of pregnancy in IDDM and NIDDM mothers. *Diabetes Res Clin Pract* 24 (Suppl):S273–S278, 1994.

Ong CYT, Liao A, Spencer K, Munim S, Nicolaides KIJ: First trimester maternal serum free beta human chorionic gonadotropin and pregnancy-associated plasma protein A as predictors of pregnancy complications. *Br J Obstet Gynecol* 107:1265–1270, 2000.

Ong CYT, Lao TT, Spencer K, Nicolaides KH: Maternal serum level of placental growth factor in diabetic pregnancies. *J Reprod Med* 49:477–480, 2004.

Oppenheimer EH, Esterly JR: Thrombosis in the newborn: comparison between diabetic and nondiabetic mothers. *J Pediatr* 67:549–556, 1965.

Ornoy A, Ratzon N, Greenbaum C, Peretz E, Soriano D, Dulitzky M: Neurobehavior of school-age children born to diabetic mothers. *Arch Dis Child Fetal Neonatal Ed* 79:94–99, 1998.

Ornoy A, Ratzon N, Greenbaum C, Wolf A, Dulitzky M: School-age children born to diabetic mothers and to mothers with gestational diabetes exhibit a high rate of inattention and fine and gross motor impairment. *J Pediatr Endocrinol Metab* 14:681–689, 2001.

Ornoy A: Growth and neurodevelopmental outcome of children born to mothers with pregestational and gestational diabetes. *Pediatr Endocrinol Rev* 3:104–113, 2005.

Ostlund E, Ulf Hanson: Antenatal non-stress test in complicated and uncomplicated pregnancies in type-1-diabetic women. *Eur J Obstet Gynecol Reprod Biol* 39:13–18, 1991.

Owen J, Yost N, Berghella V, MacPherson C, Swain M, Dildy GA III, Miodovnik M, Langer O, Sibai B; for the Maternal-Fetal Medicine Units Network, Bethesda, MD: Can shortened midtrimester cervical length predict very early spontaneous preterm birth? *Am J Obstet Gynecol* 191:298–303, 2004.

Palinski W, Napoli C: Impaired fetal growth, cardiovascular disease, and the need to move on. *Circulation* 117:341–343, 2008.

Parvin CA, Kaplan LA, Chapman JF, McManamon TG, Gronowski AM: Predicting respiratory distress syndrome using gestational age and fetal lung maturity by fluorescent polarization. *Am J Obstet Gynecol* 192:199–207, 2005.

Patel DM, Rhodes PG: Effects of insulin and hydrocortisone on lung tissue phosphatidyl choline and disaturated phosphatidyl choline in fetal rabbits in vivo. *Diabetologia* 27:478–481, 1984.

Patel D, Kalhan S: Glycerol metabolism and triglyceride-fatty acid cycling in the human newborn: effect of maternal diabetes and intrauterine growth retardation. *Pediatr Res* 31:52–58, 1992.

Pates JA, McIntyre DD, Casey BM, Leveno KJ: Predicting macrosomia. *J Ultrasound Med* 27:39–43, 2008.

Patrick J, Campbell K, Carmichael L, Natale R, Richardson B: Patterns of human fetal breathing during the last ten weeks of pregnancy. *Obstet Gynecol* 56:24–30, 1980.

Pattitt DJ, Baird HR, Aleck KA, Bennett PH, Knowler WC: Excessive obesity in offspring of Pima Indian women with diabetes during pregnancy. *N Engl J Med* 308:242–245, 1983.

Pedersen J, Molsted-Pedersen L: Prognosis of the outcome of pregnancies in diabetics. A new classification. *Acta Endocrinol* 50:70–77, 1965.

Pedersen J, Molsted-Pedersen L, Andersen B: Assessors of fetal perinatal mortality in diabetic pregnancy. Analysis of 1,332 pregnancies in the Copenhagen series, 1946–1972. *Diabetes* 23:302–306, 1974.

Pedersen JF, Molsted-Pedersen L: Early growth retardation in diabetic pregnancy. *Br Med J* 1:18–19, 1979.

Pedersen JF, Molsted-Pedersen L: Early fetal growth delay detected by ultrasound marks increased risk of congenital malformation in diabetic pregnancy. *Br Med J* 283:269–271, 1981.

Pedersen JF, Molsted-Pedersen L, Mortensen HB: Fetal growth delay and maternal hemoglobin A1C in early diabetic pregnancy. *Obstet Gynecol* 64:351–352, 1984.

Pedersen JF, Sorensen S, Molsted-Pedersen L: Serum levels of human placental lactogen, pregnancy-associated plasma protein A and endometrial secretory protein PP14 in the first trimester of diabetic pregnancy. *Acta Obstet Gynecol Scand* 77:155–158, 1998.

Peled Y, Gilboa Y, Perri T, Shohat M, Chen R, Bar J, Hod M, Pardo J: Strict glycemic control in diabetic pregnancy—implications for second trimester screening for Down syndrome. *Prenat Diagn* 23:888–890, 2003.

Penney GC, Mair G, Pearson DWM: Outcomes of pregnancies in women with type 1 diabetes in Scotland: a national population-based study. *BJOG* 110:315–318, 2003.

Perni SC, Predanic M, Kalish RB, Chervenak FA, Chasen ST: Clinical use of first-trimester aneuploidy screening in a United States population can replicate data from clinical trials. *Am J Obstet Gynecol* 194:127–130, 2006.

Perolo A, Prandstaller D, Ghi T, Gargiulo G, Leone O, Bovicelli L, Pilu G: Diagnosis and management of fetal cardiac anomalies: 10 years of experience at a single institution. *Ultrasound Obstet Gynecol* 18:615–618, 2001.

Persson B, Gentz J, Kellum M: Metabolic observations in infants of strictly controlled diabetic mothers. Plasma levels of glucose, FFA, glycerol and β-hydroxybutyrate during the first two hours after birth. *Acta Paediatr Scand* 62:465–473, 1973.

Persson B, Gentz J: Follow-up of children of insulin-dependent and gestational diabetic mothers: neuropsychological outcome. *Acta Paediatr Scand* 73:349–358, 1984.

Persson B, Hanson U: Insulin dependent diabetes in pregnancy: impact of blood glucose control on the offspring. *J Pediatr Child Health* 29:20–23, 1993.

Petersen LC, Birdi KS: The effect of fetal pulmonary surfactant production on the apparent microviscosity of amniotic fluid measured by fluorescence polarization. *Scand J Clin Lab Invest* 43:41–47, 1983.

Petersen NB, Pedersen SA, Greisen G, Pedersen JF, Molsted-Pedersen L: Early growth delay in diabetic pregnancy: relation to psychomotor development at age 4. *BMJ* 296:598–696, 1988.

Petersen MB: Status at 4–5 years in 90 children of insulin-dependent diabetic mothers. In: Sutherland HW, Stowers JM, Pearson DWM, eds. *Carbohydrate Metabolism in Pregnancy and the Newborn.* 4th ed. London: Springer-Verlag; 1989:353–361.

Peterson L, Caldwell J, Hoffman J: Insulin adsorbence to polyvinylchloride surfaces with implications for constant-infusion therapy. *Diabetes* 25:72–74, 1976.

Petrini JR, Callaghan WM, Klebanoff M, Green NS, Lackritz EM, Howse JL, Schwarz RH, Damus K: Estimated effect of 17 alpha-hydroxyprogesterone caproate on preterm birth in the United States. *Obstet Gynecol* 105:267–272, 2005.

Petry CD, Eaton MA, Wobken JA, Mills MM, Johnson DE, Georgieff MK: Liver, heart and brain iron deficiency in newborn infants of diabetic mothers. *J Pediatr* 121:109–114, 1992.

Pettitt DJ, Knowler WC, Bennett PH, Aleck KA, Baird HR: Obesity in offspring of diabetic Pima Indian women despite normal birth weight. *Diabetes Care* 10:76–80, 1987.

Pettitt DJ, Aleck KA, Baird HR, Carraher MJ, Bennett PH, Knowler WC: Congenital susceptibility to NIDDM: role of intrauterine environment. *Diabetes* 37:622–628, 1988.

Pettitt DJ, Nelson RG, Saad MF, Bennett PH, Knowler WC: Diabetes and obesity in the offspring of Pima Indian women with diabetes during pregnancy. *Diabetes Care* 16 (Suppl 1):310–314, 1993.

Philipps AF, Dubin JW, Matty PJ, Raye JR: Aterial hypoxemia and hyperinsulinemia in the chronically hyperglycemic fetal lamb. *Pediatr Res* 16:653–658, 1982a.

Philipps AF, Widness JA, Garcia JF, Raye JR, Schwartz R: Erythropoietin concentration in the chronically hyperglycemic fetal lamb. *Proc Soc Exp Biol Med* 170:42–47, 1982b.

Philipps AF, Porte PJ, Stabinsky S, Rosenkrantz TS, Raye JR: Effects of chronic fetal hyperglycemia upon oxygen consumption in the ovine uterus and conceptus. *J Clin Invest* 74:279–286, 1984.

Piazze JJ, Anceschi MM, Maranghi L, Brancato V, Marchiani E, Cosmi EV: Fetal lung maturity in pregnancies complicated by insulin-dependent and gestational diabetes: a matched cohort study. *Eur J Obstet Gynecol Reprod Biol* 83:145–150, 1999.

Pietryga M, Brazert J, Wender-Ozegowska E, Biczysko R, Dubiel M, Gudmundsson S: Abnormal uterine artery Doppler is related to vasculopathy in pregestational diabetes mellitus. *Circulation* 112:2496–2500, 2005.

Pijlman BM, de Koning WB, Wladimiroff JW, Stewart PA: Detection of fetal structural malformations by ultrasound in insulin-dependent pregnant women. *Ultrasound Med Biol* 15:541–543, 1989.

Pinette MG, Blackstone J, Wax JR, Cartin A: Fetal lung maturity indices—a plea for gestational age-specific interpretation: a case report and discussion. *Am J Obstet Gynecol* 187:1721–1722, 2002.

Piper JM, Langer O: Does maternal diabetes delay fetal pulmonary maturity? *Am J Obstet Gynecol* 168:783–786, 1993.

Piper JM, Samueloff A, Langer O: Outcome of amniotic fluid analysis and neonatal respiratory status in diabetic and nondiabetic pregnancies. *J Reprod Med* 40: 780–784, 1995.

Piper JM, Xenakis EMJ, Langer O: Delayed appearance of pulmonary maturation markers is associated with poor glucose control in diabetic pregnancies. *J Matern-Fetal Med* 7:148–153, 1998.

Piper JM: Lung maturation in diabetes in pregnancy: if and when to test. *Semin Perinatol* 26:206–209, 2002.

Plagemann A, Harder T, Kohlhoff R, Rohde W, Dorner G: Overweight and obesity in infants of mothers with long-term insulin-dependent diabetes or gestational diabetes. *Int J Obes* 21:451–456, 1997a.

Plagemann A, Harder T, Kohlhoff R, Rohde W, Dorner G: Glucose tolerance and insulin secretion in children of mothers with pregestational IDDM or gestational diabetes. *Diabetologia* 40:1094–1100, 1997b.

Platt MJ, Stanistreet M, Casson IF, Howard CV, Walkinshaw S, Pennycook S, McKendrick O: St Vincent's Declaration 10 years on: outcomes of diabetic pregnancies. *Diabet Med* 19:216–220, 2002.

Pollock RN, Buchman AS, Yaffe H, Divon MY: Obstetrical brachial plexus palsy: pathogenesis, risk factors, and prevention. *Clin Obstet Gynecol* 43:236–246, 2000.

Pometta D, Rees SB, Younger D, Kass EH: Asymptomatic bacteriuria in diabetes mellitus. *N Engl J Med* 277:1118–1121, 1967.

Prefumo F, Sebire NJ, Thilaganathan B: Decreased endovascular trophoblast invasion in first trimester pregnancies with high-resistance uterine artery Doppler indices. *Hum Reprod* 19:206–209, 2004.

Prefumo F, Celentano C, Presti F, De Biasio P, Venturini PL: Acute presentation of fetal hypertrophic cardiomyopathy in a type 1 diabetic pregnancy. *Diabetes Care* 28:2084, 2005.

Pressler JL, Hepworth JT, LaMontagne LL, Sevcik RH, Hesselink LF: Behavioral responses of newborns of insulin-dependent and nondiabetic, healthy mothers. *Clin Nurs Res* 8:103–118, 1999.

Pribylova H, Dvorakova L: Long-term prognosis of infants of diabetic mothers. Relationships between metabolic disorders in newborns and adult offspring. *Acta Diabetol* 33:30–34, 1996.

Qaseem Am, Snow V, Barry P, Hornbake ER, Rodnick JE, Tobolic T, Ireland B, Segal JB, Bass EB, Weiss KB, Green L, Owens DK; the Joint American Academy of Family Physicians/American College of Physicians Panel on Deep Venous Thrombosis/Pulmonary Embolism: Current diagnosis of venous thromboembolism in primary care: a clinical practice guideline from the American Academy of Family Physicians and the American College of Physicians. *Ann Intern Med* 146:454–458, 2007.

Quinones JN, James DN, Stamilio DM, Cleary KL, Macones GA: Thromboprophylaxis after cesarean delivery. A decision analysis. *Obstet Gynecol* 106:733–740, 2005.

Rajdl D, Racek J, Steinerova A, Novotny Z, Stozicky F, Trefil L, Siala K: Markers of oxidative stress in diabetic mothers and their infants during delivery. *Physiol Res* 54:429–436, 2005.

Rakoczi I, Tihanyi K, Cseh I, Rozsa I, Gati I, Gero G: Release of prostacyclin (PGI2) from trophoblast in tissue culture: the effect of glucose concentration. *Acta Physiol Hung* 71:545–549, 1988.

Ramanathan S, Khoo P, Arismendy J: Perioperative maternal and neonatal acid-base status and glucose metabolism in patients with insulin-dependent diabetes mellitus. *Anesth Analg* 73:105–111, 1991.

Randall P, Brealey S, Hahn S, Khan KS, Parsons JM: Accuracy of fetal echocardiography in the routine detection of congenital heart disease among unselected and low risk populations: a systematic review. *BJOG* 112:24–30, 2005.

Rasanen J, Kirkinen P: Growth and function of human fetal heart in normal, hypertensive and diabetic pregnancy. *Acta Obstet Gynecol Scand* 66:349–353, 1987.

Rasmussen MJ, Firth R, Foley M, Stronge JM: The timing of delivery in diabetic pregnancy: a 10-year review. *Aust N Z J Obstet Gynaecol* 32:313–317, 1992.

Ratzon N, Greenbaum C, Dulitzky M, Ornoy A: Comparison of the motor development of school-age children born to mothers with and without diabetes mellitus. *Phys Occup Ther Pediatr* 20:43–57, 2000.

Ray JG, Chan WS: Deep vein thrombosis during pregnancy and the puerperium: a meta-analysis of the period of risk and the leg of presentation. *Obstet Gynecol Surv* 54:265–271, 1999.

Ray JG, Vermeulen MJ, Shapiro JL, Kenshole AB: Maternal and neonatal outcomes in pregestational and gestational diabetes mellitus, and the influence of maternal obesity and weight gain: the DEPOSIT study. *QJM* 94:347–356, 2001.

Ray JG, Vermeulen MJ, Meier C, Wyatt PH: Risk of congenital anomalies detected during antenatal serum screening in women with pregestational diabetes. *QJM* 97:651–653, 2004a.

Ray P, Murphy GJ, Shutt LE: Recognition and management of maternal cardiac disease in pregnancy. *Br J Anesth* 93:428–439, 2004b.

Rayburn WF: Clinical implications from monitoring fetal activity. *Am J Obstet Gynecol* 144:967–980, 1982.

Rebarber A, Ferrara LA, Hanley ML, Istwan NB, Rhea DJ, Stanziano GJ, Saltzman DH: Increased recurrence of preterm delivery with early cessation of 17-alpha-hydroxyprogesterone caproate. *Am J Obstet Gynecol* 196:224.e1–4, 2007a.

Rebarber A, Istwan NB, Russo-Stieglitz K, Cleary-Goldman J, Rhea DJ, Stanziano GJ, Saltzman DH: Increased incidence of gestational diabetes in women receiving prophylactic 17 alpha-hydroxyprogesterone caproate for prevention of recurrent preterm delivery. *Diabetes Care* 30:2277–2280, 2007b.

Reddy UM, Mennuti MT: Incorporating first-trimester Down syndrome studies into prenatal screening. Executive Summary of the National Institute of Child Health and Human Development Workshop. *Obstet Gynecol* 107:167–173, 2006.

Reece EA, Scioscia AL, Pinter E, Hobbins JC, Green J, Mahoney MJ, Naftolin F: Prognostic significance of the human yolk sac assessed by ultrasonography. *Am J Obstet Gynecol* 159:1191–1194, 1988.

Reece EA, Winn HN, Smike C, Holford T, Nelson-Robinson L, Degennaro N, Hobbins JC: Sonographic assessment of the fetal head in diabetic pregnancies compared with normal controls. *Am J Perinatol* 7:18–22, 1990.

Reece EA, Hagay Z, Assimakopoulos E, Moroder W, Gabrielli S, DeGennaro N, Homko C, O'Connor T, Wisnitzer A: Diabetes mellitus in pregnancy and the assessment of umbilical artery waveforms using pulsed Doppler ultrasonography. *J Ultrasound Med* 12:73–80, 1994.

Reece EA, Hagay Z, Roberts AB, deGennaro N, Homko CJ, Connolly-Diamond M, Sherwin R, Tamborlane WV, Diamond MP: Fetal Doppler and behavioral responses during hypoglycemia induced with the insulin clamp technique in pregnant diabetic women. *Am J Obstet Gynecol* 172:151–155, 1995.

Reece EA, Quintela PA, Homko CJ, Sivan E: Early fetal growth delay: is it really predictive of congenital anomalies in infants of diabetic women? *J Matern-Fetal Med* 6:168–173, 1997.

Reece EA, Sivan E, Francis G, Homko CJ: Pregnancy outcomes among women with and without microvascular disease (White's classes B to FR) versus non-diabetic controls. *Am J Perinatol* 15:549–555, 1998.

Reece EA, Homko C, Miodovnik M, Langer O: A consensus report of the Diabetes in Pregnancy Study Group of North America conference. *J Matern Fetal Neonatal Med* 12:362–364, 2002.

Reece EA, Eriksson UJ: Congenital malformations: epidemiology, pathogenesis, and experimental methods of induction and prevention. In: Reece EA, Coustan DR, Gabbe SG, eds. *Diabetes in Women. Adolescence, Pregnancy, and Menopause.* 3rd ed. Philadelphia: Lippincott Williams & Wilkins; 2004:170–209.

Reller MD, Kaplan S: Hypertrophic cardiomyopathy in infants of diabetic mothers: an update. *Am J Perinatol* 5:353–358, 1988.

Remsberg KE, McKeown RE, McFarland KF, Irwin LS: Diabetes in pregnancy and cesarean section. *Diabetes Care* 22:1561–1567, 1999.

Resch BE, Gaspar R, Sonkodi S, Falkay G: Vasoactive effects of erythropoietin on human blood vessels *in vitro*. *Am J Obstet Gynecol* 188:993–996, 2003.

Richardson DK, Schwartz JS, Weinbaum PJ, Gabbe SG: Diagnostic tests in obstetrics: a method for improved evaluation. *Am J Obstet Gynecol* 152:613–618, 1985.

Righini M, Bounameaux H: Diagnosis of suspected deep venous thrombosis and pulmonary embolism during pregnancy. *Rev Med Suisse* 26:283, 286–289, 2005.

Riley LE, Tuomala RE, Heeren T, Greene MF: Low risk of post-cesarean section infection in insulin-requiring diabetic women. *Diabetes Care* 19:597–600, 1996.

Rizzo T, Freinkel N, Metzger BE, Hatcher R, Birns WJ, Barglow P: Correlations between antepartum maternal metabolism and newborn behavior. *Am J Obst Gynecol* 163:1458–1464, 1990.

Rizzo G, Arduini D, Romanini C: Cardiac function in fetuses of type I diabetic mothers. *Am J Obstet Gynecol* 164:837–843, 1991a.

Rizzo T, Metzger BE, Burns WJ, Burns K: Correlations between antepartum maternal metabolism and intelligence of offspring. *N Engl J Med* 325:911–916, 1991b.

Rizzo G, Arduini D, Romanini C: Accelerated cardiac growth and abnormal cardiac flow in fetuses of type 1 diabetic mothers. *Obstet Gynecol* 80:369–376, 1992.

Rizzo G, Arduini D, Capponi A, Romanini C: Cardiac and venous blood flow in fetuses of insulin-dependent diabetic mothers: evidence of abnormal hemodynamics in early gestation. *Am J Obstet Gynecol* 173:1775–1781, 1995a.

Rizzo G, Capponi A, Rinaldo D, Arduini D, Romanini C: Ventricular ejection force in growth-retarded fetuses. *Ultrasound Obstet Gynecol* 5:247–255, 1995b.

Rizzo G, Capponi A, Talone PE, Arduini D, Romanini C: Doppler indices from inferior vena cava and ductus venosus in predicting pH and oxygen tension in umbilical blood at cordocentesis in growth-retarded fetuses. *Ultrasound Obstet Gynecol* 7:401–410, 1996.

Rizzo T, Ogata ES, Dooley SL, Metzger BE, Cho NH: Perinatal complications and cognitive development in two- to five-year old children of diabetic mothers. *Am J Obstet Gynecol* 171:706–713, 1994.

Rizzo TA, Dooley SL, Metzger BE, Cho NH, Ogata ES, Silverman BL: Prenatal and perinatal influences on long-term psychomotor development in offspring of diabetic mothers. *Am J Obstet Gynecol* 173:1753–1758, 1995c.

Rizzo TA, Metzger BE, Dooley SL, Cho NH: Early malnutrition and child neurobehavioral development: insights from the study of children of diabetic mothers. *Child Dev* 68:26–38, 1997a.

Rizzo TA, Silverman BL, Metzger BE, Cho NH: Behavioral adjustment in children of diabetic mothers. *Acta Paediatr* 86:969–974, 1997b.

Robert MF, Neff RK, Hubbell JP, Taeusch HW, Avery ME: Association between maternal diabetes and the respiratory-distress syndrome in the newborn. *N Engl J Med* 294:357–360, 1976.

Roberts AB, Stubbs SM, Mooney R, Cooper D, Brudenell JM, Campbell S: Fetal activity in pregnancies complicated by maternal diabetes mellitus. *Br J Obstet Gynecol* 87:485–489, 1980.

Roberts JM, Gammill HS: Preeclampsia. Recent insights. *Hypertension* 46:1243–1249, 2005.

Roberts JM, Catov JM: Aspirin for preeclampsia: compelling data on benefit and risk. Editorial comment. *Lancet* 369:1765–1766, 2007.

Robertson SS, Dierker LJ: Fetal cyclic motor activity in diabetic pregnancies: sensitivity to maternal glucose. *Dev Psychobiol* 42:9–16, 2003.

Robillard JE, Sessions C, Kennedy RL, Smith FG: Metabolic effects of constant hypertonic glucose infusion in the well-oxygenated fetus. *Am J Obstet Gynecol* 130:199–203, 1978.

Robinson H, Tkatch S, Mayes DC, Bott N, Okun N: Is maternal obesity a predictor of shoulder dystocia? *Obstet Gynecol* 101:24–27, 2003.

Rodger MA, Avruch LI, Howley HE, Olivier A, Walker MC: Pelvic magnetic resonance venography reveals high rate of pelvic vein thrombosis after cesarean section. *Am J Obstet Gynecol* 194:436–437, 2006.

Romero R, Sibai BM, Sanchez-Ramos L, Valenzuela GJ, Veille JC, Tabor B, Perry KG, Varner M, Goodwin TM, Lane R, Smith J, Shangold G, Creasy GW: An oxytocin receptor antagonist (atosiban) in the treatment of preterm labor: a randomized, double-blind, placebo-controlled trial with tocolytic rescue. *Am J Obstet Gynecol* 182:1173–1183, 2000.

Ros HS, Cnattinguis S, Lipworth L: Comparison of risk factors for preeclampsia and gestational hypertension in a population-based cohort study. *Am J Epidemiol* 147 (Suppl):1062–1070, 1998.

Rosen KG, Kjellmer I: Changes in fetal heart rate and ECG during hypoxia. *Acta Physiol Scand* 93:59–66, 1975.

Rosen KG, Isaksson O: Alterations in fetal heart rate and ECG correlated to glycogen, creatine phosphate and ATP levels during graded fetal hypoxia. *Biol Neonate* 30:17–24, 1976.

Rosen KG, Dagbjartsson BA, Henriksson BA, Lagercrantz H, Kjellmer I: The relationship between circulating catecholamines and ST waveform in the fetal lamb electrocardiogram during hypoxia. *Am J Obstet Gynecol* 149:190–195, 1984.

Rosenberg TJ, Garbers S, Lipkind H, Chiasson MA: Maternal obesity and diabetes as risk factors for adverse pregnancy outcomes: differences among 4 racial/ethnic groups. *Am J Public Health* 95:1544–1551, 2005.

Rosenberg VA, Eglinton GS, Rauch ER, Skupski DW: Intrapartum maternal glycemic control in women with insulin requiring diabetes: a randomized clinical trial of rotating fluids versus insulin drip. *Am J Obstet Gynecol* 195:1095–1099, 2006.

Rosenn B, Miodovnik M, Combs CA, Khoury J, Siddiqi TA: Poor glycemic control and antepartum obstetric complications in women with insulin-dependent diabetes. *Int J Gynecol Obstet* 43:21–28, 1993.

Rosenn BM, Miodovnik M: Fetal biophysical and biochemical testing. In: Reece EA, Coustan DR, Gabbe SG, eds. *Diabetes in Women. Adolescence, Pregnancy, and Menopause.* 3rd ed. Philadelphia: Lippincott Williams & Wilkins; 2004:335–344.

Ross MG, Devoe LD, Rosen KG: ST-segment analysis of the fetal electrocardiogram improves fetal heart rate tracing interpretation and clinical decision making. *J Matern Fetal Neonatal Med* 15:181–185, 2004.

Roth JB, Thorp JA, Palmer SM, Brath PC, Walsh SW, Crandell SS: Response of placental vasculature to high glucose levels in the isolated human placental cotyledon. *Am J Obstet Gynecol* 163:1828–1830, 1990.

Rouse DJ, Owen J, Goldenberg RL, Cliver SP: The effectiveness and costs of elective cesarean delivery for fetal macrosomia diagnosed by ultrasound. *JAMA* 276:1480–1486, 1996.

Rouse DJ, Owen J, Hauth JC: Active-phase labor arrest: oxytocin augmentation for at least 4 hours. *Obstet Gynecol* 93:323–328, 1999.

Rovamo LM, Taskinen MR, Kuusi T, Raivio KO: Postheparin plasma lipoprotein and hepatic lipase activities in hyperinsulinemic infants of diabetic mothers and in large-for-date infants at birth. *Pediatr Res* 20:527–531, 1986.

Roversi GD, Pedretti E, Gargioulo M, Tronconi G: Spontaneous preterm delivery in pregnant diabetics: a high risk hitherto "unrecognized." *J Perinat Med* 10:249–253, 1982.

Rowlands S, Royston P: Estimated date of delivery from the last menstrual period and ultrasound scan: which is more accurate? *Br J Gen Pract* 43:322–325, 1993.

Rozenberg P, Chevret S, Senat M-V, Bretelle F, Bonnal AP, Sage-Femme, Ville Y: A randomized trial that compared intravaginal misoprostol and dinoprostone vaginal insert in pregnancies at high risk of fetal distress. *Am J Obstet Gynecol* 191:247–253, 2004.

Ruozi-Berretta Piazze JJ, Cosmi E, Cerekja A, Kashami A, Anceschi M: Computerized cardiotocography parameters in pregnant women affected by pregestational diabetes mellitus. *J Perinat Med* 32:426–429, 2004.

Russell JC, Cooper CM, Kethcum CH, Torday JS, Richardson DK, Holt JA, Kaplan LA, Swanson JR, Ivie WM: Multicenter evaluation of TDx test for assessing fetal lung maturity. *Clin Chem* 35:1005–1010, 1989.

Sacks DA, Chen W: Estimating fetal weight in the management of macrosomia. *Obstet Gynecol Surv* 55:229–239, 2000.

Sacks DA, Sacks A: Induction of labor versus conservative management of pregnant diabetic women. *J Matern Fetal Neonatal Med* 12:438–441, 2002.

Sacks DA: Timing and delivery of the macrosomic infant: induction versus conservative management. In: Hod M, Jovanovic L, Di Renzo GC, de Leiva A, Langer O, eds. *Textbook of Diabetes and Pregnancy.* London: Martin Dunitz; 2003:447–454.

Sacks DA: Etiology, detection, and management of fetal macrosomia in pregnancies complicated by diabetes. *Clin Obstet Gynecol* 50:980–989, 2007.

Sadler LC, Davison T, McCowan LM: A randomized controlled trial and meta-analysis of active management of labor. *Br J Obstet Gynecol* 107:909–915, 2000.

Sadovsky E, Ohel G, Havazeleth H, Steinwell A, Penchas S: The definition and significance of decreased fetal movements. *Acta Obstet Gynecol Scand* 62:409–413, 1983.

Saldeen P, Olofsson P, Parhar RS, al-Sedair S: Prostanoid production in umbilical vessels and its relation to glucose tolerance and umbilical artery flow resistance. *Eur J Obstet Gynecol Reprod Biol* 68:35–41, 1996.

Salhab WA, Wyckoff MH, Laptook AR, Perlman JM: Initial hypoglycemia and neonatal brain injury in term infants with severe fetal acidemia. *Pediatrics* 114:361–366, 2004.

Salle B, David L, Glorieux F, Delvin EE, Louis JJ, Troncy G: Hypocalcemia in infants of diabetic mothers. Studies of circulating calciotropic hormone concentrations. *Acta Paediatr Scand* 71:573–577, 1981.

Saltveldt S, Almstrom H, Kublickas M, Valentin L, Grunewald C: Detection of malformations in chromosomally normal fetuses by routine ultrasound at 12 or 18 weeks of gestation—a randomized controlled trial in 39,572 pregnancies. *BJOG* 113:664–674, 2006.

Salvesen DR, Higueras MT, Brudenell JM, Drury PL, Nicolaides KH: Doppler velocimetry and fetal heart rate studies in nephropathic diabetics. *Am J Obstet Gynecol* 167:1297–1303, 1992.

Salvesen DR, Higueras MT, Mansur CA, Freeman J, Brudenell JM, Nicolaides KH: Placental and fetal Doppler velocimetry in pregnancies complicated by maternal diabetes mellitus. *Am J Obstet Gynecol* 168:645–652, 1993a.

Salvesen DR, Freeman J, Brudenell JM, Nicolaides KH: Prediction of fetal acidaemia in pregnancies complicated by maternal diabetes mellitus by biophysical profile scoring and fetal heart rate monitoring. *Br J Obstet Gynecol* 100:227–233, 1993b.

Salvesen DR, Brudenell JM, Proudler AJ, Crook D, Nicolaides KH: Fetal pancreatic β-cell function in pregnancies complicated by maternal diabetes mellitus: relationship to fetal acidemia and macrosomia. *Am J Obstet Gynecol* 168: 1363–1369, 1993c.

Salvesen DR, Brudenell JM, Snijders RJ, Ireland RM, Nicolaides KH: Fetal plasma erythropoietin in pregnancies complicated by maternal diabetes mellitus. *Am J Obstet Gynecol* 168:88–94, 1993d.

Salvesen DR, Brudenell MJ, Nicolaides KH: Effect of delivery on fetal erythropoietin and blood gases in pregnancies with maternal diabetes mellitus. *Fetal Diagn Ther* 10:141–146, 1995.

Sardesai MG, Gray AA, McGrath MM, Ford SE: Fatal hypertrophic cardiomyopathy in the fetus of a woman with diabetes. *Obstet Gynecol* 98:925–927, 2001.

Scardo JA, Hogg BB, Newman RB: Favorable hemodynamic effects of magnesium sulfate in preeclampsia. *Am J Obstet Gynecol* 173:1249–1253, 1995.

Schaefer-Graf UM, Buchanan TA, Xiang A, Songster G, Montoro M, Kjos SL: Patterns of congenital anomalies and relationship to initial maternal fasting glucose levels in pregnancies complicated by type 2 and gestational diabetes. *Am J Obstet Gynecol* 182:313–320, 2000.

Schaefer-Graf UM, Kjos SL, Buehling KJ, Henrich W, Brauer M, Heinze T, Dudenhausen JW, Vetter K: Amniotic fluid insulin levels and fetal abdominal circumference at time of amniocentesis in pregnancies with diabetes. *Diabet Med* 20:349–354, 2003.

Schneider JM, Curet LB, Olson RW, Shay G: Ambulatory care of the pregnant diabetic. *Obstet Gynecol* 56:144–149, 1980.

Schneider H, Malek A: Lack of permeability of the human placenta for erythropoietin. *J Perinat Med* 23:71–76, 1995.

Schulte FJ, Michaelis R, Nolte R, Alber G, Parl U, Lasson U: Brain and behavioral maturation in newborn infants of diabetic mothers: I. Nerve conduction and EEG patterns. *Neuropediatrics* 1:24–55, 1969a.

Schulte FJ, Lasson U, Parl U, Nolte R, Jurgens U: Brain and behavioral maturation in newborn infants of diabetic mothers: II. Sleep cycles. *Neuropediatrics* 1:36–43, 1969b.

Schulte FJ, Albert G, Michaelis R: Brain and behavioral maturation in newborn infants of diabetic mothers: III. Motor behavior. *Neuropediatrics* 1:44–55, 1969c.

Schwartz R, Teramo KA: Effects of diabetic pregnancy on the fetus and newborn. *Semin Perinatol* 24:120–135, 2000.

Schwarze A, Gembruch U, Krapp M, Katalinic A, Germer U, Axt-Fliedner R: Qualitative venous Doppler flow waveform analysis in preterm intrauterine growth-restricted fetuses with ARED flow in the umbilical artery—correlation with short-term outcome. *Ultrasound Obstet Gynecol* 25:573–579, 2005.

Seeds AE, Leung LS, Tabor MW, Russell PT: Changes in amniotic fluid glucose, β-hydroxybutyrate, glycerol, and lactate concentrations in diabetic pregnancy. *Am J Obstet Gynecol* 135:887–895, 1979.

Seelbach-Gobel B, Heupel M, Kuhnert M, Butterwegge M: The prediction of fetal acidosis by means of intrapartum fetal pulse oxymetry. *Am J Obstet Gynecol* 180:73–81, 1999.

Segal JB, Eng J, Tamariz LJ, Bass EB: Review of the evidence on diagnosis of deep venous thrombosis and pulmonary embolism. *Ann Fam Med* 5:63–73, 2007a.

Segal JB, Streiff MB, Hoffman LV, Thornton K, Bass EB: Management of venous thromboembolism: a systematic review for a practice guideline. *Ann Intern Med* 146:211–222, 2007b.

Sells CJ, Robinson NM, Brown Z, Knopp RH: Long-term developmental follow-up of infants of diabetic mothers. *J Pediatr* 125:S9–S17, 1994.

Semmler K, Emmrich P, Kirsch G, Fuhrmann K, Heinke P: Relation of uteroplacental circulation and morphologic findings in myometrial and decidual arteries in diabetic pregnancy. *Zentralblatt fur Gynakologie* 107: 329–338, 1985.

Seppanen M, Ojanpera O, Kaapa P, Kero P: Delayed postnatal adaptation of pulmonary hemodynamics in infants of diabetic mothers. *J Pediatr* 131:545–548, 1997.

Severi FM, Rizzo G, Bocchi C, D'Antona D, Verzuri MS, Arduini D: Intrauterine growth retardation and fetal cardiac function. *Fetal Diagn Ther* 15:8–19, 2000.

Shah MPK, Farquhar JW: Children of diabetic mothers: subsequent weight. In: Camerini-Davalos RA, Cole HS, eds. *Early Diabetes in Early Life.* New York: Academic Press; 1975:587–593.

Shannon K, Davis JC, Kitzmiller JL, Fulcher SA, Koenig HM: Erythropoiesis in infants of diabetic mothers. *Pediatr Res* 20:161–165, 1986.

Sharma SK, Leveno KJ: Regional analgesia and progress of labor. *Clin Obstet Gynecol* 46:633–645, 2003.

Sheffield JS, Butler-Koster EL, Casey BM, McIntire DD, Leveno KJ: Maternal diabetes mellitus and infant malformations. *Obstet Gynecol* 100:925–930, 2002.

Sheiner E, Levy A, Walfisch A, Hallak M, Mazor M: Third degree perineal tears in a university medical center where midline episiotomies are not performed. *Arch Gynecol Obstet* 271:307–310, 2005.

Sheiner E, Levy A, Hershkowitz R, Hallak M, Hammel RD, Katz M, Kazor M: Determining factors associated with shoulder dystocia: a population-based study. *Eur J Obstet Gynecol Reprod Biol* 126:11–15, 2006.

Shields LE, Gan EA, Murphy HF, Sahn DJ, Moore TR: The prognostic value of hemoglobin A1C in predicting fetal heart disease in diabetic pregnancies. *Obstet Gynecol* 81:954–957, 1993.

Shields BM, Knight B, Hopper H, Hill A, Powell RJ, Hattersley AT, Clark PM: Measurement of cord insulin and insulin-related peptides suggests that girls are more insulin-resistant than boys at birth. *Diabetes Care* 30:2661–2666, 2007.

Shnider SM, Abboud TK, Artal R, Henriksen EH, Stefani SJ, Levinson G: Maternal catecholamines decrease during labor after lumbar epidural anesthesia. *Am J Obstet Gynecol* 147:13–15, 1983.

Sibai BM, Caritis SN, Hauth JC, MacPherson C, VanDorsten JP, Klebanoff M, Landon M, Paul RH, Meis PJ, Miodovnik M, Dombrowski MP, Thurnau GR, Moawad AH, Roberts J; for the NICHHD-MFMU: Preterm delivery in women with pregestational diabetes mellitus or chronic hypertension relative to women with uncomplicated pregnancies. *Am J Obstet Gynecol* 183:1520–1524, 2000a.

Sibai BM, Caritis SN, Hauth JC, Lindheimer M, VanDorsten JP, MacPherson C, Klebanoff M, Landon M, Miodovnik M, Paul RH, Meis PJ, Dombrowski MP, Thurnau GR, Roberts J, McNellis D; for the NICHHD-MFMU: Risks of preeclampsia and adverse neonatal outcomes among women with pregestational diabetes mellitus. *Am J Obstet Gynecol* 182:364–369, 2000b.

Sibai BM: Diagnosis, prevention, and management of eclampsia. *Obstet Gynecol* 105:402–410, 2005a.

Sibai BM: Magnesium sulfate prophylaxis in preeclampsia: evidence from randomized trials. *Clin Obstet Gynecol* 48:478–488, 2005b.

Siddappa AM, Georgieff MK, Wewerka S, Worwa C, Nelson CA, Deregnier R-A: Iron deficiency alters auditory recognition memory in newborn infants of diabetic mothers. *Pediatr Res* 55:1034–1041, 2004.

Siddiqi T, Rosenn B, Mimouni F, Khoury J, Miodovnik M: Hypertension during pregnancy in insulin-dependent diabetic women. *Obstet Gynecol* 77:514–519, 1991.

Siddiqi F, James D: Fetal monitoring in type 1 diabetic pregnancies. *Early Hum Dev* 72:1–13, 2003.

Silver RM, Lnadon MB, Rouse DJ, Leveno KJ, Spong CY, Thom EA, Moawad AH, Caritis SN, Harper M, Wapner RJ, Sorokin Y, Miodovnik M, Carpenter M, Peaceman AM, O'Sullivan MJ, Sibai B, Langer O, Thorp JM, Ramin SM, Mercer BM; the National Child Health and Human Development

Maternal-Fetal Medicine Units Network: Maternal morbidity associated with multiple repeat cesarean deliveries. *Obstet Gynecol* 107:1226–1232, 2006.

Silverman BL, Rizzo T, Green OC, Cho NH, Winter RJ, Ogata ES, Richards GE, Metzger BE: Long-term prospective evaluation of offspring of diabetic mothers. *Diabetes* 40 (Suppl 2):121–125, 1991.

Silverman BL, Landsberg L, Metzger BE: Fetal hyperinsulism in offspring of diabetic mothers: association with the subsequent development of childhood obesity. *Ann N Y Acad Sci* 699:36–45, 1993.

Silverman BL, Metzger BE, Cho NH, Loeb CA: Impaired glucose tolerance in adolescent offspring of diabetic mothers: relationship to fetal hyperinsulinism. *Diabetes Care* 18:611–617, 1995.

Silverman BL, Rizzo TA, Cho NH, Metzger BE: Long-term effects of the intrauterine environment: the Northwestern University Diabetes in Pregnancy Center. *Diabetes Care* 21 (Suppl 2):B142–B149, 1998.

Simon NV, Levisky JS, Lenko PM: The prediction of fetal lung maturity by amniotic fluid fluorescence polarization in diabetic pregnancy. *Am J Perinatol* 4:171–175, 1987.

Simpson EL, Lawrenson RA, Nightingale AL, Farmer RD: Venous thromboembolism in pregnancy and the puerperium: incidence and additional risk factors from a London perinatal database. *BJOG* 108:56–60, 2001.

Singh R, Pearson E, Avery PJ, McCarthy MI, Levy JC, Hitman GA, Sampson M, Walker M, Hattersley AT: Reduced beta cell function in offspring of mothers with young-onset type 2 diabetes. *Diabetologia* 49:1876–1880, 2006.

Skilton MR: Intrauterine risk factors for precocious atherosclerosis. *Pediatrics* 121:570–574, 2008.

Skjaeraasen J, Stray-Pedersen S: Amniotic fluid phosphatidylinositol and phosphatidylglycerol. II. Diabetic and eclamptic pregnancies. *Acta Obstet Gynecol Scand* 58:433–438, 1979.

Skupski DW, Rosenberg CR, Eglinton GS: Intrapartum fetal stimulation tests: a meta-analysis. *Obstet Gynecol* 99:129–134, 2002.

Smaill F, Hofmeyr GJ: Antibiotic prophylaxis for cesarean section. *Cochrane Database Syst Rev* 2002.

Smith BT, Giroud CJP, Robert M, Avery ME: Insulin antagonism of cortisol action on lecithin synthesis by cultured fetal lung cells. *J Pediatr* 87:953–955, 1975.

Smith RS Comstock CH, Lorenz RP, Kirk JS, Lee W: Maternal diabetes mellitus: which views are essential for fetal echocardiography? *Obstet Gynecol* 90:575–579, 1997.

Smith GCS, Stenhouse EJ, Crossley JA, Aitken DA, Cameron AD, Connor JM: Early pregnancy levels of pregnancy-associated plasma protein A and the risk of intrauterine growth restriction, premature birth, preeclampsia, and stillbirth. *J Clin Endocrinol Metab* 87:1762–1767, 2002.

Smith GCS, Shah I, Crossley JA, Aitken DA, Pell JP, Nelson SM, Cameron AD, Connor MJ, Dobbie R: Pregnancy-associated plasma protein A and alpha-fetoprotein and prediction of adverse perinatal outcome. *Obstet Gyenecol* 107:161–166, 2006.

Smith RL, Young SJ, Greer IA: The parturient with coronary heart disease. *Int J Obstet Anesth* 17:46–52, 2008.

Smythe JF, Copel JA, Kleinman CS: Outcome of prenatally detected cardiac malformations. *Am J Cardiol* 69:1471–1474, 1992.

Snow V, Qaseem A, Barry P, Hornbake ER, Rodnick JE, Tobolic T, Ireland B, Segal JB, Bass EB, Weiss KB, Green L, Owens DK; the Jount American College of Physicians/American Academy of Family Physicians Panel on Deep Venous Thrombosis/Pulmonary Embolism: Management of venous thromboembolism: a clinical practice guideline from the American College of Physicians and the American Academy of Family Physicians. *Ann Intern Med* 146:204–210, 2007b.

Snyder JM, Mendelson CR: Insulin inhibits the accumulation of the major lung surfactant apoprotein in human fetal lung explants maintained in vitro. *Endocrinology* 120:1250–1257, 1987.

Snyder JM, Kwun JE, O'Brien JA, Rosenfeld CR, Odom MJ: The concentration of the 35-kDa surfactant apoprotein in amniotic fluid from normal and diabetic pregnancies. *Pediatr Res* 24:728–734, 1988.

Snyder SW, Cardwell MS: Neuromuscular blockade with magnesium sulfate and nifedipine. *Am J Obstet Gynecol* 161:35–36, 1989.

Sobngwi E, Boudou P, Mauvais-Jarvis F, LeBlanc H, Velho G, Vexiau P, Porcher R, Hadjadj S, Pratley R, Tataranni PA, Calvo F, Gautier JF: Effect of a diabetic environment in utero on predisposition to type 2 diabetes. *Lancet* 361: 1861–1865, 2003.

Solomon CG, Seeley EW: Preeclampsia—searching for the cause. Editorial. *N Engl J Med* 350:641–642, 2004.

Soens MA, Birnbach DJ, Ranasinghe JS, van Zundert A: Obstetric anesthesia for the obese and morbidly obese patient: an ounce of prevention is worth more than a pound of treatment. *Acta Anesthesiol Scand* 52:6–19, 2008.

Sosenko IR, Kitzmiller JL, Loo SW, Blix P, Rubenstein AH, Gabbay KH: The infant of the diabetic mother: correlation of increased cord C-peptide levels with macrosomia and hypoglycemia. *N Engl J Med* 301:859–862, 1979.

Sosenko IRS, Lawson EE, Demottaz V, Frantz ID: Functional delay in lung maturation in fetuses of diabetic rabbits. *J Appl Physiol* 48:643–647, 1980.

Sosenko JM, Kitzmiller JL, Fluckiger R, Loo SW, Younger DM, Gabbay KH: Umbilical cord glycosylated hemoglobin in infants of diabetic mothers: relationships to neonatal hypoglycemia, macrosomia, and cord serum C-peptide. *Diabetes Care* 5:566–570, 1982.

Sosenko IR, Werthammer J, Cunningham MD, Frantz ID 3rd: Surfactant dysfunction in diabetic offspring: inhibitors and fatty acid lecithin content. *J Appl Physiol* 54:1097–1100, 1983.

Souka AP, Snidjers RJM, Novakov A, Soares W, Nicolaides KH: Defects and syndromes in chromosomally normal fetuses with increased nuchal translucency thickness at 10–14 weeks of gestation. *Ultrasound Obstet Gynecol* 11:391–400, 1998.

Spellacy WN, Miller S, Winegar A, Peterson PQ: Macrosomia—maternal characteristics and infant complications. *Obstet Gynecol* 66:158–161, 1985.

Spencer J, Gadalla F, Wagner W, Blake J: Cesarean section in a diabetic patient with a recent myocardial infarction. *Can J Anesth* 41:516–518, 1994.

Spencer K, Spencer CE, Power M, Dawson C, Nicolaides KH: Screening for chromosomal abnormalities in the first trimester using ultrasound and maternal serum biochemistry in a one-stop clinic: a review of three years prospective experience. *Br J Obstet Gynecol* 110:281–286, 2003a.

Spencer K, Bindra R, Nicolaides KH: Maternal weight correction of maternal serum PAPP-A and free β-hCG when screening for trisomy 21 in the first trimester of pregnancy. *Prenat Diagn* 23:851–855, 2003b.

Spencer K, Bindra R, Nix ABJ, Heath V, Nicolaides KH: Delta NT or NT MoM: which is the most appropriate for calculating accurate patient specific risks for trisomy 21 in the first trimester? *Ultrasound Obstet Gynecol* 22:142–148, 2003c.

Spencer K, Cicero S, Atzei A, Otigbah C, Nicolaides KH: Influence of maternal insulin-dependent diabetes on fetal nuchal translucency thickness and first-trimester maternal serum biochemical markers of aneuploidy. *Prenat Diag* 25:927–929, 2005.

Spinillo A, Viazzo F, Colleoni R, Chiara A, Cerbo RM, Fazzi E: Two-year infant neurodevelopmental outcome after single or multiple antenatal courses of corticosteroids to prevent complications of prematurity. *Am J Obstet Gynecol* 191:217–224, 2004.

Stamler EF, Cruz ML, Mimouni F, Rosenn B, Siddiqi T, Khoury J, Miodovnik M: High infectious morbidity in pregnant women with insulin-dependent diabetes: an understated complication. *Am J Obstet Gynecol* 163:1217–1221, 1990.

Steel JM, Johnstone SD, Corrie JET: Early assessment of gestation in diabetics. *Lancet* 2:975–976, 1984.

Steel JM, Wu PS, Johnstone FD, Muir BB, Sweeting VM, Hillier SG: Does early growth delay exist in diabetic pregnancy? *Br J Obstet Gynecol* 102:224–227, 1995.

Stehbens JA, Baker GL, Kitchell M: Outcome at ages 1, 3, and 5 of children born to diabetic women. *Am J Obstet Gynecol* 127:408–413, 1977.

Steinfeld JD, Samuels P, Bulley MA, Cohen AW, Goodman DBP, Senior MB: The utility of the TDx test in the assessment of fetal lung maturity. *Obstet Gynecol* 79:460–464, 1992.

Stenninger E, Schollin J, Aman J: Early postnatal hypoglycemia in newborn infants of diabetic mothers. *Acta Paediatr* 86:1374–1376, 1997.

Stenninger E, Flink R, Eriksson B, Sahlen C: Long-term neurological dysfunction and neonatal hypoglycemia after diabetic pregnancy. *Arch Dis Child Fetal Neonatal Ed* 79:F174–F179, 1998.

Stenninger E, Lindqvist A, Aman J, Ostlund I, Schvarcz E: Continuous Subcutaneous Glucose Monitoring System in diabetic mothers during labor and postnatal glucose adaptation of their infants. *Diabet Med* 25:450–454, 2008.

Stevenson DK, Bartoletti AL, Ostrander CR, Johnson JD: Pulmonary excretion of CO in the human infant as an index of bilirubin production. II. Infants of diabetic mothers. *J Pediatr* 94:956–958, 1976.

Stone SE, Morris TA: Pulmonary embolism during and after pregnancy. *Crit Care Med* 33 (Suppl 10):S294–S300, 2005.

Stonestreet BS, Goldstein M, Oh W, Widness JA: Effects of prolonged hyperinsulinemia on erythropoiesis in fetal sheep. *Am J Physiol* 257:R1199–R1204, 1989.

Strid H, Bucht E, Jansson T, Wennergren M, Powell TL: ATP dependent Ca2+ transport across basal membrane of human syncytiotrophoblast in pregnancies complicated by intrauterine growth restriction or diabetes. *Placenta* 24: 445–452, 2003.

Stride A, Shepherd M, Frayling TM, Bulman MP, Ellard S, Hattersley AT: Intrauterine hyperglycemia is associated with an earlier diagnosis of diabetes in HNF-1α gene mutation carriers. *Diabetes Care* 25:2287–2291, 2002.

Stuart MJ, Sunderji SG, Walenga RW, Setty BNY: Abnormalities in vascular arachidonic acid metabolism in the infant of the diabetic mother. *Br Med J* 290:1700–1702, 1985.

Stumpflen I, Stumpflen A, Wimmer M, Bernaschek G: Effect of detailed fetal echocardiography as part of routine prenatal ultrasonographic screening on detection of congenital heart disease. *Lancet* 348:854–857, 1996.

Stutchfield P, Whitaker R, Russell I; on behalf of the Antenatal Steroids for Term Elective Cesarean Section (ASTECS) Research Team: Antenatal betamethasone and incidence of neonatal respiratory distress after elective cesarean section: pragmatic randomized trial. *BMJ* 331:662–664, 2005.

Suhonen L, Hiilesmaa V, Teramo K: Glycemic control during early pregnancy and fetal malformations in women with type 1 diabetes mellitus. *Diabetologia* 43: 79–82, 2000.

Sundstrom A-K for the Swedish STAN study group: Randomized controlled trial of GTG versus CTG + ST analysis of the fetal ECG. *J Obstet Gynecol* 21:18–19, 2001.

Sykes GS, Molloy PM, Johnson P, Stirrat GM, Turnbull AC: Fetal distress and the condition of newborn infants. *Br Med J* 287:943–945, 1983.

Szymanowski K, Spaczynski M, Szpurek D, Biczysko R: Doppler evaluation of blood flow in the umbilical artery when confronted with morphologic changes in human placenta of pregnancy complicated by diabetes. *Ginekol Pol* 65: 163–170, 1994.

Tabsh KM, Brinkman CR III, Bashore RA: Lecithin/sphingomyelin ratio in pregnancies complicated by insulin-dependent diabetes mellitus. *Obstet Gynecol* 59:353–358, 1982.

Tait JF, Foerder CA, Ashwood ER, Benedetti TJ: Prospective clinical evaluation of an improved fluorescence polarization assay for predicting fetal lung maturity. *Clin Chem* 33:554–558, 1987.

Takoudes TC, Weitzen S, Slocum J, Malee M: Risk of cesarean wound complications in diabetic gestations. *Am J Obstet Gynecol* 191:958–963, 2004.

Tamura RK, Sabbagha RE, Dooley SL, Vaisrub N, Socol ML, Depp R: Real-time ultrasound determinations of weight in fetuses of diabetic gravid women. *Am J Obstet Gynecol* 153:57–60, 1985.

Tamura T, Goldenberg RL, Hou J, Johnston KE, Cliver SP, Ramey SL, Nelson KG: Cord serum ferritin concentrations and mental and psychomotor development of children at five years of age. *J Pediatr* 140:165–170, 2002.

Tan AE, Norizah WM, Rahman HA, Aziz BA, Cheah FC: Umbilical artery resistance index in diabetic pregnancies: the associations with fetal outcome and neonatal septal hypertrophic cardiomyopathy. *J Obstet Gynecol Res* 31:296–301, 2005.

Tanasijevic MJ, Winkelman JW, Wybenga DR, Richardson DK, Greene MF: Prediction of fetal lung maturity in infants of diabetic mothers using FLM S/A and disaturated phosphatidylcholine tests. *Am J Clin Pathol* 105:17–22, 1996.

Taylor PM, Wolfson JH, Bright NH, Birchard EL, Derinoz MN, Watson DW: Hyperbilirubinemia in infants of diabetic mothers. *Biol Neonate* 5:289–298, 1963.

Tchobroustsky C, Amiel-Tyson C, Cedard L, Eschwege E, Rouvillois JL, Tchobroutsky G: The lecithin/sphingomyelin ratio in 132 insulin-dependent diabetic pregnancies. *Am J Obstet Gynecol* 130:754–760, 1978.

Tchobroutsky C, Breart GL, Rambaud DC, Henrion R: Correlation between fetal defects and early growth delay observed by ultrasound. *Lancet* 2:975–976, 1985.

Teasdale F: Histomorphometry of the human placenta in Class B diabetes mellitus. *Placenta* 4:1–12, 1983.

Teasdale F: Histomorphometry of the human placenta in Class C diabetes mellitus. *Placenta* 6:69–81, 1985.

Temple RC, Aldridge V, Greenwood R, Heyburn P, Sampson M, Stanley K: Association between outcome of pregnancy and glycemic control in early pregnancy in type 1 diabetes: population-based study. *BMJ* 325:1275–1276, 2002.

Temple RC, Aldridge V, Stanley K, Murphy HR: Glycemic control throughout pregnancy and risk of preeclampsia in women with type 1 diabetes. *BJOG* 113:1329–1332, 2006.

Teramo K, Ammala P, Ylinen K, Raivio KO: Pathologic fetal heart rate associated with poor metabolic control in diabetic pregnancies. *Obstet Gynecol* 61:559–565, 1983.

Teramo KA, Widness JA, Clemons GK, Voutilainen P, McKinlay S, Schwartz R: Amniotic fluid erythropoietin correlates with umbilical plasma erythropoietin in normal and abnormal pregnancy. *Obstet Gynecol* 69:710–716, 1987.

Tcramo K, Kari MA, Eronen M, Markkanen H, Hiilesmaa V: High amniotic fluid erythropoietin levels are associated with an increased frequency of fetal and neonatal morbidity in type 1 diabetic pregnancies. *Diabetologia* 47:1695–1703, 2004.

Thacker SB, Stroup D, Chang M: Continuous electronic heart rate monitoring for fetal assessment during labor (Cochrane Review). In: *The Cochrane Library.* Issue 2. Oxford: Update Software; 2001.

Thadhani RI, Johnson RJ, Karumanchi SA: Hypertension during pregnancy. A disorder begging for pathophysiological support. *Hypertension* 46:1250–1251, 2005.

Thomas DJ, Gill B: Salbutamol-induced diabetic ketoacidosis. *Br Med J* 2:438, 1977.

Thorngren-Jerneck K, Herbst A: Perinatal factors associated with cerebral palsy in children born in Sweden. *Obstet Gynecol* 108:1499–1505, 2006.

Tincello DG, ElSapagh KM, Walkinshaw SA: Computerized analysis of fetal heart rate recordings in patients with diabetes mellitus: the Dawes-Redman criteria may not be valid indicators of fetal well-being. *J Perinat Med* 26:102–106, 1998.

Tincello D, White S, Walkinshaw S: Computerized analysis of fetal heart rate recordings in maternal type 1 diabetes mellitus. *Br J Obstet Gynecol* 108: 853–857, 2001.

Toal M, Keating S, Machin G, Dodd J, Adamson SL, Windrin RC, Kingdom JCP: Determinants of adverse perinatal outcome in high-risk women with abnormal uterine artery Doppler images. *Am J Obstet Gynecol* 198:330.e1–330.e7, 2008.

Tometzki AJ, Suda K, Kohl T, Kovalchin JP, Silverman NH: Accuracy of prenatal echocardiographic diagnosis and prognosis of fetuses with conotruncal anomalies. *J Am Coll Cardiol* 33:1696–1701,1999.

Torday J, Carson L, Lawson EE: Saturated phosphatidylcholine in amniotic fluid and prediction of the respiratory-distress syndrome. *N Engl J Med* 301:1013–1018, 1979.

Touger L, Looker HC, Krakoff J, Lindsay RS, Cook V, Knowler WC: Early growth in offspring of diabetic mothers. *Diabetes Care* 28:585–589, 2005.

Towey Ruch A, Lenke RR, Ashwood ER: Assessment of fetal lung maturity by fluorescence polarization in high risk pregnancies. *J Reprod Med* 38:133–136, 1993.

Treffers PE, Huidekoper BL, Weenink GH, Kloosterman GJ: Epidemiological observations of thrombo-embolic disease during pregnancy and in the puerperium, in 56,022 women. *Int J Obstet Gynecol* 21:327–331, 1983.

Trudinger BJ, Giles WB, Cook CM: Uteroplacental blood flow velocity-time waveforms in normal and complicated pregnancy. *Br J Obstet Gynecol* 92:39–45, 1985a.

Trudinger BJ, Giles WB, Cook CM, Bombardieri J, Collins L: Fetal umbilical artery flow velocity waveforms and placental resistance: clinical significance. *Br J Obstet Gynecol* 92:23–30, 1985b.

Tsai MY, Marshall JG: Phosphatidylglycerol in 261 samples of amniotic fluid from normal and diabetic pregnancies, as measured by one-dimensional thin-layer chromatography. *Clin Chem* 25:682–685, 1979.

Tsai MY, Josephson MW, Donhowe J: Delayed pulmonary phosphatidylglycerol synthesis and reversal by dexamethasone in fetal rats of streptozotocin-diabetic mothers. *Exp Lung Res* 4:315–323, 1983.

Tsai MY, Shultz EK, Nelson JA: Amniotic fluid phosphatidyl glycerol in diabetic and control pregnant patients at different gestational lengths. *Am J Obstet Gynecol* 149:388–392, 1984.

Tsai MY, Shultz EK, Williams PP, Bendel R, Butler J, Farb H, Wager G, Knox EG, Julian T, Thompson TR: Assay of disaturated phosphatidylcholine in amniotic fluid as a test of fetal lung maturity: experience with 2,000 analyses. *Clin Chem* 33:1648–1651, 1987.

Tsang RC, Kleinman L, Sutherland JM, Light IJ: Hypocalcemia in infants of diabetic mothers: studies in Ca, P and Mg metabolism and in parathormone responsiveness. *J Pediatr* 80:384–395, 1972.

Tsang RC, Chen IW, Friedman MA, Gigger M, Steichen J, Koffler H, Fenton L, Brown D, Pramanik A, Keenan W, Strub R, Joyce T: Parathyroid function in infants of diabetic mothers. *J Pediatr* 86:399–404, 1975.

Tsang RC, Straub R, Steichen JJ, Hartman C, Chen IW: Hypomagnesemia in infants of diabetic mothers: perinatal studies. *J Pediatr* 89:115–119, 1976.

Tsatsaris V, Papatsonis D, Goffinet F, Dekker G, Carbonne B: Tocolysis with nifedipine or beta-adrenergic agonists: a meta-analysis. *Obstet Gynecol* 97: 840–847, 2001.

Tsen LC: Anesthetic management of the parturient with cardiac and diabetic diseases. *Clin Obstet Gynecol* 46:700–710, 2003.

Tsyvian P, Malkin K, Artemieva O, Wladmiroff JW: Assessment of left ventricular filling in normally grown fetuses, growth-restricted fetuses and fetuses of diabetic mothers. *Ultrasound Obstet Gynecol* 12:33–38, 1998.

Tuncer M, Tuncer M: A long-term study of children born to diabetic mothers; with special reference to occurrence of late neurological abnormalities. *Turk J Pediatr* 16:59–69, 1974.

Tuomi T, Groop L: Intrauterine hyperglycemia modifying the development of (monogenic) diabetes? Commentary. *Diabetes Care* 26:1295–1296, 2003.

Turner LA, Cyr M, Kinch RA, Liston R, Kramer MS, Fair M, Heaman M; for the Maternal Mortality and Morbidity Study Group of the Canadian Perinatal Surveillance System: Under-reporting of maternal mortality in Canada: a question of definition. *Chronic Dis Can* 23:22–30, 2002.

Tyden O, Berne C, Ericksson U: Lung maturation in fetuses of diabetic rats. *Pediatr Res* 14:1192–1195, 1980.

Ullmo S, Vial Y, Di Bernardo S, Roth-Kleiner M, Mivelaz Y, Sekarski N, Ruiz J, Meijboom EJ: Pathologic ventricular hypertrophy in the offspring of diabetic mothers: a retrospective study. *Eur Heart J* 28:1319–1325, 2007.

Underwood MA, Gilbert WM, Sherman MP: Amniotic fluid: not just fetal urine anymore. *J Perinatol* 25:341–348, 2005.

Ursem NTC, Clark EB, Keller BB, Wladimiroff JW: Fetal heart rate and umbilical artery velocity variability in pregnancies complicated by insulin-dependent diabetes mellitus. *Ultrasound Obstet Gynecol* 13:312–316, 1999.

Usher RH, Allen AC, McLean FH: Risk of respiratory distress syndrome related to gestational age, route of delivery, and maternal diabetes. *Am J Obstet Gynecol* 111:826–832, 1971.

Vaarasmaki MS, Hartikainen A-L, Anttila M, Pramila S, Koivisto M: Factors predicting peri- and neonatal outcome in diabetic pregnancy. *Early Hum Dev* 59:61–70, 2000.

Vaarasmaki M, Anttila M, Pirttiaho H, Hartikainen A-L: Are recurrent pregnancies a risk in type 1 diabetes? *Acta Obstet Gynecol Scand* 81:1110–1115, 2002.

Valenzuela GJ, Sanchez-Ramos L, Romero R, Silver HM, Koltun WD, Millar L, Hobbins J, Rayburn W, Shangold G, Wang J, Smith J, Creasy GW: Maintenance treatment of preterm labor with the oxytocin antagonist atosiban. The Atosiban PTL-098 Study Group. *Am J Obstet Gynecol* 182:1184–1190, 2000.

van Runnard Heimel PJ, Franx A, Schobben AFAM, Huisjes AJM, Derks JB, Bruinse HW: Corticosteroids, pregnancy, and HELLP syndrome: a review. *Obstet Gynecol Surv* 60:57–70, 2004.

Vangen S, Stoltenberg C, Holan S, Moe N, Magnus P, Harris JR, Stray-Pedersen B: Outcome of pregnancy among immigrant women with diabetes. *Diabetes Care* 26:327–332, 2003.

Veille JC, Sivakoff M, Hanson R, Fanaroff AA: Interventricular septal thickness in fetuses of diabetic mothers. *Obstet Gynecol* 79:51–54, 1992.

Veille JC, Hanson R, Sivakoff M, Hoen H, Ben-Ami M: Fetal cardiac size in normal, intrauterine growth retarded, and diabetic pregnancies. *Am J Perinatol* 10: 275–279, 1993.

Vejlsgaard R: Studies on urinary infections in diabetes. III. Significant bacteriuria in pregnant diabetic patients and in matched controls. *Acta Med Scand* 193: 337–341, 1973a.

Vejlsgaard R: Studies on urinary infections in diabetes. IV. Significant bacteriuria in pregnancy in relation to age of onset, duration of diabetes. Angiopathy and urological symptoms. *Acta Med Scand* 193:343–346, 1973b.

Vejlsgaard R: Studies on urinary infections in diabetes. V. Bacteriuria in relation to various obstetrical factors, fetal outcome and mortality. *Acta Med Scand* 193: 347–352, 1973c.

Vela-Huerta MM, Vargas-Origel A, Olvera-Lopez A: Asymmetrical septal hypertrophy in newborn infants of diabetic mothers. *Am J Perinatol* 17:89–94, 2000.

Velazquez MD, Rayburn WF: Antenatal evaluation of the fetus using fetal movement monitoring. *Clin Obstet Gynecol* 45:993–1004, 2002.

Verdy M, Gagnon M-A, Caron D: Birth weight and adult obesity in children of diabetic mothers. Letter. *N Engl J Med* 290:576, 1974.

Vergani P, Roncaglia N, Locatelli A, Andreotti C, Crippa I, Pezzullo JC, Ghidini A: Antenatal predictors of neonatal outcome in fetal growth restriction with absent end-diastolic flow in the umbilical artery. *Am J Obstet Gynecol* 193:1213–1218, 2005.

Verhaeghe J, VanHerck E, Bouillon R: Umbilical cord osteocalcin in normal pregnancies and pregnancies complicated by fetal growth retardation or diabetes mellitus. *Biol Neonate* 68:377–383, 1995.

Verheijen ECJ, Critchley JA, Whitelaw DC, Tuffnell DJ: Outcomes of pregnancies in women with pre-existing type 1 or type 2 diabetes, in an ethnically mixed population. *BJOG* 112:1500–1503, 2005.

Vermillion ST, Scardo JA, Newman RB, Chauhan SP: A randomized, double-blind trial of oral nifedipine and intravenous labetalol in hypertensive emergencies of pregnancy. *Am J Obstet Gynecol* 181:858–861, 1999.

Verner AM, Manderson J, Lappin TRJ, McCance DR, Halliday HL, Sweet DG: Influence of maternal diabetes mellitus on fetal iron status. *Arch Dis Child Fetal Neonatal Ed* 92:399–401, 2007.

Villar J, Abdel-Aleem H, Merialdi M, Mathai M, Ali MM, Zavaleta N, Purwar M, Hofmeyr J, Ngoc NtN, Campodonico L, Landoulsi S, Carroli G, Lindheimer M; on behalf of the World Health Organization Calcium Supplementation for the Prevention of Preeclampsia Trial Group: World Health Organization randomized trial of calcium supplementation among low calcium intake pregnant women. *Am J Obstet Gynecol* 194:639–649, 2006a.

Villar J, Valladares E, Wojdyla D, Zavaleta N, Carroli G, Velazco A, Shah A, Camodonico L, Bataglia V, Faundes A, Langer A, Narvaez A, Donner A, Romero M, Reynoso S, de Padua KS, Giordano D, Kublickas M, Acosta A; WHO 2005 Global Survey on Maternal and Perinatal Health Research Group: Cesarean delivery rates and pregnancy outcomes: the 2005 WHO global survey on maternal and perinatal health in Latin America. *Lancet* 367:1819–1829, 2006b.

Vink JY, Poggi SH, Ghidini A, Spong CY: Amniotic fluid index and birth weight: is there a relationship in diabetic patients with poor glycemic control? *Am J Obstet Gynecol* 195:848–850, 2006.

Vintzileos AM, Nochimson DJ, Guzman EF, Knuppel RA, Lake M, Schifrin BS: Intrapartum electronic fetal heart rate monitoring versus intermittent auscultation: a meta-analysis. *Obstet Gynecol* 85:149–155, 1995a.

Vintzileos AM, Nochimson DJ, Antsaklis A, Varvarigos I, Guzman EF, Knuppel RA: Comparison of intrapartum electronic fetal heart rate monitoring versus intermittent auscultation in detecting fetal acidemia at birth. *Am J Obstet Gynecol* 173:1021–1024, 1995b.

Visalyaputra S, Rodanant O, Somboonviboon W, Tantivitayatan K, Thienthong S, Saengchote W: Spinal versus epidural anesthesia for cesarean delivery in severe preeclampsia: a prospective randomized, multicenter study. *Anesth Analg* 101:362–368, 2005.

Visser GHA, Bekedam DJ, Mulder EJH, van Ballegooie E: Delayed emergence of fetal behaviour in type-1 diabetic women. *Early Hum Dev* 12:167–172, 1985.

Visser GHA, Evers IM, Mello G: Management of the macrosomic fetus. In: Hod M, Jovanovic L, Di Renzo GC, de Leiva A, Langer O, eds. *Textbook of Diabetes and Pregnancy.* London: Martin Dunitz; 2003:455–459.

Vyas S, Nicolaides KH, Bower S, Campbell S: Middle cerebral artery flow velocity waveforms in fetal hypoxemia. *Br J Obstet Gynecol* 97:797–803, 1990.

Wager J, Fredholm BB, Lunell NO, Persson B: Metabolic and circulatory effects of oral salbutamol in the third trimester of pregnancy in diabetic and nondiabetic women. *Br J Obstet Gynecol* 88:352–361, 1981.

Waisman GD, Mayorga LM, Camera MI, Vignolo CA, Martinotti A: Magnesium plus nifedipine: potentiation of hypotensive effect in preeclampsia? *Am J Obstet Gynecol* 159:308–309, 1988.

Wald NJ, Cuckle H, Boreham J, Stirrat GM, Turnbull A: Maternal serum alpha-fetoprotein and diabetes mellitus. *Br J Obstet Gynecol* 86:101–105, 1979.

Wallace DH, Leveno KJ, Cunningham FG, Giesecke AH, Shearer VE, Sidawi JE: Randomized comparison of general and regional anesthesia for cesarean delivery in pregnancies complicated by preeclampsia. *Obstet Gynecol* 86: 193–199, 1995.

Wang R, Martinez-Frias ML, Graham JM Jr: Infants of diabetic mothers are at increased risk for the oculo-auricuolo-vertebral sequence: A case-based and case-control approach. *J Pediatr* 141:611–617, 2002.

Wapner R, Thom E, Simpson JL, Pergament E, Silver R, Filkins K, Platt L, Mahoney M, Johnson A, Hogge WA, Wilson RD, Mohide P, Hershey D, Krantz D,

Zachary J, Snijders R, Greene N, Sabbagha R, MacGregor S, Hill L, Gagnon A, Hallahan T, Jackson L; for the First Trimester Maternal Serum Biochemistry and Fetal Translucency Screening (BUN) Study Group: First trimester screening for trisomies 21 and 18. *N Engl J Med* 349:1405–1413, 2003.

Wapner R: Antenatal corticosteroids: we continue to learn. Editorial. *Am J Obstet Gynecol* 190:875, 2004.

Warburton D: Chronic hyperglycemia reduces surface-active material flux in tracheal fluid of fetal lungs. *J Clin Invest* 71:550–555, 1983a.

Warburton D: Chronic hyperglycemia with secondary hyperinsulinemia inhibits the maturational response of fetal lamb lungs to cortisol. *J Clin Invest* 72:443–440, 1983b.

Warram JH, Krolewski AS, Gottlieb MS, Kahn CR: Differences in risk of insulin-dependent diabetes in offspring of diabetic mothers and diabetic fathers. *N Engl J Med* 311:149–152, 1984.

Warram JH, Krolewski AS, Kahn CR: Determinants of IDDM and perinatal mortality in children of diabetic mothers. *Diabetes* 37:1328–1334, 1988.

Watson D, Rowan J, Neale L, Battin MR: Admissions to neonatal intensive care unit following pregnancies complicated by gestational or type 2 diabetes. *Aust N Z J Obstet Gynecol* 43:429–432, 2003.

Wax JR, Herson V, Carignan E, Mather J, Ingardia CJ: Contribution of elective delivery to severe respiratory distress at term. *Am J Perinatol* 19:81–86, 2002.

Weaver TE, Whitsett JA: Function and regulation of expression of pulmonary surfactant-associated proteins. *Biochem J* 273:249–264, 1991.

Weber HS, Copel JA, Reece A, Green J, Kleinman CS: Cardiac growth in fetuses of diabetic mothers with good metabolic control. *J Pediatr* 118:103–107, 1991.

Weiner CP: The relationship between the umbilical artery systolic/diastolic ratio and umbilical blood gas measurements in specimens obtained by cordocentesis. *Am J Obstet Gynecol* 162:1198–1202, 1990.

Weiner Z, Thaler I, Farmakides G, Barnhard Y, Maulik D, Divon MY. Fetal heart rate patterns in pregnancies complicated by maternal diabetes. *Eur J Obstet Gynecol* 70:111–115, 1996.

Weiner Z, Zloczower M, Lerner A, Zimmer E, Itskovitz-Eldor J: Cardiac compliance in fetuses of diabetic women. *Obstet Gynecol* 93:948–951, 1999.

Weiner Z, Goldstein I, Bombard A, Applewhite L, Itzkovits-Eldor J: Screening for structural fetal anomalies during the nuchal translucency ultrasound examination. *Am J Obstet Gynecol* 197:181.e1–181.e5. 2007.

Weintrob N, Karp M, Hod M: Short- and long-range complications in offspring of diabetic mothers. *J Diabetes Complications* 10:294–301, 1996.

Weiss PA, Kainer F, Haas J: Cord blood insulin to assess the quality of treatment in diabetic pregnancies. *Early Hum Dev* 51:187–195, 1998.

Weiss PAM, Scholz HS, Haas J, Tamussino KF, Seissler J, Borkenstein MH: Long-term follow-up of infants of mothers with type 1 diabetes. Evidence for hereditary and nonhereditary transmission of diabetes and precursors. *Diabetes Care* 23:905–911, 2000.

Weitz R, Laron Z: Height and weight of children born to mothers with diabetes mellitus. *Isr J Med Sci* 12:195–198, 1976.

Wells PS, Anderson DR, Bormanis J, Guy F, Mitchell M, Gray L, Clement C, Robinson KS, Lewandowski B: Value assessment of pretest probability of deep-vein thrombosis in clinical management. *Lancet* 351:1795–1798, 1997.

Welsch H, Krone HA, Wisser J: Maternal mortality in Bavaria between 1983 and 2000. *Am J Obstet Gynecol* 191:304–308, 2004.

Wen SW, Huang L, Liston R, Heaman M, Baskett T, Rusen ID, Joseph KS, Kramer MS; for the Maternal Health Study Group, Canadian Perinatal Surveillance System: Severe maternal morbidity in Canada, 1991–2001. *CMAJ* 173:759–763, 2005.

West TET, Lowy C: Control of blood glucose during labor in diabetic women with combined glucose and low-dose insulin infusion. *Br Med J* 1:1252–1254, 1977.

Westergaard HB, Langhoff-Roos J, Lingman G, Marsal K: A critical appraisal of the use of umbilical artery Doppler ultrasound in high-risk pregnancies: use of meta-analyses in evidence-based obstetrics. *Ultrasound Obstet Gynecol* 17:466–467, 2001.

Westgate J, Harris M, Curnow JSH, Greene KR: Plymouth randomized trial of cardiotocogram only versus ST waveform plus cardiotocogram for intrapartum monitoring: 2,400 cases. *Am J Obstet Gynecol* 169:1151–1160, 1993.

Westgate JA, Bennet L, Brabyn C, Williams CE, Gunn AJ: ST waveform changes during repeated umbilical cord occlusions in near-term fetal sheep. *Am J Obstet Gynecol* 184:743–751, 2001.

Westgate JA, Lindsay RS, Beattie J, Pattison NS, Gamble G, Mildenhall LFJ, Breier BH, Johnstone FD: Hyperinsulinemia in cord blood in mothers with type 2 diabetes and gestational diabetes in New Zealand. *Diabetes Care* 29:1345–1350, 2006.

Westin M, Saltvedt S, Bergman G, Kublickas M, Almstrom H, Grunewald C, Valentin L: Routine ultrasound examination at 12 or 18 gestational weeks for prenatal detection of major congenital malformations? *BJOG* 113:675–682, 2006.

White P: Childhood diabetes. Its course and influence on the second and third generations. *Diabetes* 9:345–355, 1960.

White P: Pregnancy complicating diabetes mellitus. In: Marble A, White P, Bradley RF, eds. *Joslin's Diabetes Mellitus.* 11th ed. Philadelphia: Lea & Febiger; 1971.

White E, Shy KK, Daling JR: An investigation of the relationship between cesarean section birth and respiratory distress syndrome of the newborn. *Am J Epidemiol* 121:651–663, 1985.

Whitehead SJ, Berg CJ, Chang J: Pregnancy-related mortality due to cardiomyopathy: United States, 1991–1997. *Obstet Gynecol* 102:1326–1331, 2003.

Whitelaw A: Subcutaneous fat in newborn inants of diabetic mothers: an indication of quality control. *Lancet* 1:15–18, 1977.

Whitfield CR, Sproule WB, Burdenell M: The amniotic fluid lecithin/sphingomyelin area ratio (LSAR) in pregnancies complicated by diabetes. *J Obstet Gynecol Brit Commonwl* 80:918–922, 1973.

Whittle MJ, Anderson D, Lowensohn RI, Mestman JH, Paul RH, Goebelsmann U: Estriol in pregnancy. VI. Experience with unconjugated plasma estriol assays and antepartum fetal heart rate testing in diabetic pregnancies. *Am J Obstet Gynecol* 135:764–772, 1979.

Whittle MJ, Wilson AI, Wenifield CR, Paton RD, Lugar RW: Amniotic fluid PG and the L/S ratio in the assessment of fetal lung maturity. *Br J Obstet Gynecol* 89: 727–732, 1982.

Widness JA, Susa JB, Garcia JF, Singer DB, Sehgal P, Oh W, Schwartz R, Schwartz HC: Increased erythropoiesis and elevated erythropoietin in infants born to diabetic mothers and in hyperinsulinemic rhesus fetuses. *J Clin Invest* 67: 637–642, 1981.

Widness JA, Teramo KA, Clemons GK, Voutilainen P, Stenman U-H, McKinlay SM, Schwartz R: Direct relationship of antepartum glucose control and fetal erythropoietin in human type 1 (insulin-dependent) diabetic pregnancy. *Diabetologia* 33:378–383, 1990.

Wigton TR, Sabbagha RE, Tamura RK, Cohen L, Minogue JP, Strasburger JF: Sonographic diagnosis of congenital heart disease: comparison between the four-chamber view and multiple cardiac views. *Obstet Gynecol* 82:219–224, 1993.

Wildman K, Bouvier-Colle M-H; the MOMS group: Maternal mortality as an indicator of obstetric care in Europe. *BJOG* 111:164–169, 2004.

Wilkes BM, Mento PF, Hollander AM: Reduced thromboxane receptor affinity and vasoconstrictor responses in placentae from diabetic pregnancies. *Placenta* 15:845–855, 1994.

Wilkin TJ, Murphy MJ: The gender insulin hypothesis: why girls are born lighter than boys, and the implications for insulin resistance. *Int J Obes* 30:1056–1061, 2006.

Williams PR, Sperling MA, Racasa Z: Blunting of spontaneous and alanine-stimulated glucagon secretion in newborn infants of diabetic mothers. *Am J Obstet Gynecol* 133:51–56, 1979.

Williams KP, Farquharson DF, Bebbington M, Dansereau J, Galerneau F, Wilson RD, Shaw D, Kent N: Screening for fetal well-being in a high-risk pregnant population comparing the nonstress test with umbilical artery Doppler velocimetry: a randomized controlled study. *Am J Obstet Gynecol* 188:1366–1371, 2003.

Winn-McMillan T, Karon BS: Comparison of the TDx-FLM II and lecithin to sphingomyelin ratio assays in predicting fetal lung maturity. *Am J Obstet Gynecol* 193:778–782, 2005.

Winocour PH, Taylor RJ: Early alterations of renal function in insulin-dependent diabetic pregnancies and their importance in predicting preeclamptic toxemia. *Diabetes Res* 10:159–164, 1989.

Wissler RN: Endocrine disorders. In: Chestnut DH, ed. *Obstetric Anesthesia. Principles and Practice.* 3rd ed. Philadelphia: Elsevier Mosby; 2004:734–763.

Wolf H, Hoeksma AF, Oei SL, Bleker OP: Obstetric brachial plexus injury: risk factors related to recovery. *Eur J Obstet Gynecol Reprod Biol* 88:133–138, 2000.

Wong SF, Chan FY, Cincotta RB, Oats JJ, McIntyre HD: Sonographic estimation of fetal weight in macrosomic fetuses: diabetic versus non-diabetic pregnancies. *Aust N Z J Obstet Gynecol* 41:429–432, 2001.

Wong SF, Chan FY, Oats JJN, McIntyre DH: Fetal growth spurt and pregestational diabetic pregnancy. *Diabetes Care* 25:1681–1684, 2002.

Wong SF, Chan FY, Cincotta RB, McIntyre HD, Oats JJN: Cardiac function in fetuses of poorly-controlled pre-gestational diabetic pregnancies—a pilot study. *Gynecol Obstet Invest* 56:113–116, 2003a.

Wong SF, Chan FY, Cincotta RB, McIntyre DH, Stone M: Use of umbilical artery Doppler velocimetry in the monitoring of pregnancy in women with pre-existing diabetes. *Aust N Z J Obstet Gynecol* 43:302–306, 2003b.

Wong ML, Wong WH, Cheung YF: Fetal myocardial performance in pregnancies complicated by gestational impaired glucose tolerance. *Ultrasound Obstet Gynecol* 29:395–400, 2007.

Wood SL, Jick H, Sauve R: The risk of stillbirth in pregnancies before and after the onset of diabetes. *Diabet Med* 20:703–707, 2003.

Wu PY, Modanlou H, Karelitz M: Effect of glucagon on blood glucose homeostasis in infants of diabetic mothers. *Acta Paediatr Scand* 64:441–445, 1975.

Wylie BR, Kong J, Kozak SE, Marshall CJ, Tong SO, Thompson DM: Normal perinatal mortality in type 1 diabetes mellitus in a series of 300 consecutive pregnancy outcomes. *Am J Perinatol* 19:169–176, 2002.

Yager JY, Heitjan DF, Towfighi J, Vannucci RC: Effect of insulin-induced and fasting hypoglycemia on perinatal hypoxic-ischemic brain damage. *Pediatr Res* 31:138–142, 1992.

Yajnik CS, Godbole K, Otiv SR, Lubree HG: Fetal programming of type 2 diabetes. Is sex important? Editorial. *Diabetes Care* 30:2754–2755, 2007.

Yamashita Y, Kawano Y, Kuriya N, Murakami Y, Matsuishi T, Yoshimatsu K, Kato H: Intellectual development of offspring of diabetic mothers. *Acta Paediatr* 85:1191–1196, 1996.

Yang H, Kramer MS, Platt RW, Blondel B, Breart G, Morin I, Wilkins R, Usher R: How does early ultrasound scan estimation of gestational age lead to a high rate of preterm birth? *Am J Obstet Gynecol* 186:433–437, 2002.

Yaron Y, Cherry M, Kramer RL, O'Brien JE, Hallak M, Johnson MP, Evans MI: Second-trimester maternal serum marker screening: maternal serum a-fetoprotein, b-human chorionic gonadotropin, estriol, and their various combinations as predictors of pregnancy outcome. *Am J Obstet Gynecol* 181:968–974, 1999.

Yeast JD, Porreco RP, Ginsberg HN: The use of continuous insulin infusion for the peripartum management of pregnant diabetic women. *Am J Obstet Gynecol* 131:861–864, 1978.

Yemini M, Borenstein R, Dreazen E, Apelman Z, Mogilner BM, Kessler I, Lancet M: Prevention of preterm labor by 17[alpha]-hydroxyprogesterone caproate. *Am J Obstet Gynecol* 151:574–577, 1985.

Yli BM, Kallen K, Stray-Pedersen B, Amer-Whalin I: Intrapartum fetal ECG and diabetes. *J Matern-Fetal Neonatal Med* 21:231–238, 2008.

Ylinen K: High maternal levels of hemoglobin A1C associated with delayed fetal lung maturation in insulin-dependent diabetic pregnancies. *Acta Obstet Gynecol Scand* 66:263–266, 1987.

Yogev Y, Ben-Haroush A, Chen R, Glickman H, Kaplan B, Hod M: Active induction management of labor for diabetic pregnancies at term; mode of delivery and fetal outcome—a single center experience. *Eur J Obstet Gynecol Reprod Biol* 114:166–170, 2004.

Yogman MW, Cole P, Als H, Lester BM: Behavior of newborns of diabetic mothers. *Infant Behav Dev* 5:331–340, 1982.

Yost NP, Owen J, Berghella V, MacPherson C, Swain M, Dildy GA III, Miodovnik M, Langer O, Sibai B; for the National Institute of Child Health and Human Development, Maternal-Fetal Medicine Units Network: Number and gestational age of prior preterm births does not modify the predictive value of a short cervix. *Am J Obstet Gynecol* 191:241–246, 2004.

Yssing M: Estriol excretion in pregnant diabetics related to long-term prognosis of surviving children. *Acta Endocrinol* 75 (Suppl 182):95–104, 1974.

Yssing M: Long-term prognosis of children born to mothers diabetic when pregnant. In: Camerini-Davalos RA, Cole HS, eds. *Early Diabetes in Early Life*. New York: Academic Press; 575–586, 1975.

Zhu L, Nakabayashi M, Takeda Y: Statistical analysis of perinatal outcomes in pregnancy complicated with diabetes mellitus. *J Obstet Gynecol Res* 23:555–563, 1997.

Zimmer EZ, Paz Y, Goldstick O, Beloosesky R, Weiner Z: Computerized analysis of fetal heart rate after maternal glucose ingestion in normal pregnancy. *Eur J Obstet Gynecol Reprod Biol* 93:57–60, 2000.

Zimmerman P, Kujansuu E, Tuimala R: Doppler velocimetry of the umbilical artery in pregnancies complicated by insulin-dependent diabetes. *Eur J Obstet Gynecol Reprod Biol* 47:85–93, 1992.

Zimmerman P, Kujansuu E, Tuimala R: Doppler flow velocimetry of the uterine and uteroplacental circulation in pregnancy complicatd by insulin-dependent diabetes mellitus. *J Perinat Med* 22:137–147, 1994.

Postpartum Management of Women with Preexisting Diabetes Mellitus

POSTPARTUM GLYCEMIC CONTROL AND COMPLICATIONS

—— Original contribution by Maribeth Inturrisi RN, MS, CNS, CDE and John L. Kitzmiller MD, MS

Postpartum Glycemic Control

The immediate goals of postpartum care are continuation of effective glycemic control, recognition and treatment of maternal complications, and facilitation of maternal–infant bonding and lactation. These are challenging goals in patients with high rates of CS who live with the possibility that the infant will be in a special-care nursery. In women with type 1 diabetes, it is likely that the type of insulin therapy used in pregnancy will be continued. Most women with type 2 diabetes will be converted to treatment with oral antihyperglycemic agents. It is well known that a sharp temporary drop in the maternal insulin requirement occurs immediately after delivery, with a gradual rise to 0.3–0.5 of pregnancy levels over several days (Lev-Ran 74, Kjos 00,07). For women with either type of diabetes, glycemic goals may be relaxed somewhat to approach those for nonpregnant women with diabetes: the group A1C goal is <7.0%, but encourage individual patients to strive for an A1C as close to normal (<6%) as possible without significant hypoglycemia (stay above 70 mg/dL; >3.9 mM) (ADA 05,08a); MBG <135–150 mg/dL (<7.5–8.3 mM). Useful targets are preprandial and nighttime plasma glucose <120–140 mg/dL (<6.7–7.6 mM) and 1–2-h postprandial plasma glucose <150–170 mg/dL (<8.0–9.4 mM) (Rohlfing 02, ADA 06a, Bartnik 07). SMBG should be carried out 3–7 times daily to enable women to achieve these glycemic goals consistent with low rates of postpartum complications and successful lactation for at least 6 months. The variability of plasma glucose with breast-feeding and the other challenges of infant care may suggest a role for intermittent continuous monitoring of blood glucose (Monsod 02, Garg 06, McLachlan 07, Murphy 07, Pearce 08), especially in those with hypoglycemia unawareness (ADA 08a).

We are aware that use of SMBG in type 2 diabetes patients who are not treated with insulin remains controversial (Coster 00, Karter 01, Schwedes 02, Bergenstal 05, Blonde 05, Davidson 05a, Del Prato 05, Franciosi 05, Sarol 05, Martin 06a, Chen 08) and that more adequately powered RCTs are needed to resolve the issue (Davidson 05b, Welschen 05). In 290 noninsulin- and nonacarbose-using type 2 diabetes patients, postprandial glycemic excursions played a major role in determining A1C in patients with mild or moderate hyperglycemia, but were less predictive than fasting hyperglycemia when A1C was >8.4% (Monnier 03). Analysis of quarterly 1-day glucose profiles of subjects with type 1 diabetes participating in the DCCT indicated that within-day glucose variability (Moberg 93, Brownlee 06, McCarter 06) was not an additional factor beyond MBG in the development of retinopathy (Kilpatrick 06). Pre- and post prandial glucose values were "equally predictive of the small-vessel complications of type 1 diabetes" (Kilpatrick 06). The analysis suggests that patients who balance high and low values are at no more risk than women with more steady hyperglycemia at the same mean level (Bolli 06), but does not explain why subjects in the intensive treatment arm of the DCCT had less retinopathy progression than subjects in the conventional treatment arm with equivalent A1C values (DCCT 95). Of course, DCCT subjects in intensive treatment used both pre- and postprandial daily blood glucose to monitor their response to dietary, exercise, and insulin treatment the other 90 days of each 3-month epoch and had fewer long-term cardiovascular (DCCT/EDIC 05) and microvascular complications (DCCT/EDIC 02). Because there is ample epidemiological evidence that postmeal blood glucose best predicts CVD in diabetic patients (Hanefeld 96, Bonora 01, Ceriello 05, Home 05, Monnier 06,08), analysis of the influence of within-day glucose variability on macrovascular outcomes is needed before clinicians conclude that postprandial testing is not needed in SMBG as part of intensified treatment of postpartum type 1 and type 2 diabetes.

Long-term maintenance of glycemic, BP, and lipid goals with multifactorial treatment (Gaede 99,03,08, Anselmino 08) should help protect diabetic women against development or progression of micro- and macrovascular complications and neuropathy (DCCT 95,98, UKPDS 98a,b, Stratton 00, DCCT/EDIC 00,02,05, Carter 05, Bartnik 07, Mazzone 07). Maintenance of glycemic goals should also reduce the chance of early fetal loss or major congenital malformations if there is an unexpected pregnancy (Kitzmiller 96, Temple 02, Evers 04, Jensen 04, Clausen 05, Jovanovic 05, McElduff 05, Verheijen 05, Sacks 06, Kjos 07, Reece 07, Varughese 07).

MNT, use of antihyperglycemic agents for women with type 2 diabetes, and treatment of dyslipidemia, hypertension, thyroid disease, and depression must all be tailored for the requirements of lactation. These topics are discussed in the sections titled "Lactation Nutritional Requirements and the Diabetic Food Plan" and "Drug Treatment of Diabetes and Related Disorders During Lactation."

Postpartum Complications

Data on postpartum complications in women with PDM are limited. An increase in perineal trauma is encountered with difficult vaginal deliveries (Acker 85, Casey 05). We are not aware of studies of hemorrhage or infection after vaginal deliveries of diabetic women. We also lack studies on the risk of postpartum thromboembolism after vaginal or cesarean deliveries of diabetic women. Because patients with diabetes are thought to be at increased risk for infection, especially with poor glycemic control (Rayfield 82), the rate of postcesarean endometritis and wound infections has been investigated in retrospective

TABLE IV.1 Postcesarean Complications in Women with Preexisting Diabetes Mellitus

	Diamond 1986	Stamler 1990	Riley 1996	Takoudes 2004
Cesarean deliveries	79 (24 labor or ROM)	65*	205 (all labor)	192 (106 labor)
Prophylactic antibiotics, N (%)	7 (8.9)	NA	162 (79.0)	107 (55.7)
Endometritis, N (%)	11 (13.9) pooled	5 (7.7) pooled	10 (4.9)	11 (5.7)
Wound infection, N (%)	With wound infection	With wound infection	6 (2.9)	24/186 (12.9)
Wound separation, N (%)	NA	NA	NA	18/185 (9.7)
Postpartum hemorrhage, N (%)	NA	NA	NA	23 (12.4)
Relative risk vs. controls	4.4 for endometritis + wound infection	4.8 for all PP infections	NS (endometritis in 9.2% controls)	2.5** for all wound complications
Postpartum glucose, N (%)	NA	113 ± 29 infected	218 ± 120 infected	26 >200 mg/dL (13.5)

Repeat cesarean sections only (25% in labor).
**Adjusted RR.*

NA, not available; NS, not stated; PP, postpartum; ROM, rupture of membranes; RR, relative risk.

cohort studies. Three of four studies (Diamond 86, Stamler 90, Riley 96, Takoudes 04) found increased infectious complications after cesarean deliveries of diabetic women (Table IV.1). Although assessment of predelivery and postpartum glycemic control was not optimal in these studies, investigators found no apparent relationships between postcesarean infections and glucose or glycosylated hemoglobin levels (Stamler 90, Riley 96, Takoudes 04). In the 1996 study, multiple logistic regression analysis showed that duration of labor, duration of ruptured membranes, and number of vaginal examinations were risk factors for infection. The latter two factors were more common in the randomly selected controls. Postcesarean septic pelvic thrombophlebitis was diagnosed in 5 of 205 diabetic women (2.4%) and 1 of 206 control women (0.5%) (NS) (Riley 96). In the 2004 study, multivariable subanalysis of all patients who labored showed that diabetic women were 1.9 times as likely to develop postcesarean wound complications than controls, regardless of prophylactic antibiotic use (Takoudes 04). A large number of RCTs in nondiabetic women demonstrated the value of prophylactic antibiotics in reducing postcesarean morbidity in high-risk afebrile patients with labor or ruptured membranes prior to CS (Smaill 03). A meta-analysis of four RCTs on the use of prophylactic antibiotics at CS of nondiabetic women before labor with intact membranes showed a significant decrease in endometritis (RR 0.05; 95% CI 0.01–0.38) (Chelmow 01). The risk of development of resistant organisms with single-dose therapy at CS is not well understood; the risk of anaphylaxis to the commonly used cephalosporins is <0.1% (Stiver 84, Kelkar 01, ACOG 03). Prospective controlled trials are needed in large numbers of diabetic women to determine the (1) most effective means as well as costs of preventing postcesarean infections, (2) possible interactions with glycemic control, and (3) incidence of other serious complications, such as postpartum hemorrhage and thromboembolism.

Peripartum Cardiomyopathy

PPCM with LV systolic dysfunction in the absence of prior heart disease or identifiable cause can develop during the last month of pregnancy or within 5–6 months postpartum in 1 per 3,000–4,000 deliveries (Lambert 95, Pearson 00, Kaaja 05, Sliwa 06). The frequency of occurrence is unknown with diabetes (Kaufman 03) despite increasing research on the problem of general diabetic myocardial fibrosis and cardiomyopathy, seen especially in white women (Felker 00, Trost 01, Bell 03, Bertoni 03, Cai 03, Fang 04). Further references on diabetic cardiomyopathy, LV dysfunction, and diastolic heart failure are to be found in the section titled "Heart Failure" in Part II. The pathophysiology may be different for the two types of cardiomyopathy, diabetic and peripartum. Traditional risk factors for peripartum cardiomyopathy include age, parity, hypertensive disorders, ethnicity, multifetal gestation, and perhaps inflammation and oxidative stress (Ludwig 97, Heider 99, Sundstrom 02, Bultmann 05). PPCM has a high mortality rate, and cases should be managed at high-risk perinatal centers whenever possible (Witlin 97, Pearson 00, Whitehead 03). The primary goal of therapy is to alleviate symptoms of congestive heart failure. Due to the risk of thromboembolism, anticoagulation is recommended for those with ejection fractions <35% (Pearson 00). If ventricular size and function return to normal (EF >50%), short-term prognosis is reasonable (Pearson 00), but ventricular dysfunction can recur (Sutton 91, Lambert 97, Ceci 98). The wisdom of a subsequent pregnancy with prior PPCM remains controversial (Pearson 00, Elkayam 01, Sliwa 04, Fett 06).

The separate problem of acute MI in diabetic pregnant women during the antenatal and intrapartum periods is discussed in Part II in the section titled "Coronary Heart Disease." We note here that 27–40% of all MIs associated with pregnancy occur postpartum and management is difficult (Badui 96, Roth 96, Chaithiraphan 03, James 06), but antepartum infarctions may be more common in women with PDM (Ladner 05).

Postpartum Thyroiditis

Postpartum thyroid disease (PPTD) that occurs 1–11 months after delivery is common (mean prevalence rate 5–8%, range 2–16%) in nondiabetic women (albeit subclinical in ~50–60% of subjects) (Gerstein 90, Smallridge 00a, Stagnaro-Green 00,02, Nicholson 06). Initial signs may be hypothyroidism (lethargy, poor memory, dry skin, depression) or transient thyrotoxicosis (palpitations, tremulousness, nervousness, heat intolerance) that may then progress to hypothyroidism (Ginsberg 77, Amino 82, Walfish 92, Lazarus 99). "Postpartum thyroiditis is an exacerbation of an underlying autoimmune thyroiditis, aggravated by the immunological rebound that follows the partial immunosuppression of pregnancy" (Stagnaro-Green 02). Histological studies of thyroid aspirates reveal lymphocytic infiltrate or diffuse destruction, similar to Hashimoto's thyroiditis (Jansson 84, Muller 01). Thyroid US echogenicity correlates with lymphocytic infiltration (Adams 92, Parkes 96). Hyperthyroid PPTD may result from initial release of thyroid hormone due to the autoimmune stimulation, and this phase is often diagnosed only in retrospect during work-ups for hypothyroidism (Stagnaro-Green 02).

Antimicrosomal TPOAbs are usually detected in women with postpartum thyroiditis (Jansson 84, Hayslip 88, Lazarus 96). Thyroid peroxidase antigen on the apical surface of thyroid follicular cells is involved in cell-mediated cytotoxicity (Sinclair 08). Use of TPOAb as a screening test for PPTD has a sensitivity of 0.46–0.89

and a specificity of 0.91–0.98. PPVs vary from 0.40 to 0.78 (Smallridge 00b), reflecting the "different laboratory assays used and the decrease in thyroid peroxidase that occurs during pregnancy, often to undetectable levels, followed by a postpartum rebound" (Stagnaro-Green 02). The pooled risk ratio for development of PPTD (abnormal TSH; <0.4 mIU/L or >4.5 mIU/L) in women with TPOAbs compared with women without TPOAbs is 5.7 (95% CI 5.3–6.1) based on a systematic review of 21 studies comprising 8,081 subjects. Little variance in prevalence was detected in different parts of the world (Nicholson 06). The apparent prevalence of TPOAbs is dependent on the techniques used to detect them (Sinclair 08).

One reviewer concluded that 10% of postpartum women will have significant thyroid autoantibodies, with ~50% of seropositive women requiring treatment for clinical thyroid dysfunction (TSH >10 mIU/L[μU/mL]) or symptoms of decreased energy, poor memory, dry skin, and carelessness (Stagnaro-Green 00). Once started, many experts continue treatment for hypothyroidism until 1 year after the woman has completed her family (Stagnaro-Green 02). Long-term studies of nondiabetic women with postpartum thyroiditis found that 23–59% had permanent hypothyroidism at a mean of 2.0–8.7 years follow-up, respectively (Tachi 88, Othman 90, Sakaihara 00, Lucas 05), including women who stopped T4 replacement at 1 year postpartum (Premawardhana 00, Azizi 05). Iodine supplementation (150 mcg/day) during the postpartum period to TPOAb-positive women living in an area of Denmark with mild-to-moderate iodine deficiency did not induce or worsen PPTD (Nohr 00). Selenium supplementation during pregnancy and postpartum (200 mcg/day) to TPOAb-positive women reduced the rate of PPTD (29% vs. 49%, p < 0.01) and permanent hypothyroidism (12% vs. 20%, p < 0.01) in a small RCT conducted in Italy (Negro 07).

If TSH is suppressed, an assay for TSH receptor antibody should be performed to rule out new-onset Graves' disease (Stagnaro-Green 00, Tagami 07). Graves' disease is also suggested by the presence of exopthalmos or a thyroid bruit (Stagnaro-Green 02). Among postpartum thyrotoxic patients, Graves' disease is diagnosed if thyroid radioiodine uptake is elevated, and hyperthyroid PPTD is diagnosed if uptake is suppressed (Gerstein 93). Treatment of hyperthyroid PPTD is based on symptom severity, with propranolol used to alleviate palpitations, irritability, and nervousness for typically <3 months. Antithyroid thioureas are not indicated because the hyperthyroidism is caused by a destructive thyroiditis resulting in release of preformed thyrois hormone (Stagnaro-Green 02).

It is not surprising that the risk of PPTD is increased to 18–51% in type 1 diabetes (RR 2.8–4.5 per respective control groups) (Table IV.2); the majority of cases will have subclinical hypothyroidism (Bech 91, Gerstein 93, Alvarez-Marfany 94, Weetman 94, Gallas 02, Triggiani 04). In comparison, cross-sectional studies of adolescent females with type 1 diabetes revealed a prevalence of thyroid autoimmunity of 10–15% (McKenna 90, Hansen 99, Holl 99, Kordonouri 02). A single longitudinal study of 301 young females with type 1 diabetes showed the cumulative incidence of autoimmune thyroiditis at age 18 to be 19%, with two-thirds requiring treatment with L-thyroxine (Kordonouri 05). In the 12-month postpartum studies of small numbers of women with type 1 diabetes and thyroiditis, thyroid dysfunction was usually transient (Bech 91, Alvarez-Marfany 94). During the 6-month postpartum period in Ontario, thyroid dysfunction had no statistically significant effect on indexes of glycemic control, and no patient with a normal thyroid gland by palpation at the end of pregnancy developed thyroiditis (Gerstein 93). In New York City, PPTD in diabetic women was not

TABLE IV.2 Postpartum Thyroid Studies in Type 1 Diabetic Women Without Previous Disease

N (%)	Bech 1991	Gerstein 1993	Alvarez-Marfany 1994	Gallas 2002
Site	Copenhagen, Denmark	Hamilton, Ontario	New York City, U.S.A.	Amsterdam, Netherlands
Number	57	40	28	82
Postpartum follow-up	12 months	6 months	12 months	12 months
Postpartum Graves' disease	0	1 (2.9)	1 (3.6)	1 (1.2)
Postpartum thyroid dysfunction	6 (10.5)	9 (22.5)	6 (21.4)	42 (51)
RR vs. local control nondiabetic group	3.2	4.5	2.8	5.1
Hypothyroid,* overt	4	5	3	6
Hyperthyroid,* transient	2	2	3	4
Hyperthyroid* followed by hypothyroid*	0	2	0	3
Anti-TPOAb	12 (21)	6 of 34 antimicrosomal	15 (54)	28 (34)
Thyroid replacement	0	8 (1 Graves' after Rx)	3 (1 Graves' after Rx)	NA

*Abnormal free T4 or free T3 levels.

NA, not available; RR, relative risk; Rx, radioactive iodine treatment; TPOAb, thyroid peroxidase antibody.

predicted by thyroid autoantibody status during pregnancy (in contrast to their studies of nondiabetic women), but did correlate with postpartum autoantibody levels (Alvarez-Marfany 94). The decline in TPOAb titers seen during pregnancy with a rebound at 3 months postpartum in nondiabetic women is also found in type 1 diabetes (Gallas 02). All investigators and reviewers concluded that women with type 1 diabetes should be screened at 3 months postpartum with TSH and anti-TPO levels (Weetman 94). Endocrine Society guidelines recommend that women with type 1 diabetes be screened for PPTD at 3 and 6 months postpartum (Abalovich 07).

The course of postpartum thyroiditis is not well studied in type 2 diabetes. It is unlikely that prevalence would be less than in nondiabetic women (5–7%), but would be increased in those with anti-β-cell antibodies. It is important to note that new-onset or recurrent hypothyroidism can masquerade as postpartum depression due to the overlapping of symptoms (Harris 89a, Pop 91, Harris 92, Pop 93, Custro 94, Stowe 95).

Recommendations

- Maintaining glycemic control during the postpartum period is paramount. A sharp decrease in maternal insulin requirements often occurs immediately following delivery, and the mother should be monitored and insulin adjusted accordingly. (B)

- Glycemic goals for postpartum diabetic care are based on current guidelines of the ADA for the general treatment of diabetes. The group A1C goal is <7.0%, but encourage individual patients to strive for an A1C as close to normal (<6%) as possible without significant hypoglycemia (<70 mg/dL; <3.9 mM); MBG <135–150 mg/dL (<7.5–8.3 mM); preprandial and nighttime plasma glucose <120–140 mg/dL (<6.7–7.6 mM); and 1–2-h postprandial plasma glucose <150–170 mg/dL (<8.0–9.4 mM). (A)

- SMBG should be carried out 3–7 times daily to enable women to achieve these glycemic goals that are consistent with low rates of postpartum complications and successful lactation for at least 6 months. These blood glucose goals should also reduce the chance of early fetal loss or major congenital malformations if there is an unexpected pregnancy. (E)

- Multifaceted care to prevent hyperglycemia, hypertension, and hyperlipidemia is proven to be effective in reducing diabetic complications and CVD. The use of drug therapy to achieve these goals must be adapted to the needs of lactation; those recommendations are made in the section titled "Drug Treatment of Diabetes and Related Disorders During Lactation." Any form of insulin therapy is compatible with breast-feeding. (A, B)

- Early recognition and treatment of maternal complications such as thromboembolism, hemorrhage, and cardiomyopathy is vital. The role of PDM in the risk of complications and the mortality rate need to be further studied and preventative interventions identified. (C)

- Women with PDM have a 1.9 times greater risk of infection following CS despite prophylactic antibiotic use.

- Women with type 1 diabetes have a 10–23% risk of postpartum thyroiditis and should be screened with TSH and anti-TPO levels 3 and 6 months postpartum.

- Facilitation of maternal–infant bonding and lactation is vital and can be challenging, especially if medical interventions are needed for the mother, the infant, or both. (E)

POSTPARTUM MOOD DISTURBANCES

—— Original contribution by Lisa D. Hoffman MS, LCSW and John L. Kitzmiller, MD

Transient Postpartum Emotional Lability

Transient postpartum emotional lability (misnomer: the "blues") is very common (40–60%) in women who have given birth 3–5 days previously and may last several days to weeks (Miller 02). It is unknown whether a propensity to develop postpartum emotional lability is related to diabetes, but there is evidence that the condition is unrelated to psychiatric history, environmental stressors, cultural context, breast-feeding, or parity (Hapgood 88). However, those factors "may influence whether the 'blues' lead to major depression" (Miller 02). Under conditions of high stress and inadequate support, the emotional reactivity related to puerperal hormone and neurophysiological changes may increase vulnerability to depression (Miller 02).

Postpartum Nonpsychotic Depression

Postpartum nonpsychotic depression can be identified in 7–20% of women in the U.S. or Europe within 6 months of delivery (O'Hara 96, Cooper 97, Georgiopoulos 01, Josefsson 01, Paulson 06). Depression may occur de novo postnatally or recur after previous episodes (Cox 93, Cooper 95), perhaps especially in those who relapse after discontinuing antidepressant treatment during pregnancy (Cohen 06). Postpartum depression interferes with a woman's ability to care for herself (including diabetes management) as well as her baby and contributes to later emotional, behavioral, cognitive, and interpersonal problems in her children (Jacobsen 99, Miller 02). Symptoms include despondent mood, feelings of inadequacy as a parent, impaired concentration, sleep and appetite disturbances unconnected to the baby's sleep cycle, and sometimes unwelcome thoughts of harming the infant (Miller 02). Known risk factors (Wisner 02) include a personal or family history of depression, psychosocial stress and marital conflict, increased number of stressful life events during pregnancy (including pregnancy loss) (Condon 86, Janssen 96, Neugebauer 97, Heron 04), child-care related stressors, and inadequate spousal and social support (O'Hara 91, Stowe 95, O'Hara 96, Miller 02).

A recent survey of 655 mothers delivering at an urban New York medical center suggested that adjusted ORs were 2.16 and 1.89 for postpartum depressive symptoms in African-American and Hispanic women, respectively, compared with white women (Howell 05). There are inadequate data on maternal diabetes as a specific risk factor for postpartum depression, but it is recognized that depression is a frequent comorbidity with diabetes in the general health care of women (Weissman 93, Lustman 00, Anderson 01, de Groot 01, Everson 02, Katon 04). Although the presence of anxiety or depression during pregnancy is associated with postpartum depressive episodes (O'Hara 90, Stowe 95), a recent systematic review of antenatal screening tools suggested that no measure had acceptable predictive ability to accurately identify women who will later develop postnatal depression (Austin 03).

Due to "the overlap in the normal sequelae of childbirth and the symptoms of postpartum depression" (changes in sleep, energy, weight, appetite, acceptance of affection, anxious or panicky feelings), diagnosis may be difficult (Stowe 95). Therefore, it is wise to use a screening tool at the 6-week postpartum visit to detect patients at high risk of postpartum depression (Stowe 05). The diagnosis is then made on the basis of an interview with an appropriate clinician, bearing in mind that "any emotional complaint after 14 days postpartum" or "any series of emotional complaints that are separated by more than 3 days should be considered abnormal" (Stowe 95). A recent systematic review of psychological interventions for postnatal depression concluded that identifying mothers with risk factors after delivery assisted in the prevention of postnatal depression (Dennis 04,05). The Edinburgh Postnatal Depression Scale (EPDS) is the most widely validated method to document the new mother's mood (Cox 87, Holden 91, Schaper 94, Georgiopoulis 99, Stowe 05, Gordon 06). The EPDS has evolved into a 10-question self-rating scale (Table IV.3) that can be completed and scored quickly, with four answers to each question typically ranged as always to never or never to always. The subject should answer without assistance when possible and check the answer that comes closest to how she has felt in the last 7 days. The EPDS is scored 0, 1, 2, 3 from top to bottom except for those questions marked with an asterisk, which are scored in reverse order. Maximum score is 30, and ≥12 suggests risk for depression, with sensitivity at 67–95% and specificity at 78–96% for scores of 11–12/30 (Cox 87, Harris 89b, Murray 90).

TABLE IV.3 The Edinburgh Postnatal Depression Scale

In the past 7 days:

1. I have been unable to laugh and see the funny side of things.
   - As much as I always could
   - Not quite so much now
   - Definitely not so much now
   - Not at all

2. I have looked forward with enjoyment to all things.
   - As much as I ever did
   - Rather less than I used to
   - Definitely less than I used to
   - Hardly at all

3. *I have blamed myself unnecessarily when things went wrong.
   - Yes, most of the time
   - Yes, some of the time
   - Not very often
   - No, never

4. I have been anxious or worried for no good reason.
   - No, not at all
   - Hardly ever
   - Yes, sometimes
   - Yes, very often

5. *I have felt scared or panicky for no very good reason.
   - Yes, quite a lot
   - Yes, sometimes
   - No, not much
   - No, not at all

6. *Things have been getting on top of me.
   - Yes, most of the time I haven't been able to cope at all
   - Yes, sometimes I haven't been coping as well as usual
   - No, most of the time I have coped quite well
   - No, I have been coping as well as ever

7. *I have been so unhappy that I have had difficulty sleeping.
   - Yes, most of the time
   - Yes, sometimes
   - Not very often
   - No, not at all

8. *I have felt sad or miserable.
   - Yes, most of the time
   - Yes, quite often
   - Not very often
   - No, not at all

9. *I have been so unhappy that I have been crying.
   - Yes, most of the time
   - Yes, quite often
   - Only occasionally
   - No, never

10. *The thought of harming myself has occurred to me.
    - Yes, quite often
    - Sometimes
    - Hardly ever
    - Never

Score from bottom up, 0 to 3.
Data from Cox 87, Holden 91.

Intervention is initially based on education and reassurance ("Am I the only one?") (Stowe 95). The only psychosocial/psychological intervention demonstrated to have a clear preventive effect in women at risk is intensive postpartum support provided by a health professional (Dennis 05). Couples intervention provides benefit to both partners (Misri 00); structured treatment, such as interpersonal and cognitive–behavioral psychotherapy, is of demonstrated effectiveness (Stowe 95, O'Hara 00, Miller 02, Wisne 02, Dennis 07, Grigoriadis 07). Some evidence suggests that estrogen therapy may help with delayed postpartum depression (Gregoire 96, Ahokas 00). Tricyclic or

SSRI antidepressant drugs are the mainstay of therapy (Hoffbrand 01, Miller 02), with some evidence that SSRIs are more effective in women for nonpuerperal depression (Kornstein 00). Among SSRIs, sertraline is well tolerated by postnatal women (Stowe 95), and fluoxetine and citalopram are occasionally associated with disturbances in nursing infants (see the section titled "Drug Treatment of Diabetes and Related Disorders During Lactation") (Miller 02).

Postpartum psychotic depression (unipolar depression with psychotic features: delusions, hallucinations) or bipolar disorder with mixed features (manic, depressive) occurring within 3–4 weeks of delivery are marked by disorientation, lability (Stowe 95, Miller 02), and risk of harm to the baby or mother (Attia 99). Postpartum psychotic depressions are likely to recur without maintenance treatment (Robling 00). Women with severe depression, suicidal ideation or psychosis, severe impairment of function, or failure to respond to an antidepressant should be referred for psychiatric care (Stowe 95, Miller 02).

Posttraumatic Stress Disorder

Posttraumatic stress disorder (PTSD) is defined as a sustained reaction to an event that involves actual or threatened death or serious injury or threatens damage to self or others. The response involves intense fear, helplessness or horror with persistent (at least 1 month) (a) reexperiencing of the traumatic event and (b) avoidance of stimuli associated with the event and emotional numbing. Further criteria include symptoms of increased physiological arousal and impairment in daily life (APA 94), such as diabetes self-management. Increasing attention has been given to childbirth as the stressor causing development of acute but lasting trauma symptoms (DeMier 96, Reynolds 97, Creedy 00, Soet 03, Ayers 04, Cohen 04, Wenzel 05). Although nearly one-third of women may regard their childbirth as traumatic, the prevalence of full PTSD seems to be 1.5–2% (Ayers 04). More common (2–9%) is a traumatic stress response to the pregnancy and delivery in which women have reexperiencing or avoidance symptoms in the first 6 weeks postpartum, but do not develop the full psychopathology (Ayers 04, Zaers 08). Postpartum stress symptoms can be related to stressful life events and depression as well as to pregnancy, labor, and delivery (Cohen 04) and are predicted by anxiety in late pregnancy (Zaers 08). The frequency of PTSD or traumatic stress responses in postpartum diabetic women is unknown, but it is certain that complications of pregnancy, delivery, and newborn care can be stressful and traumatic in the setting of PDM. The question as to whether diabetic women respond to such stressors in a manner different than control women deserves investigation. Clinically, it is important to be sensitive to the possible diagnoses and possibility of recurrence in a subsequent pregnancy and to refer to appropriate mental health professionals (Reynolds 97, Gamble 04). Treatment of PTSD will likely involve cognitive–behavioral therapy, often combined with pharmacological treatment, such as SSRIs (Ayers 04). We lack specific evidence on treatment of diabetic women with PTSD.

Recommendations

- Women should be closely monitored for signs of postpartum mood disturbances that may be difficult to distinguish from the normal sequelae of childbirth. It is also important to note that symptoms of hypothyroidism can mimic depression.

Research is needed on the frequency and best methods of identification and treatment of these postpartum disorders in diabetic women. (E)

- Transient postpartum emotional lability is very common, but women under high stress or lacking adequate support systems are more vulnerable to depression. (B)
- Symptoms of clinical depression can mimic the normal sequelae of childbirth. Therefore, using a screening tool, such as the EPDS, at the 6-week postpartum visit is recommended. (E)
- Postpartum depression interferes with a women's ability to care for herself, her diabetes, and her child, and the patient may become a danger to herself or the infant. Treatment should be implemented with cognitive–behavioral therapy, marital counseling, and/or tricyclic or SSRI antidepressant medications that can be used safely during breast-feeding. (E)
- Patients with postpartum psychotic depression or severe PTSD should be referred for psychiatric evaluation and treatment. (E)

BREAST-FEEDING AND DIABETES

—— *Contributed by Maribeth Inturrisi RN, CDE, Alyce Thomas RD, Jen Block RN, CDE and J Kitzmiller MD*

Benefits and Concerns of Breast-Feeding in Women with Diabetes

Breast-feeding provides health benefits to women with and without PDM as well as numerous health benefits to their offspring (Villapondo 98, Labbok 99, Newton 04, AAP 05, Schack-Nielsen 05,06, Gunderson 07a).

Maternal Effects of Lactation

Prolonged lactation is associated with increased rates of energy intake and expenditure for the energy cost of milk and lactose synthesis (Manning-Dalton 83, Sadurkis 88, Motil 90, Lovelady 93, Motil 98) and a higher rate of carbohydrate utilization consistent with the preferential noninsulin-mediated use of glucose by the mammary gland (50–60 gm/day) (Butte 99). In the fed state, dietary carbohydrate via maternal plasma glucose is the primary (80%) source of milk lactose compared with 60% from plasma glucose during short-term fasting (Sunehag 02, Tigas 02). During a 12-h overnight fast in lactating women, the glucose demand created by lactose synthesis is met by increased glycogenolysis, but not by increased lipolysis, ketogenesis, or gluconeogenesis (Tigas 02). In the fasted state, the human breast is also capable of de novo synthesis of both glucose and galactose (hexoneogenesis), with glycerol the substrate for galactose; 28% of glucose and 49% of galactose in lactose are synthesized from substrates other than plasma glucose (Sunehag 02). Estimated energy requirements of lactating women based on recently available data are derived from average rates of milk production (749 gm/day), energy density of milk (0.67 kcal/g or 2.8 kJ/g), and energy mobilization from tissues in the first 6 months (172 kcal/day or 0.72mJ/day) (Butte 01a,05). In this analysis, the energy cost of lactation was 626.2 kcal/day (2.62 mJ/day), which results in a net dietary increment of 454 kcal/day (1.9 mJ/day) over nonpregnant, nonlactating energy requirements (Butte 05). To our knowledge, separate metabolic adaptation studies have not been performed in lactating diabetic women.

Prolactin levels are higher and fasting estradiol, glucose, and insulin levels are lower 8 weeks postpartum in lactating versus nonlactating women (Lenz 81). Prolactin levels did not differ from controls at 14 or 42 days postpartum in women with PDM (Ostrom 93). Prolactin increases insulin secretion in vitro (Crepaldi 97). The insulin area under the curve in response to intravenous glucose is lower in healthy lactating women (Diniz 04). Other studies found increased insulin sensitivity during lactation (Hubinont 88, Tigas 02), and there is less glucose intolerance (Kjos 93) and improved insulin secretion (McManus 01) in lactating versus nonlactating women with previous GDM.

A clinical impression exists in some centers that many women find their diabetes more easily managed for the duration of lactation, with insulin requirements lower or no different than nonlactating women in spite of greater caloric intake with breast-feeding (Tyson 76, Miller 77, Wichelow 83, Ferris 88, Davies 89, Gagne 92, Saez-de-Ibarra 03, Stage 06). However, one group found increased episodes of hyper- and hypoglycemia in the first week of breast-feeding in mothers with type 1 diabetes (Murtaugh 98), and retrospective review of detailed clinical records in East Germany suggested that hyperglycemia was more pronounced during the first week postpartum than in the third trimester (Rodekamp 05). Interviews of women with type 1 diabetes in Denmark indicated that only 10% of women who stopped lactation during the first 4 months postpartum did so due to fluctuating blood glucose (frequent symptomatic hypoglycemia) (Stage 06). Controlled studies are needed on the metabolic effects of lactation in women with PDM. In nondiabetic women, breast-feeding episodes had no consistent effect on continuously monitored maternal glucose levels (Bentley-Lewis 07).

Women without prior GDM who reported increased duration of breast-feeding were at reduced risk of developing type 2 diabetes in the large Nurses' Health Study II (Stuebe 05). On the other hand, prolonged lactation does not reduce the recurrence rate of GDM or the high rate of development of type 2 diabetes years after GDM (MacNeill 01). Otherwise, whether prolonged, exclusive breast-feeding has specific lasting effects on glucose tolerance and insulin sensitivity has not been examined in women after weaning (Gunderson 07a). Fasting insulin and LDL-C levels increased less and HDL-C levels decreased less at 3 years in women who had lactated at least 3 months compared with parous women who never lactated (Gunderson 07b). Middle-aged women who breast-fed were less likely to have metabolic syndrome (adjusted OR 0.77 (95% CI 0.62–0.96), including significantly lower risks of elevated BP, abdominal obesity, and impaired fasting glucose. The rate of metabolic syndrome was significantly lower with increasing lifetime duration of breast-feeding (Ram 08).

Breast-feeding is inconsistently associated with maternal weight loss over 3–6 months postpartum in nondiabetic women, perhaps due to increased energy intake with lactation (Brewer 89, Dewey 93a, Kramer 93, Coitinho 01, Haiek 01). Prolactin is known to stimulate appetite (Grattan 01). Some of the variation in studies may be due to use of self-reported weight changes. Postpartum weight retention (compared with prepregnancy weight) may be greater in breast-feeding women with higher baseline body fat (Kac 04). Most (Ohlin 90, Janney 97, Olson 03, Sichieri 03), but not all (Wosje 04), prospective studies using measured weight change reported lower postpartum weight retention in lactating women, including one small study in women with type 1 diabetes (Ferris 88). Great individual variation exists in body composition changes during lactation (Sohlstrom 95, Butte 98, Chou 99). During pregnancy, body fat deposition occurs largely in the trunk and thighs, and these fat depots appear to be the main energy sources mobilized to support lactation (Wosje 04). In diabetic women, early postpartum weight loss in the first week may be greater in breast-feeding subjects (Ferris 88, Murtaugh 98), but the analysis is complicated by greater prepregnancy weight and gestational weight gain in patients choosing not to breast-feed. Evidence suggests that obese nondiabetic women are less likely to try or to continue breast-feeding (Hilson 97, Donath 00, Sebire 01, Li 02,03a, Hilson 04, Kugyelka 04, Lovelady 05, Baker 07), and the maternal prolactin response to suckling in the first week postpartum is dimished in obese women (Rasmussen 04). Prospective studies of the interactions of short or prolonged (6–12 months) breast-feeding on maternal weight, body composition, and disease indexes are lacking in diabetic women. Due to the importance of obesity on health outcomes, the effect of repeated pregnancy and breast-feeding on subsequent maternal BMI and waist circumference (a marker of visceral fat) should be studied in both nondiabetic and diabetic women (Pettitt 97, Linne 03).

In addition to maternal metabolic effects, breast-feeding for 12 months provides protection against premenopausal breast cancer, including both estrogen- and progesterone-receptor–positive and –negative tumors (Ursin 05), and the effect is greater with increasing parity (HFBC 02, Martin 05a). Epidemiological evidence also states that successful breast-feeding may be protective against epithelial ovarian cancer (Gwinn 90, Rosenblatt 93) and arthritis (Karlson 04).

Effects of Breast-Feeding on the Offspring

The WHO/United Nations Children's Fund defines lactation as follows: (1) exclusive breast-feeding, when the child receives no water, tea, juice, or food; (2) predominant breast-feeding, when the child receives water, tea, or juice but no food; (3) partial breast-feeding, when the child receives artificial milk or water, tea, juice, or food; and (4) artificial feeding, when the child receives no breast milk (WHO/UNICEF 92). Complete breast-feeding for 6 months (exclusive or predominant) in nondiabetic women has been consistently linked to a decreased incidence of a wide range of childhood infectious diseases in both developed and undeveloped countries (Pullan 80, Kovar 84, Bauchner 86, Wright 89, Howie 90, Pisacane 92, Duncan 93, Owen 93, Uhari 96, Cushing 98, Wilson 98, Raisler 99, Bertran 01, Chien 01, Davis 01, Heinig 01, Kramer 01a, WHO 01, Howie 02, Oddy 03, Marild 04, Chantry 06).

Evidence from case–control studies (possibly subject to residual confounding) and one RCT (Kramer 01a) indicates that complete breast-feeding for >4–6 months may also reduce the frequency of (1) childhood atopic eczema (vanOdjik 03, Benn 04, Laubereau 04, Stabell 04, Zutavern 04, Friedman 05, Kull 05, Ludvigsson 05, Lowe 06, Zutavern 06, Greer 08), (2) celiac disease (Auricchio 83, Greco 88, Faith-Magnusson 96, Peters 01, Ivarsson 02, D'Amico 05, Akobeng 06, Wahlberg 06, Hummel 07), and (3) sudden infant death syndrome (SIDS) (McVea 00, Alm 02) and inconsistently reduces (4) asthma (Wright 95, Gdalevich 01, Chulada 03, Kull 04, Bener 07, Miyake 08), (5) ulcerative colitis (Klement 04), and (6) leukemia–lymphomas (Shu 99, Bener 01, Beral 01, Guise 05, Kwan 05, Martin 05b, Altikaynak 06).

Calculation of a population impact number estimated that a high number of cases of asthma and celiac disease could be prevented over 7–9 years if the risk factor of "no breast-feeding" could be eliminated for 1 year in the U.K. (Akobeng 07). On the other hand, some reviewers caution that almost all data on childhood disease risk reduction with breast-feeding in developed countries "were gathered from observational studies, so one should not infer causality from these findings" (Ip 07).

The many protective effects of breast-feeding on children are independent of other factors known to be associated with rates of illness (Kramer 02a,03). There are multiple avenues by which the many bioactive breast milk components affect the infant's intestinal development and systemic immune response: maturational, antimicrobial, anti-inflammatory, and immunomodulatory polypeptide cytokines (Uauy 94, Newburg 96, Pabst 97, Xanthou 98, Hamosh 98a, Peterson 98, Garofalo 99, Kelly 00, Hamosh 01, Hoppu 01, Hamosh 02, Brandtzaeg 03, Hanson 03, Field 05, Newberg 05, Chantry 06). Immunocompetent cells in colostrum and breast milk include 40–50% macrophages, 40–50% polymorphonuclear neutrophils, and 5–10% lymphocytes (Wirt 92, Xanthou 97). With a few exceptions, we do not know whether these protective factors differ in concentration or activity in the breast milk of diabetic women. Most protective bioactive components of human breast milk are absent in bovine or soy milk-based formulas used for artificial feeding.

Breast-fed infants show higher neurodevelopmental scores on childhood follow-up (Lanting 94,98, Anderson 99, San Giovanni 00, Angelsen 01, Horwood 01, Mortensen 02, Bouwstra 03, Gustafsson 04, Daniels 05, Sacker 06, Schack-Nielsen 07); however, potentially confounding variables complicate the interpretation of these results (McCann 05). "Experimental designs involving breast-feeding are inherently limited in their ability to identify which among a number of potentially active ingredients in breast milk might be responsible for enhancement effects" (McCann 05). A large RCT that significantly enhanced exclusive breast-feeding in Belarus showed no differences in child behavior measures over a 6.5-year follow-up (Kramer 08). The demonstrated effects of maternal smoking on breast-fed infant nicotine levels and sleep patterns (Mennella 07) illustrate the difficulty of studying child development and behavior associated with breast-feeding.

Breast milk is superior to standard artificial formula in the provision of *n*-6 and *n*-3 LC-PUFAs (Koletzko 88,89, Jensen 92, Huisman 96, Koletzko 99, Mitoulis 03, Minda 04, Xiang 05, Straarup 06) that are important in neurological development (Hamosh 98b, Jensen 99, Uauy 00, Lauritzen 01, Voight 02, Das 03, Jensen 05a). The major portion of milk PUFAs is not derived directly from the short-term maternal diet, but stems from endogenous body stores, suggesting that "long-term dietary intake is of marked relevance for milk fat composition" (Koletzko 01). Formula preparations for term infants supplemented with LC-PUFAs are more expensive than standard bovine milk-based formula products, suggesting that populations most in need are less likely to use them.

The possible inverse relationship of breast-feeding infants of women with type 1 and type 2 diabetes to subsequent childhood obesity and glucose intolerance is a subject of growing and controversial study. Breast-fed infants of nondiabetic women have lower energy and protein intakes than formula-fed infants, but satisfactory growth and HC, suggesting greater metabolic efficiency with breast-feeding (Butte 84a, Axelsson 89, Butte 90, Dewey 91a,b, Heinig 93, Dewey 95, Alexy 99, Dewey 01, Koletzko 05). Formula-fed infants tend to be fatter, heavier (Dewey 92,93b, Michaelsen 94, Dewey 98a, Nielsen 98, Agostoni 99, Kramer 02b,04), and have a greater insulin response (Lucas 80,81, Ginsburg 84, Salmenpera 88, Wallensteen 91, Lonnerdal 00) than exclusively breast-fed infants. Hyperinsulinemia can retard lipolysis and enhance fat deposition (Oakley 77, Odeley 97, Liese 01). However, a questionnaire survey of 229 women with type 1 diabetes in the Netherlands showed no significant difference between breast-, formula-, or mixed-fed infants in weight and body mass index at 1 year of life (Kerssen 04).

The change in breast milk composition during feeding and lactation provides satiety signals to the infant (Hall 75), and overfeeding is more likely with volume-controlled formula-feeding by bottle (Liese 01). Evidence suggests that the volume of milk produced is influenced by the suckling infant, who can self-regulate breast milk intake (Dewey 86). Breast milk contains leptin in the milk fat globule, but leptin is removed by pasteurization and skimming in the preparation of bovine milk-based formulas (Casabiell 97, Houseknecht 97, Smith-Kirwin 98, Lyle 01, Resto 01, O'Connor 03). Indeed, breast-fed infants have higher leptin levels in early life in most (Casabiell 97, Ucar 00, Savino 02,04, Dundar 05, Savino 05a), but not all, cross-sectional studies (Lonnerdal 00). Disagreement has emerged concerning the measurement of leptin in breast milk and whether leptin is absorbed by the nursing infant. Hypotheses that early leptin intake can influence later eating behavior or that early diet can program later leptin status are being studied (Locke 02, Singhal 02, Agostini 03).

Formula-fed infants usually have a greater degree of obesity during childhood and adolescence (early studies reviwed by Butte 01b; Gillman 01, Hediger 01, Liese 01, Armstrong 02, Toschke 02a, Bergmann 03, Clifford 03, Dewey 03a, Li 03b, Parsons 03, Arenz 04, Grummer-Strawn 04, Harder 05, Kvaavik 05, Owen 05a,b, Reilly 05, Gillman 06, Harder 06, Novotny 07, Wu 08), including children of diabetic mothers (Mayer-Davis 06, Schaefer-Graf 06). Children breast-fed for ≥6 months had the lowest odds of excessive total and trunk fat mass at 9–10 years of age, and the association held after adjustment for confounders. However, there was little evidence that breast-feeding was associated with mean or threshold values of BMI (Toschke 07). Long-term follow-up studies addressing this issue should take confounders into account such as maternal education, BMI, and smoking as well as BW, timing of complementary food introduction, toddler energy intakes, and child-feeding practices (Kramer 85, Lewis 86, Agras 90, Wilson 98, Fisher 00, Spruijt-Metz 02, Toschke 02b,03, Baker 04, Bogen 04, Burke 05, Nelson 05, Schaefer-Graf 05, Gillman 06, Taveras 06). For example, a quantitative review of 11 studies that reported modestly lower BMI in individuals who were breast-fed showed that the effect was abolished after adjustment for socioeconomic status, maternal BMI, and maternal smoking during pregnancy (Owen 05b). An informative essay has been published on the strengths and limitations (residual confounding, publication bias) of a meta-analysis on breast-feeding and childhood obesity with a brief review of biological plausibility. The authors concluded that "breast-feeding has a small, but consistent, protective effect on obesity risk in childhood." This effect may have a large public health impact due to a population-attributable 7.3% of the risk for childhood overweight that could be explained by not breast-feeding (Arenz 05).

The difficulties of using large epidemiological studies to set goals for breast-feeding are illustrated in two recent reports. In the Nurses' Health Study II, 35,526 participants were followed from 1989 to 2001. They reported their body shape at ages 5 and 10 and their weight at age 18, as well as their current height and weight many years later. Their mothers answered a questionnaire on the duration of breast- or bottle-feeding and the type of milk or milk substitute in the bottle. Exclusive breast-feeding for >6 months was associated with leaner body shape at age 5 but not during adolescence or adulthood, and the duration of breast-feeding did not predict BMI category in adulthood (Michels 07). In addition to questions concerning the accuracy of distant recall of emotionally charged parameters, one wonders about the effects of behaviors during adolescence and adulthood on the outcomes. PROBIT was a huge multi-hospital RCT of breast-feeding promotion in Belarus in which 13,889 mother–infant pairs completed a

6-year follow-up. The intervention increased exclusive breast-feeding at 3 months (43.3% vs. 6.4%, p < 0.001) and reduced gastrointestinal infections and atopic eczema at 1 year (Kramer 01a), but had no effect on childhood BMI or waist circumference in a population without an epidemic of childhood obesity (Kramer 07). However, only 7.9% of the infants in the intervention group were exclusively breast-fed at 6 months (Kramer 01a). Therefore, the great majority of participants did not receive full exposure to the presumed benefit.

The relationship of breast-feeding to infant/childhood weight gain and adiposity may be important to the lifelong health of the offspring due to links to adult obesity, glucose intolerance BP, and measures of atherosclerosis (Charney 76, Parsons 99, Gou 00, AAP 03, Baird 05, Martin 05a,b, Stettler 05). Although breast-fed infants may be shorter than formula-fed infants at 12 months (Dewey 95), the effect does not persist (Martin 02). Indeed, IGF-I levels at age 7–8 years may be higher in breast-fed children (Martin 05c), even though IGF-I levels were lower during the first year of lactation compared with formula-feeding in separate studies (Savino 05a,b, Chellakooty 06). The higher protein intake with some formula-feeding might stimulate greater IGF-I production (Koletzko 05). Additional research is needed on the relationship of early infant feeding to the possible roles of GFs and adipokines in childhood growth and obesity and whether they are affected by maternal diabetes.

A relationship has been shown between breast-feeding and reduction of type 2 diabetes in Pima Indian offspring (Pettit 97,98) and perhaps in native Manitoban children (Young 02). A meta-analysis of seven studies in 76,744 subjects showed that those who were breast-fed had a lower risk of type 2 diabetes later in life than those who were formula-fed (OR 0.61; 95% CI 0.44–0.85) (Owen 06). Conversely, some individual studies in Europe demonstrated a different effect from early breast-feeding by IDMs on pediatric outcome. In the Netherlands survey of women with type 1 diabetes, maternal BMI, BW, and infant weight and BMI at 1 year of age did not differ in 39 infants who were breast-fed for 6 weeks compared with 43 infants who were given formula (Kerssen 04). In Lithuania, a cross-sectional study of oral glucose tolerance (1.75 gm/kg) at 2–5 years of age in 51 offspring of women with type 1 diabetes revealed that nine infants (17.6% vs. 4.6% in 109 controls) had 2-h glucose values of 140–198 mg/dL (7.8–11.0 mM). IGT was associated with macrosomia at birth (52.9% of diabetic offspring group, implying poor maternal glycemic control; no data were given) and BMI at 2–5 years of age. The authors claimed a positive correlation between duration of breast-feeding and 2-h glucose values. The published scattergram showed that three of nine IGT infants were breast-fed beyond 5 months compared with none of ~12 infants without IGT (Buinauskiene 04). Multivariate analysis of the risk factors for early childhood IGT was not performed.

In East Germany, data on breast and supplementary feeding during days 1–7 of life were obtained in 1980–1989 on 83 infants of women with type 1 diabetes (5 with BW >4,500 gm) and 29 infants of women with GDM (none with BW >4,500 gm). The groups were analyzed together, and the number of preterm infants was not defined. All women were encouraged to breast-feed, and infants were nonrandomly offered supplements of nondiabetic donor banked milk or formula according to the judgment of the ward pediatrician. "Thereby, all newborns in the study received differing amounts of breast milk from their biological diabetic mothers and banked donor breast milk from unrelated nondiabetic women. Because of acute nonavailability of banked breast milk, in 23 infants, short-time supplementation was necessary with standard term formula milk. During each feeding on days 1-7 postpartum, milk intake was determined using a test weighing protocol: the infant was weighed before and after every nursing by trained staff" (Plagemann 02). The weight difference (in gm) and the type of milk ingested during the meal were noted as breast milk from the biological diabetic mother (DBM), banked donor breast milk from unrelated nondiabetic mothers (BBM), or standard term formula milk. Analysis was restricted to the impact of the volume of DBM and BBM feeding in gm/day gained by the infants. At infant follow-up at a median of 2 years, relative body weight percentage was significantly higher across the tertiles (~37 infants per group) (<57, 57–124, >124 gm/day) of DBM volume: 98% ± 1.7 vs. 104% ± 1.8 vs. 109% ± 2.8 (overweight defined as 110%). Results of glucose tolerance tests did not differ in the three groups of infants, but the top tertile group of BBM volume consumed (>37 gm/day) had less IGT (1/37) and less relative body weight (99% ± 1.8) (Plagemann02). In stepwise regression analysis, DBM volume was the only factor predicting infant relative body weight at the 2-year follow-up, with BW, gestational age at delivery, gender, maternal BMI, and BBM volume excluded as nonindependent factors. The authors speculated that increased glucose and insulin concentrations in diabetic breast milk could account for their result (Plagemann 02).

Interpreting this study presents multiple problems. Data were not provided on maternal glycemic control during pregnancy or the first week postpartum or on any estimator of fetal hyperinsulinemia beyond BW. Fetal insulin production is a known determinant of later body size. No information exists on maternal nutrition during the first week postpartum. The composition of DBM and BBM was not measured, and it is impossible to determine the effect of the artificial formula given to 23 infants. Milk volumes estimated by gm/day infant gain over the first week of life were much lower than in standard investigations (Neville 88,91), but similar to decreased neonatal suckled milk volumes for the first 6 postpartum days in diabetic women in Japan (Miyake 89). The sensitivity of the scale and the techniques used to weigh the babies were not presented. A leading author states that "the validity of the determinations of human milk intake depends on the precision and accuracy of the test-weighing procedure" and describes the possible procedural errors (Butte 84a). It is possible that such precision was not obtained over 10 years of clinical care in a maternity unit (Whitfield 81, Woolridge 84). Infant weight gain over the first week could also be influenced by its suckling ability (Mathew 89, Selley 90, Richard 92), and poor suckling with breast or bottle has been described as an early morbidity in IDMs. Clean, properly controlled studies with an appropriate sample size are needed on the effect of diabetic breast milk on infant outcome.

Subsequent retrospective analysis of larger numbers of infants (152 mothers with type 1 diabetes, 90 with GDM) in this Kaulsdorf Cohort Study in 1980–1989 suggested that a different upper tertile of DBM volume consumed (81 infants: >119 gm/day infant weight gain with DBM; mean total milk intake 182 ± 50 gm/day) over the first week of life was associated with earlier development of headlifting and following with eyes by 16 weeks of life, but delay in the onset of speaking by 80 weeks. "This negative impact of DBM ingestion was not confounded by birth characteristics, total milk intake, or socioeconomic/educational status" (Plagemann 05). Another retrospective analysis of a subset of 112 infants in the cohort showed that the area under the curve of maternal blood glucose in the middle of the third trimester did not differ in 31 mothers of infants given no DBM in weeks 2–4 of life, 36 mothers of infants given some DBM, and 45 mothers of infants given only DBM. This measure of maternal glycemia did not correlate with the children's relative body weight at follow-up (Rodekamp 05). The mean duration of breast-feeding was 13 ± 1.7 weeks in the group given some DBM in the first week and 15 ± 1.7 weeks in the group given only DBM in the first week. Maternal blood glucose monitoring within 1 week postpartum (stated to be at higher glycemia levels than in the third trimester) was also not related to type of infant feeding during neonatal weeks 2–4. Infant relative body weight (percentage of ideal) at the 2-year follow-up was not affected by type of neonatal nutrition during weeks 2–4 in the infants of 83 women with type 1 diabetes and was not significantly affected (p 0.07) by the tertile of DBM ingestion during the first week of life (Rodekamp 05). Therefore, the authors recombined the type 1 diabetes and GDM groups to demonstrate that the amount of DBM milk ingested (none, some, only) during weeks 2–4 doubled the odds of being overweight at 2 years of age in multivariate analysis, including adjustment for third-trimester maternal blood glucose, but did not double the odds of being overweight when adjusted for volume of DBM ingested during the first week. Finally, logistic regression analysis revealed no significant influence of duration of breast-feeding in diabetic women on their children's overweight or 2-year IGT (Rodekamp 05).

A frequent question asked by diabetic pregnant women is, "Will my child have diabetes?" Epidemiological research for >2 decades usually has shown an association between short or zero duration of breast-feeding or earlier introduction of bovine milk and the risk of insulin/islet autoimmunity or type 1 diabetes in children of nondiabetic (Borch-Johnsen 84, Mayer 88, Dahl-Jorgensen 91, Virtanen 91,93, Fava 94; 13 early case–control studies reviewed in Gerstein 94; Perez-Bravo 96, Gimeno 97, Jones 98, Virtanen 98, Hypponen 99, McKinney 99, Wasmuth 00, EURODIAB 02, Sadauskaite-Kuehne 04, Fingerlin 06, Malcova 06, Wahlberg 06, Holmberg 07, Rosenbauer 07) and diabetic parents (Borch-Johnsen 84, Paronen 00, Kimpimaki 01). Negative epidemiological and case–control studies have also been published (Fort 86, Bodington 94, Patterson 94, Norris 96a,b, Couper 99, Hummel 00).

The question is raised as to whether the association of breast-feeding with lower risk for type 1 diabetes is due to (1) lack of ingestion of protective factors in human breast milk (Dahlquist 90, Schrezenmeir 00, Akerblom 02, Knip 05); (2) fewer enteroviral or other infections in breast-fed infants (Gibbon 97, EURODIAB 00, Pundziute-Lycka 00, Sadeharju 03, Sipetic 03, Sadeharju 07); (3) supplementation with vitamin D in northern regions (related to the antiproliferative effect of its active form, 1,25[OH]2D) (EURODIAB 99, Hypponen 01, Holick 04); (4) ingestion of harmful factors in bovine milk-based formula or cow's milk (Martin 91, Savilahti 93, Vaarala 95, Cavallo 96, Harrison 99, Vaarala 99, Muntoni 00, Virtanen 00, Monetini 01, Vaarala 02), including differences between bovine milk and human milk insulins as immunogens or tolerogens (Tittanen 06); or (5) higher weight gain (adjusted for BW) in early life with use of bottled formula milk and later overfeeding (Blom 92, Johansson 94, Khan 94, Hypponen 99, Bruining 00, Hypponen 00, Stene 01, EURODIAB 02, Libman 03, Pundziute-Lycka 04, Dahlquist 05). An additional hypothesis to be tested is that migration of bisphenol A from polycarbonate baby milk bottles into formula milk (Brede 03, Onn-Wong 05, Maragou 08) can affect insulin secretion at concentrations below the U.S. Environmental Protection Agency (EPA) oral reference dose of 50 mcg/kg/day (Adachi 05, Alonso-Magdalena 06, Ropero 08).

The association of excess infant weight gain or increased BMI at time of (earlier) diagnosis with an increased risk of type 1 diabetes or of type 2 diabetes with autoantibodies (Umpaichitra 02, Reinehr 06) leads to interesting hypotheses that the overloaded β-cells (Dahlquist 06) may have accelerated susceptibility to autoimmune damage or apoptosis (Wilkin 01, Kibiridge 03, Rosenbloom 03, Knerr 05, Dabelea 06, Wilkin 06). Recent studies suggest that the timing and quantity of introduction of soy milk (Scott 95,02, Strotmeyer 04) or other foods (cereals, fruits, roots) into the diet of high-risk infants might also play a role in the development of type 1 diabetes–related autoimmunity (Klemetti 98, Norris 03, Virtanen 03, Ziegler 03, Wahlberg 05, Virtanen 06, Wahlberg 06). A study of 1,183 children identified as high risk for type 1 diabetes (by either HLA genotype or a first-degree relative with type 1 diabetes) reported a similar association between the time of introduction of cereal (whether it contained gluten or not) and duration of breast-feeding on the risk of developing islet autoimmunity. The study found that if children at high risk were exposed to cereal at 0–3 months or >7 months of age, they were at higher risk for developing islet autoimmunity than children who were exposed at 4–6 months of age; breast-feeding at the time of cereal exposure was also found to further decrease the risk of islet autoimmunity (Ziegler 03). Another study did not find a relationship between breast-feeding and the development of celiac disease or type 1 diabetes, but did find that early introduction of gluten-containing foods increased the risk of developing islet autoantibodies (IAAs) (17.6% vs. 3.6%) in children who did not receive gluten-containing foods in the first 3 months of life (Ascher 97).

Research on this important question is continuing with the multicenter Trial to Reduce IDDM in the Genetically at Risk (TRIGR) study to test the hypothesis that weaning infants to an extensively hydrolyzed formula will delay or prevent the onset of type 1 diabetes in genetically susceptible children (Hamalainen 00, Knip 03, Akerblom 05, Rogers 05, TRIGR 07). In addition, an NIH-sponsored consortium of six international centers has been established for identification of environmental determinants of diabetes in the young (TEDDY) (NIH 04, TEDDY 07).

Given the recommendations set forth in this review that highlight the numerous health benefits of breast-feeding to both the mother and child, the need to support breast-feeding in women with type 1 and type 2 diabetes is highlighted. Recent research indicates that up to 6% of first-degree relatives of patients with type 1 diabetes are at risk of developing celiac disease (Saukkonen 01, Ziegler 03). A recent meta-analysis of major studies published between 1966 and 2004 evaluating the role of breast-feeding in the development of celiac disease found that 5 of the 6 studies reviewed demonstrated a decreased risk of celiac disease with increasing duration of breast-feeding (Akobeng 06).

Characteristics of Lactation and Breast Milk

Mammary alveolar epithelial development during pregnancy is stimulated by rising concentrations of progesterone and prolactin (and possibly human placental lactogen), while progesterone is also the major inhibitor of milk production during gestation (Neville 99,01). In addition to prolactin, insulin and corticoids are necessary to maintain synthesis of milk components in vitro (Topper 80, Neville 01). No evidence confirms that mammary development is subnormal in well-controlled diabetic women. After normal parturition with removal of the placenta, a marked decrease in progesterone level over days 1–4 and continued secretion of prolactin with blood levels near 200 ng/mL are necessary for full lactation (Neifert 81, Neville 01). A decline in mammary progesterone receptors occurs after parturition with the decline in estrogens, so progesterone administration will not inhibit postpartum milk production (Haslam 79, Neville 01).

Lactogenesis defines the transition from onset of minimal milk production in mid-pregnancy (stage I) in humans through parturition (stage II) to the copious milk secretion by day 4–5 after delivery (onset of lactation) (Neville 99,01). Colostrum is the mammary secretion product that can be obtained in late pregnancy, and especially in the first 3–4 days postpartum, during which there are rapid changes in milk volume and composition (Kunz 99, Neville 01). Colostrum has relatively high concentrations of copper, zinc, protein, secretory immunoglobulin A (sIgA), IGF-I, lactoferrin, protective oligosaccharides, LC-PUFAs, carotenoids, vitamin A (retinyl esters), vitamin B12, vitamin E, activated neutrophils, macrophages, and T-cells compared with mature milk (Wirt 92, Xanthou 97, Rodriguez-Palmero 99, Fidler 00, Picciano 01b). The concentration of sodium and chloride declines as the concentration of lactose (4–5 gm/L) and lipid increases over the first 4 days (Kunz 99, Neville 01). Early suckling contributes to immune protection of the infant and maturation of its gut. Milk removal must begin by day 3 postpartum for changes in early milk composition to occur (Kulski 81a, Neville 01). The amount of milk transferred to the infant increases from 20–200 gm/day on day 2 to 400–800 gm/day by day 8 (Neville 88,91a). As milk volume increases during lactogenesis, an increase in milk glucose concentration occurs (200–400 mg/L) due to an increase in glucose transport from the interstitial space into the alveolar cell (Neville 90,91a). Because there is continuous transition in the components of breast milk from 2 days to 4–9 months postpartum, use of the term "transitional milk" for the first 3 weeks is discouraged (Allen 91, Kunz 99).

Conditions reported to delay lactogenesis (Neville 01) include stress at parturition (Chen 98, Lau 01), placental retention (Neifert 81), perhaps CS (Procianoy 84, Sozmen 92, Rowe-Murray 02, Dewey 03b), obesity (Rasmussen 04, Lovelady 05), and possibly diabetes (Neville 88, Arthur 89, Bitman 89, Miyake 89, Neubauer 93, Hartmann 01, Plagemann 02). Regarding CS, no difference was found in milk lactose if suckling began by 12 h after delivery (Kulski 81b). A more recent study found less milk transfer to the infant born by CS on days 2–5 despite early nursing before 4 h in 73%; however, by day 6, no difference was found compared with vaginally delivered infants (Evans 03). General anesthesia for CS delays lactogenesis and maternal–infant skin contact compared with epidural anesthesia and reduces long-term breast-feeding (Lie 88, Bond 92). Studies of lactogenesis in diabetic women are difficult to interpret. Two reports of decreased early milk volume are single-case studies (Arthur 89, Bitman 89), and decreased early milk production was estimated in three larger studies based on lessened infant weight accretion after nursing, which could be influenced by inadequate suckling (Miyake 89, Neubauer 93, Plagemann 02). As noted earlier, it is recognized that early "poor feeding" with artificial or collected breast milk is a complication of some IDMs and that infant suckling is the major stimulation for milk production and let-down. Maternal obesity diminishes the prolactin response to suckling in early breast-feeding (Rasmussen 04) at a stage in which this response is more critical for milk production than in later lactation (Lovelady 05). Alternatively, obesity could be associated with poor "breast-feeding behavior" (Dewey 03b, Hilson 04) (proper latching on and adequate suckling) that results in poor prolactin response (Lovelady 05).

In one study of lactogenesis in diabetic women, no difference was found in the amounts of milk obtained by manual extraction after nursing between diabetic and control subjects, but maternal caloric intake was significantly lower in the diabetic subjects (Miyake 89). Using milk lactose as a measure of lactogenesis in two studies, its concentration was lower on day 2 in milk obtained from diabetic women, but not by day 4 (Arthur 89, Neubauer 93). In the latter, most extensive study of lactogenesis, women with type 1 diabetes had a significantly longer time interval between the last breast-feeding session and when the milk sample was obtained, and they were more likely to supplement their infants with bottle-feeding (Neubauer 93). These investigators concluded that diabetic mothers with fasting blood glucose <121 mg/dL (<6.7 mM) and postprandial blood glucose <160 mg/dL (<8.9 mM) had no differences in milk lactose, nonprotein nitrogen (NPN), or infant milk intake than controls at 2, 4, and 7 days postpartum.

Mature human milk is a complex fluid of interesting structure with caseins in colloidal dispersion, lipids mostly in emulsified globules, activated leukocytes, and carbohydrates and salts in true solution (Michaelsen 94, Xanthou 97, Jensen 99, Kunz 99, Neville 99). Most of the fat (4% of milk volume) is in membrane-bound milk fat globules of TGs and sterol esters in emulsion, with the membranes including cholesterol, phospholipids, ~5% of total milk protein, enzymes, steroid hormones, trace minerals, and fat-soluble vitamins. The globules are synthesized within the mammary alveolar cells and derive their envelopes from the alveolar cell membrane on secretion (Rodriguez-Palmero 99). The large surface area of the globules is available for binding by lipases in the infant's gastrointestinal tract, which aids efficient fat absorption (Rodriguez-Palmero 99). The casein protein micelles (with calcium phospate linkages) in colloidal dispersion constitute a small proportion of human milk (0.2–0.3%), compared with 4% in bovine milk. When caseins are precipitated, the remaining aqueousphase solution (~87% of milk volume), called "whey," contains all of the milk sugars; the major milk proteins lactoferrin, sIgA, α-lactalbumin, and serum albumin; enzymes; the nonprotein nitrogen components; minerals; salts; and most of the water-soluble minor components of milk. The whey of cow's milk is used as the base for artificial infant formula (Kunz 99, Neville 99). In early human lactation, the content of whey proteins is high compared with little amounts of casein (90:10), and the ratio changes to 60:40 or 50:50 in mature milk (Kunz 99). After full lactation is established, the process of human milk secretion is continued by the stimulus of regular removal of the milk from the gland, by prolactin to maintain four synchronized secretory processes in the alveolar cells, and by oxytocin to produce myoepithelial cell contraction and milk ejection (let-down) from the alveoli to the mammary sinuses so that the infant may suckle (Neville 99).

The complex and variable composition of breast milk and functions of the components have been extensively reviewed (Emmett 97, Xanthou 97, Picciano 98, Jensen 99, Kunz 99, Rodriguez-Palermo 99, Hamosh 01, Picciano 01a,b). Multiple clinical factors are known to affect the composition of human breast milk (Table IV.4). As a general rule, "the nutrition received by the breast-feeding infant is not dependent on the status of the maternal metabolism. For most milk components the secretory mechanisms are insulated from the regulatory mechanisms that control nutrient flux in the mother. This means that sufficient milk of adequate composition is available to the infant even in periods of inadequate food intake by the mother" (Neville 99).

The disaccharide lactose (galactose + glucose) is the major carbohydrate energy source in breast milk (40% of total kilojoules from mature milk), which also contains free galactose and glucose (with concentrations far lower than lactose: glucose 1.4–3.9 mM vs. lactose ~165 mM) (Neville 90,99). Maternal hyper- or hypoglycemia is not associated with changes in milk lactose (Tolstoi 35). Glucose clamp studies of nondiabetic lactating women show that fasting (plasma glucose at 3.8 mM; 68 mg/dL) or insulin infusion during euglycemia has little effect on milk lactose or glucose concentrations

TABLE IV.4 Factors Influencing Human Milk Composition

	Influence
Duration of gestation	Preterm: Increase in LC-PUFAs; oleic acid 24% higher than term Term: 2.6 times higher total lipid content
Stage of lactation	Lactogenesis: Increased neutrophils, polymeric IgA, hormones Early: Protein 16 g/L; increased phospholipids, cholesterol Late: Protein 8–9 g/L; increased total lipid content; larger, less dense milk fat globules; less amylase
Parity	Multigravid: Reduced FA synthesis, lower milk fat
Volume of milk	If high volume, less milk fat content
Duration of feeding	Milk fat content increases ("hind milk")
Maternal nutrition	Low-fat diet: increased mammary synthesis of FA (C6–C14) Intake of fatty acids affects *trans, n*-6, and *n*-3 fatty acids in milk High-protein diet increases protein and NPN components Low vitamin intake yields low vitamins in milk Vitamin D supplements increase vitamin D in milk and infants Dietary intake of minerals generally not reflected in milk composition
Maternal energy status	Preconception adiposity or high gestational weight gain: increased milk fat
Maternal diabetes	Less lactose, fat, and NPN at days 2–3; thereafter, not different except slightly lower LC-PUFA Hyperglycemia: Trivial increase in milk glucose (76 mg/dL vs. 7 gm/dL for lactose); milk insulin concentrations may increase with maternal hyperinsulinemia; effect on infant is unknown

Modified from Picciani 01 with data from Michaelsen 94, Rueda 98, Innis 99, Jensen 99, Kunz 99, Neville 99, Hamosh 01, Domellof 04, and Hollis 04.

FA, fatty acid; LC-PUFA, long-chain polyunsaturated fatty acid; NPN, nonprotein nitrogen.

(1.3–1.4 mM; 23–25 mg/dL), but intravenous infusion of glucose to reach plasma glucose concentrations of 8 mM (144 mg/dL) raised milk glucose to 3.9 mM (70 mg/dL) (Neville 90,93). Free oligosaccharides and glycoconjugates (glycolipids, glycoproteins) in human milk serve as important microbial and viral ligands inhibiting pathogen adhesion to gut epithelium (Kunz 99, Hamosh 01, Picciano 01a).

TGs (glycerol + fatty acids) form 97–98% of the lipid energy-yielding fraction of human breast milk (55% of total kilojoules from mature milk), and fatty acids necessary for healthy development represent ~88% of milk fat (Rueda 98, Jensen 99, Picciano 01a). Fatty acids in breast milk are derived from mobilization from endogenous stores, synthesis of fatty acids by the liver or breast tissue with excess energy intake, or from the diet (Insull 59, Jensen 96, Francois 98). SFAs make up 37% of total fatty acids in human milk, MUFAs 41%, and PUFAs 19%, including the essential LC-PUFAs linoleic acid, α-linolenic acid, and their products arachidonic acid, EPA, and DHA (Francois 98, Jensen 99). Milk fat content rises across the first 2 weeks of lactation, is variable from subject to subject and according to time of day, increases with duration of each breast-feeding session, and is decreased in the breast milk of mothers delivering preterm (Clark 82, Harzer 83, Rueda 98, Mitoulis 03, Kent 06). Provision of milk to preterm infants is a complex and important topic that will not be addressed in this document.

Milk fat content varies directly with the percentage of maternal body fat at 6–12 months postpartum, but not in earlier months (Butte 84b, Nommsen 91). Most studies show that milk total lipid concentration is unrelated to maternal dietary fat intake, but that it is increased by maternal protein intake (Nommsen 91). A relationship exists between the type of fat consumed and the fatty acid pattern of milk lipids (Lonnerdal 86, Torres 06). After ingestion of specific dietary fatty acids (lauric 12:0, stearic 18:0, *n*-9 oleic 18:1, *n*-6 linoleic 18:2, *n*-3 α-linolenic 18:3, *n*-3 EPA 20:5, *n*-3 DHA 22:6), a transfer of these fatty acids from chylomicrons into human milk occurs at 6–36 h due to activity of mammary LPL (Francois 98). Supplementation of DHA raises DHA in breast milk and infant plasma phospholipids (Harris 84, Makrides 96, Jensen 00, Francois 03, Boris 04), but use of standard fish oil capsules can cause a detrimental increase in EPA (Henderson 92, Jensen 06). No clear consensus has yet been reached regarding the effects of supplementing maternal *n*-3 fatty acid intake on infant outcome (Carlson 99, Uauy 99, Helland 03, Jensen 06), and no studies are available in diabetic women. Moderate exercise does not reduce LC-PUFA in breast milk (Bopp 05). Maternal *trans* fat intake increases potentially harmful *trans* fats in breast milk and infant plasma (Craig-Schmidt 84, Chappell 85, Koletzko 95, Innis 99, Mosley 05).

The protein constituents of breast milk provide free amino acids, urea nitrogen, and peptides for growth; protective factors such as immunoglobulins, lysozymes, lactoferrin, mucins, and cell adhesion molecules; carriers for hormones and vitamins; enzymes for digestion; casein phosphopeptides that keep minerals in solution for enhanced absorption in the gut; plus adiponectin, ghrelin, leptin, hormones, and GFs that help maturation of the newborn gut and modulate feeding behavior (Kunz 99, Hamosh 01, Picciano 01a, Lane 02, O'Connor 03, Savino 05a, Aydin 06, Martin 06b). Protective immunoglobulins, hormones, IGF-I, lactoferrin, and activated leukocytes are in highest concentration in colostrum, making early breast-feeding important (Eriksson 93, Xanthou 97, Picciano 01a). NPN compounds represent 20–25% of the total nitrogen, remain constant throughout lactation, and are much higher in concentration in human compared with bovine milk (Kunz 99). Nucleotides are an important example of these necessary compounds for infant health (Uauy 94). Micronutrients in breast milk include the fat- and water-soluble vitamins as well as the major and trace minerals. Iron and zinc in human milk have high bioavailability, and breast-fed infants have better iron absorption than those who are artificially fed (Picciano 01a). Standard bovine milk formula products have many compositional differences (Table IV.5) from breast milk of control (Koletzko 88, Nommsen 91, Huisman 96, Hamosh 98a, Garofalo 99, Hamosh 01) and diabetic women (Butte 87, Neubauer 93, vanBuesekom 93, Jackson 94, Thomas 00). Formula milk has relatively high concentrations of glucose and galactose compared with breast milk, suggesting some lactose hydrolysis (Cavalli 06), but it contains much lower concentrations of cholesterol, which is an essential component of cell membranes in the infant (Huisman 96).

Very little data have been collected on the characteristics of colostrum from diabetic women. In three investigations, mean lactose concentrations were 95–165 mM on day 2 and leveled off at 160–175 mM on days 3–5 in a total of 31 women with type 1 diabetes (Arthur 89, Neubauer 93; Cox data reported by Hartmann 01). In all three studies, lactose concentrations were less than those found in controls over the first week of breast-feeding; however, in another study of two well-controlled diabetic women, day 3-5 lactose was normal in one subject and low in another (vanBeusekom 93). Glucose levels rose to a maximum of 6.4–6.8 mM (115–122 mg/dL) in colostrum of two diabetic women on day 4 (Bitman 89, vanBeusekom 93), but remained <2 mM

TABLE IV.5 Composition of Mature (3-6 Months) Human Breast Milk from Nondiabetic and Diabetic Women Compared with Representative Bovine Milk-Based Formula and Prepared Whole Milk

Component	Control Women	Preexisting Diabetes	Bovine Formula Milk	Cow's Milk*
Lactose, gm/L	63-77 (173-202 mM)	64.5, 65.5 (188 mM)	62-71	40-52
Galactose, mg/dL	12 (45-142 μM)		0.3-1.7 mM	12
Glucose, mg/dL	19-38 (0.9-2.1 mM)	45, 71	2.6 mM	16 (0.9 mM)
Oligosaccharides, gm/L	6.5-14		Trace	1.0
Total protein, gm/L	7-14	16.3	6.9-7.3	30-40
Whey/casein ratio	60/40		60/40**	20/80
α-Lactalbumin, gm/L	2-3.3			1.2-2.0
β-Lactoglobulin, gm/L	Zero		Present	3.2-5.0
Secretory IgA, polymeric	50-100 mg/dL	82	Absent	Absent
Immunoglobulins G and M	1 mg/dL, 2 mg/dL		Absent	Absent
Lysozyme	5-25 mg/dL		Inactivated	Low
Bile salt-stimulated lipase	Present		Absent	Absent
Lactoferrin, mg/dL	50-200	145	10	Trace
Nucleotides	Present		Low***	Low
Insulin, μIU/mL	5.1-13.0	10-110	Absent	Absent
Insulin-like growth factor-1	0.13-1.1 mcg/dL		Absent	Absent
Prolactin, mcg/dL	2.0-9.0	3.4	Absent	Absent
Thyroxine, mcg/dL	0.03-1.2		Absent	Absent
Epidermal growth factor, mcg/dL	0.3-10.7		Absent	Absent
Prostaglandins			Absent	Absent
Total lipid, gm/L	24-50	37.6, 38.9, 40.3, 40.5	18.3****	33-37
Cholesterol, mg/dL	135		12-46	
Palmitic, myristic, stearic acid	16-30%	12.9 gm/L	11-24%	15.5 gm/L
Oleic acid, gm/L	10.6 (31-34%)	9.2		6.8
Trans- fatty acids, gm/L	0.6-1.9 (2-6%)			0.36
n-6 linoleic acid, gm/L	2.6-5.4 (8-18%)	3.8, 3.7 (14.4%)	0.03-0.29	0.2-0.7, as CLA
α-linolenic acid, gm/L	0.16-0.3 (0.25-1.0%)	0.45 (0.25-1.3%)	0.08-0.4	

n-6 arachidonic acid, gm/L	0.16–0 (2 0.3–0.7%)	0.16, 0.15 (0.38%)	0.02	30
n-3 docosahexanoic acid, gm/L	0.06–0.16, 0 1–0.5%	0.12, 0.12 (0.06%)	Trace	37
Vitamin A, mg/dL	30–60		100 IU	175–180
Thiamine, mcg/dL	20		33.3	0.09
Riboflavin, mcg/dL	40–60		47–50	0.046
Niacin, mg/dL	0.2–0.6		0.3–0.35	0.42
Vitamin B6, mg/dL	0.009–0.03		0.02	1.7
Vitamin B12, mcg/dL	0.05–0.1		0.08–0.1	0.06
Vitamin C, mg/dL	10		3.0	0.08
Vitamin D, mcg/dL	0.01–0.1		0.03	5.5
Vitamin E, mg/dL	0.3–0.4	0.39	0.5 IU	3.5
Folic acid, mcg/dL	8–14		5.0	
Biotin, mcg/dL	0.5–0.9		1.5	
Potassium, mg/dL	57 (11–17 mM)	42.3	35	138 (43 mM)
Sodium, mg/dL	15 (4.1–9.4 mM)	13.1	8–9	58 (15 mM)
Calcium, mg/dL	24.8 (6.3–9.0 mM)	28.6	26	125 (30 mM)
Phosphorus, mg/dL	10.7 (1.1–2.3 mM)	14.4	14	96 (11 mM)
Magnesium, mg/dL	3.4 (1.5–2.3 mM)	3.4	2.0	12 (5 mM)
Copper, mcg/dL	30	26.0	30	10–60
Iodine, mcg/dL	1.5–15			26
Iron, mcg/dL	30	22		300–600
Zinc, mcg/dL	110	140	250–330	200–600
Active leukocytes, cells/mm^3	3,000		Eliminated	Eliminated

*Fat and protein vary with breed and feed.

**Added demineralized whey or heat-treated casein.

***Can be supplemented.

****Added vegetable oils.

CLA, conjugated linoleic acid.

(36 mg/dL) in six other diabetic subjects (Arthur 89). Maternal serum and colostrum prolactin levels were lower than those found in controls on day 3 in 17 women with type 1 diabetes, but milk prolactin was similar to reference samples by day 7 (Ostrom 93). Lower colostrum prolactin levels correlated with elevated PPBG, fewer breast-feeding sessions in the first 12 h, and a longer time interval to first feeding (Ostrom 93). To our knowledge, insulin has not been evaluated in the colostrum of diabetic women.

The total protein content of colostrum has been studied in only two diabetic women (vanBeusekom 93), but total nitrogen on day 3 was 4.8 gm/L in 13 diabetic subjects compared with 3.5 gm/L in 22 controls (p < 0.05) (Neubauer 93). Colostrum TG, cholesterol, and fatty acid levels were normal in two diabetic women (vanBeusekom 93). In another study, total lipid content was reduced on day 2 in five patients compared with a reference group (8.1 vs. 11.7 gm/L, p < 0.05), but rose to 29.7 vs. 34.8 gm/L (NS), respectively, by 7 days (Jackson 94). Diabetic subjects had normal A1C levels on day 3, but PPBG values were as high as 244 mg/dL (13.6 mM). In spite of the initial reduction of total lipids in the colostrum of the diabetic women, total medium-chain fatty acids, long-chain SFAs, long-chain MUFAs, total PUFAs, and total LC-PUFAs (percentage by weight) did not differ from reference samples on days 2 or 3; *n*-6 arachidonic acid 20:4 and *n*-3 DHA levels were significantly higher than in reference samples on days 2 or 3. The probable difficulty with lactogenesis in this sample of diabetic women (most of whom had cesarean deliveries) is suggested by collection of colostrum samples in only one-half of subjects in the total diabetic study group (Neubauer 93, Jackson 94). In view of the importance of early breast-feeding to the long-term success of lactation (Dewey 03b), further investigation of clinical factors affecting the colostrum of diabetic women is indicated.

Concentrations of most nutrients in mature breast milk in women with PDM differ little from controls at a similar stage of lactation (Table IV.5) (Butte 87, Neubauer 93, vanBuesekom 93, Ferris 94, Jackson 94, Thomas 00). The major energy providers (lactose, lipids), total protein or nitrogen concentrations, and micronutrient levels are normal. Milk glucose concentrations may be elevated, but this is probably clinically insignificant because glucose accounts for only 0.4% of the total energy content of the milk (Butte 87). In a small case series in Berlin, breast milk glucose concentrations were nearly identical in 11 women with type 1 diabetes and 11 lactating controls at 1 month postpartum. Breast milk glucose concentration (range 3–29 mg/dL; 0.06–1.6 mM) did not correlate with maternal blood glucose or glycohemoglobin (Ratzmann 88). An experimental increase of plasma glucose to 16.7 mM (300 mg/dL) in seven lactating women with PDM raised the mean milk glucose concentration from a baseline of 1.3 mM (24 mg/dL) to 4.1 mM (73 mg/dL) 60–80 min after intravenous infusion (Jovanovic-Peterson 89). One study of fatty acid composition of mature breast milk found that total medium-chain fatty acids were higher and total LC-PUFAs were lower in hyperglycemic diabetic women (Jackson 94), yet another study reported equivalent values in tightly regulated diabetic and control milk samples (vanBuesekom 93). No significant correlations were found between plasma or milk glucose, dietary intake, and other nutrients analyzed in any of the studies, although relatively small sample sizes limit applicability of the data (Butte 87, Neubauer 93, vanBuesekom 93, Jackson 94).

Milk prolactin levels at day 84 were similar in diabetic subjects and controls in the single available study (Ostrom 93). We are not aware of studies of IGF-I, thyroxine, or adipokines in mature breast milk of diabetic women. Mean basal milk insulin levels at 2–5 months postpartum were 8.1 μIU/mL in nine nondiabetic lactating women compared with 47.4 μIU/mL in seven women with PDM. When the diabetic subjects were made very hyperglycemic, intravenous infusion of insulin (1 unit Regular for each increment of 25 mg/dL above baseline) raised breast milk insulin to 115 μIU/mL after a 35–50 min lag time (Jovanovic 89). Effects of such insulin levels on suckling infants are unknown. As noted earlier, additional research is needed on the influence of intensified glycemic control and MNT on nutrients, hormones, and metabolic factors in the breast milk of diabetic mothers and possible effects on the health of the offspring.

Few of the many protective bioactive factors in breast milk have been measured in diabetic women, but milk sIgA and lactoferrin did not differ from reference norms at ~3 months postpartum in one small observational study of type 1 diabetic women with slightly elevated glycosylated hemoglobin levels who were exclusively breast-feeding (Butte 87). In a separate study of 21 women with type 1 diabetes, milk tocopherol (vitamin E) levels at 7 days did not differ from reference samples, whether presented in mcg/dL or mcg/gm lipid; the levels demonstrated the expected decline from 7 to 42 days postpartum (Lammi-Keefe 95).

Special Considerations for Women with Diabetes Who Breast-Feed

The majority of well-controlled women with diabetes can successfully breast-feed with proper education, planning, and support (Walker 06, Hannula 08), although the published experience with lactation performance presents the challenges to achieving this goal (Miller 77, Whichelow 83, Picciano 87, Ferris 88,93, Webster 95, Knudsen 01, Stage 06). Breast-feeding education and training for a woman with diabetes is similar to that for a woman without diabetes, with special considerations (Fagen 98, Bradley 07). The potential problem of delayed lactogenesis in diabetic women has already been discussed. However, the major components of breast milk are normal by 3–4 days postpartum when the intensified glycemic control undergone during pregnancy is continued postpartum (vanBeusekom 93). The high rate of maternal obesity and cesarean births, plus maternal separation from infants who may be monitored in the NICU and given formula by bottle or nasogastric tube to prevent hypoglycemia, all contribute to delayed lactogenesis and reduce early breast-feeding success (Ferris 88, Neubauer 93, Evans 03, Simmons 05, Stage 06). As noted earlier, lactogenesis can be normal after cesarean delivery if infant suckling begins by 12 h postpartum (Tulski 81b). Infant sucking patterns were studied on the third day of life in infants of GDM mothers treated with insulin. These infants had fewer bursts of sucking over 5 minutes compared with infants of mothers treated with MNT and with controls. No data were provided on the quality of maternal glycemic control (Bromiker 06). We need studies on the characteristics of maternal diabetes associated with improved success on nursing of infants.

Long-term success rates for breast-feeding in diabetic women are presented in Table IV.6. The numbers for exclusive or predominant breast-feeding would be lower because 20–50% of breast-feeding diabetic women were supplementing with formula at 7 days postpartum (Ferris 93, Webster 95, Stage 06). In the 1993 study in New England, 53% of mostly well-controlled diabetic women did not attempt breast-feeding. In those women who did breast-feed, early mother–infant separation related to delays in initiation of breast-feeding and in perception of when the milk came in; diabetic mothers cited infant sleepiness as the most common infant feeding problem (none in

TABLE IV.6 Studies of Lactation Performance in Women with Preexisting Diabetes

Author (date, site)	N	3 Days	7 Days	4–8 Weeks	3–4 Months	Comments
Miller, 1977	17*	13	16	17	15	11 CS; 13 NN hypoglycemia; 11 jaundice; 6 in NICU >1 day.
Whichelow, 1983, London, UK	48	42 (87.5%)	NA	32 (66.7%) (46% in region)	27 (56%)	18 of 27 BF at 3 months put to breast <12 h vs. 5 of 15 weaned early; 16 of 42 infants had trouble suckling.
Ferris, 1988, Connecticut, U.S.	29 *25*	2 (7%) *25 (100%)*	21 (72%) *24 (95%)*	13 (45%) *13 (52%)*	NA	All study infants in NICU first 8 h; all offered formula on day 2. Mastitis in 2 PDM subjects. DM moms stop BF due to "baby poor feeder"; control moms stop BF due to "insufficient milk."
Ferris, 1993, Connecticut, U.S.	100 *33[†]*	31** (94%) *33 (100%)*	30** (91%) *32 (97%)*	23** (70%) *30 (91%)*	20** (61%) *21(64%)*	Majority of PDM chose to formula-feed; 69% of study infants were in NICU first 8 h; study infants first: breast-fed 26 h vs. 11 h in controls; 61% BF supplemented formula at 3 days vs. no controls.
Webster, 1995, Brisbane, Australia	19 *18*	16 (84%) *18 (100%)*	12 (63%) *14 (78%)*	11[s] (58%) *10[t] (56%)*	9[y] (47%) *6 (33%)*	Prospective observational study. PDM CS 68% vs. 11%; PDM infant: admitted to ward with mother 26% vs. 83%; NN hypoglycemia 89% vs. zero; timing of first BF >12 h 58% vs. 21; fed formula in nursery 93% vs. 36%.
Knudsen, 2001, Jutland, Denmark	217	215 (99%)	NA	165 (76%)	102 (47%)	Smokers less likely to BF at 4 months, 37% vs. 55%.
Stage, 2006, Copenhagen, Denmark	102	88 (86%)	NA	NA	69 (68%) *(76% in nation)*	Study infants offered breast first 2 h (47% BF), then in NICU 24 h to prevent hypoglycemia and were BF twice; 20% of BF at 4 months also on formula; exclusive BF at 4 months had more previous experience with BF and higher educational level; had less CS, smoking (9% vs. 39%), and severe NN hypoglycemia (22% vs. 40%).

Percentage success at specific times postpartum in study infants compared with controls if available, in italics.

*Nonlactating mothers excluded.

**33 of 47 BF agreed to study.

[†]*Number of controls with initial decision to formula-feed not stated.*

[s]*Supplemented in 3.*

[t]*Supplemented in 2.*

[y]*Supplemented in 1.*

BF, breast-feeding; CS, cesarean section; DM, diabetes mellitus; NA, not available; NICU, neonatal intensive care unit; NN, neonatal; PDM, preexisting diabetes mellitus.

controls) (Ferris 93). In Copenhagen by 2001–2003, 86% of women with type 1 diabetes initiated breast-feeding and 78% had long-term success despite coping with the protocol of moving their babies to the NICU after the first 2 h; 40% of those infants who were born preterm were exclusively breast-fed at 4 months (Stage 06). A recent survey of 55 diabetic pregnant women in Nashville, Tennessee, indicated that 56% planned to breast-feed compared with 62% in the control group (Johnston 06). Both figures are below national targets (75% nursing in the early postpartum period; 50% at 6 months) (Cadwell 99, USPHS 04) and suggest how much work remains to be done regarding education and motivation of parturient women.

Avoiding Neonatal Hypoglycemia with Early Breast-Feeding

Maintaining maternal normoglycemia during pregnancy and labor is the best way to avoid newborn hypoglycemia (Jovanovic 96). Betamimetic drugs, such as ephedrine (often used to treat acute hypotension associated with epidural or spinal anesthesia) or terbutaline (used acutely to stop uterine activity in the presence of fetal distress) given just before birth, can aggravate the risk for hypoglycemia in the newborn. Early breast-feeding (preferably in the first 30 min of life) repeated often (10–12 times per 24 h) may reduce this risk (ABM 99, Eidelman 01), although controlled trials have not been performed. Early suckling may at least provide the protective factors in colostrum to the infant. Newborns that are wet and cold use glucose to generate warmth; therefore, it is imperative to dry the newborn thoroughly and place the infant skin to skin with the mother to feed (Anderson 03). Women who undergo cesarean birth should not be an exception. It is possible for an otherwise healthy newborn to begin breast-feeding in the operating or recovery room. Every effort should be made to provide the care needed (physical assessment, glucose testing) by this couplet without separating them.

   Early separation of the mother/baby couplet for infant evaluation, glucose testing, or admission to the neonatal unit may delay lactogenesis (Ferris 88, Gagne 92, Ferris 93, Hartmann 01) as well as increase the likelihood that the baby will be supplemented with formula by nursing staff (Dewey 03b, Sievers 03). The couplet experiencing medically necessary separation will need extra support to establish breast-feeding. The mother can be instructed in breast pump use within the first 12 h after giving birth (Zinaman 92), although this method produces less milk transfer to the infant at 24–72 h postpartum than regular suckling (Chapman 01). Pumped colostrum or milk should be fed to the newborn, if possible, by eyedropper or feeding syringe to prevent nipple confusion (Neifert 95). Prenatal information imparted to the mother regarding the importance of frequent breast milk feeding without supplementation should be reinforced. A diabetes educator familiar with the woman's daily challenges, a readily available lactation specialist, and knowledgeable nursery and postpartum staff should be available to support the mother and baby with special needs (Wight 06, Hannula 08).

Avoiding Maternal Hypoglycemia During Nursing

Erratic patterns of glucose control include both hyper- and hypoglycemia. Because hypoglycemia is most likely to occur within 1 h after breast-feeding, this is an important time to periodically measure blood glucose (Bradley 07). Episodes of hypoglycemia induce the release of epinephrine, which can cause a temporary decrease in milk production or interfere with milk ejection. In most cases, hypoglycemia can be avoided by eating a snack containing at least 15 gm carbohydrate and some protein before or during breast-feeding. Women should be advised to avoid falling asleep and missing a snack or meal and to plan naps after (not before) meals and snacks. Nocturnal hypoglycemia may occur due to breast-feeding during the night; consequently, periodic glucose monitoring during the night is vital. If hypoglycemia is documented, the evening dose of intermediate-acting insulin should be decreased or the woman should eat an additional snack before bed or during the night.

Problems with Breast Infection

In general, a woman with hyperglycemia is more susceptible to infection of all types. For example, a yeast infection may occur on the nipples and breast tissue of a nursing mother and in the mouth of the baby. Both should seek treatment (Mass 04). Good hand washing, nipple care, and glycemic control can help reduce the incidence of yeast infections. It is important to rule out infection when unexplained blood glucose elevations occur. A diabetic woman should be trained to recognize the signs and symptoms of any infection, including mastitis (cellulitis of the interlobular connecting tissue; usually *Staphylococcus aureus,* Streptococcus, or *Escherichia coli*) (Howard 04). Cohort studies suggest that the cumulative frequency of mastitis in the first 7 weeks postpartum is ~3% (Kaufmann 91), but we lack data to prove that mastitis is more frequent in diabetic women. The health care provider should be contacted immediately to initiate treatment as early as possible to prevent progression to abscess or chronic mastitis (WHO 00a). Although mastitis changes the composition of breast milk by increasing sodium, chloride, and glucose and decreasing lactose and fat (Ramadan 72), breast-feeding can typically continue by nursing on the unaffected breast first and possibly emptying the infected breast by pump if nursing is too painful (Neifert 99, Howard 94, Mass 94).

Strategies to Enhance Breast-Feeding Success in Diabetic Women

The principles for enhancement of successful breast-feeding adopted by the WHO/UNICEF (United Nations Children's Fund) (WHO 89, WHO/UNICEF 92, WHO 98a, UNICEF 02), U.S. Office for Women's Health (DHHS 00), U.S. Public Health Service (USPHS 04), and other professional organizations (Randolph 94, ACOG 00, AAFP 02, ABM 03, ACOG 07) are listed in Table IV.7. Some of the scientific evidence supporting the Baby-Friendly Hospital Initiative (Taylor 86, Host 88, Yamouchi 90, Heacock 92, Righard 92, Perez-Escamilla 94, Freed 95, Gartner 01, Gray 02, Anderson 03, Peat 04, Poole 06, Scott 06, Zutavern 06) is presented by the initiative's major reviewers (Saadeh 96, Naylor 01, Phillip 04). The American Academy of Pediatrics (AAP) provides similar clinical and policy recommendations on breast-feeding of healthy term and high-risk infants to support its goal of exclusive breast-feeding for 4–6 months in as many infants as possible. During the early days and weeks of breast-feeding, the mother should be encouraged to have 8–12 feedings at the breast every 24 h (Gartner 05). She should offer the breasts whenever the infant shows early signs of hunger such as increased alertness, physical activity, mouthing, or rooting; crying is a late sign of hunger (Klaus 87, Gartner 05). "Formal evaluation of breastfeeding, including observation of position, latch, and milk transfer, should be undertaken by trained caregivers at least twice daily and fully documented in the record during each day in the hospital after birth" (Gartner 05). AAP guidelines include recommendations on vitamin and mineral supplements (see Table IV.7) (Kleinman 04, Gartner 05).

TABLE IV.7 Ten Steps to Successful Breast-feeding

Every facility that provides maternity services and care for newborn infants should follow these 10 steps:

1. Have a written breast-feeding policy that is routinely communicated to all health care staff.

2. *Train all pertinent health care staff in skills necessary to implement this policy.* The greater the support from health workers, the more mothers choose to breast-feed and the longer they continue the practice.

3. *Inform all pregnant women about the benefits and management of breast-feeding.* Mothers and fathers who receive appropriate prenatal counseling with accurate/sufficient information tend to maintain the practice longer.

4. *Help mothers initiate breast-feeding within 1 h of birth.* Mothers holding babies with skin-to-skin contact after delivery avoid delayed lactogenesis, breast-feed longer, and have fewer infant infections. The mother is an optimal heat source. Adapt the need for early infant treatments and routine diagnostic tests to help meet this goal.

5. *Show mothers how to breast-feed and how to maintain lactation even if they are separated from their infants.* Proper positioning of the baby at the breast is crucial to establishing breast-feeding and preventing subsidiary difficulties, including pathological breast engorgement and sore nipples that can lead to early cessation of breast-feeding. There is reduced risk of infant reflux and aspiration because gastric emptying time is shorter than with substitute feeding. For babies that must be separated, mother's milk by small cup or dropper provides advantages.

6. *Give newborn infants no food or drink other than breast milk unless medically indicated.* Supplementary feeding in the first few days after birth is not necessary for most babies, and the majority of studies show it to be associated with an increase in the risk of being weaned by 3 months postpartum. Bilirubinemia requiring treatment is most likely in infants who have been fed water or glucose water instead of breast milk and whose breast access is restricted. A hospital should pay fair market price for all formula and infant feeding supplies that it uses and should not accept free or heavily discounted formula and supplies. The same stricture should apply to outpatient clinics and offices, which should not display commercial advertising promoting use of formula. Introduce supplementary foods at 4–6 months of life.

7. *Facilitate rooming-in; encourage all mothers and infants to remain together during their hospital stay.* This facilitates the initiation and long-term establishment of breast-feeding and enhances mother/infant bonding. Infants as well as mothers may sleep better when rooming-in.

8. *Encourage breast-feeding on demand.* Infants who are permitted to self-regulate the frequency and duration of their feeds suckle more, gain weight more rapidly, and breast-feed for longer periods than infants who are restricted in their feeding patterns. Encourage mothers to have 8–12 feedings at the breast every 24 h in the early weeks.

9. *Give no artificial teats or pacifiers (also called dummies or soothers) to breast-feeding infants.* Use of these in the neonatal period may (1) condition the infant to oral actions that lead to diminished suckling strength and duration, contributing to decreased milk supply, and (2) increase exposure to infection.

10. *Foster the establishment of breast-feeding support groups and refer mothers to them on discharge from the hospital or clinic.* Helps mothers deal with breast-feeding problems and increases success and duration. Motivate fathers to encourage and support breast-feeding. Help eliminate parental smoking.

Promulgated by WHO 89,98a,02a, WHO/UNICEF 92 (Baby-Friendly Hospital Initiative), Office on Women's Health, DHHS 2000, Am Coll Obstet Gynecol 2000, and the AAFP 2002.
Adapted from Randolph 94, Saadeh 96, Naylor 01, and Phillip 04.

Use of appropriate 12-month growth charts for breast-fed infants may help reduce untoward recommendations to use early food supplements (WHO 98b, Kuczmarksi 00, Dewey 01, Powers 01). Some contraindications to breast-feeding have also been published (Lawrence 01). The American Dietetic Association strongly supports exclusive breast-feeding for 4–6 months and breast-feeding with complementary foods for at least 12 months as the ideal feeding pattern for infants (AdietA 97,01). Instituting a Baby-Friendly Hospital environment is a challenge with reference to maternal diabetes. This is a challenge worth meeting given the many maternal and infant/child benefits of prolonged breast-feeding, which may especially apply to the diabetic dyad. The concerns of prospective parents regarding breast-feeding with diabetes should be elicited and allayed in the antepartum period because studies show that the original intention of breast-feeding along with home-based peer counseling is predictive of long-term success (Wiles 84, Morrow 99, Donath 04, Scott 04). Involvement of a lactation specialist in the prenatal patient education team would be ideal. Detailed practical suggestions to accomplish successful long-term lactation and cope with breast-feeding problems are available (Neifert 99, ACOG 00, Wight 01, Berens 04, Neifert 04, Lawrence 05).

The Baby-Friendly Hospital Initiative was shown to dramatically increase breast-feeding rates in many settings; a WHO-sponsored randomized trial of the initiative's application in Belarus significantly decreased childhood illness (Kramer 01a). Commercial promotion of the use of artificial formula in healthy infants is believed to be a problem for lactation success (Howard 94, Radford 01, Weaver 06, Wright 06). A recent single-center RCT randomized 700 yet-unborn infants whose mothers intended to breast-feed to add bottle-feeding versus feeding with small plastic medicine cups if milk supplements were needed (Howard 03). Supplemental feeding was given to 481 infants during postdelivery hospitalization (33% for medical indications: hypoglycemia or excessive weight loss; 51% as a result of maternal request; 16% with no documentation). The most significant predictor of a shorter duration of breast-feeding was the receipt of supplemental feedings while in the hospital. Among women delivered by CS, breast-feeding of infants was more successful if supplemental feedings were given by small cup than by bottle (Howard 03).

An earlier trial restricted supplementary feedings to 37% in one nursery versus "traditional" formula at night along with daytime supplementation at the discretion of the nursing staff in 85% of 393 babies in the other nursery; no recorded differences were found in the percentage of mothers breast-feeding at 4 and 9 weeks. In an observational analysis of the "control" group, babies who were unsupplemented (only 15%) were far more likely to still be nursing at 4 and 9 weeks; therefore, the authors concluded that supplementation in the hospital is a marker rather than a cause of unsuccessful breast-feeding (Gray-Donald 85). Another RCT compared the effect of the supplementation of breast-feeding with 5% glucose water during the first 3 days of life (n = 83) versus initial exclusive breast-feeding (n = 87). Sustained breast-feeding (exclusive or partial) was significantly better at 4 and 16 weeks in the nonsupplemented group (Martin-Calama 97). One set of reviewers concluded that well-designed, well-conducted RCTs are needed to resolve the question concerning whether "brief exposure of breastfed infants to other liquids or feedings influences the success and/or duration of future breastfeeding" (Horvath 05), but others believe the evidence is sufficient to support the policy recommendations (AAP 05). It is perhaps self evident that a sincere attempt at breast-feeding is the best action to attain its success.

Observational studies link early use of oral pacifiers (nonnutritive sucking used to calm infants) to decreased breast-feeding duration (Barros 95, Righard 98, Riva 99). Three RCTs examined a causal association between pacifiers and breast-feeding problems. In a European 10-center RCT with negative results, 46% of 300 healthy infants randomized to "restrictive fluid supplements and avoidance of bottles and pacifiers during the first 5 days of life" violated the protocol, mostly because of maternal requests to provide a pacifier or supplements by bottle (Schubiger 97). A smaller RCT in Montreal, Quebec, regarding the effect on breast-feeding of providing anticipatory guidance to avoid pacifier use did reduce its use to 61% in the experimental group (n = 140) vs. 84% in the control group (n = 141), but did not affect cry/fuss behavior or weaning by 3 months (18.9% vs. 18.3%). The authors believed that complex breast-feeding behaviors are "heavily influenced by cultural, motivational, and psychological factors that are extremely difficult to measure, and hence to control for, in an observational study" (Kramer 01b). Because "these potent factors are likely to lead to residual confounding and reverse causality bias in observational studies" (Gray-Donald 88), the authors concluded that "pacifier use is a marker of breastfeeding difficulties or reduced motivation to breastfeed, rather than a true cause of early weaning" (Kramer 01b). A larger RCT in Rochester, NY, involved 353 breast-fed infants who were given a pacifier at 2–5 days versus use of a pacifier after 4 weeks in 345 infants. Pacifier use in the first 4 weeks of life reduced the likelihood of exclusive breast-feeding at 1 month and shortened overall breast-feeding duration (Howard 03). Studies illustrate the importance of education, motivation, and support of women intending to breast-feed. "Infants must learn to attach and suckle properly at the breast during the first few days of life to breastfeed successfully. Exposures to artificial nipples are believed to contribute to breastfeeding problems and early weaning" (Howard 03).

Effects of early discharge and postpartum home care on breast-feeding success have also been examined. Retrospective data from 20,366 automated medical records of mother/infant pairs in Massachusetts with normal vaginal deliveries were compared from a 15-month period (1994–1995) of one postpartum overnight hospitalization followed by a nurse home visit in 74% to a 27-month period (1996–1998) of state-mandated 48-h postpartum hospitalization with 45% having home visits. The rate of initiation of breast-feeding rose from 70% in 1990 to 82% in 1998, with continuation among initiators remaining constant at ~73% in the two time periods. The authors could not accurately separate out the individual effects of program components, such as home visits (Madden 03). In Ontario, Canada, 138 mother/newborn pairs delivering at ≥35 weeks were randomized to standard care and length of hospitalization versus standard hospital care with early discharge (only 7 h earlier than the standard group) and home support from nurses who were certified lactation consultants. More mothers with term newborns in the latter group were breast-feeding exclusively at the 7-day follow-up (39 of 41) compared with the control group (25 of 34) (p = 0.02), suggesting the value of the home visits (McKeever 02). Practical management guidelines for breast-feeding mothers who return to work are also available (Neilsen 04, Raju 06).

Lactation Nutritional Requirements and the Diabetic Food Plan

The goals of MNT for diabetic women during lactation (Reader 04) are to provide excellent nutrition for the infant (Allen 05), assist with effective postprandial glycemic control, and contribute to long-term risk reduction for CVD (Coulston 04, Tanasescu 04, Mozzaffarian 06). Current recommendations for the latter are to balance caloric intake and physical activity (30 min/day most days of the week) to achieve and maintain a healthy body weight; consume a diet rich in vegetables and fruits; choose whole-grain, high-fiber foods; consume fish, especially oily fish, at least twice a week; limit intake of saturated fat to <7% of energy, *trans* fat to <1% of energy, and cholesterol to <300 mg/day by choosing lean meats and vegetable alternatives and low-fat (≤1% fat) dairy products; minimize intake of partially hydrogenated fats; and choose and prepare foods with little or no salt (AHA 06, Halvorsen 06). Table 3 in the AHA 2006 Statement lists helpful practical tips to help patients implement these diet and lifestyle recommendations (AHA 06). Glycemic targets for the postpartum period are discussed earlier in the section titled "Postpartum Glycemic Control."

Hopefully, women with PDM will continue to use the MNT techniques learned during pregnancy that are detailed in Part I of this document including carbohydrate counting, occasional review of recorded food intake with nutrition clinicians, and use of between-meal and nighttime snacks at the beginning of breast-feeding sessions to prevent hypoglycemia. Even with well-balanced food intake, most diabetic lactating women will choose to take a daily vitamin/mineral supplement. Research is needed on the safe and effective use of dietary supplements for nutrients that are limited in the maternal diet during lactation, especially in diabetic women (Picciano 03). Once adequate lactation, infant growth, and maternal nutritional intake are established, it is possible for exercising and breast-feeding diabetic women to obtain gradual weight loss without harm to the baby. The ADA recently updated nutritional guidelines for the general management of diabetes, and the reader is referred to that document (ADA 08b).

The IOM published new DRIs in 2002–2004, including RDA or AI levels for energy, fiber, macronutrients, water, sodium, and potassium for lactating women of different age ranges and their breast-fed or formula-fed infants (Table IV.8) (IOM 02, Trumbo 02, IOM 04, Volpe 04). Previous reports focused on DRIs and AIs for vitamins and elements (IOM 97,98,00a,01) as well as guidance on using DRIs for planning and assessing diets for healthy people and patients (IOM 00b, Barr 02); further interpretations of the development and use of DRIs were published in the *Journal of the American Dietetic Association* (Yates 98, Monsen 00, Trumbo 01,02, Volpe 04). We define and illustrate the terms DRI, EAR, RDA, AI, and UL in Part I in the MNT section titled "Macronutrient Intake." An AI is established to probably be adequate for at least 50% of a population when data are insufficient to set a firm RDA to cover 97.5% of that population. For most recommendations in the new IOM reports, AIs were set for infants up to 1 year of age based on the average intake of the macronutrient consumed from human milk through 6 months, with the addition of complementary foods at 7–12 months (Trumbo 02). Previous reports proposed AIs for micronutrients for infants, with the exception of RDAs for iron and zinc at 7–12 months (Trumbo 02). No evidence suggests that RDIs should differ for diabetic women or their infants.

For the mother, it is important to note that the "nutritive demands of lactation are considerably greater than those of pregnancy. In the first 4–6 mo of the postpartum period, infants double their birth weight accumulated during the 9 mo of pregnancy. The milk secreted in 4 mo represents an amount of energy roughly equivalent to the total energy cost of pregnancy. However, some of the energy and many of the nutrients stored during pregnancy are available to support milk production" (Picciano 03). The EER is defined as the dietary energy intake that is predicted to maintain energy balance with TEE in healthy women of a defined age, weight, height, and level of physical activity, consistent with good health (Table IV.9) (IOM 02). Energy intakes above the EER would be expected to result in weight gain. The EER during lactation is estimated from the basic adjusted TEE using the prediction equation for adult women (which compared well with the observed TEE of lactating women) (IOM 02: Appendix Table I-5), plus milk energy output, minus energy mobilization from tissue stores. Therefore, the EER for the first 6 months of lactation is the tabular EER for the defined group plus

TABLE IV.8 Dietary Reference Intakes

Nutrient*	Lactating Female (14–18 years)	Lactating Female (19–30 years)	Lactating Female (31–50 years)	Infant (0–6 months)	Infant (7–12 months)
Water as fluids, L/day	3.1 (~13 cups)	3.1 (~13 cups)	3.1 (~13 cups)	0.7	0.6 + 0.2 food
Carbohydrate, gm/day	210	210	210	60	95
Total fiber, gm/day	29	29	29	ND	ND
Fat, gm/day	ND	ND	ND	31	30
Linoleic acid, gm/day	13	13	13	4.4	4.6
α-Linolenic acid, gm/day	1.3	1.3	1.3	0.5	0.5
Calcium, mg/day	1,300	1,000	1,000	210	210
Chromium, μg/day	44	45	45	0.2	5.5
Copper, μg/day	1,300	1,300	1,300	200	220
Fluoride, mg/day	3	3	3	0.01	0.5
Iodine, μg/day	290	290	290	110	130
Iron, mg/day	10	9	9	0.27	11
Magnesium, mg/day	360	310	320	30	75
Manganese, mg/day	2.6	2.6	2.6	0.003	0.6
Molybdenum, μg/day	50	50	50	2	3
Phosphorus, mg/day	1,250	700	700	100	275
Potassium, gm/day	5.1	5.1	5.1	0.4	0.4 + 0.3 food
Selenium, μg/day	70	70	70	15	20
Sodium, gm/day	1.5	1.5	1.5	0.12	0.12 + .25 food
Zinc, mg/day	13	12	12	2	3
Vitamin A, μg/day	1,200	1,300	1,300	400	500
Vitamin C, mg/day	115	120	120	40	50
Vitamin D, μg/day	5[a]	5[a]	5[a]	5	5
Vitamin E[b], mg/day	19	19	19	4	5
Vitamin K, μg/day	75	90	90	2.0	2.5
Thiamin, mg/day	1.4	1.4	1.4	0.2	0.3
Riboflavin, mg/day	1.6	1.6	1.6	0.3	0.4
Niacin, mg/day	17[n]	17[n]	17[n]	2[nn]	2[nn] + 2 food
Vitamin B6, mg/day	2.0	2.0	2.0	0.1	0.3
Folate, μg/day	500	500	500	65	80
Vitamin B12, μg/day	2.8	2.8	2.8	0.4	0.5
Biotin, μg/day	35	35	35	5	6
Choline, mg/day	550	550	550	125	150

Recommended intakes for lactating women in different age groups and infants at 0–6 and 7–12 months of life. Food and Nutrition Board, Institute of Medicine, National Academies 1997–2002.
RDA in ordinary type; AI in italics.
*Calculated for average individual.
[a]In the absence of adequate exposure to sunlight, 1 μg cholecalciferol = 40 IU vitamin D.
[b]As α-tocopherol.
[n]As niacin equivalents (NE):1mg of niacin = 60 mg tryptophan.
[nn]At 0–6 months preformed niacin, not NE.

ND, not determined.

TABLE IV.9 Estimated Energy Requirements (EER) for Nonpregnant Women 30 Years of Age*

Height, inches (m)	Physical Activity Level**	Weight, lb (kg) for BMI 18.5	Weight, lb (kg) for BMI 25	EER (kcal/day) for BMI 18.5	EER (kcal/day) for BMI 25
59 (1.50)	Sedentary	92 (41.6)	124 (56.2)	1,625	1,762
	Low active			1,803	1,956
	Active			2,025	2,196
	Very active			2,291	2,489
65 (1.65)	Sedentary	111 (50.4)	150 (68.0)	1,816	1,982
	Low active			2,016	2,202
	Active			2,267	2,477
	Very active			2,567	2,807
71 (1.80)	Sedentary	132 (59.9)	178 (81.0)	2,015	2,211
	Low active			2,239	2,459
	Active			2,519	2,769
	Very active			2,855	3,141

For lactation, add 500 kcal/day for milk energy output for first 6 months minus 170 kcal/day for expected weight loss from energy mobilization from tissue stores. For second 6 months, add 400 kcal/day for milk energy output minus zero expected weight loss.

**For each year below 30, add 7 kcal/day; for each year above 30, subtract 7 kcal/day.*

BMI, body mass index. BMI as kg/m².

Adapted from IOM 02, National Academy of Sciences, and Trumbo 02.

523 kcal/day (rounded to 500) for milk production (~780 mL/day; 0.67 kcal/gm milk), with the assumption that 170 kcal/day will be mobilized from energy stores accumulated during pregnancy. The EER addition for lactation at 7–12 months is 400 kcal/day because milk production rates decrease to 600 mL/day and weight stability is assumed after 6 months postpartum (IOM 02, Picciano 03). Several investigators found that basic energy intakes of ~500 kcal/day less than the recommended EERs plus exercise were compatible with good milk output and composition, healthy growth of the infants, and gradual weight loss ≥1 lb/week for overweight mothers (Butte 84b, Strode 86, Brewer 89, Lovelady 90, Dewey 94a,b, Dusdieker 94, Lovelady 95, Dewey 97,98b, Fly 98, Murtaugh 98, McCrory 99, Lovelady 00). The coupling of moderate exercise with dietary weight loss is preferred so as to preserve lean body mass (Dewey 98b, McCrory 99). Exercise results in improved cardiovascular status. Increased lactic acid in breast milk after exercise is not likely to influence the acceptance of human milk by the infant (Dewey 94a), but specific studies have not been performed in diabetic women.

The maternal lactation EAR (160 gm/day) for carbohydrate in 50% of the population is the sum of the carbohydrate secreted in human milk (60 gm/day; mostly lactose) plus the EAR for the average woman (100 gm/day). The RDA of 210 gm/day is calculated to be 130% of the EAR, which should provide "enough carbohydrate in the diet for an adequate volume of milk, to prevent ketonemia, and to maintain appropriate blood glucose levels during lactation" (Reader 04). Paying attention to the glycemic response to carbohydrate food choices and amounts has been shown to improve glycemic control (Karamlis 07, Amano 07, Barclay 08, Monro 08, Nilsson 08).

No DRI has been set for total fat intake during lactation because the amount of fat needed is dependent on the amount of energy required to maintain milk production; fat should provide 20–35% of total energy. As yet, there is no consensus on the ideal macronutrient proportions in the MNT of diabetic women. However, AIs are set for *n*-6 linoleic acid and *n*-3 α-linolenic acid during lactation because PUFAs in the maternal diet are crucial for infant brain and retinal development (Reader 04). Several guidelines and methods are available on methods to increase PUFA intake and limit consumption of cholesterol, saturated, and *trans* fats in the interest of long-term maternal health (ADietA 07, Johnson 07, Wylie-Rosett 07, Chardigny 08, St-Onge 08). "Food environments and health messages should be designed to encourage intake of fruits and vegetables, whole grains, nuts, fish, and low-fat dairy foods and discourage intake of fatty meats and processed foods that are low in fiber and high in saturated and trans fat" (Nettleton 07). There is no consensus on the benefit/risk of supplementing long-chain *n*-3 fatty acids to lactating women, but a study in adult nondiabetic females demonstrated that consuming two servings of fatty fish (salmon and albacore tuna) per week enriched blood lipids with *n*-3 fatty acids as much as did use of one to two fish oil capsules (DHA-rich [like fish] rather than EPA-rich) per day over 4–16 weeks. The frequency of fishy aftertaste was frequent in the capsule group (Harris 07).

The EAR for additional protein in lactation is based on the output of total protein and nonprotein nitrogen in human milk and is calculated to be +0.39 gm protein per kilogram body weight per day or 21.2 gm/day additional protein for the reference woman. This is added to the usual female EAR for protein of 0.66 gm/kg/day. The RDA of 71 gm/day is equal to the EAR (covers 50% of the population) plus 24% to cover 97.5% of the population. The RDA is estimated to promote the conservation of skeletal muscle while maintaining good milk production (Reader 04), with total protein concentrations of 7–14 gm/L and infant protein intake of ~1 gm/kg/day compared with 1.8 gm/kg/day in infants fed formula milk (Heinig 93). As noted earlier, there is concern that infants receiving the highest-protein formulas may have an elevation of insulin-stimulating amino acids in their plasma (Janas 85, Axelsson 89), and increased insulin could result in obesity (Koletzko 05).

Total water intake includes drinking water, water in beverages, and water as part of food (~22%). An AI of total water (3.8 L/day in lactation vs. 3.0 L/day for pregnancy) is set to prevent the effects of dehydration (IOM 04). No evidence suggests that renal function and hydration status differ during lactation in most diabetic women. The lactation AI is based on median total water intakes during lactation estimated in the NHANES III survey (IOM 04). To sum the nonpregnant total water need for females aged 14–18 years (2.3 L/day), 19–30 years (2.7 L/day), and 31–50 years (2.9 L/day) with the water content of the average daily milk output during the first 6 months of lactation (0.78 L milk × 87% = 0.68 L water) generates estimated total water needs of 2.9, 3.4, and 3.6 L/day, respectively (IOM 04).

Sodium and chloride are required to maintain extracellular volume and plasma osmolality, and the AI is set "to ensure that the overall diet provides an adequate intake of other important nutrients and to cover sodium sweat losses in unacclimatized individuals who are exposed to high temperatures or who become physically active" (IOM 04). No evidence suggests that the sodium requirements of lactating women differ from those of nonlactating women, although a small amount of sodium is secreted into the milk each day (0.12 gm/day) (IOM 04). Because the estimated median energy intake of lactating women (2,066 kcal/day) falls within the range of energy consumed by young nonpregnant women (IOM 02), the AI for sodium for lactating women (1.5 gm/day: all ages, same as for pregnancy; 3.8 gm/day NaCl) is set to be equal to that of young, nonlactating women. The tolerable UL for maternal sodium intake in lactation is set to be 2.3 gm/day to reduce hypertension (IOM 04). The AI for chloride is set at an equal equimolar amount based on the AI for sodium (IOM 04). As the major intracellular cation in the body, potassium is required for normal cellular function. The AI is set to maintain lower BP levels, reduce the adverse effects of sodium chloride intake on BP, reduce the risk of kidney stones, and possibly decrease bone loss (IOM 04). The AI of 5.1 gm/day (vs. 4.7 gm/day for pregnant and nonpregnant women, all ages) is based on the output of 0.4 gm/day in human milk, assuming near 100% conversion of dietary potassium to milk (IOM 04). No UL is set for potassium, but caution is warranted in diabetic women using supplements while on drug therapy or in the presence of nephropathy (IOM 04). Evidence states that U.S. adults often consume more sodium and less potassium than the respective AI recommendations (IOM 04), but we lack adequate dietary intake data on diabetic lactating women.

Recommended intakes for several elements and vitamins are higher in lactation than in pregnancy (Picciano 03, Allen 05). Therefore, the energy density of the diabetic mother's diet is important because the estimated increased need for other nutrients is greater than the estimated increase in energy needs (Picciano 03). Authorities stress that maternal micronutrient deficiencies can cause a major reduction in the concentration of some of these nutrients in breast milk, with subsequent infant depletion (Allen 05). "Priority" micronutrients that may be deficient in lactating women and breast milk include thiamine, riboflavin, vitamin A, vitamins B-6 and B-12, and iodine. Evidence suggests that improved maternal dietary intake (marine and land animal source foods, fruits, vegetables) or use of multiple micronutrient supplements can reverse this problem (Allen 05).

Tables listing food sources for nutrients that are most likely to be deficient in the diets of lactating women are available (IOM 91, Howard 04). However, poor maternal diet does not typically negate the many benefits of breast-feeding because nutrients are drawn from maternal stores (IOM 91, Lawrence 01). Introduction of complementary feedings before 4–6 months of age generally does not increase total caloric intake or rate of growth and only substitutes foods that lack the protective components of human milk (Gartner 05). The iron content of breast milk declines from 0.9 mg/L in early milk to 0.3 mg/L by 5 months; term infants only absorb <0.05 mg/kg/day. However, iron deficiency is unlikely in full-term breast-fed infants because iron stores in the body are sufficient to meet requirements (Calvo 92, Pisacane 95, Griffen 01); the degree to which this is true in IDMs is unclear (Georgieff 90), and additional research is needed. Iron may be administered by drops while continuing exclusive breast-feeding (Dewey 04, Gartner 05). In most cases, primary prevention of iron-deficiency anemia in exclusively breast-fed infants depends on the introduction of iron-fortified foods by 4–6 months of age. If supplementary milk feeds are required, iron-fortified formulas should be used (Griffen 01).

Evidence suggests that the RDA for maternal vitamin B6 intake is inadequate to achieve breast milk vitamin B6 levels consistent with normal behavioral functioning in infants (Kang-Yoon 92, Heiskanen 96, Lovelady 01, Chang 02, Ooylan 02). Diabetic women on strict vegetarian diets should be counseled about potential nutritional deficits in their milk (Thomas 79, Sanders 99, ADietA 03), and vitamin B12 should be supplemented (IOM 91, Allen 02). The recommended AI of vitamin D cannot be met for the breast-feeding infant with human milk as the sole source (Gartner 03). There-fore, the AAP recommends that all breast-fed infants should receive 200 IU of oral vitamin D drops daily beginning during the first 2 months of life and continuing until the daily consumption of vitamin D–fortified milk or formula is 500 mL due to the risks of exposing young children to sunlight (Gartner 05). Newborn infants of mothers with dark skin or who wear concealing clothes have a high prevalence of vitamin D deficiency (Dawadu 07, Dijkstra 07). Higher-dose maternal vitamin D supplements (100 µg/day = 4,000 IU/day) are required to elevate 25(OH)D2 concentrations in nursing infants (Hollis 04). Vitamin K is given intramuscularly after the initial feeding but within the first 6 h of life; fluoride should not be supplemented during the first 6 months (Gartner 05).

Concerning beverages, alcohol freely and quickly passes into breast milk at levels approaching those of maternal plasma (Mennella 91, Howard 99). Peak levels appear in maternal plasma in 15 min, at 30–60 min in breast milk, or at 60–90 min if the mother drinks alcohol with food (da Silva 93, Lawrence 05). Acute alcohol consumption changes the hormonal milieu of lactating women in that prolactin levels are enhanced, but oxytocin release is attenuated during breast stimulation (Mennella 05); the milk ejection reflex can be partially blocked by ingestion of >1 gm/kg absolute alcohol (Cobo 73). "Old wives tales" to the contrary, use of alcohol actually induces lower milk yield (Mennella 98a). Ingestion of <1 gm/kg of absolute alcohol produces low breast milk alcohol levels that usually do not affect the infant (Lawton 85, Lawrence 05). Infant psychomotor development can be affected by long-term maternal consumption of two drinks per day (Little 89). However, short-term exposure to alcohol in breast milk can cause the infant to sleep less in the 3–4 h after nursing (Mennella 98b). Alcohol use should be minimized in diabetic lactating women, and nursing should be delayed for 4 h after its ingestion. If a nursing mother drinks >6 cups/day of a caffeine-containing beverage, caffeine can accumulate in the infant and result in wakeful, hyperactive babies (Lawrence 05).

Environmental toxins appearing in breast milk are a concern to nursing mothers (AAP 01, Pronczuk 02). Human milk "may contain certain components that either prevent intestinal absorption of xenobiotics or inactivate them" (Berlin 05). No data exist to indicate whether the protection or risk differs in diabetic women and their infants. The average woman is not likely to be exposed to chemicals such as herbicides, pesticides, and heavy metals, and levels in human milk are very low (Giroux 92, Rogan 94, Lawrence 01). Biomonitoring of human milk can provide exposure information about the mother and breast-fed infant. Technical workshops are convened regularly to review human milk surveillance for environmental chemicals in the U.S. The expert panel of the most recent workshop concluded that there is little evidence for adverse health effects in breast-fed infants due to background levels of environmental chemicals in human milk, and there is need for a greater number of systematic studies (Berlin 05). Lead crosses the placenta to a greater degree than it appears in human milk unless the maternal lead level is >40 µg/dL (Lawrence 01, Gundacker 02, Dorea 04). Women exposed to mercury in seafood or from dental amalgams (Drasch 98, Drexler 98) are at a theoretical risk (Oskarsson 96, Sakamoto 02, Bjornberg 05), but no neurodevelopmental impairment related to breast-feeding was found in the Faroe Islands (Jensen 05b) or the Seychelles (Meyers 95, Davidson 98), where mothers are exposed to mercury in fish. In fact, breast-fed infants were more advanced than those fed by formula. The current chronic oral reference dose (daily intake that is likely to be without appreciable risk of deleterious effects during a lifetime) for methylmercury set by the EPA is

0.1 μg/kg/day (Rice 03), with some evidence for a reference dose of 0.2–0.4 μg/kg/day due to pharmacokinetic or site-specific variation (Clewell 99, Shipp 00).

It is important for women with celiac disease to breast-feed because convincing data show that an increased duration of breast-feeding decreases infant risk of developing celiac disease. Children who were breast-fed for <90 days were five times more likely to develop celiac disease than children who were breast-fed for >90 days (Peters 01), there was a 63% reduction in the risk of developing celiac disease in children who were breast-fed for >2 months (Faith-Magnusson 96), and infants who were breast-fed for <30 days were four times more likely to develop celiac disease than those who were breast-fed for >30 days (Ivarsson 02). An additional study examined the relationship of exclusive versus partial breast-feeding on the risk of developing celiac disease and found that the median time of exclusive breast-feeding in children with celiac disease was 2.5 months and partial breast-feeding was 3.9 months versus 4 months of exclusive breast-feeding and 6 months of partial breast-feeding in control subjects without celiac disease (Auricchio 83). The accuracy of the data in these case–control studies is subject to recall bias, and they lacked control of other variables that may contribute to development of celiac disease. Additionally, mean follow-up time in these studies was a limitation. Long-term prospective studies are necessary to further distinguish whether breast-feeding does indeed offer protection from celiac disease or whether it delays the appearance of symptoms or age of onset (Akobeng 06).

Several studies evaluated the impact and timing of the introduction of gluten in the diet in relation to breast-feeding and the development of celiac disease in children. Two large studies found a decreased prevalence of celiac disease in children who were breast-fed at the time that gluten was introduced in their diet (Auriccho 83, Faith-Magnusson 96). A population-based study in Sweden confirmed the reduction in the risk of celiac disease in children <2 years of age if they were still being breast-fed when gluten was introduced into their diet; there was a greater protective effect if they continued to breast-feed following the introduction of gluten. However, the risk of developing celiac disease was greater if gluten was introduced in the diet in large amounts (Barker 06). Studies need to be performed in diabetic women to distinguish whether the same effects will occur and whether breast-feeding plus gluten at 4 months of age delays the onset of celiac disease or has a stronger protective effect (Akobeng 06).

Additional support for mothers with celiac disease is needed to ensure successful breast-feeding and adequate nutrition during breast-feeding. The principles of MNT for diabetic women with celiac disease are described in Part I of this document. With intensified management of celiac disease, the duration of breast-feeding was significantly longer for women with celiac disease (7.03 ± 1.17 months) than in an untreated control population (2.77 ± 0.52 months; $p < 0.0003$) (Ciacci 96). Regarding undiagnosed or untreated maternal celiac disease, malabsorption of iron, folate, vitamin B12, or the fat-soluble vitamins A, D, E, and K is possible and could affect the nutritional status of the breast-fed infant.

Additionally, as outlined earlier with reference to breast-feeding in women with diabetes, there is a call for further research on the metabolic effects of lactation in women with PDM and celiac disease. Conflicting data have arisen on the impact of celiac disease on glycemic control (Acerini 98, Kaukinen 99, Mohn 01, Amini 02, Hill 02, Chand 06), but this has not been studied in the postpartum period.

Recommendations

- Beginning in the preconception period, diabetic women and their families should be educated about the tremendous benefits of long-term breast-feeding of their infants, with increased emphasis during prenatal care. It is ideal to provide specific lactation counseling in the third trimester. Diabetes and pregnancy caregivers should facilitate the application of provisions of the Baby-Friendly Hospital Initiative and incorporate its principles into outpatient care. Collaboration with pediatric caregivers is important to facilitate the early breast-feeding of IDMs and minimize neonatal hypoglycemia and jaundice. (A, E)

- Breast-feeding should be strongly encouraged for women with diabetes. Human milk is the preferred food for all infants, with rare exceptions. Early suckling provides optimal protective factors that reduce infections in infants and improve the health of children. Exclusive breast-feeding is ideal nutrition and sufficient to support optimal growth and development for the first 4–6 months after birth. Supplementation of cereals is suggested at 4–6 months as breast-feeding continues. It is recommended that breast-feeding continue for at least 12 months and thereafter for as long as mutually desired. (A, B)

- Once lactation is established, balancing caloric intake with physical activity to achieve a weight loss of ≤4.4 lb/month (≤2 kg/month) appears to be safe for women who are initially overweight. Lean women may be at risk for impaired lactation performance if energy intake is restricted. Breast-feeding women are advised to consume ≥1,800 kcal/day (≥7.53 MJ/day) and to avoid liquid diets and weight loss medications. Intake of carbohydrates, fat, and protein according to DRIs should provide adequate nutrition for the infant and assist with good glycemic control of the diabetic mother. (A, E)

- Whether supplements of specific vitamins and elements are needed in diabetic mothers and their infants during the first 4–6 months of exclusive breast-feeding requires additional research. Consideration should be given to providing vitamin B6 supplements for the mother. All breast-fed infants should receive vitamin D supplements. Infants of strict vegetarian mothers should be supplemented with vitamin B12. IDMs should be tested for iron deficiency and treated accordingly. (E)

- Exercise during lactation appears to be safe for most diabetic women when precautions are taken to avoid maternal hypoglycemia. (A, E)

- Alcohol consumption while breast-feeding may have adverse effects on the infant's feeding and behavior as well as on glycemic control. (B)

- Women with celiac disease need special nutritional support because they can be at a higher risk of nutritional deficiencies of iron; fat-soluble vitamins A, D, E, and K; vitamin B12; and folate, especially if they are undiagnosed or not adhering to a gluten-free diet. (B)

- Women with celiac disease should be counseled on the potential impact of breast-feeding on the reduction of risk of celiac disease in children and that the introduction of gluten into the infant diet in small to moderate amounts between 4 and 6 months of age will maximize the benefit. (B)

DRUG TREATMENT OF DIABETES AND RELATED DISORDERS DURING LACTATION

—— *Contributed by Maribeth Inturrisi RN, MS, CDE, RH Knopp MD,*
Martin Montoro MD, and J Kitzmiller MD

Characteristics of Drug Transfer into Breast Milk and the Infant

The reader will note that investigators usually refer to the passage of nutrients into breast milk as "secretion" and to the passage of drugs as "excretion." We have attempted to follow this convention.

Passage of a drug into breast milk is influenced by the following factors: size of the molecule and its concentration in maternal plasma (dose–level), degree of ionization and pH of the substrate (plasma 7.4; milk 6.8), solubility in lipids and water, degree of binding to plasma proteins compared with milk proteins, and specific pharmacokinetic characteristics influencing the passive or carrier-mediated diffusion rates of the drug or active metabolites. Some drugs enter breast milk by active transport against a concentration gradient (Lawrence 05, Anderson 06). Drugs of a molecular weight <200 daltons are expected to diffuse into breast milk (subject to other influences) (Lawrence 05), and drugs >500 daltons have restricted transfer (Hale 04). Ionized compounds are excreted into breast milk to a lesser degree than non-ionized compounds. Drugs that are weak acids are ionized to a greater extent in the plasma and transfer more poorly. Drugs that are weak bases become more ionized in the more acid substrate of the milk; thus, the amount in the milk will exceed that in plasma (ion trapping) (Wilson 83, Atkinson 88a, Howard 99).

Transfer of water-soluble drugs and ions is inhibited by the hydrophobic glycophospholipid membrane of the alveolar epithelial cells, so they must pass through water-filled pores in the membrane and paracellular spaces (Lawrence 05). Non-ionized lipid-soluble drugs usually dissolve and pass through the lipid phase of the basal membrane and then through the apical membrane. Highly lipid-soluble drugs will equilibrate in plasma and milk, and those with lower lipid solubility "will clear the plasma at a constant rate, but the clearance curve for the milk will peak lower and later, and the drug will linger in the milk" [like metformin] (Lawrence 05). The mammary alveolar epithelium is most permeable during the first week postpartum. Drugs that are highly bound to plasma proteins will generally have less transfer to milk because the unbound free fraction of drug is low (Riant 86). The influence of milk proteins and lipids on the concentration of drugs in whole breast milk is controversial (Atkinson 90, Larsen 03, Lawrence 05). Drugs are much less bound to milk proteins in the whey fraction (very low binding to milk albumin and lactoferrin; none to α-lactalbumin) than to plasma proteins, but there is drug binding to the casein fraction (Atkinson 88b, Stebler 90).

The breast milk/plasma (M/P) drug ratio has been used by clinicians to gauge possible exposure to the infant. The M/P ratio expresses the concentration of the drug in milk versus the concentration in maternal plasma at the same time, but this does not remain constant (Lawrence 05). Time-dependent variations of drug concentrations in milk demand a pharmacokinetic model for the study of drugs in breast milk (Wilson 85). The M/P ratio of a drug is "only valuable when the time of the measurement is known in relation to the dosing of the mother" (Lawrence 05).

The amount of drug transferred into the circulation of the infant is the most important question, but it has received less attention due to the difficulty of the investigation. Oral bioavailability of a drug affects absorption from the baby's gastrointestinal tract, but is difficult to measure in vivo. Another important factor is the infant's ability to detoxify and excrete a given drug. "What dosages and blood levels are safe? These latter two questions are more critical than the pharmacokinetic theory. The ultimate question is: Can this infant be safely exposed to this chemical as it appears in breast milk without a risk that exceeds the tremendous benefits of being breastfed?" (Lawrence 05).

Use of Antihyperglycemic Agents During Lactation

Lactating women with type 2 diabetes may be switched from insulin therapy to oral agents after delivery. In a single-dose study (5 or 10 mg) of eight women with type 2 diabetes, glyburide remained beneath the level of detectability in 29 samples of breast milk over an 8-h period (Feig 05). In a related daily-dose study of five breast-feeding women treated with glyburide or glipizide over the first 16 days postpartum, neither drug was found in breast milk when using a less sensitive assay, and plasma glucose was normal in their infants (Feig 05). The lack of transfer of glyburide to milk may be related to its unusually high degree of protein binding (99.9%) in maternal plasma because the older sulfonylurea drugs chlorpropamide and tolbutamide are secreted into breast milk (Briggs 05a) or possibly to glyburide back-transfer to maternal plasma via an unknown transporter as demonstrated in the placenta (Kraemer 06). Three studies of metformin in a total of 17 lactating diabetic women showed limited transfer of metformin into breast milk with mean milk-to-maternal plasma ratios of 0.35, 0.54, and 0.63, respectively, and mean milk metformin concentrations of 0.27, 0.27, and 0.42 mg/L in a prolonged, flat profile (Hale 02, Gardiner 03, Briggs 05b). Metformin is a highly polar drug with poor lipid solubility (Hale 04). Mean infant exposure to the drug was only 0.21%, 0.28%, and 0.65% of the weight-normalized maternal dose, respectively; only two of six infants had detectable plasma metformin concentrations of 0.05 and 0.08 mg/L 2.5 h after a maternal dose of 500 mg and normal plasma glucose levels (Hale 02, Gardiner 03, Briggs 05b). The authors concluded that the limited mother-to-baby transfer of metformin seemed to be clinically insignificant and that metformin is compatible with breast-feeding. Continued study of exposed infants will be necessary to detect any long-term effects. A larger experience has been recorded in 61 metfomin-treated, lactating, nondiabetic women with polycystic ovary syndrome whose infants were studied at 3 and 6 months of age compared with 50 formula-fed infants of similar mothers. No exposure-related effects were detected on infant weight, height, aggregate motor–social development scores, or intercurrent illnesses (Glueck 06).

Because <2% of acarbose is absorbed as active drug in adults (systemic absorption of metabolites = 34%), "the amount of unmetabolized drug available for transfer to the milk is probably clinically insignificant," and it is listed as probably compatible with breast-feeding (Briggs 05a). No human data are available on its use in lactation, but small amounts of acarbose or its metabolites are secreted into the milk of lactating rats (Briggs 05a). The effect of TZD agents ("glitazones"; activators of nuclear PPARγ) on nursing infants is unknown, but transfer into milk is expected due to the low molecular weight of the compounds. TZDs or their three active metabolites have been detected in the milk of lactating rats (Briggs 05a).

Treating Dyslipidemias in the Postpartum Period

Postpartum Lipid Testing

Lipid and lipoprotein levels return to the nonpregnant baseline at different times. Plasma TG, HDL-C, and Apo A$_1$ levels return to the prepregnancy baseline by approximately 6 weeks. However, total-C and LDL-C levels approach baseline much more slowly (Figure IV.1) as does apo B in the LDL fraction, reflecting the mobilization of cholesterol from involuting maternal organs such as breast, uterus, and fat stores (Montes 84). Testing for cholesterol elevations in the postpartum period must take this physiological adaptation into account or wait almost 1 year for comparison with age-specific reference lipid values in nonpregnant women (LRCP 80). Otherwise, unexplained hyperlipidemia postpartum might be due to postpartum hypothyroidism.

Effect of Lactation on Postpartum Maternal Lipids

Lactation is associated with a tendency toward lowered TG and raised HDL-C levels, with no change in LDL-C (Knopp 85, Erkolla 86). In one study shown in Table IV.10, plasma TG levels are 20 mg/dL lower and HDL-C levels are 14 mg/dL higher with lactation, in which lactating and nonlactating subjects had identical lipid levels in late gestation. The effect of diabetes on lipoprotein or fatty acid response to lactation has not been studied to our knowledge, but one might expect similar differences at equivalent levels of diabetic control. Total and individual fatty acids in plasma phospholipids decline significantly over 16 weeks postpartum, probably reflecting the postpartum decline in HDL that is rich in phospholipids. The decline in fatty acids is unaffected by lactation with the exception of higher EPA levels with breast-feeding (Otto 01).

Postpartum Lipid Therapy

The goals of lipid therapy in diabetic women without overt CVD are to maintain LDL-C <100 mg/dL (<2.6 mM), HDL-C >50 mg/dL (>1.4 mM), and lower TGs to <150 mg/dL (1.7 mM). Annual testing (or more often if needed) should be performed for lipid disorders to achieve goals (ADA 08a). MNT can be used by lactating women to help attain these goals by limiting the intake of saturated fat to <7% of energy, *trans* fat to <1% of energy, and cholesterol to <300 mg/day by choosing lean meats and vegetable alternatives, fat-free (skim) or low-fat (1% fat) dairy products, and minimizing the intake of partially hydrogenated fats (AHA 06). Table 3 of the 2006 AHA Scientific Statement provides helpful practical dietary tips to assist women in achieving these goals (AHA 06). Increasing physical activity by exercising 30 min daily on most days of the week has been shown to improve the lipid profile in diabetic women (ADA 08a).

Due to the potential for adverse effects in infants, statins should not be used during breast-feeding (Briggs 05a). Gemfibrozil is probably excreted into breast milk due to low molecular weight, but there are no studies of its use in human lactation. A leading reference states: "The drug should probably not be used in breastfeeding women because of the potential for severe toxicity, including tumors, in the nursing infants" (Briggs 05a). Niacin, the precursor to niacinamide, is needed in breast milk, and the dietary RDA for lactating women is 17 mg/day (IOM 97). We lack studies of the use of niacin in the treatment of hypertriglyceridemia during the postpartum period in diabetic lactating women. High-potency fish oil that is refined free of possible mercury content would be a reasonable treatment for hypertriglyceridemia during lactation when TG levels are >1,000 mg and there is risk for pancreatitis. Due to restrictions on

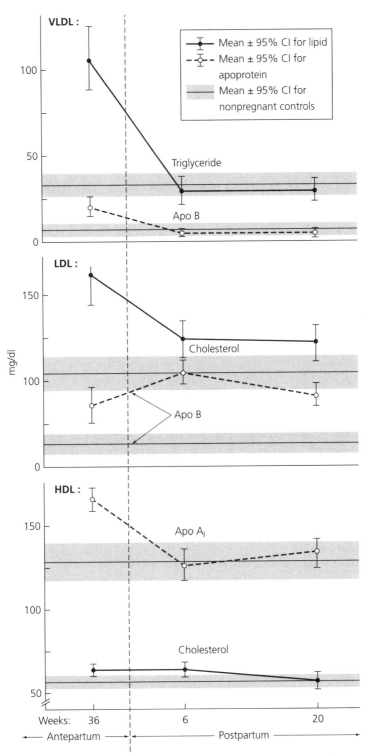

FIGURE IV.1 Postpartum changes in cholesterol, triglycerides, and apoproteins in normal pregnancy. Apo, apolipoprotein; CI, confidence interval; HDL, high-density lipoprotein; LDL, low-density lipoprotein; VLDL, very-low-density lipoprotein.

TABLE IV.10 Effect of Postpartum Lactation on Lipoprotein Levels

	Mean ± 1 Standard Deviation (mg/dL)			
	Lactating	Nonlactating	Difference	P Value
Number	56	16		
Triglyceride	92 ± 71	112 ± 56	−20	0.02
Cholesterol (-C)	207 ± 31	188 ± 29	−19	0.007
LDL-C	129 ± 31	121 ± 30	8	0.27
HDL-C	65 ± 15	51 ± 8	14	0.0004
Apo B	76 ± 28	66 ± 20	10	0.27
Apo A-I	142 ± 23	126 ± 19	16	0.02

Six weeks postpartum. Adapted from Knopp 85.
APO, apolipoprotein; HDL-C, high-density lipoprotein cholesterol; LDL-C, low-density lipoprotein cholesterol.

drug therapy during lactation and considering the severity of dyslipidemia as well as the presence or absence of CVD, clinician and patient must weigh the maternal risk of no pharmacotherapy for the short term with the tremendous benefit to the infant of exclusive breast-feeding for at least 4 months.

Antihypertensive Therapy During Lactation

Current definitions of hypertension (≥130/80) are discussed in Part II in the section titled "Blood Pressure Control." Due to the risks of CVD, nephropathy, and retinopathy, the goals of BP control in diabetic women are to keep systolic pressure <130 mmHg and diastolic pressure <80 mmHg (ADA 06a, AHA 06). Use of multiple drugs and self-monitoring of BP is often necessary to reach these goals. Lifestyle intervention (diet as noted earlier in MNT for lactation and 30 min exercise daily on most days of the week) is recommended. Patients should choose and prepare foods with little or no salt (AHA 06).

Antihypertensive drugs with proven safety records in breast-feeding mothers include methyldopa, low-dose thiazides, ACE inhibitors, CCBs, and selected β-adrenergic blockers (Hale 04). Table IV.11 presents the degree of protein binding, M/P ratios, percentage of adult dose, and maximum drug concentration in human milk for selected antihypertensive agents used in diabetic women (Howard 99). α-Methyldopa is a relatively weak antihypertensive with limiting side effects; theoretically, it can decrease milk production via direct effects on the pituitary (Lawrence 05). Methyldopa appears in low amounts in milk at average levels of 0.02–1.14 μg/mL, with peak appearance 3-6 h after the maternal dose. The infant is believed to receive 195 μg daily, 0.02% of the maternal dose, or <3% of the newborn therapeutic (effective) dose (White 85). Low plasma levels were detected in 2 of 4 infants studied without apparent harmful effects (Hauser 85, White 85). A fact to be noted is the persistence for some days of methyldopa in the newborn infants of late pregnancy-treated women who did not nurse their babies. The drug is slowly eliminated by excretion in the urine after metabolism to the sulphate conjugate (Jones 79). Large doses of short-acting thiazides or usual doses of long-acting thiazides and loop diuretics can cause suppression of lactation (Howard 99), but low-dose thiazides do not. Hydrochlorothiazides and

TABLE IV.11 Characteristics of Selected Antihypertensive Drugs Found in Breast Milk

Drug	Oral Availability (% ± SD)	Plasma Protein Bound (%)	Milk/ Plasma Ratio	Adult Dose in Milk (%)	Maximum Amount in Milk (mg/L)
Atenolol	56 ± 30	5–16	1.3–6.8	12.4 ± 6.8	1.8
Captopril	60–75% absorbed	30 ± 6	0.006–0.6	0.002–0.014	0.008
Chlorthalidone	64 ± 10	75 ± 1	0.03–0.05	6.7	36
Clonidine	87 ± 12	20	1.5–4.0	7.9 ± 0.1	0.002
Diltiazem	80–90% absorbed	70–86	0.98–1	0.9	0.22
Enalapril	53–74% absorbed	<50	0.14–0.78		0.002
Hydrochlorothiazide	72 ± 7	58 ± 17	0.25–0.43		0.125
Labetalol	10–80	45–55	0.4–2.6	0.004–0.07	0.662
Methyldopa	8–62	1–16	0.19–0.34	0.02–0.09	1.36
Metoprolol	42.5 ± 18.5	8–11.5	2.0–4.8	1.7–5.0	0.225
Nifedipine	31–92	90–98	1.0	<0.004	0.053
Propranolol	2–54	87 ± 6	0.05–2.0	0.05–1.0	0.16
Verapamil	>90% absorbed	90 ± 2	0.23–0.94	0.01–0.84	0.026

Adapted from Howard 99 and used with permission.

chlorthalidone are minimally excreted in human milk at <4% of the newborn therapeutic dose, with peak thiazide levels 7.5 h after the maternal dose (Lawrence 05). Of the ACE inhibitors, captopril and enalapril are found in very low concentrations in human milk (Devlin 81, Redman 90), and no untoward clinical effects have been described in nursing infants (Huutunen 89, Shannon 00a, Hale 04). Time to peak appearance in milk for captopril is 3.8 ± 0.6 h at only 0.1% of the newborn effective therapeutic dose (Lawrence 05). Experience with angiotensin II receptor blockers is not described during human lactation, but losartan and an active metabolite appear in rat milk in significant concentrations (Lawrence 05).

Of the CCBs, nifedipine and verapamil are transferred into breast milk in small amounts at <5% and <1% of the newborn effective doses, with peak levels at 0.8 and 1.3 h after the maternal dose, respectively (Miller 86, Ehrenkranz 89, Penny 89, Manninen 91, Howard 99). In case studies of two breast-feeding women using verapamil 240 mg/day, milk concentrations were 23% and 60% of maternal plasma levels, respectively. Infant serum level was 2.1 ng/mL with no effects observed in one infant, and verapamil was undetectable in the other (Andersen 83, Anderson 87). It may be of interest that verapamil is an inhibitor of the placental drug transporter P-glycoprotein, which is also expressed in lactating rat mammary tissue (Edwards 05). Limited human evidence demonstrates that diltiazem may pass more freely into human milk (Okada 85, Atkinson 88a, Briggs 05a), but diltiazem, verapamil, and nifedipine are considered compatible with breast-feeding by the AAP (Shannon 00b). Diltiazem undergoes hepatic metabolism, and time to peak appearance in milk is 2.5 ± 0.5 h after oral dosing (Lawrence 05). Concern exists that long-acting preparations of CCBs might lead to more drug accumulation in the infant. There are no data available to evaluate the effect of amlodipine in breast-feeding.

The β-blockers acebutalol and atenolol have been associated with case reports of bradycardia, hypotension, and cyanosis in infants (Boutroy 86, Schimmel 89). Atenolol's peak concentration in milk (469–630 ng/mL) is 5 ± 3 h after an oral dose at equivalent or higher concentrations than maternal plasma, but the infant serum concentration is only 0.1% of the mother's concentration (Liedholm 81, Thorley 83, Kulas 84, Lawrence 05). Propranolol, metoprolol, and labetalol are considered compatible with breast-feeding because no untoward effects have been reported in infants of treated mothers (Taylor 81, Hale 04). Propranolol's peak concentration in milk occurs 2–4 h after a maternal dose at 0.4–6% of the newborn therapeutic dose; 5–10% of Caucasians are poor metabolizers (Levitan 73, Bauer 79, Smith 83, Lawrence 05). Its high degree of plasma protein binding may protect the infant (Riant 86). Metoprolol undergoes first-pass metabolism, but the metabolites are active. Metoprolol concentrates in milk with peak levels 4 ± 2 h after the maternal dose, with an increased half-life in the infant (Lawrence 05). Although no harmful neonatal effects have been described in infants (Sandstrom 80, Liedholm 81, Kulas 84, Lindeberg 84), they should be monitored for signs of β-blockade (Howard 99, Shannon 00c). Plasma concentrations of metoprolol in infants were negligible when nursing was not undertaken earlier than 4 h after a maternal dose (Kulas 84). Labetalol undergoes extensive first-pass metabolism and peaks in breast milk at 2.7 ± 0.6 h, with a mean level of 33 ng/mL with typical maternal doses. Labetalol was identified in plasma of some, but not all, infants (Lunell 85, Lawrence 05).

Clonidine was detected in breast milk at concentrations of ~2 ng/mL in the first, second, and seventh week postpartum (compared with ~1 ng/mL in maternal serum) and was less concentrated in the serum of infants of nine nursing mothers using mean daily doses of 200–400 μg. None of the infants were hypotensive (Hartikainen-Sorri 87). According to the manufacturer, prazocin is secreted into human milk in small amounts at concentrations of 1–4% of the newborn therapeutic dose, but no reports of its use during lactation were located (Briggs 05a, Lawrence 05).

Treatment of Thyroid Disease and Lactation

Because low prolactin levels can occur in a thyroid-deficient state, diabetic women with hypothyroidism should be treated with thyroid hormone to ensure full lactation (Lawrence 05). A small amount of physiological thyroid hormone appears in the milk of healthy women (Sack 77, Mizuta 83). Levothyroxine and tri-iodothyronine levels in the milk are too low for replacement doses to produce changes in thyroid function in the infant (Varma 78, Hale 04). Graves' disease may worsen in the postpartum period, and antithyroid drugs will be needed (Mandel 01). The milk-to-maternal plasma ratio for PTU is 0.1 after maternal ingestion of 200 mg; 0.025% of the administered dose appears in breast milk over 4 h (Low 79, Kampmann 80). Calculations showed that treatment with PTU 200 mg three times daily would transmit 149 μg/day to the infant, equivalent to a subtherapeutic daily dose of 3 mg for a 70-kg adult (Kampmann 80). A higher proportion of oral doses of methimazole or its precursor carbimazole appear in breast milk as 0.1–0.17% of an orally administered dose (Johansen 82). PTU is more extensively protein bound and more ionized in plasma than methimazole (Mandel 01). However, breast-fed infants of thyrotoxic mothers treated with methimazole 20–30 mg daily had low subtherapeutic serum levels <0.03 μg/mL 2 h after the mother ingested the dose (Azizi 00). Several investigators (reviewed in Mandel 01) studied the thyroid function of breast-fed infants during maternal treatment with PTU up to 450 mg/day or methimazole 20 mg/day and found normal TSH and free T4 levels, even when the mother became hypothyroidal during treatment (Azizi 96). Verbal and performance IQ scores and somatic growth of children followed 48–74 months after maternal treatment with methimazole during lactation did not differ from controls (Azizi 00). Maternal antithyroid drug treatment seems safe whether continued after delivery or started in the postpartum period (Mandel 01, Lawrence 05). A lactating mother with thyroid disease should not be given iodine for any reason because iodine is concentrated in the milk (Lawrence 05).

Antidepressant Drugs During Lactation

Depression in the postpartum period occurs in 10–15% of mothers and is at least as common in women with PDM. Because clinical depression can interfere with effective parenting and produce significant neurobehavioral delay in infants, antidepressants may need to be continued or initiated (Wisner 96, Howard 99, Hale 04, Gentile 05, Lawrence 05, Eberhard-Gran 06). Neonatal antidepressant withdrawal is well described (TerHorst 08), but treatment of severe maternal depression is of more benefit than risk (ACOG 06a). Recommended drugs during lactation have included the tricyclic antidepressants amitriptyline, nortriptyline, and desipramine; clomipramine; dothiepin; or the SSRIs sertraline and paroxetine (Wisner 96, Berle 04). The Committee on Drugs of the AAP lists these and eight other antidepressants as "drugs for which the effect on nursing infants is unknown but may be of concern" because they "could conceivably alter short-term and long-term central nervous system function" (AAP 01). The AAP 2001 statement and a later review (Eberhard-Gran 06) cite references indicating no reported infant effects except for colic, irritability, feeding and sleep disorders, and slow weight gain with maternal fluoxetine and citalopram. High infant concentrations of the main metabolite of doxepin were associated with sedation and respiratory depression in breast-fed infants (AAP 01, Eberhard-Gran 06).

The AAP committee notes that sertraline is concentrated in human milk relative to simultaneous maternal plasma concentrations (AAP 01), although it is 98–99% plasma protein bound (Berle 04, Lawrence 05). In studies of 56 mother–infant pairs, the highest concentration of sertraline was detected in the hindmilk 8–9 h after maternal ingestion. Sertraline was detected in 19.6% of infant sera, but desmethylsertraline was detected in 46% of infants tested for the metabolite (Stowe 97, Hendrick 01, Stowe 03), which has a half-life of 66 h compared with 25 h for sertraline (Howard 99). Sertraline is a potent inhibitor of serotonin transporter function in platelets as well as the CNS, and one report found minimal effect on platelet serotonin transport in nursing infants (Epperson 01). At least one case report found neurological withdrawal symptoms in a 3-week-old infant whose nursing mother abruptly stopped the drug (Kent 95). Exposure to paroxetine in breast milk has produced no reported adverse effects in infants (Hendrick 01, Eberhard-Gran 06). Paroxetine is 95% plasma protein bound, with the usual plasma peak at 4.8–5.6 h after dosing and an M/P ratio of 1.0, but it is usually not detectable in the infant (Hendrick 01, Berle 04, Weissman 04, Lawrence 05). Limited studies of fluvoxamine during breast-feeding reveal 77% binding to plasma proteins, an M/P ratio of 0.3–1.3, 0.5% of the adult dose in breast milk, and no detectable medication or drug effects in 14 infants (Wright 91, Yoshida 97, Arnold 00, Hendrick 01, Piontek 01, Kristensen 02, Haag 03, Lawrence 05).

The tricyclic antidepressants amitriptyline, nortriptyline, and desipramine are excreted into milk, with M/P ratios of 0.5–1.7, 0.6–3.7, and 0.4–1.2, respectively, but are usually are not detected in infant serum (Lawrence 05). These drugs have not caused observable effects in breast-fed infants; however, use of the secondary amines nortriptyl-ine and desipramine (metabolites of amitriptyline and imipramine, respectively) and administration of a single dose at bedtime with substitute feedings during the night may minimize infant exposure (Howard 99). Use of tricyclic antidepressants may be limited by maternal anticholinergic side effects (Eberhard-Gran 06). Clomipramine is 96.5–98.6% plasma protein bound, with an M/P ratio of 0.8–1.6 but only 0.4% of the maternal dose found in milk, and is usually not detected in infant serum (Lawrence 05). Dothiepin has an M/P ratio of 0.3–1.6 with 0.15–0.58% of the maternal dose in breast milk, but no drug detected in infant sera (Lawrence 05). A 3–5-year follow-up study of 15 children exposed to dothiepin in breast milk revealed no differences in cognitive scores compared with controls (Buist 95). Bupropion is excreted into breast milk (Briggs 93), and bupropion or its metabolite was not detected in only two infants eval-uated (Baab 02). Case reports describe neonatal seizures possibly related to bupropion use by the breast-feeding mother (Chaudron 04, Bup. 05).

Recommendations

- Following delivery, women with type 2 diabetes may be switched from insulin therapy to oral antihyperglycemic agents. Careful consideration of the type of agent is needed in the lactating mother. Glipizide, glyburide, metformin, and acarbose are considered compatible with breast-feeding. (B, E)

- Clinicians should recognize the effects of time from delivery and presence of lactation on maternal lipid levels. The goal of lipid therapy in diabetic women is to maintain: (A)
  - LDL-C <100 mg/dL
  - HDL-C >50 mg/dL
  - TGs <150 mg/dL

- There is no known contraindication to breast-feeding in the presence of hyperli-pidemia. Use of gemfibrozil and statins should be avoided in lactating women. Niacin and fish oil capsules can be used for severe hypertriglyceridemia. (E)

- Lifestyle modification should be used to manage hyperlipidemia. (A)
  - Limit saturated fat to <7% of energy intake
  - Limit *trans* fats to <1% of energy intake
  - Limit cholesterol to <300 mg/day
  - Increase physical activity with at least 30 min of exercise on most days

- The goal of BP control in women with diabetes is to keep BP <130/ 80 mmHg. Use of multiple drugs and self-monitoring of BP is often necessary to reach the goal. Every attempt to maximize lifestyle modification should be made in lactating women (diet, exercise, lipids as stated earlier). The effect of limitation of salt intake on diabetic lactating women is unknown. (A)

- The antihypertensive agents methyldopa, low-dose thiazides, ACE inhibitors (captopril, lisinopril), CCBs, and selected β-adrenergic blockers (labetalol, metoprolol, propranolol) are considered compatible with breast-feeding. (C)

- Lactating women with diabetes should be treated for thyroid deficiency because low prolactin levels can occur in the thyroid-deficient state. Antithyroid drug treatment appears to be safe whether continued after delivery or started in the postpartum period. Iodine is an exception because it is concentrated in breast milk and should never be given to a lactating mother. (E)

- Depression can interfere with a mother's ability to care for herself, her diabetes, and her child and should be treated. Based on very limited studies, recommended therapy may include the following medications, although the AAP advises: "Use with caution due to possible unknown long-term effects." (E)
  - Tricyclic antidepressants: amytriptyline, nortriptyline, desipramine, clomipramine, dothiepin
  - SSRI antidepressents: fluvoxamine, paroxetine

CONTRACEPTION FOR BREAST-FEEDING DIABETIC WOMEN

Original contribution by Siri L. Kjos, MD and Martin Montoro, MD

Contraception for diabetic women is considered and chosen in the context of general reproductive health. Planning future pregnancies is highly important to reduce the risk of early fetal wastage and major congenital malformations. Breast-feeding is highly important to improve the health of the child as well as provide benefits to the diabetic mother. Today, diabetic women have a wide variety of options for controlling fertility that are more safe and effective (Skouby 86a, Kjaer 92, Skouby 93, Gibb 94, Gupta 97, Lawrenson 99, Kjos 04; European surveys cited in Napoli 05, Schwartz 06, Visser 06). While more prospective clinical trials are needed, existing studies in diabetic women and extrapolation from prospective studies in healthy women support the use of most contraceptive methods. This section first presents the principles of reproductive health and lifestyle counseling for diabetic women. We then provide an overview of contraceptive methods, followed by answers to a series of questions with reference to contraception during the first 4–6 months of exclusive breast-feeding as well as contraception in diabetic women with and without complications in the interpregnancy period. A stepwise approach will be outlined for the postpartum/breast-feeding period and the interpregnancy period to help identify which contraceptive methods are best suited to each woman based on her disease state and lifestyle. The goal will be to enable the clinician to provide individualized counseling by considering diabetic sequelae and comorbidities, contraceptive metabolic effects and risks, and individual lifestyle demands particular to each woman.

Reproductive Health and Lifestyle Counseling

Counseling should be a collaborative process involving a patient's internist or medical specialist, her obstetrician/gynecologist or perinatologist and the patient herself. To be successful, counseling must consider the patient's desires for pregnancy. Together, a plan to optimize her health, timing of pregnancy if desired, and contraceptive method should be developed. Pregnancy and contraceptive counseling should be reviewed at every medical visit during the reproductive life of a woman with diabetes. The principles of reproductive health counseling for diabetic women are set out in Table IV.12.

Lifestyle is an important element of pregnancy planning and contraceptive counseling. Providing a woman with positive lifestyle goals to achieve prior to pregnancy encourages her to actively participate and enables her to control her own and her future child's health. Her desire to achieve a healthy pregnancy can be greatly improved by changing her lifestyle to engage in daily exercise, achieve a healthy weight, and follow diabetic nutritional guidelines. Conversely, harmful lifestyle factors must be addressed

TABLE IV.12 Reproductive Counseling for Women with Diabetes (or Prediabetes)

Reproductive counseling for women with diabetes (or prediabetes) should:

- Occur at each medical visit during reproductive life
- Identify the risks associated with pregnancy related to diabetes and diabetic sequelae
  - ○ Maternal morbidity/mortality risk: e.g., complications from or acceleration of retinopathy, nephropathy, hypertension
  - ○ Obstetrical risks, e.g., congenital anomalies, miscarriage, growth disturbances, prematurity, postnatal complications
  - ○ Possible teratogenic risks from medication or uncontrolled disease
- Identify an optimal time to plan pregnancy with respect to diabetes and personal life
- Discuss how to preserve and optimize health before pregnancy:
  - ○ Establish therapeutic goals to be reached before conception, e.g., glycemic targets, blood pressure control, renal function, healthy weight
  - ○ Identify which, if any, evaluations or procedures should be completed before conception: e.g., retinal examination or surgery, cardiovascular evaluation
- Review the risks of an unwanted or unplanned pregnancy and termination
- Identify any risks of possible interactions with contraceptive selection:
  - ○ Possible complications resulting from interaction of method and diabetic disease process or other coexisting risk factors or diabetic comorbidities
  - ○ Possible beneficial interactions or changes from specific contraceptive methods
- Recognize that there may not be an entirely risk-free and highly effective contraceptive choice
- Recognize that avoiding or delaying pregnancy with an effective contraceptive may be a preferable and lesser net risk than unplanned pregnancy
- Individualize contraceptive options to select the safest choice that is acceptable to the patient and her lifestyle
- Identify lifestyle factors that she could positively alter to improve her general health and preparation for pregnancy
  - ○ Take daily vitamin supplement containing 0.4 mg/day folic acid: reduces risk of neural tube defects
  - ○ Encourage smoking cessation: increases risk of growth restriction in fetus and SIDS in newborn, worsens vascular disease risk
  - ○ Achieve healthy weight
  - ○ Engage in a daily exercise program
  - ○ Stop unnecessary drug use/abuse: alcohol, illicit, prescription
  - ○ Avoid high-risk sexual behavior

SIDS, sudden infant death syndrome.

in the discussion of pregnancy planning and contraceptive choice. Not only do they influence contraceptive choice, but they can have a relatively greater adverse impact on maternal–child health than suboptimal compliance with medical care. Cigarette smoking—an independent risk factor for MI, vascular disease, and hypertension and an absolute contraindication for combination oral contraceptive (COC) use after the age of 35—is also the greatest and most preventable cause of IUGR and has been associated with newborn SIDS. A summary of key points concerning diabetic reproductive health counseling is presented in Table IV.13.

TABLE IV.13 Specific Reproductive Health Counseling Regarding Type of Diabetes, Risk of Pregnancy to Mother and Fetus, and Possible Disease Interactions with Contraceptives

	Risk of Pregnancy and Risk to Fetus/Neonate	Risks and Health Surveillance for Possible Disease Interactions with Contraceptive Prescription
Type 1 Diabetes Mellitus **Type 2 Diabetes Mellitus** **Type 1 or 2 Diabetes with Vascular Sequelae**	Pregnancy: —Risk dependent on glycemic control and presence of micro- or macrovascular complications Health surveillance to reduce pregnancy risk: —Lifestyle: Achieve ideal body weight prior to pregnancy, exercise daily, follow individualized medical nutritional therapy Fetal/Neonate: —Risk of major anomalies: Related to glycemic control during embryogenesis; overall rate: 6–10%, increasing to 22–25% —Risk of fetal loss, stillbirth, and newborn morbidities related to glycemic control Health surveillance to reduce fetal/neonatal risk: —Achieve good glycemic control prior to conception and during pregnancy —Control hypertension, lipid abnormalities, and glucose to minimize/limit retinal and renal damage as well as cardiovascular complications —Avoid teratogenic medications: ACE inhibitors and ARBs are contraindicated during embryogenesis and pregnancy; sulfonylureas (2nd generation) and metformin acceptable	General risks to consider: —Worsening of glucose intolerance (progestin effect) —Increasing weight gain —Development or exacerbation of hyperlipidemia (hormonal contraception) —Development or exacerbation of hypertension (estrogen effect) —Development of thromboembolic disease (estrogen effect) —Development of sexually transmitted disease and potentially life-threatening infection (IUD) Health surveillance to reduce risk: —Monitor BP, weight, and glycosylated hemoglobin each visit (every 4–6 months) —Daily self-monitoring of blood glucose —Annual fasting lipid profile —Monitor hemoglobin (IUD) —Lifestyle: Counseling and interventions for medical nutritional therapy, achieve healthy body weight, and daily exercise —Lifestyle and medical therapy to control hyperglycemia, hypertension, and/or lipid abnormalities —Control hypertension, lipid abnormalities, and glucose to minimize retinal and renal damage as well as cardiovascular complications

Other Cardiovascular Disease Risk Factors
 	
Hypertension
Hyperlipidemia
 	
Obesity:BMI >30 kg/m²
 	
Older age (>35 years)
 	
Smoking
    <35 years
    ≥35 years
	Pregnancy:
	—Risk dependent on severity and medical control of condition, number of risk factors, presence of other coexisting disease or morbidity
	—Possible significant morbidity/mortality
	
	Health surveillance to reduce maternal risk:
	—Lifestyle: Achieve ideal body weight, exercise daily, individualized medical nutritional therapy
	—Counseling with individualized medical nutritional therapy
	—Smoking cessation program
	
	Fetal/Neonate:
	—Risk of intrauterine growth retardation (smoking, vascular disease), prematurity, fetal loss, placental abruption, low birth weight
	—Risk of aneuploidy (>35 years)
	—Exposure to medical therapy
		General risks to consider:
		—Risk of thromboembolism, thrombosis, stroke, myocardial infarction
		—Exacerbation of medical condition (hypertension, hyperlipidemia, fluid retention, weight gain)
		—Interaction with medications
		
		Health surveillance:
		—Monitor BP, weight, and cardiovascular status (baseline assessment and evaluation of symptoms each visit)
		—Metabolic syndrome screening
		—Lifestyle: Counseling and interventions for medical nutritional therapy, achieve healthy body weight, and daily exercise
		—Smoking cessation program

ACE, angiotensin-converting enzyme; ARB, angiotensin-receptor blocker; BP, blood pressure; IUD, intrauterine device.

Overview of Contraceptive Methods with Reference to Diabetes

Barrier Methods

Barrier methods, such as male and female condoms, diaphragms, and spermicides, produce no metabolic side effects and have no contraindications to their use. Their typical failure rate is relatively high because successful contraception is dependent on proper application with each coitus and may expose a diabetic woman to an unacceptable pregnancy risk. Condoms have been demonstrated to decrease the risk of HIV and sexually transmitted disease (STD) transmission. All women in nonmonogamous relationships should be encouraged to use condoms irrespective of contraceptive benefits to reduce this risk.

Hormonal Contraceptives

Hormonal contraceptives contain either a progestin compound alone or in conjunction with estrogen. They can be administered orally, intramuscularly, transdermally, or transvaginally. Table IV.14 provides an overview of metabolic effects on glucose tolerance, serum lipids, BP, and coagulation factors (Spellacy 71, Scrivasteva 75, Steel 78a, Knopp 82, Meade 82, Wilson 84, Deslypere 85, Perlman 85, Godsland 90, Speroff 93, Godsland 96, Lopez 07, Xiang 07).

In addition to "the pill," several newer methods and routes of delivery for hormonal contraceptives have become available. Hormonal contraception containing estrogen and progestin can be administered via injection, transdermally, or intravaginally. These newer methods lack long-term epidemiological safety data, and limited studies have detailed their metabolic effects. Thus, they will be considered similar to COCs in their risks and benefits (Steel 78b, Rosenberg 97, Pettitti 03). Limited data from short-term studies in healthy women show a neutral effect on BP, coagulation factors, and lipid metabolism with combination injectable contraception (CIC) (Haiba 89, Kesseru 91). Minimal information is available regarding metabolic effects of the transdermal patch or vaginal ring (Smallwood 01). Data are also lacking regarding the newer progestin-only implant containing etonogestrel; therefore, it will be considered together with the well-studied levonorgestrel (LVN) implant and injectable depomedroxy-progesterone

TABLE IV.14 Metabolic Effects of Hormonal Contraceptive Components

	Oral Estrogen	Oral Progestin	Progestin Intramuscular Injections and Implants	Intrauterine Device
Glucose tolerance	Neutral	↑ Insulin resistance ↑ Glucose tolerance	↑ Insulin resistance ↑ Glucose tolerance	Neutral
Serum lipids	↑ HDL-Cholesterol ↓ LDL-Cholesterol ↑ Triglyceride	↓ HDL-Cholesterol ↑ LDL-Cholesterol	↓ Triglyceride Minimal effect on HDL-Cholesterol and cholesterol	Neutral
Blood pressure	Slight ↑	Neutral	Neutral	Neutral
Coagulation factors	↑ Globulins: dose-dependent ↑	Neutral	Neutral	Neutral

↑ *Increase.*
↓ *Decrease. HDL, high-density lipoprotein; LDL, low-density lipoprotein.*

acetate (DMPA) (Fajumi 83, Shaaban 84a,b, Liew 85, Fahreus 86, Fahmy 91, Konje 92, Singh 92, Diab 00, Kim 01, Rogovskaya 05). Finally, studies examining contraception in diabetic women are limited and mostly retrospective (Shawe 03, ACOG 06b), necessitating the extrapolation of information from clinical trials, epidemiological data in healthy women, and the WHO classification of categories of risk (WHO 04).

Intrauterine Devices

Intrauterine devices (IUDs) have been investigated in diabetic women for three decades and have generally been found to be safe and effective as long as clinical guidelines are followed. Use of IUDs is discussed below in the following section.

Breast-Feeding and Postpartum Contraception: Stepwise Questions

Question 1. Is contraception necessary for a diabetic woman during the postpartum period while she is breast-feeding?

During pregnancy, elevated levels of progesterone and estrogen produced by the placenta block the effect of prolactin on the breast. After delivery, estrogen and progesterone levels drop drastically, removing the inhibitory effect of prolactin and permitting breast milk production. Breast engorgement and full milk secretion begins 3–4 days after delivery. Newborn suckling further stimulates the release of prolactin, sustaining milk production and interrupting the cyclic release of pulsatile gonadotropin-releasing hormone (GnRH) from the hypothalamus. This in turn interrupts the pulsatile release of leutinizing hormone (LH), blocking follicle-stimulating hormone (FSH)–mediated stimulation of the ovary and ovulation. The earliest return of ovulation after delivery in nonbreast-feeding women has been documented to be 25 days (Campbell 93). Thus, fertility can return by 4 weeks after delivery, thereby necessitating the need for contraception.

In women who are exclusively breast-feeding, ovulation is reliably delayed for up to 6 months, providing 98% efficacy in pregnancy protection (Kennedy 89, Perez 92, Labbok 94, WHO 00b). Because breast-feeding delays ovulation, all contraceptive methods used during this period have a low failure rate when used correctly; it is assumed that this applies to diabetic women as well. Exclusive breast-feeding when used as birth control is called the lactation amenorrhea method (LAM). To be used effectively, women should start exclusive breast-feeding immediately postpartum, breast-feed at least every 4 h during daytime and 6 h during nighttime, and avoid milk supplementation. If menses return or if women are >6 months postpartum or are supplementing feeding, another contraceptive method should be used. The cumulative pregnancy rate at 6 months with LAM is up to 1.2% (95% CI, 0–2.4%) (Truit 03).

During the newborn period, contraceptive needs are often reduced because intercourse is less frequent with the demands of motherhood. Furthermore, women may be reluctant to take any medication while breast-feeding. Encouraging the use of LAM plus condoms during this period will effectively provide pregnancy protection and encourage exclusive breast-feeding, which has tremendous benefits for the newborn.

Question 2. Can hormonal contraception be used during breast-feeding?

For women who desire hormonal contraception, they can be reassured that the level of hormone transferred to breast milk, <1% of the maternal dose, is comparable with hormone levels observed during ovulatory cycles. A recent review of limited, older studies comparing the effect of COCs and progestin-only oral contraceptives (POCs) on breast milk found that POC use during the first 6 weeks postpartum had no effect on breast milk volume (Truit 03). The evidence was inconclusive for COC use, with two studies showing a decrease in volume and two other studies showing no difference. No effect has been found on infant growth and weight with either POC or COC use or with progestin implants.

Lacking good evidence-based studies, recommendations for when to initiate hormonal contraception in breast-feeding women come from expert committees (WHO 02, ACOG 04, FFP 04, ACOG 06). In breast-feeding women, POCs can be started on day 21 postpartum without additional protection, with the notation that the use of POC before 6 weeks is outside of the product license (FFP 04). The ACOG states that COCs should not be started before 6 weeks postpartum after lactation is well established and the infant's nutritional status is well monitored. The WHO supports COC use after 6 months and states that it can be used between 6 weeks and 6 months only if acceptable alternatives are not available. Again, the use of COCs while breast-feeding is outside product licenses. The prescription of estrogen-containing methods should also be delayed for six weeks to avoid further increasing the elevated risk of postpartum thromboembolic events.

Progestin-only injectable methods, such as DMPA, are also not recommended until 6 weeks postdelivery (ACOG 04), but may be given as early as 21 days postpartum if the risk of immediate pregnancy is high (FFP 04). Emergency contraception, given within 72 h of unprotected coitus, is not indicated before 21 days postpartum, after which time the standard use guidelines can be followed that summarize contraceptive choices and their timing of use during breast-feeding (Table IV.15).

Question 3: When should other forms of contraception be started after delivery?

The copper-medicated IUD and other nonmedicated IUDs can be inserted directly after delivery within 48 h, or their insertion should be delayed until 4 weeks after delivery. The levonorgestrel intrauterine system (LVN-IUS) may be inserted

TABLE IV.15 When to Initiate Postpartum Contraception

When to Initiate	Contraceptive Method for Breast-Feeding Women
Immediately postpartum	Lactation amenorrhea method (exclusive breast-feeding) Postpartum bilateral tubal ligation Copper intrauterine device (<48 h) Condoms and spermicide
<4 weeks postpartum	Progestin-only oral contraceptives (day 21) Progestin-only implant (day 28) Emergency contraception (day 21)
After 4 weeks postpartum	Intrauterine device (copper-medicated and nonmedicated) Levonorgestrel intrauterine system
After 6 weeks postpartum	Progestin-only injectables (DMPA) Combination oral contraceptives (after established breast-feeding) Diaphragm and cervical caps (after uterine involution) Interval sterilization

DMPA, depomedroxy-progesterone acetate.

4 weeks after delivery. Diaphragms and cervical caps should not be fitted or used until 6 weeks postpartum to allow for uterine involution and proper fitting. IUDs are also effective when inserted as emergency contraception after unprotected intercourse (FFP 04).

Question 4: What are special concerns about prescribing contraceptives to breast-feeding women with diabetes?

All postpartum women should be given information about hormonal and nonhormonal methods. Counseling for postpartum contraceptive options must consider a woman's attitudes, beliefs, and preferences as well as her diabetes. No method will be effective unless she is satisfied and compliant with the method. Her need for contraception should consider the expected frequency of intercourse, her recovery from delivery, and breast-feeding patterns. Women are often reluctant to use medication when breast-feeding for fear of affecting their baby. Encouraging breast-feeding in diabetic women should be a priority for physicians. Studies in diabetic women found that only one-half had received information about breast-feeding during pregnancy (Stage 06). Thus, promoting LAM with condom use offers excellent pregnancy protection, promotes exclusive breast-feeding, and removes the woman's worry of ingesting additional medication.

When hormonal or IUD methods are desired by diabetic women, they should be initiated according to the standard guidelines described in Tables IV.13 and IV.15. To determine which hormonal method or IUD is best suited for women with diabetes, the guideline questions for nonbreast-feeding women can be used (Table IV.16). Contraindications to methods arise when vascular sequelae, hypertension, smoking, or serious comorbidities are present in women with type 1 and type 2 diabetes (see Question 6). Injectable DMPA use in women with prior GDM was associated with an increased risk of developing diabetes compared with COC use (annual incidence rate 19% vs. 12%, hazard ratio 1.58, 95% CI 1.00–2.50) over 6–108 months (median: 12 months). DMPA interacted with baseline serum TG levels and, separately, with breast-feeding to increase diabetes risk (Xiang 06).

Contraception After the 6-Month Puerperium with or without Continued Breast-Feeding: Stepwise Questions

Question 5: Is the diabetic woman a candidate for hormonal contraception?

Reproductive-age women produce estrogen and progesterone, and it is therefore not surprising that most women with diabetes can safely use hormonal contraception. Few exceptions exist, and they are generally unrelated to diabetes. These include liver disease (active hepatitis, cirrhosis, cholestasis associated with prior hormonal contraception use), malignant or benign liver tumors (focal nodular hyperplasia, adenomas), or estrogen- or progesterone-sensitive malignancies, such as breast cancer.

Question 6: Is the woman a candidate for estrogen-containing contraception?

Estrogen is added to hormonal contraception to decrease intermenstrual bleeding. It produces a dose-dependent increase in globulin production, increasing coagulation factors and angiotensin II levels that increase thromboembolic risk and mean arterial BP, respectively. Estrogens produce desirable effects on HDL-C and LDL-C levels and no effect on insulin resistance (Table IV.14) (ACOG 06). However, they also can increase serum TG levels, which often are elevated in women with type 2 diabetes. When elevations in serum TGs occur, switching to a lower estrogen dose (20 mcg) of

TABLE IV.16 Specific Considerations for Various Types of Contraceptives

	Combination Estrogen/ Progestin Contraceptives (Oral, Injectable, Transdermal, Transvaginal)	Progestin-Only Oral Contraceptives	Injectable or Implanted Progestin Contraception	Copper IUD and Levonorgestrel- IUS
Type 1 Diabetes Mellitus	**Acceptable with risk:** Choose the lowest dose of estrogen ($\downarrow$ thrombotic risk and minimize BP effect) and lowest dose and potency of progestin ($\downarrow$ effect on insulin resistance and lipid metabolism)	**Acceptable with risk:** Short-term use of POP in type 1 diabetes found no deterioration in diabetes control or indicators	**Acceptable with risk:** No data available	**No restriction:** Cu-IUD: metabolically neutral; no evidence of $\uparrow$ risk of PID **Acceptable:** LVN-IUS, no data
Type 2 Diabetes Mellitus	**Acceptable with risk:** No data available. —Choose the lowest dose of estrogen ($\downarrow$ thrombotic risk and minimize BP effect) and lowest dose and potency of progestin ($\downarrow$ effect on insulin resistance and lipid metabolism)	**Acceptable with risk:** No data available	**Acceptable with risk:** Avoid: DMPA	**No restriction:** Cu-IUD: metabolically neutral **Acceptable:** LVN-IUS, no data
Type 1 or 2 Diabetes with Vascular Sequelae	**Avoid:** No evidence that low-dose COCs accelerate retinopathy **Contraindicated:** With macrovascular disease	**Acceptable with risk:** No data available	**Acceptable with risk:** No data available	**No restriction:** Cu-IUD: metabolically neutral
CVD Risk Factors **Hyperlipidemia** **Obesity: BMI >30 kg/m²** **Older Age (>35 years)** **Smoking** **<35 years** **≥35 years**	**Avoid:** Multiple risk factors significantly $\uparrow$ risk for CVD —Can consider use in women with 1 risk factor with close monitoring along with implementation of lifestyle changes and/or therapy **Acceptable with risk:** <35 years **Avoid:** Light smokers ≥35 years **Contraindicated:** Heavy smokers ≥35 years	**Acceptable with risk:** —Multiple risk factors significantly $\uparrow$ risk for CVD —Monitor lipids, BP, diabetes screening No restrictions No restrictions	**Acceptable with risk:** —Multiple risk factors significantly $\uparrow$ risk for CVD. —Monitor lipids, BP **Avoid DMPA:** Possible $\uparrow$ weight gain, $\downarrow$ bone mineral density No restrictions	**No restrictions:** Cu-IUD: Metabolically neutral **Acceptable:** LVN-IUS, no data —Encourage healthy lifestyle changes —Irregular bleeding: recommend biopsy, consider LVN-IUS

BMI, body mass index; BP, blood pressure; COCs, combination oral contraceptives; Cu-IUD, copper-medicated intrauterine device; CVD, cardiovascular disease; DMPA, depomedroxy-progesterone acetate; LVN-IUS, levonorgestrel intrauterine system; PID, pelvic inflammatory disease; POP, progestin-only pills.

COCs or POCs may be helpful, in addition to dietary changes and evaluation of thyroid status. Diabetic women with uncontrolled dyslipidemia are advised to use other methods (Knopp 93, Diab 00).

Due to adverse effects on coagulation and BP, diabetic women with hypertension and/or CVD should use not estrogen-containing contraceptives. Also, diabetic women who smoke or have migraines should avoid COCs (Table IV.16) (Lidegaard 95). Several population studies demonstrate that COC use in hypertensive women compared with nonusers increased risk of MI, stroke, and PAD (WHO 95, Lewis 97, Gillum 00, Tanis 01, Khader 03, Siritho 03, VandenBosch 03, Chan 04, Martijn 08). Currently, no studies exist that examine COC use in women with type 2 diabetes who often have other cardiovascular risk factors and coexisting metabolic syndrome. In such women with several risk factors for arterial and venous thromboembolic disease, an estrogen-containing oral contraceptive is not a first-choice method because it could further increase thrombotic risk and BP. A progestin-only method would be preferable. If there is a strong reason for COC use, women should have regular monitoring of serum lipids, BP, and renal function in addition to glycemic monitoring (Table IV.13). Lifestyle changes to reduce cardiovascular risk should be implemented in all women with diabetes or PDM.

COC formulations have not generally been recommended when diabetic microvascular disease is present. However, retrospective cross-sectional studies (Klein 90) and case–control trials (Garg 94) did not find an increased risk of diabetic sequelae (retinopathy, renal disease, hypertension) or their progression with past or current use of COCs. Limited available studies present contrasting results on the effects of COCs on DN. Two case–control analyses associated COC use with microalbuminuria (Ribstein 99, Monster 01). A prospective 20-year follow-up study of 33 diabetic COC users (median duration 8 years) compared with 81 diabetic nonusers found increased development of macroalbuminuria (18% vs. 2%; p = 0.003; adjusted RR 8.9) when adjusted for other covariables (Ahmed 05). On the other hand, a preliminary 14-year follow-up study of 216 women with type 1 diabetes observed a protective effect from COC use on the development of clinical DN (Coustaco 06). Clearly, more research is needed to determine the effects of hormonal contraception on the renal manifestations of diabetes. RCTs are necessary to negate the effects of residual confounding on the analyses.

There is evidence that nondiabetic COC users exhibit elevated angiotensin II levels and angiotensin II type 1 receptor expression (Ribstein 99, Kang 01, Ahmed 04), as well as a significant increase in the vasodilating renal plasma flow response to an ACE inhibitor (Ahmed 05). The renal and systemic consequences to activation of the renin-angiotensin system (RAS) are considered to be minimal in nondiabetic women (Cherney 07). The possibility of increased vasodilatory activity counteracting the effect of RAS activaton is supported by increased skin endothelial NO synthase mRNA levels in COC users, reflected by a blunted renal hemodynamic response to l-arginine infusion (Cherney 07). Diabetic subjects without COC showed enhanced angiotensin-dependent control of the renal circulation compared with controls (Lansang 01). COC users showed an even greater enhancement that was marked by an increased renal vasodilation response to an ACE inhibitor, indicating a more activated RAS with a greater response to inhibition. The authors suggested that caution and surveillance should be applied to COC use in the context of diabetes (Ahmed 05).

Diabetic women without micro- or macrovascular disease are candidates for COCs. The lowest possible dose/potency of both estrogen and progestin should be selected. Short-term (<1 year) prospective studies in women with type 1 diabetes have evaluated lower doses of older progestins—norethindrone (NET, ≤0.75 mg mean daily dose) or triphasic LVN preparations—and newer progestins (gestodene, desogestrel). All studies demonstrated no or minimal effect on glycemic parameters, serum lipids (Radberg 81, Skouby 85a,86b), and cardiovascular risk factors (Petersen 94,95).

Because contraceptive data are scarce on women with type 2 diabetes, we must examine studies of women with prior GDM and IGT who share many risk factors with type 2 diabetes. In such women, short-term prospective studies have not demonstrated an adverse effect of low-dose/potency COCs on glucose or lipid metabolism (Skouby 85b,87, Kjos 90). A long-term controlled study in Latinas found that continued use of two COCs, one with monophasic NET (40 g) and the other with triphasic LVN (50–125 g), did not influence the development of diabetes, with virtually identical 3-year cumulative incidence rates for those using oral contraceptives (25.4%) compared with nonhormonal methods (26.5%) (Kjos 98). Thus, COCs do not appear to increase diabetes rates in women at high risk to develop type 2 diabetes. In the prospective, observational CARDIA (Coronary Artery Risk Development in Young Adults) study of 1,940 young women of mixed ethnicity in 1985–1986, use of COCs was not associated with higher rates of incident diabetes (Kim 02), confirming older large prospective studies (Rimm 92, Chasan-Taber 97).

It is currently unclear whether the monthly injectable combination contraceptive (Lunelle; estradiol cypionate 5 mg/medroxyprogesterone 25 mg), the weekly transdermal patch (OrthoEvra, norelgestromin 6 mg/ethinyl estradiol 0.75 mg), or the 3-week intravaginal ring (NuvaRing, etonogestrel 125 g/ethinyl estradiol 15 g) offer any metabolic advantages over COCs. The benefit of these methods is their longer duration of protection due to less frequent application. No studies have evaluated these methods in diabetic women. Thus, the route of combination contraceptives should be based on patient preference and expected reliability in administration of method (daily, weekly, monthly). Clinical and metabolic monitoring guidelines are presented in Tables IV.13 and IV.16.

Question 7: What is the best dose and formulation of oral progestin if the woman is a candidate for COCs?

COCs contain a wide variety of progestin formulations and doses. Most progestins are testosterone derivatives and have varying degrees of androgenic effects such as decreasing sex-binding globulin, increasing insulin resistance, and adverse changes in serum lipids (Godsland 90). Newer formulations of oral progestins (desogestrel, gestodene) or older, lower-dose/potency NET preparations minimize androgenic side effects and therefore generally should be selected. Estrogen-dominant COC formulations with newer progestins may improve metabolic states in women in whom increased insulin resistance, unfavorable lipid profiles, and hirsutism should be minimized, such as those with prior GDM and polycystic ovarian syndrome.

Question 8: Which women should use progestin-only contraception?

Women desiring hormonal contraception but who are unable to use estrogen are candidates for progestin-only methods. Because progestin-only formulations do not increase BP (Wilson 84, Chasan-Taber 96, Hussain 04) or coagulation factors (Meade 82, Shaaban 84b, Haiba 89), these methods offer an important option for diabetic women with vascular disease, hypertension, and cardiovascular/thromboembolic risk factors.

Two formulations of POCs are taken continuously with no pill-free intervals, with one containing NET (0.35 mg/day) and the other LVN (0.75 mg/day). Longer-acting options include an injection every 3 months (DMPA) or every month (NET or EN), an implant (etonogestrel) every 3 years, or an intrauterine system containing LVN (LVN-IUS) every 5 years. The LVN implant (Norplant) that is currently off the U.S. market has an excellent safety record.

Few studies compare the metabolic effects of the various routes of administration in either healthy or diabetic women. DMPA appears to have a less desirable effect on serum lipids and insulin resistance (Fajumi 83, Liew 85, Fahmy 91) compared with Norplant (Konje 92, Singh 92, Diab 00). DMPA has also been associated with weight gain and bone demineralization. A recent observational study compared DMPA with COC use in women with prior GDM for up to 9 years after delivery and found higher annual diabetes incidence rates in DMPA users (19% vs. 12%). However, women with an initial higher risk were selected for DMPA administration. After adjusting for baseline imbalances of BMI, breast-feeding, family history of diabetes, HDL-C and TG levels, and weight gain, differences in development of diabetes were no longer significant, thus pointing out the importance of RCTs to minimize bias (Xiang 06). In contrast, oral progestins have been widely studied in healthy and diabetic women (Radberg 81), have a documented safety profile, and can be rapidly discontinued if side effects occur. However, in select patients in whom daily compliance is problematic, such as a sexually active teenager with type 1 diabetes, a highly efficacious long-acting method may be preferable. When prescribing these methods in either diabetic or prediabetic women, periodic glucose and lipid monitoring similar to those recommended for oral contraceptives are recommended (Tables IV.13 and IV.16).

Question 9: Is the diabetic woman a candidate for an intrauterine device?

In general, guidelines for the use of IUDs in women with diabetes follow the same guidelines as in healthy parous women, such as those at low risk for sexually transmitted infections and without recent pelvic inflammatory disease (PID). Because IUDs have little or no systemic effects and are metabolically neutral, they offer an ideal method for diabetic women with vascular disease such as hypertension, retinopathy, or hyperlipidemia. Thus, many women with well-controlled diabetes are excellent candidates for IUDs.

General gynecological principles should be followed for proper patient selection, insertion, and monitoring in diabetic women. None of the studies involving diabetic women used prophylactic antibiotics with insertion or removal, and it seems unlikely that prophylaxis would add any benefit.

Question 10: What are the advantages/disadvantages of the copper-containing intrauterine device versus the levonorgestrel-containing intrauterine system?

The copper-medicated IUD (Cu-IUD) is metabolically neutral and highly efficacious. It has minimal problems when patients are properly selected to be at low risk for STDs and an aseptic insertion technique is followed. In a large meta-analysis of several prospective WHO trials, the overall incidence of PID associated with Cu-IUD use was 1.6 per 1,000 women-years of IUD use (Farley 92). The one drawback of the Cu-IUD is increased menstrual blood loss that can be counteracted by daily iron supplementation or multivitamin. In spite of a difficult early experience (Steel 78b, Gosden 82), no prospective studies examining Cu-IUDs or nonmedicated devices in diabetic women, whether type 1 or type 2 diabetes, have found any evidence for an increased rate of pelvic infection or decreased efficacy with IUD use (Wiese 77, Lawless 82, Skouby 84, Kimmerle 93, Kjos 94). However, caution must be exercised: due to the low incidence of PID, it is unlikely that a substantial study in diabetic women will be conducted to demonstrate the absence of an increased risk of pelvic infection (Farley 92). The great advantage of the Cu-IUD is its 10-year duration, high efficacy, and metabolic neutrality that allows its use in nearly all diabetic women (Table IV.16).

The second intrauterine system containing levonorgestrel (LVN-IUS) releases LVN into the uterine cavity and reaches a plasma level equal to 5% of what would be reached with a 105-mcg dose of oral LVN. Its systemic metabolic effects are minimal, but it exerts a local progestin effect on the endometrium, thereby decreasing menstrual blood loss (Stewart 01). This action makes LVN-IUS desirable in conditions in which anemia occurs, such as diabetic renal disease. Due to a lack of studies examining the LVN-IUS in women with medical disease, its use is considered by the WHO to be "acceptable with risk" or "avoid" in women with increased medical risk, such as diabetes (WHO 04). In a recent RCT in women with type 1 diabetes, use of an LVN-releasing device compared favorably with the copper T 380A IUD and had no adverse effct on glucose metabolism (Rogovskaya 05).

Recommendations

- Contraception and pregnancy planning for diabetic women should be reviewed at every nonprenatal medical visit during the reproductive age. Specific, detailed counseling on contraception, breast-feeding, and future pregnancy planning should occur in the third trimester of pregnancy and again in the early postpartum period. (E)
- Breast-feeding should be strongly encouraged in women with diabetes. (A, E)
- The LAM and barrier methods are acceptable and effective in diabetic women. (E)
- Low-dose COCs and POCs can be prescribed in most diabetic women with close monitoring. (E)
- The lowest dose and potency of progestin should be selected to minimize adverse effects on carbohydrate and lipid metabolism. (B)
- Non-orally administered hormonal contraceptive methods are considered second-line contraceptive choices due to the absence of data and experience. (E)
- The IUD is an excellent contraceptive method for properly selected diabetic women at low risk for STDs. (E)
- Due to adverse effects on coagulation and BP, diabetic women with microvascular sequelae, hypertension, and/or CVD should not use estrogen-containing contraceptives. Additional prospective, controlled studies are needed so as to strengthen this conservative recommendation. (B)
- Diabetic women who smoke or have migraines should avoid COCs. (B)

STRATEGIES TO IMPROVE DIABETES CARE
FOR FUTURE PREGNANCIES

In spite of the usual motivation of patients and their families to deliver healthy babies and the demonstration by centers of excellence that near-normal perinatal outcome can be achieved by intensified treatment before and throughout pregnancy, implementation of the standards of care for diabetes is suboptimal in the health care system (Resnick 06). Surveys of large populations of pregnant diabetic women (both type 1 and type 2 diabetes) continue to show increased perinatal mortality and morbidity with effects on long-term development and health of the offspring (see the "Introduction" to

Part I). Loss of contact with the diabetes care team after pregnancy and/or discontinuation of frequent self-monitoring of blood glucose can lead to worsening of long-term glycemic control (Feig 06).

The lack of continuity of care impedes the opportunity to apply effective preconception care of diabetes (Klinke 03, DPG 05, Sacks 06, Villamore 06, Kjos 07, Leguizamon 07, Reece 07, Varughese 07, Modder 08). As noted throughout this book, the level of control of blood glucose, BP, albuminuria, weight, smoking, and thyroid function (and perhaps lipids) at the onset of pregnancy strongly influences perinatal outcome and child development. Increased access of underserved populations (Glazier 06) to intensified primary care and diabetes self-management and behavioral intervention programs (Peyrot 07,08) will be necessary to achieve these goals. Increasingly the awareness of the implications of unplanned pregnancy in young women with diabetes and their use of contraception as needed is also of vital importance (Charron-Prochownik 06).

The challenge is to implement interventions with strategies to improve patient, provider, payor, and system adherence to guidelines of care and find mechanisms to translate research into practice (Shojanian 06, Pogach 07). Abundant RCT data on the reduction of diabetes and CVD complications are cited in the "Introduction" to Part II. Multifaceted approaches to diabetes care intervention and patient skills management training in the community as well as in the referral center offer hope for improved results (Anderson 95, Olivarius 01, Siminario 04, Nielsen 06, Piatt 06). Systems allowing physician-supported clinicians to provide feedback and decisions regarding medication dosing and changes in food plan and exercise achieve the best results (Farmer 05, Ziemer 06). Actively engaging patients in treatment decision-making and monitoring can improve control (Heisler 03, Naik 08).

Study the methods of eliciting patient information and negotiating for management options in a cross-cultural context (Carrillo 99). Consider the LEARN approach when caring for patients with diverse cultural backgrounds: Listen to the woman's perspective, express Empathy, Acknowledge the wisdom of family and folk traditions, Recommend a treatment plan, and Negotiate a treatment plan with which all can agree. Educate translators about program goals and the methods to achieve them. For further discussion, refer to Section 12 on Cultural Competency, Sweet Success Guidelines for Care – 2002, California Diabetes and Pregnancy Program, California Department of Health, from which this approach is taken with permission.

The suggested strategies listed here supplement those discussed in the Standards of Medical Care in Diabetes (Funnell 08). Similar multifactorial interventions, including sustained patient education, improve BP control (Roumie 06). The routes to success are to help our patients control glucose, BP, lipids, albuminuria, and smoking so as to attain a long and healthy life, as well as to anticipate uncomplicated pregnancies and undamaged children—a sweet result indeed.

Recommendations

- Recruit and refer patients for preconception care of diabetes because this model of care has been demonstrated to prevent major congenital malformations and improve other perinatal outcomes in a cost-effective manner. (E)
- Develop and fund research on novel interventions based on laboratory studies of the biochemical mechanisms of diabetic embryopathy and later fetal maldevelopment. (E)

- Continually educate clinicians in the community on program goals and means to achieve them, and provide updates based on local outcome data analysis to encourage the participation ("buy-in") of referring doctors. Their encouragemant toward their patients is essential for success. (A) Diabetes and Pregnancy Team members must market their services to these clinicians and develop effective means of communicating with their offices.

- Emphasize cultural competency in the staff, focus on the individual patient and significant others at the center of the management team, and explore both social and cultural factors. (E)

- Work to solve patient transportation problems, and disperse team services into both rural and urban communities. Develop telephone and online methods of communication with patients and their families. Recruit living partners to understand, assist, and encourage the diabetes self-management plan.

- Develop networks to market team services in contracting with third-party payors, providing them with local outcome data and negotiating ways to reduce health care costs. Work with patients and their insurance plans to secure coverage for the crucial components of diabetes self-management.

AFTERWORD: LOOKING INTO THE FUTURE WITH MUCH ANTICIPATION!

E. Albert Reece MD, PhD, MBA

We have made great strides over the past decades in the treatment and care of diabetes. We understand better than ever before the effects of glucose and insulin on the body, and we have a variety of options at our fingertips to help us achieve optimal control. Although we have not yet perfected a cure for diabetes, what used to be a death knell for many patients is becoming, in many cases, a very manageable chronic illness.

Today, a patient diagnosed with type 1 diabetes can be treated by using a variety of insulin formulations, and patients with type 2 diabetes have access to a rapidly expanding armamentarium of oral drugs, each with the ability to further fine-tune glycemic control. New medications are continually being developed and improved. Perhaps more significantly, our understanding of the biological and genetic mechanisms underlying the development of diabetes is improving rapidly as scientists and clinicians continue to extend the boundaries of our knowledge on several fronts. New developments are on the horizon, ranging from inhaled insulin to islet transplantation and from automated glucose monitoring to gene and stem cell therapy.

However, even as we continue these remarkable advances in treatment, the threat of diabetes looms even larger as the number of patients who live with the disease continues to soar. Specifically, we are witnessing a frightening increase in the prevalence of type 2 diabetes, which is occurring, on average, at least 20 years earlier in a person's lifespan; an increasing number of teens and young children are being diagnosed (Alberti 04, Permutt 05). In fact, in the U.S., up to 45% of those who are newly diagnosed with diabetes in the pediatric age group have type 2 diabetes, which may currently be more common in children and adolescents than type 1 diabetes (Alberti 04).

Direct medical expenditures and lost productivity due to diabetes were estimated to cost the U.S. $132 billion in 2002 (Hogan 03). It is clear that, as more people are faced with the detrimental effects of this disease for a greater portion of their lifespan, we will see a resultant increase in morbidity and mortality unless we rapidly find more effective means to treat, prevent, and hopefully cure what can be termed our society's newest epidemic.

Clinical and basic research is already forging ahead on several fronts in this urgent quest to eradicate diabetes. Translation of these many and varied research projects from bench to bedside will be rapid, as each new discovery and application leads to a greater understanding of the causes and development of diabetes.

Critical to our understanding, and thus to our treatment, of diabetes is its relationship to obesity. While epidemiological studies show a clear relationship between diabetes and obesity (Zimmer 99, Hu 01), the molecular and physiological relationships between them are not fully understood. However, much progress has already been made to improve our understanding of the regulation of energy homeostasis. This progress has led to the identification of molecules such as the enteric hormone ghrelin that has been shown to increase food intake, downregulate energy expenditure, and conserve body fat (Helmling 06). In addition, studies of plasma adiponectin, a fat-derived protein that influences the body's utilization of sugars and production of lipids, may eventually help us to explain the clustering of disorders known as "metabolic syndrome" (Martin 05c). Clearly, the obesity–diabetes relationship is an area of intense investigation (Speakman 04) that promises to deliver a means to ameliorate obesity (Ozcan 04) and thus greatly reduce the incidence of diabetes.

Within our reach are several developments that will improve and simplify existing treatments. Recent dramatic advances in diabetes medications continue, allowing us to achieve even more accurate glycemic control for our patients. New insulin analogs are constantly evolving that absorb faster and last longer, and they may soon become indistinguishable from natural pancreatic insulin secretion (Langer 02, Lapolla 05). In addition, insulin administration will see widespread change over the next several years as oral, inhaled, and even transdermal insulins (Zahn 05) replace the less convenient injected insulin that currently predominates. With these new types of insulin, patients will likely see improved glycemic profiles with reduced fasting and postprandial glucose levels, as well as decreased complications and fewer hypoglycemic episodes.

In addition to insulin, several other new drugs for the management of diabetes are under development, including the very promising incretin mimetic agents (Lebovitz 06). Many other agents that act on fundamental abnormalities, such as energy imbalance, inflammation, and vascular biological conditions, are in the early stages of development and are likely to become available during the next 5–10 years (Lebovitz 06).

Continuous glucose monitoring systems that are currently in the experimental stages will soon eliminate the need for patients to perform a finger stick to check glucose levels. These monitoring systems are being designed to measure interstitial glucose levels via a skin patch and transmit the measurements to a wireless handheld display device. On the heels of this technology will most certainly follow a two-in-one automated system that will monitor and evaluate glucose levels and then deliver medication as needed.

One day in the not too distant future, even this sort of automated medicine administration may become obsolete. Research is currently being conducted on a remarkable system that delivers insulin via an intestinal patch (Mitragotri 03). Administered orally in a capsule that would remain intact through the stomach and then dissolve in the intestines, the patch would adhere to the intestinal wall and slowly release insulin into the intestinal membrane.

But why wait until a person develops diabetes before treating it? Gene therapy is ripe with potential, and we may soon see the day when we have the means to genetically alter the progression of diabetes before symptoms actually develop. Even now, animal studies are being conducted that explore the feasibility of inserting genes into the pancreas that prevent fat storage because excess pancreatic fat destroys insulin-producing cells (Kruse 05). In addition, ongoing studies of embryonic stem cells may soon yield a greater understanding of how pancreatic precursor cells and islet hormone-producing cells develop from the endoderm and thus determine how the mammalian pancreas forms (Odorico 05). Finally, new studies suggest that immune defects may play a role in the pathogenesis of diabetic embryopathy and that, by stimulating the maternal immune system, we may be able to counteract these effects even before they develop (Reece 05).

The ultimate manifestation of such genetic manipulation would be, of course, to prevent diabetes in utero or even prior to conception. Although genetic manipulation cannot yet offer such salvation, it may in truth already exist—in the form of nutritional supplements. Today, preventive measures are of the utmost importance in early prevention, and we already know that excellent preconception and first-trimester glucose control can greatly reduce, if not eliminate, the risk of diabetes-related birth defects from developing in the child (Fuhrmann 83). In addition, studies in animals have demonstrated that in the diabetic state, an excess of free oxygen radicals induces fetal maldevelopment and that vitamin E, a known antioxidant, can reduce the incidence of neural tube malformations in the offspring of diabetic rats (Reece 05).

Dietary supplements or vitamin therapy offer a potential adjunctive and/or alternative approach to preconception care for women with diabetes who wish to conceive. Multiple experimental studies in animal models have successfully blocked diabetes-induced dysmorphogenesis by using such agents (Pinter 86, Reece 89,94, Huyhn 95, Reece 96, Eriksson 00, Baron 03, Carney 04). Supplementing the diet with myoinositol, arachidonic acid, prostaglandins, and antioxidant compounds has diminished the growth retardation, high embryonic absorption rates, and neural tube defects elicited by hyperglycemia in animal models. Further study is most certainly warranted to determine whether similar reductions in malformations in the offspring of women with diabetes may be achieved through dietary supplementation and/or antioxidant therapy.

These remarkable possibilities do not by any means encompass all of the work being done by the many scientists and clinicians who are dedicated to breaking the stranglehold of this tenacious disease. As we gain a more complete understanding of the pathogenesis of diabetes as well as its metabolic and biochemical markers, science will lead us with increasing certainty down the path to a cure. Indeed, it can even be anticipated that, as a result of this demonstrated dedication and ingenuity of our researchers and physicians, the diabetes epidemic will be completely eradicated within the next generation.

Part 4 Reference

AAFP—American Academy of Family Physicians: AAFP policy statement on breastfeeding 2002. Available at: http://www.aafp.org/x6633.xml. Accessed March 12, 2008.

AAP—American Academy of Pediatrics, Committee on Drugs: The transfer of drugs and other chemicals into human milk. *Pediatrics* 108:776–789, 2001.

AAP—American Academy of Pediatrics, Committee on Nutrition: Prevention of pediatric overweight and obesity. Policy statement. *Pediatrics* 112:424–430, 2003.

AAP—American Academy of Pediatrics, Section on Breastfeeding: Breastfeeding and the use of human milk. Policy statement. *Pediatrics* 115:496–506, 2005.

Abalovich M, Amino N, Barbour LA, Cobin RH, De Groot L, Glinoer D, Mandel SJ, Stagnaro-Green: Management of thyroid dysfunction during pregnancy and postpartum: an Endocrine Society clinical practice guideline. *J Clin Endocrinol Metab* 92 (Suppl):S1–S47, 2007.

ABM—Academy of Breastfeeding Medicine: Guidelines for glucose monitoring and treatment of hypoglycemia in term breastfed neonates. Clinical protocol #1. *ABM News Views* 5:12–13, 1999.

ABM—Academy of Breastfeeding Medicine: Peripartum breastfeeding management for the healthy mother and infant at term. Clinical Protocol #5. *ABM News Views* 9:6–7, 2003.

Acerini CL, Ahmed ML, Ross KM, Sullivan PB, Bird G, Dunger DB: Celiac disease in children and adolescents with IDDM: clinical characteristics and response to gluten free diet. *Diabet Med* 15:38–44, 1998.

ACOG—American College of Obstetricians and Gynecologists: Breastfeeding: maternal and infant aspects. Educational bulletin #258. *Obstet Gynecol* 96:rear pages 1–16, 2000.

ACOG—American College of Obstetricians and Gynecologists: Prophylactic antibiotics in labor and delivery. Practice bulletin #47. Clinical management guidelines for obstetrician-gynecologists. *Obstet Gynecol* 102:875–882, 2003.

ACOG—American College of Obstetricians and Gynecologists, Committee on Obstetric Practice: Treatment with selective serotonin reuptake inhibitors during pregnancy. Committee Opinion #354. *Obstet Gynecol* 108:1601–1603, 2006a.

ACOG—American College of Obstetricians and Gynecologists: Use of hormonal contraception in women with coexisting medical conditions. ACOG practice bulletin #73. *Obstet Gynecol* 107:1453–1472, 2006b.

ACOG—American College of Obstetricians and Gynecologists, Committee on Health Care for Underserved Women, Committee on Obstetric Practice: Breastfeeding: maternal and infant aspects. Committee Opinion # 361. *Obstet Gynecol* 109:479–480, 2007.

ADA—American Diabetes Association, Workgroup on Hypoglycemia: Defining and reporting hypoglycemia in diabetes. A report from the American Diabetes Association Workgroup on Hypoglycemia. *Diabetes Care* 28:1245–1249, 2005.

ADA—American Diabetes Association: Standards of medical care in diabetes—2006. *Diabetes Care* 29 (Suppl 1):S4–S42, 2006a.

ADA—American Diabetes Association: Nutrition recommendations and interventions for diabetes—2006. A position statement of the American Diabetes Association. *Diabetes Care* 29:2140–2157, 2006b.

ADA—American Diabetes Association: Standards of medical care in diabetes—2008. Position statement. *Diabetes Care* 31 (Suppl 1):S12–S54, 2008a.

ADA—American Diabetes Association: Nutrition recommendations and interventions for diabetes. A position statement of the American Diabetes Association. *Diabetes Care* 31:S61–S78, 2008b.

Adachi T, Yasuda K, Mori C, Yoshinaga M, Aoki N, Tsujimoto G, Tsuda K: Promoting insulin secretion in pancreatic islets by means of bisphenol A and nonylphenol via estrogen receptors. *Food Chem Toxicol* 43:713–719, 2005.

Adams H, Jones M, Othman S, Lazarus JH, Parkes AB, Hall R: The sonographic appearances in postpartum thyroiditis. *Br Med J* 305:152–156, 1992.

ADietA—American Dietetic Association: Promotion of breastfeeding. Position statement. *J Am Diet Assoc* 97:662–666, 1997.

ADietA—American Dietetic Association: Breaking the barriers to breastfeeding. Position statement. *J Am Diet Assoc* 101:1213–1220, 2001.

ADietA—American Dietetic Association; Dietitians of Canada: Position of the American Dietetic Association and the Dietitians of Canada: vegetarian diets. *J Am Diet Assoc* 103:748–765, 2003; also *Can J Diet Practice Res* 64:62–81, 2003.

ADietA—American Dietetic Association: Position of the American Dietetic Association and Dietitians of Canada: dietary fatty acids. *J Am Diet Assoc* 107:1599–1611, 2007.

Agostoni C, Grandi F, Gianni ML, Silano M, Torcoletti M, Giovanni M, Riva E: Growth patterns of breast fed and formula fed infants in the first 12 months of life: an Italian study. *Arch Dis Child* 81:395–399, 1999.

Agostini C, Verduci E: Early nutrition and programming: too little, too much, or ? *Pediatr Res* 54:151, 2003.

Agras WS, Kraemer HC, Berkowitz RI, Hammer LD: Influence of early feeding style on adiposity at 6 years of age. *J Pediatr* 116:805–809, 1990.

AHA—American Heart Association Nutrition Committee, Lichtenstein AH, Appel LJ, Brands M, Carnethon M, Daniels S, Franch HA, Franklin B, Kris-Etherton P, Harris WS, Howard B, Karanja N, Lefevre M, Rudel L, Sacks F, Van Horn L, Winston M, Wylie-Rosett J: Diet and lifestyle recommendations revision 2006. A scientific statement from the American Heart Association Nutrition Committee. *Circulation* 114:82–96, 2006.

Ahmed SB, Kang AK, Burns KD, Kennedy CR, Lai V, Cattran DC, Scholey JW, Miller JA: Effects of oral contraceptive use on the renal and systemic vascular response to angiotensin II infusion. *J Am Soc Nephrol* 15:780–786, 2004.

Ahmed SB, Hovind P, Parving H-H, Rossing P, Price DA, Laffel LM, Lansang MC, Stevanovic R, Fisher NDL, Hollenberg NK: Oral contraceptives, angiotensin-dependent renal vasoconstriction, and risk of diabetic nephropathy. *Diabetes Care* 28:1988–1994, 2005.

Ahokas A, Aito M, Rimon R: Positive treatment effect of estradiol in postpartum psychosis: a pilot study. *J Clin Psychiatr* 61:166–169, 2000.

Akerblom HK, Vaarala O, Hyoty H, Ilonen J, Knip M: Environmental factors in the etiology of type 1 diabetes. *Am J Med Genet* 115:18–29, 2002.

Akerblom HK, Virtanen SM, Ilonen J, Savilahti E, Vaarala O, Reunanen A, Teramo K, Hamalainen T, Paronen J, Riikjarv MA, Ormisson A, Ludvigsson J, Dosch HM, Hakulinen T, Knip M; the Finnish TRIGR Study Group: Dietary manipulation of beta-cell autoimmunity in infants at increased risk of type 1 diabetes: a pilot study. *Diabetologia* 48:829–837, 2005.

Akobeng AK, Ramanan AV, Buchan I, Heller RF: Effect of breast feeding on risk of celiac disease: a systematic review and meta-analysis of observational studies. *Arch Dis Child* 91:39–43, 2006.

Akobeng AK, Heller RF: Assessing the population impact of low rates of breast feeding on asthma, celiac disease and obesity: the use of a new statistical method. *Arch Dis Child* 92:483–485, 2007.

Alexy U, Kersting M, Sichert-Hellert W, Manz F, Schoch G: Macronutrient intake of 3- to 36-month-old German infants and children: results of the DONALD Study. *Ann Nutr Metab* 43:14–22, 1999.

Allen JC, Keller RP, Archer P, Neville MC: Studies in human lactation: milk composition and daily secretion rates of macronutrients in the first year of life. *Am J Clin Nutr* 54:69–80, 1991.

Allen LH: Impact of vitamin B-12 deficiency during lactation on maternal and infant health. *Adv Exp Med Biol* 503:57–67, 2002.

Allen LH: Multiple micronutrients in pregnancy and lactation: an overview. *Am J Clin Nutr* 81 (Suppl):1206S–1212S, 2005.

Alm B, Wennergren G, Norvenius SG, Skjaerven R, Lagercrantz H, Helweg-Larsen K, Irgens LM: Breast-feeding and the sudden infant death syndrome in Scandinavia, 1992–1995. *Arch Dis Child* 86:400–402, 2002.

Alonso-Magdalena P, Morimoto S, Ripoll C, Fuentes E, Nadal A: The estrogenic effect of bisphenol A disrupts pancreatic beta-cell function in vivo and induces insulin resistance. *Environ Health Perspect* 114:106–112, 2006.

Altinkaynak S, Selimoglu MA, Turgut A, Kilicasian B, Ertekin V: Breast-feeding duration and childhood acute leukemia and lymphomas in a sample of Turkish children. *J Pediatr Gastroenterol Nutr* 42:568–572, 2006.

Alvarez-Marfany M, Roman SH, Drexler AJ, Robertson C, Stagnaro-Green A: Long-term prospective study of postpartum thyroid dysfunction in women with insulin dependent diabetes mellitus. *J Clin Endocrinol Metab* 79:10–16, 1994.

Amano Y, Sugiyama M, Lee JS, Kawakubo K, Mori K, Tang AC, Akabayashi A: Glycemic index-based nutritional education improves blood glucose control in Japanese adults. A randomized controlled trial. *Diabetes Care* 30:1874–1876, 2007.

Amini R, Murphy N, Edge J, Ahmed M, Accrini C, Dunger D: A longitudinal study of the effects of a gluten- free diet on glycemic control and weight gain in subjects with type 1 diabetes and celiac disease. *Diabetes Care* 25: 1117–1122, 2002.

Amino N, Mori H, Iwatami Y, Tanizawa O, Kawashima M, Tsuge I, Ibaragi K, Kumahara Y, Miyai K: High prevalence of transient postpartum thyrotoxicosis and hypothyroidism. *N Engl J Med* 306:849–852, 1982.

Andersen HJ: Excretion of verapamil in human milk. *Eur J Clin Pharmacol* 25: 279–280, 1983.

Anderson P, Bondesson U, Mattiasson I, Johansson BW: Verapamil and norverapamil in plasma and breast milk during breast feeding. *Eur J Clin Pharmacol* 31: 625–627, 1987.

Anderson RM, Funnell MM, Butler PM, Arnold MS, Fitzgerald JT, Feste C: Patient empowerment: results of a randomized controlled trial. *Diabetes Care* 18: 943–949, 1995.

Anderson JW, Johnstone BM, Remley DT: Breast-feeding and cognitive development: a meta-analysis. *Am J Clin Nutr* 70:525–535, 1999.

Anderson RJ, Freedland KE, Clouse RE, Lustman PJ: The prevalence of comorbid depression in adults with diabetes: a meta-analysis. *Diabetes Care* 24:1069–1078, 2001.

Anderson GC, Moore E, Hepworth J, Bergman N: Early skin-to-skin contact for mothers and their healthy newborn infants. *Cochrane Database Syst Rev* 2003;(2): CD003519.

Anderson GD: Using pharmacokinetics to predict the effects of pregnancy and maternal-infant transfer of drugs during lactation. *Expert Opin Drug Metab Toxicol* 2:947–960, 2006.

Angelsen NK, Vik T, Jacobsen G, Bakketeig LS: Breast feeding and cognitive development at age 1 and 5 years. *Arch Dis Child* 85:183–188, 2001.

Anselmino M, Malmberg K, Ohrvik J, Ryden; the Euro Heart Survey Investigators: Evidence-based medication and revascularization: powerful tools in the management of people with diabetes and coronary artery disease: a report from the Euro Heart Survey on diabetes and the heart. *Eur J Cardiovasc Prev Rehabil* 15:216–223, 2008.

APA—American Psychiatric Association Committee on Nomenclature and Statistics: *Diagnosis and Statistical Manual of Mental Disorders.* 4th ed. Washington, DC: American Psychiatric Association; 1994:424–429.

Arenz S, Ruckerl R, Koletzko B, von Kries R: Breast-feeding and childhood obesity: a systematic review. *Int J Obes Relat Metab Disord* 28:1247–1256, 2004.

Arenz S, von Kries R: Protective effect of breastfeeding against obesity in childhood. Can a meta-analysis of observational studies help to validate the hypothesis? *Adv Exp Biol Med* 569:40–48, 2005.

Armstrong J, Reilly JJ: Breastfeeding and lowering the risk of childhood obesity. *Lancet* 359:2003–2004, 2002.

Arnold LM, Suckow RF, Lichtenstein PK: Fluvoxamine concentrations in breast milk and in maternal and infant sera. *J Clin Psychopharmacol* 20:491–493, 2000.

Arthur PG, Smith M, Hartmann PE: Milk lactose, citrate, and glucose as markers of lactogenesis in normal and diabetic women. *J Pediatr Gastroenterol Nutr* 9:488–496, 1989.

Ascher H, Krantz I, Rydberg L, Nordin P, Kristiansson B: Influence of infant feeding and gluten intake on celiac disease. *Arch Dis Child* 76:113–117, 1997.

Atkinson HC, Begg EJ, Darlow BA: Drugs in human milk: clinical pharmacokinetic considerations. *Clin Pharmacokinet* 14:217–240, 1988a.

Atkinson HC, Begg EJ: The binding of drugs to major human milk whey proteins. *Br J Clin Pharmacol* 26:107–109, 1988b.

Atkinson HC, Begg EJ: Prediction of drug distribution into human milk from physicochemical characteristics. *Clin Pharmacokinet* 18:151–167, 1990.

Attia E, Downey J, Oberman M: Postpartum psychoses. In: Miller LJ, ed. *Postpartum Mood Disorders*. Washington, DC: American Psychiatric Press; 1999:99–117.

Auricchio S, Follo D, DeRitis G, Guinta A, Marzorati D, Prampolini L, Ansoldi N, Levi P, dell'Olio D, Bossi A: Does breastfeeding protect against the development of clinical symptoms of celiac disease in children? *J Pediatr Gastroenterol Nutr* 2:428–433, 1983.

Austin M, Lumley J: Antenatal screening for postnatal depression: a systematic review. *Acta Psychiatr Scand* 107:10–17, 2003.

Axelsson IE, Ivarsson SA, Raiha NC: Protein intake in early infancy: effects on plasma amino acid concentrations, insulin metabolism, and growth. *Pediatr Res* 26:614–617, 1989.

Aydin S, Aydin S, Ozkan Y, Kumru S: Ghrelin is present in human colostrum, transitional and mature milk. *Peptides* 27:878–882, 2006.

Ayers S: Delivery as a traumatic event: prevalence, risk factors, and treatment for postnatal posttraumatic stress disorder. *Clin Obstet Gynecol* 47:552–567, 2004.

Azizi F: Effect of methimazole treatment of maternal thyrotoxicosis on thyroid function in breastfeeding infants. *J Pediatr* 128:855–858, 1996.

Azizi F, Khoshniat M, Bahrainian M, Hedayati M: Thyroid function and intellectual development of infants nursed by mothers taking methimazole. *J Clin Endocrinol Metab* 85:3233–3238, 2000.

Azizi F: The occurrence of permanent thyroid failure in patients with subclinical postpartum thyroiditis. *Eur J Endocrinol* 153:367–371, 2005.

Baab SW, Peindl KS, Piontek CM, Wisner KL: Serum bupropion levels in 2 breastfeeding mother-infant pairs. *J Clin Psychiatry* 63:910–911, 2002.

Badui E, Enciso R: Acute myocardial infarction during pregnancy and puerperium: a review. *Angiology* 47:739–756, 1996.

Baird J, Fisher D, Lucas P, Kleijnen J, Roberts H, Law C: Being big or growing fast: systematic review of size and growth in infancy and later obesity. *BMJ* 331: 929–931, 2005.

Baker JL, Michaelsen KF, Rasmussen KM, Sorensen TIA: Maternal prepregnant body mass index, duration of breastfeeding, and timing of complementary food introduction are associated with infant weight gain. *Am J Clin Nutr* 80: 1579–1588, 2004.

Baker JL, Michaelsen KF, Sorensen TIA, Rasmussen KM: High prepregnant body mass index is associated with early termination of full and any breastfeeding in Danish women. *Am J Clin Nutr* 86:404–411, 2007.

Barclay AW, Petocz P, McMillan-Price J, Flood VM, Prvan T, Mitchell P, Brand-Miller JC: Glycemic index, glycemic load, and chronic disease risk—a meta-analysis of observational studies. *Am J Clin Nutr* 87:627–637, 2008.

Barker J: Type 1 diabetes-associated autoimmunity: natural history, genetic associations, and screening. *J Clin Endocrinol Metab* 91: 1210–1217, 2006.

Barr SI, Murphy SP, Poos MI: Interpreting and using the Dietary Reference Intakes in dietary assessment of individuals and groups. *J Am Diet Assoc* 102:780–788, 2002.

Barros FC, Victora CG, Semer TC, Tonioli Filho S, Tomasi E, Weiderpass E: Use of pacifiers is associated with decreased breastfeeding duration. *Pediatrics* 95: 497–499, 1995.

Bartnik M, Norhammar A, Ryden L: Hyperglycemia and cardiovascular disease. Symposium based on 2007 guidelines from the Task Force on Diabetes and Cardiovascular Diseases of the European Society of Cardiology and the European Association for the Study of Diabetes. *J Intern Med* 262:145–156, 2007.

Bauchner H, Leventhal JM, Shapiro ED: Studies of breast-feeding and infections: how good is the evidence? *JAMA* 256:887–892, 1986.

Bauer JH, Pape B, Zajicek J, Groshong T: Propranolol in human plasma and breast milk. *Am J Cardiol* 43:860–862, 1979.

Bech K, Hoier-Madsen M, Feldt-Rasmussen U, Jensen BM, Molsted-Pedersen L, Kuhl C: Thyroid function and autoimmune manifestations in insulin-dependent diabetes mellitus during and after pregnancy. *Acta Endocrinol (Copenh)* 124: 534–539, 1991.

Bell DSH: Diabetic cardiomyopathy. Editorial. *Diabetes Care* 26:2949–2951, 2003.

Bener A, Denic S, Galadari S: Longer breast-feeding and protection against childhood leukemia and lymphomas. *Eur J Cancer* 37:234–238, 2001.

Bener A, Ehlayel MS, Alsowaidi S, Sabbah A: Role of breast feeding in primary prevention of asthma and allergic diseases in a traditional society. *Eur Ann Allergy Clin Immunol* 39:337–343, 2007.

Benn CS, Wohlfahrt J, Aaby P, Westergaard T, Benfeldt E, Michaelsen KF, Bjorksten B, Melbye M: Breast feeding and risk of atopic dermatitis during the first 18 months of life by parental history of allergy. *Am J Epidemiol* 160: 217–223, 2004.

Bentley-Lewis R, Goldfine AB, Green DE, Seely EW: Lactation after normal pregnancy is not associated with blood glucose fluctuations. *Diabetes Care* 30:2792–2793, 2007.

Beral V, Fear NT, Alexander F, Appleby P: Breastfeeding and childhood cancer. *Br J Cancer* 85:1685–1694, 2001.

Berens PD: Applied physiology in the peripartum management of lactation. *Clin Obstet Gynecol* 47:643–655, 2004.

Bergenstal RM, Gavin JR 3rd; Global Consensus Conference on Glucose Monitoring Panel: The role of self-monitoring of blood glucose in the care of people with diabetes: report of a global consensus conference. *Am J Med* 118 (Suppl 9A): 1S–6S, 2005.

Bergmann KE, Bergmann RL, von Kries R, Bohm O, Richter R, Dudenhausen JW, Wahn U: Early determinants of childhood overweight and adiposity in a birth cohort study: role of breast-feeding. *Int J Obes Relat Metab Disord* 27:162–172, 2003.

Berle JO, Steen VM, Aamo TO, Breilid H, Zahlsen K, Spigset O: Breastfeeding during maternal antidepressant treatment with serotonin reuptake inhibitors: infant exposure, clinical symptoms, and cytochrome p450 genotypes. *J Clin Psychiatry* 65:1228–1234, 2004.

Berlin CM Jr, LaKind JS, Fenton SF, Wang RY, Bates MN, Brent RL, Condon M, Crase BL, Dourson ML, Ettinger AS, Foos B, Furst P, Giacola GP, Goldstein DA, Haynes SG, Hench KD, Kacew S, Koren G, Lawrence RA, Mason A, McDiarmid MA, Moy G, Needham LL, Paul IM, Pugh LC, Qian Z, Salamone L, Selevan SG, Sonawane B, Tarzian AJ, Tully MR, Uhl K: Conclusions and recommendations of the Expert Panel: Technical Workshop on Human Milk Surveillance and Biomonitoring for Environmental Chemicals in the United States. *J Toxicol Environ Health A* 68:1825–1831, 2005.

Bertoni AG, Tsai A, Kasper EK, Brancatti FL: Diabetes and idiopathic cardiomyopathy. A nationwide case-control study. *Diabetes Care* 26:2791–2795, 2003.

Bertran AP, de Onis M, Lauer JA, Villar J: Ecological study of effect of breast feeding on infant mortality in Latin America. *BMJ* 323:303–306, 2001.

Bitman J, Hamosh M, Hamosh P, Lutes V, Neville MC, Seacat J, Wood DL: Milk composition and volume during the onset of lactation in a diabetic mother. *Am J Clin Nutr* 50:1364–1369, 1989.

Bjornberg KA, Vahter M, Berglund B, Niklasson B, Blennow M, Sandborgh-Englund G: Transport of methylmercury and inorganic mercury to the fetus and breastfed infant. *Environ Health Perspect* 113:1381–1385, 2005.

Blom L, Persson LA, Dahlquist G: A high linear growth is associated with an increased risk of childhood diabetes. *Diabetologia* 35:528–533, 1992.

Blonde L, Karter AJ: Current evidence regarding the value of self-monitored blood glucose testing. *Am J Med* 118 (Suppl 9A):20S–26S, 2005.

Bodington ZMJ, McNally PG, Burden AC: Cow's milk and type 1 childhood diabetes: no increase in risk. *Diabet Med* 11:663–665, 1994.

Bogen DL, Hanusa BH, Whitaker RC: The effect of breast-feeding with and without formula use on the risk of obesity at 4 years of age. *Obes Res* 12:1527–1535, 2004.

Bolli GB: Glucose variability and complications. Editorial. *Diabetes Care* 29:1707–1709, 2006.

Bond GM, Holloway AM: Anesthesia and breastfeeding—the effect on mother and infant. *Anaesth Intensive Care* 20:426–430, 1992.

Bonora E, Muggio M: Postprandial blood glucose as a risk factor for cardiovascular disease in type II diabetes: the epidemiological evidence. *Diabetologia* 44:2107–2114, 2001.

Bopp M, Lovelady C, Hunter C, Kinsella T: Maternal diet and exercise: effects on long-chain polyunsaturated fatty acid concentrations in breast milk. *J Am Diet Assoc* 105:1103–1104, 2005.

Borch-Johnsen K, Mandrup-Poulsen T, Zachau-Christiansen B, Joner G, Christy M, Kastrup K, Nerup J: Relation between breast-feeding and incidence rates of insulin-dependent diabetes mellitus. A hypothesis. *Lancet* 2:1083–1086, 1984.

Boris J, Jensen B, Salvig JD, Secher NJ, Olsen SF: A randomized controlled trial of the effect of fish oil supplementation in late pregnancy and early lactation on the n-3 fatty acid content in human breast milk. *Lipids* 39:1191–1196, 2004.

Boutroy MJ, Bianchetti G, Dubroc C, Vert P, Morselli PL: To nurse when receiving acebutolol: is it dangerous for the neonate? *Eur J Clin Pharmacol* 30:737–739, 1986.

Bouwstra H, Boersma ER, Boehm G, Dijck-Brouwer DAJ, Muskiet FAJ, Hadders-Algra M: Exclusive breastfeeding of healthy term infants for at least 6 weeks improves neurological condition. *J Nutr* 133:4243–4245, 2003.

Bradley C: Managing diabetes while breast-feeding. *Diabetes Self Manag* 24:87–89, 2007.

Brandtzaeg P: Mucosal immunity: integration between mother and the breast-fed infant. *Vaccine* 21:3382–3388, 2007.

Brede C, Fjeldal P, Skjevrak I, Herikstad H: Increased migration levels of bisphenol A from polycarbonate baby bottles after dishwashing, boiling and brushing. *Food Add Contam* 20:684–689, 2003.

Brandtzaeg P: Mucosal immunity: integration between mother and the breast-fed infant. *Vaccine* 21:3382–3388, 2003.

Brewer MM, Bates MR, Vannoy LP: Postpartum changes in maternal weight and body fat depots in lactating vs nonlactating women. *Am J Clin Nutr* 49:259–265, 1989.

Briggs GG, Samson JH, Ambrose PJ, Schroeder DH: Excretion of bupropion in breast milk. *Ann Pharmacother* 27:431–433, 1993.

Briggs GG, Freeman RK, Yaffe SJ: *Drugs in Pregnancy and Lactation*. 7th ed. Philadelphia: Lippincott Williams & Wilkins; 2005a.

Briggs GG, Ambrose PJ, Nageotte MP, Padilla G, Wan S: Excretion of metformin into breast milk and the effect on nursing infants. *Obstet Gynecol* 105:1437–1441, 2005b.

Bromiker R, Rachamm A, Hammerman C, Schimmel M, Kaplan M, Medoff-Cooper B: Immature sucking patterns in infants of mothers with diabetes. *J Pediatr* 149:640–643, 2006.

Brownlee M, Hirsch IB: Glycemic variability: a hemoglobin A1C–independent risk factor for diabetic complications. Editorial. *JAMA* 295:1707–1708, 2006.

Bruining GJ: Association between infant growth before onset of juvenile type 1 diabetes and autoantibodies to IA-2. *Lancet* 356:655–656, 2000.

Buinauskiene J, Baliutaviciene D, Zalinkevicius R: Glucose tolerance of 2- to 5-yr-old offspring of diabetic mothers. *Pediatr Diabetes* 5:143–146, 2004.

Buist A, Janson H: Effect of exposure to dothiepin and northiaden in breast milk on child development. *Br J Psychiatry* 167:370–373, 1995.

Bultmann BD, Klingel K, Nabauer M, Wallwiener D, Kardolf R: High prevalence of viral genomes and inflammation in peripartum cardiomyopathy. *Am J Obstet Gynecol* 193:363–365, 2005.

Burke V, Beilin LJ, Simmer K, Oddy WH, Blake KV, Doherty D, Kendall GE, Newnham JP, Landau LI, Stanley FJ: Breastfeeding and overweight: longitudinal analysis in an Australian birth cohort. *J Pediatr* 147:56–61, 2005.

Butte NF, Garza C, Smith EO, Nichols BL: Human milk intake and growth in exclusively breast-fed infants. *J Pediatr* 104:187–195, 1984a.

Butte NF, Garza C, Stuff JE, O'Brian Smith E, Nichols BL: Effect of maternal diet and body composition on lactational performance. *Am J Clin Nutr* 39:296–306, 1984b.

Butte NF, Garza C, Burr R, Goldman AS, Kennedy K, Kitzmiller JL: Milk composition of insulin-dependent diabetic women. *J Pediatr Gastroenterol Nutr* 6:936–941, 1987.

Butte NF, Smith ED, Garza C: Energy utilization of breast-fed and formula-fed infants. *Am J Clin Nutr* 51:350–358, 1990.

Butte NF, Hopkinson JM: Body composition changes during lactation are highly variable among women. *J Nutr* 128:381S–385S, 1998.

Butte NF, Hopkinson JM, Mehta N, Moon JK, O'Brian-Smith E: Adjustments in energy expenditure and substrate utilization during late pregnancy and lactation. *Am J Clin Nutr* 69:299–307, 1999.

Butte NF, Wong WW, Hopkinson JM: Energy requirements of lactating women derived from doubly labelled water and milk energy output. *J Nutr* 131:53–58, 2001a.

Butte NF: The role of breastfeeding in obesity. *Pediatr Clin North Am* 48:189–198, 2001b.

Butte NF, King JC: Energy requirements during pregnancy and lactation. *Public Health Nutr* 8:1010–1027, 2005.

Cadwell K: Reaching the goals of "Healthy People 2000" regarding breastfeeding. *Clin Perinatol* 26:527–537, 1999.

Cai L, Kang YJ: Cell death and diabetic cardiomyopathy. *Cardiovasc Toxicol* 3: 219–228, 2003.

Calvo EB, Galindo AC, Aspres NB: Iron status in exclusively breast-fed infants. *Pediatrics* 90:375–379, 1992.

Campbell OM, Gray RH: Characteristics and determinants of postpartum ovarian function in women in the United States. *Am J Obstet Gynecol* 169:55–60, 1993.

Carlson SE: Long-chain polyunsaturated fatty acids and development of human infants. *Acta Paediatr* 430 (Suppl):72–77, 1999.

Carrillo JE, Green AR, Betancourt JR: Cross-cultural primary care: a patient-based approach. *Ann Intern Med* 130:829–834, 1999.

Carter RE, Lackland DT, Cleary PA, Yim E, Lopes-Virella MF, Gilbert GE, Orchard TJ; the DCCT/EDIC Study Research Group: Intensive treatment of diabetes is associated with a reduced rate of peripheral arterial calcification in the Diabetes Control and Complications Trial. *Diabetes Care* 30:2646–2648, 2007.

Casabiell X, Piniero V, Tome MA, Peino R, Dieguez C, Casanueva FF: Presence of leptin in colostrum and/or breast milk from lactating mothers: a potential role in the regulation of neonatal food intake. *J Clin Endocrinol Metab* 82:4270–4273, 1997.

Casey BM, Schaffer JI, Bloom SL, Heartwell SF, McIntire DD, Leveno KJ: Obstetric antecedents for postpartum pelvic floor dysfunction. *Am J Obstet Gynecol* 192:1655–1662, 2005.

Cavalli C, Teng C, Battaglia FC, Bevilacqua G: Free sugar and sugar alcohol concentrations in human breast milk. *J Pediatr Gastroenterol Nutr* 42:215–221, 2006.

Cavallo MG, Fava D, Monetini L, Barone F, Pozilli P: Cell-mediated immune response to beta casein in recent-onset insulin-dependent diabetes: implications for disease pathogenesis. *Lancet* 348:926–928, 1996.

Ceci O, Berardesca C, Caradonna F, Corsano P, Guglielmi R, Nappi L: Recurrent peripartum cardiomyopathy. *Eur J Obstet Gynecol Reprod Biol* 76:29–30, 1998.

Ceriello A: Postprandial hyperglycemia and diabetes complications: is it time to treat? *Diabetes* 54:1–7, 2005.

Chaithiraphan V, Gowda RM, Khan IA, Reimers CD: Peripartum acute myocardial infarction: management perspective. *Am J Ther* 10:75–77, 2003.

Chan W, Ray J, Wai E, Ginsburg S, Hannah M, Corey P, Ginsberg J: Risk of stroke in women exposed to low-dose Ocs: a critical evaluation of the evidence. *Arch Intern Med* 164:741–747, 2004.

Chand N, Minas AA: Celiac disease: current concepts in diagnosis and treatment. *J Clin Gastroenterol* 40: 3–14, 2006.

Chang SJ, Kirksey A: Vitamin B-6 status of breast-fed in infants in relation to pyridoxine HCl supplementation of mothers. *J Nutr Sci Vitaminol (Tokyo)* 48:10–17, 2002.

Chantry CJ, Howard CR, Auinger P: Full breastfeeding duration and associated decrease in respiratory tract infection in U.S. children. *Pediatrics* 117:425–432, 2006.

Chapman DJ, Young S, Ferris AM, Perez-Escamilla R: Impact of breast pumping on lactogenesis stage II after cesarean delivery: a randomized clinical trial. *Pediatrics* 107:E94, 2001.

Chappell JE, Clandinin MT, Kearney-Volpe C: Trans fatty acids in human milk lipids: influence of maternal diet and weight loss. *Am J Clin Nutr* 42:49–56, 1985.

Chardigny J-M, Destaillats F, Malpuech-Brugere C, Moulin J, Bauman DE, Lock AL, Barbano DM, Mensink RP, Bezelgues J-P, Chaumont P, Combe N, Cristiani I, Joffe F, German JB, Dioisi F, Boirie Y, Sebedio J-L: Do *trans* fatty acids from industrially produced sources and from natural sources have the same effect on cardiovascular disease risk factors in healthy subjects? Results of the *trans* Fatty Acids Collaboration (TRANSFACT) study. *Am J Clin Nutr* 87:558–566, 2008.

Charney E, Goodman HC, McBride M, Lyon B, Pratt R: Childhood antecedents of adult obesity. Do chubby infants become obese adults? *N Engl J Med* 295:6–9, 1976.

Charron-Prochownik D, Sereika SM, Falsetti D, Wang SL, Becker D, Jacober S, Mansfield J, White NH: Knowledge, attitudes and behaviors related to sexuality and family planning in adolescent women with and without diabetes. *Pediatr Diabetes* #7:267–273, 2006.

Chasan-Taber L, Willett WC, Manson JE, Spiegelman D, Hunter DJ, Curhan G, Colditz GA, Stampfer MJ: Prospective study of oral contraceptives and hypertension among women in the United States. *Circulation* 94:483–489, 1996.

Chasan-Taber L, Willett W, Stampfer M, Hunter D, Colditz G, Spiegelman D, Manson J: A prospective study of oral contraceptives and NIDDM among U.S. women. *Diabetes Care* 20:330–335, 1997.

Chaudron LH, Schoenecker CJ: Bupropion and breastfeeding: a case of a possible infant seizure. *J Clin Psychiatry* 65:881–882, 2004.

Chellakooty M, Juul A, Boisen KA, Damgaard IN, Kai CM, Schmidt IM, Petersen IM, Skakkebaek NE, Main KM: A prospective study of serum insulin-like growth factor I (IGF-I) and IGF-binding protein-3 in 942 healthy infants: associations with birth weight, gender, growth velocity, and breastfeeding. *J Clin Endocrinol Metab* 91:820–826, 2006.

Chelmow D, Ruehli MS, Huang E: Prophylactic use of antibiotics for nonlaboring patients undergoing cesarean delivery with intact membranes: a meta-analysis. *Am J Obstet Gynecol* 184:656–661, 2001.

Chen DC, Nommsen-Rivers L, Dewey KG, Lonnerdal B: Stress during labor and delivery and early lactation performance. *Am J Clin Nutr* 68:335–344, 1998.

Chen HS, Wu TE, Jap TS, Lin SH, Hsiao LC, Lin HD: Improvement of glycemia control in subjects with type 2 diabetes by self-monitoring of blood glucose: comparison of two management programs adjusting bedtime dosage. *Diabetes Obes Metab* 10:34–40, 2008.

Cherney DZ, Scholey JW, Cattran DC, Kang AK, Zimplemann J, Kennedy C, Lai V, Burns KD, Miller JA: The effect of oral contraceptives on the nitric oxide system and renal function. *Am J Physiol* 293:F1539–F1544, 2007.

Chien PF, Howie PW: Breast milk and the risk of opportunistic infection in infancy in industrialized and non-industrialized settings. *Adv Nutr Res* 10:69–104, 2001.

Chou T, Chan GM, Moyer-Mileur L: Postpartum body composition changes in lactating and nonlactating primiparas. *Nutrition* 15:481–484, 1999.

Chulada PC, Arbes SJ Jr, Dunson D, Zeldin DC: Breast-feeding and the prevalence of asthma and wheeze in children: analyses from the Third National Health and Nutrition Examination Survey, 1988–1994. *J Allergy Clin Immunol* 111: 328–336, 2003.

Ciacci C, Cirillo M, Auriemma G, Di Dato G, Sabbatini F, Mazzacca G: Celiac disease and pregnancy outcome. *Am J Gastroenterol* 91: 718–722, 1996.

Clark RM, Ferris AM, Fey M, Brown PB, Hundrieser KE, Jensen RG: Changes in the lipids of human milk from 2 to 16 weeks postpartum. *J Pediatr Gastroenterol Nutr* 1:311–315, 1982.

Clewell HJ, Gearhart JM, Gentry PR, Covington TR, VanLandingham CB, Crump KS, Shipp AM: Evaluation of the uncertainty in an oral reference dose for methylmercury due to interindividual variability in pharmacokinetics. *Risk Anal* 19:547–558, 1999.

Clifford TJ: Breast feeding and obesity. Editorial. *BMJ* 327:879–880, 2003.

Cobo E: Effect of different doses of ethanol on the milk-ejecting reflex in diabetic women. *Am J Obstet Gynecol* 115:817–821, 1973.

Cohen MM, Ansara D, Schei B, Stuckless N, Stewart DE: Posttraumatic stress disorder after pregnancy, labor, and delivery. *J Women's Health* 13:315–324, 2004.

Cohen LS, Alrtshuler LL, Harlow BL, Nonacs R, Newport DJ, Viguera AC, Suri R, Burt VK, Handrick V, Reminick AM, Longhead A, Vitonis AF, Stowe ZN: Relapse of major depression during pregnancy in women who maintain or discontinue antidepressant treatment. *JAMA* 295:499–507, 2006.

Coitinho DC, Sichieri R, D'Aquino Benicio MH: Obesity and weight change related to parity and breast-feeding among parous women in Brazil. *Public Health Nutr* 4:865–870, 2001.

Condon JT: Management of established pathological grief reaction after stillbirth. *Am J Psychiatry* 143:987–992, 1986.

Cooper PJ, Murray L: Course and recurrence of postnatal depression. Evidence for the specificity of the diagnostic concept. *Br J Psychiatr* 166:191–195, 1995.

Cooper P, Murray L: Prediction, detection, and treatment of postnatal depression. *Arch Dis Child* 77:97–99, 1997.

Costaco T, Ellis D, Orchard TJ: Oral contraceptive use and overt nephropathy in women with type diabetes. *Diabetes* 55 (Suppl 1):A7, 2006.

Coster S, Gulliford MC, Seed PT, Powrie JK, Swaminathan R: Self-monitoring in type 2 diabetes mellitus: a meta-analysis. *Diabet Med* 17:755–761, 2000.

Coulston AM: Cardiovascular disease risk in women with diabetes needs attention. Editorial. *Am J Clin Nutr* 79:931–932, 2004.

Couper JJ, Steele C, Beresford S, Powell T, McCaul K, Pollard A, Gellert S, Tait B, Harrison LC, Colman PG: Lack of association between duration of breast-feeding or introduction of cow's milk and development of islet autoimmunity. *Diabetes* 48:2145–2149, 1999.

Cox JL, Holden JM, Sagovsky R: Development of the 10-item Edinburgh Postnatal Depression Scale. *Br J Psychiatry* 150:782–786, 1987.

Cox JL, Murray D, Chapman G: A controlled study of the onset, duration and prevalence of postnatal depression. *Br J Psychiatry* 163:27–31, 1993.

Craig-Schmidt MC, Weete JD, Faircloth SA, Wickwire MA, Livant EJ: The effect of hydrogenated fat in the diet of nursing mothers on lipid composition and prostaglandin content of human milk. *Am J Clin Nutr* 39:778–786, 1984.

Creedy DK, Shocet IM, Horsfall J: Childbirth and the development of acute trauma symptoms: incidence and contributing factors. *Birth* 27:104–111, 2000.

Crepaldi SC, Carniero EM, Boschero AC: Long-term effect of prolactin treatment on glucose-induced insulin secretion in cultured neonatal rat islets. *Horm Metab Res* 29:220–224, 1997.

Cushing AH, Samet JM, Lambert WE, Skipper BJ, Hunt WC, Young SA, McLaren LC: Breastfeeding reduces risk of respiratory illness in infants. *Am J Epidemiol* 147:863–870, 1998.

Custro N, Scafidi V, Lo Baido R, Nastri L, Abbate G, Cuffaro MP, Gallo S, Vienna G, Notarbartolo A: Subclinical hypothyroidism resulting from autoimmune thyroiditis in female patients with endogenous depression. *J Endocrinol Invest* 17:641–646, 1994.

D'Amico MA, Holmes J, Stavropoulos SN, Frederick M, Levy J, DeFelice AR, Kazlow PG, Green PH: Presentation of pediatric celiac disease in the United States: prominent effect of breastfeeding. *Clin Pediatr (Phila)* 44:249–258, 2005.

da Silva VA, Malheiros LR, Moraes-Santos AR, Barzano MA, McLean AE: Ethanol pharmacokinetics in lactating women. *Braz J Med Biol Res* 26:1097–1103, 1993.

Dabelea D, D'Agostino RB, Mayer-Davis EJ, Pettitt DJ, Imperatore G, Dolan LM, Pihoker C, Hillier TA, Marcovina SM, Linder B, Ruggiero AM, Hamman RF; SEARCH for Diabetes in Youth Study Group: Testing the accelerator hypothesis. Body size, β-cell function, and age at onset of type 1 (autoimmune) diabetes. *Diabetes Care* 29:290–294, 2006.

Dahl-Jorgensen K, Joner G, Hanssen KF: Relationship between cow's milk consumption and incidence of IDDM in childhood. *Diabetes Care* 17:1488–1490, 1991.

Dahlquist GG, Blom LG, Persson LA, Sandstrom AI, Wall SG: Dietary factors and the risk of developing insulin dependent diabetes in childhood. *BMJ* 300:1302–1306, 1990.

Dahlquist GG, Pundziute-Lycka A, Nystrom L; Swedish Childhood Diabetes Study Group; Diabetes Incidence Study in Sweden (DISS) Group: Birthweight and risk of type 1 diabetes in children and young adults: a population-based register study. *Diabetologia* 48:1114–1117, 2005.

Dahlquist G: Can we slow the rising incidence of childhood-onset autoimmune diabetes? The overload hypothesis. *Diabetologia* 49:20–24, 2006.

Daniels MC, Adair LS: Breast-feeding influences cognitive development in Filipino children. *J Nutr* 135:2589–2595, 2005.

Das UN: Long-chain polyunsaturated fatty acids in the growth and development of the brain and memory. *Nutrition* 19:62–65, 2003.

Davidson PW, Myers GJ, Cox C, Axtell C, Shamlave C, Sloane-Reeves J, Cernichiari E, Needham L, Choi A, Wang Y, Berlin M, Clarkson TW: Effects of prenatal and postnatal methylmercury exposure from fish consumption on neurodevelopment: outcomes at 66 months of age in the Seychelles Child Development Study. *JAMA* 280:701–707, 1998.

Davidson J: Strategies for improving glycemic control: effective use of glucose monitoring. *Am J Med* 118 (Suppl 9A):27S–32S, 2005a.

Davidson MB: Editor's response to self-monitoring of blood glucose in patients with type 2 diabetes who are not using insulin. *Diabetes Care* 28:2597, 2005b.

Davies HA, Clark JDA, Dalton KJ, Edwards OM: Insulin requirements of diabetic women who breast feed. *BMJ* 298:1357–1358, 1989.

Davis, MK: Breastfeeding and chronic disease in childhood and adolescence. *Pediatr Clin North Am* 48:125–141. 2001.

Dawodu A, Wagner CL: Mother-child vitamin D deficiency: an international perspective. *Arch Dis Child* 92:737–740, 2007.

DCCT—Diabetes Control and Complications Trial Research Group: Effect of intensive therapy on the development and progression of neuropathy. *Ann Intern Med* 113:49–51, 1995.

DCCT—Diabetes Control and Complications Trial Research Group: The effect of intensive diabetes therapy on measures of autonomic nervous system function in the Diabetes Control and Complications Trial (DCCT). *Diabetologia* 41: 416–423, 1998.

DCCT—Diabetes Control and Complications Trial Research Group: The relationship of glycemic exposure (HbA1C) to the risk of development and progression of retinopathy in the Diabetes Control and Complications trial. *Diabetes* 44:968–983, 2005.

DCCT/EDIC—The Diabetes Control and Complications Trial/Epidemiology of Diabetes Interventions and Complications Research Group: Retinopathy and nephropathy in patients with type 1 diabetes four years after a trial of intensive therapy. *N Engl J Med* 342:381–389, 2000.

DCCT/EDIC—The Diabetes Control and Complications Trial/Epidemiology of Diabetes Interventions and Complications Research Group, Writing Team: Effect of intensive therapy on the microvascular complications of type 1 diabetes mellitus. *JAMA* 287:2563–2569, 2002.

DCCT/EDIC—The Diabetes Control and Complications Trial/Epidemiology of Diabetes Interventions and Complications Research Group: Intensive diabetes treatment and cardiovascular disease in patients with type 1 diabetes. *N Engl J Med* 353:2643–2653, 2005.

de Groot M, Anderson R, Freedland KE, Clouse RE, Lustman PJ: Association of depression and diabetes complications: a meta-analysis. *Psychosom Med* 63: 619–630, 2001.

Del Prato S, Felton AM, Munro N, Nesto R, Zimmet P, Zinman B; Global Partnership for Effective Diabetes Management: Improving glucose management: ten steps to get more patients with type 2 diabetes to glycemic goal. *Int J Clin Pract* 59:1345–1355, 2005.

DeMier RL, Hynan MT, Harris HB, Manniello RL: Perinatal stressors as predictors of symptoms of post-traumatic stress in mothers of infants at high risk. *J Perinatol* 16:276–280, 1996.

Dennis CL, Creedy D: Psychosocial and psychological interventions for preventing postpartum depression. *Cochrane Database Syst Rev* 2004;(4):CD001134.

Dennis C-L: Psychosocial and psychological interventions for prevention of postnatal depression: systematic review. *BMJ* 331:15–18, 2005.

Dennis CL, Hodnett E: Psychosocial and psychological interventions for treating postpartum depression. *Cochrane Database Syst Rev* 2007;(4):CD006116.

Deslypere JP, Thiery N, Vermeulen A: Effect of long-term hormonal contraception on plasma lipids. *Contraception* 31:633–642, 1985.

Devlin RG, Fleiss PM: Captopril in human blood and breast milk. *Eur J Clin Pharmacol* 21:110–113, 1981.

Dewey KG, Lonnerdal B: Infant self-regulation of breast milk intake. *Acta Paediatr Scand* 75:893–898, 1986.

Dewey KG, Heinig MJ, Nommsen LA, Lonnerdal B: Maternal versus infant factors related to breast milk intake and residual milk volume: the DARLING study. *Pediatrics* 87:829–837, 1991a.

Dewey KG, Heinig MJ, Nommsen LA, Lonnerdal B: Adequacy of energy intake among breastfed infants in the DARLING study: relationships to growth velocity, morbidity and activity levels. *J Pediatr* 119:538–547, 1991b.

Dewey KG, Heinig MJ, Nommsen LA, Peerson JM, Lonnerdal B: Growth of breast-fed and formula-fed infants from 0 to 18 months: the DARLING study. *Pediatrics* 89:1035–1041, 1992.

Dewey KG, Heinig MJ, Nommsen LA: Maternal weight loss patterns during prolonged lactation. *Am J Clin Nutr* 58:162–166, 1993a.

Dewey KG, Heinig MJ, Nommsen LA, Peerson JM, Lonnerdal B: Breast-fed infants are leaner than formula-fed infants at 1 year of age: the DARLING study. *Am J Clin Nutr* 57:140–145, 1993b.

Dewey KG, McCrory MA: Effects of dieting and physical activity on pregnancy and lactation. *Am J Clin Nutr* 59 (Suppl):446S–453S, 1994a.

Dewey KG, Lovelady CA, Nommsen-Rivers LA, McCrory MA, Lonnerdal B: A randomized study of the effects of aerobic exercise by lactating women on breast-milk volume and composition. *N Engl J Med* 330:449–453, 1994b.

Dewey KG, Peerson JM, Brown KH, Krebs NF, Michaelsen KF, Persson LA, Salmenpera L, Whitehead RG, Yeung DL; World Health Organization Working Group on Infant Growth: Growth of breast-fed infants deviates from current reference data: a pooled analysis of U.S., Canadian, and European data sets. *Pediatrics* 96:495–503, 1995.

Dewey KG: Energy and protein requirements during lactation. *Annu Rev Nutr* 17:19–36, 1997.

Dewey KG: Growth characteristics of breast-fed compared to formula-fed infants. *Biol Neonate* 74:94–105, 1998a.

Dewey KG: Effects of caloric restriction and exercise during lactation. *J Nutr* 128:386S–389S, 1998b.

Dewey KG: Nutrition, growth, and complementary feeding of the breastfed infant. *Pediatr Clin North Am* 48:87–104, 2001.

Dewey KG: Is breastfeeding protective against childhood obesity? *J Hum Lact* 19:9–18, 2003a.

Dewey KG, Nommsen-Rivers LA, Heinig MJ, Cohen RJ: Risk factors for suboptimal infant breastfeeding behavior, delayed onset of lactation, and excess neonatal weight loss. *Pediatrics* 112:607–619, 2003b.

Dewey KG, Cohen RJ, Brown KH: Exclusive breast-feeding for 6 months, with iron supplementation, maintains adequate micronutrient status among term, low-birthweight, breast-fed infants in Honduras. *J Nutr* 134:1091–1098, 2004.

DHHS—U. S. Department of Health and Human Services, Office on Women's Health: HHS blueprint for action on breastfeeding. Washington, DC: 2000; 1–31. Available at: www.4woman.gov/breastfeeding/bluprntbk2.pdf. Accessed May 1, 2008.

Diab KM, Zaki MM: Contraception in diabetic women: comparative metabolic study of Norplant, depot medroxyprogesterone acetate, low dose oral contraceptive pill and CuT380a. *J Obstet Gynecol Res* 26:17–26, 2000.

Diamond MP, Entmann SS, Salyer SL, Vaughn WK, Boehm FH: Increased risk of endometritis and wound infection after cesarean section in insulin-dependent diabetic women. *Am J Obstet Gynecol* 155:297–300, 1986.

Dijkstra SH, van Beek A, Janssen JW, de Vleeschouwer LHM, Huysman WA, van der Akker ELT: High prevalence of vitamin D deficiency in newborn infants of high-risk mothers. *Arch Dis Child* 92:750–753, 2007.

Diniz JMM, Da Costa THM: Independent of body adiposity, breast-feeding has a protective effect on glucose metabolism in young adult women. *Br J Nutr* 92:905–912, 2004.

Domellof M, Lonnerdal B, Dewey KG, Cohen RJ, Hernell O: Iron, zinc, and copper concentrations in breast milk are independent of maternal milk status. *Am J Clin Nutr* 79:111–115, 2004.

Donath SM, Amir LH: Does maternal obesity adversely affect breastfeeding initiation and duration? *J Pediatr Child Health* 36:482–486, 2000.

Donath SM, Amir LH; ALSPAC Study Team: Relationship between prenatal infant feeding intention and initiation and duration of breastfeeding: a cohort study. *Acta Paediatr* 92:352–356, 2004.

Dorea JG: Mercury and lead during breast-feeding. *Br J Nutr* 92:21–40, 2004.

DPG—Diabetes and Pregnancy Group: Knowledge about preconception care in French women with type 1 diabetes. *Diabetes Metab* 31:443–447, 2005.

Drasch G, Aigner S, Roider G, Staiger F, Lipowsky G: Mercury in human colostrum and early breast milk. Its dependence on dental amalgam and other factors. *J Trace Elem Med Biol* 12:23–27, 1998.

Drexler H, Schaller KH: The mercury concentration in breast milk resulting from amalgam fillings and dietary habits. *Environ Res* 77:124–129, 1998.

Duncan B, Ely J, Holberg CJ, Wright AL, Martinez FD, Taussig LM: Exclusive breastfeeding for at least 4 months protects against otitis media. *Pediatrics* 91:867–872, 1993.

Dundar NO, Anal O, Dundar B, Ozkan H, Caliskan S, Buyukgebiz A: Longitudinal investigation of the relationship between breast milk leptin levels and growth in breast-fed infants. *J Pediatr Endocrinol Metab* 18:181–187, 2005.

Dusdieker LB, Hemingway DL, Stumbo PJ: Is milk production impaired by dieting during lactation? *Am J Clin Nutr* 59:833–840, 1994.

Eberhard-Gran M, Eskild A, Opjordsmoen S: Use of psychotropic medications in treating mood disorders during lactation. Practical recommendations. *CNS Drugs* 20:187–198, 2006.

Edwards JE, Alcorn J, Savolainen J, Anderson BD, McNamara PJ: Role of P-glycoprotein in distribution of nelfinavir across the blood-mammary tissue barrier and blood-brain barrier. *Antimicrob Agents Chemother* 49:1626–1628, 2005.

Ehrenkranz RA, Ackerman BA, Hulse JD: Nifedipine transfer into human milk. *J Pediatr* 114:478–480, 1989.

Eidelman AI: Hypoglycemia and the breastfed neonate. *Pediatr Clin North Am* 48:377–387, 2001.

Elkayam U, Tummala PP, Rao K, Akhter MW, Karaalp IS, Wani OR, Hameed A, Gviazda I, Shotan A: Maternal and fetal outcomes of subsequent pregnancies in women with peripartum cardiomyopathy. *N Engl J Med* 344:1567–1571, 2001.

Emmett PM, Rogers IS: Properties of human milk and their relationship with maternal nutrition. *Early Hum Dev* 49 (Suppl):S7–S28, 1997.

Epperson N, Czarkowski KA, Ward-O'Brien D, Weiss E, Gueorguieva R, Jatlow P, Anderson GM: Maternal sertraline treatment and serotonin transport in breast-feeding mother-infant pairs. *Am J Psychiatry* 158:1631–1637, 2001.

Eriksson U, Duc G, Froesch ER, Zapf J: Insulin-like growth factors (IGF) I and II and IGF binding proteins (IGFBPs) in human colostrum/transitory milk during the first week postpartum: comparison with neonatal and maternal serum. *Biochem Biophys Res Commun* 196:267–273, 1993.

Erkolla R, Viikari J, Irjala K, Solakivi-Jaakkola T: One-year followup of lipoprotein metabolism after pregnancy. *Biol Res Pregnancy* 7:47–51, 1986.

EURODIAB Substudy 2 Study Group: Vitamin D supplement in early childhood and risk for type 1 (insulin-dependent) diabetes mellitus. *Diabetologia* 42:51–54, 1999.

EURODIAB Substudy 2 Study Group: Infections and vaccinations as risk factors for childhood type 1 (insulin-dependent) diabetes mellitus: a multicenter case-control investigation. *Diabetologia* 43:47–53, 2000.

EURODIAB Substudy 2 Study Group: Rapid early growth is associated with increased risk of childhood type 1 diabetes in various European populations. *Diabetes Care* 25:1755–1760, 2002.

Evans KC, Evans RG, Royal R, Esterman AJ, James SL: Effects of cesarean section on breast milk transfer to the normal term newborn over the first week of life. *Arch Dis Child Fetal Neonatal Ed* 88:F380–F382, 2003.

Everson SA, Maty SC, Lynch JW, Kaplan GA: Epidemiologic evidence for the relation between socioeconomic status and depression, obesity, and diabetes. *J Psychosom Res* 53:891–895, 2002.

Fagen C: Preparing pregnant women with diabetes for special breast-feeding challenges. Practice Points: translating research into practice. *J Am Diet Assoc* 98:648, 1998.

Fahmy K, Abdel-Razik, Shaaraway M, al-Kholy G, Saad S, Wagdi A, al-Azzony M: Effect of long-acting progestagen-only injectable contraceptives on carbohydrate metabolism and its hormonal profile. *Contraception* 44:419–430, 1991.

Fahreus L, Sydsjo A, Wallentin L: Lipoprotein changes during treatment of pelvic endometriosis with medroxyprogesterone acetate. *Fertil Steril* 45:501–506,1986.

Faith-Magnusson K, Franzen L, Jansson G, Laurin P, Stenhammar L: Infant feeding history shows distinct differences between Swedish celiac and reference children. *Pediatr Allergy Immunol* 7:1–5, 1996.

Fajumi JO: Alterations in blood lipids and side effects induced by depo-provera in Nigerian women. *Contraception* 27:161–175, 1983.

Fang ZY, Prins JB, Marwick TH: Diabetic cardiomyopathy: evidence, mechanisms, and therapeutic implications. *Endocr Rev* 25:543–567, 2004.

Farley TMM, Rosenberg MJ, Rowe PJ, Chen J-H, Meirek O: Intrauterine devices and pelvic inflammatory disease: an international perspective. *Lancet* 339:785–788, 1992.

Farmer AJ, Gibson OJ, Dudley C, Bryden K, Hayton PM, Tarassenko L, Neil A: A randomized controlled trial of the effect of real-time telemedicine support on glycemic control in young adults with type 1 diabetes (ISRCTN 46889446). *Diabetes Care* 28:2697–2702, 2005.

Fava D, Leslie RD, Pozzilli P: Relationship between dairy product consumption and incidence of IDDM in childhood in Italy. *Diabetes Care* 17:1488–1490, 1994.

Feig DS, Briggs GG, Kraemer JM, Ambrose PJ, Moskovitz DN, Nageotte M, Donat DJ, Padilla G, Wan S, Klein J, Koren G: Transfer of glyburide and glipizide into breast milk. *Diabetes Care* 28:1851–1855, 2005.

Feig DS, Cleave B, Tomlinson G: Long-term effects of a diabetes and pregnancy program. Does the education last? *Diabetes Care* 29:526–530, 2006.

Felker GM, Thompson RE, Hare JM, Hruban RH, Clemetson DE, Howard DL, Baughman KL, Kasper EK: Underlying causes and long-term survival in patients with initially unexplained cardiomyopathy. *N Engl J Med* 342:1077–1084, 2000.

Ferris AM, Dalidowitz CK, Ingardia CM, Reece EA, Fumia FD, Jensen RG, Allen LH: Lactation outcome in insulin-dependent diabetic women. *J Am Diet Assoc* 88:317–322, 1988.

Ferris AM, Neubauer SH, Bendal RB, Green KN, Ingardia CJ, Reece EA: Perinatal lactation protocol and outcome in mothers with and without insulin-dependent diabetes mellitus. *Am J Clin Nutr* 58:43–48, 1993.

Ferris AM, Reece EA: Nutritional consequences of chronic maternal conditions during pregnancy and lactation: lupus and diabetes. *Am J Clin Nutr* 59 (Suppl):465S–473S, 1994.

Fett JD, Christie LG, Murphy JG: Outcomes of subsequent pregnancy after peripartum cardiomyopathy: a case series from Haiti. *Ann Intern Med* 145:30–34, 2006.

FFP—Faculty of Family Planning and Reproductive Health Care Clinical Effectiveness Unit: Contraceptive choices for breastfeeding women. Family planning and reproductive health care guidance (July 2004). *J Fam Plan Reprod Health Care* 30:181–189, 2004.

Fidler N, Koletzko B: The fatty acid composition of human colostrum. *Eur J Nutr* 39:31–37, 2000.

Field CJ: The immunological components of human milk and their effect on immune development in infants. *J Nutr* 135:1–4, 2005.

Fingerlin TE, Brady HL, Steck AK, Bugawan TL, Blair A, Redondo MJ, Erlich HA, Rewers MJ, Norris JM: Increased risk of islet autoimmunity due to gene-environment interaction between polymorphisms in the IL-4R gene and infant diet. *Diabetes* 55 (Suppl 1):A20, 2006.

Fisher JO, Birch LL, Smiciklas-Wright H, Picciano MF: Breast-feeding through the first year predicts maternal control in feeding and subsequent toddler energy intakes. *J Am Diet Assoc* 100:641–646, 2000.

Fly AD, Uhlin KL, Wallace JP: Major mineral concentrations in human milk do not change after maximal exercise testing. *Am J Clin Nutr* 68:345–349, 1998.

Fort P, Lanes R, Dahlem S, Recker B, Weyman-Daum M, Pugliese M, Lifshitz F: Breastfeeding and insulin-dependent diabetes in children. *J Am Coll Nutr* 5: 439–441, 1986.

Francois CA, Connor SL, Wander RC, Connor WE: Acute effects of dietary fatty acids on the fatty acids of human milk. *Am J Clin Nutr* 67:301–308, 1998.

Francois CA, Connor SL, Bolewicz LC, Connor WE: Supplementing lactating women with flaxseed oil does not increase docosahexaenoic acid in their milk. *Am J Clin Nutr* 77:226–233, 2003.

Francoisi M, Pellegrini F, De Berardis G, Belfiglio M, Di Nardo B, Greenfield S, Kaplan SH, Rossi MC, Sacco M, Tognoni G, Valentini M, Nicolucci A; QuED Study Group—Quality of Care and Outcomes in Type 2 Diabetes: Self-monitoring of blood glucose in non-insulin-treated diabetic patients: a longitudinal evaluation of its impact on metabolic control. *Diabet Med* 22: 900–906, 2005.

Freed GL, Clark SJ, Lohr JA, Sorenson JR: Pediatrician involvement in breast-feeding promotion: a national study of residents and practitioners. *Pediatrics* 96:490–494, 1995.

Friedman NJ, Zeiger RS: The role of breast-feeding in the development of allergies and asthma. *J Allergy Clin Immunol* 115:1238–1248, 2005.

Funnell MM, Brown TL, Childs BP, Haas LB, Hosey GM, Jensen B, Maryniuk M, Peyrot M, Piette JD, Reader D, Siminerio LM, Weinger K, Weiss MA: National standards for diabetes self-management education. *Diabetes Care* 31 (Suppl 1): S97–S104, 2008.

Gaede P, Vedel P, Parving H-H, Pedersen O: Intensified multifactorial intervention in patients with type 2 diabetes mellitus and microalbuminuria: the Steno type 2 randomized study. *Lancet* 353:617–622, 1999.

Gaede P, Vedel P, Larsen N, Jensen GVH, Parving H-H, Pedersen O: Multifactorial intervention and cardiovascular disease in patients with type 2 diabetes. *N Engl J Med* 348:383–393, 2003.

Gaede P, Lund-Anderson H, Parving HH, Pedersen O: Effect of a multifactorial intervention on mortality in type 2 diabetes. *N Engl J Med* 358:580–591, 2008.

Gagne MP, Leff EW, Jefferis SC: The breastfeeding experience of women with type 1 diabetes. *Health Care Women Intl* 13:249–260, 1992.

Gallas PR, Stolk RP, Bakker K, Endert E, Wiersinga WM: Thyroid dysfunction during pregnancy and in the first postpartum year in women with diabetes mellitus type 1. *Eur J Endocrinol* 147:443–451, 2002.

Gamble J, Creedy D: Content and processes of postpartum counseling after a distressing birth experience: a review. *Birth* 31:213–218, 2004.

Gardiner SJ, Kirkpatrick CM, Begg EJ, Zhang M, Moore MP, Saville DJ: Transfer of metformin into human milk. *Clin Pharmacol Ther* 73:71–77, 2003.

Garg SK, Chase HP, Marshal G, Hoops S, Holmes DL, Jackson WE: Oral contraceptives and renal and retinal complications in young women with insulin-dependent diabetes mellitus. *JAMA* 271:1099–1102, 1994.

Garg S, Zisser H, Schwartz S, Bailey T, Kaplan R, Ellis S, Jovanovic L: Improvement in glycemic excursions with a transcutaneous, real-time continuous glucose sensor. A randomized controlled trial. *Diabetes Care* 29:44–50, 2006.

Garofalo RP, Goldman AS: Expression of functional immunomodulating and anti-inflammatory factors in human milk. *Clin Perinatol* 26:361–377, 1999.

Gartner LM, Herschel M: Jaundice and breastfeeding. *Pediatr Clin North Am* 48:389–399, 2001.

Gartner LM, Greer FR; the Section on Breastfeeding and Committee on Nutrition, American Academy of Pediatrics: Prevention of rickets and vitamin D deficiency: new guidelines for vitamin D intake. *Pediatrics* 111:908–910, 2003.

Gartner LM, Morton J, Lawrence RA, Naylor AJ, O'Hare D, Schanler RJ, Eidelman AI; American Academy of Pediatrics, Section on Breastfeeding: Breastfeeding and the use of human milk. Policy statement. *Pediatrics* 115:496–506, 2005.

Gdalevich M, Mimouni D, Mimouni M: Breast-feeding and the risk of bronchial asthma in childhood: a systematic review with meta-analysis of prospective studies. *J Pediatr* 139:261–266, 2001.

Gentile S: The safety of newer antidepressants in pregnancy and breastfeeding. *Drug Saf* 28:137–152, 2005.

Georgiopoulis AM, Bryan TL, Yawn BP, Houstan MS, Rummans TA, Therneau TM: Population-based screening for postpartum depression. *Obstet Gynecol* 93:653–657, 1999.

Georgiopoulos AM, Bryan TL, Wollan P, Yawn BP: Routine screening for postpartum depression. *J Fam Pract* 50:117–122, 2001.

Gerstein HC: How common is postpartum thyroiditis? A methodologic overview of the literature. *Arch Intern Med* 150:1397–1400, 1990.

Gerstein HC: Incidence of postpartum thyroid dysfunction in patients with type 1 diabetes mellitus. *Ann Intern Med* 118:419–423, 1993.

Gerstein HC: Cow's milk exposure and type 1 diabetes mellitus: a critical overview of the clinical literature. *Diabetes Care* 17:13–19, 1994.

Gibb D, Hockey S, Brown LJ, Lunt H: Attitudes and knowledge regarding contraception and prepregnancy counseling in insulin-dependent diabetes. *N Z Med J* 107:484–486, 1994.

Gibbon C, Smith T, Egger P, Betts P, Phillips D: Early infection and subsequent insulin dependent diabetes. *Arch Dis Child* 77:384–385, 1997.

Gillman MW, Rifas-Shiman SL, Camargo CA, Berkey CS, Frazier AL, Rocketts HRH, Field AE, Colditz GA: Risk of overweight among adolescents who were breastfed as infants. *JAMA* 285:2461–2467, 2001.

Gillman MW, Rifas-Shiman SL, Berkey CS, Frazier AL, Rockett HRH, Camargo CA Jr, Field AE, Colditz GA: Breast-feeding and overweight in adolescence. *Epidemiology* 17:112–114, 2006.

Gillum LA, Mamidipudi SK, Johnston SC: Ischemic stroke risk with oral contraceptives: a meta-analysis. *JAMA* 284:72–78, 2000.

Gimeno SGA, de Souza JMP: IDDM and milk consumption. A case-control study in Sao Paulo, Brazil. *Diabetes Care* 20:1256–1260, 1997.

Ginsberg J, Walfish PG: Postpartum transient thyrotoxicosis with painless thyroiditis. *Lancet* 1:1125–1128, 1977.

Ginsburg BE, Lindblad BS, Lundsjo A, Persson B, Zetterstrom R: Plasma valine and urinary C-peptide in breast-fed and artificially fed infants up to six months of age. *Acta Paediatr Scand* 73:213–217, 1984.

Giroux D, Lapointe G, Baril M: Toxicological index and the presence in the workplace of chemical hazards for workers who breast-feed infants. *Am Ind Hyg Assoc* 53:471–474, 1992.

Glazier RH, Bajcar J, Kennie NR, Willson K: A systematic review of interventions to improve diabetes care in socially disadvantaged populations. *Diabetes Care* 29:1675–1688, 2006.

Glueck CJ, Salehi M, Sieve L, Wang P: Growth, motor, and social development in breast- and formula-fed infants of metformin-treated women with polycystic ovary syndrome. *J Pediatr* 148:628–632, 2006.

Godsland IF, Crook D, Simpson R, Proudler T, Felton C, Lees B, Anyaoku V, Devenport M, Wynn V: The effects of different formulations of oral contraceptive agents on lipid and carbohydrate metabolism. *N Engl J Med* 323:1375–1381, 1990.

Godsland I: The influence of female sex steroids on glucose metabolism and insulin action. *J Intern Med* 240:1–65, 1996.

Gordon TEJ, Cardone IA, Kim JJ, Gordon SM, Silver RK: Universal perinatal depression screening in an academic medical center. *Obstet Gynecol* 107:342–347, 2006.

Gosden C, Steel J, Ross A, Springerbett A: Intrauterine contraception in diabetic women. *Lancet* 1:530–535, 1982.

Gou SS, Huang C, Maynard LM, Demerath E, Towne B, Chumlea WC, Siervogel RM: Body mass index during childhood, adolescence and young adulthood in relation to adult overweight and adiposity: the Fels Longitudinal Study. *Int J Obes Relat Metab Disord* 24:1628–1635, 2000.

Grattan DR: The actions of prolactin in the brain during pregnancy and lactation. *Prog Brain Res* 133:153–171, 2001.

Gray L, Miller LW, Philipp BL, Blass EM: Breastfeeding is analgesic in healthy newborns. *Pediatrics* 109:590–593, 2002.

Gray-Donald K, Kramer MS, Munday S, Leduc DG: Effect of formula supplementation in the hospital on the duration of breast-feeding: a controlled clinical trial. *Pediatrics* 75:514–518, 1985.

Gray-Donald K, Kramer MS: Causality inference in observational vs. experimental studies: an empirical comparison. *Am J Epidemiol* 127:885–892, 1988.

Greco L, Auricchio S, Mayer M, Grinoldi M: Case-control study on nutritional risk factors in celiac disease. *J Pediatr Gastroenterol Nutr* 7:395–399, 1988.

Greer FR, Sicherer SH, Burks AW; the Committee on Nutrition and Section on Allergy and Immunology, American Academy of Pediatrics: Effects of early nutritional interventions on the development of atopic disease in infants and children: the role of maternal dietary restriction, breastfeeding, timing of introduction of complementary foods, and hydrolyzed formulas. *Pediatrics* 121:183–191, 2008.

Gregoire AJ, Kumar R, Everitt B, Henderson AF, Studd JW: Transdermal estrogen for treatment of severe postnatal depression. *Lancet* 347:930–933, 1996.

Griffen IJ, Abrams SA: Iron and breastfeeding. *Pediatr Clin North Am* 48:401–413, 2001.

Grigoriadis S, Ravitz P: An approach to interpersonal psychotherapy for postpartum depression: focusing on interpersonal changes. *Can Fam Physician* 53: 1469–1475, 2007.

Grummer-Strawn LM, Mei Z: Does breastfeeding protect against pediatric overweight? Analysis of longitudinal data from the Centers for Disease Control and Prevention Pediatric Nutrition Surveillance System. *Pediatrics* 113:e81–e86, 2004 [DOI: 10.1542/peds.113.2.e81].

Guise J-M, Austin D, Morris CD: Review of case-control studies related to breastfeeding and reduced risk of childhood leukemia. *Pediatrics* 116:e724–e731, 2005.

Gundacker C, Pietschnig B, Wittmann KJ, Lischka A, Salzer H, Hohenauer L, Schuster E: Lead and mercury in breast milk. *Pediatrics* 110:873–878, 2002.

Gunderson EP: Breastfeeding after gestational diabetes pregnancy: subsequent obesity and type 2 diabetes mellitus in women and their offspring. *Diabetes Care* 30 (Suppl 2):S161–S168, 2007a.

Gunderson EP, Lewis CE, Wei GS, Whitmer RA, Quesenberry CP, Sidney S: Lactation and changes in maternal metabolic risk factors. *Obstet Gynecol* 109:729–738, 2007b.

Gupta S: Clinical guidelines on contraception and diabetes. *Eur J Contracept Reprod Health Care* 2:167–171, 1997.

Gustafsson PA, Duchen K, Birberg U, Karlsson T: Breastfeeding, very long polyunsaturated fatty acids (PUFA) and IQ at 6 1/2 years of age. *Acta Paediatr* 93:1280–1287, 2004.

Gwinn ML, Lee NC, Rhodes PH, Layde PM, Rubin GL: Pregnancy, breastfeeding, and oral contraceptives and the risk of epithelial ovarian cancer. *J Clin Epidemiol* 43:559–568, 1990.

Haag S, Granberg K, Carleborg L: Excretion of fluvoxamine into breast milk. *Br J Pharmacol* 49:P286–P288, 2003.

Haiba NA, el-Habashy MA, Said SA, Darwish EA, Abdel-Sayed WS, Nayel SE: Clinical evaluation of two monthly injectable contraceptives and their effects on some metabolic parameters. *Contraception* 39:619–632, 1989.

Haiek LN, Kramer MS, Ciampi A, Tirado R: Postpartum weight loss and infant feeding. *J Am Board Fam Pract* 14:85–94, 2001.

Hale TW, Kristensen JH, Hackett LP, Kohan R, Ilett KF: Transfer of metformin into human milk. *Diabetologia* 45:1509–1514, 2002.

Hale TW: Maternal medications during breastfeeding. *Clin Obstet Gynecol* 47:696–711, 2004.

Hall B: Changing composition of human milk and early development of an appetite control. *Lancet* 1:779–781, 1975.

Halvorsen BL, Carlsen MH, Phillips KM, Bohn SK, Holte K, Jacobs DR Jr, Blomhoff R: Content of redox-active compounds (ie, antioxidants) in foods consumed in the United States. *Am J Clin Nutr* 84:95–135, 2006.

Hamalainen AM, Ronkainen MS, Akerblom HK, Knip M: Postnatal elimination of transplacentally acquired disease-associated antibodies in infants born to families with type 1 diabetes: the Finnish TRIGR Study Group trial to reduce IDDM in the genetically at risk. *J Clin Endocrinol Metab* 85:4249–4253, 2000.

Hamosh M: Protective functions of proteins and lipids in human milk. *Biol Neonate* 74:163–176, 1998a.

Hamosh M, Salem N Jr: Long-chain polyunsaturated fatty acids. *Biol Neonate* 74:106–120, 1998b.

Hamosh M: Bioactive factors in human milk. *Pediatr Clin North Am* 48:69–86, 2001.

Hamosh M: The milky way: from mammary gland to milk to newborn—Macy-Gyorgy Award presentation (1999). *Adv Exp Med Biol* 503:17–25, 2002.

Hanefeld M, Fischer S, Julius U, Schilze J, Schwanebeck U, Schmechel H, Zirgelasch HJ, Lindner J: Risk factors for myocardial disease and death in newly detected NIDDM: the Diabetes Intervention Study, 11-year follow-up. *Diabetologia* 39:1577–1583, 1996.

Hannula L, Kaunonen M, Tarkka MT: A systematic review of professional support interventions for breastfeeding. *J Clin Nurs* 17:1132–1143, 2008.

Hansen D, Bennedbaek FN, Hansen LK, Houer-Madsen M, Jacobsen BB, Hegedus L: Thyroid function, morphology and autoimmunity in young patients with insulin-dependent diabetes mellitus. *Eur J Endocrinol* 140:512–518, 1999.

Hanson LA, Korotkova M, Lundin S, Haversen L, Silfverdal SA, Mattsby-Baltzer I, Strandvik B, Telemo E: The transfer of immunity from mother to child. *Ann N Y Acad Sci* 987:199–206, 2003.

Hapgood CC, Elkind GS, Wright JJ: Maternity blues: phenomena and relationship to later postpartum depression. *Aust N Z J Psychiatry* 22:299–306, 1988.

Harder T, Bergmann R, Kallischnigg G, Plagemann A: Duration of breastfeeding and risk of overweight: a meta-analysis. *Am J Epidemiol* 162:397–403, 2005.

Harder T, Schellong K, Plagemann A: Differences between meta-analyses on breastfeeding and obesity support causality of the association. Letter. *Pediatrics* 117:987–988, 2006.

Harris WS, Connor WE, Lindsey S: Will dietary ω-3 fatty acids change the composition of human milk? *Am J Clin Nutr* 40:780–785, 1984.

Harris B, Fung H, Johns S, Kologlu M, Bhatti R, McGregor AM, Richards CJ, Hall R: Transient postpartum thyroid dysfunction and postnatal depression. *J Affect Disord* 17:243–249, 1989a.

Harris B, Huckle P, Thomas R, Johns S, Fung H: The use of rating scales to identify postnatal depression. *Br J Psychiatry* 154:813–817, 1989b.

Harris B, Othman S, Davies JA, Weppner GJ, Richards CJ, Newcombe RG, Lazarus JH, Parkes AB, Hall R, Phillips DI: Association between postpartum thyroid dysfunction and thyroid antibodies and depression. *BMJ* 305:152–156, 1992.

Harris WS, Pottala JV, Sands SA, Jones PG: Comparison of the effects of fish and fish-oil capsules on the *n*-3 fatty acid content of blood cells and plasma phospholipids. *Am J Clin Nutr* 86:1621–1625, 2007.

Harrison LC, Honeyman MC: Cow's milk and type 1 diabetes. The real debate is about mucosal immune function. *Diabetes* 48:1501–1507, 1999.

Hartikainen-Sorri A-L, Heikkinen JE, Koivisto M: Pharmacokinetics of clonidine during pregnancy and nursing. *Obstet Gynecol* 69:598–600, 1987.

Hartmann P, Cregan M: Lactogenesis and the effects of insulin-dependent diabetes mellitus and prematurity. *J Nutr* 131:3016S–3020S, 2001.

Harzer G, Haug M, Dieterich I, Gentner PR: Changing patterns of human milk lipids in the course of lactation and during the day. *Am J Clin Nutr* 37:612–621, 1983.

Haslam SZ, Shyamala G: Effect of estradiol on progesterone receptors in normal mammary glands and its relationship with lactation. *Biochem J* 182:127–131, 1979.

Hauser GJ, Almog S, Tirosh M, Spirer Z: Effect of alpha-methyldopa excreted in human milk on the breast-fed infant. *Helv Pediatr Acta* 40:83–86, 1985.

Hayslip CC, Fein HG, O'Donnell VM, Friedman DS, Klein TA, Smallridge RC: The value of serum antimicrosomal antibody testing in screening for symptomatic postpartum thyroid dysfunction. *Am J Obstet Gynecol* 159:203–209, 1988.

Heacock HJ, Jeffery HE, Baker JL, Page M: Influence of breast versus formula milk on physiological gastroesophageal reflux in healthy newborn infants. *J Pediatr Gastroenterol Nutr* 14:41–46, 1992.

Hediger ML, Overpeck MD, Kuczmarski RJ, Ruan WJ: Association between infant breastfeeding and overweight in young children. *JAMA* 285:2453–2460, 2001.

Heider AL, Kuller JA, Strauss RA, Wells SR: Peripartum cardiomyopathy: a review of the literaure. *Obstet Gynecol Surv* 54:526–531, 1999.

Heinig MJ, Nommsen LA, Peerson JM, Lonnerdal B, Dewey KG: Energy and protein intakes of breast-fed and formula-fed infants during the first year of life and their association with growth velocity: the DARLING study. *Am J Clin Nutr* 58:152–161, 1993.

Heinig MJ: Host defense benefits of breastfeeding for the infant. Effect of breastfeeding duration and exclusivity. *Pediatr Clin North Am* 48:105–123, 2001.

Heiskanen K, Siimes MA, Perheentupe J, Salmenpera L: Risk of low vitamin B-6 status in infants breast-fed exclusively beyond six months. *J Pediatr Gastroenterol Nutr* 23:38–44, 1996.

Heisler M, Vijan S, Anderson RM, Ubel PA, Bernstein SJ, Hofer TP: When do patients and their physicians agree on diabetes treatment goals and strategies, and what difference does it make? *J Gen Intern Med* 18:893–902, 2003.

Helland IB, Smith L, Saarem K, Saugstad OD, Drevon CA: Maternal supplementation with very-long-chain n-3 fatty acids during pregnancy and lactation augments children's IQ at 4 years of age. *Pediatrics* 111:e39–e44, 2003.

Henderson RA, Jensen RG, Lammi-Keefe CJ, Ferris AM, Dardick KR: Effect of fish oil on the fatty acid composition of human milk and maternal and infant erythrocytes. *Lipids* 27:863–869, 1992.

Hendrick V, Fukuchi A, Altshuler L, Widawski M, Wertheimer A, Brunhuber MV: Use of sertraline, paroxetine and fluvoxamine by nursing women. *Br J Psychiatry* 179:163–166, 2001.

Heron J, O'Connor TG, Evans J, Golding J, Glover V; the ALSPAC Study Team: The course of depression through pregnancy and the postpartum in a community sample. *J Affect Disord* 80:65–73, 2004.

HFBC—Hormonal Factors in Breast Cancer Collaborative Group: Breast cancer and breastfeeding: collaborative reanalysis of individual data from 47 epidemiological studies in 30 countries, including 50,302 women with breast cancer and 96,973 women without the disease. *Lancet* 360:187–195, 2002.

Hill ID, Bhatnagar S, Cameron DJ, De Rosa S, Maki M, Russell GJ, Troncone R: Celiac disease: Working Group report of the First World Congress of Pediatric Gastroenterology, Hepatology, and Nutrition. *J Pediatr Gastroenterol Nutr* 35:78–88, 2002.

Hilson JA, Rasmussen KM, Kjolhede CL: Maternal obesity and breast-feeding success in a rural population of Caucasian women. *Am J Clin Nutr* 66:1371–1378, 1997.

Hilson JA, Rasmussen KM, Kjolhede CL: High prepregnant body mass index is associated with poor lactation outcomes among white, rural women independent of psychosocial and demographic correlates. *J Hum Lact* 20:18–29, 2004.

Hoffbrand S, Howard L, Crawley H: Antidepressant drug treatment for postnatal depression. *Cochrane Database Syst Rev* 2001; (2):CD002018.

Holden JM: Postnatal depression: its nature, effects, and identification using the Edinburgh Postnatal Depression Scale. *Birth* 18:211–221, 1991.

Holick MF: Vitamin D: importance in the prevention of cancers, type 1 diabetes, heart disease, and osteoporosis. *Am J Clin Nutr* 79:362–371, 2004.

Holl RW, Boehm B, Loos U, Grabert M, Heinze E, Homoki J: Thyroid autoimmunity in children and adolescents with type 1 diabetes mellitus. Effect of age, gender and HLA type. *Horm Res* 52:113–118, 1999.

Hollis BW, Wagner CL: Vitamin D requirements during lactation: high-dose maternal supplementation as therapy to prevent hypovitaminosis D for both the mother and the nursing infant. *Am J Clin Nutr* 80 (Suppl 6):1752S–1758S, 2004.

Holmberg H, Wahlberg J, Vaarala O, Ludvigsson J; ABIS Study Group: Short duration of breastfeeding as a risk factor for beta-cell autoantibodies in 5-year-old children from the general population. *Br J Nutr* 97:111–116, 2007.

Home P: Contributions of basal and postprandial hyperglycemia to micro- and macrovascular complications in people with type 2 diabetes. *Curr Med Res Opin* 21:989–998, 2005.

Hoppu U, Kalliomaki M, Laiho K, Isolauri E: Breast milk—immunomodulatory signals against allergic diseases. *Allergy* 56 (Suppl 67):23–26, 2001.

Horvath A, Koletzko B, Kalisz M, Szajewska H: The effect of supplemental fluids or feedings during the first days of life on the success and duration of breastfeeding: a systematic review of randomized controlled trials. *Arch Pediatr Adolesc Med* 159:597–598, 2005.

Horwood LJ, Darlow BA, Mogridge N: Breast milk feeding and cognitive ability at 7–8 years. *Arch Dis Child Fetal Neonatal Ed* 84:F23–F27, 2001.

Host A, Husby S, Osterballe O: A prospective study of cow's milk allergy in exclusively breastfed infants. Incidence, pathogenetic role of early inadvertent exposure to cow's milk formula, and characterization of bovine milk protein in human milk. *Acta Paediatr Scand* 77:663–670, 1988.

Houseknecht KL, McGuire MK, Portocarrero CP, McGuire MA, Beerman K: Leptin is present in human milk and is related to maternal plasma leptin concentration and adiposity. *Biochem Biophys Res Commun* 240:742–747, 1997.

Howard CR, Howard FM, Weitzman M, Lawrence R: Antenatal formula advertising: another potential threat to breastfeeding. *Pediatrics* 94:102–104, 1994.

Howard CR, Lawrence RA: Drugs and breastfeeding. *Clin Perinatol* 26:447–478, 1999.

Howard CR, Howard FM, Lanphear B, Eberly S, deBlieck EA, Oakes D, Lawrence RA: Randomized clinical trial of pacifier use and bottle-feeding or cupfeeding and their effect on breastfeeding. *Pediatrics* 111:511–518, 2003.

Howard CR, Howard FM: Management of breastfeeding when the mother is ill. *Clin Obstet Gynecol* 47:683–695, 2004.

Howell EA, Mora PA, Horowitz CR, Leventhal H: Racial and ethnic differences in factors associated with early postpartum depressive symptoms. *Obstet Gynecol* 105:1442–1450, 2005.

Howie PW, Forsyth JS, Ogston SA, Clark A, Florey CD: Protective effect of breastfeeding against infection. *BMJ* 300:11–16, 1990.

Howie PW: Protective effect of breastfeeding against infection in the first and second six months of life. *Adv Exp Med Biol* 503:141–147, 2002.

Hubinont CJ, Balasse H, Dufrane SP, Leclercq-Meyer V, Sugar J, Schwers J, Malaisse WJ: Changes in pancreatic B cell function during late pregnancy, early lactation and postlactation. *Gynecol Obstet Invest* 25:89–95, 1988.

Huisman M, van Beusekom CM, Lanting CI, Nijeboer HJ, Muskiet FA, Boersma ER: Triglycerides, fatty acids, sterols, mono- and disaccharides and sugar alcohols in human milk and current types of infant formula milk. *Eur J Clin Nutr* 50:255–260, 1996.

Hummel M, Fuchtenbusch M, Schenker M, Ziegler AG: No major association of breast-feeding, vaccinations, and childhood viral diseases with early islet autoimmunity in the German BABYDIAB Study. *Diabetes Care* 23:969–974, 2000.

Hummel S, Hummel M, Banholzer J, Hanak D, Mollenhauer U, Bonifacio E, Ziegler AG: Development of autoimmunity to transglutaminase C in children of patients with type 1 diabetes: relationship to islet autoantibodies and infant feeding. *Diabetologia* 50:390–394, 2007.

Hussain SF: Progestogen-only pills and high blood pressure: is there an association? A literature review. *Contraception* 69:89–97, 2004.

Huutunen K, Gronhagen-Riska C, Fyhrquist F: Enalapril treatment of a nursing mother with slightly impaired renal function. *Clin Nephrol* 31:278, 1989.

Hypponen E, Kenward MG, Virtanen SM, Piitlainen A, Virta-Autio P, Tuomilehto J, Knip M, Akerblom HK; the Childhood Diabetes in Finland (DIME) Study Group: Infant feeding, early weight gain, and risk of type 1 diabetes. *Diabetes Care* 22:1961–1999, 1999.

Hypponen E, Virtanen S, Kenward M, Knip M, Akerblom H; Childhood Diabetes in Finland Study Group: Obesity, increased linear growth and risk of type 1 diabetes in children. *Diabetes Care* 23:1755–1760, 2000.

Hypponen E, Laara E, Reunanen A, Jarvelin MR, Virtanen SM: Intake of vitamin D and risk of type 1 diabetes: a birth cohort study. *Lancet* 358:1500–1503, 2001.

Innis SM, King DJ: *trans* fatty acids in human milk are inversely associated with concentrations of essential *all-cis* n-6 and n-3 fatty acids and determine *trans*, but not n-6 and n-3, fatty acids in plasma lipids of breast-fed infants. *Am J Clin Nutr* 70:383–390, 1999.

Insull W, Hirsch T, James T, Ahrens EH: The fatty acids of human milk. II. Alterations produced by manipulation of caloric balance and exchange of dietary fats. *J Clin Invest* 38:443–450, 1959.

IOM—Institute of Medicine: *Nutrition During Lactation.* Washington, DC: National Academies Press; 1991. Available at: http://www.nap.edu/catalog.php?record_id=1577. Accessed March 12, 2008.

IOM—Institute of Medicine, Food and Nutrition Board: *Dietary Reference Intakes for Calcium, Phosphorus, Magnesium, Vitamin D, and Fluoride.* Washington, DC: National Academies Press; 1997. Available at: http://www.nap.edu/catalog.php?record_id=5776. Accessed March 12, 2008.

IOM—Institute of Medicine, Food and Nutrition Board: *Dietary Reference Intakes for Thiamin, Riboflavin, Niacin, Vitamin B-6, Folate, Vitamin B-12, Pantothenic Acid, Biotin, and Choline.* Washington, DC: National Academies Press; 1998. Available at: http://www.nap.edu/catalog.php?record_id=6015. Accessed March 12, 2008.

IOM—Institute of Medicine, Food and Nutrition Board: *Dietary Reference Intakes for Vitamin C, Vitamin E, Selenium, and Carotenoids.* Washington, DC: National Academies Press; 2000a. Available at: http://www.nap.edu/catalog.php?record_id=9810. Accessed March 12, 2008.

IOM—Institute of Medicine, Food and Nutrition Board: *Dietary Reference Intakes: Applications in Dietary Assessment.* Washington, DC: National Academies Press; 2000b. Available at: http://www.nap.edu/catalog.php?record_id=9956. Accessed March 12, 2008.

IOM—Institute of Medicine, Food and Nutrition Board: *Dietary Reference Intakes for Vitamin A, Vitamin K, Arsenic, Boron, Chromium, Copper, Iodine, Iron, Manganese, Molybdenum, Nickel, Silicon, Vanadium, and Zinc.* Washington, DC: National Academies Press; 2001. Available at: http://www.nap.edu/catalog.php?record_id=10026. Accessed March 12, 2008.

IOM—Institute of Medicine, Food and Nutrition Board: *Dietary Reference Intakes for Energy, Carbohydrate, Fiber, Fat, Fatty Acids, Cholesterol, Protein and Amino Acids (Macronutrients).* Washington, DC: National Academies Press; 2002. Available at: http://www.nap.edu/catalog.php?record_id=10490. Accessed March 12, 2008.

IOM—Institute of Medicine, Food and Nutrition Board: *Dietary Reference Intakes for Water, Potassium, Sodium, Chloride, and Sulfate.* Washington, DC: National Academies Press; 2004. Available at: http://www.nap.edu/catalog.php?record_id=10925. Accessed March 12, 2008.

Ip S, Chung M, Raman G, Chew P, Magula N, DeVine D, Trikalinos T, Lau J: Breastfeeding and maternal and infant health outcomes in developed countries. *Evid Rep Technol Assess (Full Rep)* (153):1–186, 2007.

Ivarsson A, Hernell O, Stenlund H, Persson LA: Breast-feeding protects against celiac disease. *Am J Clin Nutr* 75:914–921, 2002.

Jackson MB, Lammi-Keefe CJ, Jensen RG, Couch SC, Ferris AM: Total lipid and fatty acid composition of milk from women with and without insulin-dependent diabetes mellitus. *Am J Clin Nutr* 60:353–361, 1994.

Jacobsen T: Effects of postpartum disorders on parenting and on offspring. In: Miller LJ, ed. *Postpartum Mood Disorders.* Washington, DC: American Psychiatric Press; 1999:119–139.

Janney CA, Xhang D, Sowers M: Lactation and weight retention. *Am J Clin Nutr* 66:1116–1124, 1997.

Janssen HJEM, Cuisinier MCJ, Hoogduin KAL, de Graauw KP: Controlled prospective study on the mental health of women after pregnancy loss. *Am J Psychiatry* 153:226–230, 1996.

Jansson R, Bernander S, Karlsson A, Levin K, Nilsson G: Autoimmune thyroid dysfunction in the postpartum period. *J Clin Endocrinol Metab* 58:681–687, 1984.

Jensen RG, Ferris AM, Lammi-Keefe CJ: Lipids in human milk and infant formulas. *Annu Rev Nutr* 12:417–441, 1992.

Jensen RG: The lipids in human milk. *Prog Lipid Res* 35:53–92, 1996.

Jensen RG: Lipids in human milk. *Lipids* 34:1243–1271, 1999.

Jensen CL, Maude M, Anderson RE, Heird WC: Effect of docosahexaenoic acid supplementation of lactating women on the fatty acid composition of breast milk lipids and maternal and infant plasma lipids. *Am J Clin Nutr* 71 (Suppl): 292S–299S, 2000.

Jensen CL, Voight RG, Prager TC, Zou YL, Fraley JK, Rozelle JC, Turcich MR, Llorente AM, Anderson RE, Heird WC: Effects of maternal docosahexaenoic acid intake on visual function and neurodevelopment in breastfed term infants. *Am J Clin Nutr* 82:125–132, 2005a.

Jensen TK, Grandjean P, Jorgensen EB, White RF, Debes F, Weihe P: Effects of breast feeding on neuropsychological development in a community with methylmercury exposure from seafood. *Expo Anal Environ Epidemiol* 15: 423–430, 2005b.

Jensen CL: Effects of n-3 fatty acids during pregnancy and lactation. *Am J Clin Nutr* 83:S1452–S1457, 2006.

Johansen K, Andersen AN, Kampmann JP, Hansen JM, Mortensen HB: Excretion of methimazole in human milk. *J Clin Pharmacol* 23:339–341, 1982.

Johansson C, Samuelsson U, Ludvigsson J: A high weight gain early in life is associated with an increased risk of type 1 (insulin-dependent) diabetes mellitus. *Diabetologia* 37:91–94, 1994.

Johnson GH, Keast DR, Kris-Etherton PM: Dietary modeling shows that the substitution of canola oil for fats commonly used in the United States would increase compliance with dietary recommendations for fatty acids. *J Am Diet Assoc* 107:1726–1734, 2007.

Johnston M, Craves C, Arbogast PG, Cooper WO: Feeding attitudes of pregnant women with diabetes. *Diabetes Care* 29:1457–1458, 2006.

Jones HM, Cummings AJ, Setchell KD, Lawson AM: A study of the disposition of alpha-methyldopa in newborn infants following its administration to the mother for the treatment of hypertension during pregnancy. *Br J Clin Pharmacol* 8: 433–440, 1979.

Jones ME, Swerdlow AJ, Gill LE, Goldacre MJ: Pre-natal and early life risk factors for childhood onset diabetes mellitus: a record linkage study. *Int J Epidemiol* 27: 444–449, 1998.

Josefsson A, Berg G, Nordin C, Sydsjo G: Prevalence of depressive symptoms in late pregnancy and postpartum. *Acta Obstet Gynecol Scand* 80:251–255, 2001.

Jovanovic L, ed. *Medical Management of Pregnancy Complicated by Diabetes.* 3rd ed. Alexandria, VA: American Diabetes Association; 1996:67–86.

Jovanovic-Peterson L, Fuhrmann K, Hedden K, Walker L, Peterson CM: Maternal milk and plasma glucose and insulin levels: studies in normal and diabetic subjects. *J Am Coll Nutr* 8:125–131, 1989.

Julius S, Nesbitt SD, Egan BM, Weber MA, Michelson EL, Kaciroti N, Black HR, Grimm RH, Messerli FH, Oparil S, Schork MA; Trial of Preventing Hypertension (TROPHY) Study Investigators: Feasibility of treating prehypertension with an angiotensin-receptor blocker. *N Engl J Med* 354: 1685–1697, 2006.

Kaaja RJ, Greer IA: Manifestations of chronic disease during pregnancy. *JAMA* 294:2751–2757, 2005.

Kac G, Benicio MHDA, Velasquez-Melendez G, Valente JG, Struchiner CJ: Breastfeeding and postpartum weight retention in a cohort of Brazilian women. *Am J Clin Nutr* 79:487–493, 2004.

Kampmann JP, Johansen K, Hansen JM, Helweg J: Propylthiouracil in human milk. *Lancet* 1:736–738, 1980.

Kang AK, Duncan JA, Cattran DC, Floras JS, Lai V, Scholey JW, Miller JA: Effect of oral contraceptives on the rennin-angiotensin system and renal function. *Am J Physiol* 280:R807–R813, 2001.

Kang-Yoon SA, Kirksey A, Giacoia G, West K: Vitamin B-6 status of breast-fed neonates: influence of pyridoxine supplementation on mothers and neonates. *Am J Clin Nutr* 56:548–558, 1992.

Karamanlis A, Chaikomin R, Doran S, Bellon M, Bartholomeusz FD, Wishart JM, Jones KL, Horowitz M, Rayner CK: Effects of protein on glycemic and incretin responses and gastric emptying after oral glucose in healthy subjects. *Am J Clin Nutr* 86:1364–1368, 2007.

Karlson EW, Mandl LA, Hanknison Grodstein F: Do breast-feeding and other reproductive factors influence future risk of rheumatoid arthritis? Results from the Nurses' Health Study. *Arthritis Rheum* 50:3458–3467, 2004.

Karter AJ, Ackerson LM, Darbinian JA, D'Agostino RB, Ferrara A, Liu J, Selby JV: Self-monitoring of blood glucose levels and glycemic control: the Northern California Kaiser Permanente Diabetes Registry. *Am J Med* 111:1–9, 2001.

Katon W, Von Korff M, Ciechanowski P, Russo J, Lin E, Simon G, Ludman E, Walker E, Bush T, Young B: Bahavioral and clinical factors associated with depression among individuals with diabetes. *Diabetes Care* 27:914–920, 2004.

Kaufman I, Bondy R, Benjamin A: Peripartum cardiomyopathy and thromboembolism; anesthetic management and clinical course of an obese, diabetic patient. *Can J Anesth* 50:161–165, 2003.

Kaufmann R, Foxman B: Mastitis among lactating women: occurrence and risk factors. *Soc Sci Med* 33:701–705, 1991.

Kaukinen K, Salmi J, Lahtela J, Siljamaki-Ojansuu U, Koivisto AM, Oksa H, Collin P: No effect of gluten-free diet on the metabolic control of type 1 diabetes in patients with diabetes and celiac disease. *Diabetes Care* 22: 1747–1748, 1999.

Kelkar PS, Li JT: Cephalosporin allergy. *N Engl J Med* 345:804–809, 2001.

Kelly D, Coutts AGP: Early nutrition and the development of immune function in the neonate. *Proc Nutr Soc* 59:177–185, 2000.

Kennedy KI, Rivera R, McNeilly AS: Consesus statement on the use of breastfeeding as a family planning method. *Contraception* 39:477–496, 1989.

Kent LS, Laidlaw JD: Suspected congenital sertraline dependence. *Br J Psychiatry* 167:412–413, 1995.

Kent JC, Mitoulas LR, Cregan MD, Ramsay DT, Doherty DA: Volume and frequency of breastfeedings and fat content of breast milk throughout the day. *Pediatrics* 117:e387–e395, 2006.

Kerssen A, Evers IM, de Valk HW, Visser GH: Effect of breast milk of diabetic mothers on bodyweight of the offspring in the first year of life. *Eur J Clin Nutr* 58:1429–1431, 2004.

Kesseru EV, Aydinlik S, Etchepareborda JJ, Kaufmann J: A multicentered, two-year, phase III clinical trial of norethisterone enanthate 50 mg plus estradiol valerate 5 mg as a monthly injectable contraceptive. *Contraception* 44: 589–598, 1991.

Khader YS, Rice J, John L, Abueita O: Oral contraceptives use and the risk of myocardial infarction: a meta-analysis. *Contraception* 2003, 68:11–17, 2003.

Khan N, Couper JJ: Low-birth-weight infants show earlier onset of IDDM. *Diabetes Care* 17:653–656, 1994.

Kibiridge M, Metcalf B, Renuka R, Wilkin TJ: Testing the accelerator hypothesis. The relationship between body mass and age at diagnosis of type 1 diabetes. *Diabetes Care* 26:2865–2870, 2003.

Kilpatrick ES, Rigby AS, Atkin SL: The effect of glucose variability on the risk of microvascular complications in type 1 diabetes. *Diabetes Care* 29:1486–1490, 2006.

Kim C, Seidel KW, Begier EA, Kwok YS: Diabetes and depot medroxyprogesterone contraception in Navajo women. *Arch Intern Med* 161:1766–1771, 2001.

Kim C, Siscovick DS, Sidney S, Lewis CE, Kiefe CI, Koepsell TD: Oral contraceptive use and association with glucose, insulin, and diabetes in young adult women. The CARDIA Study. *Diabetes Care* 25:1027–1032, 2002.

Kimmerle R, Weiss R, Berger M, Kurz K-H: Effectiveness, safety and acceptablilty of a copper intrauterine device (CU Safe 300) in type I diabetic women. *Diabetes Care* 16:1227–1230, 1993.

Kimpimaki T, Erkkola M, Korhonen S, Kupila A, Virtanen SM, Ilonen J, Simell O, Knip M: Short-term exclusive breastfeeding predisposes young children with increased genetic risk of type I diabetes to progressive beta-cell autoimmunity. *Diabetologia* 44:63–69, 2001.

Kjaer K, Hagen C, Sando SH, Eshoj O: Contraception in women with IDDM: an epidemiological study. *Diabetes Care* 15:1585–1590, 1992.

Kjos SL, Shoupe D, Douyan S, Friedman RL, Bernstein GS, Mestman JH, Mishell DR Jr: Effect of low-dose oral contraceptives on carbohydrate and lipid metabolism in women with recent gestational diabetes: results of a controlled, randomized, prospective study. *Am J Obstet Gynecol* 163:1822–1827, 1990.

Kjos SL, Henry O, Lee RM, Buchanan TA, Mishell DR Jr: The effect of lactation on glucose and lipid metabolism in women with recent gestational diabetes. *Obstet Gynecol* 82:451–455, 1993.

Kjos SL, Ballagh SA, La Cour M, Xiang A, Mishell DR, Jr: The copper T380A intrauterine device in women with type II diabetes mellitus. *Obstet Gynecol* 84:1006–1009, 1994.

Kjos SL, Peters RK, Xiang A, Thomas D, Schaefer U, Buchanan TA: Contraception and the risk of type 2 diabetes mellitus in Latina women with prior gestational diabetes mellitus. *JAMA* 280:533–538, 1998.

Kjos SL: Postpartum care of the woman with diabetes. *Clin Obstet Gynecol* 43:75–86, 2000.

Kjos SL, Buchanan TA: Postpartum management, lactation, and contraception. In: Reece EA, Coustan DR, Gabbe SG, eds. *Diabetes in Women. Adolescence, Pregnancy, and Menopause.* Philadelphia: Lippincott Williams & Wilkins; 2004:441–449.

Kjos SL: After pregnancy complicated by diabetes: postpartum care and education. *Obstet Gynecol Clin North Am* 34:335–349, 2007.

Klaus MH: The frequency of suckling. A neglected but essential ingredient of breast-feeding. *Obstet Gynecol Clin North Am* 14:623–633, 1987.

Klein BEK, Moss SE, Klein R: Oral contraceptives in women with diabetes. *Diabetes Care* 13:895–898, 1990.

Kleinman RE: Complementary feeding. In: *Pediatric Nutrition Handbook.* 5th ed. Elk Grove Village, IL: American Academy of Pediatrics; 2004:103–115.

Klement E, Cohen RV, Boxman J, Joseph A, Reif S: Breastfeeding and risk of inflammatory bowel disease: a systematic review with meta-analysis. *Am J Clin Nutr* 80:1342–1352, 2004.

Klemetti P, Savilahti E, Ilonen J, Akerblom HK, Vaarala O: T-cell reactivity to wheat gluten in patients with insulin-dependent diabetes mellitus. *Scand J Immunol* 47:48–53, 1998.

Klinke J, Toth EL: Preconception care for women with type 1 diabetes. *Can Fam Physician* 49:769–773, 2003.

Knerr I, Wolf J, Reinehr T, Stachow R, Grabert M, Schober E, Rascher W, Holl RW; DPV Scientific Initiative of Germany and Austria: The 'accelerator hypothesis': relationship between weight, height, body mass index and age at diagnosis in a large cohort of 9,248 German and Austrian children with type 1 diabetes mellitus. *Diabetologia* 48:2501–2504, 2005.

Knip M: Cow's milk and the new trials for prevention of type 1 diabetes. *J Endocrinol Invest* 26:265–267, 2003.

Knip M, Akerblom HK: Early nutrition and later diabetes risk. *Adv Exp Med Biol* 569:142–150, 2005.

Knopp RH, Walden CE, Wahl PW, Hoover JJ: Effects of oral contraceptives on lipoprotein triglyceride and cholesterol: relationships to estrogen and progestin potency. *Am J Obstet Gynecol* 142:725–731, 1982.

Knopp RH, Walden CE, Wahl PW, Bergelin RO, Chapman M, Irvine S, Albers JJ: Effect of postpartum lactation on lipoprotein lipids and apoproteins. *J Clin Endocrinol Metab* 60:542–547, 1985.

Knopp RH, LaRosa JC, Burkman RT Jr: Contraception and dyslipidemia. *Am J Obstet Gynecol* 168:1994–2005, 1993.

Knudsen A, Pedersen H, Klebe JG: Impact of smoking on the duration of breastfeeding in mothers with insulin-dependent diabetes mellitus. *Acta Paediatr* 90:926–930, 2001.

Kodonouri O, Klinghammer A, Lang EB, Gruters-Kieslich A, Grabert M, Holl RW: Thyroid autoimmunity in children and adolescents with type 1 diabetes mellitus; a multicenter survey. *Diabetes Care* 25:1346–1350, 2002.

Kodonouri O, Hartmann R, Deiss D, Wilms M, Gruters-Kieslich A: Natural course of autoimmune thyroiditis in type 1 diabetes: association with gender, age, diabetes duration, and puberty. *Arch Dis Child* 90:411–414, 2005.

Koletzko B, Mrotzek M, Bremer HJ: Fatty acid composition of mature human milk in Germany. *Am J Clin Nutr* 47:954–959, 1988.

Koletzko B, Bremer HJ: Fat content and fatty acid composition of infant formulas. *Acta Pediatr Scand* 78:513–521, 1989.

Koletzko B: Potential adverse effects of trans fatty acids in infants and children. *Eur J Med Res* 1:123–125, 1995.

Koletzko B, Rodriguez-Palmiero M: Polyunsaturated fatty acids in human milk and their role in early infant development. *J Mammary Gland Biol Neoplasia* 4: 269–284, 1999.

Koletzko B, Rodriguez-Palmero M, Demmelmair H, Fidler N, Jensen R, Sauerwald T: Physiological aspects of human milk lipids. *Early Hum Dev* 65 (Suppl): S3–S18, 2001.

Koletzko B, Broekaert I, Demmelmair H, Franke J, Hannibal I, Oberle D, Schiess S, Baumann BT, Verwied-Jorky S; on behalf of the EU Childhood Obesity Project: Protein intake in the first year of life: a risk factor for later obesity? *Adv Exp Med Biol* 569:69–79, 2005.

Konje JC, Otolorin EO, Ladipo AO: The effect of continuous subdermal levonorgestrel (Norplant) on carbohydrate metabolism. *Am J Obstet Gynecol* 166:15–19, 1991.

Kornstein SG, Schatzberg AF, Thase ME, Yonkers KA, McCullough JP, Keitner GI, Gelenberg AJ, Davis SM, Harrison WM, Keller MB: Gender differences in treatment response to sertraline versus imipramine in chronic depression. *Am J Psychiatry* 157:1445–1452, 2000.

Kovar MG, Serdula MK, Marks JS, Fraser DW: Review of the epidemiological evidence for an association between infant feeding and infant health. *Pediatrics* 74:615–638, 1984.

Kraemer J, Klein J, Lubetsky A, Koren G: Perfusion studies of glyburide transfer across the human placenta: implications for fetal safety. *Am J Obstet Gynecol* 195:270–274, 2006.

Kramer MS, Barr RG, Leduc DG, Boisjoly C, Pless IB: Infant determinants of childhood weight and adiposity. *J Pediatr* 107:104–107, 1985.

Kramer FM, Stunkard AJ, Marshall KA, McKinney S, Liebschutz J: Breast-feeding reduces maternal lower-body fat. *J Am Diet Assoc* 93:429–433, 1993.

Kramer MS, Chalmers B, Hodnett ED, Sevkovskaya Z, Dzikovich I, Shapiro S, Collet J-P, Vanilovich I, Mezen I, Ducruet T, Shishko G, Zubovich V, Mknuik D, Gluchanina E, Dombrovskiy V, Ustinovitch A, Kot T, Bogdanovich N, Ovchinikova L, Helsing E; for the PROBIT Study Group: Promotion of Breastfeeding Intervention Trial (PROBIT). A randomized trial in the Republic of Belarus. *JAMA* 285:413–420, 2001a.

Kramer MS, Barr RG, Dagenais S, Yang H, Jones P, Ciofani L, Jane F: Pacifier use, early weaning, and cry/fuss behavior: a randomized controlled trial. *JAMA* 286:322–326, 2001b.

Kramer MS, Kakuma R: The optimal duration of exclusive breastfeeding. *Cochrane Database Syst Rev* 2002a;(3):CD003517.

Kramer MS, Guo T, Platt RW, Shapiro S, Collet J-P, Chalmers B, Hodnett E, Sevkovskaya Z, Dzikovich I, Vanilovich I; for the PROBIT Study Group: Breastfeeding and infant growth: biology or bias? *Pediatrics* 110:343–347, 2002b.

Kramer MS, Guo T, Platt RW, Sevskokaya Z, Dzikovich I, Collet J-P, Shapiro S, Chalmers B, Hodnett E, Vanilovich I, Mezen I, Ducruet T, Shishko G, Bogdanovich N: Infant growth and health outcomes associated with 3 compared with 6 mo of exclusive breastfeeding. *Am J Clin Nutr* 78:291–295, 2003.

Kramer MS, Guo T, Platt RW, Vanilovich I, Sevkovskaya Z, Dzikovich I, Michaelsen KF, Dewey K; Promotion of Breastfeeding Intervention Trial Study Group: Feeding effects on growth during infancy. *J Pediatr* 145:600–605, 2004.

Kramer MS, Matush L, Vanilovich I, Platt RW, Bogdanovich N, Sevkovskaya Z, Dzikovich I, Shishko G, Collet J-P, Martin RM, Smith GD, Gillman MW, Chalmers B, Hodnett E, Shapiro S; the Promotion of Breastfeeding Intervention Trial (PROBIT) Study Group: Effects of prolonged and exclusive breastfeeding on child height, weight, adiposity, and blood pressure at age 6.5 y: evidence from a large randomized trial. *Am J Clin Nutr* 86:1717–1721, 2007.

Kramer MS, Fombonne E, Igumov S, Matush L, Mironova E, Bogdanovich N, Tremblay RE, Chalmers B, Zhang X, Platt RW; the Promotion of Breastfeeding Intervention (PROBIT) Study Group: Effects of prolonged and exclusive breastfeeding on child behavior and maternal adjustment: evidence from a large, randomized trial. e.435–e.440 abstract. *Pediatrics* 121:591, 2008.

Kristensen JH, Hackett LP, Kohan R, Paech M, Ilett KF: The amount of fluvoxamine in milk is unlikely to be a cause of adverse effects in breastfed infants. *J Hum Lact* 18:138–143, 2002.

Kuczmarksi RJ, Ogden CL, Grummer-Strawn LM, Flegal KM, Guo SS, Wei R, Mei Z, Curtin LR, Roche AF, Johnson CL: CDC growth charts: United States. Advance data from vital and health statistics: #314. Hyattsville, MD: National Center for Health Statistics; 2000.

Kugyelka JG, Rasmussen KM, Frongillo EA: Maternal obesity is negatively associated with breastfeeding success among Hispanic but not Black women. *J Nutr* 134:1746–1753, 2004.

Kulas J, Lunell NO, Rosing U, Steen B, Rane A: Atenolol and metoprolol. A comparison of their excretion into human breast milk. *Acta Obstet Gynecol Scand* 118 (Suppl):65–69, 1984.

Kull I, Almqvist C, Lilja G, Pershagen G, Wickman M: Breast-feeding reduces the risk of asthma during the first 4 years of life. *J Allergy Clin Immunol* 114: 755–760, 2004.

Kull I, Boehme M, Wahlgren C-F, Nordvall L, Pershagen G, Wickman M: Breast-feeding reduces the risk for childhood eczema. *J Allergy Clin Immunol* 116: 657–661, 2005.

Kulski JK, Hartmann PE: Changes in human milk composition during the initiation of lactation. *Aust J Exp Biol Med Sci* 59:101–114, 1981a.

Kulski JK, Smith M, Hartmann PE: Normal and cesarean section delivery and the initiation of lactation in women. *Aust J Exp Biol Med Sci* 59:405–412, 1981b.

Kunz C, Rodriguez-Palmiero M, Koletzko B, Jensen R: Nutritional and biochemical properties of milk, part I: general aspects, proteins, and carbohydrates. *Clin Perinatol* 26:307–333, 1999.

Kvaavik E, Tell GS, Klepp K-I: Surveys of Norwegian youth indicated that breast feeding reduced subsequent risk of obesity. *J Clin Epidemiol* 58:849–855, 2005.

Kwan ML, Buffler PA, Wiemels JL, Metayer C, Selvin S, Dulore JM, Block G: Breastfeeding patterns and risk of childhood acute lymphoblastic leukemia. *Br J Cancer* 93:379–384, 2005.

Labbok M, Perez A, Valdes V, Sevilla F, Wade K, Laukaran VH, Cooney KA, Coly S, Sanders C, Queenan JT: The Lactational Amenorrhea Method (LAM): a postpartum introductory family planning method with policy and program implications. *Adv Contracept* 10:93–109, 1994.

Labbok MH: Health sequelae of breastfeeding for the mother. *Clin Perinatol* 26:491–503, 1999.

Lambert M, Weinert L, Hibbard J, Korcarz C, Lindheimer M, Lang RM: Contractile reserve in patients with peripartum cardiomyopathy and recovered left ventricular function. *Am J Obstet Gynecol* 176:189–195, 1997.

Lammi-Keefe CJ, Jonas CR, Ferris AM, Capacchione CM: Vitamin E in plasma and milk of lactating women with insulin-dependent diabetes mellitus. *J Pediatr Gastroenterol Nutr* 20:305–309, 1995.

Lampert MB, Lang RM: Peripartum cardiomyopathy. *Am Heart J* 130:860–870, 1995.

Lane RH, Dvorak B, MacLennan NK, Dvorakova K, Halpern MD, Pham TD, Philipps AF: IGF alters jejunal glucose transporter expression and serum glucose levels in immature rats. *Am J Physiol* 283:R1450–R1560, 2002.

Lanting C, Fidler V, Huisman M, Touwen BC, Boersma ER: Neurological differences between 9-year old children fed breast-milk or formula-milk as babies. *Lancet* 344:1319–1322, 1994.

Lanting CI, Patandin S, Weisglas-Kuperus N, Touwen BCL, Boersma ER: Breastfeeding and neurological outcome at 42 months. *Acta Paediatr* 87:1224–1229, 1998.

Larsen LA, Ito S, Koren G: Prediction of milk/plasma concentration ratio of drugs. *Ann Pharmacother* 37:1299–1306, 2003.

Lau C: Effects of stress on lactation. *Pediatr Clin North Am* 48:221–234, 2001.

Laubereau B, Brockow I, Zirngibl A, Koletzko S, Gruebl A, von Berg A, Filipiak-Pittroff B, Berdel D, Bauer CP, Reinhardt D, Heinrich J, Wichmann HE: the GINI Study Group: Effect of breast-feeding on the development of atopic dermatitis during the first 3 years of life—results from the GINI–birth cohort study. *J Pediatr* 144:602–607, 2004.

Lauritzen L, Hansen HS, Jorgensen MH, Michaelsen KF: The essentiality of long-chain *n*-3 fatty acids in relation to development and function of the brain and retina. *Prog Lipid Res* 40:1–94, 2001.

Lawless M, Vessey MP: Intrauterine device use by diabetic women. *Br J Fam Plan* 7:110–111, 1982.

Lawrence RM, Lawrence RA: Given the benefits of breastfeeding, what contraindications exist? *Pediatr Clin North Am* 48:235–251, 2001.

Lawrence RA, Lawrence RM: *Breastfeeding. A Guide for the Medical Profession.* 6th ed. New York: Elsevier Mosby; 2005.

Lawrenson RA, Leydon GM, Williams TJ, Newsom RB, Feher MD: Patterns of contraception in UK women with type 1 diabetes mellitus: a GP data base study. *Diabet Med* 16:395–399, 1999.

Lawton ME: Alcohol in breast milk. *Aust N Z J Obstet Gynecol* 25:71–73, 1985.

Lazarus JH, Hall R, Othman S, Parkes AB, Richards CJ, McCulloch B, Harris B: The clinical spectrum of postpartum thyroid disease. *QJM* 89:429–435, 1996.

Lazarus JH: Clinical manifestations of postpartum thyroid disease. *Thyroid* 9:685–689, 1999.

Leguizamon G, Igarzabal ML, Reece EA: Periconceptional care of women with diabetes mellitus. *Obstet Gynecol Clin North Am* 34:225–239, 2007.

Lenz S, Kuhl C, Hornnes PJ, Hagen C: Influence of lactation on oral glucose tolerance in the puerperium. *Acta Endocrinol (Copenh)* 98:428–431, 1981.

Levitan AA, Manion JC: Propranolol therapy during pregnancy and lactation. *Am J Cardiol* 32:247, 1973.

Lev-Ran A: Sharp temporary drop in insulin requirement after cesarean section in diabetic patients. *Am J Obstet Gynecol* 120:905–908, 1974.

Lewis DS, Bertrand HA, McMahon CA, McGill HC, Carey KD, Masoro EJ: Preweaning food intake influences the adiposity of young adult baboons. *J Clin Invest* 78:899–905, 1986.

Lewis MA, Heinemann LA, Spitzer WO, MacRae KD, Bruppacher R: The use of oral contraceptives and the occurrence of acute myocardial infarction in young women. Results from the Transnational Study on Oral Contraceptives and the Health of Young Women. *Contraception* 56:129–140, 1997.

Li R, Ogden C, Ballew C, Gillespie C, Grummer-Strawn LM: Prevalence of exclusive breastfeeding among U.S. infants: the Third National Health and Nutrition Examination Survey (Phase II, 1991–1994). *Am J Public Health* 92:1107–1110, 2002.

Li R, Jewell S, Grummer-Strawn L: Maternal obesity and breast-feeding practices. *Am J Clin Nutr* 77:931–936, 2003a.

Li L, Parsons TJ, Power C: Breast feeding and obesity in childhood: cross sectional study. *BMJ* 327:904–905, 2003b.

Libman IM, Pietropaolo M, Arslanian SA, LaPorte RE, Becker DJ: Changing prevalence of overweight children and adolescents at onset of insulin-treated diabetes. *Diabetes Care* 26:2871–2875, 2003.

Lidegaard O: Oral contraceptives, pregnancy and the risk of cerebral thromboembolism: the influence of diabetes, hypertension, migraine and previous thrombotic disease. *Br J Obstet Gynecol* 102:153–159, 1995.

Lie B, Juul J: Effect of epidural vs. general anesthesia on breastfeeding. *Acta Obstet Gynecol Scand* 67:207–209, 1988.

Liedholm H, Melander A, Bitzen PO, Helm G, Lonnerholm G, Mattiasson I, Nilsson B, Wahlin-Boll E: Accumulation of atenolol and metoprolol in human breast milk. *Eur J Clin Pharmacol* 20:229–231, 1981.

Liese AD, Hirsch T, von Mutuis E, Keil U, Leupold W, Weiland SK: Inverse association of overweight and breastfeeding in 9 to 10-y-old children in Germany. *Int J Obes* 25:1644–1650, 2001.

Liew DFM, Ng CSA, Yong YM, Ratnam SS: Long term effects of depo-provera on carbohydrate and lipid metabolism. *Contraception* 31:51–64,1985.

Lindeberg S, Sandstrom B, Lundborg P, Regardh CG: Disposition of the adrenergic blocker metoprolol in the late-pregnant woman, the amniotic fluid, the cord blood and the neonate. *Acta Obstet Gynecol Scand* 118 (Suppl):61–64, 1984.

Linne Y, Dye L, Barkeling B, Rossner S: Weight development over time in parous women—the SPAWN study—15 years follow-up. *Int J Obes Relat Metab Disord* 27:1516–1522, 2003.

Little RE, Anderson KW, Ervin CH, Worthington-Roberts B, Clarren SK: Maternal alcohol use during breastfeeding and infant mental and motor development at one year. *N Engl J Med* 321:425–430, 1989.

Locke R: Preventing obesity—the breast milk-leptin connection. *Acta Paediatr* 91:891–896, 2002.

Lonnerdal B: Effects of maternal dietary intake on human milk composition. *J Nutr* 116:499–513, 1986.

Lonnerdal B, Havel PJ: Serum leptin concentrations in infants: effects of diet, sex, and adiposity. *Am J Clin Nutr* 72:484–489, 2000.

Lopez LM, Grimes DA, Schulz KF: Steroidal contraceptives effect on carbohydrate metabolism in women without diabetes mellitus. *Cochrane Database Syst Rev* 2007 (2):CD006133.

Lovelady CA, Lonnerdal B, Dewey KG: Lactation performance of exercising women. *Am J Clin Nutr* 52:103–109, 1990.

Lovelady CA, Meredith CN, McCrory MA, Nommsen LA, Joseph LJ, Dewey KG: Energy expenditure in lactating women: a comparison of doubly labelled water and heart rate-monitoring methods. *Am J Clin Nutr* 57:512–518, 1993.

Lovelady CA, Nommsen-Rivers LA, McCrory MA, Dewey KG: Effects of exercise on plasma lipids and metabolism of lactating women. *Med Sci Sports Exerc* 27: 22–28, 1995.

Lovelady CA, Garner KE, Moreno KL, Williams JP: The effect of weight loss in overweight, lactating women on the growth of their infants. *N Engl J Med* 342:449–453, 2000.

Lovelady CA, Williams JP, Garner KE, Moreno KL, Taylor ML, Leklem JE: Effect of energy restriction and exercise on vitamin B-6 status of women during lactation. *Med Sci Sports Exerc* 33:512–518, 2001.

Lovelady CA: Is maternal obesity a cause of poor lactation performance? *Nutr Rev* 63:352–355, 2005.

Low LCK, Lang J, Alexander WD: Propylthiouracil in breast milk. *Lancet* 2:1011, 1979.

Lowe AJ, Carlin JB, Bennett CM, Abramson MJ, Hosking CS, Hill DJ, Dharmage SC: Atopic disease and breast feeding—cause or consequence? *J Allergy Clin Immunol* 117:682–687, 2006.

LRCP—Lipid Research Clinics Program: *The Lipid Research Clinics Population Studies Data Book.* Lipid Metabolism Branch, Division of Heart and Vascular Diseases, National Heart, Lung, and Blood Institute. Bethesda, MD: Department of Health and Human Services, Public Health Service, National Institutes of Health; 1980.

Lucas A, Adrian TE, Blackburn AN, Sarson DL, Aynsley-Green A, Bloom SR: Breast vs bottle: endocrine responses are different with formula feeding. *Lancet* 1: 1267–1269, 1980.

Lucas A, Bowes S, Bloom SR, Aynsley-Green A: Metabolic and endocrine responses to a milk feed in six-day-old term infants: differences between breast and cow's milk formula feeding. *Acta Paediatr Scand* 70:195–200, 1981.

Lucas A, Pizarro E, Granada ML, Salinas I, Roca J, Sanmarti A: Postpartum thyroiditis: a long-term follow-up. *Thyroid* 15:1177–1181, 2005.

Ludvigsson JF, Mostrom M, Ludvigsson J, Duchen K: Exclusive breastfeeding and risk of atopic dermatitis in some 8300 infants. *Pediatr Allergy Immunol* 16:201–208, 2005.

Ludwig P, Fischer E: Peripartum cardiomyopathy. *Aust N Z J Obstet Gynecol* 37:156–160, 1997.

Lunell NO, Kulas J, Rane A: Transfer of labetalol into amniotic fluid and breast milk in lactating women. *Eur J Clin Pharmacol* 28:597–599, 1985.

Lustman PJ, Anderson RJ, Freedland KE, deGroot M, Carney RM, Clouse RE: Depression and poor glycemic control: a meta-analytic review of the literature. *Diabetes Care* 23:934–942, 2000.

Lyle RE, Kincaid SC, Bryant JC: Human milk contains detectable levels of immunoreactive leptin. *Adv Exp Med Biol* 501:87–92, 2001.

MacNeill S, Dodds L, Hamilton DC, Armson BA, VandenHof M: Rates and risk factors for recurrence of gestational diabetes. *Diabetes Care* 24:659–662, 2001.

Madden JM, Soumerai SB, Lieu TA, Mandl KD, Zhang F, Ross-Degnan D: Effects on breastfeeding of changes in maternity length-of-stay policy in a large health maintenance organization. *Pediatrics* 111:519–524, 2003.

Makrides M, Neumann MA, Gibson RA: Effect of maternal docosahexaenoic acid (DHA) supplementation on breast milk composition. *Eur J Clin Nutr* 50:352–357, 1996.

Malcova H, Sumnik Z, Drevinek P, Venhacova J, Lebl J, Cinek O: Absence of breast-feeding is associated with the risk of type 1 diabetes: a case-contol study in a population with rapidly increasing incidence. *Eur J Pediatr* 165:114–119, 2006.

Mandel SJ, Cooper DS: The use of antithyroid drugs in pregnancy and lactation. Commentary. *J Clin Endocrinol Metab* 86:2354–2359, 2001.

Manninen AK, Juhakoski A: Nifedipine concentrations in maternal and umbilical serum, amniotic fluid, breast milk and urine of mothers and offspring. *Int J Clin Pharmacol Res* 11:231–236, 1991.

Manning-Dalton C, Allen LH: The effects of lactation on energy and protein consumption, postpartum weight change and body composition of well nourished North American women. *Nutr Res* 3:293–308, 1983.

Maragou NC, Makri A, Lampi EN, Thomaidis NS, Koupparis MA: Migration of bisphenol A from polycarbonate baby bottles under real use conditions. *Food Addit Contam* 25:373–383, 2008.

Marild S, Hansson S, Jodal U, Oden A, Svedberg K: Protective effect of breastfeeding against urinary tract infection. *Acta Paediatr* 93:164–168, 2004.

Martijn Pruissen DO, Slooter AJC, Rosendaal FR, van der Graaf Y, Algra A: Coagulation factor XIII gene variation, oral contraceptives, and risk of ischemic stroke. *Blood* 111:1282–1286, 2008.

Martin JM, Trink B, Daneman D, Dosch HM, Robinson B: Milk proteins in the etiology of insulin-dependent diabetes mellitus (IDDM). *Ann Med* 23:447–452, 1991.

Martin RM, Smith GD, Mangtani P, Frankel S, Gunnell D: Association between breast feeding and growth: the Boyd-Orr cohort study. *Arch Dis Child Fetal Neonatal Ed* 87:F193–F201, 2002.

Martin RM, Middleton N, Gunnell D, Owen CG, Smith GD: Breast-feeding and cancer: the Boyd-Orr cohort and a systematic review with meta-analysis. *J Natl Cancer Inst* 97:1446–1457, 2005a.

Martin RM, Gunnell D, Owen CG, Smith GD: Breast-feeding and childhood cancer: a systematic review with meta-analysis. *Int J Cancer* 117:1020–1031, 2005b.

Martin RM, Holly JM, Smith GD, Ness AE, Emmett P, Rogers I, Gunnell D; ALSPAC Study Team: Could associations between breastfeeding and insulin-like growth factors underlie associations of breastfeeding with adult chronic disease? The Avon Longitudinal Study of Parents and Children. *Clin Endocrinol* 62: 728–737, 2005c.

Martin RM, Ebrahim S, Griffin M, Davey Smith G, Nicolaides AN, Georgiou N, Watson S, Frankel S, Holly JM, Gunnell D: Breastfeeding and atherosclerosis: intima-media thickness and plaques at 65-year follow-up of the Boyd Orr cohort. *Aterioscler Thromb Vasc Biol* 25:1482–1488, 2005d.

Martin RM, Gunnell D, Smith GD: Breastfeeding in infancy and blood pressure in later life: systematic review and meta-analysis. *Am J Epidemiol* 161:15–26, 2005e.

Martin S, Schneider B, Heinemann L, Lodwig V, Kurth HJ, Kolb H, Scherbaum WA: Self-monitoring of blood glucose in type 2 diabetes and long term outcome: an epidemiological cohort study. *Diabetologia* 49:271–278, 2006a.

Martin LJ, Woo JG, Geraghty SR, Altaye M, Davidson BS, Banach W, Dolan LM, Ruiz-Palacios GM, Morrow AL: Adiponectin is present in human milk and is associated with maternal factors. *Am J Clin Nutr* 83:1106–1111, 2006b.

Martin-Calama J, Bunuel J, Valero MT, Labay M, Lasarte JJ, Valle F, de Miguel C: The effect of feeding gluose water to breastfeeding newborns on weight, body temperature, blood glucose, and breastfeeding duration: a randomized controlled trial. *J Hum Lact* 13:209–213, 1997.

Mass S: Breast pain: engorgement, nipple pain and mastitis. *Clin Obstet Gynecol* 47:676–682, 2004.

Mathew OP, Bhatia J: Sucking and breathing pattern during breast- and bottle-feeding in term neonates. *AJDC* 143:588–592, 1989.

Mayer EJ, Hamman RF, Gay EC, Lezotte DC, Savitz DA, Klingensmith GJ: Reduced risk of IDDM among breast-fed children: the Colorado IDDM Registry. *Diabetes* 37:1625–1632, 1988.

Mayer-Davis EJ, Rifas-Shiman S, Zhou L, Hu FB, Colditz GA, Gillman MW: Breast-feeding and risk for childhood obesity. Does maternal diabetes or obesity matter? *Diabetes Care* 29:2231–2237, 2006.

Mazzone T: Prevention of macrovascular disease in patients with diabetes mellitus: opportunities for intervention. *Am J Med* 120:S26–S32, 2007.

McCann JC, Ames BN: Is docohexaenoic acid, an *n*-3 long-chain polyunsaturated fatty acid, required for development of normal brain function? An overview of evidence from cognitive and behavioral tests in humans and animals. *Am J Clin Nutr* 82:281–295, 2005.

McCarter RJ, Hempe JM, Chalew SA: Mean blood glucose and biological variation have greater influence on HbA1C levels than glucose instability. An analysis of data from the Diabetes Control and Complications Trial. *Diabetes Care* 29: 352–355, 2006.

McCrory MA, Nommsen-Rivers LA, Mole PA, Lonnerdal B, Dewey KG: Randomized trial of the short-term effects of dieting compared with dieting plus exercise on lactation performance. *Am J Clin Nutr* 69:959–967, 1999.

McKeever P, Stevens B, Miller KL, MacDonell JW, Gibbins S, Guerriere D, Dunn MS, Coyte PC: Home versus hospital breastfeeding support for newborns: a randomized controlled trial. *Birth* 29:258–265, 2002.

McKenna MJ, Herskowitz R, Wolfsdorf JI: Screening for thyroid disease in children with IDDM. *Diabetes Care* 13:801–803, 1990.

McKinney PA, Parslow R, Gurney KA, Law GR, Bodansky I IJ, Williams R: Perinatal and neonatal determinants of childhood type 1 diabetes. A case-control study in Yorkshire, UK. *Diabetes Care* 22:928–932, 1999.

McLachlan K, Jenkins A, O'Neal D: The role of continuous glucose monitoring in clinical decision-making in diabetes in pregnancy. *Aust N Z J Obstet Gynecol* 47:186–190, 2007.

McManus RM, Cunningham I, Watson A, Harker L, Finegood DT: Beta-cell function and visceral fat in lactating women with a history of gestational diabetes. *Metabolism* 50:715–719, 2001.

McVea KL, Turner PD, Peppler DK: The role of breastfeeding in sudden infant death syndrome. *J Hum Lact* 16:13–20, 2000.

Meade TW. Oral contraceptives, clotting factors and thrombosis. *Am J Obstet Gynecol* 142;758–761, 1982.

Mennella JA, Beauchamp GK: The transfer of alcohol to human milk: effects on flavor and the infant's behavior. *N Engl J Med* 325:981–985, 1991.

Mennella JA: Short-term effects of maternal alcohol consumption on lactational performance. *Alcohol Clin Exp Res* 22:1389–1392, 1998a.

Mennella JA, Gerrish CJ: Effects of exposure to alcohol in mother's milk on infant sleep. *Pediatrics* 101:e2, 1998b.

Mennella JA, Pepino Y, Teff KL: Acute alcohol consumption disrupts the hormonal milieu of lactating women. *J Clin Endocrinol Metab* 90:1979–1985, 2005.

Mennella JA, Yourshaw LM, Morgan LK: Breastfeeding and smoking: short-term effects on infant feeding and sleep. *Pediatrics* 120:497–502, 2007.

Meyers GJ, Marsh DO, Davidson PW, Shamlaye CF, Tanner M, Choi A, Cernichiari E, Choisy O, Clarkson TW: Main neurodevelopmental study of Seychellois children following in utero exposure to methylmercury from a maternal fish diet: outcome at six monhs. *Neurotoxicology* 16:653–664, 1995.

Michaelsen KF, Larsen PS, Thomsen BL, Samuelson G: The Copenhagen cohort study on infant nutrition and growth: breast-milk intake, human milk macronutrient content, and influencing factors. *Am J Clin Nutr* 59:600–611, 1994.

Michels KB, Willett WC, Graubard BI, Vaidya RL, Cantwell MM, Sansbury LB, Forman MR: A longitudinal study of infant feeding and obesity throughout life course. *Int J Obes (Lond)* 31:1078–1085, 2007.

Miller DL: Birth and long-term unsupplemented breastfeeding in 17 insulin-dependent diabetic mothers. *Birth Fam J* 4:65–70, 1977.

Miller MR, Withers R, Bhamra R, Holt DW: Verapamil and breastfeeding. *Eur J Clin Pharmacol* 30:125–126, 1986.

Miller LJ: Postpartum depression. *JAMA* 287:762–765, 2002.

Minda H, Kovacs A, Funke S, Szasz M, Burus I, Molnar S, Marosvolgyi T, Decsi T: Changes of fatty acid composition of human milk during the first month of lactation: a day-to-day approach in the first week. *Ann Nutr Metab* 48:202–209, 2004.

Misri S, Kostaras X, Fox D, Kostaras D: The impact of partner support in the treatment of postpartum depression. *Can J Psychiatry* 45:554–558, 2000.

Mitoulos LR, Gurrin LC, Doherty DA, Sherriff JL, Hartmann PE: Infant intake of fatty acids from human milk over the first year of lactation. *Br J Nutr* 90: 979–986, 2003.

Miyake A, Tahara M, Koike K, Tanizawa O: Decrease in neonatal suckled milk volume in diabetic women. *Eur J Obstet Gynecol Reprod Biol* 33:49–53, 1989.

Miyake Y, Tanaka K, Sasaki S, Kiyohara C, Ohya Y, Fukushima W, Yokoyama T, Hirota Y; the Osaka Maternal and Child Health Study Group: Breastfeeding and the risk of wheeze and asthma in Japanese infants: the Osaka Maternal and Child Health Study. *Pediatr Allergy Immunol* Feb 11 2008 (Epub ahead of print).

Mizuta H, Amino N, Ichihara K, Harada T, Nose O, Tanizawa O, Mivai K: Thyroid hormones in human milk and their influence on thyroid function of breast-fed babies. *Pediatr Res* 17:468–471, 1983.

Moberg E, Kollind M, Lins PE, Adamson U: Estimation of blood-glucose variability in patients with insulin-dependent diabetes mellitus. *Scand J Clin Lab Invest* 53:507–514, 1993.

Modder J: Diabetes in pregnancy: can we make a difference? *BJOG* 115:419–420, 2008.

Mohn A, Cerruto M, Lafusco D, Prisco F, Tumini S, Stoppoloni O, Chiarelli F: Celiac disease in children and adolescents with type I diabetes: importance of hypoglycemia. *J Pediatr Gastroenterol Nutr* 32:37–40, 2001.

Monetini L, Cavallo MG., Stefanini L, Ferrazzoli F, Bizzarri C, Marietti G., Curro V, Cervoni M, Pozzilli P; IMDIAB Group: Bovine beta-casein antibodies in breast- and bottle-fed infants: their relevance in type 1 diabetes. *Diabetes Metab Res Rev* 17:51–54, 2001.

Monnier L, Lapinski H, Colette C: Contributions of fasting and postprandial plasma glucose increments to the overall diurnal hyperglycemia of type 2 diabetic patients. Variations with increasing levels of HbA1C. *Diabetes Care* 26:881–885, 2003.

Monnier L, Mas E, Ginet C, Michel F, Villon L, Cristol J-P, Colette C: Activation of oxidative stress by acute glucose fluctuations compared with sustained chronic hyperglycemia in patients with type 2 diabetes. *JAMA* 295:1681–1687, 2006.

Monnier L, Colette C: Glycemic variability: should we and can we prevent it? *Diabetes Care* 31 (Suppl 2):S150–S154, 2008.

Monro JA, Shaw M: Glycemic impact, glycemic glucose equivalents, glycemic index, and glycemic load: definitions, distinctions, and implications. *Am J Clin Nutr* 87 (Suppl):237S–243S, 2008.

Monsen ER: Dietary reference intakes for antioxidant vitamins: Vitamin C, Vitamin E, selenium, and carotenoids. *J Am Diet Assoc* 100:637–640, 2000.

Monsod TP, Flanagan DE, Rife DE, Saenz R, Caprio S, Sherwin RS, Tamborlane WV: Do sensor glucose levels accurately predict plasma glucose concentrations during hypoglycemia and hyperinsulinemia? *Diabetes Care* 25:889–893, 2002.

Monster TB, Janssen WM, de Jong PE, de Jong-van den Berg LT: Oral contraceptive use and HRT are associated with microalbuminuria. *Arch Intern Med* 161: 2000–2005, 2001.

Montes A, Walden CE, Knopp RH, Cheung M, Chapman MB, Albers JJ: Physiologic and supraphysiologic increases in lipoprotein lipids and apoproteins in late pregnancy and postpartum. Possible markers for the diagnosis of "prelipemia." *Arteriosclerosis* 4:407–417, 1984.

Morrow AL, Guerrero ML, Shults J, Valva JJ, Lutter C, Bravo J, Ruiz-Palacios G, Morrow RC, Butterfoss FD: Efficacy of home-based peer counseling to promote exclusive breastfeeding: a randomized controlled trial. *Lancet* 353:1226–1231, 1999.

Mortensen EL, Michaelsen KF, Sanders SA, Reinisch JM: The association between duration of breastfeeding and adult intelligence. *JAMA* 287:2365–2371, 2002.

Mosley EE, Wright AL, McGuire MK, McGuire MA: *trans* Fatty acids in milk produced by women in the United States. *Am J Clin Nutr* 82:1292–1297, 2005.

Motil KJ, Montandon CM, Garza C: Basal and postprandial metabolic rates in lactating and nonlactating women. *Am J Clin Nutr* 52:610–615, 1990.

Motil KJ, Sheng H, Kertz BL, Montandon CM, Ellis KJ: Lean body mass of well-nourished women is preserved during lactation. *Am J Clin Nutr* 67:292–300, 1998.

Mozaffarian D, Katan MB, Ascherio A, Stampfer MJ, Willett WC: Trans fatty acids and cardiovascular disease. *N Engl J Med* 354:1601–1613, 2006.

Muller AF, Drexhage HA, Bergout A: Postpartum thyroiditis and autoimmune thyroiditis in women of childbearing age: recent insights and consequences for antenatal and postnatal care. *Endocr Rev* 22:605–630, 2001.

Muntoni S, Cocco P, Aru G, Cucca F, Muntoni S: Nutritional factors and worldwide incidence of childhood type 1 diabetes. *Am J Clin Nutr* 71:1525–1529, 2000.

Murphy HR, Rayman G, Duffield K, Lewis KS, Kelly S, Johal B, Fowler D, Temple RC: Changes in the glycemic profiles of women with type 1 and type 2 diabetes during pregnancy. *Diabetes Care* 30:2785–2791, 2007.

Murray L, Carothers AD: The validation of the Edinburgh Postnatal Depression Scale on a community sample. *Br J Psychiatry* 157:288–290, 1990.

Murtaugh MA, Ferris AM, Capacchione CM, Reece EA: Energy intake and glycemia in lactating women with type 1 diabetes. *J Am Diet Assoc* 98:642–648, 1998.

Napoli A, Colatrella A, Botta R, Di Cianni G, Fresa R, Gambea S, Italia S, Mannino D, Piva I, Suraci C, Tonutti L, Torlone E, Tortul C, Lapolla A; Italian Diabetic Pregnancy Study Group (SID): Contraception in diabetic women: an Italian study. *Diabetes Res Clin Pract* 67:267–272, 2005.

Nappi C, Colace G, Affinito P, Taglialatela M, Di Renzo GF, Montemagno U, Annunziato L: Ibopamine-induced reduction of serum prolactin level and milk secretion in puerperal women. *Eur J Clin Pharmacol* 39:133–135, 1990.

Naylor AJ: Baby-Friendly Hospital Initiative. Protecting, promoting, and supporting breastfeeding in the twenty-first century. *Pediatr Clin North Am* 48:475–483, 2001.

Negro R, Greco G, Mangieri T, Pezzarossa A, Dazzi D, Hassan H: The influence of selenium supplementation on postpartum thyroid status in pregnant women with thyroid peroxidase autoantibodies. *J Clin Endocrinol Metab* 92:1263–1268, 2007.

Neifert MR, McDonough SL, Neville MC: Failure of lactogenesis associated with placental retention. *Am J Obstet Gynecol 140*:477–478, 1981.

Neifert M, Lawrence RA, Seacat J: Nipple confusion: toward a formal definition. *J Pediatr* 126:S125–S129, 1995.

Neifert MR: Clinical aspects of lactation. Promoting breastfeeding success. *Clin Perinatol* 26:281–306, 1999.

Neifert MR: Breastmilk transfer: positioning, latch-on, and screening for problems in milk transfer. *Clin Obstet Gynecol* 47:656–675, 2004.

Neilsen J: Return to work: practical management of breastfeeding. *Clin Obstet Gynecol* 47:724–733, 2004.

Nelson MC, Gordon-Larsen P, Adair LS: Are adolescents who were breast-fed less likely to be overweight? Analyses of sibling pairs to reduce confounding. *Epidemiology* 16:247–253, 2005.

Nettleton JA: Striving to increase compliance with dietary guidelines for fatty acid intake: a call for a multifaceted dietary approach. *J Am Diet Assoc* 107: 1723–1725, 2007.

Neubauer SH, Ferris AM, Chase CG, Fanelli J, Thompson CA, Lammi-Keefe CJ, Clark RM, Jensen RG, Bendel RW, Green KW: Delayed lactogenesis in women with insulin-dependent diabetes mellitus. *Am J Clin Nutr* 58:54–60, 1993.

Neugebauer R, Kline J, Shrout P, Skodol A, O'Connor P, Geller PA, Stein Z, Sussner M: Major depressive disorder in the 6 months after miscarriage. *JAMA* 277: 383–388, 1997.

Neville MC, Keller RP, Seacat J, Lutes V, Neifert MR, Casey C, Allen JA, Archer P: Studies in human lactation: milk volumes in lactating women during the onset of lactation and full lactation. *Am J Clin Nutr* 48:1375–1386, 1988.

Neville MC, Hay WW Jr, Fennessey P: Physiological significance of the concentration of human milk glucose. *Protoplasma* 159:118–128, 1990.

Neville MC, Allen JC, Archer P, Casey CE, Seacat J, Keller RP, Lutes V, Rasbach J, Neifert M: Studies in human lactation: milk volume and nutrient composition during weaning and lactogenesis. *Am J Clin Nutr* 54:81–92, 1991.

Neville MC, Sawicki VS, Hay WW Jr: Effects of fasting, elevated plasma glucose, and plasma insulin concentrations on milk secretion in women. *J Endocrinol* 139:165–173, 1993.

Neville MC: Physiology of lactation. *Clin Perinatol* 26:251–279, 1999.

Neville MC, Morton J, Umemura S: Lactogenesis. The transition from pregnancy to lactation. *Pediatr Clin North Am* 48:35–52, 2001.

Newburg DS: Oligosaccharides and glycoconjugates of human milk: their role in host defense. *J Mammary Gland Biol Neoplasia* 1:271–283, 1996.

Newburg DS, Ruiz-Palacios GM, Morrow AL: Human milk glycans protects infants against enteric pathogens. *Annu Rev Nutr* 25:37–58, 2005.

Newton ER: Breastmilk: the gold standard. *Clin Obstet Gynecol* 47:632–642, 2004.

Nicholson WK, Robinson KA, Smallridge RC, Ladenson PW, Powe NR: Prevalence of postpartum thyroid dysfunction: a quantitative review. *Thyroid* 16:573–582, 2006.

Nielsen G, Thomsen B, Michaelsen K: Influence of breast feeding and complementary food on growth between 5 and 10 months. *Acta Paediatr* 87:911–917, 1998.

Nielsen ABS, de Fine Olivarius N, Gannik D, Hindsberger C, Hollnagel H: Structured personal diabetes care in primary health care affects only women's HbA1C. *Diabetes Care* 29:963–969, 2006.

NIH—National Institutes of Health: Consortium for identification of the environmental determinants of diabetes in the young (TEDDY). Available at: http://t1diabetes.nih.gov/consortia/TEDDY.pdf. Accessed Apr 25, 2008.

Nilsson AC, Ostman EM, Granfeldt Y, Bjorck IME: Effect of cereal test breakfasts differing in glycemic index and content of indigestible carbohydrates on daylong glucose tolerance in health subjects. *Am J Clin Nutr* 87:645–654, 2008.

Nohr SB, Jorgensen A, Pedersen KM, Laurberg P: Postpartum thyroid dysfunction in pregnant thyroid peroxidase antibody-positive women living in an area with mild to moderate iodine deficiency: is iodine supplementation safe? *J Clin Endocrinol Metab* 85:3191–3198, 2000.

Nommsen LA, Lovelady CA, Heinig MJ, Lonnerdal B, Dewey KG: Determinants of energy, protein, lipid, and lactose concentrations in human milk during the first 12 mo of lactation: the DARLING Study. *Am J Clin Nutr* 53:457–465, 1991.

Norris JM, Scott FW: A meta-analysis of infant diet and insulin-dependent diabetes: do biases play a role? *Epidemiology* 7:87–92, 1996a.

Norris JM, Beaty B, Klingensmith G, Yu L, Hoffman M, Chase P, Erlich HA, Hamman RF, Eisenbarth GS, Rewers M: Lack of association between early exposures to cow's milk protein and β-cell autoimmunity. Diabetes Autoimmunity Study in the Young (DAISY). *JAMA* 276:609–614, 1996b.

Norris JM, Barriga K, Klingensmith G, Hoffman M, Eisenbarth GS, Erlich HA, Rewers M: Timing of initial cereal exposure in infancy and risk of islet autoimmunity. *JAMA* 290:1713–1720, 2003.

Novotny R, Coleman P, Tenorio L, Davison N, Camacho T, Ramirez V, Vijayadeva V, Untalan P, Diaz Tudela MD: Breastfeeding is associated with lower body mass index among children of the Commonwealth of the Northern Mariana Islands. *J Am Diet Assoc* 107:1743–1746, 2007.

O'Connor D, Funanage V, Locke R, Spear M, Leef K: Leptin is not present in infant formulas. *J Endocrinol Invest* 26:490, 2003.

O'Hara MW, Zekoski EM, Phillips LH, Wright EJ: Controlled prospective study of postpartum mood disorders: comparison of childbearing and non-child-bearing women. *J Abnorm Psychol* 99:3–15, 1990.

O'Hara MW, Schlechte JA, Lewis DA, Varner MW: Controlled prospective study of postpartum mood disorders: psychological, environmental, and hormonal variables. *J Abnorm Psychol* 100:63–73, 1991.

O'Hara M, Swain A: Rates and risk of postpartum depression—a meta-analysis. *Int Rev Psychiatry* 8:37–54, 1996.

O'Hara MW, Stuart S, Gorman LL, Wenzel A: Efficacy of interpersonal psychotherapy for postpartum depression. *Arch Gen Psychiatry* 57:1039–1045, 2000.

Oakley JR: Differences in subcutaneous fat in breast- and formula-fed infants. *Arch Dis Child* 52:79–80, 1977.

Oddy WH, Sly PD, De Klerk NH, Landau LI, Kendall GE, Holt PG, Stanley FJ: Breast feeding and respiratory morbidity in infancy: a birth cohort study. *Arch Dis Child* 88:224–228, 2003.

Odeley OE, de Courten M, Pettitt DJ, Ravussin E: Fasting hyperglycemia is a predictor of increased body weight gain and obesity in Pima Indian children. *Diabetes* 46:1341–1345, 1997.

Ohlin A, Rossner S: Maternal body weight development after pregnancy. *Int J Obes* 14:159–173, 1990.

Okada M, Inoue H, Nakamura H, Kishimoto M, Suzuki T: Excretion of diltiazem in human milk. *N Engl J Med* 312:992–993, 1985.

Olivarius N, Beck-Nielsen H, Andreasen AH, Horder M, Pedersen PA: Randomized controlled trial of structured personal care of type 2 diabetes mellitus. *BMJ* 323:970–975, 2001.

Olson CM, Stawderman MS, Hinton PS, Pearson TA: Gestational weight gain and postpartum behaviors associated with weight change from early pregnancy to one year postpartum. *Int J Obes Relat Metab Disord* 27:117–127, 2003.

Onn-Wong K, Woon-Leo L, Leng-Seah H: Dietary exposure assessment of infants to bisphenol A from the use of polycarbonate baby milk bottles. *Food Addit Contam* 22:280–288, 2005.

Ooylan LM, Hart S, Porter KB, Driskell JA: Vitamin B-6 content of breast milk and neonatal behavioral functioning. *J Am Diet Assoc* 102:1433–1438, 2002.

Oskarsson A, Schiltz A, Skerfving S, Hallen IP, Ohlin B, Lagerkvist BJ: Total and inorganic mercury in breast milk in relation to fish consumption and amalgam in lactating women. *Arch Environ Health* 51:234–241, 1996.

Ostrom KM, Ferris AM: Prolactin concentrations in serum and milk of mothers with and without insulin-dependent diabetes mellitus. *Am J Clin Nutr* 58:49–53, 1993.

Othman S, Phillips DIW, Parkes AB, Richards CJ, Harris B, Fung H, Darke C, John R, Hall R, Lazarus JH: A long-term follow-up of postpartum thyroiditis. *Clin Endocrinol* 32:559–564, 1990.

Otto SJ, van Houwelingen AC, Badart-Smook A, Hornstra G: Comparison of the peripartum and postpartum phospholipid polyunsaturated fatty acid profiles of lactating and nonlactating women. *Am J Clin Nutr* 73:1074–1079, 2001.

Owen MJ, Baldwin CD, Swank PR, Pannu AK, Johnson DL, Howie VM: Relation of infant feeding practices, cigarette smoke exposure, and group child care to the onset and duration of otitis media with effusion in the first two years of life. *J Pediatr* 123:702–711, 1993.

Owen CG, Martin RM, Whincup PH, Smith GD, Cook DG: Effect of infant feeding on the risk of obesity across the life course: a quantitative review of published evidence. *Pediatrics* 115:1367–1377, 2005a.

Owen CG, Martin RM, Whincup PH, Davey-Smith G, Gillman MW, Cook DG: The effect of breastfeeding on mean body mass index throughout life: a quantitative review of published and unpublished observational evidence. *Am J Clin Nutr* 82:1298–1307, 2005b.

Owen CG, Martin RM, Whincup PH, Smith GD, Cook DG: Does breastfeeding influence risk of type 2 diabetes in later life? A quantitative analysis of published evidence. *Am J Clin Nutr* 84:1043–1054, 2006.

Pabst HF, Spady DW, Pilarski LM, Carson MM, Beeler JA, Krezolek M: Differential modulation of the immune response by breast- or formula-feeding of infants. *Acta Paediatr* 86:1291–1297, 1997.

Parkes AB, Adams H, Othman S, Hall R, John R, Lazarus JH: The role of complement in the pathogenesis of postpartum thyroiditis. *Eur J Endocrinol* 133:210–215, 1996.

Paronen J, Knip M, Savilahti E, Virtanen SM, Ilonen J, Akerblom HK, Vaarala O; Finnish Trial to Reduce IDDM in the Genetically at Risk Study Group (TRIGR): Effect of cow's milk exposure and maternal type 1 diabetes on cellular and humoral immunization to dietary insulin in infants at genetic risk for type 1 diabetes. *Diabetes* 49:1657–1665, 2000.

Parsons TJ, Power C, Logan S, Summerbell CD: Childhood predictors of adult obesity: a systematic review. *Int J Obes* 23 (Suppl 8):S1–S107, 1999.

Parsons TJ, Power C, Manor O: Infant feeding and obesity through the life course. *Arch Dis Child* 88:793–794, 2003.

Patterson CC, Carson DJ, Hadden DR, Waugh NR, Cole SK: A case-control investigation of perinatal risk factors for childhood IDDM in North Ireland and Scotland. *Diabetes Care* 17:376–381, 1994.

Paulson JF, Dauber S, Leiferman JA: Individual and combined effects of postpartum depression in mothers and fathers on parenting behavior. *Pediatrics* 118: 659–668, 2006.

Pearce KL, Noakes M, Keogh J, Clifton PM: Effect of carbohydrate distribution on postprandial glucose peaks with the use of continuous glucose monitoring in type 2 diabetes. *Am J Clin Nutr* 87:638–644, 2008.

Pearson GD, Veille J-C, Rahimtoola S, Hsia J, Oakley CM, Hosenpud JD, Ansari A, Baughman KL: Peripartum cardiomyopathy. National Heart, Lung, and Blood Institute and Office of Rare Diseases (National Institutes of Health) Workshop Recommendations and Review. *JAMA* 283:1183–1188, 2000.

Peat J, Allen J, Nguyen N, Hayen A, Oddy W, Mihrshahi S: Motherhood meets epidemiology: measuring risk factors for breast-feeding cessation. *Public Health Nutr* 7:1033–1037, 2004.

Penny WJ, LewisMJ: Nifedipine is excreted in human milk. *Eur J Clin Pharmacol* 36:427–428, 1989.

Perez A, Labbok MH, Queenan JT: Clinical study of the lactational amenorrhoea method for family planning. *Lancet* 339:968–70, 1992.

Perez-Bravo F, Carrasco E, Gutierrez-Lopez MD, Martinez MT, Lopez G, Garcia de los Rios M: Genetic predisposition and environmental factors leading to the development of insulin-dependent diabetes mellitus in Chilean children. *J Mol Med* 74:105–109, 1996.

Perez-Escamilla R, Pollitt E, Lonnerdal B, Dewey KG: Infant feeding policies in maternity wards and their effect on breastfeeding success: an analytic overview. *Am J Public Health* 84:89–97, 1994.

Perlman JA, Russell-Briefel R, Ezzati T, Lieberknecht: Oral glucose tolerance and the potency of contraceptive progestins. *J Chronic Dis* 338:857–864, 1985.

Peters U, Schneeweiss S, Trautwein EA, Erbersdobler HF: A case-control study of the effect of infant feeding on celiac disease. *Ann Nutr Metab* 45:135–142, 2001.

Petersen KR, Skouby SO, Sidelmann J, Molsted-Pedersen L, Jespersen J: Effects of contraceptive steroids on cardiovascular risk factors in women with insulin-dependent diabetes mellitus. *Am J Obstet Gynecol* 171:400–405, 1994.

Petersen KR, Skouby SO, Vedel P, Haaber AB: Hormonal contraception in women with IDDM. *Diabetes Care* 18:800–806, 1995.

Peterson JA, Patton S, Hamosh M: Glycoproteins of the human milk fat globule in the protection of the breast-fed infant against infections. *Biol Neonate* 74: 143–162, 1998.

Petitti DB: Combination estrogen-progestin oral contraceptives. *N Engl J Med* 349:1443–1450, 2003.

Pettitt DJ, Forman MR, Hanson RL, Knowler WC, Bennett PH: Breastfeeding and incidence of non-insulin-dependent diabetes mellitus in Pima Indians. *Lancet* 350:166–168, 1997.

Pettitt DJ, Knowler WC: Long-term effects of the intrauterine environment, birth weight and breast-feeding in Pima Indians. *Diabetes Care* 21 (Suppl 2): B138–B141, 1998.

Peyrot M, Rubin RR: Behavioral and psychosocial interventions in diabetes. A conceptual review. *Diabetes Care* 30:2433–2440, 2007.

Peyrot M, Rubin RR: Access to diabetes self-management education. *Diabetes Educ* 34:90–97, 2008.

Phillip BL, Merewood A: The Baby-Friendly way: the best breastfeeding start. *Pediatr Clin North Am* 51:761–783, 2004.

Piatt GA, Orchard TJ, Emerson S, Simmons D, Songer TJ, Brooks MM, Korytkowski M, Simerio LM, Ahmad U, Zgibor JC: Translating the chronic care model into the community. Results from a randomized controlled trial of a multifaceted diabetes care intervention. *Diabetes Care* 29:811–817, 2006.

Picciano MF: Insulin-dependent diabetes and lactational performance. *J Pediatr Gastroenterol Nutr* 6:838–840, 1987.

Picciano MF: Human milk: nutritional aspects of a dynamic food. *Biol Neonate* 74:84–93, 1998.

Picciano MF: Nutrient composition of human milk. *Pediatr Clin North Am* 48: 53–67, 2001a.

Picciano MF: Representative values for constituents of human milk (table). *Pediatr Clin North Am* 48:263–264, 2001b.

Picciano MF: Pregnancy and lactation: physiological adjustments, nutritional requirements and the role of dietary supplements. *J Nutr* 133:1997S–2002S, 2003.

Piontek CM, Wisner KL, Perel JM, Peindl KS: Serum fluvoxamine levels in breastfed infants. *J Clin Psychiatry* 62:111–113, 2001.

Pisacane A, Graziano L, Mazzarella G, Scarpellino B, Zona G: Breastfeeding and urinary tract infection. *Acta Paediatr* 120:87–89, 1992.

Pisacane A, De Vizia B, Valiante A, Vaccaro F, Russo M, Grillo G, Giustardi A: Iron status in breast-fed infants. *J Pediatr* 127:429–431, 1995.

Plagemann A, Harder T, Franke K, Kohlhoff R: Long-term impact of neonatal breast-feeding on body weight and glucose tolerance in children of diabetic mothers. *Diabetes Care* 25:16–22, 2002.

Plagemann A, Harder T, Kohlhoff R, Rodekamp E, Franke K, Dudenhausen JW: Impact of early neonatal breast-feeding on psychomotor and neurophysiological development in children of diabetic mothers. *Diabetes Care* 28:573–578, 2005.

Pogach L, Engelgau M, Aron D: Measuring progress toward achieving hemoglobin A1C goals in diabetes care. Pass/fail or partial credit. *JAMA* 297:520–523, 2007.

Poole JA, Barriga K, Leung DYM, Hoffman M, Eisenbarth GS, Rewers M, Norris JM: Timing of initial exposure to cereal grains and the risk of wheat allergy. *Pediatrics* 117:2175–2182, 2006.

Pop VJ, de Rooy HA, Vader HL, van der Heide D, van Son M, Komproe IH, Essed GG, de Geus CA: Postpartum thyroid dysfunction and depression in an unselected population. *N Engl J Med* 324:1815–1816, 1991 [erratum *N Engl J Med* 325:371, 1991].

Pop VJM, de Rooy HAM, Vader HL, van der Heide D, van Som MM, Komproe IH: Microsomal antibodies during gestation in relation to postpartum thyroid dysfunction and depression. *Acta Endocrinol* 129:26–30, 1993.

Powers NG: How to assess slow growth in the breastfed infant. Birth to 3 months. *Pediatr Clin North Am* 48:345–363, 2001.

Premawardhana LDKE, Parkes AB, Ammari F, John R, Darke C, Adams H, Lazarus JH: Postpartum thyroiditis and long-term thyroid status: prognostic influence of thyroid peroxidase antibodies and ultrasound echogenicity. *J Clin Endocrinol Metab* 85:71–75, 2000.

Procianoy RS, Fernandes-Filho PH, Lazaro L, Sartori NC: Factors affecting breastfeeding: the influence of cesarean section. *J Trop Pediatr* 30:39–42, 1984.

Pronczuk J, Akre J, Moy G, Vallenas C: Global perspectives in breast milk contamination: infectious and toxic hazards. *Environ Health Perspect* 110: A349–A351, 2002.

Pullan CR, Toms GL, Martin AJ, Gardner PS, Webb JKG, Appleton DR: Breast-feeding and respiratory syncytial virus infection. *Br Med J* 281:1034–1036, 1980.

Pundziute-Lycka A, Urbonaite B, Dahlquist G: Infections and risk of type 1 (insulin-dependent) diabetes mellitus in Lithuanian children. *Diabetologia* 43: 1229–1234, 2000.

Pundziute-Lycka A, Persson LA, Cedermark G, Jansson-Roth A, Nilsson U, Westin V, Dahlquist G: Diet, growth and the risk for type 1 diabetes in childhood. A matched case-referent study. *Diabetes Care* 12:2784–2789, 2004.

Radberg T, Gustafson A, Skryten A, Karlsson K: Oral contraception in diabetic women. Diabetes control, serum and high density lipoprotein lipids during low-dose progestogen, combined oestrogen/progestogen and non-hormonal contraception. *Acta Endocrinol* 98:246–251, 1981.

Radford A, Southall DP: Successful application of the Baby-Friendly Hospital Initiative contains lessons that must be applied to the control of formula feeding in hospitals in industrialized countries. *Pediatrics* 108:766–768, 2001.

Raisler J, Alexander C, Camp P: Breast-feeding and infant illness: a dose-response relationship? *Am J Public Health* 89:25–30, 1999.

Raju TNK: Continued barriers for breast-feeding in public and the workplace. *J Pediatr* 148:677–679, 2006.

Ram KT, Bobby P, Hailpern SM, Lo JC, Schocken M, Skurnick J, Santoro N: Duration of lactation is associated with lower prevalence of the metabolic syndrome in midlife—SWAN, the study of women's health across the nation. *Am J Obstet Gynecol* 198:268.e1–268.e6, 2008.

Ramadan MA, Salah MM, Eid SZ: The effect of breast infection on the composition of human milk. *J Reprod Med* 9:84–87, 1972.

Randolph L, Cooper L, Fonseca-Becker F, York M, McIntosh M: *Baby-Friendly Hospital Initiative Feasibility Study: Final Report.* Healthy Mothers, Healthy Babies National Coalition Expert Work Group. Alexandria, VA: HMHB; 1994.

Rasmussen KM, Kjolhede CL: Prepregnant overweight and obesity diminish the prolactin response to suckling in the first week postpartum. *Pediatrics* 113: e465–e471, 2004 [DOI: 10.1542/peds.113.5.e465].

Ratzmann KP, Steindel I, Hildebrandt R, Kohloff R: Is there a relationship between metabolic control and glucose concentration in breast milk of type I (insulin-dependent) diabetic mothers? *Exp Clin Endocrinol* 92:32–36, 1988.

Rayfield EJ, Ault MJ, Keusch GT, Brothers MJ, Nechemias C, Smith H: Infection and diabetes: the case for glucose control. *Am J Med* 72:439–450, 1982.

Reader D, Franz MJ: Lactation, diabetes, and nutrition recommendations. *Curr Diabetes Rep* 4:370–376, 2004.

Redman CWG, Kelly JG, Cooper WD: The excretion of enalapril and enaliprat in human breast milk. *Eur J Clin Pharmacol* 38:99, 1990.

Reece EA, Homko CJ: Prepregnancy care and the prevention of fetal malformations in the pregnancy complicated by diabetes. *Clin Obstet Gynecol* 50:990–997, 2007.

Reilly JJ, Armstrong J, Dorosty AR, Emmett PM, Ness A, Rogers I, Steer C, Sheriff A; for the Avon Longitudinal Study of Parents and Children Study Team: Early life risk factors for obesity in childhood: cohort study. *BMJ* 330:1357–1362, 2005.

Reinehr T, Schober E, Wiegand S, Thon A, Holl R; the DPV-Wiss Study: β-cell autoantibodies in children with type 2 diabetes mellitus: subgroup or misclassification? *Arch Dis Child* 91:473–477, 2006.

Resnick HE, Foster GL, Bardsley J, Ratner RE: Achievement of American Diabetes Association clinical practice recommendations among U.S. adults with diabetes, 1999–2002. The National Health and Nutrition Examination Survey. *Diabetes Care* 29:531–537, 2006.

Resto M, O'Connor D, Leef K, Funanage V, Spear M, Lock R: Leptin levels in preterm human breast milk and infant formula. *Pediatrics* 108:e15, 2001.

Reynolds JL: Posttraumatic stress disorder after childbirth: the phenomenon of traumatic birth. *Can Med Assoc J* 156:831–835, 1997.

Riant P, Urien S, Albengres E, Duche JC, Tillement JP: High plasma protein binding as a parameter in the selection of beta-blockers for lactating women. *Biochem Pharmacol* 35:4579–4581, 1986.

Ribstein J, Halimi JM, du Cailar G, Mimran A: Renal characteristics and effect of angiotensin suppression in oral contraceptive users. *Hypertension* 33:90–95, 1999.

Rice DC, Schoeny R, Mahaffey K: Methods and rationale for derivation of a reference dose for methylmercury by the U.S. EPA. *Risk Anal* 23:107–115, 2003.

Richard L, Alade MO: Sucking technique and its effect on success of breastfeeding. *Birth* 19:185–189, 1992.

Righard L: Are breastfeeding problems related to incorrect breastfeeding technique and the use of pacifiers and bottles? *Birth* 25:40–44, 1998.

Riley LE, Tuomala RE, Heeren T, Greene MF: Low risk of post-cesarean section infection in insulin-requiring diabetic women. *Diabetes Care* 19:597–600, 1996.

Rimm E, Manson J, Stampfer M, Colditz G, Willett W, Rosner B, Hennekens C, Speizer F: Oral contraceptive use and the risk of type 2 diabetes mellitus in a large prospective study of women. *Diabetologia* 35:967–972, 1992.

Riva E, Banderali G, Agostoni C, Silano M, Radaelli G, Giovannini M: Factors associated with initiation and duration of breastfeeding in Italy. *Acta Paediatr* 88:411–415, 1999.

Robling SA, Paykel ES, Dunn NJ, Abbott R, Katona C: Long-term outcome of severe puerperal psychiatric illness. *Psychol Med* 30:1263–1271, 2000.

Rodekamp E, Harder T, Kohlhoff R, Franke K, Dudenhausen JW, Plagemann A: Long-term impact of breast-feeding on body weight and glucose tolerance in children of diabetic mothers. Role of the late neonatal period and early infancy. *Diabetes Care* 28:1457–1462, 2005.

Rodriguez-Palmero M, Koletzko B, Kunz C, Jensen R: Nutritional and biochemical properties of human milk. Part II. Lipids, micronutrients and bioactive factors. *Clin Perinatol* 26:335–359, 1999.

Rogan WJ, Ragan NB: Chemical contaminants, pharmacokinetics, and the lactating mother. *Environ Health Perspect* 102 (Suppl 11):89–95, 1994.

Rogers LM, Jovanovic L, Becker DJ: Should she or shouldn't she? The relationship between infant feeding practices and type 1 diabetes in the genetically at risk. Commentary. *Diabetes Care* 28:2809, 2005.

Rogovskaya S, Rivera R, Grimes DA, Chen P-L, Pierre-Louis B, Prilepskaya V, Kulakov V: Effect of a levonorgestrel intrauterine system on women with type 1 diabetes: a randomized trial. *Obstet Gynecol* 105:811–815, 2005.

Rohlfing CL, Wiedmeyer H-M, Little RR, England JD, Tennill A, Goldstein DE: Defining the relationship between plasma glucose and HbA1C: analysis of glucose profiles and HbA1C in the Diabetes Control and Complications Trial. *Diabetes Care* 25:275–278, 2002.

Ropero AB, Alonso-Magdalena P, Garcia-Garcia E, Ripoll C, Fuentes E, Nadal A: Bisphenol-A disruption of the endocrine pancreas and blood glucose homeostasis. *Int J Androl* 31:194–200, 2008.

Rosenbauer J, Herzig P, Kaiser P, Giani G: Early nutrition and risk of type 1 diabetes mellitus—a nationwide case-control study in preschool children. *Exp Clin Endocrinol Diabetes* 115:502–508, 2007.

Rosenberg L, Palmer JR, Sands MI, Grimes D, Bergman U, Daling J, Mills A: Modern oral contraceptives and cardiovascular disease. *Am J Obstet Gynecol* 177:707–715, 1997.

Rosenblatt KA, Thomas DB; WHO Collaborative Study of Neoplasia and Steroid Contraceptives: Lactation and the risk of epithelial ovarian cancer. *Int J Epidemiol* 22:192–197, 1993.

Rosenbloom AL: Obesity, insulin resistance, β-cell autoimmunity, and the changing clinical epidemiology of childhood diabetes. Editorial. *Diabetes Care* 26: 2954–2956, 2003.

Roth A, Elkayam U: Acute myocardial infarction associated with pregnancy. *Ann Intern Med* 125:751–762, 1996.

Roumie CL, Elasy TA, Greevy R, Griffin MR, Liu X, Stone WJ, Wallston KA, Dittus RS, Alverez V, Cobb J, Speroff T: Improving blood pressure control through provider education, provider alerts, and patient education. A cluster randomized trial. *Ann Intern Med* 145:165–175, 2006.

Rowe-Murray HJ, Fisher JRW: Baby friendly hospital practices: cesarean section is a persistent barrier to early initiation of breast-feeding. *Birth* 29:124–136, 2002.

Rueda R, Ramirez M, Garcia-Salmeron JL, Maldonado J, Gil A: Gestational age and origin of human milk influence total lipid and fatty acid contents. *Ann Nutr Metab* 42:12–22, 1998.

Saadeh R, Akre J: Ten steps to successful breastfeeding: a summary of the rationale and scientific evidence. *Birth* 23:154–160, 1996.

Sack J, Amado O, Lunenfeld B: Thyroxine concentration in human milk. *J Clin Endocrinol Metab* 45:171–173, 1977.

Sacker A, Quigley MA, Kelly YJ: Breastfeeding and developmental delay: findings from the millennium cohort study. *Pediatrics* 118:e682–e689, 2006.

Sacks DA: Preconception care for diabetic women: background, barriers, and strategies for effective implementation. *Curr Diabetes Rev* 2:147–161, 2006.

Sadauskaite-Kuehne V, Ludvigsson J, Padaiga Z, Jasinkiene E, Samuelsson U: Longer breastfeeding is an independent protective factor against development of type I diabetes mellitus in childhood. *Diabetes Metab Res Rev* 20:150–157, 2004.

Sadeharju K, Hamalainen AM, Knip M, Lonnrot M, Koskela P, Virtanen SM, Ilonen J, Akerblom HK, Hyoty H; Finnish TRIGR Study Group: Enterovirus infections as a risk factor for type 1 diabetes: virus analyses in a dietary intervention trial. *Clin Exp Immunol* 132:271–277, 2003.

Sadeharju K, Knip M, Virtanen SM, Savilahti E, Tauriainen S, Koshela P, Akerblom HK, Hyoty H; Finnish TRIGR Study Group: Maternal antibodies in breast milk protect the child from enterovirus infections. *Pediatrics* 119:941–946, 2007.

Sadurkis A, Kabir N, Wager J, Forsum E: Energy metabolism, body composition, and milk production in healthy Swedish women during lactation. *Am J Clin Nutr* 48:44–49, 1988.

Saez-de-Ibarra L, Gaspar R, Obesso A, Herranz L: Glycemic behavior during lactation: postpartum practical guidelines for women with type 1 diabetes. *Pract Diabetes Int* 20:271–275, 2003.

Sakaihara M, Yamada H, Kato EH, Ebina Y, Shimada S, Kobashi G, Fukushi M, Fujimoto S: Postpartum thyroid dysfunction in women with normal thyroid function during pregnancy. *Clin Endocrinol (Oxf)* 53:487–492, 2000.

Sakamoto M, Kubota M, Matsumoto S, Nakano A, Akagi H: Declining risk of methylmercury exposure to infants during lactation. *Environ Res* 90:185–189, 2002.

Salmenpera L, Perheentupa J, Siimes MA, Adrian TE, Bloom SR, Aynsley-Green A: Effects of feeding regimen on blood glucose and plasma concentrations of pancreatic hormones and gut regulatory peptides at 9 months of age: comparison between infants fed with milk formula and infants exclusively breast-fed from birth. *J Pediatr Gastroenterol Nutr* 7:651–666, 1988.

San Giovanni J, Berkey C, Dwyer J, Colditz G: Dietary essential fatty acids, long-chain polyunsaturated fatty acids, and visual resolution acuity in healthy fullterm infants: a systematic review. *Early Hum Dev* 57:165–188, 2000.

Sanders TA: Essential fatty acid requirements of vegetarians in pregnancy, lactation, and infancy. *Am J Clin Nutr* 70:555S–559S, 1999.

Sandstrom B, Regardh CG: metoprolol excretion into breast milk. *Br J Clin Pharmacol* 9:518–519, 1980.

Sarol JN Jr, Nicodemus NA Jr, Tan KM, Grava MB: Self-monitoring of blood glucose as part of a multi-component therapy among non-insulin-requiring type 2 diabetes patients: a meta-analysis (1996–2004). *Curr Med Res Opin* 21:173–183, 2005.

Saukkonen T, Ilonen J, Akerblom HK, Savilahti E. Prevalence of celiac disease in siblings of patients with type 1 diabetes is related to the prevalence of DQB1*02 allele. *Diabetelogia* 44:1051–1053, 2001.

Savilahti E, Saukonnen T, Virtala ET, Tuomilehto J, Akerblom HK; the Childhood Diabetes in Finland Study Group: Increased levels of cow's milk and β-lactoglobulin antibodies in young children with newly diagnosed IDDM. *Diabetes Care* 16:984–989, 1993.

Savino F, Costamagna M, Prino A, Oggero R, Silvestro L: Leptin levels in breast-fed and formula-fed infants. *Acta Paediatr* 91:897–902, 2002.

Savino F, Nanni GE, Maccario S, Costamagna M, Oggero R, Silvestro L: Breast-fed infants have higher leptin values than formula-fed infants in the first four months of life. *J Pediatr Endocrinol Metab* 17:1527–1532, 2004.

Savino F, Fissore MF, Grassino EC, Nanni GE, Oggero R, Silvestro L: Ghrelin, leptin and IGF-I levels in breast-fed and formula-fed infants in the first years of life. *Acta Paediatr* 94:531–537, 2005a.

Savino F, Nanni GE, Maccario S, Oggero R, Mussa GC: Relationships between IGF-I and weight Z-score, BMI, tricipital skinfold thickness, and type of feeding in healthy infants in the first five months of life. *Ann Nutr Metab* 49:83–87, 2005b.

Schack-Nielsen L, Larnkjoer A, Michaelsen KF: Long-term effects of breastfeeding on the infant and mother. *Adv Exp Med Biol* 569:16–23, 2005.

Schack-Nielsen L, Michaelsen KF: Breast feeding and future health. *Curr Opin Clin Nutr Metab Care* 9:289–296, 2006.

Schack-Nielsen L, Michaelsen KF: Advances in our understanding of the biology of human milk and its effects on the offspring. *J Nutr* 137:503S–510S, 2007.

Schaefer-Graf UM, Pawliczak J, Passow D, Hartmann R, Rossi R, Buhrer C, Harder T, Plagemann A, Vetter K, Kordonouri O: Birth weight and parental BMI predict overweight in children from mothers with gestational diabetes. *Diabetes Care* 28:1745–1750, 2005.

Schaefer-Graf UM, Hartmann R, Pawliczak J, Passow D, Abou-Dakn M, Vetter K, Kordonouri O: Association of breast-feeding and early childhood overweight in children from mothers with gestational diabetes mellitus. *Diabetes Care* 29: 1105–1107, 2006.

Schaper AM, Rooney BL, Kay NR, Silva PD: Use of the Edinburgh Postnatal Depression Scale to identify postpartum depression in a clinical setting. *J Reprod Med* 620–624, 1994.

Schimmel MS, Eidelman AJ, Wilschanski MA, Shaw D Jr, Ogilvie RJ, Koren G: Toxic effects of atenolol consumed during breast feeding. *J Pediatr* 114:476–478, 1989.

Schrezenmeir J, Jagla A: Milk and diabetes. *J Am Coll Nutr* 19 (Suppl):176S–190S, 2000.

Schubiger G, Schwarz U, Tonz O; Neonatal Study Group: UNICEF/WHO baby-friendly hospital initiative: does the use of bottles and pacifiers in the neonatal nursery prevent successful breastfeeding? *Eur J Pediatr* 156:874–877, 1997.

Schwarz EB, Maselli J, Gonzales R: Contraceptive counseling of diabetic women of reproductive age. *Obstet Gynecol* 107:1070–1074, 2006.

Schwedes U, Siebolds M, Mertes G; the SMBG Study Group: Meal-related structured self-monitoring of blood glucose. Effect on diabetes control in non-insulin-treated type 2 diabetic patients. *Diabetes Care* 25:1928–1932, 2002.

Scott FW: AAP recommendations on cow milk, soy, and early infant feeding. *Pediatrics* 96:515–518, 1995.

Scott FW, Rowsell P, Wang G-S, Burghardt K, Kolb H, Flohe S: Oral exposure to diabetes-promoting food or immunomodulators in neonates alters gut cytokines and diabetes. *Diabetes* 51:73–78, 2002.

Scott J, Shaker I, Reid M: Parental attitudes toward breastfeeding: their association with feeding outcome at hospital discharge. *Birth* 31:125–131, 2004.

Scott JA, Binns CW, Oddy WH, Graham KI: Predictors of breastfeeding duration: evidence from a cohort study. *Pediatrics* 117:e646–e655, 2006.

Scrivasteva MC, Oakley NW, Thomkins CV, Sonksen PH, Wynn V: Insulin metabolism, insulin sensitivity and hormonal response to insulin infusion in patients taking oral contraceptive steroids. *Eur J Clin Invest* 5:425–435, 1975.

Sebire NJ, Jolly M, Harris JP, Wadsworth J, Joffe M, Beard RW, Regan L, Robinson S: Maternal obesity and pregnancy outcome: a study of 287,213 pregnancies in London. *Int J Obes Relat Metab Disord* 25:1175–1182, 2001.

Selley WG, Ellis RE, Flack FC, Brooks WA: Coordination of sucking, swallowing and breathing in the newborn: its relationship to infant feeding and normal development. *Br J Disord Comm* 25:311–327, 1990.

Shaaban MM, Elwan SI, Abdalla SA, Darwish HA: Effect of subdermal levonorgestrel contraceptive implants, Norplant, on serum lipids. *Contraception* 30:413–419, 1984a.

Shaaban M, Elwan SI, el-Kabsh MY, Farghaly SA, Thabet N: Effect of levonorgestrel contraceptive implants, Norplant, on blood coagulation. *Contraception* 30: 421–430, 1984b.

Shannon ME, Malecha SE, Cha AJ: Angiotensin converting enzyme inhibitors (ACEIs) and angiotensin II receptor blockers (ARBs) and lactation: an update. *J Hum Lact* 16:152–155, 2000a.

Shannon ME, Malecha SE, Cha AJ: Calcium channel antagonists and lactation: an update. *J Hum Lact* 16:60–64, 2000b.

Shannon ME, Malecha SE, Cha AJ: Beta blockers and lactation: an update. *J Hum Lact* 16:240–245, 2000c.

Shawe J, Lawrenson R: Hormonal contraception in women with diabetes mellitus: special considerations. *Treat Endocrinol* 2:321–330, 2003.

Shipp AM, Gentry PR, Lawrence G, Van Landingham C, Covington T, Clewell HJ, Gribben K, Crump K: Determination of a site-specific reference dose for methylmercury for fish-eating populations. *Toxicol Ind Health* 16:335–438, 2000.

Shojanian KG, Ranji SR, McDonald KM, Grimshaw JM, Sundaram V, Rushakoff RJ, Owens DK: Effects of quality improvement strategies for type 2 diabetes on glycemic control. A meta-regression analysis. *JAMA* 296:427–440, 2006.

Shu XO, Linet MS, Steinbuch M, Wen WQ, Buckley JD, Neglia JP, Potter JD, Reaman GH, Robison LL: Breast-feeding and risk of childhood acute leukemia. *J Natl Cancer Inst* 91:1765–1772, 1999.

Sichieri R, Field AE, Rich-Edwards J, Willett WC: Prospective assessment of exclusive breastfeeding in relation to weight change in women. *Int J Obes Relat Metab Disord* 27:815–820, 2003.

Sievers E, Haase S, Oldigs HD, Schaub J: The impact of peripartum factors on the onset and duration of lactation. *Biol Neonate* 83:246–252, 2003.

Siminario LM, Zgibor JC, Solano FX: Implementing the chronic care model for improvements in diabetes practice and outcomes in primary care: the University of Pittsburgh Medical Center experience. *Clin Diabet* 22:54–58, 2004.

Simmons D, Conroy C, Thompson CF: In-hospital breast feeding rates among women with gestational diabetes and pregestational type 2 diabetes in South Auckland. *Diabet Med* 22:177–181, 2005.

Sinclair D: Analytical aspects of thyroid antibodies estimation. *Autoimmunity* 41: 46–54, 2008.

Singh K, Viegas OA, Koh SC, Ratnam SS: The effect of long-term use of Norplant implants on haemostatic function. *Contraception* 45:141–53, 1992.

Singhal A, Farooqi IS, O'Rahilly SO, Cole TJ, Fewtrell M, Lucas A: Early nutrition and leptin concentrations in later life. *Am J Clin Nutr* 75:993–999, 2002.

Sipetic S, Vlajinac H, Kocev N, Badmanovic S: The Belgrade childhood diabetes study: associations of infections and vaccinations on diabetes in childhood. *Ann Epidemiol* 13:645–651, 2003.

Siritho S, Thrift AG, McNeil JJ, You RX, Davis SM, Donnan GA: Risk of ischemic stroke among users of the oral contraceptive pill: the Melbourne Risk Factor Study (MERFS) Group. *Stroke* 34:1575–1580, 2003.

Skouby SO, Molsted-Pedersen L, Kosonen A: Consequences of intrauterine contraception in diabetic women. *Fertil Steril* 42:568–572, 1984.

Skouby SO, Jensen BM, Kuhl C, Molsted-Pedersen L, Svenstrup B, Nielsen J: Hormonal contraception in diabetic women: acceptability and influence on diabetes control of a nonaldekylated estrogen/progestogen compound. *Contraception* 32:23–31, 1985a.

Skouby SO, Kuhl C, Molsted-Pedersen L, Petersen K, Christensen MS: Triphasic oral contraception: metabolic effects in normal women and those with previous gestational diabetes. *Am J Obstet Gyncol* 153:495–500, 1985b.

Skouby SO, Molsted-Pedersen L, Kuhl C: Contraception in diabetic women. *Acta Endocrinol* 277 (Suppl):125–129, 1986a.

Skouby SO, Molsted-Pedersen, Kuhl C, Bennett P: Oral contraceptives in diabetic women: metabolic effects of four compounds with different estrogen/progestogen profiles: *Fertil Steril* 1986; 46:858–864, 1986b.

Skouby SO, Anderson O, Saurbrey N, Kuhl C: Oral contraception and insulin sensitivity: in vivo assessment in normal women and women with previous gestational diabetes. *J Clin Endocrinol Metab* 64:519–523, 1987.

Skouby SO, Petersen KR: Oral contraception in diabetic women. *Gynecol Endocrinol* 7 (Suppl):1–4, 1993.

Sliwa K, Forster O, Zhanje F, Candy G, Kachope J, Essop R: Outcome of subsequent pregnancy in patients with documented peripartum cardiomyopathy. *Am J Cardiol* 93:1441–1443, 2004.

Sliwa K, Fett J, Elkayam U: Peripartum cardiomyopathy. *Lancet* 368:687–693, 2006.

Smaill F, Hofmeyr GJ: Antibiotic prophylaxis for cesarean section (Cochrane Review). In: *The Cochrane Library.* Issue 2. Oxford: Update Software; 2003.

Smallridge RC: Disclosing subclinical thyroid diseases. An approach to mild laboratory abnormalities and vague or absent symptoms. *Postgrad Med* 107: 143–146, 149–152, 2000a.

Smallridge RC: Postpartum thyroid disease: a model of immunologic dysfunction. *Clin Appl Immunol Rev* 1:89–103, 2000b.

Smallwood GH, Meador ML, Lenihan JP, Shangold GA, Fisher AC, Creasy GW; ORTHO EVRA/EVRA 002 Study group: Efficacy and safety of a transdermal contraceptive system. *Obstet Gynecol* 98:799–805, 2001.

Smith MT, Livingstone I, Hooper WD, Eadie MJ, Triggs EJ: Propranolol, propranolol glucuronide, and napthoxylactic acid in breast milk and plasma. *Ther Drug Monitor* 5:87–93, 1983.

Smith-Kirwin SM, O'Connor DM, Johnston J, deLancey J, Hassink SG, Funanage VL: Leptin expression in human mammary cells and breast milk. *J Clin Endocrinol Metab* 83:1810–1813, 1998.

Soet JE, Brack GA, Dilorio C: Prevalence and predictors of women's experiences of psychological trauma during childbirth. *Birth* 30:36–46, 2003.

Sohlstrom A, Forsum E: Changes in adipose tissue volume and distribution during reproduction in Swedish women as assesses by magnetic resonance imaging. *Am J Clin Nutr* 61:287–295, 1995.

Sozmen M: Effects of early suckling of cesarean-born babies on lactation. *Biol Neonate* 62:67–68, 1992.

Spellacy WN, Buhi WC, Birk SA: The effect of estrogens on carbohydrate metabolism: glucose, insulin and growth hormone studies on one hundred seventy-one women ingesting premarin, mestranol and ethinyl estradiol for six months. *Am J Obstet Gynecol* 114:388–392, 1971.

Speroff L, DeCherney A: Evaluation of a new generation of oral contraceptives. The Advisory Board of the New Progestins. *Obstet Gynecol* 81:1034–1047, 1993.

Spruijt-Metz D, Lindquist CH, Birch LL, Fisher JO, Goran MI: Relation between mothers' child-feeding practices and children's adiposity. *Am J Clin Nutr* 75: 581–586, 2002.

Stabell BC, Wohlfahrt J, Aaby P: Breastfeeding and risk of atopic dermatitis, by parental history of allergy, during the first 18 months of life. *Am J Epidemiol* 160:217–223, 2004.

Stage E, Norgard H, Damm P, Mathiesen E: Long-term breast-feeding in women with type 1 diabetes. *Diabetes Care* 29:771–774, 2006.

Stagnaro-Green A: Recognizing, understanding, and treating postpartum thyroiditis. *Endocrinol Metab Clin North Am* 29:417–430, 2000.

Stagnaro-Green A: Postpartum thyroiditis. Clinical review 152. *J Clin Endocrinol Metab* 87:4042–4047, 2002.

Stebler T, Guentert TW: Binding of drugs in milk: the role of casein in milk protein binding. *Pharm Res* 7:633–637, 1990.

Steel JM, Duncan LJP: The effect of oral contraceptives on insulin requirements in diabetic women. *Br J Fam Plan* 3:77–78, 1978a.

Steel JM, Duncan LJP: Serious complications of oral contraception in insulin-dependent diabetes. *Contraception* 17:291–295, 1978b.

Stene LC, Magnus P, Lie RT, Sovik O, Joner G: Birth weight and childhood onset type 1 diabetes: population-based cohort study. *BMJ* 322:889–892, 2001.

Stettler N, Stallings VA, Troxel AB, Zhao J, Schinnar R, Nelson SE, Ziegler EE, Strom BL: Weight gain in the first week of life and overweight in adulthood. A cohort study of European American subjects fed infant formula. *Circulation* 111:1897–1903, 2005.

Stewart A, Cummins C, Gold L, Jordan R, Phillips W: The effectiveness of the levonorgestrel-releasing intrauterine systems in menorrhagia: a systemic review. *BJOG* 108:74–86, 2001.

Stiver HG, Forward KR, Tyrell DL, Krip G, Livingstone RA, Fugere P, Lemay M, Verschelden G, Hunter JD, Carson GD: Comparative cervical microflora shifts after cefoxitin or cefazolin prophylaxis against infection following cesarean section. *Am J Obstet Gynecol* 149:718–721, 1984.

St-Onge M-P, Bosarge A: Weight-loss diet that includes consumption of medium-chain triacylglycerol oil leads to a greater rate of weight and fat mass loss than does olive oil. *Am J Clin Nutr* 87:621–626, 2008.

Stowe ZN, Nemeroff CB: Women at risk for postpartum-onset major depression. *Am J Obstet Gynecol* 173:639–645, 1995.

Stowe ZN, Owens MJ, Landry JC, Kilts CD, Ely T, Llewellyn A, Nemeroff CB: Sertraline and desmethylsertraline in human breast milk and nursing infants. *Am J Psychiatry* 154:1255–1260, 1997.

Stowe ZN, Hostetter AL, Owens MJ, Ritchie JC, Sternberg K, Cohen LS, Nemeroff CB: The pharmacokinetics of sertraline excretion into human breast milk: determinants of infant serum concentrations. *J Clin Psychiatry* 64:73–80, 2003.

Stowe ZN, Hostetter AL, Newport DJ: The onset of postpartum depression: implications for clinical screening in obstetrical and primary care. *Am J Obstet Gynecol* 192:522–526, 2005.

Straarup EM, Lauritzen L, Faerk J, Hoy C-E, Michaelsen KF: The stereospecific triacylglycerol structures and fatty acid profiles of human milk and infant formulas. *J Pediatr Gastroenterol Nutr* 42:293–299, 2006.

Stratton IM, Adler AI, Neil HA, Matthews DR, Manley SE, Cull CA, Hadden D, Turner RC, Holman RR: Association of glycemia with macrovascular and microvascular complications of type 2 diabetes (UKPDS) 35): prospective observational study. *BMJ* 321:405–412, 2000.

Strode MA, Dewey KG, Lonnerdal B: Effects of short-term caloric restriction on lactational performance of well-nourished women. *Acta Paediatr Scand* 75: 222–229, 1986.

Strotmeyer ES, Yang Z, LaPorte RE, Chang Y-F, Steenkiste AR, Pietropaolo M, Nucci AM, Shen S, Wang L, Wang B, Dorman JS: Infant diet and type 1 diabetes in China. *Diabetes Res Clin Pract* 65:283–292, 2004.

Stuebe AM, Rich-Edwards JW, Willett WC, Manson JE, Michels KB: Duration of breast-feeding and incidence of type 2 diabetes. *JAMA* 294:2601–2610, 2005.

Sundstrom JB, Fett JD, Carraway RD, Ansari AA: Is peripartum cardiomyopathy an organ-specific autoimmune disease? *Autoimmun Rev* 1:73–77, 2002.

Sunehag AL, Louie K, Bier JL, Tigas S, Haymond MW: Hexoneogenesis in the human breast during lactation. *J Clin Endocrinol Metab* 87:297–301, 2002.

Sutton MS, Cole P, Plappert M, Saltzman D, Goldhaber S: Effects of subsequent pregnancy on left ventricular function in peripartum cardiomyopathy. *Am Heart J* 121:1776–1778, 1991.

Tachi J, Amino N, Tamaki H, Aozasa M, Aotani Y, Miyai K: Long-term follow-up and HLA association in patients with postpartum thyroiditis. *J Clin Endocrinol Metab* 66:480–484, 1988.

Tagami T, Hagiwara H, Kimura T, Usui T, Shimatsu A, Naruse M: The incidence of gestational hyperthyroidism and postpartum thyroiditis in treated patients with Graves' disease. *Thyroid* 17:767–772, 2007.

Takoudes TC, Weitzen S, Slocum J, Malee M: Risk of cesarean wound complications in diabetic gestations. *Am J Obstet Gynecol* 191:958–963, 2004.

Tanasescu M, Cho E, Manson JE, Hu FB: Dietary fat and cholesterol and the risk of cardiovascular disease among women with type 2 diabetes. *Am J Clin Nutr* 79:999–1005, 2004.

Tanis BC, van den Bosch MA, Kemmeren JM, Cats VM, Helmerhorst FM, Algra A, van der Graaf Y, Rosendaal FR: Oral contraceptives and the risk of myocardial infarction. *N Engl J Med* 345:1787–1793, 2001.

Taveras EM, Rifas-Shiman SL, Scanlon KS, Grummer-Strawn LM, Sherry B, Gillman MW: To what extent is the protective effect of breastfeeding on future overweight explained by decreased maternal feeding restriction? *Pediatrics* 118:2341–2348, 2006.

Taylor EA, Turner P: Anti-hypertensive therapy with propranolol during pregnancy and lactation. *Postgrad Med J* 57:427–430, 1981.

Taylor P, Malani J, Brown D: Early suckling and prolonged breastfeeding. *Am J Dis Child* 140:51–54, 1986.

TEDDY—TEDDY Study Group: The Environmental Determinants of Diabetes in the Young (TEDDY) study: study design. *Pediatr Diabetes* 8:286–298, 2007.

TerHorst PG, Jansman FG, van Lingen RA, Smit JP, de Jong-van den Berg LT, Brouwers JR: Pharmacological aspects of neonatal antidepressant withdrawal *Obstet Gynecol Surv* 63:267–279, 2008.

Thomas MR, Kawamoto J: Dietary evaluation of lactating women with or without vitamin and mineral supplementation. *J Am Diet Assoc* 74:669–672, 1979.

Thomas B, Ghebremeskel K, Offley-Shore B, Lowy C, Crawford MA: Fatty acid composition of maternal milk from insulin-dependent diabetic, gestational diabetic and healthy control women. *Proc Nutr Soc* 59:59A, 2000.

Thorley KJ: Pharmacokinetics of atenolol in pregnancy and lactation. *Drugs* 25 (Suppl 2): 216–217, 1983.

Tigas S, Sunehag A, Haymond MW: Metabolic adaptation to feeding and fasting during lactation in humans. *J Clin Endocrinol Metab* 87:302–307, 2002.

Tittanen M, Paronen J, Savilahti E, Virtanen SM, Ilonen J, Knip M, Akerblom HK, Vaarala O; Finnish TRIGR Study Group: Dietary insulin as an immunogen and tolerogen. *Pediatr Allergy Immunol* 17:538–543, 2006.

Tolstoi E: The relationship of the blood glucose to the concentration of lactose in the milk of lactating diabetic women. *J Clin Invest* 14:863–866, 1935.

Topper YJ, Freeman CS: Multiple hormone interactions in the developmental biology of the mammary gland. *Physiol Rev* 60:1049–1099, 1980.

Torres AG, Ney JC, Meneses F, Trugo NMF: Polyunsaturated fatty acids and conjugated linoleic acid isomers in breast milk are associated wirh plasma non-esterified and erythrocyte membrane fatty acid composition in lactating women. *Br J Nutr* 95:517–524, 2006.

Toschke AM, Vignerova J, Lhotska L, Osancova K, Koletzko B, von Kries R: Overweight and obesity in 6- to 14-year old Czech children in 1991: a protective effect of breast-feeding. *J Pediatr* 141:764–769, 2002a.

Toschke AM, Koletzko B, Slikker W Jr, Hermann M, von Kries R: Childhood obesity is associated with maternal smoking in pregnancy. *Eur J Pediatr* 161:445–448, 2002b.

Toschke AM, Montgomery SM, Pfeiffer U, von Kries R: Early intrauterine exposure to tobacco-inhaled products and obesity. *Am J Epidemiol* 158:1068–1074, 2003.

Toschke AM, Martin RM, von Kries R, Wells J, Smith GD, Ness AR: Infant feeding method and obesity: body mass index and dual-energy X-ray absorptiometry measurements at 9–10 y of age from the Avon Longitudinal Study of Parents and Children (ALSPACT). *Am J Clin Nutr* 85:1578–1585, 2007.

Triggiani V, Ciampolillo A, Guastamacchia E, Licchelli B, Fanelli M, Resta F, Tafaro E: Prospective study of post-partum thyroid immune dysfunctions in type 1 diabetic women and in a healthy control group living in a mild iodine deficient area. *Immunopharmacol Immunotoxicol* 26:215–224, 2004.

TRIGR—TRIGR Study Group: Study design of the Trial to Reduce IDDM in the Genetically at Risk (TRIGR). *Pediatr Diabetes* 8:117–137, 2007.

Trost S, LeWinter M: Diabetic cardiomyopathy. *Curr Treat Options Cardiovasc Med* 3:481–492, 2001.

Truit ST, Fraser AB, Grimes DA, Gallo MF, Kchulz KF: Combined hormonal versus nonhormonal versus progestin-only contraception in lactation. *Cochrane Database Syst Rev* 2003;(2):CDC003988.

Trumbo P, Yates A, Schlicker S, Poos M: Dietary reference intakes: vitamin A, vitamin K, arsenic, boron, chromium, copper, iodine, iron, manganeses, molybdenum, nickel, silicon, vanadium, and zinc. *J Am Diet Assoc* 101:294–301, 2001.

Trumbo P, Schlicker S, Yates AA, Poos M: Dietary reference intakes for energy, carbohydrate, fiber, fat, fatty acids, cholesterol, protein and amino acids. *J Am Diet Assoc* 102:1621–1631, 2002.

Tyson JE, Hock RA: Gestational and pregestational diabetes: an approach to therapy. *Am J Obstet Gynecol* 125:1009–1027, 1976.

Uauy R, Quan R, Gil A: Role of nucleotides in intestinal development and repair: implications for infant nutrition. *J Nutr* 124:1436S–1441S, 1994.

Uauy R, Peirano P: Breast is best: human milk is the optimal food for brain development. *Am J Clin Nutr* 70:433–444, 1999.

Uauy R, Mena P, Rojas C: Essential fatty acids in early life: structural and functional role. *Proc Nutr Soc* 59:3–15, 2000.

Ucar B, Kirel B, Bor O, Sultan Kilic F, Dogruel N, Durmas Aydogdu S, Tekin N: Breast milk leptin concentrations in initial and terminal milk samples: relationships to maternal and infant plasma leptin concentrations, adiposity, serum glucose, insulin, lipid and lipoprotein levels. *J Pediatr Endocrinol Metab* 13:149–156, 2000.

Uhari M, Mantysaari K, Niemela M: A meta-analytic review of the risk factors for acute otitis media. *Clin Infect Dis* 22:1079–1083, 1996.

UKPDS 33—UK Prospective Diabetes Study Group: Intensive blood-glucose control with sulphonylureas or insulin compared with conventional treatment and risk of complications in patients with type 2 diabetes. *Lancet* 352:837–853, 1998a.

UKPDS 34—UK Prospective Diabetes Study Group: Effect of intensive blood-glucose control with metformin on complications in overweight patients with type 2 diabetes. *Lancet* 352:854–865, 1998b.

Umpaichitra V, Banerji MA, Castells S: Autoantibodies in children with type 2 diabetes mellitus. *J Pediatr Endocrinol Metab* 15:525–530, 2002.

UNICEF—United Nations Children's Fund,United States Committee: Barriers and solutions to the global ten steps to successful breastfeeding: a summary of in-depth interviews with hospitals participating in the WHO-UNICEF Baby-Friendly Hospital Initiative interim program in the United States. Washington, DC: Office of Public Policy and Government Relations; 2002.

Ursin G, Bernstein L, Lord SJ, Karim R, Deapen D, Press MF, Daling JR, Norman SA, Liff JM, Marchbanks PA, Folger SG, Simon MS, Strom BL, Burkman RT, Weiss LK, Spirtas R: Reproductive factors and subtypes of breast cancer defined by hormone receptor and histology. *Br J Cancer* 93:364–371, 2005.

USPHS: U.S. Public Health Service's healthy people 2010. 2004. Available at http://www.healthypeople.gov. Accessed March 12, 2008.

Vaarala O, Saukkonen T, Savilahti E, Klemola T, Akerblom HK: Development of immune response to cow's milk proteins in infants receiving cow's milk or hydrolyzed formula. *J Allergy Clin Immunol* 96:917–923, 1995.

Vaarala O, Knip M, Paronen J, Hamalainen A, Muona P, Vaatainen M, Ilonen J, Simell O, Akerblom HK: Cow's milk formula feeding induces primary immunization to insulin in infants at genetic risk for type 1 diabetes. *Diabetes* 48:1389–1394, 1999.

Vaarala O: The gut immune system and type 1 diabetes. *Ann N Y Acad Sci* 958: 39–46, 2002.

vanBuesekom CM, Zeegers TA, Martini IA, Velvis HJR, Visser GHA, van Doormal JJ, Muskiet FAJ: Milk of patients with tightly controlled insulin-dependent diabetes mellitus has normal macronutrient and fatty acid composition. *Am J Clin Nutr* 57:938–943, 1993.

VandenBosch MA, Kemmeren JM, Tanis BC, Mali WP, Helmerhorst FM, Rosendaal FR, Algra A, Van Der Graaf Y: The RATIO study: oral contraceptives and the risk of peripheral arterial disease in young women. *J Thromb Haemost* 1: 439–444, 2003.

vanOdjik J, Kull I, Borres MP, Brandtzaeg P, Edberg U, Hanson LA, Host A, Kultunen M, Olsen SF, Skerfving S, Sundell J, Wille S: Breastfeeding and allergic disease: a multidisciplinary review of the literature (1966–2001) on the mode of early feeding in infancy and its impact on later atopic manifestations. *Allergy* 58:833–843, 2003.

Varma SK, Collins M, Row A, Haller WS, Varma K: Thyroxine, tri-iodothyronine, and reverse tri-iodothyronine concentrations in human milk. *J Pediatr* 93: 803–806, 1978.

Varughese GI, Chowdhury SR, Warner DP, Barton DM: Preconception care of women attending adult general diabetes clinics—are we doing enough? *Diabetes Res Clin Pract* 76:142–145, 2007.

Villamore E, Cnattingius S: Interpregnancy weight change and risk of adverse pregnancy outcomes: a population-based study. *Lancet* 368:1164–1170, 2006.

Villapondo S, Hamosh M: Early and late effects of breast-feeding: does breast-feeding really matter? *Biol Neonate* 74:177–191, 1998.

Virtanen SM, Rasanen L, Aro A, Lindstrom J, Sippola H, Lounamaa R, Toivanen L, Tuomilehto J, Akerblom HK; Childhood Diabetes in Finland Study Group: Infant feeding in Finnish children <7 yr of age with newly diagnosed IDDM. *Diabetes Care* 14:415–417, 1991.

Virtanen SM, Rasanen L, Ylonen K, Aro A, Clayton D, Langholz B, Pitkaniemi J, Savilahti E, Lounamaa R, Tuomilehto J, Akerblom HK; Childhood Diabetes in Finland Study Group: Early introduction of dairy products associated with increased risk of IDDM in Finnish children. *Diabetes* 42:1786–1790, 1993.

Virtanen SM, Hypponen E, Laara E, Vahasalo P, Kulmala P, Savola K, Rasanen L, Aro A, Knip M, Akerblom HK; the Childhood Diabetes in Finland Study Group: Cow's milk consumption, disease-associated autoantibodies and type 1 diabetes mellitus: a follow-up study in siblings of diabetic children. *Diabet Med* 15:730–738, 1998.

Virtanen SM, Laara E, Hypponen E, Reijonen H, Rasanen L, Aro A, Knip M, Ilonen J, Akerblom HK; Childhood Diabetes in Finland Study Group: Cow's milk consumption, HLA-DQB1 genotype and IDDM. A nested case-control study of siblings of children with diabetes. *Diabetes* 49:912–917, 2000.

Virtanen SM, Knip M: Nutritional risk predictors of β-cell autoimmunity and type 1 diabetes at a young age. *Am J Clin Nutr* 78:1053–1067, 2003.

Virtanen SM, Kenward MG, Erkkola M, Kautiainen S, Kronberg-Kippila C, Hakulinen T, Ahonen S, Uusitalo L, Niinisto S, Veijola R, Simell O, Ilonen J, Knip M: Age at introduction of new foods and advanced beta cell autoimmunity in young children with HLA-conferred susceptibility to type 1 diabetes. *Diabetologia* 49:1512–1521, 2006.

Visser J, Snel M, Van Vliet HA: Hormonal versus non-hormonal contraceptives in women with diabetes mellitus type 1 and 2. *Cochrane Database Syst Rev* 2006 (4): CD003990.

Voight RG, Jensen CL, Fraley JK, Rozelle JC, Brown FR 3rd, Heird WC: Relationship between omega 3 long-chain polyunsaturated fatty acid status during early infancy and neurodevelopmental status at 1 year of age. *J Hum Nutr Diet* 15:111–120, 2002.

Volpe SL: Serving on the Institute of Medicine's Dietary Reference Intake Panel for Electrolytes and Water. *J Am Diet Assoc* 104:1885–1887, 2004.

Wahlberg J, Fredriksson J, Nikolic E, Vaarala O, Ludvigsson J; ABIS-Study Group: Environmental factors related to the induction of beta-cell autoantibodies in 1-year old healthy children. *Pediatr Diabetes* 6:199–205, 2005.

Wahlberg J, Vaarala O, Ludvigsson J; ABIS-study group: Dietary risk factors for the emergence of type 1 diabetes-related autoantibodies in 21/2-year-old Swedish children. *Br J Nutr* 95:603–608, 2006.

Walfish PG, Meyerson J, Provias JP, Vargas MT, Papsin FR: Prevalence and characteristics of postpartum thyroid dysfunction: results of a survey from Toronto, Canada. *J Endocrinol Invest* 15:265–272, 1992.

Walker M; International Lactation Consultant Association: Breastfeeding with diabetes: yes you can! *J Hum Lact* 22:345–346, 2006.

Wallensteen M, Lindblad BS, Zetterstrom R, Persson B: Acute C-peptide, insulin and branched chain amino acid response to feeding in formula and breast-fed infants. *Acta Paediatr Scand* 80:143–148, 1991.

Wasmuth HE, Kolb H: Cow's milk and immune-mediated diabetes. *Proc Nutr Soc* 59:573–579, 2000.

Weaver LT: Relationships between pediatricians and infant milk formula companies. Commentary on infant nutrition. *Arch Dis Child* 91:386–387, 2006.

Webster J, Moore K, McMullen A: Breastfeeding outcomes for women with insulin-dependent diabetes. *J Hum Lact* 11:195–200, 1995.

Weetman AP: Insulin-dependent diabetes mellitus and postpartum thyroiditis: an important association. Editorial. *J Clin Endocrinol Metab* 79:7–9, 1994.

Weissman MM, Bland R, Joyce PR, Newman S, Wells JE, Wittchen H-U: Sex differences in rates of depression: cross-national perspectives. *J Affect Dis* 29: 77–84, 1993.

Weissman AM, Levy BT, Hartz AJ, Bentler S, Donohue M, Ellingrod VL, Wisner KL: Pooled analysis of anti-depressant levels in lactating mothers, breast milk, and nursing infants. *Am J Psychiatry* 161:1066–1078, 2004.

Welschen LM, Bloemendal E, Nijpels G, Dekker JM, Heine RJ, Stalman WA, Bouter LM: Self-monitoring of blood glucose in patients with type 2 diabetes who are not using insulin: a systematic review. *Diabetes Care* 28:1510–1517, 2005.

Wenzel A, Haugen EN, Jackson LC, Brendle JR: Anxiety symptoms and disorders at eight weeks postpartum. *Anxiety Disord* 19:295–331, 2005.

White WB, Andreoli JW, Cohn RD: Alpha-methyldopa disposition in mothers with hypertension and in their breastfed infants. *Clin Pharmacol Ther* 37:387–390, 1985.

Whitehead SJ, Berg CJ, Chang J: Pregnancy-related mortality due to cardiomyopathy: United States, 1991–1997. *Obstet Gynecol* 102:1326–1331, 2003.

Whitfield M, Kay R, Stevens S: Validity of routine clinical test weighing as a measure of intake of breast-fed infants. *Arch Dis Child* 56:919–921, 1981.

WHO—World Health Organization Family and Reproductive Health, Division of Child Health and Development: *Protecting, Promoting and Supporting Breastfeeding: The Special Role of Maternity Services.* A joint WHO/UNICEF statement. Publication # WHO/CHD/98.9. Geneva, Switzerland: World Health Organization; 1989.

WHO—World Health Organization Collaborative Study of Cardiovascular Disease and Steroid Hormone Contraception Writing Group: Venous thromboembolic disease and combined oral contraceptives: results of international multicentre case-control study. *Lancet* 346:1575–1582, 1995.

WHO—World Health Organization: *Evidence for Ten Steps to Successful Breastfeeding.* Revised ed. WHO/CHD/98.9 Geneva, Switzerland: World Health Organization; 1998a.

WHO—World Health Organization Working Group on the Growth Reference Protocol: *A Growth Curve for the 21st Century: The WHO Multicenter Growth Reference Study.* Geneva, Switzerland: World Health Organization; 1998b.

WHO—World Health Organization and Department of Child and Adolescent Health and Development: *Mastitis: Causes and Management.* Geneva, Switzerland: World Health Organization; 2000a:1–45.

WHO—World Health Organization. Quality Care in Family Planning. In: *Medical Eligibility Criteria for Contraceptive Use.* Geneva, Switzerland: World Health Organization Reproductive Health and Research; 2000b.

WHO—World Health Organization Collaborative Study Team on the Role of Breastfeeding on the Prevention of Infant Mortality: Effect of breastfeeding on infant and child mortality due to infectious diseases in less developed countries: a pooled analysis. *Lancet* 355:451–455, 2001.

WHO—World Health Organization: *Selected Practice Recommendations for Contraceptive Use.* Geneva, Switzerland: World Health Organization; 2002.

WHO—World Health Organization: *Medical Eligibility Criteria for Contraceptive Use.* 3rd ed. Geneva, Switzerland: World Health Organization; 2004.

WHO/UNICEF—World Health Organization/United Nations Children's Fund: Indicators for assessing health facility practices that affect breastfeeding. Report of the Joint WHO/UNICEF Informal Interagency Meeting. Geneva, Switzerland: WHO/UNICEF; 1992.

Wichelow MJ, Doddridge MC: Lactation in diabetic women. *BMJ* 287:649–650, 1983.

Wiese J: Intrauterine contraception in diabetic women. *Fertil Steril* 28:422–425, 1977.

Wight NE: Management of common breastfeeding issues. *Pediatr Clin North Am* 48:321–344, 2001.

Wight NE: Hypoglycemia in breastfed neonates. *Breastfeeding Med* 1:253–262, 2006.

Wiles LS: The effect of prenatal breastfeeding education on breastfeeding success and the maternal perception of the infant. *J Obstet Gynecol Neonatal Nurs* 13:253–257, 1984.

Wilkin TJ: The accelerator hypothesis: weight gain as the missing link between type I and type II diabetes. *Diabetologia* 44:914–922, 2001.

Wilkin TJ: The great weight gain experiment, accelerators, and their implications for autoantibodies in diabetes. *Arch Dis Child* 91:456–458, 2006.

Wilson JT: Determinants and consequences of drug excretion in breast milk. *Drug Metab Rev* 14:619–652, 1983.

Wilson ES, Cruickshank J, McMaster M, Weir RJ: A prospective controlled study of the effect on blood pressure of contraceptive preparations containing different types of dosages and progestogen. *Br J Obstet Gynecol* 91:1254–1260, 1984.

Wilson JT, Brown RD, Hinson JL, Dailey JW: Pharmacokinetic pitfalls in the estimation of the breast milk/plasma ratio for drugs. *Annu Rev Pharmacol Toxicol* 25:667–689, 1985.

Wilson AC, Forsyth JS, Greene SA, Irvine L, Hau C, Howie PW: Relation of infant diet to childhood health: seven-year follow-up of cohort children in Dundee infant feeding study. *BMJ* 316:21–25, 1998.

Wirt DP, Adkins LT, Palkowetz KH, Schmalstieg FC, Goldman AS: Activated and memory T lymphocytes in human milk. *Cytometry* 13:282–290, 1992.

Wisner KL, Perel JM, Findling RL: Antidepressant treatment during breastfeeding. *Am J Psychiatry* 153:1132–1137, 1996.

Wisner KL, Parry BL, Piontek CM: Postpartum depression. *N Engl J Med* 347: 194–199, 2002.

Witlin AG, Mable WC, Sibai BM: Peripartum cardiomyopathy: an ominous diagnosis. *Am J Obstet Gynecol* 176:182–188, 1997.

Woolridge MW, Butte N, Dewey KG: Methods for the measurement of milk volume intake of the breast-fed infant. In: Jensen RG, Neville MC, eds. *Human Lactation: Milk Components Methodologies.* New York: Plenum Press; 1984:5–21.

Wosje KS, Kalkwarf HJ: Lactation, weaning, and calcium supplementation: effects on body composition in postpartum women. *Am J Clin Nutr* 80:423–429, 2004.

Wright AL, Holberg CJ, Martinez FD, Morgan WJ, Taussig LM; Group Health Medical Associates: Breastfeeding and lower respiratory tract illness in the first year of life. *BMJ* 299:945–949, 1989.

Wright S, Dawling S, Ashford JJ: Excretion of fluvoxamine in breast milk. *Br J Clin Pharmacol* 31:209, 1991.

Wright AL, Holberg CJ, Taussig LM, Martinez FD: Relationship of infant feeding to recurrent wheezing at age 6 years. *Arch Pediatr Adolesc Med* 149:758–763, 1995.

Wright CM, Waterston AJR: Relationships between pediatricians and infant formula milk companies. Commentary on infant nutrition. *Arch Dis Child* 91:383–385, 2006.

Wylie-Rosett J, Albright AA, Apovian C, Clark NG, Delahanty L, Franz MJ, Hoogwerf B, Kulkarni K, Lichtenstein AH, Mayer-Davis E, Mooradian AD, Wheeler M: 2006–2007 American Diabetes Association nutrition recommendations: issues for practice translation. *J Am Diet Assoc* 107: 1296–1304, 2007.

Xanthou M: Human milk cells. *Acta Paediatr* 86:1288–1290, 1997.

Xanthou M: Immune protection of human milk. *Biol Neonate* 74:121–133, 1998.

Xiang M, Harbige LS, Zetterstrom R: Long-chain polyunsaturated fatty acids in Chinese and Swedish mothers: diet, breast milk and infant growth. *Acta Paediatr* 94:1543–1549, 2005.

Xiang AH, Kawakubo M, Kjos SL, Buchanan TA: Long-acting injectable progestin contraception and risk of type 2 diabetes in Latino women with prior gestational diabetes mellitus. *Diabetes Care* 29:613–617, 2006.

Xiang AH, Kawakubo M, Buchanan TA, Kjos SL: A longitudinal study of lipids and blood pressure in relation to method of contraception in Latino women with prior gestational diabetes mellitus. *Diabetes Care* 30:1952–1958, 2007.

Yamouchi Y, Yamanouchi I: The relationship between rooming-in/not rooming-in and breastfeeding variables. *Acta Paediatr Scand* 79:1017–1022, 1990.

Yates AA, Schlicker SA, Suitor CW: Dietary reference intakes: the new basis for recommendations for calcium and related nutrients, B vitamins, and choline. *J Am Diet Assoc* 98:699–706, 1998.

Yoshida K, Smith B, Kumar RC: Fluvoxamine in breast-milk and infant development. *Br J Clin Pharmacol* 44:210–211, 1997.

Young TK, Martens PJ, Taback SP, Sellers EAC, Dean HJ, Cheang M, Flett B: Type 2 diabetes mellitus in children-prenatal and early infancy risk factors among native Canadians. *Arch Pediatr Adolesc Med* 156:651–655, 2002.

Zaers S, Waschke M, Ehlert U: Depressive symptoms and symptoms of post-traumatic stress disorder in women after childbirth. *Psychosom Obstet Gynecol* 29:61–71, 2008.

Ziegler AG, Schmid S, Huber D, Hummel M, Bonifacio E: Early infant feeding and risk of developing type 1 diabetes-associated autoantibodies. *JAMA* 290: 1721–1772, 2003.

Ziemer DC, Doyle JP, Barnes CS, Branch WT Jr, Cook CB, el-Kebbi IM, Gallina DL, Kolm P, Rhee MK, Phillips LS: An intervention to overcome clinical inertia and improve diabetes mellitus control in a primary care setting. Improving primary care of African Americans with diabetes. *Arch Intern Med* 166:507–513, 2006.

Zinaman MJ, Hughes V, Queenan JT, Labbok MH, Albertson B: Acute prolactin and oxytocin responses and milk yield to infant suckling and artificial methods of expression in lactating women. *Pediatrics* 89:437–440, 1992.

Zutavern A, von Mutius E, Harris J, Mills P, Moffatt S, White C, Cullinan P: The introduction of solids in relation to asthma and eczema. *Arch Dis Child* 89: 303–308, 2004.

Zutavern A, Brockow I, Schaaf B, Bolte G, von Berg A, Diez U, Borte M, Herbarth O, Wichmann HE, Heinrich J; LISA Study Group: Timing of solid food introduction in relation to atopic dermatitis and atopic sensitization: results from a prospective birth cohort study. *Pediatrics* 117:401–411, 2006.

Index

Methionine, metabolism of, 66

Methyl group transfer, B-complex vitamins, and homocysteine, 68–71

Methyldopa, 350

Methylmercury, 74–75

Microalbuminuria, during diabetic pregnancy, 380–381

Micronutrient intake, 42–68

Miglitol, 103

Milk
glycemic index for, 31
See also Breast milk

Minerals, and trace elements, 44–55

Moderately active, defined, 105

Monoamine oxidase inhibitors, 114

Monounsaturated fatty acids (MUFAs), defined, 36

Montoro, Martin N. 284, 374, 728, 737

Mood disturbances, postpartum, 693–697

Morbidity, neonatal, 603

Mortality, maternal, 607–610

Multiple daily injections (MDIs), 89–90, 95

Nateglinide, 103

Neonatal care, 605

Neonatal hypoglycemia, avoiding, with early breast-feeding, 715

Neotame, 71

Nephropathy. *See* Diabetic nephropathy (DN)

Niacin, 60, 372–373

Nonalcoholic fatty liver disease, 84–86

Nonnutritive sweeteners. *See* Sugar substitutes

Nonstress test (NST), 569–571

Normoglycemia, during pregnancy, 9–10

NPH insulin, 91

Nuchal translucency (NT) thickness, 564

Nursing. *See* Breast-feeding

Nutrient intake
sources of information, 24
See also Macronutrient intake, Micronutrient intake

Nutritional circumstances, special, 77–87

Nutrition management. *See* Medical nutrition therapy (MNT)

Obesity, and post-bariatric surgery pregnancy, 87

Ogata, Edward S., 601

Oral medications
α-glucosidase inhibitors, 103
biguanides, 99–101
incretins, 104
meglitinide analogs, 103
recommendations, 104–105
sulfonylureas, 97–99

thiazolidinediones, 101–103
for type 2 diabetes in pregnancy, 96–105
See also Contraception

Organochlorines, 75–76

Panic disorders, 116

Paramsothy, Pathmaja, 294, 355

PCBs. *See* Polychlorinated biphenyls and dioxins

Pediatrician, communication with, 604–605

Perinatal outcome, and studies of maternal glucose profiles, 5

Peripartum cardiomyopathy, 690

Peripheral arterial disease. *See* Lower extremity arterial disease (LEAD)

Pesticides, 75–76

Phenformin, 99

Phosphorus, 45

Physical activity
and CVD management, 331
for managing dyslipidemias, 371–372
and pregnant women with diabetes, 105–111

Physical examination
for CHD, 318–319
infant, 605
initial, 1–3

Placental-fetal iron balance, 52–53

Plant sterols, 373

Plasma anhydro-D-glucitol, 14

Plasma lipids, effects of diabetes on, 367–369
Polychlorinated biphenyls and dioxins, 75–76

Polyunsaturated fatty acids (PUFAs), 36, 40–41

Postpartum emotional lability, transient, 693

Postpartum lipid testing, 730

Postpartum lipid therapy, 730, 732

Postpartum management
breast-feeding and contraception, 741–743
glycemic control and complications, 687–693
mood disturbances, 693–697
peripartum cardiomyopathy, 690
recommendations for maintaining glycemic control, 692–693

Postpartum nonpsychotic depression, 694–696

Postpartum psychotic depression, 696

Postpartum thyroiditis, 690–692

Posttraumatic stress disorder (PTSD), 696

Potassium, 44
and management of DKA, 274

Prazosin, 354

Preeclampsia, 342
managing, 581–583
and trials using vitamins C and E, 57